Decision Making in Emergency Critical Care
An Evidence-Based Handbook

EDITOR

John E. Arbo, MD
Assistant Professor of Emergency Medicine and Critical Care Medicine
New York-Presbyterian Hospital/Weill Cornell Medical Center
New York, New York

ASSOCIATE EDITORS

Stephen J. Ruoss, MD
Professor of Pulmonary and Critical Care Medicine
Co-Chief, Division of Pulmonary and Critical Care Medicine
Stanford University Medical Center
Stanford, California

Geoffrey K. Lighthall, MD
Associate Professor of Anesthesia and Critical Care Medicine
Stanford University Medical Center
Stanford, California

Michael P. Jones, MD
Assistant Professor of Emergency Medicine
Associate Program Director – Jacobi/Montefiore Emergency Medicine Residency Program
Albert Einstein College of Medicine
New York, New York

SPECIAL EDITOR: NEUROLOGY SECTION

Joshua Stillman, MD, MPH
Assistant Professor of Medicine
Emergency Medicine Director of the Stroke Center at New York-Presbyterian Hospital/Columbia University Medical Center
New York, New York

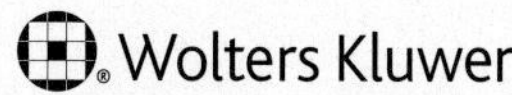
Wolters Kluwer

Philadelphia • Baltimore • New York • London
Buenos Aires • Hong Kong • Sydney • Tokyo

Acquisitions Editor: Jamie M. Elfrank
Product Development Editor: Ashley Fischer
Production Project Manager: David Orzechowski
Manufacturing Manager: Beth Welsh
Marketing Manager: Stephanie Manzo
Design Coordinator: Teresa Mallon
Production Service: SPi Global

Two Commerce Square
2001 Market Street
Philadelphia, PA 19103 USA
LWW.com

Printed in China

978-1-4511-8689-5
1-4511-8689-4
Library of Congress Cataloging-in-Publication Data available upon request

---

To purchase additional copies of this book, call our customer service department at (800) 638-3030 or fax orders to (301) 223-2320. International customers should call (301) 223-2300.

Visit Lippincott Williams & Wilkins on the Internet: at LWW.com. Lippincott Williams & Wilkins customer service representatives are available from 8:30 am to 6 pm, EST.

10 9 8 7 6 5 4 3

RRS1604

To John and Marlene for a lifetime of support, to Rani for her editorial genius, and to Morgan for never letting me forget the bigger picture

CONTRIBUTORS

Darryl Abrams, MD
Assistant Professor of Medicine
Division of Pulmonary, Allergy, and Critical Care
Department of Medicine
Columbia University Medical Center
Assistant Attending Physician
Division of Pulmonary, Allergy, and Critical Care
Department of Medicine
New York-Presbyterian Hospital
New York, New York

Cara Agerstrand, MD
Assistant Professor of Medicine
Department of Medicine
Columbia College of Physicians and Surgeons and the New York-Presbyterian Hospital
New York, New York

John E. Arbo, MD
Assistant Professor of Clinical Medicine
Department of Medicine
Weill Cornell Medical College
Attending Physician
Division of Emergency Medicine and Pulmonary Critical Care Medicine
New York-Presbyterian Hospital/Weill Cornell Medical College
New York, New York

Anne-Sophie Beraud, MD, MS
Consulting Instructor
Division Cardiovascular Medicine
Stanford University School of Medicine
Stanford, California
Staff Cardiologist
Cardiovascular Medicine
Clinique Pasteur
Toulouse, France

Rana Biary, MD
Assistant Professor
Department of Emergency Medicine
Division of Medical Toxicology
New York University Medical Center
New York, New York

Nicole Bouchard, MD, BSc
Assistant Clinical Professor
Director of Medical Toxicology
Division of Emergency Medicine
New York-Presbyterian Hospital/Columbia University Medical Center
New York, New York

Daniel Brodie, MD
Associate Professor of Medicine
Department of Medicine
Columbia College of Physicians and Surgeons and the New York-Presbyterian Hospital
New York, New York

Carlos Brun, MD
Clinical Instructor
Department of Anesthesiology, Perioperative, and Pain Medicine
Stanford University School of Medicine
Stanford, California
Attending and Intensivist
Anesthesiology and Perioperative Care Service
VA Palo Alto Health Care System
Palo Alto, California

Carla M. Carvalho, MD
Surgical Critical Care Fellow
Stanford University Medical Center
Stanford, California

Betty C. Chen, MD
Acting Instructor
Division of Emergency Medicine
Department of Medicine
University of Washington School of Medicine
Attending Physician
Division of Emergency Medicine
Department of Medicine
Harborview Medical Center
Seattle, Washington

Glenn Chertow, MD, MPH
Norman S. Coplon/Satellite Healthcare
Professor of Medicine
Chief, Division of Nephrology
Stanford University School of Medicine
Palo Alto, California

Jey K. Chung, MD
Fellow
Division of Pulmonary and Critical Care Medicine
Stanford University Medical Center
Stanford, California

Nicholas J. Connors, MD
Medical Toxicology Fellow
Division of Medical Toxicology
Department of Emergency Medicine
New York University School of Medicine
New York, New York

J. Randall Curtis, MD, MPH
A. Bruce Montgomery–American Lung Association Endowed Chair in Pulmonary and Critical Care Medicine
Division of Pulmonary & Critical Care Medicine
University of Washington
Professor of Medicine, Section Head
Division of Pulmonary & Critical Care
Harborview Medical Center
Seattle, Washington

Christopher Davis, MD, DTMH
Assistant Professor
Department of Emergency Medicine
Altitude Research Center
University of Colorado School of Medicine
Aurora, Colorado

Katy M. Deljoui
Critical Care Medicine Fellow
Department of Pulmonary and Critical Care Medicine
University of Maryland Medical Center
Baltimore, Maryland

Rachel H. Dotson, MD
Attending Physician
Division of Pulmonary and Critical Care Medicine
Department of Medicine
California Pacific Medical Center
San Francisco, California

E. Wesley Ely, MD, MPH
Professor
Division of Allergy, Pulmonary, and Critical Care
Department of Internal Medicine
Vanderbilt University Medical Center
Nashville, Tennessee

Morgan Eutermoser, MD, DTMH
Wilderness Medicine Fellow
Department of Emergency Medicine
University of Colorado
Aurora, Colorado

Jose Evangelista III, MD
Assistant Professor
Department of Emergency Medicine
Division of Undersea and Hyperbaric Medicine
University of California San Diego
San Diego, California

Brandon Foreman, MD
Clinical Fellow in Neurocritical Care/EEG
Division of Neurocritical Care
Department of Neurology
Columbia University College of Physicians and Surgeons
New York-Presbyterian Hospital
New York, New York

Shai Friedland, MD
Assistant Professor
Stanford University School of Medicine
Staff Physician
Gastroenterology
Stanford University Hospital and Veteran Affairs Hospital Palo Alto
Palo Alto, California

Samuel Gerson, MD
Assistant Clinical Professor
School of Medicine
University of California San Diego
La Jolla, California
Attending Physician
Emergency Medicine
University of California San Diego Medical Center
San Diego, California

Laleh Gharahbaghian, MD
Clinical Assistant Professor
Division of Emergency Medicine
Department of Surgery
Stanford University School of Medicine
Director, Emergency Ultrasound Program and Fellowship
Division of Emergency Medicine
Department of Surgery
Stanford University Medical Center
Stanford, California

Alberto Goffi, MD
Clinical Fellow
Interdepartmental Division of Critical Care
University of Toronto
Intensivist, Medical-Surgical and Neuro-Intensive Care Unit
University Health Network–Toronto Western Hospital
Toronto, Ontario, Canada

M. Cristina Vazquez-Guillamet, MD
Infectious Disease Fellow
University of New Mexico Hospital
Albuquerque, New Mexico

Francois Haddad, MD, FAHA
Director Biomarker and Phenotypic Core Laboratory
Stanford Cardiovascular Institute
Stanford University Medical Center
Stanford, California

Alexis Halpern, BA, MD
Assistant Professor of Clinical Medicine
Assistant Director, Geriatric Emergency Medicine Fellowship
Department of Medicine
Weill Cornell Medical College
Attending Physician
Division of Emergency Medicine
New York-Presbyterian Hospital/Weill Cornell Medical College
New York, New York

Jin H. Han, MD, MSc
Assistant Professor
Department of Emergency Medicine
Vanderbilt University School of Medicine
Nashville, Tennessee

Lawrence A. Ho, BS, MD
Clinical Assistant Professor
Center for Interstitial Lung Disease, Pulmonary and Critical Care
University of Washington
Seattle, Washington

Joe L. Hsu, MD, MPH
Instructor of Medicine
Department of Medicine
Stanford University School of Medicine
Attending
Department of Medicine
Stanford University Medical Center
Stanford, California

Catherine T. Jamin, MD
Assistant Professor, Chief of Emergency Medicine Critical Care
Division of Pulmonary and Critical Care
Department of Emergency Medicine
NYU Langone Medical Center
Assistant Professor, Chief of Emergency Medicine Critical Care
Division of Pulmonary and Critical Care
Department of Emergency Medicine
Bellevue Hospital Center
New York, New York

Michael P. Jones, MD
Assistant Professor
Department of Emergency Medicine
Albert Einstein College of Medicine
Associate Residency Director
Department of Emergency Medicine
Jacobi Medical Center
Bronx, New York

Shawn K. Kaku, MD
Fellow
Division of Pulmonary and Critical Care Medicine
Stanford University Medical Center
Stanford, California

Jon-Emile S. Kenny, MD
Fellow
Division of Pulmonary and Critical Care Medicine
Stanford University Medical Center
Stanford, California

Feras Khan, MD
Clinical Assistant Professor
Department of Emergency Medicine
University of Maryland School of Medicine
Baltimore, Maryland

Hong K. Kim, MD, MPH
Assistant Professor
Department of Emergency Medicine
University of Maryland School of Medicine
Attending Physician
Department of Emergency Medicine
Mercy Medical Center
Baltimore, Maryland

Michael Klompas, MD, MPH, FRCPC, FIDSA
Associate Professor
Department of Population Medicine
Harvard Medical School and Harvard Pilgrim Health Care Institute
Associate Hospital Epidemiologist
Brigham and Women's Hospital
Boston, Massachusetts

James Lantry III, MD
Critical Care Fellow
Department of Medicine
University of Maryland
Baltimore, Maryland

Cappi Lay, MD
Assistant Clinical Professor
Department of Emergency Medicine/Neurocritical Care
University of Washington
Assistant Clinical Professor
Department of Emergency Medicine/Neurocritical Care
Harborview Medical Center
Seattle, Washington

Jarone Lee, MD, MPH
Instructor in Surgery
Department of Surgery
Harvard Medical School
Quality Director, Surgical Critical Care
Trauma, Emergency Surgery, Surgical Critical Care
Massachusetts General Hospital
Boston, Massachusetts

Jay Lemery, MD
Associate Professor
Department of Emergency Medicine
University of Colorado School of Medicine
Attending Physician
Department o Emergency Medicine
University of Colorado Hospital
Aurora, Colorado

Geoffrey K. Lighthall, MD, PhD
Associate Professor, Anesthesia and Critical Care Department of Anesthesia
Stanford University School of Medicine
Stanford, California
Staff Physician Anesthesia and Critical Care Department of Anesthesia
Veteran Affairs Hospital
Palo Alto, California

Glen A. Lutchman, MD, MHSc
Clinical Assistant Professor of Medicine
Division of Gastroenterology and Hepatology
Stanford University Medical Center
Stanford, California

Chad M. Meyers, MD
Associate Chief, Emergency Critical Care
Assistant Director, Emergency ICU
Department of Emergency Medicine
NYU School of Medicine
New York, New York

Paul Maggio, MD, MBA, FACS
Assistant Professor of Surgery
Co-Director Critical Care Medicine
Stanford University Medical Center
Stanford, California

Thomas "Tom" Mailhot, MD
Clinical Assistant Professor
Department of Emergency Medicine
Keck School of Medicine of the University of Southern California
Director Emergency Ultrasound Fellowship
LAC + USC Medical Center
Los Angeles, California

Diku P. Mandavia, MD, FACEP, FRCPC
Attending Staff Physician
Department of Emergency Medicine
University of Southern California
Department of Emergency Medicine
LAC+USC Medical Center
Los Angeles, California

Jeffrey Manko, MD
Program Director, Emergency Medicine Residency
Department of Emergency Medicine
NYU/Bellevue Medical Center
New York, New York

A.L.O. Manoel, MD
Clinical Fellow
Interdepartmental Division of Critical Care
University of Toronto
Clinical and Research Fellow
Department of Critical Care
Department of Medical Imaging
St. Michael's Hospital
Toronto, Ontario, Canada

David M. Maslove, MD, MS, FRCPC
Assistant Professor
Department of Medicine and Critical Care Program
Queen's University
Kingston General Hospital
Internal Medicine and Critical Care
Kingston General Hospital
Kingston, Ontario, Canada

Michael T. McCurdy, MD
Assistant Professor
Departments of Medicine and Emergency Medicine
University of Maryland School of Medicine
Program Director
Critical Care Medicine Fellowship
University of Maryland Medical Center
Baltimore, Maryland

Anil Mendiratta, MD
Associate Professor
Comprehensive Epilepsy Center
Department of Neurology
Columbia University College of Physicians and Surgeons
Attending Physician
Department of Neurology
New York-Presbyterian Hospital/Columbia University Medical Center
New York, New York

Venu Menon, MD
Staff Physician
Department of Cardiovascular Medicine
Cleveland Clinic
Cleveland, Ohio

Tsuyoshi Mitarai, MD, FACEP
Clinical Assistant Professor
Division of Emergency Medicine
Department of Surgery
Stanford University School of Medicine
Attending Physician
Medical Intensive Care Unit
Emergency Department
Stanford University Medical Center
Stanford, California

Paul K. Mohabir, MD
Clinical Associate Professor of Medicine
Division of Pulmonary and Critical Care Medicine
Stanford University School of Medicine
Stanford, California

Joshua J. Mooney, MD
Fellow
Division of Pulmonary and Critical Care
Department of Medicine
Stanford University Medical Center
Stanford, California

Mary R. Mulcare, MD
Assistant Professor of Clinical Medicine
Department of Medicine
Weill Cornell Medical College
Attending Physician
Division of Emergency Medicine
New York-Presbyterian/Weill Cornell Medical College
New York, New York

Parvathi A. Myer, MD, MHS
Attending Physician
Department of Gastroenterology
Kaiser Permanente
Irvine, California

Margaret J. Neff, MD, MSc
Clinical Associate Professor of Medicine
Division of Pulmonary & Critical Care Medicine
Department of Medicine
Stanford University School of Medicine
Stanford, California
Medical Director, Medical-Surgical ICU
Critical Care Service
VA Palo Alto Health Care System
Palo Alto, California

Lewis S. Nelson, MD
Professor and Medical Toxicology Fellowship Director
Department of Emergency Medicine
New York University School of Medicine
Attending Physician
Department of Emergency Medicine
NYU Langone Medical Center and Bellevue Hospital Center
New York, New York

Pratik Pandharipande, MD, MSCI
Professor of Anesthesiology and Surgery
Department of Anesthesiology
Vanderbilt University Medical Center
Nashville, Tennessee

Walter G. Park, MD, MS
Assistant Professor of Medicine
Department of Medicine
Stanford University School of Medicine
Medical Director, Pancreas Clinic
Department of Medicine
Stanford University Medical Center
Stanford, California

Phillips Perera, MD, RDMS
Clinical Associate Professor, Emergency Medicine
Department of Surgery
Stanford University Medical Center
Stanford, California

Thomas B. Perera, MD
Associate Professor
Department of Emergency Medicine
Albert Einstein College of Medicine
Residency Director
Department of Emergency Medicine
Jacobi/Montefiore Medical Centers
Bronx, New York

Jane Marie Prosser, MD
Assistant Professor of Clinical Medicine
Consult, Medical Toxicology
Department of Medicine
Weill Cornell Medical College
Attending Physician
Division of Emergency Medicine
New York-Presbyterian Hospital/Weill Cornell Medical College
New York, New York

Susan Y. Quan, MD
Fellow
Division of Gastroenterology
Stanford University Medical Center
Stanford, California

Rama B. Rao, MD
Assistant Professor of Clinical Medicine
Director, Medical Toxicology
Department of Medicine
Weill Cornell Medical College
Attending Physician
Division of Emergency Medicine
New York-Presbyterian Hospital/Weill Cornell Medical College
New York, New York

Vidya K. Rao, MD, MBA
Clinical Instructor
Department of Anesthesiology, Perioperative and Pain Medicine
Divisions of Cardiac Anesthesia and Critical Care Medicine
Stanford University School of Medicine
Stanford, California

Catherine S. Reid
Clinical Instructor
Department of Anesthesia
Stanford University School of Medicine
Stanford, California

Chanu Rhee, MD
Research Fellow
Department of Population Medicine
Harvard Medical School/Harvard Pilgrim Health Care Institute
Associate Physician
Division of Infectious Diseases
Department of Medicine
Brigham and Women's Hospital
Boston, Massachusetts

Robert M. Rodriguez, MD
Professor of Emergency Medicine
Department of Emergency Medicine
School of Medicine
University of California San Francisco
San Francisco, California

Daniel Runde, MD
Assistant Residency Director
Department of Emergency Medicine
University of Iowa Hospitals and Clinics
Assistant Professor
Department of Emergency Medicine
University of Iowa Hospitals and Clinics
Iowa City, Iowa

Stephen Ruoss, MD
Professor of Medicine
Department of Medicine, Division of Pulmonary and Critical Care Medicine
Stanford University School of Medicine
Professor of Medicine
Department of Medicine, Division of Pulmonary and Critical Care Medicine
Stanford University Medical Center
Stanford, California

Tara Scherer, MD
Assistant Professor
Department of Emergency Medicine
Vanderbilt University
Nashville, Tennessee

Michael C. Scott, MD
Fellow, Combined Emergency Medicine/Internal Medicine/Critical Care Program
Departments of Internal Medicine, Emergency Medicine and Critical Care
University of Maryland Medical Center
Baltimore, Maryland

Daniel Sedehi, MD
Cardiology Fellow
Department of Cardiovascular Medicine
Cleveland Clinic
Cleveland, Ohio

Zina Semenovskaya, MD
Wilderness Medicine Fellow
Division of Emergency Medicine
Stanford University
Stanford, California
Associate Clinical Instructor
Department of Emergency Medicine
San Francisco General Hospital
San Francisco, California

Sam Senturia, MD
Assistant Professor of Clinical Medicine
Department of Medicine
Weill Cornell Medical College
Attending Physician
Division of Emergency Medicine
New York-Presbyterian Hospital/Weill Cornell Medical College
New York, New York

Nina Patel Shah, DO
Fellow
Division of Pulmonary and Critical Care Medicine
Stanford University Medical Center
Stanford, California

Lauren K. Shawn, MD
Attending Physician
Emergency Medicine
Mt Sinai St Luke's Roosevelt
New York, New York

Paul Singh, MD, MPH
Neuroendovascular Surgery Fellow
Department of Neurosurgery
New York Presbyterian Hospital/Weill Cornell Medical Center
New York, New York

Corey Slovis, MD
Professor of Emergency Medicine and Medicine
Chairman Department of Emergency Medicine
Vanderbilt University School of Medicine
Chief of Emergency Services
Vanderbilt University Hospital
Nashville, Tennessee

Silas W. Smith, MD
Assistant Professor
Department of Emergency Medicine
Division of Medical Toxicology
NYU School of Medicine
Bellevue Hospital Center
New York, New York

Deborah M. Stein, MD, MPH
Associate Professor of Surgery
Department of Surgery
Chief of Trauma and Medical Director, Neurotrauma Critical Care
Program in Trauma
University of Maryland School of Medicine
Associate Professor of Surgery
Department of Surgery
Chief of Trauma and Medical Director, Neurotrauma Critical Care
R Adams Cowley Shock Trauma Center
University of Maryland Medical Center
Baltimore, Maryland

Michael E. Stern, MD
Assistant Professor of Clinical Medicine
Director, Geriatric Emergency Medicine Fellowship
Department of Medicine
Weill Cornell Medical College
Attending Physician
Division of Emergency Medicine
New York-Presbyterian Hospital/Weill Cornell Medical College
New York, New York

Joshua Sternbach, MD
Fellow
Division of Pulmonary and Critical Care Medicine
Stanford University Medical Center
Stanford, California

Joshua Stillman, MD, MPH
Assistant Professor of Medicine
Division of Emergency Medicine
Emergency Medicine Director of the Stroke Center at New York-Presbyterian Hospital/Columbia University Medical Center
New York, New York

Matthew C. Strehlow, MD
Clinical Associate Professor of Emergency Medicine
Department of Surgery
Stanford University School of Medicine
Clinical Associate Professor of Emergency Medicine
Department of Surgery
Stanford University Medical Center
Stanford, California

Mark Su, MD, MPH
Clinical Associate Professor
Department of Emergency Medicine
New York University School of Medicine
Attending Physician
Department of Emergency Medicine
Bellevue Hospital Center
New York, New York

Payal Sud, MD
Assistant Professor of Emergency Medicine
Hofstra North Shore-LIJ School of Medicine at Hofstra University
Hempstead, New York
Medical Toxicologist, Emergency Physician
Department of Emergency Medicine
North Shore University Hospital and
Long Island Jewish Medical Center
Manhasset, New York and
New Hyde Park, New York

Anand Swaminathan, MD, MPH, FACEP, FAAEM
Assistant Residency Director
Department of Emergency Medicine
New York University Hospital
Assistant Professor
Department of Emergency Medicine
New York University/Bellevue Emergency Department
New York, New York

Mai Takematsu, MD
Physician
Division of Medical Toxicology
Department of Emergency Medicine
New York University School of Medicine
Physician
Department of Emergency Medicine
Bellevue Hospital Center
New York, New York

Mohamed Teleb, MD
Clinical Instructor
Department of Neurology
Medical College of Wisconsin
Clinical Instructor
Department of Neurology
Froedtert Hospital and Medical College of Wisconsin
Milwaukee, Wisconsin

Martina Trinkaus, MD, BSc, BPHE
Assistant Professor
Divisions of Hematology and Medical Oncology
Department of Medicine
University of Toronto
Staff Hematologist
Divisions of Hematology and Medical Oncology
St. Michael's Hospital
Toronto, Ontario, Canada

D. Turkel-Parrella, MD
Clinical Fellow
Department of Neurology
University of Toronto
Clinical Fellow, Vascular and Interventional Neurology
Division of Neurology
Department of Medical Imaging
St. Michael's Hospital
Toronto, Ontario, Canada

Christina Ulane, MD, PhD
Assistant Professor of Neurology
Department of Neurology
The Neurological Institute, Columbia University Medical Center
Attending Physician
Department of Neurology
New York Presbyterian Hospital, Columbia University Medical Center
New York, New York

Eduard E. Vasilevskis, MD, MPH
Assistant Professor
Division of General Internal Medicine and Public Health
Department of Internal Medicine
Vanderbilt University Medical Center
Nashville, Tennessee

Audrey K. Wagner
Critical Care Medicine Fellow
Department of Pulmonary and Critical Care Medicine
University of Baltimore Maryland Medical Center
Baltimore, Maryland

Richard Ward, MBBS
Assistant Professor
Division of Hematology
Department of Medicine
University of Toronto
Staff Physician
Division of Medical Oncology and Hematology
Department of Medicine
University Health Network
Toronto, Ontario, Canada

Scott Weingart, MD, FCCM
Associate Clinical Professor
Director of Emergency Department Critical Care
Emergency Medicine
Mount Sinai School of Medicine
Elmhurst Hospital Center
New York, New York

Emilee Willhem-Leen, MD, MS
Fellow
Division of Nephrology
Stanford University Medical Center
Stanford, California

Sarah R. Williams, MD
Associate Program Director
Stanford/Kaiser Emergency Medicine Residency
Co-Director
Stanford EM Ultrasound Fellowship
Clinical Associate Professor of Surgery/Emergency Medicine
Department of Surgery, Division of Emergency Medicine
Stanford University School of Medicine
Stanford, California

Michael E. Winters, MD
Associate Professor of Emergency Medicine and Medicine
Departments of Emergency Medicine and Medicine
University of Maryland School of Medicine
Medical Director, Adult Emergency Department
Co-Director, Combined Emergency Medicine/Internal Medicine/Critical Care Program
University of Maryland Medical Center
Baltimore, Maryland

Robert J. Wong, MD, MS
Gastroenterology and Hepatology Fellow
Division of Gastroenterology and Hepatology
Stanford University School of Medicine
Stanford, California

Randall Wood, MD
Attending Physician
Unity Point Health-Saint Lukes Hospital
Sioux City, Iowa

PREFACE: FROM THE EDITOR

Emergency physicians are caring for a growing number of critically ill patients. This increase in ED-critical care volume, coupled with prolonged patient stays, has placed new demands on the emergency physician. He or she must now provide not only acute resuscitative care, but also extended management of complex cardiac, pulmonary, and neurologic emergencies.

Leadership in the field of emergency medicine has embraced this broadening ED-ICU overlap in a timely and skillful manner. Residency program directors are placing new emphasis on critical care medicine in resident education and clinical training. Nationally, emergency departments have become a focus for evidence-based trials in goal-directed therapy for the critically ill. And finally, in a much-anticipated collaboration, the American Board of Emergency Medicine (ABEM) and the American Board of Internal Medicine (ABIM) have agreed to allow graduates of emergency medicine residencies to sit for board certification in critical care medicine following fellowship training.

Decision Making in Emergency Critical Care: An Evidence-Based Handbook is a portable guide to diagnosis and treatment in emergency critical care for the resident and attending emergency physician. Its collaborating authors include fellows and attending physicians in the fields of emergency medicine, pulmonary and critical care medicine, cardiology, gastroenterology, and neurocritical care. It is not intended as a guide to what emergency physicians already do best; namely, recognize and correct acute life-threatening conditions. Rather, it details the fundamentals of critical care medicine for the emergency physician who must make sustained data-driven decisions for the critically ill patient in an often chaotic and resource-limited environment.

Each chapter provides a streamlined review of a common problem in critical care medicine, evidence-based guidelines for management, and a summary of relevant literature. The result, we hope, is a valuable guide to rational clinical decision making in the challenging—and changing—world of emergency critical care.

John E. Arbo, MD

CONTENTS

Section 8 Sepsis and Septic Shock 394

Section 9 Disorders of Acid-Base, Electrolytes, and Fluid Balance 491

Section 10 Endocrine Critical Care 543

Section 11 Toxicologic Critical Care 587

Section 12 Environmental Critical Care 680

Section 13 Sedation and Delirium 704

Section 14 Geriatrics and Palliative Care 741

Section 15 The ED-ICU Transfer of Care 762

SECTION 1
Introduction

1

Emergency Critical Care

Robert M. Rodriguez

THE GROWTH OF EMERGENCY DEPARTMENT CRITICAL CARE

Emergency physicians are assuming an ever-expanding role in the care of critically ill patients. The emergency department (ED) is the hospital entry point for virtually all trauma admissions, over 70% of adult sepsis admissions, and the vast majority of patients with acute myocardial infarction, acute stroke, and major gastrointestinal bleeding.[1]

More than a quarter of all patients admitted to the hospital from the ED are critically ill at their time of presentation.[2,3] While some of these patients are admitted to the ICU, many more are resuscitated and stabilized in the ED. Because of increases in ED boarding and delays in ICU transfer, however, EDs are being asked to provide extended ICU-level care.[4] This new volume of ED-based critical care has not only demanded an increasingly solid foundation in critical care medicine from the emergency physician but also given rise to a new specialist: the emergency intensivist. As experts on the presenting phase of critical illness, these physicians are valued members of the critical care team and are uniquely suited to provide a seamless patient transition from the ED to the ICU.

Physicians with dual training in emergency and critical care medicine have successfully combined careers in the ED and ICU for decades; but only in the past several years has there been a formal EM/critical care certification pathway. Historically, emergency physicians who wanted critical care medicine certification had to complete a second residency in addition to fellowship training (usually through an EM/internal medicine/critical care medicine combination). Years of intense lobbying have finally resulted in a more practical certification pathway for the EP. After completing an EM residency and an approved 2-year critical care medicine fellowship, emergency physicians can now be certified in critical care medicine through the American Board of Internal Medicine. This cohort, which began as a handful of triple-trained EM critical care physicians, now encompasses more than 200 EM physicians certified in critical care medicine in the United States.[6]

This surge of EM intensivists has been paralleled by exciting innovations in ED-based diagnosis and therapy. Given that patient physiology changes most rapidly during the first few hours of patient presentation, it is not surprising that these new approaches are profoundly affecting morbidity and mortality in the critically ill.[3] ED-based landmark trials have revolutionized approaches to resuscitation, sepsis, and trauma and have had an impact on many critical care disciplines.

EARLY IDENTIFICATION AND RESUSCITATION OF CRITICAL ILLNESS

One of the most important ED-centered concepts, ushered in by Rivers' landmark study of early goal-directed therapy (EGDT), is that outcomes are improved by early recognition of critical illness and by prompt, aggressive resuscitation.[7] An excellent example of this paradigm of timely, structured ED critical care is the current ED sepsis "bundle" of care (i.e., early identification of septic patients, prompt antibiotic delivery, and aggressive hemodynamic resuscitation) endorsed by the Society of Critical Care Medicine and other international organizations.[8] ED protocols incorporating sepsis bundles have been shown not only to significantly improve survival outcomes but also to decrease the rate of ICU admission by approximately 11%.[2,8]

To continue the example, the first step in ED sepsis protocols is rapid identification and risk stratification, which is accomplished using algorithms that incorporate triage vital signs and lactate point-of-care devices.[9,10] Following identification of severe sepsis, computer-generated and other automatic flagging systems may speed up and ensure reliable activation of sepsis bundle protocols. To further accelerate this process, EM investigators have recently proposed less invasive alternatives for determining central venous oxygen saturation measurement ($SCvO_2$) and central venous pressure, facilitating implementation of EGDT. In a recent study, clearance of >10% of venous blood lactate was found to be an equivalent resuscitative endpoint as achieving an $SCvO_2$ > 70%, effectively reducing the need for placement of central venous catheters.[11] New minimally invasive techniques for assessing intravascular volume status and volume responsiveness have also been introduced, including systolic pressure and pulse pressure variation arterial waveform analysis, physiologic response to passive leg raising, and respirophasic changes in inferior vena cava diameter as measured by bedside ultrasound.[12–16] ED-based research networks and studies, such as the Protocolized Care for Early Septic Shock (ProCESS) trial, continue to refine optimal emergency sepsis management.[17]

Structured early identification and risk-stratification protocols have improved ED care for many other critical disease processes as well. Rapid identification of ST-segment elevation MI (STEMI) via point-of-first-contact electrocardiogram analysis is now standard practice in order to reduce reperfusion (door-to-balloon) times. Many emergency medical systems have also implemented prehospital wireless transmission of 12-lead ECGs to facilitate early identification of STEMI patients and timely transport to dedicated cardiac care centers.[18]

Similarly, in acute stroke management, ED protocols that incorporate early stroke scale examinations are improving diagnosis and management. Many emergency physicians have trained their paramedics to screen patients with abbreviated stroke detection instruments in the field, in order to direct at-risk patients to comprehensive stroke centers for potential reperfusion therapy.[19]

Improved ED-staging algorithms also help identify patients with impending respiratory failure due to pneumonia, COPD, and other respiratory illnesses.[10,20] These tools promote early delivery of appropriate antibiotics, timely initiation of ventilatory support and judicious triage of ICU beds. Analogous to early hemodynamic fluid resuscitation in patients with shock, timely, aggressive respiratory support with non-invasive positive pressure ventilation (NIPPV) in the ED has been shown to improve outcomes and, in many cases, to avert endotracheal intubation and ICU admission.[21] Formerly limited to use in patients with COPD, NIPPV has now been shown to decrease respiratory distress and improve outcomes in a broad spectrum of pulmonary disorders.[21,22]

THE ED–ICU TEAM APPROACH

Protocols emphasizing a team-oriented approach have transformed the delivery of ED critical care. Based on the "golden hour" model of trauma resuscitation, emergency physicians and intensivists have developed ED-based critical care collaborations for treating acute coronary syndrome, stroke, and sepsis. Enhanced communication and structured, automated activation of protocols are the keys to the success of these endeavors. The first step in these protocols is early recognition of critical illness, which ideally begins in the prehospital setting. After recognition of acute disease, prompt notification of key consultants (STEMI team, stroke team, or sepsis team) mobilizes resources and brings critical care personnel to the ED for a timely, orchestrated resuscitation and a smooth transition to the cardiac catheterization laboratory, endovascular suite, or other critical care unit.

Just as ED-derived critical care concepts can benefit ICU practice, so too can ICU-centered concepts improve outcomes in the ED, especially in the setting of extended wait times for transfer to the ICU. For example, with the reported 20% increase in risk of ventilator-associated pneumonia (VAP) per hour spent in the ED, simple ICU VAP reduction measures (head of bed elevation, oral chlorhexidine application, and oral gastric tube decompression) should now be the standard of care in the ED.[26–28] Likewise, ED application of ICU-derived ventilator management standards, such as ARDSnet protocols, should be fully implemented. The lung-protective ventilation strategies outlined in the ARDSnet protocols have recently been demonstrated to benefit a broader population of patients without adult respiratory distress syndrome, making early consideration of these protocols in a broader ED population a logical extension of ICU care.[29]

FUTURE DIRECTIONS

The expanded delivery of critical care in the ED opens fertile ground for emergency physician and intensivist research collaboration on a number of unresolved management issues. In sepsis, for example, the best choice (if there is a best choice) of a first-line vasopressor for patients with septic shock has yet to be clearly determined. Similarly, the adrenal suppression effects of etomidate have raised debate as to whether it should continue to be used as an intubation induction agent in patients with sepsis.[30,31]

A number of unresolved issues also remain for cardiac arrest patients receiving postresuscitation care in the ED. For example, the optimal timing and temperature goals for therapeutic hypothermia (or avoidance of hyperthermia) are unclear, as is the question of whether the neuroprotective benefits extend to patient populations beyond those resuscitated from ventricular fibrillation. Likewise, the potential detrimental effects of postresuscitation hyperoxia and hyperglycemia are undetermined,[32] as are optimal blood pressure targets and glucose control in patients with traumatic brain injury. Collaboration between emergency physicians and intensivists will be needed to address these questions.

Optimal care of the critically ill patient begins with early recognition of disease and aggressive resuscitation in the ED, and is followed by a well-coordinated, multidisciplinary effort to facilitate a smooth transition from ED to the ICU. The ED–ICU partnership has never been stronger and will continue to grow as more EM-trained physicians embark on critical care fellowships. This text provides the emergency physician with the foundation necessary to provide our sickest patients with both immediate and ongoing care.

REFERENCES

1. Wunsch H, Angus DC, Harrison DA, et al. Comparison of medical admissions to intensive care units in the United States and United Kingdom. *Am J Respir Crit Care Med.* 2011;183:1666–1673.
2. Nguyen HB, Rivers EP, Havstad S, et al. Critical care in the emergency department: a physiologic assessment and outcome evaluation. *Acad Emerg Med.* 2000;7:1354–1361.
3. Rivers EP, Nguyen HB, Huang DT, et al. Critical care and emergency medicine. *Curr Opin Crit Care.* 2002;8:600–606.
4. Chalfin DB, Trzeciak S, Likourezos A, et al. Impact of delayed transfer of critically ill patients from the emergency department to the intensive care unit. *Crit Care Med.* 2007;35:1477–1483.
5. Wang HE, Shapiro NI, Angus DC, et al. National estimates of severe sepsis in United States emergency departments. *Crit Care Med.* 2007;35:1928–1936.
6. SAEM
7. Rivers E, Nguyen B, Havstad S, et al. Early goal-directed therapy in the treatment of severe sepsis and septic shock. *N Engl J Med.* 2001;345:1368–1377.
8. Levy MM, Dellinger RP, Townsend SR, et al. The Surviving Sepsis Campaign: results of an international guideline-based performance improvement program targeting severe sepsis. *Crit Care Med.* 2010;38:367–374.
9. Goyal M, Pines JM, Drumheller BC, et al. Point-of-care testing at triage decreases time to lactate level in septic patients. *J Emerg Med.* 2010;38:578–581.
10. Howell MD, Donnino MW, Talmor D, et al. Performance of severity of illness scoring systems in emergency department patients with infection. *Acad Emerg Med.* 2007;14:709–714.
11. Jones AE, Shapiro NI, Trzeciak S, et al. Lactate clearance vs central venous oxygen saturation as goals of early sepsis therapy: a randomized clinical trial. *JAMA.* 2010;303:739–746.
12. Nagdev AD, Merchant RC, Tirado-Gonzalez A, et al. Emergency department bedside ultrasonographic measurement of the caval index for noninvasive determination of low central venous pressure. *Ann Emerg Med.* 2010;55:290–295.
13. Feissel M, Michard F, Faller JP, et al. The respiratory variation in inferior vena cava diameter as a guide to fluid therapy. *Intensive Care Med.* 2004;30:1834–1837.
14. Barbier C, Loubieres Y, Schmit C, et al. Respiratory changes in inferior vena cava diameter are helpful in predicting fluid responsiveness in ventilated septic patients. *Intensive Care Med.* 2004;30:1740–1746.
15. Marik PE, Baram M, Vahid B. Does central venous pressure predict fluid responsiveness? A systematic review of the literature and the tale of seven mares. *Chest.* 2008;134:172–178.
16. Marik PE, Cavallazzi R, Vasu T, et al. Dynamic changes in arterial waveform derived variables and fluid responsiveness in mechanically ventilated patients: a systematic review of the literature. *Crit Care Med.* 2009;37:2642–2647.
17. The ProCESS Investigators. A Randomized trial of protocol-based care for early septic shock. *NEJM* 2014. Epub ahead of print.

18. Moyer P, Ornato JP, Brady WJ Jr, et al. Development of systems of care for ST-elevation myocardial infarction patients: the emergency medical services and emergency department perspective. *Circulation.* 2007;116:e43–e48.
19. Acker JE III, Pancioli AM, Crocco TJ, et al. Implementation strategies for emergency medical services within stroke systems of care: a policy statement from the American Heart Association/American Stroke Association Expert Panel on Emergency Medical Services Systems and the Stroke Council. *Stroke.* 2007;38:3097–3115.
20. Charles PG, Wolfe R, Whitby M, et al. SMART-COP: a tool for predicting the need for intensive respiratory or vasopressor support in community-acquired pneumonia. *Clin Infect Dis.* 2008;47:375–384.
21. Hill NS, Brennan J, Garpestad E, et al. Noninvasive ventilation in acute respiratory failure. *Crit Care Med.* 2007;35:2402–2407.
22. Antro C, Merico F, Urbino R, et al. Non-invasive ventilation as a first-line treatment for acute respiratory failure: "real life" experience in the emergency department. *Emerg Med J.* 2005;22:772–777.
23. Leifer D, Bravata DM, Connors JJ III, et al. Metrics for measuring quality of care in comprehensive stroke centers: detailed follow-up to Brain Attack Coalition comprehensive stroke center recommendations: a statement for healthcare professionals from the American Heart Association/American Stroke Association. *Stroke.* 2011;42:849–877.
24. Sattin JA, Olson SE, Liu L, et al. An expedited code stroke protocol is feasible and safe. *Stroke.* 2006;37:2935–2939.
25. Nolan JP, Soar J. Postresuscitation care: entering a new era. *Curr Opin Crit Care.* 2010;16:216–222.
26. Carr BG, Kaye AJ, Wiebe DJ, et al. Emergency department length of stay: a major risk factor for pneumonia in intubated blunt trauma patients. *J Trauma.* 2007;63:9–12.
27. Grap MJ, Munro CL, Unoki T, et al. Ventilator-associated Pneumonia: the Potential Critical Role of Emergency Medicine in Prevention. *J Emerg Med.* 2012;42:353–362.
28. Wood S, Winters ME. Care of the intubated emergency department patient. *J Emerg Med.* 2011;40:419–427.
29. Serpo Neto A, Cardoso SO, Manetta JA, et al. Association between use of lung-protective ventilation with lower tidal volumes and clinical outcomes among patients without acute respiratory distress syndrome. *JAMA.* 2012;308:1651–1659.
30. Chan CM, Mitchell AL, Shorr AF. Etomidate is associated with mortality and adrenal insufficiency in sepsis: a meta-analysis*. *Crit Care Med.* 2012;40(11):2945–2953.
31. Cuthbertson BH, Sprung CL, Annane D, et al. The effects of etomidate on adrenal responsiveness and mortality in patients with septic shock. *Intensive Care Med.* 2009;35:1868–1876.
32. Kilgannon JH, Jones AE, Shapiro NI, et al. Association between arterial hyperoxia following resuscitation from cardiac arrest and in-hospital mortality. *JAMA.* 2010;303:2165–2171.
33. Duchesne JC, Kimonis K, Marr AB, et al. Damage control resuscitation in combination with damage control laparotomy: a survival advantage. *J Trauma.* 2010;69(1):46–52.
34. Goldstein RS. Management of the critically ill patient in the emergency department: focus on safety issues. *Crit Care Clin.* 2005;21:81–89.

SECTION 2
Hemodynamic Monitoring

2

Tissue Oxygenation and Cardiac Output

Geoffrey K. Lighthall and Catherine S. Reid

BACKGROUND

The two principle determinants of tissue perfusion are, (1) a mean arterial pressure (MAP) sufficient to maintain constant blood flow within key organs (i.e., within the autoregulatory range); and, (2) tissue oxygen delivery in excess of metabolic demand. Deliberate evaluation of these physiologic relationships can help define an individual's risk for organ dysfunction and shock, as well as establish end points of resuscitation.

The balance between oxygen utilization (VO_2) and oxygen delivery (DO_2) provides a conceptual framework for understanding the development of organ dysfunction and for the formation of resuscitation strategies. DO_2 is the product of cardiac output (CO) and arterial oxygen content and may be determined using the calculations in Table 2.1. Under normal conditions, global VO_2 is approximately 25% of the delivered quantity, demonstrated by mixed venous oxyhemoglobin saturations of 70% to 75%. Factors that unilaterally increase VO_2 or decrease DO_2, therefore, increase the oxygen extraction ratio (VO_2/DO_2) and lower the body's overall oxygen reserves. In extreme cases, when DO_2 falls below a critical threshold (Fig. 2.1A), DO_2 limits oxygen consumption. Below this point, oxygen consumption becomes supply-dependent, mitochondrial respiration is impaired, and lactic acidosis often manifests.[1–3] The curve is a snapshot of a dynamic situation; infection and stress raise oxygen demand, while hemorrhage, hypovolemia, or impaired cardiac function compromises DO_2.

Most clinicians are accustomed to thinking of shock, organ failure, and perfusion not in terms of the VO_2/DO_2 relationship, but rather in terms of changes in blood pressure, or MAP. In the case of cellular function, these two physiologic parameters overlap significantly. When MAP drops below the autoregulatory threshold for a given organ (Fig. 2.1B), regional imbalances between VO_2 and DO_2 occur, yet may escape detection. Note that deficits in DO_2 can occur in the setting of an apparently normal MAP—a condition termed cryptic shock[4]—and that a desirable level of total-body DO_2 can exist in conjunction with an inadequate MAP.

Resuscitation from shock states focuses on moving the patient to within the normal range on these curves (Fig. 2.1A and B). Careful inspection of the determinants underlying DO_2

TABLE 2.1 Determinants of Tissue Oxygenation

Variable	Calculation
MAP	CO · SVR
DO_2	$CO \times CaO_2$
VO_2	$CO \cdot (CaO_2 - CvO_2)$
CaO_2	$(1.34 \cdot Hb \times SaO_2) + 0.0031 \cdot PaO_2$
O_2ER	$VO_2/DO_2 = (CaO_2 - CvO_2/CaO_2)$

MAP, mean arterial pressure; CO, cardiac output; SVR, systemic vascular resistance; VO_2, oxygen utilization; CaO_2, arterial oxygen content; CvO_2, mixed venous oxygen content; Hb, hemoglobin; SaO_2, hemoglobin saturation; DO_2, oxygen delivery; PaO_2, partial pressure of arterial oxygen; O_2ER, oxygen extraction ratio.

and MAP (Table 2.1, Fig. 2.1A) reveals the common factor of CO. As the sole factor whose improvement leads to increases in both MAP and DO_2, CO optimization is typically the focus of patient examination and monitoring, fluid replacement, and other resuscitative measures. Pursuit of resuscitative targets other than CO is of less clear benefit. For example, in the wrong situation, raising MAP with alpha-adrenergic agonists may actually worsen CO and have disastrous consequences for DO_2 and tissue perfusion. Similarly, raising hemoglobin levels with aggressive transfusion does not necessarily improve DO_2,

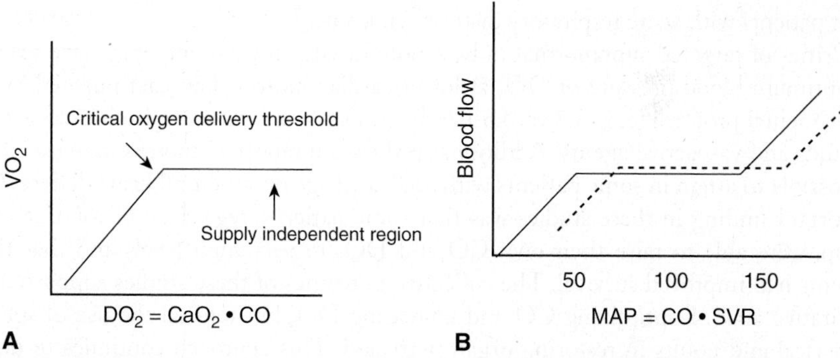

FIGURE 2.1 The key determinants of organ perfusion are depicted. In **(A)**, the relationship between oxygen consumption (VO_2) and delivery (DO_2) is indicated. Patients usually function on the rightward side of the curve, where an excess of oxygen is supplied relative to demand. As delivery decreases relative to consumption, the patient moves left on the curve. A decrease in central venous oxygen saturation accompanies leftward movement on the curve. In severe cases where delivery is unable to meet metabolic demands, the patient slips beneath the critical DO_2 threshold, where oxygen consumption is limited by delivery. Organ dysfunction and lactic acidosis are regarded as evidence of pathologic oxygen supply. In **(B)**, the autoregulatory curve describing constancy of organ blood flow over a broad range of MAP is shown. Some patients with chronic hypertension have curves shifted to the right relative to the normotensive curve as shown with the dashed line. For both relationships shown, the flat horizontal portions indicate safe ranges, indicative of adequate organ blood flow and intact homeostatic mechanisms. Movement to the down-sloping portions on the left indicates decompensation, placing the patient at risk for organ failure. VO_2, oxygen uptake/minute; CaO_2, oxygen content of arterial blood [mainly hemoglobin]; CO, cardiac output; MAP, mean arterial pressure; SVR, systemic vascular resistance; DO_2, oxygen delivery.

can produce volume overload, and can precipitate acute lung injury. For these reasons, the critical care community pays close attention to interventions that modulate CO and to monitoring systems that capture these changes. This chapter provides a review of the evolution of our understanding of these concepts; details of the evidence from specific studies of these subjects are presented in the Literature Tables of Chapters 3, 4, and 5.

HISTORICAL PERSPECTIVE

Modern hemodynamic monitoring and resuscitation have evolved significantly from decades ago, when manipulation of CO and DO_2 indices to supranormal values was believed to improve patient survival. In the early 1970s, enhanced ventricular performance and increased DO_2 and consumption were predicted to improve survival in trauma patients.[5] Subsequent studies in surgical patients appeared to confirm the survival benefit of using a pulmonary artery catheter (PAC) to facilitate increases in CO and DO_2.[6–10] Deliberate augmentation of DO_2 in medical and surgical ICU patients was the natural next step; however, therapy designed to achieve such supranormal indices repeatedly failed to improve outcomes in this patient population.[11–14] The difference in outcomes was believed to be due to the use of less stringent and, in some cases, clinician-generated, resuscitative end points in larger and better-controlled studies comparing pulmonary artery and CVP catheters. These studies demonstrated no advantage of pursuing supranormal indices in high-risk surgical patients,[15] in patients with shock and sepsis,[16] or in adult patients with acute respiratory distress syndrome.[17]

Critics of targeted supranormal indices noted that some patients may have reached an optimum blood pressure or DO_2 at lower cardiac indices than that pursued by the experimental protocol (e.g., 3.3 vs. 4.5 L/min/m^2) and suffered harm from excessive use of fluids and vasoactive agents. Additionally, these supranormal indices may have been impossible to attain in some patients with advanced age or structural heart disease. One important finding in these studies was that some patients, regardless of the treatment group, were able to raise their own CO and DO_2 to very high levels and that these patients had improved survival. The collective outcomes of these studies supported the qualitative goal of optimizing CO and increasing DO_2 but refuted the use of specific numerical end points in restoring organ perfusion. This approach continues to define critical care resuscitative philosophy.

OPTIMIZATION OF CARDIAC OUTPUT

CO is the product of heart rate and stroke volume. In healthy individuals, stoke volume is normally a function of preload; however, with any acute or chronic disease, stroke volume is also sensitive to ventricular performance (contractility) and afterload. Optimization of tissue perfusion requires the provider to answer four questions: (1) Is the patient fluid responsive (i.e., will a fluid challenge increase stroke volume)? (2) Is contractility adequate (i.e., does the patient need an inotrope)? (3) Does the patient need a vasopressor? and (4) Does the patient need a blood transfusion? If the patient has adequate MAP (achieved using vasopressors if needed), hemoglobin within normal range and constant across serial measurements, and a relatively static demand for oxygen (VO_2), then the provider need addresses only fluid responsiveness and contractility to optimize CO. Techniques used to monitor these parameters will vary by clinical circumstance and available resources; whereas some suit initial evaluation in the ED, others with greater trending capabilities may be preferred in the ICU.

FLUID RESPONSIVENESS

Fluid responsiveness describes the ability of the heart to increase its stroke volume—and consequently CO—in response to infusion of fluids. From a patient management perspective, fluid responsiveness determines the extent to which circulatory homeostasis can be maintained with fluids alone, without the addition of inotropes or vasopressors. The decision to give a patient more fluids requires an understanding of the concepts demonstrated by the Frank-Starling curve, which describes how stroke volume responds to changes in preload (Fig. 2.2). The ascending portion of the Frank-Starling curve corresponds to the fluid-responsive phase of resuscitation, seen as a fairly linear increase in CO. Once the left ventricle reaches the plateau phase of the curve, additional fluid administration will not further improve CO and may lead to adverse consequences such as hydrostatic pulmonary edema.

Methods of interpreting intravascular volume range from clinical assessments (e.g., inspection of veins or a passive leg-raising test), to more invasive methods (e.g., central venous and pulmonary artery catheterization), and to newer and technically sophisticated methods (e.g., echocardiography and analysis of flow parameters). When evaluating these techniques, it is helpful to consider their ability to predict a state of fluid responsiveness versus euvolemia and how their unique characteristics may be paired with different clinical situations to yield accurate and meaningful information.

Passive Leg-Raising

The passive leg-raising test (PLR), in which the legs of a supine patient are elevated to 45 degrees, delivers a reversible endogenous fluid challenge by increasing venous return; the effect on blood pressure and heart rate is subsequently evaluated. When PLR is used in concert with an existing arterial line, changes in preload leading to increased

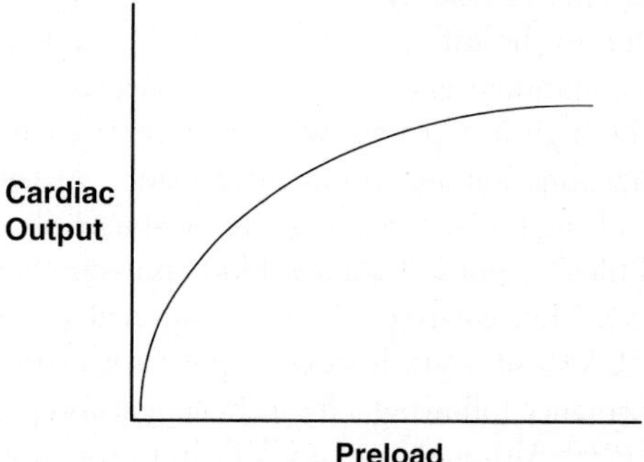

FIGURE 2.2 The Frank-Starling curve describing the relationship between cardiac output (CO) and preload. Volume responsiveness describes the steep portion of the curve in which modest changes in preload result in significant increases in CO and hence MAP. In the upper region of the curve, a similar change in preload would result in a negligible change in CO.

CO and blood pressure are immediately apparent. Because fluid bolus administration is the primary alternative to a PLR, the PLR can quickly identify patients for whom fluid infusion would be of no benefit and potentially harmful. The PLR has shown good correspondence with other derived indices in predicting fluid responsiveness in patients with sepsis and pancreatitis[18] and has been compared favorably with transthoracic echo[19] and esophageal Doppler[20] in mechanically ventilated patients. PLR is a valuable technique in early patient assessment, as it requires little technical skill and does not rely on the presence of a central venous and pulmonary arterial catheter for preload assessment.

Central Venous Pressure Monitoring

Central venous pressure (CVP) is the measurement of pressure within the thorax in the superior vena cava and serves as a reasonable surrogate for right atrial pressure. Historically, CVP was widely used to estimate intravascular volume in critically ill patients,[21] with the implication that CVP served as a reasonable surrogate for left ventricular preload and that some correspondence between measured values and CO existed.

The standard test for volume responsiveness was to give a fluid challenge that increases the CVP by 2 mm Hg and then determine whether it increased CO.[22] A study of 83 ICU patients showed that patients with an increase in CVP of 2 mm Hg following a bolus of approximately 500 mL of isotonic crystalloids over 10 to 30 minutes had a cardiac index increase of 300 mL/min/m^2. Two additional findings of the study were important: (1) only 4.5 % of the patients with a CVP more than 10 mm Hg responded to a fluid challenge; and (2) of patients who had increase in CO, 42% only had a simultaneous increase in blood pressure. The study concluded that, first, patients with a CVP of more than 10 mm Hg responded poorly to volume infusion and that 10 mm Hg likely represented euvolemia in most individuals; and second, that blood pressure increase was not a good indicator of cardiac response to a fluid challenge.[23] These data, which supported the notion that CVPs in the 8 to 12 mm Hg range indicated volume repletion, were incorporated into early goal-directed therapy and subsequently into the initial versions of the Surviving Sepsis Guidelines.[24,25]

More recent examination of central pressures has shown CVP to be a poor indicator of intravascular volume. A healthy person may have a CVP of less than zero in an upright position (due to the influence of negative intrathoracic pressure generated during spontaneous respirations) and still have an adequate CO and be euvolemic. Conversely, CVP can be high in a patient with poor ventricular function and low CO or with good ventricular function and volume overload.[26] As these common scenarios illustrate, values derived from pressure readings are most usefully considered in conjunction with a dynamic clinical response—such as blood pressure or urine output—or with another measure of CO. Meta-analyses show no difference between fluid responders and nonresponders at CVPs of a given value; a poor correlation between changes in CVP and cardiac performance following a fluid challenge; and poor correlation between blood volume and CVP.[27,28] Although use of CVPs in resuscitation persists, the recommendation for their application has softened in the latest Surviving Sepsis Guidelines,[29] and many believe the practice of targeted CVPs should be abandoned completely.[28] Despite the inability of CVP to represent the dynamic range of fluid responsiveness, a low CVP (<5 mm Hg) in a critically ill patient is generally assumed to correlate with hypovolemia.[29] Ideally, however, significant hypovolemia should be suspected clinically and acted upon empirically, without the need for invasive pressure monitoring.

Pulmonary Artery Catheterization

In the setting of cardiac and lung pathology, aberrations in right heart compliance and pulmonary vascular resistance can drastically alter the relationship between CVP and left atrial pressure. In critically ill patients with such underlying pathology, pulmonary artery catheterization remains a reasonable option for measuring both right and left heart and pulmonary artery pressures. As with the CVP, however, pulmonary artery occlusion pressure (PAOP, or "wedge" pressure) measurements are dependent on myocardial compliance. Multiple studies of ICU patients with acute illness have shown PAOP to correlate poorly or inconsistently with left ventricular end-diastolic volume (LVEDV).[30–33] Studies in mechanically ventilated patients receiving positive-end expiratory pressure (PEEP) show that PEEP drastically alters the relationship between PAOP and recruitable stoke volume, and surprisingly, that a right heart parameter (right ventricular end-diastolic volume; RVEDV) correlated more reliably with changes in the cardiac index.[34,35]

As noted, use of the PAC was historically justified by the assumption that it was desirable to target improvements in physiologic parameters to supranormal end points in critically ill patients. Use of PACs for this purpose has fallen over the last 10 years because of the reasons cited, because of relative success with CVP-based methods for resuscitation in septic shock,[36] and because of unique complications of the PAC, including ventricular arrhythmias, right bundle-branch block, thromboembolism, pulmonary artery rupture,[37–39] and frequent misinterpretation of PAC-generated data.[40,41] Despite these issues, debate continues as to whether the PAC can assist in fluid and hemodynamic management in patients with severe cardiac or pulmonary pathology. A number of randomized trials have assessed protocols for fluid and inotrope management, both with and without the PA catheter in patients undergoing major surgery,[15] in patients with congestive heart failure,[42] shock and ARDS,[16,39] and in general ICU populations,[43–45] and have demonstrated no hospital or mortality benefit ascribable to the device. Future research is needed to demonstrate whether the PAC retains a useful niche in the management of the very few critically ill patients (e.g., those with severe pulmonary hypertension) in whom maintenance of CO requires careful manipulation of pulmonary artery pressures.

CARDIAC CONTRACTILITY

Central Venous Oxygen Saturation and Lactate Clearance

While a central venous catheter is of limited value in assessing fluid responsiveness and of no use in direct measurement of CO, analysis of CVP-derived central venous oxygen saturation ($ScvO_2$) can provide insight into the adequacy of cardiac contractility and CO. $ScvO_2$ provides a dynamic measure of the VO_2/DO_2 relationship; $ScvO_2$ values of >70% are consistent with an adequate CO and perfusion status. When VO_2 is constant among several serial Fick equation measurements (i.e., all obtained with the patient at a similar level of activity and with a similar body temperature), increases and decreases in $ScvO_2$ indicate horizontal movement along the VO_2/DO_2 curve (Fig. 2.1A) and thus indicate a change in CO or hemoglobin, or both. If the hemoglobin is also constant during serial measurements of $ScvO_2$, then changes in the latter value (again, indicating horizontal movement along the curve) indicate changes in CO. In the absence of significant bradycardia, CO problems are typically due to inadequate stroke volume, either from low preload or from problems with contractility. Continuing with the condition in which VO_2 and hemoglobin are constant along several measurements, if a patient is on the upper reaches of the Starling curve, and therefore is euvolemic, then abnormalities in $ScvO_2$ are indicative of inadequate contractility and suggest the need for inotropic support. The $ScvO_2$ target of 70% is an integral part of the Surviving Sepsis campaign's resuscitation bundle for severe sepsis,[36] and careful inspection of the algorithm reveals the logic detailed above, in which $ScvO_2$ is used to judge adequacy of contractility. Intermittent blood samplings via CVP, dialysis, or peripherally inserted central catheters lines, or the use of catheters with oximetric sensors are equally valid means of analyzing $ScvO_2$.

Central vein oximetry is based on the assumption that the cellular machinery responsible for oxygen uptake and utilization functions normally and that changes in measured values reflect oxygen supply and demand. This is not, however, always the case. In sepsis, mitochondrial function can be impaired as a result of depletion of high-energy substrates related to the inflammatory burst; in this case, oxygen consumption is disrupted in the setting of high demand—a state termed cytopathic hypoxia.[46,47] Under these conditions, central venous saturation will be deceptively normal because tissues cannot fully utilize the oxygen delivered. Organ function and adequacy of blood flow should therefore be simultaneously assessed. To this end, lactate clearance has recently been studied as an assessment of cellular function during resuscitation. In two recent multicenter trials, patient inability to normalize lactate with resuscitation was found to be an independent predictor of mortality.[48,49] In a recent landmark trial, a lactate clearance of 10% was found to be equivalent to $ScvO_2$ as both the resuscitative end point and predictor of mortality.[50] Importantly, resuscitation to a $ScvO_2$ saturation of >70% can still be associated with lactate nonclearance for the reasons stated above; in these instances, clinical assessment of organ function and lactate clearance should be used to guide ongoing resuscitation.[49]

Echocardiography

Transthoracic echocardiography (TEE), with its increased portability and affordability, has found a place in all acute care settings, and the modern intensivist and emergency physician are expected to be skilled in its use. Where the PAC uses pressure measurements to make volume determinations, echocardiography relies on direct visualization of the cardiac anatomy and flow dynamics. In patients with overlapping causes of circulatory failure, echocardiography can evaluate structural abnormalities, contractility, and intravascular volume in a single efficient exam.

In the last decade, the improved image quality of portable echocardiography machines has made TTE a popular tool for intravascular fluid assessment. Right heart preload can be reliably obtained by direct measurement of variation in the diameter of the inferior vena cava (IVC) with respiration and by measurement of right and left ventricular end-diastolic volumes. In one study, a 50% decrease in IVC diameter (caval index), seen in the subcostal views with spontaneous breathing, correlated with an RA pressure of <10 mm Hg (mean SD 6±5) as measured by CVP.[51] Recent studies in ED settings found caval index measurement to be a useful noninvasive tool for initial estimation of CVP and, more importantly, fluid responsiveness.[52] In mechanically ventilated patients, an IVC variation of 12% with respiration (delta IVC) differentiated fluid responders from nonresponders.[53] In another study of mechanically ventilated septic patients, the CVP and the IVC diameter increase on inspiration (distensibility index [dIVC]) was measured before and after a gelatin fluid challenge of 7 mL/kg. Response was measured as an increase in cardiac index (CI) of 15% or more. A dIVC of >18% predicted fluid responsiveness with a sensitivity and specificity of 90%. Changes in CVP, however, correlated poorly with changes in CI or dIVC.[54] Although it can be challenging to visualize the IVC in patients who are obese or post–abdominal surgery, TTE is usually able to provide a quick, noninvasive, and reliable method of assessing intravascular volume status and fluid responsiveness in most patients.

TTE is also a promising tool for noninvasive measurements of global cardiac contractility and left ventricular function. A goal-oriented exam can provide a rapid assessment of the adequacy of contractility and aid in resuscitation decision making.[55,56] While this technique (discussed in detail in Chapter 6) requires an initial investment in training of medical staff, it has a subsequent high success rate and requires little time to perform. Studies have demonstrated that after initial training—including basic echocardiography, review of images, and demonstration of image acquisition and interpretation techniques—intensivists were able to successfully perform and interpret (84% correct) a limited TTE in a mean time of 11 minutes.[56] Goal-directed TTE can also aid in the diagnosis of specific pathologies contributing to a patient's hemodynamic instability. TTE is safe and noninvasive, which make it an ideal tool for repeated assessment of hemodynamic variables that change as a result of interventions or the disease process itself.

As noted above, fluid responsiveness and contractility are the key factors influencing CO; an emergency physician experienced in TTE can evaluate both without the need for CVP monitoring. For the many patients who do receive central catheter placement—to facilitate safe administration of vasopressors or serial assessment of $ScvO_2$—the volumetric views provided by echocardiography may help contextualize waveform or catheter-based values.

INFLUENCE OF CARDIOPULMONARY INTERACTIONS ON CARDIAC OUTPUT

Cardiac output and MAP interact with the respiratory system in a predictable manner. With positive pressure ventilation, venous return to the left ventricle is initially augmented, causing a rise in cardiac output and MAP during early inspiration. Following this, a decrease in RV preload caused by positive intrathoracic pressure will manifest as a drop in LV preload. The varying effects of positive pressure ventilation on preload and cardiac output are influenced by the patient's intravascular volume status. For example, with hypovolemia, the myocardium is on the steep portion of the Frank-Starling curve, such that minor variations in left ventricular preload with inspiration or expiration can cause appreciable changes in CO and MAP.

In mechanically ventilated patients, changes in arterial pressure waveforms and Doppler analysis of aortic blood flow during the respiratory cycle can be used to evaluate euvolemia and fluid responsiveness. Where CVP and other pressure-based measures of fluid responsiveness are suspect in these patients, flow-based measurements

TABLE 2.2 Hemodynamic Monitoring Devices

Device or Modality	Ability to Evaluate or Measure:								
	Invasiveness	Pre-load	Contractility	Euvolemia	Fluid Responsiveness	CO	VO_2/DO_2	Training Needs	Limitations or Artifacts
CVP	Central vein	RA pressure	Indirect, from $ScVO_2$	Yes	Generally, if low	Indirect via $ScVO_2$	$ScVO_2$	+	Prone to respiratory artifacts
Pulmonary Artery	Central vein	LA pressure	Starling curves from TDCO	Plateau of Starling curve	CO responsive to dPAWP	Direct measurement	SvO_2	+++	Prone to respiratory and valvular artifacts
Arterial Line	Art line	No	No	Lack of PPV, SPV	Lack of SPV	No	No	+	SPV depends on MV
TTE	None	Visual	Visual	Yes	Visual estimate	No	No	+++	Image quality, non-continuous device
Esophageal Doppler	Nasoesophageal probe	Flow analysis	Wave analysis	Yes	Wave analysis during MV	Via assumptions	No	++	Probe focus and position, requires MV

Common means of circulatory monitoring are listed and compared for their ability to estimate intravascular volume, contractility, and cardiac output.
CO, cardiac output; MV, mechanical ventilation; PPV, pulse pressure variation; SPV, systolic pressure variation; dPAWP, change in (delta) pulmonary artery wedge pressure; TDCO, thermodilution cardiac output.

using Doppler achieve their highest accuracy. Similarly proven are several indices of fluid responsiveness derived from the interaction between positive pressure ventilation and arterial blood pressure waveforms (e.g., systolic and pulse pressure variation). Measurement of these indices is described in Table 2.2 and discussed fully in Chapter 3. Reliable parameters for predicting fluid responsiveness have not been developed for patients breathing spontaneously.

CONCLUSION

Optimization of CO is central to the maintenance of circulatory homeostasis. The emergency and critical care communities have moved away from resuscitation based on targeted values of CO and toward resuscitation based on adequacy of CO. Evaluating adequacy of CO requires assessment of fluid responsiveness and contractility. A number of invasive and noninvasive tools can be used in a flexible manner to provide rapid answers to these fundamental questions.

REFERENCES

1. Astiz ME, et al. Oxygen delivery and consumption in patients with hyperdynamic septic shock. *Crit Care Med.* 1987;15(1):26–28.
2. Astiz ME, et al. Relationship of oxygen delivery and mixed venous oxygenation to lactic acidosis in patients with sepsis and acute myocardial infarction. *Crit Care Med.* 1988;16(7):655–658.
3. Shibutani K, et al. Critical level of oxygen delivery in anesthetized man. *Crit Care Med.* 1983;11(8):640–643.
4. Puskarich MA, et al. Outcomes of patients undergoing early sepsis resuscitation for cryptic shock compared with overt shock. *Resuscitation.* 2011;82(10):1289–1293.
5. Shoemaker WC, Montgomery ES, Kaplan E, et al. Physiologic patterns in surviving and nonsurviving shock patients. Use of sequential cardiorespiratory variables in defining criteria for therapeutic goals and early warning of death. *Arch Surg.* 1973(106):630–636.
6. Rady MY, Edwards JD, Nightingale P. Early cardiorespiratory findings after severe blunt thoracic trauma and their relation to outcome. *Br J Surg.* 1992;79(1):65–68.
7. Tuchschmidt J, et al. Early hemodynamic correlates of survival in patients with septic shock. *Crit Care Med.* 1989;17(8):719–723.
8. Shoemaker WC, et al. Prospective trial of supranormal values of survivors as therapeutic goals in high-risk surgical patients. *Chest.* 1988;94(6):1176–1186.
9. Boyd O, Grounds RM, Bennett ED. A randomized clinical trial of the effect of deliberate perioperative increase of oxygen delivery on mortality in high-risk surgical patients. *JAMA.* 1993;270(22):2699–2707.
10. Bishop MH, et al. Prospective, randomized trial of survivor values of cardiac index, oxygen delivery, and oxygen consumption as resuscitation endpoints in severe trauma. *J Trauma.* 1995;38(5):780–787.
11. Gattinoni L, et al. A trial of goal-oriented hemodynamic therapy in critically ill patients. SvO_2 Collaborative Group. *N Engl J Med.* 1995;333(16):1025–1032.
12. Tuchschmidt J, et al. Elevation of cardiac output and oxygen delivery improves outcome in septic shock. *Chest.* 1992;102(1):216–220.
13. Yu M, et al. Effect of maximizing oxygen delivery on morbidity and mortality rates in critically ill patients: a prospective, randomized, controlled study. *Crit Care Med.* 1993;21(6):830–838.
14. Hayes MA, et al. Elevation of systemic oxygen delivery in the treatment of critically ill patients. *N Engl J Med.* 1994;330(24):1717–1722.
15. Sandham JD, et al. A randomized, controlled trial of the use of pulmonary-artery catheters in high-risk surgical patients. *N Engl J Med.* 2003;348(1):5–14.
16. Richard C, et al. Early use of the pulmonary artery catheter and outcomes in patients with shock and acute respiratory distress syndrome: a randomized controlled trial. *JAMA.* 2003;290(20):2713–2720.
17. Wheeler AP, et al. Pulmonary-artery versus central venous catheter to guide treatment of acute lung injury. *N Engl J Med.* 2006;354(21):2213–2224.

18. Preau S, et al. Passive leg raising is predictive of fluid responsiveness in spontaneously breathing patients with severe sepsis or acute pancreatitis. *Crit Care Med.* 2010;38(3):819–825.
19. Lamia B, et al. Echocardiographic prediction of volume responsiveness in critically ill patients with spontaneously breathing activity. *Intensive Care Med.* 2007;33(7):1125–1132.
20. Monnet X, et al. Passive leg raising predicts fluid responsiveness in the critically ill. *Crit Care Med.* 2006;34(5):1402–1407.
21. Boldt J, et al. Volume replacement strategies on intensive care units: results from a postal survey. *Intensive Care Med.* 1998;24(2):147–151.
22. Magder SA, Georgiadis GS, Cheong T. Respiratory variations in right atrial pressure predict response to fluid challenge. *J Crit Care.* 1992;7:76–85.
23. Magder S, Bafaqeeh F. The clinical role of central venous pressure measurements. *J Intensive Care Med.* 2007;22(1):44–51.
24. Dellinger RP, et al. Surviving sepsis campaign guidelines for management of severe sepsis and septic shock. *Crit Care Med.* 2004;32(3):858–873.
25. Dellinger RP, et al. Surviving sepsis campaign: international guidelines for management of severe sepsis and septic shock: 2008. *Crit Care Med.* 2008;36(1):296–327.
26. Magder S. How to use central venous pressure measurements. *Curr Opin Crit Care.* 2005;11(3):264–270.
27. Marik PE, Baram M, Vahid B. Does central venous pressure predict fluid responsiveness? A systematic review of the literature and the tale of seven mares. *Chest.* 2008;134(1):172–178.
28. Marik PE, Cavallazzi R. Does the central venous pressure predict fluid responsiveness? An updated meta-analysis and a plea for some common sense. *Crit Care Med.* 2013;41(7):1774–1781.
29. Dellinger RP, et al. Surviving sepsis campaign: international guidelines for management of severe sepsis and septic shock: 2012. *Crit Care Med.* 2013;41(2):580–637.
30. Fontes ML, et al. Assessment of ventricular function in critically ill patients: limitations of pulmonary artery catheterization. Institutions of the McSPI Research Group. *J Cardiothorac Vasc Anesth.* 1999;13(5):521–527.
31. Spinelli L, et al. Losartan treatment and left ventricular filling during volume loading in patients with dilated cardiomyopathy. *Am Heart J.* 2002;143(3):433–440.
32. Tousignant CP, Walsh F, Mazer CD. The use of transesophageal echocardiography for preload assessment in critically ill patients. *Anesth Analg.* 2000;90(2):351–355.
33. Hansen RM, et al. Poor correlation between pulmonary arterial wedge pressure and left ventricular end-diastolic volume after coronary artery bypass graft surgery. *Anesthesiology.* 1986;64(6):764–770.
34. Cheatham ML, et al. Right ventricular end-diastolic volume index as a predictor of preload status in patients on positive end-expiratory pressure. *Crit Care Med.* 1998;26(11):1801–1806.
35. Diebel L, et al. End-diastolic volume versus pulmonary artery wedge pressure in evaluating cardiac preload in trauma patients. *J Trauma.* 1994;37(6):950–955.
36. Rivers E, et al. Early goal-directed therapy in the treatment of severe sepsis and septic shock. *N Engl J Med.* 2001;345(19):1368–1377.
37. Coulter TD, Wiedemann HP. Complications of hemodynamic monitoring. *Clin Chest Med.* 1999;20(2):249–267. vii.
38. Hadian M, Pinsky MR. Evidence-based review of the use of the pulmonary artery catheter: impact data and complications. *Crit Care.* 2006;10(suppl 3):S8.
39. Wheeler AP, Bernard GR, Thompson BT, et al. Pulmonary-artery versus central venous catheter to guide treatment of acute lung injury. *N Engl J Med.* 2006;354(21):2213–2224.
40. Jacka MJ, et al. Pulmonary artery occlusion pressure estimation: how confident are anesthesiologists? *Crit Care Med.* 2002;30(6):1197–1203.
41. Summerhill EM, Baram M. Principles of pulmonary artery catheterization in the critically ill. *Lung.* 2005;183(3):209–219.
42. Binanay C, et al. Evaluation study of congestive heart failure and pulmonary artery catheterization effectiveness: the ESCAPE trial. *JAMA.* 2005;294(13):1625–1633.
43. Guyatt G. A randomized control trial of right-heart catheterization in critically ill patients. Ontario Intensive Care Study Group. *J Intensive Care Med.* 1991;6(2):91–95.
44. Harvey S, et al. Assessment of the clinical effectiveness of pulmonary artery catheters in management of patients in intensive care (PAC-Man): a randomised controlled trial. *Lancet.* 2005;366(9484):472–477.
45. Rhodes A, et al. A randomised, controlled trial of the pulmonary artery catheter in critically ill patients. *Intensive Care Med.* 2002;28(3):256–264.
46. Fink MP. Bench-to-bedside review: cytopathic hypoxia. *Crit Care.* 2002;6(6):491–499.
47. Fink M. Cytopathic hypoxia in sepsis. *Acta Anaesthesiol Scand Suppl.* 1997;110:87–95.

48. Puskarich MA, et al. Whole blood lactate kinetics in patients undergoing quantitative resuscitation for severe sepsis and septic shock. *Chest.* 2013;143(6):1548–1553.
49. Arnold RC, et al. Multicenter study of early lactate clearance as a determinant of survival in patients with presumed sepsis. *Shock.* 2009;32(1):35–39.
50. Jones AE, et al. Lactate clearance vs central venous oxygen saturation as goals of early sepsis therapy: a randomized clinical trial. *JAMA.* 2010;303(8):739–746.
51. Kircher BJ, Himelman RB, Schiller NB. Noninvasive estimation of right atrial pressure from the inspiratory collapse of the inferior vena cava. *Am J Cardiol.* 1990;66(4):493–496.
52. Nagdev AD, et al. Emergency department bedside ultrasonographic measurement of the caval index for noninvasive determination of low central venous pressure. *Ann Emerg Med.* 2010;55(3):290–295.
53. Feissel M, et al. The respiratory variation in inferior vena cava diameter as a guide to fluid therapy. *Intensive Care Med.* 2004;30(9):1834–1837.
54. Barbier C, Loubières Y, Schmit C. Respiratory changes in inferior vena cava diameter are helpful in predicting fluid responsiveness in ventilated septic patients. *Intensive Care Med.* 2004;30:1740–1746.
55. Jensen MB, et al. Transthoracic echocardiography for cardiopulmonary monitoring in intensive care. *Eur J Anaesthesiol.* 2004;21(9):700–707.
56. Manasia AR, et al. Feasibility and potential clinical utility of goal-directed transthoracic echocardiography performed by noncardiologist intensivists using a small hand-carried device (SonoHeart) in critically ill patients. *J Cardiothorac Vasc Anesth.* 2005;19(2):155–159.

3

Noninvasive Hemodynamic Monitoring

Chad M. Meyers

BACKGROUND

The provision of optimal medical care presents a dilemma in emergency medicine. As the importance of early resuscitation continues to be reinforced, the role and responsibilities of the emergency physician continue to expand.[1,2] Unfortunately, overcrowded emergency departments and overextended staff weaken the emergency physician's ability to provide the highest level of care to the sickest patients.[3–5] This concerning trend is exemplified in the early management of severe sepsis, in which full realization of the benefits of aggressive goal-directed therapy is often constrained by the requirement for invasive monitoring.[6,7] Knowledge of noninvasive hemodynamic monitoring modalities enables the emergency physician to improve diagnostic efficiency and more effectively deliver care to the critically ill.[8] This chapter reviews the noninvasive monitoring devices available to the emergency physician and discusses their clinical applicability.

CARDIAC OUTPUT MONITORING

As discussed in detail in Chapter 2, tissue oxygenation is maintained during periods of rising metabolic demand by the modulation of cardiac output and tissue oxygen extraction. If cardiac output or arterial oxygen content is suboptimal, the delivery of oxygen, or tissue perfusion, may drop below a critical threshold, and the body's oxygen consumption becomes supply dependent. If this supply-dependent phase is not rapidly corrected, tissues enter a dysoxic state and a shock ensues (Fig. 3.1).

The ability of physicians to make reliable clinical estimates of cardiac output is limited. Emergency physicians, intensivists, and surgeons were consistently unable to provide accurate clinical assessment of hemodynamics when compared to invasive and noninvasive determination of cardiac output and systemic vascular resistance.[9–13] This limitation likely reflects an overdependence on measurements such as blood pressure and heart rate, neither of which are reliable indicators of cardiac output or critical illness.[14,15] A significant number of critically ill patients will present with normal vital signs despite having global tissue hypoxia, identified by an elevated lactate or abnormal central venous oxygen saturation (Scv02).[16] Noninvasive cardiac monitors enable the emergency physician to identify concerning trends in cardiac function present in critically ill patients prior to the development of significant hemodynamic instability; importantly, this information not only helps guide management but also has been shown to predict outcome.[17–19]

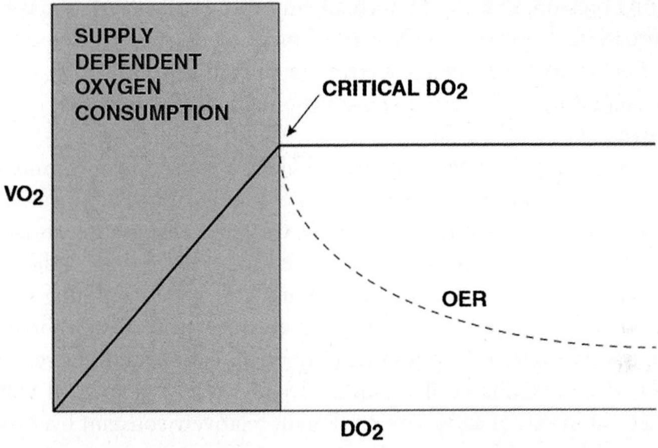

FIGURE 3.1 The relationship between oxygen delivery (DO_2), oxygen consumption (VO_2), and oxygen extraction ratio (OER). As DO_2 decreases, tissue OER increases in order to maintain constant VO_2. However, beyond a certain critical DO_2 at which OER is maximized, VO_2 becomes supply dependent, oxygen deficit accumulates, and a shock state ensues. Figure courtesy of Chad M. Meyers, MD.

Management of compromised cardiac output requires a basic understanding of the determinants of cardiac function. Cardiac output is the product of stroke volume and heart rate. Stroke volume, in turn, is dependent on preload, afterload, and the quality of cardiac contractility.[20] Each of these variables may be estimated and manipulated to optimize forward flow. For example, an echocardiogram with evidence of poor contractility may prompt the administration of inotropic agents. The most common initial therapeutic strategy, however, is restoration of homeostasis, which typically begins with an assessment of preload and an attempt to determine fluid responsiveness.

IMPORTANCE OF FLUID RESPONSIVENESS

The importance of fluid resuscitation in the management of the critically ill patient cannot be overstated. Fluid resuscitation using objective endpoints has been found to improve clinical outcomes in various clinical settings, while overzealous resuscitation has been found to increase mortality.[7,21–30] Ultimately, the decision to administer fluid to a patient in shock is driven by the goal of improving cardiac output as a means of restoring adequate tissue perfusion. This concept is referred to as fluid responsiveness and implies residence on the ascending portion of the Frank-Starling curve. Historically, the determination of fluid responsiveness relied on static estimates of preload such as central venous pressure (CVP) and pulmonary artery occlusion pressure (PAOP). However, as discussed in Chapter 2, static pressure–based measurements have repeatedly been shown to be poor predictors of fluid responsiveness.[31–36] While the adequacy of preload largely determines response to fluid administration, the interplay between venous return and cardiac output is also dependent on the contractile state of the heart and afterload, both of which change unpredictably in patients with critical illness. Thus, an increase in right-sided filling pressure that would normally improve cardiac output may correspond to the flat, nonrecruitable portion of the cardiac function curve in the same patient with critical illness associated as pathologic alterations in cardiac contractility (Fig. 3.2).[37–40] In this circumstance, further fluid resuscitation would do little to improve cardiac output and risk fluid overload.

In contrast to static measurements of preload like CVP that provide limited information regarding the potential for fluids to enhance forward flow, noninvasive monitors attempt to measure, either directly or indirectly, dynamic changes in cardiac output as a function of filling pressure. The calculations used to generate these indices are predicated on heart–lung interactions in which venous return, cardiac filling pressure, and cardiac output change as a result of increasing and decreasing intrathoracic pressure during the respiratory cycle. The reproducibility of these indices, however, is currently limited to sedated and mechanically ventilated patients in whom tidal volumes, and therefore changes in intrathoracic pressure, remain relatively constant over time. While useful indices of fluid responsiveness in spontaneously breathing patients do exist, nearly all studies demonstrating reliable prediction of fluid responsiveness have done so in ventilated patients without spontaneous breathing and with tidal volumes of >8 mL/kg.

THE SCIENCE OF DEVICE ASSESSMENT

The evaluation of a novel noninvasive cardiac output monitor requires assessment of both the reliability of its measurements and the validity of its clinical application. Since the inception of the pulmonary artery catheter (PAC), thermodilution-based measurements of cardiac output are the standard to which new devices are compared and reliability assessed. Early studies comparing cardiac monitors used linear regression and correlation in their analysis. The error of such methods is that they focused on the relationship between measurements and not their agreement; that is, two monitors might correlate well but produce substantially different measurements. Bland and Altman realized the limitation of such methodology and introduced the concepts of bias and precision when comparing a new method of clinical measurement to a standard reference.[41,42] This type of analysis provides more useful information regarding the interchangeability of two measurement devices.

What is considered an acceptable limit of agreement, however, is controversial.[43–45] A 1999 meta-analysis of noninvasive cardiac output monitors proposed that a percentage error of ± 30% be adopted as the acceptable limit of error between a novel cardiac monitor and bolus thermodilution.[44] The reliability of thermodilution, however, is itself disputed.[46] One intraoperative study using magnetic aortic flowmetry—the original gold standard for cardiac output—noted the percent error of PAC thermodilution for measuring cardiac output to be as high as 46%.[47] Ultimately, very few cardiac monitors have consistently achieved the 30% threshold for acceptable reliability, arguably because of the limitations of PAC thermodilution to which they are being compared. To accommodate this variability, it was proposed that the standard for acceptable level of agreement for a novel cardiac output monitor be increased to ± 45%.[45] The implications of such a wide range of agreement are, however, considerable, and discussion regarding

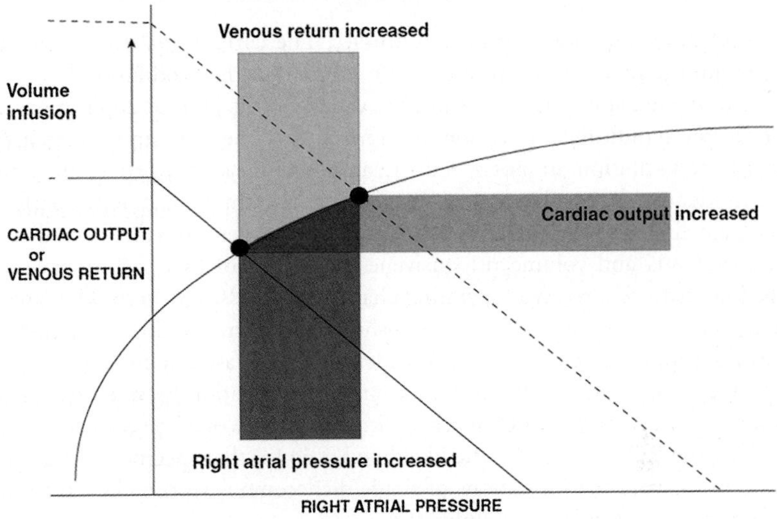

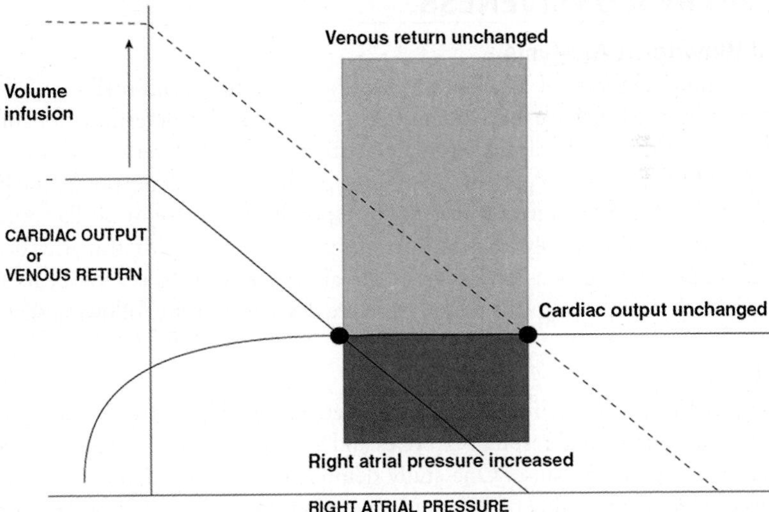

FIGURE 3.2 In Guyton's depiction of cardiocirculatory function, the intersection of the two curves represents the current cardiac output and right atrial pressure for any given combination of venous return and cardiac function states. In the patient with normal cardiac function who is operating on the ascending fluid-responsive portion of the Frank-Starling curve, the infusion of volume results in a rightward shift of the venous return curve, with subsequent increase in venous return, preload, right atrial pressure, and, ultimately, cardiac output. In contrast, in the patient with decreased cardiac performance whose venous return/cardiac function intersection already lies on the flat unresponsive portion of the Frank-Starling curve, further infusion of volume will not result in increased cardiac output, instead only resulting in increased resistive right atrial filling pressures and likely volume overload. Figure courtesy of Chad M. Meyers, MD.

what constitutes acceptable reliability continues. The current goal for a novel cardiac output monitor remains 30% agreement with PAC bolus thermodilution.[48]

While device reliability is important, the validity of its clinical application is arguably of greater significance. It is now recognized that the most important indicators of adequate resuscitation are not specific quantitative measures, per se, but rather the qualitative adequacy of cardiac output. To this end, assessment of monitor performance is increasingly linked to the ability to predict physiologic determinants of cardiac output such as euvolemia and volume responsiveness. Analysis of this performance is often described in terms of a receiver operating characteristic (ROC) curve. The "area under the curve," or AUC, represents the relationship between true and false positives over a range of thresholds of positivity and provides an overall assessment of device performance. AUC values range between 0.5 (a random association between test result and outcome) and 1, a perfect prediction. In addition, the slope of a line connecting any two points along the ROC represents the likelihood ratio for that specific interval, allowing the clinician to avoid the limitations of single dichotomous yes/no clinical cutoffs and improving context-specific applicability.[49–51]

PRINCIPALS OF MINIMALLY INVASIVE ASSESSMENT OF FLUID RESPONSIVENESS

Arterial Waveform Analysis

Various dynamic methods of arterial waveform analysis, both minimally invasive and completely noninvasive, have been identified to assist in the determination of fluid responsiveness in the mechanically ventilated patient. As venous return decreases with positive pressure ventilation, a patient functioning on the ascending portion of the Frank-Starling curve will demonstrate a transient corresponding decrease in cardiac output. If arterial pressure is continuously transduced in the presence of sinus rhythm, this decrease in cardiac output manifests as a change in the arterial waveform several beats later.[52] Several calculations capturing this relationship are described in the following sections.

Delta-down

Delta-down (d-down) is defined as the difference, in mm Hg, between the minimum systolic pressure over several respiratory cycles and a reference systolic pressure measured during an end-expiratory pause. One study demonstrated that a d-down >5 mm Hg had a positive predictive value of 95% and a negative predictive value of 93% for fluid responders and nonresponders, respectively. The magnitude of the d-down correlated linearly with the corresponding increase in cardiac output achieved with additional fluids.[53]

Pulse Pressure Variation

Pulse pressure variation (PPV) is defined as the difference between the maximal and minimal pulse pressures that occurs during the respiratory cycle (Fig. 3.3). Various diagnostic PPV thresholds are described, with two studies demonstrating values of >13% or >11% to have a positive predictive value of 94% or 100% and a negative predictive value of 96% and 93%, respectively.[54,55] In a meta-analysis comparing intravascular arterial

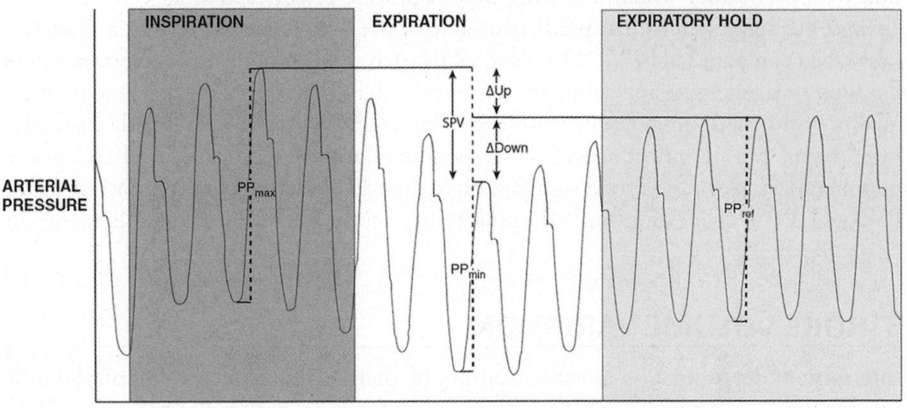

FIGURE 3.3 Various methods of arterial waveform analysis can assist with the determination of fluid responsiveness in mechanically ventilated patients without spontaneous breathing. PPV is the difference between maximal (PP_{max}) and minimal (PP_{min}) pulse pressure over the respiratory cycle. Delta-down (ΔDown) is defined as the difference between the systolic pressure of a reference pulse pressure (PP_{ref}) measured during an expiratory hold and the minimal systolic pressure during the respiratory cycle. SPV is defined as the total change in systolic pressure over the respiratory cycle and is the sum of delta-down and delta-up (ΔUp). Figure courtesy of Chad M. Meyers, MD.

modalities, PPV had the greatest diagnostic accuracy for fluid-responsive states, when compared to other such measures including systolic pressure variation (SPV) and pulse contour estimates of stroke volume variation (SVV), to be discussed below.[53]

Pulse Oximeter Waveform Analysis

The photoplethysmogram, or waveform, displayed by transmission pulse oximeters represents the variation in light intensity transmitted through the fingertip or ear lobe. The intensity of this transmitted light is inversely related to intravascular blood volume. Similar in appearance to arterial blood pressure waveforms, the pulse oximeter waveform is traditionally used by the clinician to distinguish between physiologic and noisy waveforms, in order to determine the reliability of arterial oxygen saturation measurements.[56]

Photoplethysmographic waveforms also permit the calculation of several completely noninvasive indices that have been shown to correlate with fluid responsiveness in ventilated patients without spontaneous respirations. A respiratory variation in pulse oximetry plethysmographic waveform amplitude, or d-POP, of >13% was found to predict fluid responsiveness with 80% sensitivity and 90% specificity when compared to its intravascular physiologic correlate PPV.[57] Another photoplethysmographic measure, the perfusion index (PI), describes the relationship between the pulsatile and nonpulsatile plethysmographic signal. Changes in PI are monitored over the respiratory cycle using a specialized pulse oximeter (Masimo Corp, Irvine, CA) and are displayed as the plethysmographic variability index (PVI), allowing for continuous assessment of fluid responsiveness. In a series of 25 patients after induction of general anesthesia, a PVI >14% was found to discriminate responders with 81% sensitivity and 100% specificity.[58]

A meta-analysis of 10 studies investigating d-POP and PVI found inferior correlation with each other when predicting the magnitude of corresponding cardiac output change, but suggested similar predictive value in the determination of fluid responsiveness when compared to PPV.[59] However, while such simple noninvasive determinants of fluid responsiveness are appealing, the accuracy of d-POP and PVI are dependent on the quality of the plethysmographic waveform. Two studies observing ICU patients receiving norepinephrine infusions with corresponding vasoactive drug-induced changes in peripheral vascular tone found significantly reduced correlation between both d-POP/PVI and PPV, suggesting limited applicability in the critically ill hemodynamically unstable patient.[60,61]

STROKE VOLUME VARIATION

Intermittent determination of cardiac output by methods such as bolus thermodilution provide the clinician with broad trends in cardiac function, but are limited in periods of rapid hemodynamic change common in critical illness. Cardiac output monitors capable of continuous beat-to-beat stroke volume assessment not only assist the emergency physician with earlier recognition of sudden changes in cardiovascular function but also provide a unique dynamic marker of fluid responsiveness. A meta-analysis of 23 studies investigating the relationship between fluid responsiveness and SVV as determined by a variety of devices (PiCCO, LiDCO, FloTrac, and USCOM) found a pooled sensitivity and specificity of 81% and 80%, respectively, and an area under the receiver operating characteristic curve (AUC) of 0.84.[62] A similar meta-analysis supported these findings, but demonstrated slightly weaker predictive values when comparing SVV to PPV and SPV, the AUC of which were 0.94 and 0.86, respectively.[53] While most of these studies were performed in the operating room under general anesthesia, eight were performed in the ICU with heterogeneous mechanically ventilated patient populations without spontaneous breathing. In another study that investigated intubated septic shock patients spontaneously breathing on the mechanical ventilator, the AUC was reduced to 0.52, prompting investigators to conclude that SVV is not of value in spontaneously breathing patients.[63] Additionally, nearly all studies demonstrating the utility of arterial waveform measures (PPV, SPV, SVV) in ventilated patients did so in patients receiving tidal volumes of >8 mL/kg.[53,62] In studies in which patients received tidal volumes of <8 mL/kg (typically acute respiratory distress syndrome [ARDS] patients following low TV protocols), this relationship was not maintained.[64,65]

ULTRASOUND INDICES

Inferior Vena Cava

Echocardiographic evaluation of the inferior vena cava (IVC) using the subcostal view provides the clinician with a noninvasive estimation of right heart filling pressure and fluid responsiveness in mechanically ventilated patients. As intrathoracic pressure increases and decreases with positive pressure ventilation, low venous return and low right-sided filling pressures (i.e., low intravascular volume) result in an increase in both right atrial and IVC compliance, which manifests as respirophasic change in the diameter of the IVC.[38] A study measuring cardiac output in septic patients before and after volume expansion with colloids demonstrated that a distensibility index of the IVC (dIVC) of >18% has a sensitivity of 90% and specificity of 90% for the determination of fluid responsiveness (Table 3.1). A second study, also evaluating fluid responsiveness, demonstrated a dIVC of >12% to have a positive predictive value of 93% and negative predictive value of 92%.[66,67] Of note, the application of IVC ultrasound may be limited in obese or postoperative laparotomy patients.

Brachial Artery Peak Velocity Variation

Similar to arterial waveform analysis, noninvasive Doppler assessment of brachial artery flow over the respiratory cycle can identify volume-responsive patients. This technique requires the patient be mechanically ventilated without spontaneous breathing and in sinus rhythm. When brachial artery maximum and minimum velocities were recorded during standardized ventilation with a handheld ultrasound device, a brachial artery peak velocity variation (d-$Vpeak_{brach}$) >16% was found to correlate with PPV.[68] In a separate case series, d-$Vpeak_{brach}$ > 10% was found to predict fluid responsiveness with a sensitivity of 74% and specificity of 95%.[69]

MEASUREMENTS OF VOLUME RESPONSIVENESS IN SPONTANEOUSLY BREATHING PATIENTS

The reliance of dynamic indices on positive changes in intrathoracic pressure limits their applicability in spontaneously breathing patients. While a single study found that a drop in right atrial pressure >1 mm Hg (as measured by CVP) during inspiration predicted volume response in spontaneously breathing patients, most other studies have not duplicated these findings.[31] One study found that SVV in mechanically ventilated patients who were breathing spontaneously with pressure support did not have value in predicting fluid responsiveness, with an AUC of 0.52.[63] In spontaneously breathing patients who are significantly volume depleted, these indices may still be of some value. In a study of hemodynamically unstable and clinically volume-depleted patients, PPV >12% was found to be 92% specific for identifying volume responsiveness, but

TABLE 3.1 Formulas and Thresholds for the Determination of Fluid Responsiveness

Modality	Formula	Fluid Response Threshold
Pulse pressure variation (PPV)	$PPV(\%) = 100 \times \frac{(PPV_{max} - PPV_{min})}{(PPV_{max} + PPV_{min} / 2)}$	>13% or >11%
Pulse oxymetry plethysmographic waveform amplitude (ΔPOP)	$\Delta POP(\%) = 100 \times \frac{(POP_{max} - POP_{min})}{(POP_{max} + POP_{min} / 2)}$	>13%
Distensibility index of the IVC (dIVC)	$dIVC = \frac{\text{Inspiratory diameter} - \text{Expiratory diameter}}{\text{Inpiratory diameter}}$	>12% or >18%
Brachial artery peak velocity variation($\Delta Vpeak_{brach}$)	$\Delta Vpeak_{brach}(\%) = 100 \times \frac{(Vpeak_{max} - Vpeak_{min})}{(Vpeak_{max} + Vpeak_{min} / 2)}$	>10% or >16%

the absence of PPV had poor sensitivity (63%) for excluding hypovolemia.[70] Significant IVC variation may also have value in identification of fluid responsiveness. In a study of 40 hemodynamically unstable patients, IVC collapse of >40% had a sensitivity and specificity of 70% and 80%, respectively, for fluid responders.[71]

Passive Leg Raise

The simplest provocative test of fluid responsiveness is to administer a fluid bolus and then measure whether an appropriate increase in cardiac output has occurred. This fluid challenge can be extrinsic, in the form of a bolus of crystalloid or colloid fluids, or intrinsic, in the form of autotransfused lower extremity blood volume achieved by passive leg raise (PLR). PLR is performed by elevating the lower extremities 30 to 45 degrees relative to the upper body in supine position for a period of 1 to 5 minutes and then measuring cardiac output invasively or noninvasively. An increase in cardiac output of 10% to 15% after PLR predicts fluid responsiveness.[72–81]

The PLR-induced change in cardiac output (PLR-cCO) technique is capable of accurately determining fluid responsiveness in mechanically ventilated or spontaneously breathing patients and is not affected by the presence of cardiac dysrhythmias. In one meta-analysis, which reviewed the applicability of PLR-cCO in the ICU—and included patients spontaneously breathing or mechanically ventilated—the pooled sensitivity and specificity for fluid-responsive patients were 89.4% and 91.4%, respectively, with an AUC of 0.95.[77]

PLR-induced changes in arterial pulse pressure (PLR-cPP) have also been evaluated for their ability to determine fluid responsiveness in spontaneously breathing patients with normal sinus rhythm. In a case series of 34 nonintubated patients, PLR-induced changes in radial pulse pressure >9% were shown to predict fluid responsiveness with a sensitivity of 79% and specificity of 85%.[76] However, in a meta-analysis, including both spontaneously breathing and mechanically ventilated patients, PLR-cPP demonstrated significantly lower predictive value for fluid responsiveness than PLR-cCO, with a pooled sensitivity and specificity of 59.5% and 86.2%, respectively, and an AUC of 0.76.[77]

End-Tidal CO_2

In mechanically ventilated patients with stable minute ventilation and stable tissue carbon dioxide (CO_2) production, continuous capnometry may provide a simple method to determine fluid response. Two studies demonstrated that an end-tidal CO_2 ($EtCO_2$) increases >5% in response to PLR-predicted fluid response with a sensitivity of 71% and 90.5% and a specificity of 100% and 93.7%, respectively.[82,83]

SPECIFIC DEVICES AND TECHNIQUES FOR THE ASSESSMENT OF CARDIAC OUTPUT

Pulse Contour Analysis

Several devices are available that indirectly estimate cardiac output by changes in the contour of the arterial waveform over the cardiac cycle. Derived from Otto Frank's Windkessel model published in 1899, pulse contour analysis estimates beat-to-beat cardiac output based on the relationship between blood pressure, stroke volume, arterial compliance, and vascular resistance.[84,85] While each device uses a different method to calculate the variables in the Windkessel relationship, they can be broadly divided into two main categories: calibrated and uncalibrated.[86]

The two calibrated devices, the Pulse Contour Cardiac Output, or PiCCO (Pulsion Medical Systems SE, Munich, Germany), and Lithium Detected Cardiac Output, or LiDCO (LiDCO Ltd, London, UK), compensate for individual differences in vascular impedance by intermittent direct determination of cardiac output using indicator dilution techniques. Beat-to-beat cardiac output is then calculated using continuous measurement of the area under the systolic portion of the arterial pulse wave.[87] PiCCO uses transpulmonary thermodilution to determine cardiac output, a method that requires both central venous and central arterial cannulation.[88] The LiDCO monitor uses lithium bolus dilution and uses an arterial catheter paired with either a peripheral or central venous catheter.[89,90] Both devices require recalibration via indicator dilution every 4 to 6 hours or whenever a change in patient status occurs.[91,92]

Uncalibrated devices determine cardiac output by mathematically estimating aortic impedance and vascular resistance. Beat-to-beat cardiac output is then calculated in a similar manner as calibrated devices. The most widely tested of the uncalibrated devices, the FloTrac (Edwards Lifesciences, Irvine, CA), requires only peripheral artery catheterization and standard patient characteristics to estimate large-vessel compliance and estimate cardiac output.[93,94] An additional uncalibrated device, Nexfin (Edwards Lifesciences, Irvine, CA), uses the volume-clamp principle to estimate arterial pressure via an inflatable finger cuff, calculating cardiac output via an updated Modelflow algorithm that allows for a completely noninvasive monitoring modality.[95,96]

When compared to PAC thermodilution, the reliability of pulse contour analysis for the estimation of cardiac output varies greatly. PiCCO device estimates of cardiac output have been found to correlate acceptably with thermodilution; however, these studies have shown conflicting results during periods of hemodynamic instability.[91,97,98] One study demonstrated that PiCCO remained reliable when compared to transpulmonary thermodilution in septic patients with circulatory failure.[99] However, two additional studies demonstrated a percentage error of >30% if the device was not recalibrated hourly during periods of hemodynamic instability or following therapeutic maneuvers such as fluid challenge.[100,101]

The LiDCO system has been found to correlate well with thermodilution both intra- and postoperatively, but has not been well studied during periods of hemodynamic instability.[89,90,102] The FloTrac device has been studied widely given its simplicity, minimal invasiveness, and ease of use; however, results have been inconsistent and mostly disappointing.[86] Despite several generations of software and hardware updates, the FloTrac has generally shown an unacceptable cardiac output agreement with PAC thermodilution.[45,86,103–108] Although a meta-analysis of 16 prospective investigations found an improvement in the accuracy and precision of the FloTrac when comparing earlier versions of the device and more recent versions, the review was criticized for excluding studies that evaluated hemodynamically unstable patients.[45,109] A subgroup analysis of the newer generation of FloTrac devices found a percentage error of 44.7% when compared to PAC thermodilution when septic and critically ill patient populations were included.[45]

A meta-analysis of 24 studies in mixed patient populations comparing PiCCO, LiDCO, and FloTrac with PAC thermodilution found a pooled percentage error of 41.3% for all three pulse contour monitors.[45] In another comparative study of LiDCO, PiCCO, and FloTrac, LiDCO was found to have the best overall agreement when compared to PAC thermodilution, with a percentage agreement of 29%, compared to 41% and 59% for PiCCO and FloTrac, respectively.[106,110] The Nexfin has not been extensively studied, but preliminary results are promising when compared to thermodilution intraoperatively and in the cardiac ICU.[111–113]

Ultimately, while the simplicity of uncalibrated devices such as FloTrac makes application in the ED attractive, the poor performance of the current models limits their applicability. The calibrated PiCCO and LiDCO devices demonstrate improved reliability when compared to thermodilution, but are limited by the need for frequent recalibration during periods of hemodynamic instability or following therapeutic intervention. In addition, the PiCCO device requires central venous and central arterial cannulation for calibration by transpulmonary thermodilution, which limits its applicability.

Ultrasound

Esophageal Doppler

Esophageal Doppler allows continuous estimation of stroke volume by recording the velocity of blood flow in the descending aorta with a flexible ultrasound probe—roughly the size of a nasogastric tube—placed either nasally or orally in a mechanically ventilated patient. The accurate assessment of stroke volume via esophageal measurement relies on two assumptions: (1) the presence of a stable cephalic-to-caudal blood flow ratio, which may be inconsistent in certain patients, and (2) a homogenous cross-sectional area of the aorta. Aortic measurement is estimated either by calculations based on height, weight, and age or directly via real-time motion-mode (M-mode) Doppler on capable models.[114] While esophageal Doppler is highly operator dependent, it is quickly performed, and one study suggests no more than 12 placements are needed to become proficient.[114] In a prospective study in the emergency department (ED), mean time until optimal Doppler signal was obtained was 5.7 minutes.[115]

The reliability of esophageal Doppler to estimate cardiac output when compared to PAC thermodilution is, however, not encouraging. Two separate meta-analyses demonstrated limits of agreement of ± 65% and 42.1%, respectively.[44,45] A meta-analysis of 11 validation studies also found limited agreement in cardiac output values when compared to PAC thermodilution, but improved results when following trends. The limited number of studies included in the review does make it difficult to draw conclusions regarding the accuracy of these findings.[116] Analyzed separately, studies comparing M-mode–capable esophageal Doppler with PAC thermodilution have revealed better agreement and may provide the clinician with a valuable method to continuously measure cardiac output in the mechanically ventilated patient.[117–119]

USCOM Cardiac Monitor

The ultrasonic cardiac output monitor, or USCOM (USCOM LTD, Sydney, Australia), is a completely noninvasive cardiac output monitoring system that uses transthoracic Doppler to measure either transaortic or transpulmonary blood flow. Stroke volume is calculated by measurement of the velocity time integral (VTI) and the cross-sectional area of the outflow tract.[86,120] Clinical trials comparing USCOM with thermodilution have shown conflicting results.[121–124] In one meta-analysis, the range of percentage error in the 10 studies reviewed was between 14% and 56%, with a pooled percentage error of 42.7%.[120] In addition, like esophageal Doppler, the USCOM device is user dependent, with a failure rate to obtain measurements ranging from 5% to 24% across studies.[120,122,124–126]

Transthoracic Echocardiography

Transthoracic echocardiography (TTE) provides the emergency physician with indispensable clinical information regarding left and right cardiac function, ventricular dilation, pericardial effusion, and valvular competence.[86,127,128] As with the USCOM device, TTE can provide intermittent quantitative estimation of cardiac output using Doppler assessment of the left ventricular outflow tract (LVOT) and VTI calculations. Basic qualitative information regarding adequacy of cardiac filling and global function is also easily obtained. While providing no numerical data regarding cardiac output, a brief and focused qualitative exam can often identify patients that need more fluid versus those that are euvolemic and distinguish between patients needing inotropes from those with normal function. A detailed discussion of echocardiographic evaluation of the critically ill patients is presented in Chapter 6.

While the utility of transthoracic LVOT assessment to follow cardiac output changes is limited given the necessity of repeat measurements and time-consuming nature of the study, it may have a role in the absence of other specialized devices.

Transthoracic Electrical Bioimpedance

Transthoracic electrical bioimpedance (TEB) estimates cardiac output by measuring resistance in the thorax to high-frequency, low-magnitude current to determine changes in total thoracic fluid content over the cardiac cycle. First introduced in the 1970s, cardiac bioimpedance monitors use skin electrodes applied to the neck and thorax, allowing for quick and completely noninvasive cardiac monitoring.[129,130] TEB is limited in its ability to assess cardiac output in patients with dysrhythmias or pulmonary edema.[87,129,131] In two studies evaluating critically ill ED patients, estimation of cardiac output using TEB agreed well with PAC thermodilution, but accuracy was compromised in the presence of pulmonary edema, pleural effusions, chest wall edema, or chest tubes.[18,132] However, when clinical studies comparing TEB with PAC thermodilution were systematically reviewed, the findings were less favorable. A 1999 meta-analysis estimated the percentage error of TEB compared with PAC thermodilution to be ± 38%.[44] A more recent meta-analysis echoed the limitation of TEB, estimating an overall mean percent error of ± 42.9%.[45] A newer noninvasive cardiac output monitor, or NICOM device (NICOM, Cheetah Medical Inc., Wilmington, DE), using the related principle of bioreactance, has been less rigorously studied. It is unclear at this time whether it shares the same limitations as TEB.[133–136]

Carbon Dioxide and the Fick Principle

The Fick equation, which is based on the conservation of mass, allows for the calculation of cardiac output (or alveolar blood flow) by measuring the arteriovenous difference in oxygen consumption. The Fick principle may be applied to any gas diffusing through the lungs, including carbon dioxide.[8] These concepts are discussed in detail in Chapter 2.

The noninvasive cardiac output device, or NICO (Novametrix Medical Systems Inc., Wallingford, CT), uses a partial carbon dioxide rebreathing technique in intubated patients to estimate CO_2 elimination (VCO_2) and uses the changes in venous and arterial CO_2 $EtCO_2$ to calculate the aretiorvenous difference in CO_2. However, to accurately assess cardiac output by expired CO_2, pulmonary capillary blood flow must also be known. To determine this, pulmonary shunting is estimated using SpO_2 and FiO_2; thus, the NICO provides a noninvasive determination of cardiac output using mainstream capnometry, a differential pressure pneumotachometer, and pulse oximetry.[137] One shortcoming of this technique is that $EtCO_2$ provides unreliable estimates of $PaCO_2$ in unstable patients due to the variability of V/Q mismatch in the critically ill. Estimating pulmonary capillary blood flow can compensate for this, but several studies have demonstrated the calculated pulmonary shunt fraction by NICO differs considerably from traditionally calculated shunt fraction by blood gas analysis.[138,139] In light of this, cardiac output calculated by NICO was typically only considered accurate when limited to stable patients with normal pulmonary function or when monitoring trends.[87] This was supported by a pooled analysis of 167 measurements from 8 studies performed in various patient populations, which found a mean percentage error of ± 44.5% for partial CO_2 rebreathing method.[45] At this time, the NICO may be more appropriate for anesthetized patients in the operating room rather than in the stabilization of critically ill patients in the ED.

A PRACTICAL FLUID STRATEGY IN SEVERE SEPSIS

Despite evidence of significant reduction in mortality when used to guide therapy in patients with severe sepsis and septic shock, the adoption of early goal-directed therapy (EGDT) is not widespread.[6,140–142] One barrier to implementation is the requirement for central venous access and specialized monitoring equipment.[6,140] In hemodynamically stable patients who meet the criteria for severe sepsis by elevated lactate alone, and who do not require central access for vasopressor support, adherence to the EGDT algorithm's requirement for central access is understandably reduced.[143,144] Central venous catheterization is not a benign procedure, and the clinical information gained by knowledge of the CVP and central venous O_2 ($ScvO_2$) saturation must be balanced with the inherent risk of invasive monitoring.[145–147] Furthermore, in a recent landmark study, lactate clearance compared favorably with $ScvO_2$ as a final resuscitative endpoint in patients with severe sepsis.[148]

Aggressive fluid therapy, however, remains a cornerstone of management in sepsis, and despite the well-documented limitations of CVP in predicting fluid responsiveness, its use has been found to significantly increase the volume of fluid administered in the first 6 hours of therapy.[7] The additional fluids given in the EGDT trial's experimental group are thought to have played a central role in the observed positive impact on mortality. In the trial, the control group resuscitated empirically received on average 3.5 ± 2.4 L crystalloid, compared with the experimental group guided by a target CVP of 8 to 12 mm Hg, which received 4.9 ± 2.9 L.[7] Other studies have found a similar disparity between empiric and targeted volume resuscitation in severe sepsis.[143] Importantly, despite the significantly larger volume of fluid given, respiratory failure requiring mechanical ventilation was not more frequent in the EGDT group. Therefore, while CVP does not adequately predict fluid responsiveness, it may demonstrate the concept of fluid tolerance: A patient with severe sepsis who is not volume overloaded will likely benefit from additional fluid therapy.

Using measures of fluid responsiveness to guide therapy in sepsis is ideal. However, indices of fluid responsiveness can be cumbersome, time consuming, and often require the patient to be mechanically ventilated without spontaneous respirations. In contrast, fluid tolerance can be quickly assessed with an ultrasound survey of the IVC, heart, and lungs and is a valuable initial assessment tool. While IVC variation has limited capability to predict fluid responsiveness in spontaneously breathing patients, a collapse of >50% has been demonstrated to correlate well with CVP <8 mm Hg.[149,150] In patients in whom adequate visualization of the IVC is difficult, ultrasound of the bilateral apical three interspaces provides an alternative approach to estimating cardiac filling pressures. One study—while investigating fluid tolerance in the ICU—demonstrated that <3 b-lines (a comet tail artifact indicating subpleural interstitial edema) per interspace identified a pulmonary artery opening pressure, or PAOP, of <18 mm Hg with a PPV of 97%.[151] It should be noted, while the absence of lung ultrasound b-lines is indicative of low filling pressures, their presence is too sensitive and does not accurately reflect high filling pressures.[151] Therefore, while the development of b-lines should prompt caution, it may not accurately reflect the transition past the upper inflection point of the Frank-Starling curve.

Indicators of fluid tolerance are not meant to replace those of fluid responsiveness. Instead, they are meant to supplement the preliminary clinical evaluation and increase the clinician's confidence in initial volume resuscitation. If, during the administration of fluid, the patient develops clinical evidence of volume overload—or indices of fluid tolerance are lost and a subsequent repeat serum lactate has not normalized—then more time-intensive measures of fluid responsiveness are justified to guide fluid therapy.

Finally, qualitative assessment of ejection fraction with early standardized echocardiography is always recommended as it provides the clinician with an overall estimate of cardiac function and has been demonstrated to improve survival and ventilator-free days when performed in the ICU.[152]

CONCLUSION

While knowledge of hemodynamics plays an important role in the ED resuscitation of the critically ill, the determination of cardiac function has historically been limited to the intensivist. With the advent of noninvasive hemodynamic monitoring, emergency physicians can now quickly and efficiently assess cardiac output and fluid responsiveness at a stage in the care of the critical patient in which goal-directed therapy is most crucial. A familiarity with these advanced techniques, as well as their appropriate application and limitations, will assist the emergency physician in meeting resuscitative endpoints.

LITERATURE TABLE

TRIAL	DESIGN	RESULT
Fluid Responsiveness		
Arterial Waveform Analysis		
Michard et al., *Am Respir Crit Care Med.* 2000[52]	Prospective observational study of 40 patients with sepsis, mechanically ventilated, without spontaneous breathing and in normal sinus rhythm	PPV > 13% predicted fluid response with 94% sensitivity and 96% specificity
Marik et al., *Crit Care Med.* 2009[53]	Systematic review of 29 studies, enrolling 685 patients, investigating PPV, SPV, SVV and CVP in the OR and ICU. Patients were mechanically ventilated, without spontaneous breathing and in normal sinus rhythm	AUC for PPV 0.94 (CI, 0.93–0.95) AUC for SPV 0.86 (CI, 0.86–0.90) AUC for SVV 0.72 (CI, 0.78–0.88) AUC for CVP 0.55 (CI, 0.48–0.62)
Kramer et al., *Chest.* 2004[54]	Prospective observational study of 21 patients undergoing CABG, mechanically ventilated, without spontaneous breathing and in normal sinus rhythm	PPV > 11% predicted fluid response with 100% sensitivity and 93% specificity
Sandroni et al., *Intensive Care Med.* 2012[59]	Systematic review of 10 studies, enrolling 233 patients, investigating POP and PVI in the OR and ICU. Patients were mechanically ventilated, without spontaneous breathing and in normal sinus rhythm	Pooled AUC for POP and PVI 0.85 (CI, 0.79-0.92) Pooled sensitivity 80% (CI, 0.74-0.85) Pooled specificity 76% (CI, 0.68-0.82)
Stroke Volume Variation		
Zhang et al., *J Anesth.* 2011[62]	Systematic review of 23 studies, enrolling 568 patients, in the OR and ICU. Patients were mechanically ventilated, without spontaneous breathing and in normal sinus rhythm	AUC for SVV 0.84 (CI, 0.81–0.87) Pooled sensitivity 81% Pooled specificity 80%
Perner et al., *Acta Anaesthesiol Scand.* 2006[63]	Prospective observational study of 30 consecutive patients with septic shock. Patients were mechanically ventilated but spontaneously breathing	AUC for SVV in spontaneously breathing patients was 0.52 (CI, 0.30–0.73)
Inferior Vena Cava Index		
Feissel et al., *Intensive Care Med.* 2004[66]	Prospective observational study of 39 patients in the MICU with septic shock. Patients were mechanically ventilated and without spontaneous breathing.	dIVC > 12% predicted fluid response with positive predictive value of 93% and a negative predictive value of 92%
Barbier et al., *Intensive Care Med.* 2004[67]	Prospective observational study of 23 patients in the ICU with sepsis. Patients were mechanically ventilated and without spontaneous breathing.	dIVC > 18% predicted fluid response with 90% sensitivity and 90% specificity
Brachial Artery Peak Velocity Variation		
Brennan et al., *Chest.* 2007[68]	Prospective observational study of 30 patients, mechanically ventilated with tidal volume >8 mL/kg, without spontaneous respiration, and in sinus rhythm	$\Delta Vpeak_{brach}$ > 16% predicted fluid response with 91% sensitivity and 95% specificity

LITERATURE TABLE *(Continued)*

TRIAL	DESIGN	RESULT
Monge et al., *Crit Care.* 2009[69]	Prospective observational study of 38 patients in the ICU. Patients were mechanically ventilated without spontaneous respiration, and in sinus rhythm	$\Delta Vpeak_{brach}$ > 10% predicted fluid response with 74% sensitivity and 95% specificity
Passive Leg Raise		
Cavallaro et al., *Intensive Care Med.* 2010[77]	Systematic review of 9 studies enrolling 353 patients investigating cardiac output changes induced by PLR in the ICU. Patients were mechanically ventilated with and without spontaneous respirations or spontaneously breathing off the ventilator.	AUC for PLR was 0.95 (CI, 0.92–0.97) Pooled sensitivity 89.4% (CI, 0.84–0.93) Pooled specificity 91.4% (CI, 0.85–0.95)
Cardiac Output Monitors		
Critchley and Critchley, *J Clin Monit Comput.* 1999[44]	Meta-analysis of 25 studies comparing transthoracic bioimpedance or esophageal Doppler to bolus thermodilution in the OR, ICU, pediatrics or animals.	Percent error for bioimpedance ±37% Percent error for Doppler ±65%
Peyton et al., *Anesthesiology.* 2010[45]	Meta-analysis of 47 studies investigating pulse contour, esophageal Doppler, partial carbon dioxide rebreathing, and transthoracic bioimpedance with bolus thermodilution in the OR and ICU	Percent error for pooled pulse contour ±41.3% Percent error for FloTrac ± 44.7% Percent error for bioimpedance ±42.9% Percent error for Doppler ± 42.1% Percent error for partial CO_2 rebreathing ±44.5%
Marik et al., *J Cardiothorac Vasc Anesth.* 2013[86]	Review article and meta-analysis of 45 studies investigating the FloTrac during cardiac surgery and in the ICU	Percent error for FloTrac during cardiac surgery ±37% Percent error for FloTrac in ICU ± 47%
Hadian et al., *Crit Care.* 2010[106]	Prospective observational study in 17 postoperative cardiac surgery patients comparing LiDCO, PiCCO, FloTrac and PAC thermodilution	Percent error for LiDCO ±29% Percent error for PiCCO ±41% Percent error for FloTrac ±59%
Mayer et al., *Cardiothorac Vasc Anesth.* 2009[109]	Meta-analysis of 16 studies representing 3,372 data points comparing FloTrac and bolus thermodilution in patients in the OR and ICU without hemodynamic instability	Percent error for first gen FloTrac ± 44% Percent error for second gen FloTrac ± 30%

CI, confidence interval.

REFERENCES

1. Dellinger RP, Levy MM, Rhodes A, et al. Surviving sepsis campaign: international guidelines for management of severe sepsis and septic shock: 2012. *Crit Care Med.* 2013;41:580–637.
2. Nelson M, Waldrop RD, Jones J, et al. Critical care provided in an urban emergency department. *Am J Emerg Med.* 1998;16:56–59.
3. Magid DJ, Sullivan AF, Cleary PD, et al. The safety of emergency care systems: results of a survey of clinicians in 65 US emergency departments. *Ann Emerg Med.* 2009;53:715 e711–723 e711.
4. Warden G. *Hospital-Based Emergency Care: At the Breaking Point.* Washington, DC: The National Academies Press; 2006.
5. Richardson DB. Increase in patient mortality at 10 days associated with emergency department overcrowding. *Med J Aust.* 2006;184:213–216.
6. Jones AE, Kline JA. Use of goal-directed therapy for severe sepsis and septic shock in academic emergency departments. *Crit Care Med.* 2005;33:1888–1889; author reply 1889–1890.

7. Rivers E, Nguyen B, Havstad S, et al. Early goal-directed therapy in the treatment of severe sepsis and septic shock. *N Engl J Med.* 2001;345:1368–1377.
8. Meyers C, Weingart S. Critical care monitoring in the emergency department. *Emerg Med Pract.* 2007;9:1–29.
9. Nowak RM, Sen A, Garcia AJ, et al. The inability of emergency physicians to adequately clinically estimate the underlying hemodynamic profiles of acutely ill patients. *Am J Emerg Med.* 2012;30:954–960.
10. Stevenson LW, Perloff JK. The limited reliability of physical signs for estimating hemodynamics in chronic heart failure. *JAMA.* 1989;261:884–888.
11. Eisenberg PR, Jaffe AS, Schuster DP. Clinical evaluation compared to pulmonary artery catheterization in the hemodynamic assessment of critically ill patients. *Crit Care Med.* 1984;12:549–553.
12. Veale WN Jr, Morgan JH, Beatty JS, et al. Hemodynamic and pulmonary fluid status in the trauma patient: are we slipping? *Am Surg.* 2005;71:621–625; discussion 625–626.
13. Neath SX, Lazio L, Guss DA. Utility of impedance cardiography to improve physician estimation of hemodynamic parameters in the emergency department. *Congest Heart Fail.* 2005;11:17–20.
14. Wo CC, Shoemaker WC, Appel PL, et al. Unreliability of blood pressure and heart rate to evaluate cardiac output in emergency resuscitation and critical illness. *Crit Care Med.* 1993;21:218–223.
15. Rady MY, Smithline HA, Blake H, et al. A comparison of the shock index and conventional vital signs to identify acute, critical illness in the emergency department. *Ann Emerg Med.* 1994;24:685–690.
16. Rady MY, Rivers EP, Nowak RM. Resuscitation of the critically ill in the ED: responses of blood pressure, heart rate, shock index, central venous oxygen saturation, and lactate. *Am J Emerg Med.* 1996;14:218–225.
17. Dunham CM, Chirichella TJ, Gruber BS, et al. Emergency department noninvasive (NICOM) cardiac outputs are associated with trauma activation, patient injury severity and host conditions and mortality. *J Trauma Acute Care Surg.* 2012;73:479–485.
18. Shoemaker WC, Wo CC, Chien LC, et al. Evaluation of invasive and noninvasive hemodynamic monitoring in trauma patients. *J Trauma.* 2006;61:844–853; discussion 853–844.
19. Lu KJ, Chien LC, Wo CC, et al. Hemodynamic patterns of blunt and penetrating injuries. *J Am Coll Surg.* 2006;203:899–907.
20. Marino PM. Circulatory blood flow. In: Zinner S, ed. *The ICU Book.* 1998:3–18.
21. Kern JW, Shoemaker WC. Meta-analysis of hemodynamic optimization in high-risk patients. *Crit Care Med.* 2002;30:1686–1692.
22. Polonen P, Ruokonen E, Hippelainen M, et al. A prospective, randomized study of goal-oriented hemodynamic therapy in cardiac surgical patients. *Anesth Analg.* 2000;90:1052–1059.
23. Lopes MR, Oliveira MA, Pereira VO, et al. Goal-directed fluid management based on pulse pressure variation monitoring during high-risk surgery: a pilot randomized controlled trial. *Crit Care.* 2007;11:R100.
24. Gan TJ, Soppitt A, Maroof M, et al. Goal-directed intraoperative fluid administration reduces length of hospital stay after major surgery. *Anesthesiology.* 2002;97:820–826.
25. Wakeling HG, McFall MR, Jenkins CS, et al. Intraoperative oesophageal Doppler guided fluid management shortens postoperative hospital stay after major bowel surgery. *Br J Anaesth.* 2005;95:634–642.
26. Noblett SE, Snowden CP, Shenton BK, et al. Randomized clinical trial assessing the effect of Doppler-optimized fluid management on outcome after elective colorectal resection. *Br J Surg.* 2006;93:1069–1076.
27. Hamilton MA, Cecconi M, Rhodes A. A systematic review and meta-analysis on the use of preemptive hemodynamic intervention to improve postoperative outcomes in moderate and high-risk surgical patients. *Anesth Analg.* 2011;112:1392–1402.
28. Boyd JH, Forbes J, Nakada TA, et al. Fluid resuscitation in septic shock: a positive fluid balance and elevated central venous pressure are associated with increased mortality. *Crit Care Med.* 2011;39:259–265.
29. de-Madaria E, Soler-Sala G, Sanchez-Paya J, et al. Influence of fluid therapy on the prognosis of acute pancreatitis: a prospective cohort study. *Am J Gastroenterol.* 2011;106:1843–1850.
30. Rosenberg AL, Dechert RE, Park PK, et al. Review of a large clinical series: association of cumulative fluid balance on outcome in acute lung injury: a retrospective review of the ARDSnet tidal volume study cohort. *J Intensive Care Med.* 2009;24:35–46.
31. Magder S. Respiratory variations in right atrial pressure predict response to fluid challenge. *J Crit Care.* 1992;7:76–85.
32. Tavernier B, Makhotine O, Lebuffe G, et al. Systolic pressure variation as a guide to fluid therapy in patients with sepsis-induced hypotension. *Anesthesiology.* 1998;89:1313–1321.
33. Wiesenack C, Fiegl C, Keyser A, et al. Continuously assessed right ventricular end-diastolic volume as a marker of cardiac preload and fluid responsiveness in mechanically ventilated cardiac surgical patients. *Crit Care.* 2005;9:R226–R233.

34. Wiesenack C, Fiegl C, Keyser A, et al. Assessment of fluid responsiveness in mechanically ventilated cardiac surgical patients. *Eur J Anaesthesiol.* 2005;22:658–665.
35. Rex S, Brose S, Metzelder S, et al. Prediction of fluid responsiveness in patients during cardiac surgery. *Br J Anaesth.* 2004;93:782–788.
36. Marik PE, Baram M, Vahid B. Does central venous pressure predict fluid responsiveness? A systematic review of the literature and the tale of seven mares. *Chest* 2008;134:172–178.
37. Feihl F, Broccard AF. Interactions between respiration and systemic hemodynamics. Part I: basic concepts. *Intensive Care Med.* 2009;35:45–54.
38. Feihl F, Broccard AF. Interactions between respiration and systemic hemodynamics. Part II: practical implications in critical care. *Intensive Care Med.* 2009;35:198–205.
39. Henderson WR, Griesdale DE, Walley KR, et al. Clinical review: Guyton--the role of mean circulatory filling pressure and right atrial pressure in controlling cardiac output. *Crit Care.* 2010;14:243.
40. Magder S. Point: the classical Guyton view that mean systemic pressure, right atrial pressure, and venous resistance govern venous return is/is not correct. *J Appl Physiol.* 2006;101:1523–1525.
41. Bland JM, Altman DG. Statistical methods for assessing agreement between two methods of clinical measurement. *Lancet.* 1986;1:307–310.
42. Bland JM, Altman DG. Agreed statistics: measurement method comparison. *Anesthesiology.* 2012;116:182–185.
43. Cecconi M, Rhodes A, Poloniecki J, et al. Bench-to-bedside review: the importance of the precision of the reference technique in method comparison studies—with specific reference to the measurement of cardiac output. *Crit Care.* 2009;13:201.
44. Critchley LA, Critchley JA. A meta-analysis of studies using bias and precision statistics to compare cardiac output measurement techniques. *J Clin Monit Comput.* 1999;15:85–91.
45. Peyton PJ, Chong SW. Minimally invasive measurement of cardiac output during surgery and critical care: a meta-analysis of accuracy and precision. *Anesthesiology.* 2010;113:1220–1235.
46. Stetz CW, Miller RG, Kelly GE, et al. Reliability of the thermodilution method in the determination of cardiac output in clinical practice. *Am Rev Respir Dis.* 1982;126:1001–1004.
47. Botero M, Kirby D, Lobato EB, et al. Measurement of cardiac output before and after cardiopulmonary bypass: comparison among aortic transit-time ultrasound, thermodilution, and noninvasive partial CO_2 rebreathing. *J Cardiothorac Vasc Anesth.* 2004;18:563–572.
48. Critchley LA. Bias and precision statistics: should we still adhere to the 30% benchmark for cardiac output monitor validation studies? *Anesthesiology.* 2011;114:1245; author reply 1245–1246.
49. Brown MD, Reeves MJ. Evidence-based emergency medicine/skills for evidence-based emergency care. Interval likelihood ratios: another advantage for the evidence-based diagnostician. *Ann Emerg Med.* 2003;42:292–297.
50. Feldman JM. Is it a bird? Is it a plane? The role of patient monitors in medical decision making. *Anesth Analg.* 2009;108:707–710.
51. Gallagher EJ. Evidence-based emergency medicine/editorial. The problem with sensitivity and specificity. *Ann Emerg Med.* 2003;42:298–303.
52. Michard F, Teboul JL. Using heart-lung interactions to assess fluid responsiveness during mechanical ventilation. *Crit Care.* 2000;4:282–289.
53. Marik PE, Cavallazzi R, Vasu T, et al. Dynamic changes in arterial waveform derived variables and fluid responsiveness in mechanically ventilated patients: a systematic review of the literature. *Crit Care Med.* 2009;37:2642–2647.
54. Kramer A, Zygun D, Hawes H, et al. Pulse pressure variation predicts fluid responsiveness following coronary artery bypass surgery. *Chest.* 2004;126:1563–1568.
55. Michard F, Boussat S, Chemla D, et al. Relation between respiratory changes in arterial pulse pressure and fluid responsiveness in septic patients with acute circulatory failure. *Am J Respir Crit Care Med.* 2000;162:134–138.
56. Reisner A, Shaltis PA, McCombie D, et al. Utility of the photoplethysmogram in circulatory monitoring. *Anesthesiology.* 2008;108:950–958.
57. Cannesson M, Attof Y, Rosamel P, et al. Respiratory variations in pulse oximetry plethysmographic waveform amplitude to predict fluid responsiveness in the operating room. *Anesthesiology.* 2007;106:1105–1111.
58. Cannesson M, Desebbe O, Rosamel P, et al. Pleth variability index to monitor the respiratory variations in the pulse oximeter plethysmographic waveform amplitude and predict fluid responsiveness in the operating theatre. *Br J Anaesth.* 2008;101:200–206.
59. Sandroni C, Cavallaro F, Marano C, et al. Accuracy of plethysmographic indices as predictors of fluid responsiveness in mechanically ventilated adults: a systematic review and meta-analysis. *Intensive Care Med.* 2012;38:1429–1437.

60. Biais M, Cottenceau V, Petit L, et al. Impact of norepinephrine on the relationship between pleth variability index and pulse pressure variations in ICU adult patients. *Crit Care.* 2011;15:R168.
61. Landsverk SA, Hoiseth LO, Kvandal P, et al. Poor agreement between respiratory variations in pulse oximetry photoplethysmographic waveform amplitude and pulse pressure in intensive care unit patients. *Anesthesiology.* 2008;109:849–855.
62. Zhang Z, Lu B, Sheng X, et al. Accuracy of stroke volume variation in predicting fluid responsiveness: a systematic review and meta-analysis. *J Anesth.* 2011;25:904–916.
63. Perner A, Faber T. Stroke volume variation does not predict fluid responsiveness in patients with septic shock on pressure support ventilation. *Acta Anaesthesiol Scand.* 2006;50:1068–1073.
64. Reuter DA, Bayerlein J, Goepfert MS, et al. Influence of tidal volume on left ventricular stroke volume variation measured by pulse contour analysis in mechanically ventilated patients. *Intensive Care Med.* 2003;29:476–480.
65. De Backer D, Heenen S, Piagnerelli M, et al. Pulse pressure variations to predict fluid responsiveness: influence of tidal volume. *Intensive Care Med.* 2005;31:517–523.
66. Feissel M, Michard F, Faller JP, et al. The respiratory variation in inferior vena cava diameter as a guide to fluid therapy. *Intensive Care Med.* 2004;30:1834–1837.
67. Barbier C, Loubieres Y, Schmit C, et al. Respiratory changes in inferior vena cava diameter are helpful in predicting fluid responsiveness in ventilated septic patients. *Intensive Care Med.* 2004;30:1740–1746.
68. Brennan JM, Blair JE, Hampole C, et al. Radial artery pulse pressure variation correlates with brachial artery peak velocity variation in ventilated subjects when measured by internal medicine residents using hand-carried ultrasound devices. *Chest.* 2007;131:1301–1307.
69. Monge Garcia MI, Gil Cano A, Diaz Monrove JC. Brachial artery peak velocity variation to predict fluid responsiveness in mechanically ventilated patients. *Crit Care.* 2009;13:R142.
70. Soubrier S, Saulnier F, Hubert H, et al. Can dynamic indicators help the prediction of fluid responsiveness in spontaneously breathing critically ill patients? *Intensive Care Med.* 2007;33:1117–1124.
71. Muller L, Bobbia X, Toumi M, et al. Respiratory variations of inferior vena cava diameter to predict fluid responsiveness in spontaneously breathing patients with acute circulatory failure: need for a cautious use. *Crit Care.* 2012;16:R188.
72. Monnet X, Teboul JL. Passive leg raising. *Intensive Care Med.* 2008;34:659–663.
73. Monnet X, Bleibtreu A, Ferre A, et al. Passive leg-raising and end-expiratory occlusion tests perform better than pulse pressure variation in patients with low respiratory system compliance. *Crit Care Med.* 2012;40:152–157.
74. Monnet X, Dres M, Ferre A, et al. Prediction of fluid responsiveness by a continuous non-invasive assessment of arterial pressure in critically ill patients: comparison with four other dynamic indices. *Br J Anaesth.* 2012;109:330–338.
75. Monnet X, Rienzo M, Osman D, et al. Passive leg raising predicts fluid responsiveness in the critically ill. *Crit Care Med.* 2006;34:1402–1407.
76. Preau S, Saulnier F, Dewavrin F, et al. Passive leg raising is predictive of fluid responsiveness in spontaneously breathing patients with severe sepsis or acute pancreatitis. *Crit Care Med.* 2010;38:819–825.
77. Cavallaro F, Sandroni C, Marano C, et al. Diagnostic accuracy of passive leg raising for prediction of fluid responsiveness in adults: systematic review and meta-analysis of clinical studies. *Intensive Care Med.* 2010;36:1475–1483.
78. Lamia B, Ochagavia A, Monnet X, et al. Echocardiographic prediction of volume responsiveness in critically ill patients with spontaneously breathing activity. *Intensive Care Med.* 2007;33:1125–1132.
79. Thiel SW, Kollef MH, Isakow W. Non-invasive stroke volume measurement and passive leg raising predict volume responsiveness in medical ICU patients: an observational cohort study. *Crit Care.* 2009;13:R111.
80. Biais M, Vidil L, Sarrabay P, et al. Changes in stroke volume induced by passive leg raising in spontaneously breathing patients: comparison between echocardiography and Vigileo/FloTrac device. *Crit Care.* 2009;13:R195.
81. Maizel J, Airapetian N, Lorne E, et al. Diagnosis of central hypovolemia by using passive leg raising. *Intensive Care Med.* 2007;33:1133–1138.
82. Chalak LF, Barber CA, Hynan L, et al. End-tidal $CO(_2)$ detection of an audible heart rate during neonatal cardiopulmonary resuscitation after asystole in asphyxiated piglets. *Pediatr Res.* 2011;69: 401–405.
83. Monnet X, Bataille A, Magalhaes E, et al. End-tidal carbon dioxide is better than arterial pressure for predicting volume responsiveness by the passive leg raising test. *Intensive Care Med.* 2013;39:93–100.
84. Frank O. The basic shape of the arterial pulse. First treatise: mathematical analysis. 1899. *J Mol Cell Cardiol.* 1990;22:255–277.

85. Montenij LJ, de Waal EE, Buhre WF. Arterial waveform analysis in anesthesia and critical care. *Curr Opin Anaesthesiol.* 2011;24:651–656.
86. Marik PE. Noninvasive cardiac output monitors: a state-of the-art review. *J Cardiothorac Vasc Anesth.* 2013;27:121–134.
87. Chaney JC, Derdak S. Minimally invasive hemodynamic monitoring for the intensivist: current and emerging technology. *Crit Care Med.* 2002;30:2338–2345.
88. Sakka SG, Reinhart K, Wegscheider K, et al. Is the placement of a pulmonary artery catheter still justified solely for the measurement of cardiac output? *J Cardiothorac Vasc Anesth.* 2000;14:119–124.
89. Linton R, Band D, O'Brien T, et al. Lithium dilution cardiac output measurement: a comparison with thermodilution. *Crit Care Med.* 1997;25:1796–1800.
90. Sundar S, Panzica P. LiDCO systems. *Int Anesthesiol Clin.* 2010;48:87–100.
91. Goedje O, Hoeke K, Lichtwarck-Aschoff M, et al. Continuous cardiac output by femoral arterial thermodilution calibrated pulse contour analysis: comparison with pulmonary arterial thermodilution. *Crit Care Med.* 1999;27:2407–2412.
92. Pearse RM, Ikram K, Barry J. Equipment review: an appraisal of the LiDCO plus method of measuring cardiac output. *Crit Care.* 2004;8:190–195.
93. Langewouters GJ, Wesseling KH, Goedhard WJ. The static elastic properties of 45 human thoracic and 20 abdominal aortas in vitro and the parameters of a new model. *J Biomech.* 1984;17:425–435.
94. Geerts BF, Aarts LP, Jansen JR. Methods in pharmacology: measurement of cardiac output. *Br J Clin Pharmacol.* 2011;71:316–330.
95. Truijen J, van Lieshout JJ, Wesselink WA, et al. Noninvasive continuous hemodynamic monitoring. *J Clin Monit Comput.* 2012;26:267–278.
96. Wesseling KH, Jansen JR, Settels JJ, et al. Computation of aortic flow from pressure in humans using a nonlinear, three-element model. *J Appl Physiol.* 1993;74:2566–2573.
97. Zollner C, Haller M, Weis M, et al. Beat-to-beat measurement of cardiac output by intravascular pulse contour analysis: a prospective criterion standard study in patients after cardiac surgery. *J Cardiothorac Vasc Anesth.* 2000;14:125–129.
98. Rodig G, Prasser C, Keyl C, et al. Continuous cardiac output measurement: pulse contour analysis vs thermodilution technique in cardiac surgical patients. *Br J Anaesth.* 1999;82:525–530.
99. Monnet X, Anguel N, Naudin B, et al. Arterial pressure-based cardiac output in septic patients: different accuracy of pulse contour and uncalibrated pressure waveform devices. *Crit Care.* 2010;14:R109.
100. Hamzaoui O, Monnet X, Richard C, et al. Effects of changes in vascular tone on the agreement between pulse contour and transpulmonary thermodilution cardiac output measurements within an up to 6-hour calibration-free period. *Crit Care Med.* 2008;36:434–440.
101. Muller L, Candela D, Nyonzyma L, et al. Disagreement between pulse contour analysis and transpulmonary thermodilution for cardiac output monitoring after routine therapeutic interventions in ICU patients with acute circulatory failure. *Eur J Anaesthesiol.* 2011;28:664–669.
102. Costa MG, Della Rocca G, Chiarandini P, et al. Continuous and intermittent cardiac output measurement in hyperdynamic conditions: pulmonary artery catheter vs. lithium dilution technique. *Intensive Care Med.* 2008;34:257–263.
103. Staier K, Wiesenack C, Gunkel L, et al. Cardiac output determination by thermodilution and arterial pulse waveform analysis in patients undergoing aortic valve replacement. *Can J Anaesth.* 2008;55: 22–28.
104. De Backer D, Marx G, Tan A, et al. Arterial pressure-based cardiac output monitoring: a multicenter validation of the third-generation software in septic patients. *Intensive Care Med.* 2011;37:233–240.
105. Cannesson M, Attof Y, Rosamel P, et al. Comparison of FloTrac cardiac output monitoring system in patients undergoing coronary artery bypass grafting with pulmonary artery cardiac output measurements. *Eur J Anaesthesiol.* 2007;24:832–839.
106. Hadian M, Kim HK, Severyn DA, et al. Cross-comparison of cardiac output trending accuracy of LiDCO, PiCCO, FloTrac and pulmonary artery catheters. *Crit Care.* 2010;14:R212.
107. Hamm JB, Nguyen BV, Kiss G, et al. Assessment of a cardiac output device using arterial pulse waveform analysis, Vigileo, in cardiac surgery compared to pulmonary arterial thermodilution. *Anaesth Intensive Care.* 2010;38:295–301.
108. Tsai YF, Su BC, Lin CC, et al. Cardiac output derived from arterial pressure waveform analysis: validation of the third-generation software in patients undergoing orthotopic liver transplantation. *Transplant Proc.* 2012;44:433–437.
109. Mayer J, Boldt J, Poland R, et al. Continuous arterial pressure waveform-based cardiac output using the FloTrac/Vigileo: a review and meta-analysis. *J Cardiothorac Vasc Anesth.* 2009;23:401–406.

110. Critchley LA. Pulse contour analysis: is it able to reliably detect changes in cardiac output in the hemodynamically unstable patient? *Crit Care.* 2011;15:106.
111. Bogert LW, Wesseling KH, Schraa O, et al. Pulse contour cardiac output derived from non-invasive arterial pressure in cardiovascular disease. *Anaesthesia.* 2010;65:1119–1125.
112. Sokolski M, Rydlewska A, Krakowiak B, et al. Comparison of invasive and non-invasive measurements of haemodynamic parameters in patients with advanced heart failure. *J Cardiovasc Med (Hagerstown).* 2011;12:773–778.
113. Broch O, Renner J, Gruenewald M, et al. A comparison of the Nexfin(R) and transcardiopulmonary thermodilution to estimate cardiac output during coronary artery surgery. *Anaesthesia.* 2012;67:377–383.
114. Laupland KB, Bands CJ. Utility of esophageal Doppler as a minimally invasive hemodynamic monitor: a review. *Can J Anaesth.* 2002;49:393–401.
115. Rodriguez RM, Berumen KA. Cardiac output measurement with an esophageal Doppler in critically ill Emergency Department patients. *J Emerg Med.* 2000;18:159–164.
116. Dark PM, Singer M. The validity of trans-esophageal Doppler ultrasonography as a measure of cardiac output in critically ill adults. *Intensive Care Med.* 2004;30:2060–2066.
117. Bein B, Worthmann F, Tonner PH, et al. Comparison of esophageal Doppler, pulse contour analysis, and real-time pulmonary artery thermodilution for the continuous measurement of cardiac output. *J Cardiothorac Vasc Anesth.* 2004;18:185–189.
118. Lafanechere A, Albaladejo P, Raux M, et al. Cardiac output measurement during infrarenal aortic surgery: echo-esophageal Doppler versus thermodilution catheter. *J Cardiothorac Vasc Anesth.* 2006;20:26–30.
119. Moxon D, Pinder M, van Heerden PV, et al. Clinical evaluation of the HemoSonic monitor in cardiac surgical patients in the ICU. *Anaesth Intensive Care.* 2003;31:408–411.
120. Chong SW, Peyton PJ. A meta-analysis of the accuracy and precision of the ultrasonic cardiac output monitor (USCOM). *Anaesthesia.* 2012;67:1266–1271.
121. Horster S, Stemmler HJ, Strecker N, et al. Cardiac output measurements in septic patients: comparing the accuracy of USCOM to PiCCO. *Crit Care Res Pract.* 2012;2012:270631.
122. Boyle M, Steel L, Flynn GM, et al. Assessment of the clinical utility of an ultrasonic monitor of cardiac output (the USCOM) and agreement with thermodilution measurement. *Crit Care Resusc.* 2009;11:198–203.
123. Tan HL, Pinder M, Parsons R, et al. Clinical evaluation of USCOM ultrasonic cardiac output monitor in cardiac surgical patients in intensive care unit. *Br J Anaesth.* 2005;94:287–291.
124. Thom O, Taylor DM, Wolfe RE, et al. Comparison of a supra-sternal cardiac output monitor (USCOM) with the pulmonary artery catheter. *Br J Anaesth.* 2009;103:800–804.
125. Chand R, Mehta Y, Trehan N. Cardiac output estimation with a new Doppler device after off-pump coronary artery bypass surgery. *J Cardiothorac Vasc Anesth.* 2006;20:315–319.
126. Corley A, Barnett AG, Mullany D, et al. Nurse-determined assessment of cardiac output. Comparing a non-invasive cardiac output device and pulmonary artery catheter: a prospective observational study. *Int J Nurs Stud.* 2009;46:1291–1297.
127. Vincent JL, Rhodes A, Perel A, et al. Clinical review: update on hemodynamic monitoring—a consensus of 16. *Crit Care.* 2011;15:229.
128. Salem R, Vallee F, Rusca M, et al. Hemodynamic monitoring by echocardiography in the ICU: the role of the new echo techniques. *Curr Opin Crit Care.* 2008;14:561–568.
129. Raaijmakers E, Faes TJ, Scholten RJ, et al. A meta-analysis of three decades of validating thoracic impedance cardiography. *Crit Care Med.* 1999;27:1203–1213.
130. Critchley LA, Lee A, Ho AM. A critical review of the ability of continuous cardiac output monitors to measure trends in cardiac output. *Anesth Analg.* 2010;111:1180–1192.
131. Critchley LA, Calcroft RM, Tan PY, et al. The effect of lung injury and excessive lung fluid, on impedance cardiac output measurements, in the critically ill. *Intensive Care Med.* 2000;26:679–685.
132. Shoemaker WC, Belzberg H, Wo CC, et al. Multicenter study of noninvasive monitoring systems as alternatives to invasive monitoring of acutely ill emergency patients. *Chest.* 1998;114:1643–1652.
133. Raval NY, Squara P, Cleman M, et al. Multicenter evaluation of noninvasive cardiac output measurement by bioreactance technique. *J Clin Monit Comput.* 2008;22:113–119.
134. Marque S, Cariou A, Chiche JD, et al. Comparison between Flotrac-Vigileo and Bioreactance, a totally noninvasive method for cardiac output monitoring. *Crit Care.* 2009;13:R73.
135. Fagnoul D, Vincent JL, Backer DD. Cardiac output measurements using the bioreactance technique in critically ill patients. *Crit Care.* 2012;16:460.
136. Squara P, Denjean D, Estagnasie P, et al. Noninvasive cardiac output monitoring (NICOM): a clinical validation. *Intensive Care Med.* 2007;33:1191–1194.

137. Jaffe MB. Partial CO_2 rebreathing cardiac output—operating principles of the NICO system. *J Clin Monit Comput.* 1999;15:387–401.
138. Nilsson LB, Eldrup N, Berthelsen PG. Lack of agreement between thermodilution and carbon dioxide-rebreathing cardiac output. *Acta Anaesthesiol Scand.* 2001;45:680–685.
139. Odenstedt H, Stenqvist O, Lundin S. Clinical evaluation of a partial CO_2 rebreathing technique for cardiac output monitoring in critically ill patients. *Acta Anaesthesiol Scand.* 2002;46:152–159.
140. Stoneking L, Denninghoff K, Deluca L, et al. Sepsis bundles and compliance with clinical guidelines. *J Intensive Care Med.* 2011;26:172–182.
141. Kuo YW, Chang HT, Wu PC, et al. Compliance and barriers to implementing the sepsis resuscitation bundle for patients developing septic shock in the general medical wards. *J Formos Med Assoc.* 2012;111:77–82.
142. Zhu Y, Tao RJ, Shi W, et al. A study of rate of compliance with sepsis bundle in patients with severe sepsis and septic shock in emergency department. *Zhongguo Wei Zhong Bing Ji Jiu Yi Xue.* 2011;23:138–141.
143. Mikkelsen ME, Gaieski DF, Goyal M, et al. Factors associated with nonadherence to early goal-directed therapy in the ED. *Chest.* 2010;138:551–558.
144. Kang MJ, Shin TG, Jo IJ, et al. Factors influencing compliance with early resuscitation bundle in the management of severe sepsis and septic shock. *Shock.* 2012;38:474–479.
145. Parienti JJ, du Cheyron D, Timsit JF, et al. Meta-analysis of subclavian insertion and nontunneled central venous catheter-associated infection risk reduction in critically ill adults. *Crit Care Med.* 2012;40:1627–1634.
146. Ruesch S, Walder B, Tramer MR. Complications of central venous catheters: internal jugular versus subclavian access—a systematic review. *Crit Care Med.* 2002;30:454–460.
147. Eisen LA, Narasimhan M, Berger JS, et al. Mechanical complications of central venous catheters. *J Intensive Care Med.* 2006;21:40–46.
148. Jones AE, Shapiro NI, Trzeciak S, et al. Lactate clearance vs central venous oxygen saturation as goals of early sepsis therapy: a randomized clinical trial. *JAMA.* 2010;303:739–746.
149. Kircher BJ, Himelman RB, Schiller NB. Noninvasive estimation of right atrial pressure from the inspiratory collapse of the inferior vena cava. *Am J Cardiol.* 1990;66:493–496.
150. Nagdev AD, Merchant RC, Tirado-Gonzalez A, et al. Emergency department bedside ultrasonographic measurement of the caval index for noninvasive determination of low central venous pressure. *Ann Emerg Med.* 2010;55:290–295.
151. Lichtenstein DA, Meziere GA, Lagoueyte JF, et al. A-lines and B-lines: lung ultrasound as a bedside tool for predicting pulmonary artery occlusion pressure in the critically ill. *Chest.* 2009;136:1014–1020.
152. Kanji H. Early standardized echocardiography improves survival in patients with shock. abstract. *Crit Care Med.* 2012;40:18.

4

Arterial Blood Pressure Monitoring

Vidya K. Rao and John E. Arbo

BACKGROUND

Arterial blood pressure (ABP) is an essential cardiovascular vital sign and monitoring parameter for all critically ill patients. ABP may be measured indirectly using an inflatable external cuff or directly by cannulation of a peripheral artery.

Indirect ABP measurement is performed noninvasively and requires the use of an external expandable cuff and a pressure gauge, known as a sphygmomanometer. The cuff is wrapped around an extremity overlying an artery and inflated to a pressure that temporarily occludes arterial blood flow. The cuff is then gradually deflated, and blood pressure is determined by auscultation of Korotkoff sounds or by an automated system that measures oscillations as blood flow resumes.

While inexpensive and easy to perform, indirect ABP measurement has limitations that make it unsuitable for critically ill patients. Auscultation is cumbersome in a busy environment and is impaired by ambient noise. The patient's body habitus as well as improper cuff size, position, or external compression can prevent an accurate measurement.[1–3] In critically ill patients, the principal disadvantage of indirect ABP measurement is the inability to provide continuous measurement, which is useful in hemodynamic compromise or vasopressor administration. Indirect measurements also frequently fail to correlate with direct pressure monitoring, especially in times of rapidly changing or unstable hemodynamics.[4,5] Finally, repetitive cycling of the blood pressure cuff can result in arm pain, limb edema, ischemia, neuropathy, and, in rare cases, compartment syndrome.[6–8]

Direct ABP monitoring, in which a catheter is inserted into a peripheral artery and continuously transduced, is the benchmark for arterial pressure measurement and is considered standard of care for most critically ill patients. An ABP catheter enables dynamic monitoring and provides continual vascular access when repetitive blood sampling is required. As discussed later in this chapter, the arterial pressure waveform also offers a wealth of diagnostic information.

GENERAL DEFINITIONS

Systolic blood pressure (SBP) is the peak pressure generated by ventricular contraction, and diastolic blood pressure (DBP) is the lowest pressure observed during ventricular filling. Pulse pressure (PP) is defined as the difference between the systolic and diastolic pressures.

Mean arterial pressure (MAP) is the time-weighted average of arterial pressures in a single cardiac cycle, and represents systemic perfusion pressure. MAP is calculated using the following formula:

$$\text{MAP} = \left(\frac{1}{3}\right) \times \text{SBP} + \left(\frac{2}{3}\right) \times \text{DBP}$$

Noninvasive blood pressure measurement determines SBP, DBP, and MAP by comparison of oscillatory characteristics to cuff pressures, where MAP is the point of maximal oscillations during cuff deflation.[9] Direct ABP measurement produces an arterial waveform that consists of a systolic peak and a diastolic trough. MAP is then determined by integrating the area under the curve.[10]

DIRECT BLOOD PRESSURE MONITORING

Indications

Direct ABP monitoring provides continuous, beat-to-beat arterial pressure measurement, which is essential in the management of patients who are hemodynamically unstable, have advanced cardiovascular disease or significant dysrhythmia, require vasopressor support, or whose condition necessitates targeted blood pressure control (Table 4.1). Waveform analysis can also provide significant insight into a patient's physiology, including intravascular volume status, volume responsiveness, and the presence of valvular abnormalities. As previously mentioned, this modality provides dependable vascular access and is indicated in patients with pulmonary compromise or significant

TABLE 4.1 Comparison of Invasive and Noninvasive Blood Pressure Monitoring in Critically Ill Patients

	Advantages	Disadvantages
Invasive monitoring	Continuous measurement of ABP	Technical skill required to obtain access
	Utility in titration of vasoactive infusions	Complications associated with procedure
	Continuous vascular access when repetitive blood sampling is required	Site-specific considerations with regard to accuracy of measurement
	Additional data regarding pathophysiology and hemodynamics provided by arterial waveform analysis	Inaccuracy associated with monitoring system and equipment
Noninvasive monitoring	Avoidance of a procedure and associated complications	Inability to provide continuous measurement
	Ease of performance	Impairment of accuracy from cuff mismatch, body habitus, position, and external compression
		Poor correlation with gold standard invasive measurement in hemodynamically unstable patients
		Complications associated with compression from repetitive cycling of cuff

acid–base derangements where frequent blood sampling is required. Peripheral arterial catheters may also be placed in patients prior to the administration of thrombolytic therapy to facilitate the collection of laboratory studies.

Site Selection

Factors that must be considered in site selection include the presence of adequate collateral circulation and patient comfort, as well as the phenomenon of distal pulse amplification that causes distal SBP measurements to be higher than central SBP, without significant differences in DBP or MAP.

The radial artery is the most commonly used vessel for ABP monitoring due to its superficial location, ease of cannulation, presence of collateral flow, and low risk of complications.[11] However, due to its small caliber, this site carries the highest incidence of temporary arterial occlusion, reported to occur in over 25% of procedures performed.[11–13] Despite its high incidence, temporary occlusion of the artery does not appear to have serious sequelae in most cases.[11] Given its peripheral location, a radial artery catheter provides a less accurate measurement of aortic pressure than do more centrally placed catheters due to distal pulse wave amplification.

The femoral artery is the second most commonly used site. The central location of this vessel allows for more accurate measurement of aortic blood pressure, particularly in patients requiring high-dose vasopressor administration, and its larger caliber mitigates the risk of temporary arterial occlusion seen with radial catheters.[11] However, clinicians must be cognizant of—and monitor for—retroperitoneal hemorrhage following cannulation. Historically, there has been reluctance to use this site given its proximity to the anogenital region and the concern that it carries an increased risk of infection. However, published studies do not uniformly substantiate or refute this concern.[14,15]

The axillary artery has gained popularity in recent decades as it permits measurement of central pressure using a cannulation site that is considered to be in a cleaner location. This approach is more technically challenging than are others, and is often avoided due to the theoretical risk of cerebral embolic events given its proximity to the carotid artery. The incidence of major complications associated with this cannulation site was similar to that of radial and femoral catheterization.[11]

Complications

Arterial catheterization is generally considered to be a safe procedure, but complications can and do occur, and must be factored into site selection (Table 4.2). Risks include temporary arterial occlusion, ischemia, pseudoaneurysm, arteriovenous fistula, infection, bleeding, air embolism, and hematoma.[11,16] Patients with preexisting vascular disease,

TABLE 4.2 Complications of Arterial Lines

• Hematoma/Bleeding	• Pseudoaneurysm
• Local infection	• Arteriovenous fistula formation
• Nerve injury	• Sepsis
• Temporary arterial occlusion	• Compartment syndrome
• Permanent arterial occlusion/limb ischemia	• Equipment defect

arterial injury, high-dose vasopressor administration, and long-term cannulation may be at higher risk for adverse events.[10] Fortunately, serious complications occur in <1% of cases.[11] Use of the Allen test does not minimize complications associated with arterial artery cannulation and has been abandoned.

Contraindications

Contraindications are generally relative, site specific, and based upon consideration of risk and benefit. Relative contraindications include significant peripheral vascular disease and Raynaud syndrome due to the associated risk of limb ischemia, and severe coagulopathy or use of thrombolytics given the risk of bleeding. Placement of intra-arterial catheters should also be avoided at sites with signs of obvious infection, burns, vascular trauma, or previous vascular surgery or grafts.[17,18] Cannulation ipsilateral to arteriovenous dialysis shunts will yield false results and should be avoided.

THE MONITORING SYSTEM

Components of the Monitoring System

Data from the monitoring system must be converted into a waveform that can be visualized on the patient's monitor. Monitoring systems consist of several parts beyond the arterial cannula, including a fluid-filled system, transducer, flushing assembly, microprocessor, amplifier, and display.

- The fluid-filled system creates a column of fluid, usually heparinized saline, between the arterial cannula and the transducer, known as hydraulic coupling. To minimize waveform distortion, the tubing must be noncompliant, as short as possible, and free of air bubbles, blood clots, and extraneous three-way stopcocks. It is imperative that the tubing be clearly labeled to avoid inadvertent intra-arterial injection of medications.
- A flushing assembly that often contains heparinized saline pressurized to 300 mm Hg is attached to the fluid tubing to help maintain patency of the cannula. The system also allows high-pressure fluid flushes through the tubing system in order to keep it clear of clot and debris.
- The transducer converts pressure into an electrical signal. Changes in arterial pressure are transferred via the fluid in the tubing to a flexible diaphragm contained in the transducer. Movement of the diaphragm causes an imbalance by stretching or compressing four strain gauges that are incorporated into a Wheatstone bridge circuit. The imbalance creates an electrical current.
- Once pressure is converted into an electrical signal in the transducer, it is transmitted through an electrical cable to a microprocessor to be filtered, and then through an amplifier, after which the waveform is shown on an on-screen display.

The Physics of the Arterial Pressure Waveform

The arterial pressure waveform is composed of a fundamental wave and a series of harmonic waves. The fundamental wave frequency is equivalent to the pulse rate, and the frequencies of the harmonic waves are multiples of the fundamental frequency. Fourier analysis, the process by which the complex arterial waveform is constructed

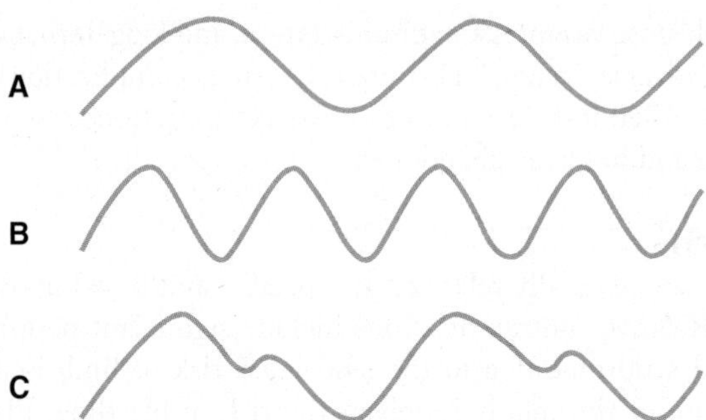

FIGURE 4.1 The arterial pressure waveform **(C)** is a sum of a fundamental wave **(A)** and six to eight harmonic waves **(B)**. Summation is performed by Fourier analysis. From Pittman JA, Ping JS, Mark JB. Arterial and central venous pressure monitoring. *Int Anesthesiol Clin.* 2004;42:13–30.

from these component waves, is performed by the microprocessor, and the arterial waveform is then amplified and visually displayed on the monitor (Fig. 4.1).[19]

The dynamic response of the ABP monitoring system is determined by resonant frequency and damping.[10,20] Resonant (or natural) frequency is defined as the frequency at which a given material oscillates when disrupted. When a system is stimulated by a frequency that is close to its own resonant frequency, it oscillates and amplifies the incoming signal.[9,21] Thus, if the frequencies of the fundamental or harmonic waves of an ABP waveform approach, coincide with, or overlap with the resonant frequency of the ABP monitoring system, amplification occurs and results in elevated SBP and PP measurements. The resonant frequency of the monitoring system is designed to be at least five to eight multiples above the fundamental frequency, and is determined by the physical properties of the system's components. Increasing tubing diameter while reducing tubing length, compliance, and density of the fluid in the system can increase the natural frequency of the monitoring system.

In addition to having a high resonant frequency, the ABP monitoring system must also be properly damped. Damping occurs when the energy in an oscillating system is reduced.[21] While some degree of damping, termed critical damping, is essential in the monitoring system, overdamping and underdamping can result in inaccurate measurement of ABP. Overdamping may occur when the system contains excess tubing, stopcocks, occlusion, and air, and can be identified by examining the arterial waveform for a slurred upstroke, absent dicrotic notch, and loss of fine detail.[9] Overdamped waves display falsely lower SBPs, falsely higher DBPs, and a narrowed PP, though MAP may still be accurate. Conversely, underdamping results in increased oscillations and therefore a falsely elevated SBP and PP. A patient's physiology can also result in underdamping; tachycardia increases the fundamental frequency given the high pulse rate. As the fundamental frequency approaches the resonant frequency of the monitoring system, oscillations are amplified and the system becomes underdamped.

The "square wave" or "fast flush" test evaluates the dynamic response of the monitoring system and helps predict signal distortion by determining the system's natural frequency and degree of damping. This test is performed by briefly opening the continuous flush valve and increasing the flow of fluid to 30 mL/h, which generates a square wave

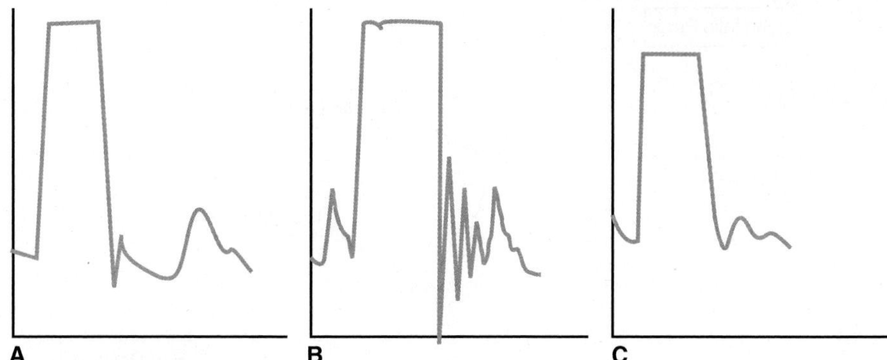

FIGURE 4.2 Square flush test. **A:** Optimal damping as evidenced by one to two oscillations prior to the return of the waveform. **B:** Underdamped: excessive oscillation and overestimation of the SBP. **C:** Overdamped: minimal oscillation and underestimation of the SBP.

that can be seen on the patient's monitor. Once the valve is closed, the resulting oscillations on the waveform are examined. The system's natural frequency is inversely proportional to the time between successive oscillation peaks; if the oscillation cycle is shorter, the system has a higher natural frequency. The degree of damping is determined by evaluating the ratio of the amplitudes of adjacent oscillation peaks. The amplitude ratio is then referenced with a graph that contains the corresponding damping coefficient. In an underdamped system, the amplitude ratio of successive oscillation peaks will be higher, and the system will have a lower damping coefficient. Conversely, overdamped systems will have lower amplitude ratios, and an elevated damping coefficient (Fig. 4.2).

Leveling and Zeroing

Following cannulation and connection to the pressure transducer tubing, the ABP monitoring system must be leveled and zeroed in order to provide consistent and accurate ABP measurements.

Leveling is the process of eliminating the influence of hydrostatic pressure on the measured BP. The transducer is leveled to the phlebostatic axis, defined as the intersection of the 4th intercostal space and the midaxillary line. This external location correlates to the anatomic position of the right atrium, which reflects central blood pressure. If positioned too low, the transducer will produce a deceptively high-pressure reading; if positioned too high, it will produce a deceptively low reading. Occasionally, the transducer is placed at the level of the tragus when cerebral perfusion pressure is the primary concern.

Zeroing is the process of eliminating the effects of atmospheric pressure on measured BP. To zero the system, it is opened to atmospheric pressure and set to a pressure of zero. This ensures that atmospheric pressure is the starting value.

ARTERIAL PRESSURE WAVEFORM ANALYSIS

The Arterial Waveform

The arterial waveform consists of five main elements: systolic upstroke, systolic peak, systolic decline, dicrotic notch, and the point of end diastole (Fig. 4.3).

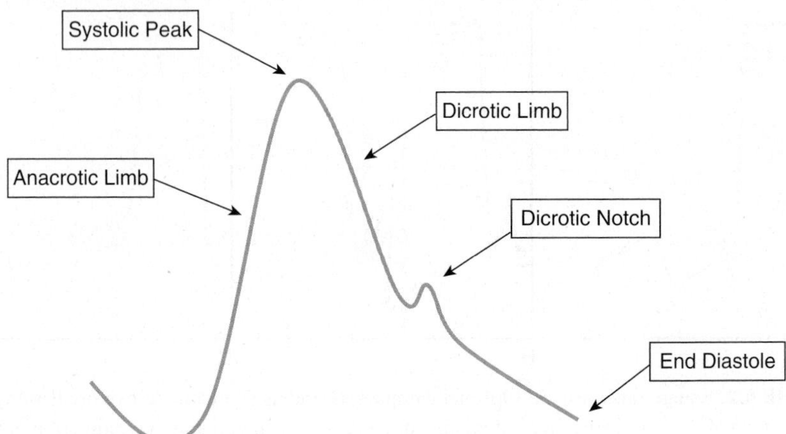

FIGURE 4.3 Arterial pressure waveform.

- The systolic upstroke, or anacrotic limb, begins with the opening of the aortic valve and appears as a rapid rise in the arterial waveform. Data regarding degree of contractility and left ventricular (LV) stroke volume may be inferred from the rate of ascent and height of the anacrotic limb.
- The systolic peak is the highest point of the waveform and marks the SBP, or the maximum pressure generated by the left ventricle during contraction.
- The systolic decline, or dicrotic limb, immediately follows the systolic peak and represents a decrease in blood flow out of the left ventricle.
- The dicrotic notch is seen during the course of the dicrotic limb and represents the closure of the aortic valve and the start of diastole.
- The point of end diastole is the lowest point of the waveform and marks the diastolic pressure.

Waveform Abnormalities

Close examination of the arterial line waveform can provide diagnostic clues regarding cardiac pathology, such as cardiac tamponade, aortic valvular disease, LV failure, and hypertrophic cardiomyopathy (Fig. 4.4A–D).

- *Pulsus tardus* and *pulsus parvus* are seen in aortic stenosis due to the fixed outflow obstruction imposed on the LV by the stenotic valve. This waveform is marked by a slow systolic rise (pulsus tardus), a late peak, and diminished amplitude (pulsus parvus), often mimicking an overdamped waveform (Fig. 4.4B).
- A *bisferiens pulse* is seen in aortic regurgitation and is characterized by two systolic peaks secondary to the large volume of blood ejected from the LV during systole. The first peak, or percussion wave, arises from ventricular ejection. The second peak, or tidal wave, arises from a wave reflected from the peripheral circulation as well as elastic recoil of the aorta. A bisferiens pulse will also demonstrate a sharp systolic upstroke, a low diastolic pressure, and a widened PP because of a backflow of blood into the LV during diastole (Fig. 4.4C).

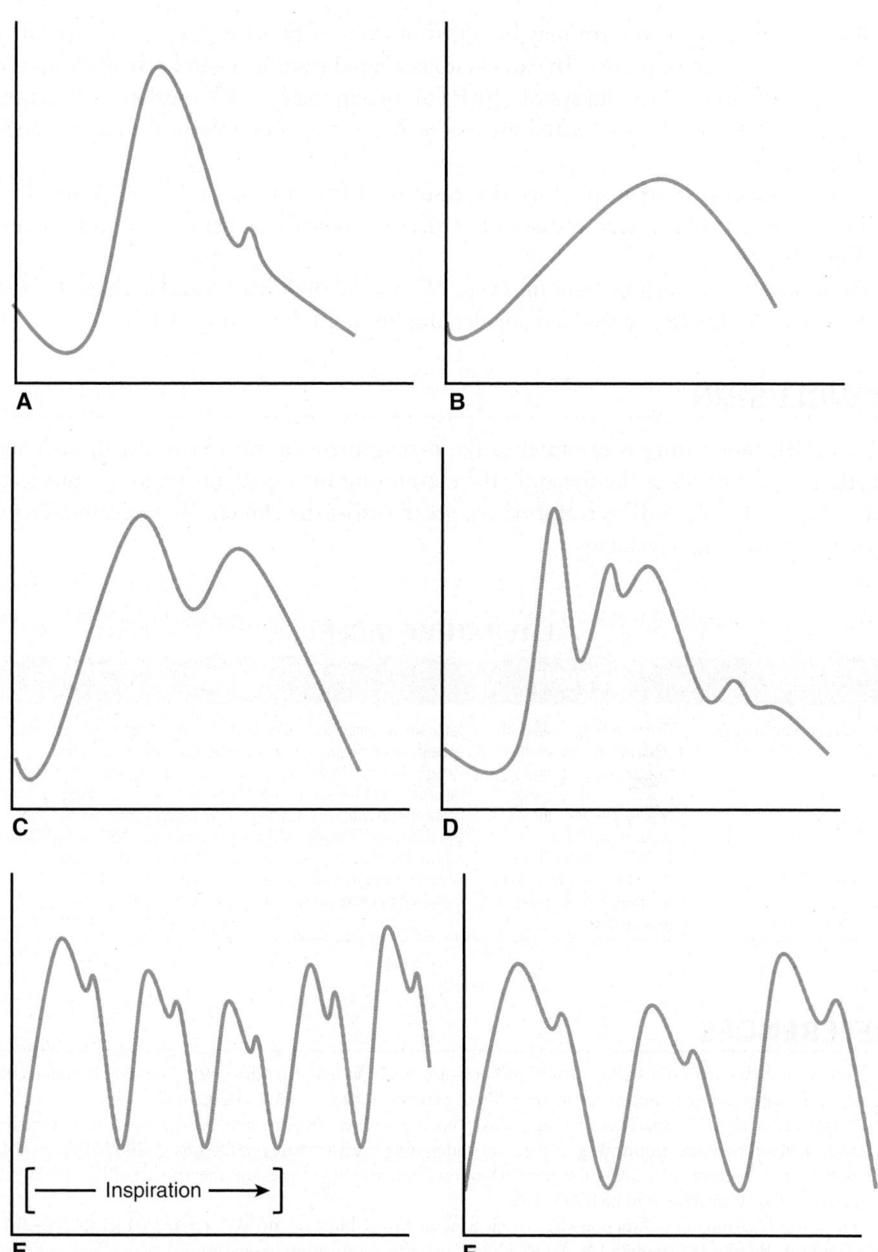

FIGURE 4.4 **A:** Normal arterial waveform. **B:** Pulsus parvus and pulsus tardus. **C:** Bisferiens pulse. **D:** Spike-and-dome. **E:** Pulsus paradoxus. **F:** Pulsus alternans.

- A *spike-and-dome* waveform may be noted in cases of hypertrophic cardiomyopathy and consists of three phases. In early systole, a rapid systolic upstroke arises from the forceful LV ejection. In mid systole, SBP falls precipitously as LV outflow obstruction occurs. In late systole, a reflected wave is seen, creating a double-peaked appearance (Fig. 4.4D).[22]
- *Pulsus paradoxus* is an inspiratory decrease in SBP in excess of 10 to 12 mm Hg. This finding may be seen in cases of cardiac tamponade or pericardial constriction (Fig. 4.4E).
- *Pulsus alternans* is seen in cases of severe LV systolic dysfunction and is characterized by regular, alternating larger and smaller amplitude PP beats (Fig. 4.4F).

CONCLUSION

Direct ABP monitoring is essential in the management of most critically ill patients. In addition to providing the dynamic BP monitoring these patients require, a nuanced appreciation of arterial BP waveforms can greatly assist the clinician in understanding a patient's underlying physiology.

LITERATURE TABLE

TRIAL	DESIGN	RESULT
Lehman et al., *Crit Care Med.* 2013[23]	Retrospective, single-center study of patients admitted to intensive care units at a tertiary medical center requiring invasive arterial pressure monitoring. 27,022 simultaneously measured invasive arterial/noninvasive blood pressure pairs recorded	Noninvasive modalities overestimate systolic pressure in hypotensive patients when compared to invasive blood pressure monitoring. Patients in whom NIBP readings were <70 mm Hg systolic had higher rates of acute kidney injury and ICU mortality when compared to patients with direct ABP readings in the same range ($p = 0.008$ and $p < 0.001$, respectively). MAP measurements from NIBP and IABP were similar, and there were no significant differences in the incidences of acute kidney injury or ICU mortality in patients with MAP < 60 measured by either modality ($p = 0.28$ and $p = 0.76$, respectively)

REFERENCES

1. Bur A, et al. Accuracy of oscillometric blood pressure measurement according to the relation between cuff size and upper-arm circumference in critically ill patients. *Crit Care Med.* 2000;28:371–376.
2. Hager H, et al. A comparison of noninvasive blood pressure measurement on the wrist with invasive arterial blood pressure monitoring in patients undergoing bariatric surgery. *Obes Surg.* 2009;19:717–724.
3. Bur A, et al. Factors influencing the accuracy of oscillometric blood pressure measurement in critically ill patients. *Crit Care Med.* 2003;31:793–799.
4. Horowitz D, Amoateng-Adjepong Y, Zarich S, et al. Arterial line or cuff BP? *Chest.* 2013;143:270–271.
5. Araghi A, Bander JJ, Guzman JA. Arterial blood pressure monitoring in overweight critically ill patients: invasive or noninvasive? *Crit Care.* 2006;10:R64.
6. Jeon YS, Kim YS, Lee JA, et al. Rumpel-Leede phenomenon associated with noninvasive blood pressure monitoring—a case report. *Korean J Anesthesiol.* 2010;59:203–205.
7. Lin CC, Jawan B, de Villa MV, et al. Blood pressure cuff compression injury of the radial nerve. *J Clin Anesth.* 2001;13:306–308.
8. Alford JW, Palumbo MA, Barnum MJ. Compartment syndrome of the arm: a complication of noninvasive blood pressure monitoring during thrombolytic therapy for myocardial infarction. *J Clin Monit Comput.* 2002;17:163–166.

9. Ward M, Langton J. Blood pressure measurement. *Contin Educ Anaesth Crit Care Pain.* 2007;7(4).
10. Schroeder R, Barbeito A, Bar-Yosef S, et al. *Miller's Anesthesia.* USA: Churchill Livingstone; 2009.
11. Scheer B, Perel A, Pfeiffer UJ. Clinical review: complications and risk factors of peripheral arterial catheters used for haemodynamic monitoring in anaesthesia and intensive care medicine. *Crit Care.* 2002;6:199–204.
12. Soderstrom CA, Wasserman DH, Dunham CM, et al. Superiority of the femoral artery of monitoring. A prospective study. *Am J Surg.* 1982;144, 309–312.
13. Bedford RF. Wrist circumference predicts the risk of radial-arterial occlusion after cannulation. *Anesthesiology.* 1978;48:377–378.
14. Frezza EE, Mezghebe H. Indications and complications of arterial catheter use in surgical or medical intensive care units: analysis of 4932 patients. *Am Surg.* 1988;64:127–131.
15. Lorente L, Santacreu R, Martin MM, et al. Arterial catheter-related infection of 2,949 catheters. *Crit Care.* 2006;10:R83.
16. Salmon AA, et al. Analysis of major complications associated with arterial catheterisation. *Qual Saf Health Care.* 2010;19:208–212.
17. Milzma D, Janchar T. Arterial puncture and cannulation. In: Roberts J, Hedges J, eds. *Clinical Procedures in Emergency Medicine.* Philadelphia, PA: WB Saunders; 2004:384–400.
18. Stroud S, Rodriguez R. Arterial puncture and cannulation. In: Reichman E, Simon R, eds. *Emergency Medicine Procedures.* New York, NY: McGraw Hill; 2003:298–410.
19. Pittman JA, Ping JS, Mark JB. Arterial and central venous pressure monitoring. *Int Anesthesiol Clin.* 2004;42:13–30.
20. Gilbert M. Principles of pressure transducers, resonance, damping and frequency response. *Anaest Intens Care Med.* 2012;13:1.
21. Boutros A, Albert S. Effect of the dynamic response of transducer-tubing system on accuracy of direct blood pressure measurement in patients. *Crit Care Med.* 1983;11:124–127.
22. Roth JV. The spike-and-dome arterial waveform pattern. *J Cardiothorac Vasc Anesth.* 1994;8:484.
23. Lehman L, Saeed M, Talmor D, et al. Methods of blood pressure measurement in the ICU. *Crit Care Med.* 2013;41:33–40.

5

The Central Venous and Pulmonary Artery Catheter

Carlos Brun and Geoffrey K. Lighthall

BACKGROUND

Since their inception, both central venous and pulmonary artery catheters (PACs) have been influential in the management of critically ill patients. Bedside use of a central venous catheter (CVC) was first clearly described by Wilson[1] in 1962, who noted the clinical importance of bedside volume assessment and described CVC indications and techniques. Wilson explained the association between extremes of central venous pressures (CVPs) and volume status in the settings of normal or inadequate circulation. He further noted that, although the CVP indicated the circulating blood volume in relation to the pumping capacity of the heart at a given point in time, to maintain a CVP at a "predetermined level" would be clinically misguided.

Bedside use of a flow-directed, balloon-tipped catheter to measure right heart pressures was described in 1970 by Swan and Ganz.[2] Early studies in critically ill patients showed improved survival with PAC use in targeting supranormal cardiac output (CO) and oxygen delivery indices; later, more carefully designed studies demonstrated no benefit with this strategy.[3–5] Recent studies in geriatric, high-risk surgery, and lung injury patients have also shown no benefit of fluid management based on PAC measurements.[6,7]

The lack of survival benefit with PAC use may be partially attributable to misinterpretation of waveforms, misguided correlations with preload, and resuscitation to predetermined numeric end points rather than measures of adequate circulation.[8–10] The declining use of these invasive monitors has led to decreased familiarity with waveform analysis and a lack of appreciation of the full set of information that can be obtained from these devices. This chapter aims to provide a basic understanding of the information that can be obtained through accurate interpretation of the waveforms and numerical data generated by central venous and PACs and to identify each catheter's appropriate clinical application.

CENTRAL VENOUS CATHETERS

Indications

CVCs have traditionally been inserted to assess circulatory volume, to provide intravenous access for vasopressors, and to facilitate simultaneous delivery of multiple medications. CVCs also allow assessment of central venous oxyhemoglobin saturation ($ScvO_2$), a value used to assess the adequacy of oxygen delivery relative to consumption (DO_2/VO_2). When accurately interpreted, CVP waveforms yield a wealth of hemodynamic data, as well as information about a patient's cardiac health, and can help identify a number of disease states commonly seen in the critically ill. Patient benefits from CVCs are likely maximized in scenarios in which clinicians are versed in the full range of quantitative and qualitative information available from the catheter.

Qualitative Waveform Analysis

Qualitative analysis of CVP waveforms yields information analogous to the examination of jugular venous pulsation (JVP), but with greater ease and visibility. Insight into both structural and electrical functions of the heart is obtained by analysis of characteristic waveforms present during each cardiac cycle.

Each CVP tracing contains *a*, *c*, and *v* waves and *x* and *y* descents. These waves and descents represent the spikes and troughs in pressure that occur in the right atria during each cardiac cycle. The *a* wave reflects atrial contraction and occurs after the ECG P wave at end diastole. Following atrial contraction, atrial pressures begin to fall due to atrial relaxation and downward right ventricular movement during systole. This fall in pressure—represented by the *x* descent—is briefly interrupted in early systole by isovolumetric contraction of the right ventricle (RV) against a closed tricuspid valve—represented by the *c* wave. The time between *a* and *c* waves peaks is identical to the PR interval, albeit 80 to 100 ms later than the corresponding ECG.

The *v* wave follows the *x* descent and reflects passive atrial filling, which begins at the end of systole and peaks in early diastole. The *y* descent indicates atrial diastolic emptying and passive ventricular filling.[12] While this discussion centers on the CVP, the PAC in the "wedged" position produces identical-appearing waves, but reflects left atrial activity (discussed below). Some examples of the variability of CVP waveforms and their ability to indicate pathology are highlighted below (Fig. 5.1).

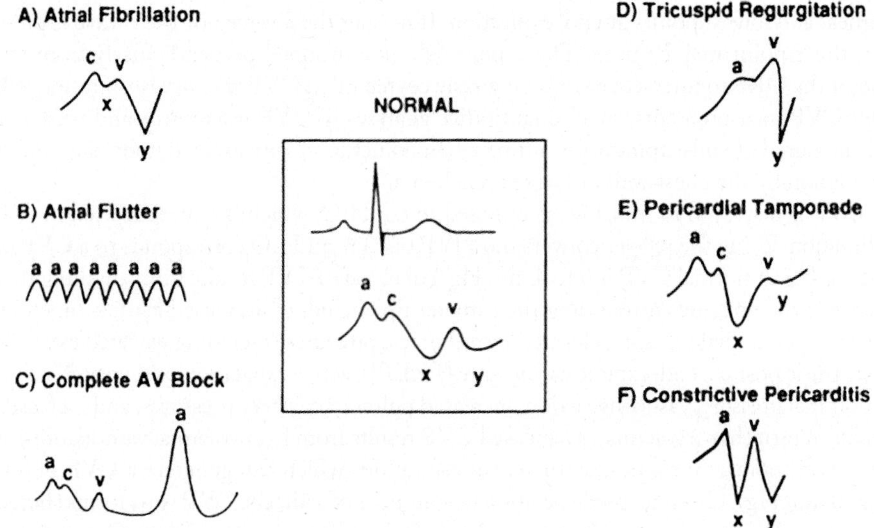

FIGURE 5.1 **Center:** Normal EKG to CVP waveform relationship. **A–F:** CVP waveform changes seen with specified pathology.

Pathologies that can be detected by analysis of CVP waveforms include the following:

A. Atrial fibrillation: lack of coordinated atrial activity leads to absence of *a* waves.
B. Atrial flutter: atrial activity leads to high-frequency *a* waves.
C. AV dissociation: intermittent atrial contraction against a closed tricuspid valve leads to large "cannon" *a* waves.
D. Tricuspid valve dysfunction: tricuspid valve regurgitation leads to prominent *v* waves or fusion of the *c* and *v* waves without an *x* descent. In tricuspid stenosis, the mean CVP will be high with large *a* waves and small slurred *y* descents due to a continuously elevated atrial diastolic pressure.
E. Pericardial tamponade: CVP values reflect pericardial pressures and change as the size of the heart changes during the cardiac cycle. During diastole, as the heart enlarges, pericardial pressures increase and limit passive ventricular filling; thus, the *y* descent is impaired. As blood is ejected during systole, the heart becomes smaller, pericardial pressures exert less influence, and the CVP falls, resulting in an isolated *x* descent.
F. Restrictive and constrictive diseases: pathologies, including constrictive pericarditis, myocarditis, infiltrative diseases, hypertrophy, and ischemia, are typified by high mean filling pressures (tall *a* and *v* waves) and short, steep *x* and *y* descents, which create an "M" or "W" pattern. The "square root sign" describes an abrupt *y* descent followed by a plateau when the diastolic pressure limit is met.

Quantitative Central Venous Pressure Analysis

Since pressure-based estimates of preload attempt to estimate ventricular volume, CVP is measured when there is a continuous column of fluid between the catheter tip and the ventricle. During the cardiac cycle, this continuity exists when the atrioventricular valves are open and corresponds to the pressure at the end of the *a* wave just prior to the *c* wave. If the *c* wave is not seen, CVP can be inferred from the mean of the *a* wave's highest and lowest points at end-expiration. If neither the *a* wave nor the *c* wave is present, the *z* point may be used. The *z* point is a line dropped perpendicularly from the end of the QRS to intersect a simultaneously co-recorded CVP tracing. Respiration will alter CVP measurements, so all quantitative analyses of CVP waveforms and pressures are measured at end-expiration—a time when no net forces are exerted upon the central circulation by the chest wall or lung parenchyma.

CVP is displayed in mm Hg, as opposed to cm H_2O, which is generally used in JVP estimation. Using the proper conversion, a JVP of 13.6 cm H_2O corresponds to a CVP of 10 mm Hg. A normal CVP is 0 to 4 mm Hg. An elevated CVP results from anything that increases the pressure surrounding the catheter tip, including decreased cardiac function, elevated pericardial pressure, elevated intrathoracic pressures (including elevated extrinsic or intrinsic positive end-expiratory pressure [PEEP]), active exhalation or increased intra-abdominal pressure, vasoconstriction, increased pulmonary artery pressures, and increased venous return (hypervolemia). Decreased CVP results from hypovolemia, vasodilation, or decreased thoracic pressure due to active inspiration (which can generate a CVP of less than 0 mm Hg). Given its predisposition to a number of artifacts, CVP waveforms should be analyzed over several respiratory cycles—ideally using a printout from the monitor. All principles discussed here for CVP, as well as Figure 5.1, are equally applicable to measurements of 'wedge' or pulmonary artery occlusion pressure (PAOP) using a PAC.

Many intensivists have used CVP to guide fluid therapy in septic patients.[11,13,14] Traditionally, the CVP was thought to be a reliable indicator of fluid responsiveness of the left ventricle.[1,15] The belief was that if CVP reflected right ventricular preload and therefore stroke volume, CVP should ultimately predict left ventricular preload and stroke volume. The fact that CVP does not accurately reflect the Starling curve of the left ventricle is due to the complex nature of venous return as it relates to CO. Venous return to the right heart is determined by the difference between mean circulatory filling pressure and right atrial pressure; the pressure gradient for left heart filling is affected by transpulmonary pressure, pulmonary venous pressure, and interventricular septal function. Since addition of fluid sufficient to raise CVP does not always augment CO, its role as the measure of preload has been questioned. CVP changes have not been shown to correlate reliably with corresponding changes in blood volume, left heart preload, or fluid responsiveness.[8,10,16] In a meta-analysis of 24 ICU-based studies, a poor relationship between CVP (or changes in CVP) and changes in cardiac index following fluid administration were observed (pooled correlation coefficient between CVP and change in cardiac index, 0.18).[8] Furthermore, a "normal" CVP does not necessarily reflect euvolemia, as splanchnic circulation allows the venous system to accommodate approximately a 10% intravascular volume gain or loss without a change in CVP. Research has also shown that in critically ill patients, a CVP > 12 mm Hg does not substantially increase CO, suggesting that this value corresponds to the upper, non–fluid-responsive portion of the Starling curve.[17,18] Despite good rationale to abandon CVP as a marker of fluid responsiveness, CVP-guided resuscitation persists. The 2012 Surviving Sepsis Campaign (SSC) guidelines continue to endorse CVP as a tool to assure adequate intravascular volume during fluid administration. While acknowledging that "there are limitations to CVP as a marker of intravascular volume status and response to fluid," the guidelines conclude, "a low CVP generally can be relied upon as supporting a positive response to fluid loading."[14]

In managing hemodynamically unstable patients, current clinical evidence calls for avoiding static measures of intravascular pressure such as CVP and PAOP in favor of more accurate indicators of volume responsiveness (see Chapter 3). Monitoring techniques based on dynamic cardiopulmonary interactions—such as pulse pressure, stroke volume variation, and indices derived from Doppler measurements—are better predictors of volume responsiveness and are used increasingly in critical care.[10]

Central Venous Oximetry

CVCs allow measurement of the oxyhemoglobin saturation of superior vena caval blood ($ScvO_2$), thus providing an ability to assess the relationship between VO_2 and DO_2. While the gold standard for this VO_2/DO_2 assessment is mixed venous oxygen saturation (SvO_2) measured in the pulmonary artery, $ScvO_2$ has been demonstrated to provide a reliable surrogate in septic patients.[18] Changes in $ScvO_2$ can be used to estimate adequacy of CO and thus to gauge efforts to reverse deficits in tissue perfusion. A decrease in $ScvO_2$ should prompt examination of the components of oxygen delivery (see Chapter 2); if fluid status and hematocrit are determined to be adequate, cardiac contractility should be evaluated and inotropic support initiated when indicated to help normalize DO_2/VO_2.[14] $ScvO_2$ may also be a marker for cardiopulmonary reserve. For example, a decrease in $ScvO_2$ of >4.5% during a spontaneous breathing trial was reported as a sensitive and specific predictor of reintubation in difficult-to-wean patients.[19]

Complications

Significant complications attributable to CVC insertion include infection; arterial or venous injury or fistula; venous thrombosis; DVT/pulmonary embolism; hematoma; hemothorax; pneumothorax; chylothorax; nerve injury; knotting or dislocation of other implanted catheters or equipment; air embolus; and dysrhythmias.[20,21] Catheter placement should be justified by a sound physiologic rationale for use, and removal should occur as soon as these indications cease to exist.[22]

Contraindications

Relative contraindications to CVC placement include coagulopathy, infection at the insertion site, right heart ventricular assist devices, and recent pacemaker placement. Some of these obstacles can be managed by placement of the CVC at an alternative anatomic site (e.g., internal jugular vs. subclavian in the case of coagulopathy). Absolute contraindications are vascular occlusion and patient refusal.

Practical Considerations

Ultrasound guidance should be used wherever available when placing a CVC. Use of continuous ultrasound guidance for insertion of CVC improves first-pass success, decreases procedure duration, and minimizes number of needle passes.[20,21] Placement of a CVC should occur concurrently with therapeutic maneuvers and not delay empiric treatment of extremes in intravascular volume or blood pressure.

PULMONARY ARTERY CATHETERS

PACs are not typically employed as resuscitative or analytic tools in the ED; their use is generally seen in the ICU, operating room, and cardiac catheterization lab. The PAC is capable of providing simultaneous assessment of CO, SvO_2, left-sided filling pressures, and continuous right-sided pressures. The PAC is available in thermodilution, pacing, or continuous CO/SvO_2 models. The ability to measure SvO_2 allows evaluation of adequacy of DO_2 in the context of CO measurements. PAC insertion should not delay either resuscitation or ICU admission.

As with CVP, no absolute PAOP has been shown to predict fluid responsiveness, as euvolemic pressures are dependent upon each individual's left ventricular function and compliance.[10,23] Thus, the usefulness of the PAC may be limited to specific situations not fully addressed in randomized trials where PAC use failed to show any benefit. In 53 Japanese hospitals, the ATTEND registry showed an in-hospital mortality benefit for patients with acute nonischemic heart failure managed with a PAC (PAC 1.4% vs. non-PAC 4.4%).[24] Rationale for PAC placement in registry patients was cardiogenic shock, shock and pulmonary edema, and diagnosis of type of shock; patients were managed individually without a generalized treatment protocol. In a retrospective analysis of the National Trauma Data Bank, a mortality benefit with PAC use was seen in severely injured patients in shock (base deficit ≤ -11) except in patients aged 41 to 60.[25] Interestingly, patients older than 60 with severe injury had decreased mortality even with base deficit of -6 to -10, possibly signifying that PAC placement at admission in severely injured patients was associated with earlier resuscitation.

A unique characteristic of the PAC is its ability to provide continuous measurement of pulmonary artery pressures. The ability to titrate pulmonary vasodilators and monitor CO changes remains an attractive advantage of the PAC, although it has not been addressed experimentally. In patients with cardiogenic shock, PACs may help following reperfusion therapy to gauge response to supportive interventions.[26] A recent review on left ventricular assist devices advocated use of the PAC to differentiate between right and left heart failure when investigating causes of hypotension in the setting of adequate filling pressures.[13] Many of the recent studies on PACs excluded patients that received a PAC based on physician preference—including patients with severe heart failure or pulmonary vascular disease—and thus may have some selection bias against potential beneficiaries of the device.[24,27,28,29,31]

Indications

There are no clear indications regarding PAC use in the emergency department or ICU; in lieu of clinical evidence, existing personal or institutional practices and preferences dictate use. It is not uncommon for institutions to employ PACs in postoperative cardiac surgery patients to provide a broad set of physiologic parameters, allowing practitioners to distinguish between hypovolemia, vasoplegia, and inadequate cardiac contractility.

Insertion and Data Interpretation

A PAC may be inserted through any large vein, but the right internal jugular and left subclavian veins are optimal for maintaining the catheter's curvature and are likely the best locations for easy flotation of the tip. Waveform recognition (Fig. 5.2) is typically sufficient for guiding the catheter to its resting position in a central branch of the pulmonary artery. However, fluoroscopy and echocardiography are occasionally used if this approach is unsuccessful. A plain radiograph should be obtained to confirm final position and to rule out right ventricular coiling, aberrant placement, overinsertion, or mechanical complications such as pneumothorax and hemothorax.

Device-specific problems during PAC insertion include failure to zero the transducer, misconnections of pressure tubing and transducer wires to pulmonary artery (PA) and CVP ports causing erroneous display of waveforms, failure to inflate the balloon, advancing too slowly or quickly, and misinterpretation of waveforms. The larger introducer catheter also increases risks of bleeding and carotid injury.

The normal pulmonary arterial tracing has an arterial-like waveform with systolic pulmonary pressures in the 15 to 25 mm Hg range. The PAOP or "wedge" waveform reflects left atrial filling and is recognized by disappearance of the PA waveform and appearance of a CVP-like waveform during catheter advancement. When compared to the CVP tracing, the PAOP tracing normally has two prominent peaks (*a* and *v* waves) instead of three. The PAOP should be measured at end-expiration as the average of the *a* wave's peak and nadir pressures.

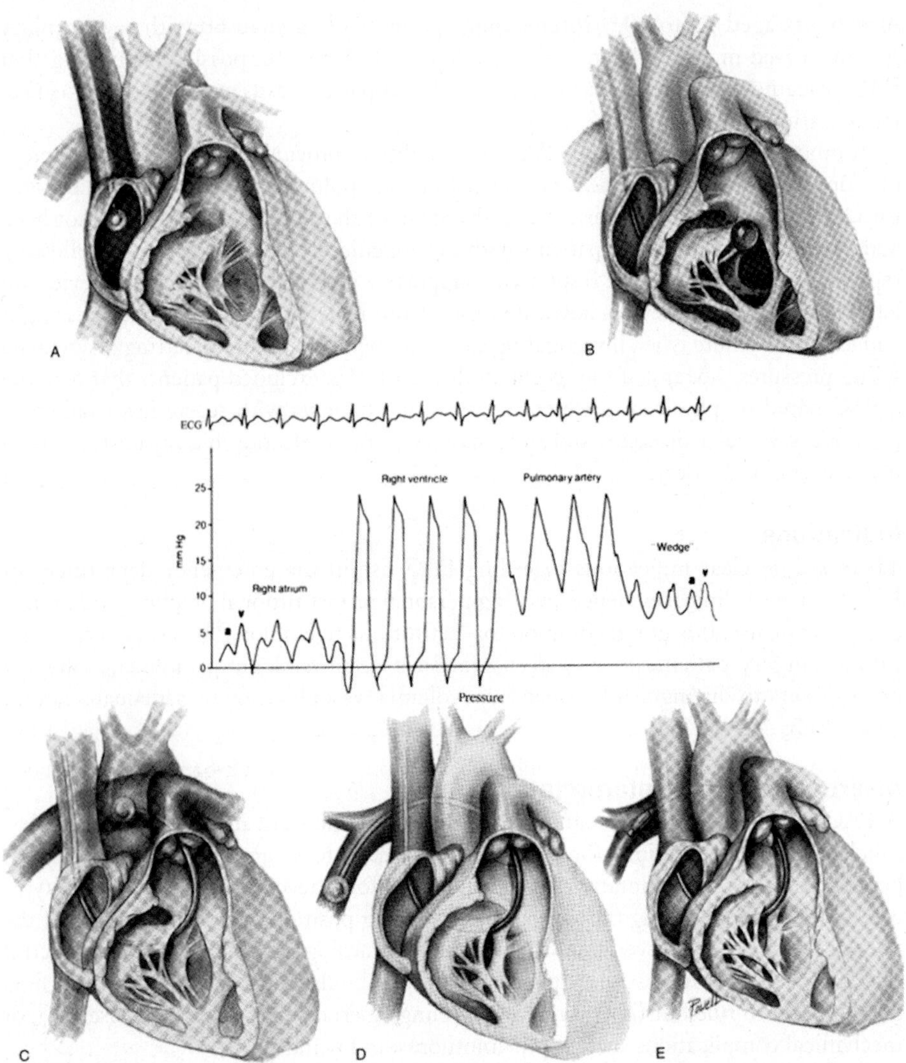

FIGURE 5.2 **A:** With the PAC tip in the right atrium, the balloon is inflated. **B:** The catheter is advanced into the right ventricle with the balloon inflated, and right ventricle pressure tracings are obtained. **C:** The catheter is advanced through the pulmonary valve into the pulmonary artery. A rise in diastolic pressure should be noted. **D:** The catheter is advanced to the "wedge" or PAOP position. A typical PAOP tracing should be noted with A and V waves. **E:** The balloon is deflated. Phasic pulmonary artery pressure should reappear on the monitor. Center: Waveform tracings generated as the balloon-tipped catheter is advanced through the right heart chambers into the pulmonary artery. Adapted from Wiedmann HP, Matthay MA, Matthey RA. Cardiovascular pulmonary monitoring in the intensive care unit (Part 1). *Chest.* 1984;85:537.

In a patient with normal pulmonary vascular resistance (PVR), the PA diastolic pressure (PAD) will be 8 to 15 mm Hg and only slightly higher (1 to 4 mm Hg) than the PAOP. This normal PAD–PAOP gradient often allows the practitioner to follow trends in PAD as estimates of LV filling pressures and eliminates the need for balloon inflation and repeated catheter "wedging." PAD pressures that are higher than normal (>20 mm Hg) raise concern for either elevated left heart pressures or elevated PVR. For example, with a PAD of 22 mm Hg, a similar PAOP (say 18 mm Hg) would point to elevated left-sided filling pressures as the cause of pulmonary venous hypertension. A PAD of 22 with a PAOP of 10 indicates that the left heart and related structures are not responsible for the elevated pulmonary artery pressure and that the pressure likely comes from high PVR. Elevations in PAOP may also be due to atrial myxomas, mitral valvulopathy, and high PEEP.

As with the CVC, qualitative information regarding left ventricular pump and electrical function can be obtained through the study of waveforms and their intervals. The discussion in the CVP section above is equally applicable here, except that the *a* and *c* waves of the PAOP tend to be fused, and an abnormally large v wave would reflect mitral valve regurgitation or poor LV compliance.

PACs had a historical role in defining the hemodynamic profiles associated with prototypic shock states (Table 5.1). Hypovolemic shock is readily recognized by decreased right- and left-sided filling pressures with decreased CO and a high SVR. Cardiogenic shock typically refers to LV failure, which is identified by increased right- and left-sided pressures, decreased CO, and increased SVR. Pure right heart failure is observed with elevated CVP, decreased PAOP and CO, and increased SVR. While a common cause of RV failure is LV failure, other possible etiologies include RV ischemia, pulmonary embolism, and pulmonary hypertension. Distributive shock from sepsis has been clinically described as progressive from an "early" or "warm" to a "late" or "cold" state. A change in measured CO via the PAC can differentiate the prototypically high CO in warm shock versus the low CO of cold distributive shock. This is relevant, as the latter condition may require inotropes while the former may not.

TABLE 5.1 Shock State Identification by PAC Hemodynamic Parameters (Normal Values for Each Parameter Noted in Parentheses)

Shock State	CVP (0–4 mm Hg)	PAP (15–25/8–15) PAOP (8–12 mm Hg)	Cardiac Index (2.2–4.2 L/min/m^2)	SVR (700–1,200 Dynes–s/cm^{-5})
Hypovolemic	↓	↓	↓	↑
Cardiogenic or obstructive left heart	↑	↑	↓	↑
Obstructive right heart	↑	↓	↓	↑
Distributive early	↓	↓	↑	↓
Distributive late	↓	↓	↓	↓

Complications

Complications from pulmonary artery catheterization include those of CVC placement, as well as more PAC-specific problems such as misinterpretation of data, higher likelihood of arrhythmia, pulmonary artery injury, pulmonary infarction, valvular injury, and catheter knotting or tangling with other devices. Of note, misinterpretation of respiratory cycle and corresponding wedge pressures can lead to large over- or underestimates of filling pressures. As with any central catheter, there is always a risk of infection, which is dependent on the length of time a PAC/introducer is maintained and the sterility of the techniques used to place it.

PAC placement is often difficult in patients with pulmonary artery hypertension, where tricuspid regurgitation and a large RV size impede flotation through the right heart. The catheter may coil in the RV, leading to arrhythmias and prolonged insertion times. Pulmonary artery injury can result from spontaneous wedging (also called "over wedging") (Fig. 5.3). Spontaneous wedging is evident when the PA waveform transitions to a "wedged" waveform without deliberate catheter advancement or balloon inflation. Over wedging occurs because of inadvertent migration of the catheter tip or occlusion of the PAC tip against a vessel wall.

Contraindications

Contraindications to PAC placement include left bundle branch block (LBBB) (given the ~5% risk of inducing right bundle branch block [RBBB]), right-sided cardiac mass, or right-sided infectious endocarditis. Contraindications listed for CVCs are also applicable. Attention should be paid to each particular PAC inserted, as several

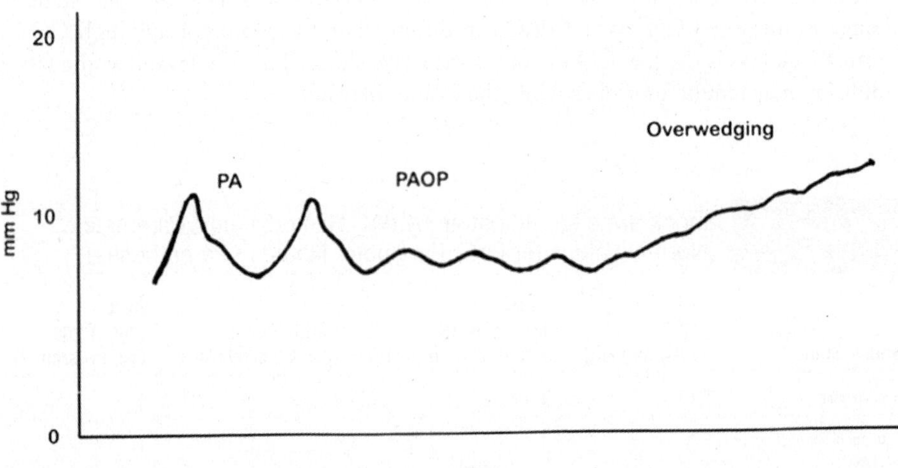

FIGURE 5.3 Overwedging. This condition should be suspected with a rise in PA pressures above known occlusion pressure values. A balloon inflated in this position could lead to pulmonary artery rupture. After assuring balloon deflation, catheters should be withdrawn to the main pulmonary artery and readvanced if necessary. Rarely, a PAC tip thrombus can produce an "overwedging" waveform. Adapted from Civetta GA. *Taylor & Kirby's Critical Care*. W. W. Philadelphia, PA: Norton & Company; 2009:175.

models contain heparin and/or latex and therefore would be contraindicated in patients with heparin-induced thrombocytopenia or a latex allergy. Risks of complications from insertion, manipulation, and interpretation are further increased with operator inexperience.

CONCLUSION

Invasive pressure monitoring is most useful when a change in hemodynamic status demands further clarification and assessment of adequacy of perfusion. CVCs enable the safe administration of vasoconstrictors and measurement of $ScvO_2$ and, with proper interpretation of their waveforms, provide a wealth of hemodynamic data. The PAC's ability to continuously monitor pulmonary artery pressures, CO, and SvO_2 remains useful in the management of complex patients, yet awaits a clearly defined population or protocol that demonstrates a clinical benefit. These "upstream" indicators of perfusion, however, have idiosyncrasies and inherent limitations. Careful examination of these capabilities over the last 30 years demonstrates that end points of resuscitation should also include evaluation of "downstream" variables, such as organ function and oxidative metabolism (e.g., lactate). Given the still widespread use of invasive pressure monitoring, understanding the full array of data available from CVC and PAC numerical and waveform data is important in assuring that the patient will derive the greatest benefit from his or her exposure to the risks of catheterization. The clinician at the bedside, not the devices, determines patient outcome.

LITERATURE TABLE

TRIAL	DESIGN	RESULT
CVP		
Marik et al., *Chest.* 2008[8]	Meta-analysis of 24 ICU-based studies to determine the ability of CVP, or changes in CVP, to predict fluid responsiveness	No relationship between CVP and changes in CVP with changes in cardiac index (CI) following fluid administration. Pooled correlation coefficient between CVP and change in CI = 0.18 (95% CI, 0.08–0.28). The pooled area under the ROC curve = 0.56 (95% CI, 0.51–0.61)
Michard and Teboul, *Chest.* 2002[10]	Meta-analysis of 334 ICU patients to evaluate prediction of change in SV or CI with fluid administration from change in CVP	No CVP threshold to identify fluid responsiveness. Only inspiratory decrease in change in CVP was equivalent to other dynamic parameters ("delta-down" arterial systolic blood pressure, pulse pressure variation, and change in aortic blood flow velocity) in ability to predict change in CI with fluid administration. Results seen in two studies of spontaneously breathing patients showed inspiratory decrease of CVP $\geq$ 1 mm Hg correlated with change in CO after fluid challenge. Those two studies reported positive predictive values of 77% and 84% and negative predictive values of 81% and 93%, respectively
Kumar et al., *Crit Care Med.* 2004[28]	Prospective, nonrandomized, nonblinded interventional study of 44 patients in cardiac catheterization and echocardiography lab to predict change in CI with fluid administration based on change in CVP	No relationship between change in CI and change in CVP with fluid administration. Pearson correlation coefficient = 0.32 ($p = 0.31$)

(*Continued*)

LITERATURE TABLE *(Continued)*

TRIAL	DESIGN	RESULT
PAC Studies		
Sandham et al., *N Engl J Med.* 2003[7]	Prospective, multicenter, nonblinded RCT of 1,994 elderly, high-risk (ASA 3 or 4) patients comparing goal directed therapy (GDT) with PAC vs. standard care without PAC perioperative optimization. Optimization was defined as utilization of supranormal hemodynamic parameter goals of CI of 3.5–4.5, MAP > 70, PAOP of 18, HR < 120, and HCT > 27	Six-month mortality was unchanged with PAC GDT vs. standard care (12% vs. 13%, $p = 0.93$). Weaknesses include atypical GDT (supranormal hemodynamic goals) and low overall mortality
Shah et al., *JAMA.* 2005[9]	Meta-analysis of 13 RCT of 5,051 patients with ARDS, severe heart failure, sepsis, general ICU treatment, or high-risk surgery, and the impact of PAC use on outcome	No mortality benefit comparing PAC use to no PAC use (combined OR = 1.04, CI = 0.90–1.2). PAC use was associated with increased use of inotropes (OR = 1.58, CI = 1.19–2.12) and vasodilators (OR = 2.35, CI = 1.75–3.15). Weaknesses include no GDT strategies and no specific criteria for PAC placement
Sotomi et al., *Int J Cardiol.* 2014[24]	Prospective, observational, multicenter cohort trial reporting the association of PAC use and mortality in 1,004 patients with acute heart failure syndrome	Decreased mortality with PAC use (1.4% vs. 4.4%, $p = 0.006$). Weaknesses included exclusion of patients with acute coronary syndrome, creatinine >3.5, or prior use of dopamine/dobutamine
Wheeler et al., *N Engl J Med.* 2006[29]	Prospective, multicenter, nonblinded RCT of 1,000 patients' 60-day mortality comparing PAC vs. CVP to guide hemodynamic management in ALI	No mortality difference using PAC vs. CVP (27% vs. 26%, $p = 0.69$). Also no significant difference in length of mechanical ventilation. Weaknesses included broad exclusion criteria and PAC management starting 40 h after admission
Harvey et al., *Lancet.* 2005[30]	Prospective, multicenter, nonblinded RCT of 1,041 patients to compare PAC use to usual care in reducing mortality in critically ill patients	No significant difference in mortality was found comparing PAC to usual care (68% vs. 66%, $p = 0.39$). No difference in ICU length of stay (12 d with PAC vs. 11 d without PAC, $p = 0.26$). Weaknesses included delay in randomization (16 h), no GDT, and high overall mortality
Richard et al., *JAMA.* 2003[31]	Prospective, multicenter, nonblinded RCT of 676 patients comparing early PAC use in shock and ARDS to usual care. Early use was defined as PAC placement within 12 h of ARDS or shock diagnosis	No difference in 14 d mortality comparing PAC vs. no PAC (50% vs. 51%, $p = 0.7$). Weaknesses included frequent use of echocardiography to guide therapy (64% of patients with PAC and 78% of patients without PAC received echocardiography)

CI, confidence interval; HR, hazard ratio; OR, odds ratio.

REFERENCES

1. Wilson JN, et al. Central venous pressure in optimal blood volume maintenance. *Arch Surg.* 1962;85:563–578.
2. Swan HJ, et al. Catheterization of the heart in man with use of a flow-directed balloon-tipped catheter. *N Engl J Med.* 1970;283(9):447–451.
3. Hayes MA, et al. Elevation of systemic oxygen delivery in the treatment of critically ill patients. *N Engl J Med.* 1994;330(24):1717–1722.
4. Gattinoni L, et al. A trial of goal-oriented hemodynamic therapy in critically ill patients. SvO2 Collaborative Group. *N Engl J Med.* 1995;333(16):1025–1032.
5. Boyd O, Hayes M. The oxygen trail: the goal. *Br Med Bull.* 1999;55(1):125–139.
6. Wiedemann HP, et al. Comparison of two fluid-management strategies in acute lung injury. *N Engl J Med.* 2006;354(24):2564–2575.
7. Sandham JD, et al. A randomized, controlled trial of the use of pulmonary-artery catheters in high-risk surgical patients. *N Engl J Med.* 2003;348(1):5–14.
8. Marik PE, Baram M, Vahid B. Does central venous pressure predict fluid responsiveness? A systematic review of the literature and the tale of seven mares. *Chest.* 2008;134(1):172–178.

9. Shah MR, et al. Impact of the pulmonary artery catheter in critically ill patients: meta-analysis of randomized clinical trials. *JAMA.* 2005;294(13):1664–1670.
10. Michard F, Teboul JL. Predicting fluid responsiveness in ICU patients: a critical analysis of the evidence. *Chest.* 2002;121(6):2000–2008.
11. Rivers E, et al. Early goal-directed therapy in the treatment of severe sepsis and septic shock. *N Engl J Med.* 2001;345(19):1368–1377.
12. Pittman JA, Ping JS, Mark JB. Arterial and central venous pressure monitoring. *Int Anesthesiol Clin.* 2004;42(1):13–30.
13. McIntyre LA, et al. A survey of Canadian intensivists' resuscitation practices in early septic shock. *Crit Care.* 2007;11(4):R74.
14. Dellinger RP, et al. Surviving sepsis campaign: international guidelines for management of severe sepsis and septic shock: 2012. *Crit Care Med.* 2013;41(2):580–637.
15. Hughes RE, Magovern GJ. The relationship between right atrial pressure and blood volume. *AMA Arch Surg.* 1959;79(2):238–243.
16. Magder S. Bench-to-bedside review: an approach to hemodynamic monitoring—Guyton at the bedside. *Crit Care.* 2012;16(5):236.
17. Magder S. More respect for the CVP. *Intensive Care Med.* 1998;24(7):651–653.
18. Walley KR. Use of central venous oxygen saturation to guide therapy. *Am J Respir Crit Care Med.* 2011;184(5):514–520.
19. Teixeira C, et al. Central venous saturation is a predictor of reintubation in difficult-to-wean patients. *Crit Care Med.* 2010;38(2):491–496.
20. Troianos CA, et al. Guidelines for performing ultrasound guided vascular cannulation: recommendations of the American Society of Echocardiography and the Society of Cardiovascular Anesthesiologists. *J Am Soc Echocardiogr.* 2011;24(12):1291–1318.
21. Wigmore TJ, et al. Effect of the implementation of NICE guidelines for ultrasound guidance on the complication rates associated with central venous catheter placement in patients presenting for routine surgery in a tertiary referral centre. *Br J Anaesth.* 2007;99(5):662–665.
22. Pronovost P, et al. An intervention to decrease catheter-related bloodstream infections in the ICU. *N Engl J Med.* 2006;355(26):2725–2732.
23. Tousignant CP, Walsh F, Mazer CD. The use of transesophageal echocardiography for preload assessment in critically ill patients. *Anesth Analg.* 2000;90(2):351–355.
24. Sotomi Y, et al. Impact of pulmonary artery catheter on outcome in patients with acute heart failure syndromes with hypotension or receiving inotropes: from the ATTEND Registry. *Int J Cardiol.* 2014;171(2):165–172.
25. Friese RS, Shafi S, Gentilello LM. Pulmonary artery catheter use is associated with reduced mortality in severely injured patients: a National Trauma Data Bank analysis of 53,312 patients. *Crit Care Med.* 2006;34(6):1597–1601.
26. Chatterjee K. The Swan-Ganz catheters: past, present, and future. A viewpoint. *Circulation.* 2009;119(1):147–152.
27. Hamilton MA, Cecconi M, Rhodes A. A systematic review and meta-analysis on the use of preemptive hemodynamic intervention to improve postoperative outcomes in moderate and high-risk surgical patients. *Anesth Analg.* 2011;112(6):1392–1402.
28. Kumar A, et al. Pulmonary artery occlusion pressure and central venous pressure fail to predict ventricular filling volume, cardiac performance, or the response to volume infusion in normal subjects. *Crit Care Med.* 2004;32(3):691–699.
29. Wheeler AP, et al. Pulmonary-artery versus central venous catheter to guide treatment of acute lung injury. *N Engl J Med.* 2006;354(21):2213–2224.
30. Harvey S, et al. Assessment of the clinical effectiveness of pulmonary artery catheters in management of patients in intensive care (PAC-Man): a randomised controlled trial. *Lancet.* 2005;366(9484):472–477.
31. Richard C, et al. Early use of the pulmonary artery catheter and outcomes in patients with shock and acute respiratory distress syndrome: a randomized controlled trial. *JAMA.* 2003;290(20):2713–2720.

SECTION 3
Critical Care Ultrasonography

6

Principles of Critical Care Ultrasonography

Phillips Perera, Laleh Gharahbaghian, Thomas "Tom" Mailhot, Sarah R. Williams, and Diku P. Mandavia

BACKGROUND

Traditionally, clinicians have divided shock into four distinct categories. In each category, there are several subtypes (Table 6.1).

Rapidly determining the type of shock state in the critically ill patient and initiating the appropriate resuscitative measures can lower patient mortality.[1,2] With the decreased reliance on invasive monitoring tools for shock assessment, focused bedside ultrasonography, or ultrasound (US), has evolved to become a key means for evaluation. As US allows for the rapid assessment of both the anatomy and physiology of the shock patient, multiple resuscitation protocols have been created.

The major resuscitation US protocols in critically ill medical and trauma patients include ACES,[3] BEAT,[4] BLEEP,[5] Boyd ECHO,[6] EGLS,[7] Elmer/Noble Protocol,[8] FALLS,[9] FATE,[10] FAST,[11] extended FAST,[12] FEEL resuscitation,[13] FEER,[14] FREE,[15] POCUS (FAST and RELIABLE),[16] RUSH-HIMAP,[17] RUSH (pump/tank/pipes),[18–20] Trinity,[21] and UHP.[22] These algorithms have many similar components but differ in the sequence of exam performance (Table 6.2).

The RUSH protocol, named for Rapid Ultrasound in Shock, offers one easily remembered and comprehensive resuscitation protocol first to identify the shock state and then to monitor targeted therapy.

SOCIETY SUPPORT FOR FOCUSED ULTRASOUND IN CRITICALLY ILL PATIENTS

The use of focused US, including the individual components of the RUSH exam, has been supported by the major emergency medicine organizations. These organizations include the American College of Emergency Physicians (ACEP), the Society for Academic Emergency Medicine, and the Council of Emergency Medicine Residency Directors (CORD).[23–26] Critical care societies have endorsed both training in and the

TABLE 6.1 Categories of Shock States

1. Distributive: sepsis, anaphylaxis, neurogenic
2. Hypovolemic: hemorrhagic, severe volume loss
3. Obstructive: pulmonary embolism, cardiac tamponade, tension PTX
4. Cardiogenic: cardiac pump failure (mechanical, chronotropic), valvular disease

clinical use of bedside US. US has become an increasingly important diagnostic modality for this specialty.[27–30] In 2010, an important collaborative paper was published jointly between the American Society of Echocardiography (ASE) and ACEP that endorsed focused echocardiography (echo) for a defined set of emergent conditions.[31] These exam indications and goals include the core exam components of the RUSH exam (Tables 6.3 to 6.5).

In addition, other components of the RUSH exam, including the FAST, lung, aorta, and deep venous thrombosis (DVT) US exams, are supported by ACEP as core applications for use by the emergency physician.[23]

PERFORMANCE OF THE RUSH EXAMINATION: BASIC CONCEPTS

Ultrasound Probe Selection

A phased array probe at 2 to 3 MHz is used for the cardiac and thoracic components of the exam. A curvilinear probe at 2 to 3 MHz can be used for the abdominal components (FAST and aorta). A linear array probe at 8 to 12 MHz is used for the more superficial vascular components (DVT, internal jugular (IJ) veins).

Ultrasound Presets

The heart moves rapidly in reference to other body structures. For this reason, selection of a high frame rate on the US machine settings will allow for optimal imaging. This is done by selecting the cardiac preset, which is preloaded on most current US machines. The abdominal preset is best for the FAST and aorta exams. The vascular or venous preset is best for the DVT and IJ vein exams.

B-Mode Ultrasound

The RUSH US exam utilizes modalities that can image both critical anatomy and physiology.[32] This is done by first employing two-dimensional B-mode imaging. B-mode imaging projects the body as a continuum of color in the gray spectrum, termed echogenicity. Echogenicity results from the fact that the US probe first acts as a transducer that sends sound waves into the body. The sound waves then penetrate into the body, traveling a distance until they are bounced back to the probe. Different tissues will have varying resistance to the movement of sound. Higher-density (hyperechoic) structures will reflect an increasing amount of the sound back to the probe, resulting in a brighter appearance (i.e., a calcified heart valve, diaphragm). Fluid-filled structures (hypoechoic or anechoic) will allow for increased propagation of sound through the body, leading to a darker appearance (i.e., blood, body fluids) (Fig. 6.10).

TABLE 6.2 Ultrasound Resuscitation Protocols and Examination Components

Protocol:	ACES	BEAT	BLEEP	Boyd: ECHO	EGLS	Elmer/ Noble	FATE	FAST	FALLS	E-FAST	FEEL: RESUS	FEER	FREE	POCUS	RUSH: HIMAP	RUSH: Pump Tank Pines	Trinity	UHP
Cardiac	1	1	1	1	2	1	1	2	3	2	1	1	1	3	1	1	1	3
IVC	2	2	2	2	3	2			4					4	2	2		
FAST-A/P	4					3		1		1				1	3	3	3	1
Aorta	3													5	4	7	2	2
Lungs-PTX					1	4			2	4				2	5	6		
Lungs-effusion	5						2			3						4		
Lungs-edema					4	5			1					6		5		
DVT														7		8		
Ectopic pregnancy														8				

Numbers indicate order of exam sequence for each protocol.

TABLE 6.3 ACEP/ASE Consensus Guidelines for Ultrasound Exam—Clinical Indications

American College of Emergency Physicians and American Society of Echocardiography Consensus Guidelines on Focused Echocardiography
Recognized clinical indications for ultrasound examination:

1. Cardiac trauma: Focused assessment with sonography in trauma (FAST) exam
2. Cardiac arrest
3. Hypotension/shock
4. Dyspnea/shortness of breath
5. Chest pain

M-Mode Ultrasound

M-mode or "motion" mode illustrates an "ice pick" image of movement across a defined anatomical axis in relation to time. This generates a gray-scale illustration of movement over time that can be used to easily document motion on a static image (Figs. 6.11 and 6.12).

Doppler Ultrasound

Doppler US allows for the evaluation of motion within the body. The Doppler shift is defined as the movement of body structures relative to the position of the US probe. A positive Doppler shift results from structures (such as blood cells) moving toward the probe and a negative Doppler shift from movement away from the probe. The Doppler shift can be interpreted in several imaging modalities, two of which are discussed below.

Color-Flow Doppler

This modality demonstrates directionality of flow both toward and away from the probe and is often used in echo and vascular applications. Movement toward the probe results in a shorter frequency of sound. It is traditionally represented as red on the US image. Movement away from the probe results in a longer frequency of sound and is typically represented as blue. The scale that displays the color-flow Doppler setting should be set high (>70 cm/s) for echo to best capture the fast flow of the blood traveling through the heart. A lower scale can be used for the evaluation of the aorta and other vascular applications (DVT, IJ veins).

Pulsed-Wave Doppler

Pulsed-wave Doppler allows for assessment of flow velocity in a waveform that identifies the specific speed of blood flow over time. This modality is often used in advanced echo to define the velocity of blood flow through cardiac valves.

TABLE 6.4 ACEP/ASE Consensus Guidelines for Core Ultrasound Exam—Clinical Goals

American College of Emergency Physicians and American Society of Echocardiography Consensus Guidelines on Focused Echocardiography
Core echocardiography indications:

1. Assessment for pericardial effusions and pericardial tamponade
2. Assessment of global cardiac systolic function
3. Identification of marked right ventricular and left ventricular enlargement
4. Assessment of intravascular volume
5. Guidance of pericardiocentesis
6. Confirmation of transvenous pacemaker wire placement

TABLE 6.5	ACEP/ASE Consensus Guidelines for Advanced Ultrasound Exam—Exam Goals

American College of Emergency Physicians and American Society of Echocardiography Consensus Guidelines on Focused Echocardiography

The following conditions may be suspected on focused echocardiography:
(Additional imaging should be obtained if possible.)

1. Intracardiac masses
2. Cardiac chamber thrombus
3. Regional wall motion abnormalities
4. Endocarditis
5. Aortic dissection

Orientation of Indicator on Machine and Probe

Historically, there has been practice variation between different US exams with regard to the orientation of the indicator dot on the screen and the marker on the probe. The reason for this being that the first widespread applications used in emergency medicine practice, such as the FAST and OB/GYN exams, were oriented based on traditional radiology practice, with the US screen indicator dot oriented to the left. Emergency medicine-practiced echo was therefore configured similarly. This differs from traditional cardiology practice, where the indicator dot is oriented to the right on the US screen. Despite this difference, the standard practice has been to orient the US probe (at a 180-degree variance, depending on screen orientation), so that the cardiac images obtained with the screen indicator dot on either side display the heart in the same configuration. In this chapter, the probe orientation for all RUSH exam components, including the cardiac views, will be described with the screen indicator dot located to the left side. This convention avoids having to flip the screen marker dot between different exams.

THE RUSH EXAM: PROTOCOL COMPONENTS

The RUSH exam involves a 3-part bedside physiologic patient assessment, which is simplified as "the pump," "the tank," and "the pipes."

RUSH STEP 1: THE PUMP

Clinicians caring for the patient in shock should begin with assessment of "the function of the pump," which is a goal-directed echo exam looking specifically for:

1. The degree of left ventricular contractility
2. Detection of pericardial effusion and cardiac tamponade
3. The presence of right ventricular enlargement

In addition, other cardiac pathology may be detected on bedside echo. A confirmatory test should generally be ordered if more advanced pathology is seen on bedside US, in accordance with the joint ACEP/ASE guidelines. The information gained by this exam can also allow a better assessment of the need for an emergent cardiac procedure. If indicated, US can then allow more accurate guidance of both the pericardiocentesis procedure and placement of a transvenous pacemaker wire.

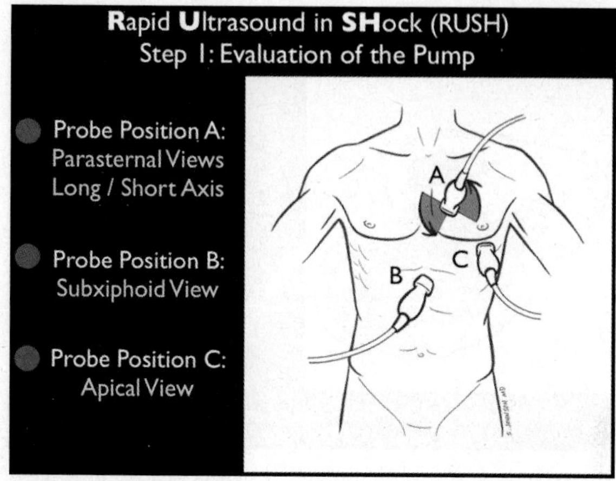

FIGURE 6.1 RUSH step 1, standard windows for cardiac ultrasound.

Performance of the Echocardiography Examination

There are three traditional windows used for performance of cardiac US. These are the parasternal (long- and short-axis views), subxiphoid, and apical views (Fig. 6.1).

The Parasternal Long-Axis View

Patient Position This view can be performed with the patient in a supine position. Turning the patient into a left lateral decubitus position will often improve this view by moving the heart away from the sternum and closer to the chest wall. This displaces the lung from the path of the sound waves.

Probe Position The probe should initially be positioned just lateral to the sternum at about the third intercostal space. The probe position can then be adjusted for optimal imaging by moving the probe up or down one additional intercostal space. The probe indicator should be oriented toward the patient's left elbow (Fig. 6.2).

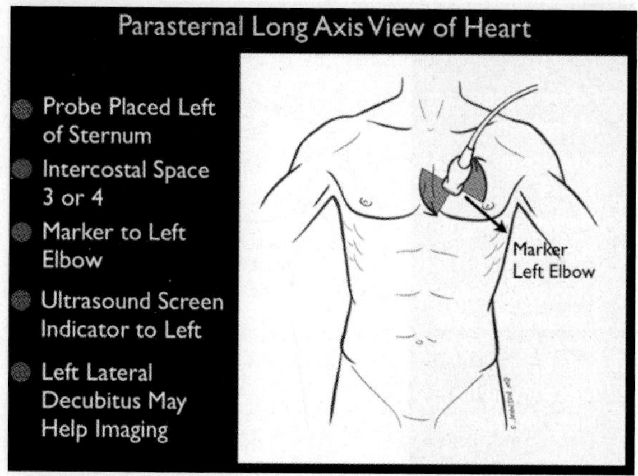

FIGURE 6.2 Parasternal long axis, probe position.

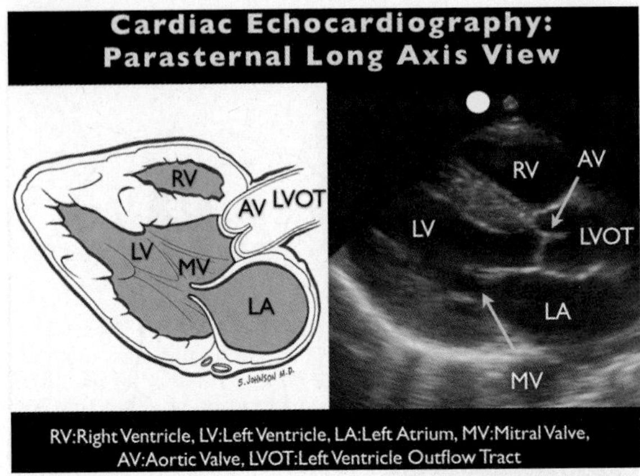

FIGURE 6.3 Parasternal long axis, anatomy.

Anatomic and Sonographic Correlation The parasternal long-axis view will visualize three cardiac chambers and the aorta. The right atrium is not seen from this view. Optimally, the parasternal long-axis images have both the aortic and mitral valves in the same view. The aortic valve and aortic root can be visualized as the area known as the left ventricular outflow tract (Fig. 6.3).

Parasternal Short-Axis View

Probe Position This view is obtained by first identifying the heart in the parasternal long-axis view and then rotating the probe 90 degrees clockwise. The probe indicator dot is aligned toward the patient's right hip (Fig. 6.4).

Anatomic and Sonographic Correlation The short-axis view visualizes the left and right ventricles in cross section and is known as the ring, or doughnut view, of the heart (Fig. 6.5). The traditional view is of the left ventricle at the level of the mitral

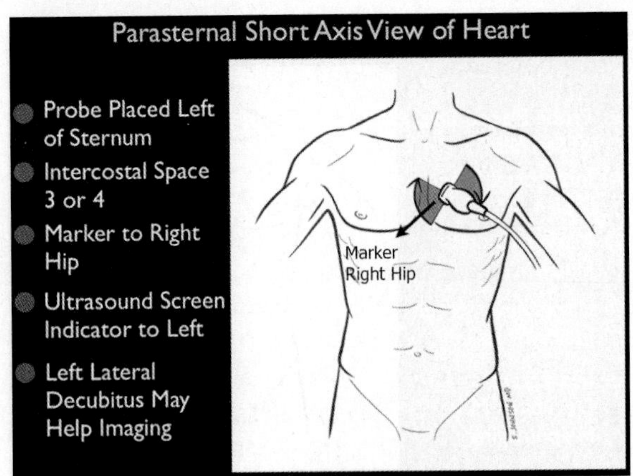

FIGURE 6.4 Parasternal long axis, probe position.

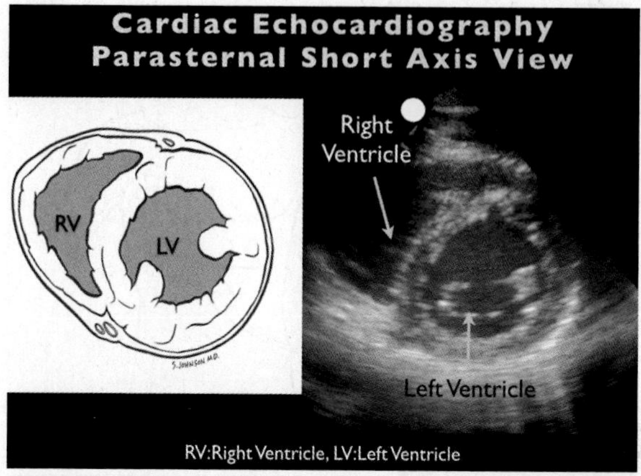

FIGURE 6.5 Parasternal short axis, anatomy.

valve, which appears as a "fish mouth" opening and closing during the cardiac cycle. Visualizing the heart as a cylinder with the US beam cutting tangentially through different levels, one can look as far inferiorly as the apex of the left ventricle and superiorly to the level of the aortic valve.

To best evaluate left ventricular contractility, the probe is moved inferiorly to the level of the papillary muscles, allowing confirmation of the assessment taken from the parasternal long-axis view. In addition, cardiologists routinely evaluate for segmental wall motion abnormalities on this view. If the probe is angled superiorly and medially from the above location, the aortic valve and right ventricular outflow tract will come into view. The aortic valve should appear as the "Mercedes-Benz sign" with a normal tricuspid configuration. A calcified bicuspid valve that may be prone to stenosis and pathology can be identified here.[33]

Subxiphoid Window

Patient Position This view is performed with the patient supine. Bending the patient's knees will relax the abdominal muscles and can improve imaging.

Probe Position Place the probe just inferior to the xiphoid tip of the sternum, with the indicator oriented toward the patient's right side (Fig. 6.6). Flattening and pushing down on the probe will aim the US beam up and under the sternum to best image the heart. If gas-filled stomach or intestine impedes imaging, one can move the probe to the patient's right while simultaneously aiming the probe toward the patient's left shoulder, to utilize more of the blood-filled liver as an acoustic window.

Anatomic and Sonographic Correlation The liver, which will be seen anteriorly, will act as the acoustic window to the heart from the subxiphoid view, allowing all four cardiac chambers to be seen. Because of the superior ability to visualize the right side of the heart from the subxiphoid window, it is often employed when close assessment of these chambers is needed (Fig. 6.7).

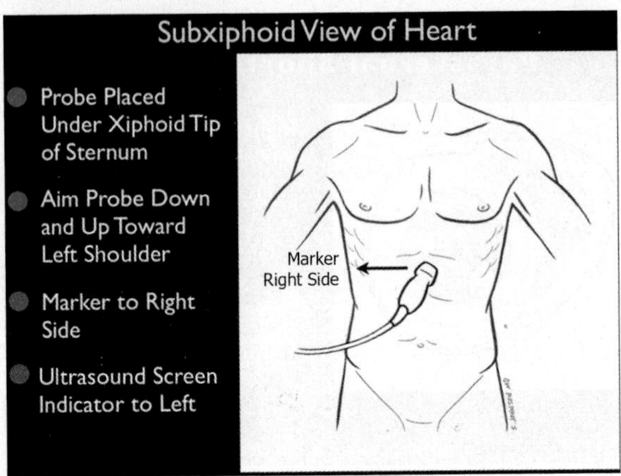

FIGURE 6.6 Subxiphoid view, probe position.

Apical Window

Patient Position Roll the patient into the left lateral decubitus position to bring the heart closer to the lateral chest wall, and obtain optimal imaging from this view.

Probe Position Palpate the point of maximal impulse on the lateral chest wall and place the transducer at this point. This is generally just below the nipple line in men and under the breast in women. For the apical view, the probe marker will be oriented toward the patient's right elbow (Fig. 6.8).

Anatomic and Sonographic Correlation The apical window allows for detailed assessment of the sizes and movements of all four cardiac chambers in relation to one another (Fig. 6.9). The apical four-chamber view is the first traditional view from this window.

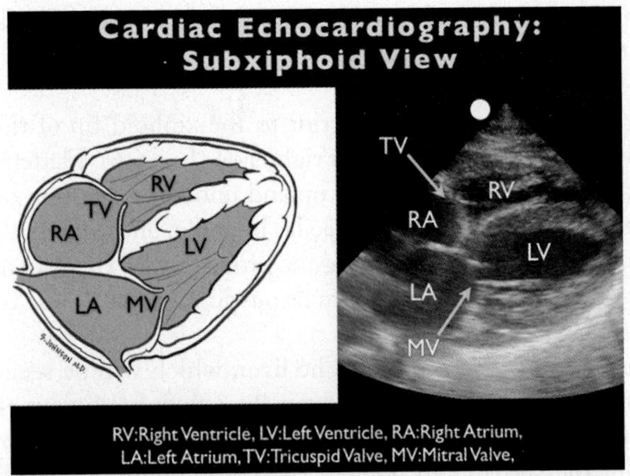

FIGURE 6.7 Subxiphoid view, anatomy.

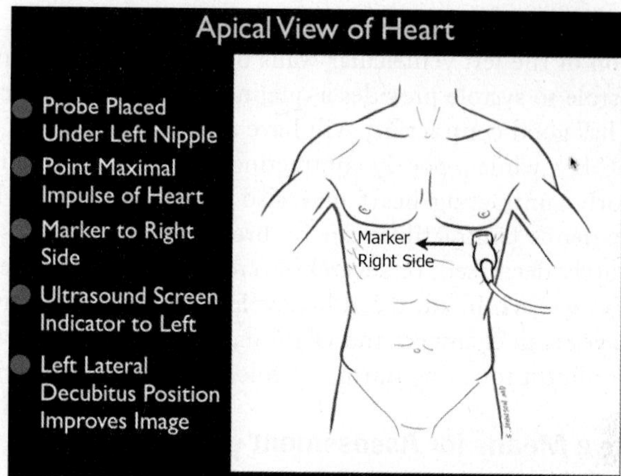

FIGURE 6.8 Apical view, probe position.

The optimal views from this position have both the mitral and tricuspid valves in the image. From this position, the probe can then be angled more superiorly to obtain the apical 5-chamber view. The "5th chamber" will be the aortic valve and aortic outflow tract in the middle of the image.

RUSH STEP 1a: ASSESSMENT OF CARDIAC CONTRACTILITY

Background

A relatively high percentage of critical patients may have compromised cardiac function contributing to their shock state, which may be diagnosed with bedside echo.[34] Published studies have demonstrated that emergency physicians with focused training can accurately evaluate left ventricular contractility.[35]

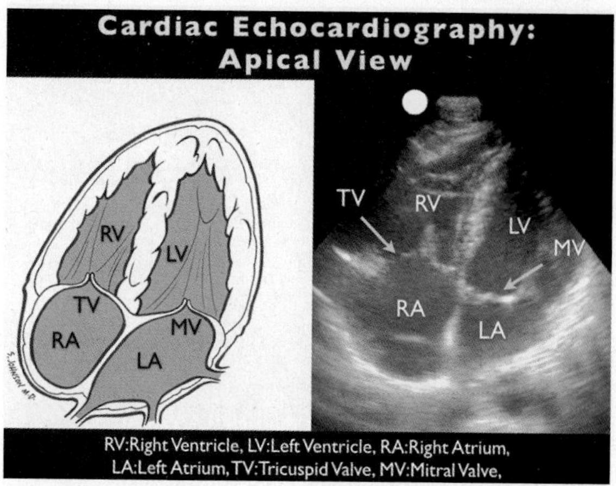

FIGURE 6.9 Apical view, anatomy.

Qualitative Evaluation of Left Ventricular Contractility

Evaluating motion of the left ventricular walls by a visual estimation of the volume change from diastole to systole provides a qualitative assessment of contractility.[34–36] A ventricle that has good contractility will have a large-volume change between the two cycles (Fig. 6.10), while a poorly contracting heart will have a small percentage change. The poorly contracting heart may also be dilated in size. Based on these assessments, a patient's contractility can be broadly categorized as being normal, mildly to moderately decreased, or severely decreased. A fourth category, known as hyperdynamic, can be seen in advanced hypovolemia or in distributive shock states. The heart will have small chambers and vigorous, hyperkinetic contractions with the endocardial walls almost touching during systole.

Semiquantitative Means for Assessment of Contractility

Fractional Shortening

M-mode can be used to graphically depict the movements of the left ventricular walls through the cardiac cycle. In the parasternal long-axis view, the M-mode cursor is placed across the left ventricle beyond the tips of the mitral valve leaflets at about the midventricle area. The resulting tracing allows a two-dimensional length-based measurement of the chamber diameters over time. Fractional shortening is calculated according to the following formula:

$$(\text{EDD} - \text{ESD}) / \text{EDD} \times 100$$

where ESD is the end-systolic diameter, measured at the smallest dimension between the ventricular walls, and EDD is the end-diastolic diameter, where the distance is greatest (Fig. 6.11).

In general, fractional shortening above 35% to 40% correlates to a normal ejection fraction.[37] Compared to the comprehensive volumetric assessment required for measuring ejection fraction, fractional shortening is a semiquantitative method for determining systolic function that is relatively fast and easy to perform.[38]

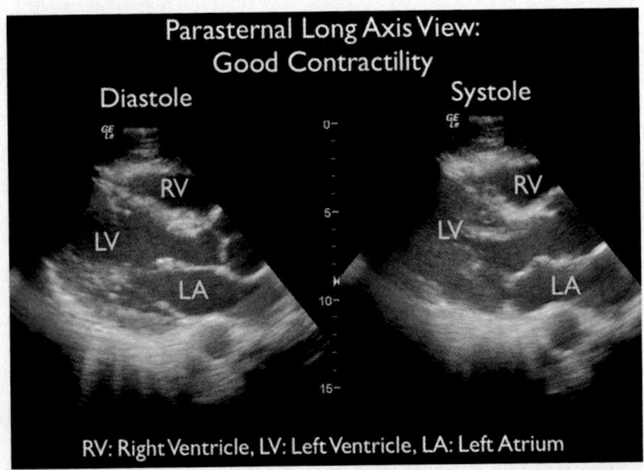

FIGURE 6.10 Left ventricle, good contractility.

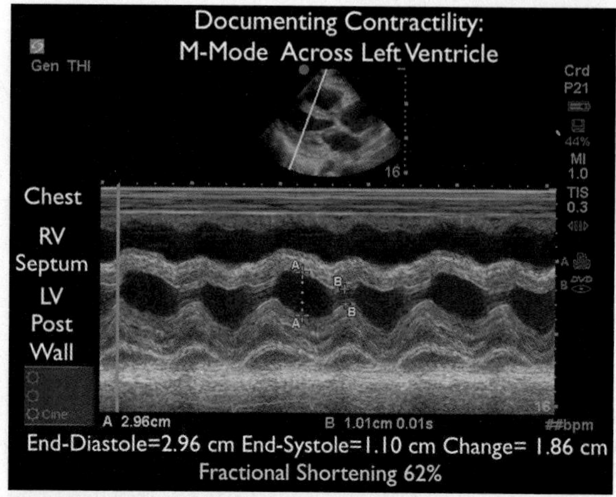

FIGURE 6.11 M-mode, good contractility.

E-Point Septal Separation

Motion of the anterior leaflet of the mitral valve in the parasternal long-axis view can also be used to assess left ventricular contractility. In the early diastolic phase of a normal contractile cycle, the anterior mitral leaflet can be observed to fully open to a position close to the septal wall. This is with the caveat that mitral valve abnormalities (stenosis, regurgitation), aortic regurgitation, and extreme left ventricle hypertrophy are not present. Early diastolic opening of the mitral valve is represented on M-mode US as the E-point. The distance measured between the E-point, representing the position of the fully open mitral valve, and the septum is known as the E-point septal separation or EPSS.[39] To measure the EPSS, the M-mode cursor is placed over the tip of the anterior mitral valve leaflet. In a normal contractile state, the EPSS will be <7 mm, as the mitral valve will almost approximate the septum during early diastolic filling.[39–41] As left ventricular contractility decreases, diastolic flow through the valve will diminish. This results in decreased mitral valve opening to a position relatively farther from the septum and a corresponding increase in the EPSS (Fig. 6.12). Further research is ongoing to determine the accuracy of correlation between EPSS and fractional shortening.[42]

RUSH STEP 1b: DIAGNOSIS OF PERICARDIAL EFFUSION AND CARDIAC TAMPONADE

Pathophysiology

Published studies have documented that pericardial effusions may be found relatively commonly in critical patients presenting with acute shortness of breath, respiratory failure, shock, and cardiac arrest.[43,44] Fortunately, the literature also indicates that emergency physicians with focused echo training can accurately identify effusions.[45] Pericardial effusions may result in hemodynamic instability as the pressure in the pericardial sac acutely increases, resulting in reduced cardiac filling.[46] Acute pericardial effusions (as

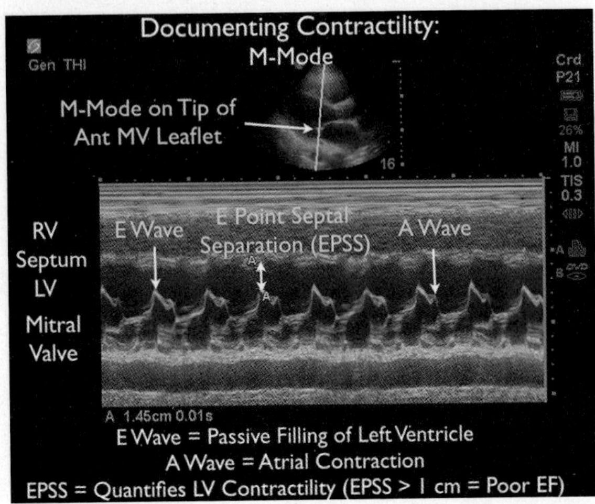

FIGURE 6.12 Mitral valve, E-point septal separation.

small as 50 cc) may result in tamponade. This pathology may quickly compromise the trauma patient. Conversely, in chronic conditions, the pericardium may slowly stretch to accommodate large effusions over time without tamponade.[47]

Sonographic Appearance of Pericardial Effusions

Pericardial effusions are generally recognized by a dark, or anechoic, appearance. However, inflammatory or infectious conditions may result in effusions with a brighter, or more echogenic, appearance. In addition, traumatic pericardial effusions will take on a more echogenic appearance over time as blood clots.

Grading Scale for the Size of Pericardial Effusions

One scale for describing the size of the effusion is shown below (Table 6.6).[48]

Specific Echocardiographic Windows for Evaluating Pericardial Effusions

Parasternal Long-Axis View

Size and Location of Effusions Smaller effusions will first layer posteriorly behind the heart. As effusions grow in size, they will surround the heart in a circumferential manner, moving into the anterior pericardial space.[47] Most effusions are free flowing in the pericardial sac. However, occasionally loculated effusions may occur. These typically occur in postoperative cardiac surgery patients and in inflammatory conditions.[49]

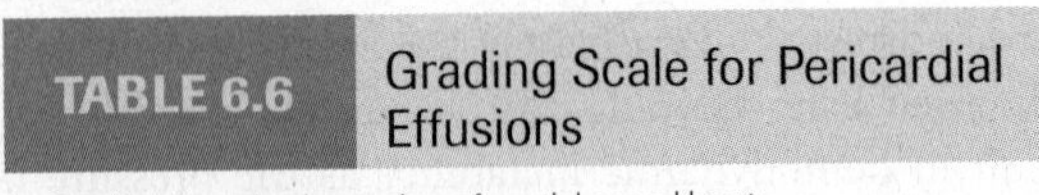

TABLE 6.6 Grading Scale for Pericardial Effusions

A. **Small:** <1 cm depth, noncircumferential around heart
B. **Moderate:** <1 cm depth, circumferential around heart
C. **Large:** >1 cm depth, circumferential around the heart

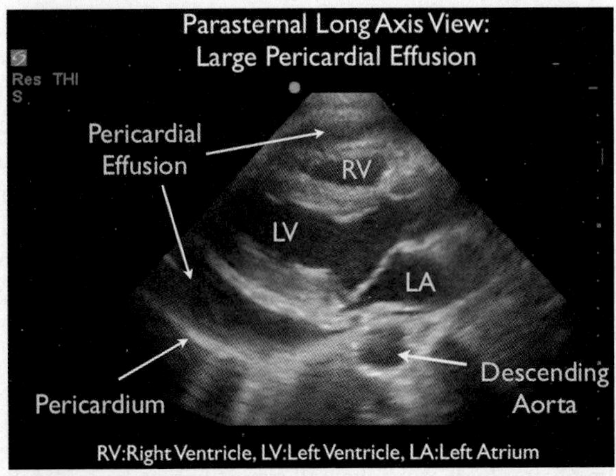

FIGURE 6.13 Pericardial fluid.

Differentiation of Pleural from Pericardial Fluid The critical landmarks for detection of a pericardial effusion are the descending aorta and the posterior pericardial reflection. The descending aorta will appear as a circle directly behind the left atrium, posterior to the mitral valve (Fig. 6.13). The posterior pericardial reflection will be identified as a hyperechoic structure immediately anterior to the descending aorta. First, select the appropriate depth of the US image, so that the descending aorta and pericardial reflection are adequately visualized posteriorly on the screen. Pericardial effusions will be located anterior to the descending aorta and above the posterior pericardial reflection (Fig. 6.13). In contrast, pleural effusions will be located posterior to the descending aorta and below the posterior pericardial reflection (Fig. 6.14). To further confirm the presence of a left pleural effusion, the probe can be moved to a lateral position on the chest wall as for the FAST views and aimed above the diaphragm to visualize the lower thoracic cavity (Fig. 6.17).

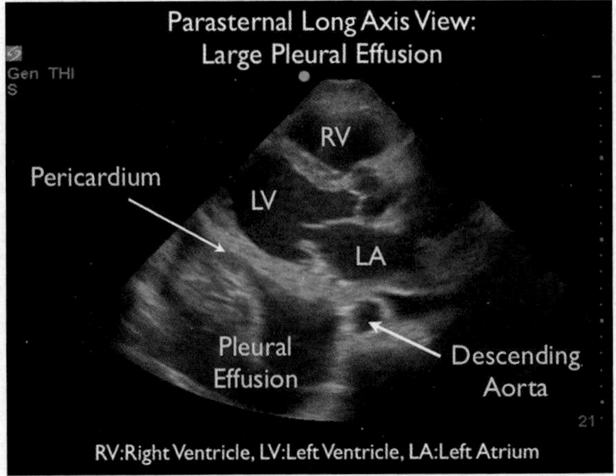

FIGURE 6.14 Pleural fluid.

Pericardial Fat Pad A pericardial, or epicardial, fat pad may at times be confused with a pericardial effusion. The typical location for this structure is in the area just deep to the near-field pericardial reflection and anterior to the heart. The fat pad often has a classic appearance, with an interspersed speckling of bright, or hyperechoic, regions. From the parasternal views, an isolated anterior "echo-dense" structure is more suggestive of a fat pad and not of an effusion. For an effusion to be visualized anteriorly on the parasternal views, a circumferential effusion would usually be present (with the exception of the presence of a rarer loculated pericardial effusion). From the subxiphoid view, the fat pad would be seen closer to the probe, located just beneath the near-field pericardial reflection and anterior to the heart.

Subxiphoid View

Size and Location of Effusions Because the subxiphoid window is taken from a position inferior to the heart, small effusions will typically first layer out with gravity along the near-field pericardial reflection. This is especially noted in cases where the patient has been in an upright position. Larger effusions will spread to surround the heart circumferentially.

Differentiation of Pericardial Effusion from Ascites Ascites may be confused with a pericardial effusion. To help differentiate between the two, ascites will be seen nearer to the probe, anterior to the near-field pericardial reflection, outside the pericardial sac, and surrounding the liver within the abdominal cavity. In contrast, a pericardial effusion is located posterior to the near-field pericardium, adjacent to the heart, and within the pericardial sac.

Echocardiographic Diagnosis of Cardiac Tamponade

Ultrasound Findings

As pericardial effusions accumulate, the pressure in the pericardial sac rises and will first compromise the lower pressure circuit of the right heart. This is best recognized sonographically as an inability of these chambers to fully expand during the relaxation phase of the cardiac cycle. Cardiac tamponade is thus classically defined on US as diastolic collapse of either the right atrium or the right ventricle. While both right heart chambers should be evaluated, diastolic collapse of the right ventricle is a more specific finding. This is because as tamponade progresses, the right atrium may take on an appearance of a "furiously contracting chamber" with hyperdynamic contractions. This can at times make differentiation of atrial systolic contraction from diastolic collapse more difficult.

Diastolic collapse of the right ventricle in tamponade is best understood as a spectrum of US findings, from a subtle serpentine deflection of the wall to complete chamber compression (Fig. 6.15).[50] One important pitfall to this general diagnostic strategy is seen in the patient with pulmonary hypertension, where diastolic collapse of the right heart may occur late in the disease process.

Advanced Strategies in the Identification of Tamponade

There are several more advanced strategies used to document diastolic compression of the right heart in tamponade.[51] The first is to attach an EKG monitoring lead to the US machine to allow for simultaneous display of both the US and electrical phases. Systole

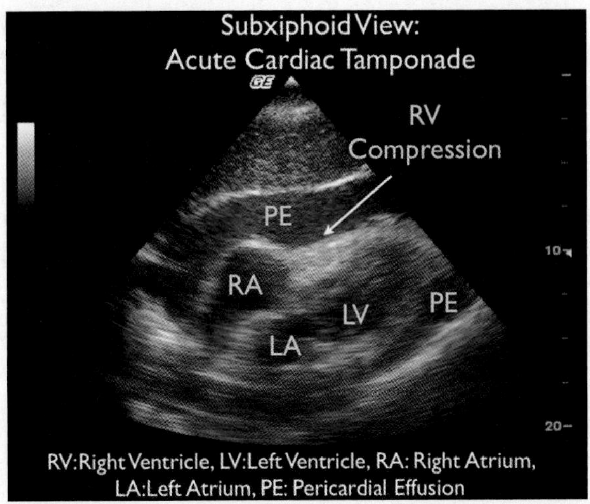

FIGURE 6.15 Cardiac tamponade, right ventricular collapse. PE, pericardial effusion.

will be identified immediately following the QRS, and diastole will follow later in the electrical cycle, just prior to the next P–QRS complex. Slowing the video down and scrolling through the echo with simultaneous attention to both the EKG phase and the US will allow discrimination of systolic from diastolic movements of the right atrium and ventricle. In tamponade, right atrial diastolic collapse may be noted first, occurring directly after atrial systole and early after the QRS complex. Right ventricular diastolic collapse will be noted later as tamponade progresses. This will be seen on EKG later in the electrical cycle and just before the following P–QRS complex.

Evaluation of the inferior vena cava (IVC) may also be performed to confirm tamponade physiology. A dilated, or plethoric, IVC without respiratory collapse implies tamponade.[52] A more advanced exam using Doppler US allows for one of the most sensitive tests to evaluate for tamponade. From the apical 4-chamber view, color-flow Doppler can first be used to identify the flow of blood through the tricuspid and mitral valves. Pulsed-wave Doppler is then used to identify the augmented respiratory variation in the flow velocities across these valves, which is noted in tamponade. In inspiration, an increase in blood flow through the tricuspid valve and a decrease in flow through the mitral valve will be seen. Flow variations >25% across the tricuspid valve and >15% across the mitral valve are considered abnormal.[53]

Ultrasound Guidance of Pericardiocentesis

In cases of cardiac tamponade and shock, an emergent pericardiocentesis is generally indicated. Emergency physicians have classically been taught the subxiphoid approach for pericardiocentesis. However, a large review from the Mayo Clinic included 1,127 pericardiocentesis procedures and found that the optimal position for placement of the needle was the apical position in 80% of patients.[54] The subxiphoid approach was only chosen in 20% of these procedures, due to the interposition of the liver. US allows for accurate guidance of the pericardiocentesis needle and guidewire into the pericardial sac. In addition, agitated saline can be used as a form of US contrast to confirm proper needle placement in the pericardial space.[55,56]

RUSH STEP 1c: ECHOCARDIOGRAPHY IN PULMONARY EMBOLUS AND EVALUATION FOR RIGHT VENTRICULAR ENLARGEMENT

Background

While a CT scan is typically thought of as the current diagnostic standard for pulmonary embolism, focused echo can identify one of the more serious complications of this disease, right ventricular strain. This finding correlates with a poorer prognosis and the need for more immediate treatment.[57,58] Right ventricular enlargement on focused echo may also suggest this pathology in the undifferentiated patient presenting in shock, potentially leading to more timely diagnosis and treatment.

Echocardiography Literature for Pulmonary Embolus

Studies have previously evaluated the use of echo for the diagnosis of pulmonary embolus, specifically looking for the presence of right ventricular enlargement due to acute cardiac strain. The documented sensitivity of this test in all patients with pulmonary embolus is only moderate. Therefore, echo cannot be used to rule out a pulmonary embolus, especially in those patients who are hemodynamically stable. However, identification of right ventricular enlargement can be of increased diagnostic utility in cases of hypotension with suspected thromboembolic disease, where it will have a higher specificity and positive predictive value.[59–64]

The traditional treatment of patients with a pulmonary embolus has been with anticoagulation. However, more recent guidelines recommend the combined use of anticoagulants and fibrinolytics in cases of severe pulmonary embolism.[65–68] This is defined as the presence of acute right heart strain and clinical signs and symptoms of hypotension, severe shortness of breath, or altered mental status.

Echocardiographic Findings of Hemodynamically Significant Pulmonary Embolism

Parasternal Views

The relative sizes of the left and right ventricles can be evaluated from this window. A normal ratio of the right to the left ventricle is defined as 0.6:1 with a greater than 1:1 ratio indicating right ventricular dilatation.[69,70] A higher relative ratio, combined with deflection of the interventricular septum from right to left, indicates the right ventricular strain that may be seen in a severe pulmonary embolus. In acute right ventricular strain, the chamber wall will typically be thin, due to the lack of time for compensatory hypertrophy. Conversely, in cases of chronic pulmonary strain seen in conditions of long-standing pulmonary artery hypertension, the right ventricle will compensate with hypertrophy. This will result in a thicker wall, typically measuring >5 mm.[48,71] These findings can allow the clinician to further differentiate the US findings of acute from chronic right heart enlargement. On the parasternal short-axis view, the interventricular septum may be seen to bow from right to left with high right-side pressures. This can result in a finding known as the left ventricular "D-shaped cup," or "D-sign," as the septum is pushed down and away from the right ventricle (Fig. 6.16).[72]

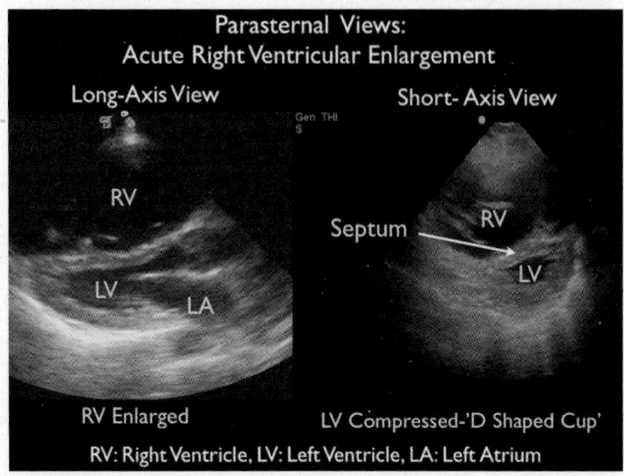

FIGURE 6.16 Parasternal views, RV strain.

Subxiphoid and Apical Views

The subxiphoid view may also be used in the assessment of right ventricular strain: however, one must take care to aim the probe to capture the widest chamber size, avoiding underestimation of dimensions by imaging the right ventricle off-axis. The apical window is another excellent view for visualization of both right ventricular enlargement and septal bowing. In addition to findings of right ventricular strain, occasionally clot may be visualized within the heart.[73]

RUSH STEP 1 - OTHER USES: THE PATIENT WITH HEART BLOCK AS CAUSE FOR SHOCK: ULTRASOUND GUIDANCE OF TRANSVENOUS PACEMAKER PLACEMENT

In cases of cardiogenic shock due to pump failure from bradycardia, immediate transvenous pacemaker placement may be indicated in cases unresponsive to medications. US guidance of transvenous pacemaker placement can be performed from either the subxiphoid or apical window. The pacing wire should be observed to pass from the right atrium through the tricuspid valve and into the right ventricle. Optimally, the wire can be observed to float up against the electrically active right ventricular septum and mechanical capture then confirmed with US.

RUSH STEP 2: THE TANK

The second part of the RUSH protocol focuses on the determination of the effective intravascular volume status, referred to as "the tank" (Fig. 6.17). This information, in conjunction with evaluation of cardiac status, provides a key guide to fluid management in the critical patient. The evaluation of "the tank" is composed of three components: (1) "Tank Fullness", (2) "Tank Leakiness", and (3) "Tank Compromise."

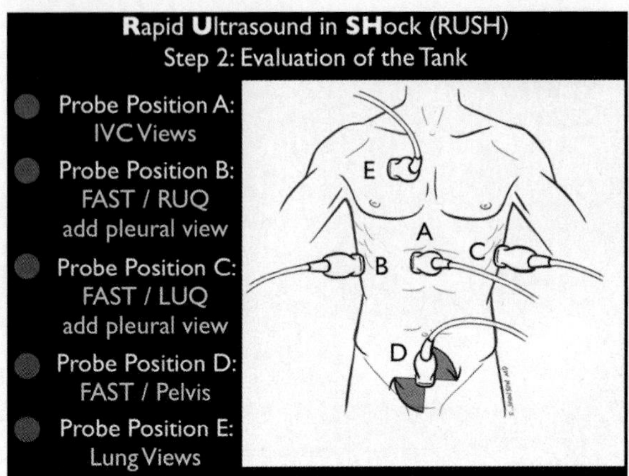

FIGURE 6.17 RUSH step 2, evaluation of the "tank."

1) "Fullness of the Tank": Inferior Vena Cava and Internal Jugular (IJ) Veins

Following evaluation of the heart and quantification of contractility, assessment of the central venous pressure (CVP) or "fullness of the tank" should be performed. The IVC will typically be the primary structure evaluated to give this information (Fig. 6.17, position A). However, if the IVC cannot be seen well in a given patient, evaluation of the IJ veins can provide an alternate means for volume assessment.

Ultrasound Evaluation of the Inferior Vena Cava

Patient Position The IVC is best evaluated with patient in the supine position.

Probe Position From the subxiphoid window, there are several variant views that are utilized in the imaging of the IVC. First, identify the right atrium in the four-chamber subxiphoid view and angle the probe inferiorly toward the spine to visualize the IVC as it joins this chamber. The IVC can then be followed inferiorly as it runs from the right atrium through the liver to the confluence with the three hepatic veins. Next, rotate the probe from the subxiphoid four-chamber view to the subxiphoid two-chamber view, by orienting the probe with the indicator oriented superiorly toward the ceiling. This allows for imaging of the right ventricle above the left ventricle, with the aorta typically seen in a long-axis orientation inferior to the heart. Moving the probe toward the patient's right side will then bring the IVC into view.

Anatomic and Sonographic Correlation Current recommendations for the measurement of the IVC are at the point just inferior to the confluence with the hepatic veins. This is approximately 2 cm from the junction of the right atrium and the IVC.[74] Examining the IVC first as a circular structure in a short-axis plane is recommended. This can avoid slicing the US beam to the side of IVC and resulting in a falsely low measurement, in a pitfall known as the cylinder tangent effect. The probe can then be rotated to image the IVC in a longitudinal plane. This will allow confirmation of the accuracy of vessel measurements.

Differentiation of IVC from Aorta The aorta and the IVC may be confused with one another. The aorta can be identified as a thicker-walled and pulsatile structure, with more prominent branch vessels and a location to the patient's left side. In contrast, the IVC has thinner walls, is often compressible with the probe, can be seen to move through the liver, and is located to the patient's right side. While the IVC may have pulsations due to its proximity to the aorta, Doppler US will allow differentiation of arterial pulsations from the phasic movement of IVC blood with respirations.

Ultrasound Evaluation of the IVC for Volume Status A noninvasive estimation of the patient's intravascular volume can be determined by examining both the relative size and the respiratory dynamics of the IVC. The assessment of the IVC should follow the determination of cardiac contractility, allowing the clinician to evaluate both parameters together to more accurately gauge the volume status. As the patient breathes, the IVC will have a normal pattern of inspiratory collapse. This respiratory variation can be further accentuated by having the patient sniff, or inspire forcefully. M-mode US, positioned in both the short- and long-axis planes of the IVC, can graphically document these dynamic respiratory changes in vessel size. Previous studies have demonstrated a positive correlation between the size and respiratory change of the IVC taken simultaneously with the patient's measured CVP, in an examination termed sonospirometry (Figs. 6.18 and 6.19).[75–83] Changes in the size and respiratory variation of the IVC and/or IJ veins can then be followed over time as fluid is given to the patient in shock, to assess for a therapeutic response. Clinical decisions to continue fluid loading, or to start vasopressor agents, can be assisted through knowledge of the "fullness of the tank."

Newer published guidelines by the ASE support this general use of the evaluation of IVC size and respiratory change in assessment of CVP, but suggest more specific ranges for the pressure measurements (Table 6.7).[84]

In intubated patients, the respiratory dynamics of the IVC will be reversed. In these patients, the IVC becomes less compliant and more distended in both respiratory phases. However, important physiologic data can still be obtained in these patients, as fluid

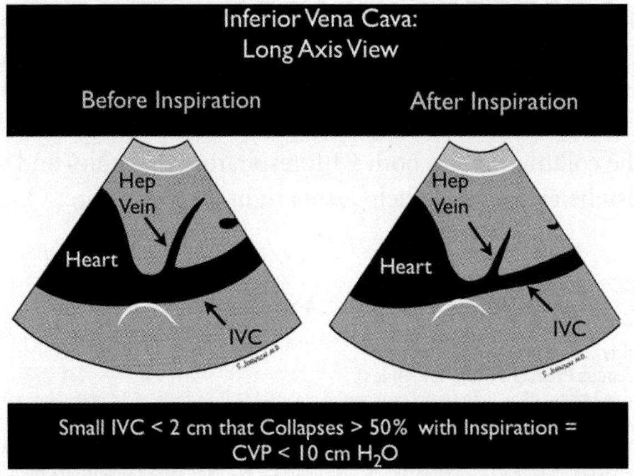

FIGURE 6.18 IVC evaluation, low CVP.

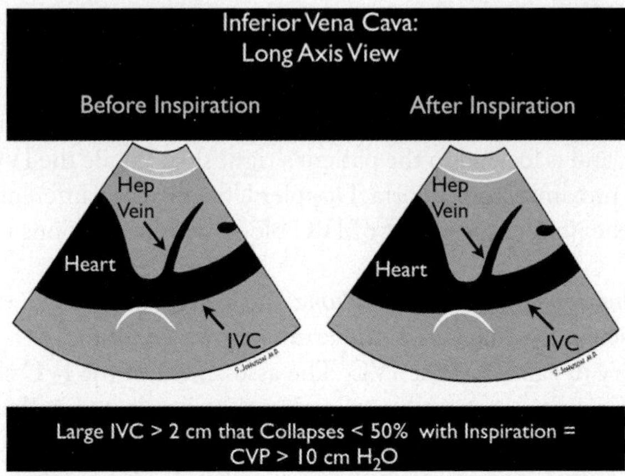

FIGURE 6.19 IVC evaluation, high CVP.

responsiveness has been correlated with an increase in IVC diameter over time.[85] This highlights the importance of serial examinations of the IVC in the shock patient to better assess response to therapy. In the nonintubated patient, the size and percentage respiratory collapse of the IVC can be used to assess for changes in CVP with fluid loading. In the intubated patient, the absolute size of the IVC may be a better indicator of CVP and successful fluid loading will be seen as a progressively larger IVC noted on serial US exams.

Evaluation of the Internal Jugular Vein

The IJ veins may be evaluated as an alternative means of volume assessment. This is helpful in the patient in whom a gas-filled stomach or intestine prohibits imaging of the IVC. The patient should be positioned with the head of the bed elevated to 30 degrees. A high-frequency linear array probe is recommended for this exam. For volume assessment, one should examine both the relative fullness and the height of the vessel column in the neck. Both short- and long-axis views of the vein can be utilized (Figs. 6.20 and 6.21). The US measurement for jugular venous distention has been performed by identifying the absolute vertical height of the column of blood in the IJ vein at end expiration as measured above the sternal angle. To this measurement is added 5 cm, which is the distance from the right atrium to the sternal notch.

Jugular venous distention measured >8 cm has been predictive of elevated CVP.[86,87] The change in the column height, both with respiratory dynamics and with the Valsalva maneuver, can also be evaluated to help assess right atrial pressure. One study looked at

TABLE 6.7 IVC Correlation to CVP, ASE Guidelines

IVC Size and Collapsibility
Correlation to Central Venous Pressure (ASE Guidelines):

A. IVC diameter < 2.1 cm, collapses >50% with sniff: Correlates to a normal CVP pressure of 3 mm Hg (range 0–5 mm Hg) (While a normal measurement in the healthy patient, this would be considered low in the critically ill patient)
B. IVC diameter > 2.1 cm, collapses <50% with sniff: Correlates to a high CVP pressure of 15 mm Hg (range 10–20 mm Hg)
C. Scenarios in which the IVC diameter and collapse do not fit these indices: An intermediate value of 8 mm Hg (range 5–10 mm) may be used

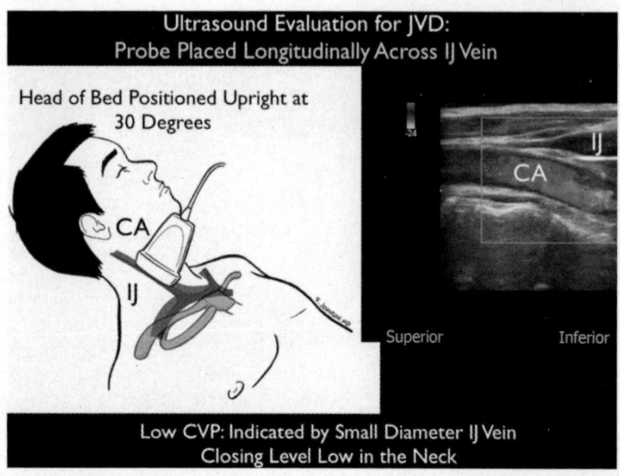

FIGURE 6.20 Internal jugular vein, low CVP. CA, carotid artery.

the percentage change in the cross-sectional area of the vein during Valsalva and found a decreased measurement to be present with elevated right atrial pressure, suggesting a more plethoric and less compliant vein.[86–88] Another study looked at the maximal IJ vein diameters (IJV max diam) in both expiration and inspiration to measure a collapsibility index.[89]

This was defined as follows:

IJV max diam (expiration) – IJV max diam (inspiration) / IJV max diam (expiration)

A collapsibility index >39% correlated best with hypovolemia, with a sensitivity of 87.5% and specificity of 100%.

2) "Leakiness of the Tank": FAST and Thoracic Ultrasound

Once a patient's intravascular volume status has been determined, the next step is to assess for "leakiness of the tank." This refers to hemodynamic compromise due to a loss of fluid from the core vascular circuit. This assessment is initiated with the Extended Focused Assessment

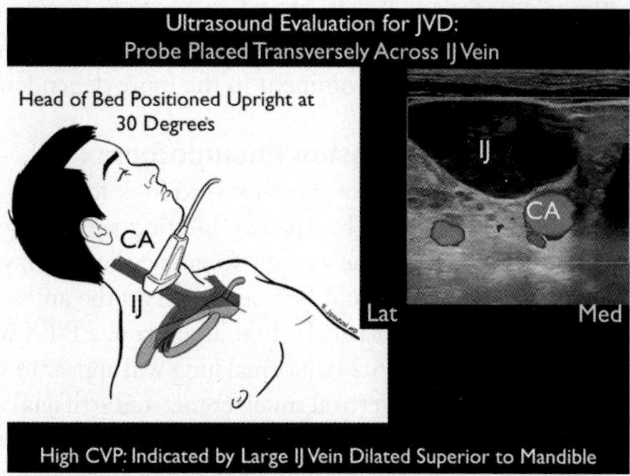

FIGURE 6.21 Internal jugular vein, high CVP.

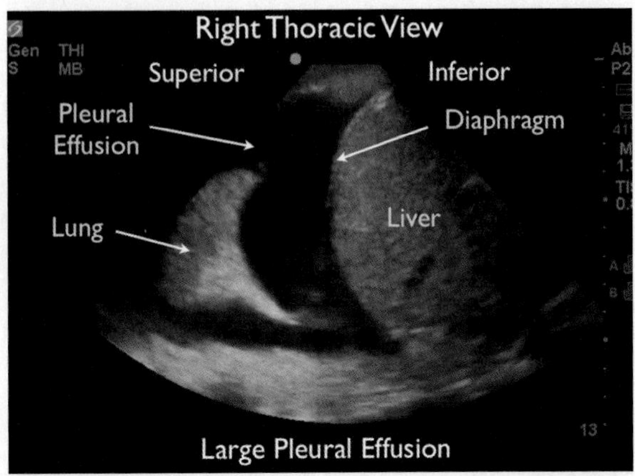

FIGURE 6.22 Pleural effusion.

with Sonography for Trauma exam.[11,12] The traditional FAST exam will identify fluid collections in the abdominal and pelvic cavities (Fig. 6.17, positions B, C, D). The extended FAST exam includes evaluation of the thoracic cavity for fluid and for pneumothorax (PTX).

A thoracic fluid collection, either a pleural effusion or hemothorax depending on the clinical scenario, can be identified by aiming the probe above the diaphragm from the standard right and left upper quadrant views (Fig. 6.22). Traumatic conditions resulting in hemothorax or hemoperitoneum cause hypovolemic shock due to a "hole in the tank." This in combination with a hyperdynamic heart and flat IVC correlates with hypovolemic shock. In a female patient of childbearing age presenting in shock, this may reflect a ruptured ectopic pregnancy, resulting in physiology effectively similar to a traumatic condition. Conversely, medical conditions causing pleural effusions and ascites often occur due to "tank overload." This occurs when there is failure of the heart, kidneys, or liver. Finally, lung US can identify pulmonary edema, a sign often indicative of both "tank overload" and "tank leakiness," with fluid accumulation in the lung parenchyma.[90–92] This exam is performed by placing the phased array probe over the thorax to look for US B-lines, or "lung rockets" (Fig. 6.23). Optimally, the clinician should inspect both anterior (Fig. 6.17, position E) and lateral areas of the thorax to increase exam sensitivity, as edema in the supine patient may be increasingly prominent in the more dependent lateral areas.[93]

3) "Compromise of the Tank": Tension Pneumothorax

The third component of the assessment of the tank is to look for "tank compromise." A tension PTX may result in hypotension by severely limiting venous return to the heart within the superior and inferior venae cavae. A high-frequency linear array probe is optimal for use in the PTX exam. The probe should first be placed on the anterior chest at about the second intercostal space in the midclavicular line, as air from a PTX will first collect in this location in the supine patient (Fig. 6.24). Normal lung will appear to slide horizontally back and forth as the patient breathes. Vertical small "comet-tail artifacts" will also be noted to extend a short distance posteriorly off the pleura. These findings result from the US appearance of the normally apposed pleural line, made up of the combined inner visceral pleura of the lung and the outer parietal pleural layer of the thoracic cavity (Fig. 6.25).

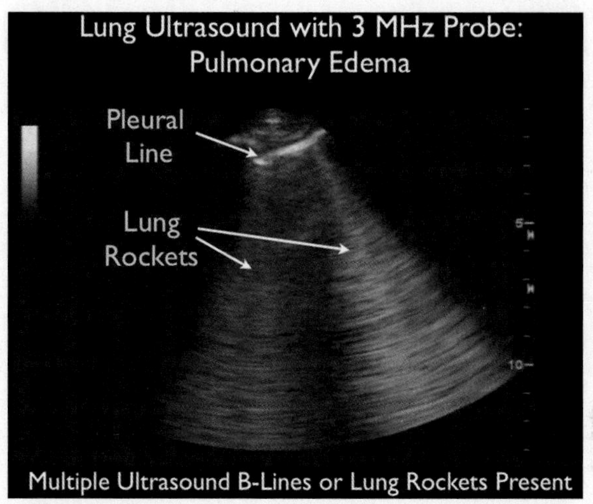

FIGURE 6.23 Ultrasound B-lines, lung rockets.

In a PTX, air will collect within the thoracic cavity and will split the normally touching parietal and visceral layers. On US, a single line that represents the solitary parietal pleura will be seen, as the visceral pleura will be obscured by air. This single line will not slide back and forth with respirations, and vertical comet tails will not be seen.[94–97]

In an incomplete PTX, a portion of the lung may still be inflated and will touch up against the outer parietal pleura. The lead point, or transition point, is the area where the lung in an incomplete PTX makes contact with the outer pleural layer. This may be seen on US as an area where lung sliding is seen on one side of the image, while no sliding is seen on the other. The transition point of lung sliding may be observed to move across the US field as the patient breathes. To find the transition point, the probe is moved progressively more laterally on the chest wall from the midclavicular line toward the midaxillary line.

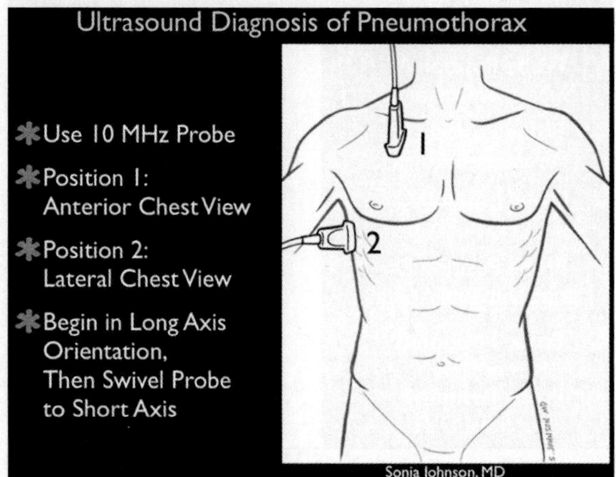

FIGURE 6.24 Probe position, pneumothorax exam.

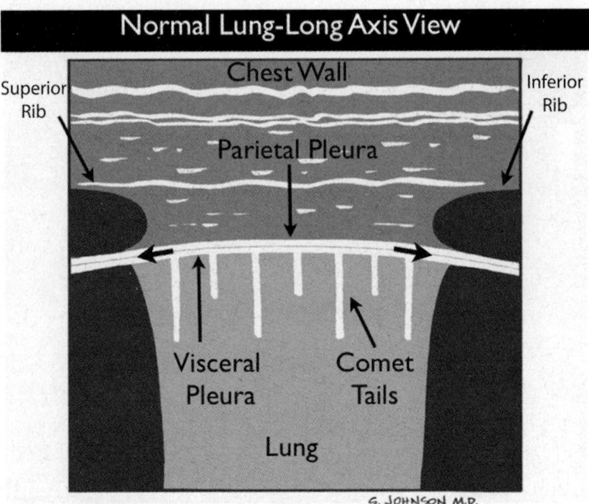

FIGURE 6.25 Normal lung on US.

M-mode US can confirm the B-mode US findings of a PTX. Normal lung sliding gives the appearance of "waves on the beach" or "the seashore sign." In PTX, the loss of lung sliding will result in the "stratosphere" or "the bar-code" signs.

An emergent needle decompression can then be performed rapidly in patient in shock where a PTX is identified on US, especially in cases where there may be a delay in obtaining a chest radiograph.

RUSH STEP 3: THE PIPES

The third and final step in the RUSH exam is to examine "the pipes," or the major arterial and venous structures (Fig. 6.26).

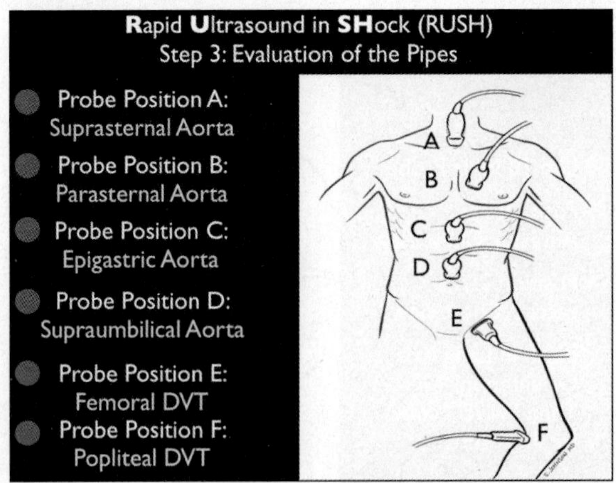

FIGURE 6.26 RUSH step 3, evaluation of the "pipes."

The first part of this exam is to assess the arterial side of the circulatory system. Vascular catastrophes, such as a ruptured abdominal aortic aneurysm (AAA) or an aortic dissection, are life-threatening causes of hypotension that may be accurately diagnosed with bedside US.[98]

AAA may be diagnosed by detection of an aorta larger than 3 cm in diameter. As most AAAs rupture into the retroperitoneal space, it may not be possible to visualize the actual area of aortic rupture. This is because the retroperitoneal area can be difficult to image with US. However, in the patient presenting in shock where AAA is diagnosed and rupture is clinically suspected, emergency surgical consultation and expedited therapy should be pursued. In the chest, dilation of the aortic root to a size >3.8 cm may be seen with a proximal, or Stanford class A, thoracic aortic dissection. This is measured just distal to the aortic valve.[99] An intimal flap may at times be seen here, confirming dissection.[100,101]

The evaluation of the major venous structures would then be indicated if right ventricular enlargement is identified on echo and a thromboembolic etiology for shock is suspected. In this scenario, imaging of the veins of the lower extremities for a DVT would be indicated. The limited leg compression DVT examination can be performed rapidly by evaluation of a targeted portion of the proximal femoral and popliteal veins, where the majority of thrombi are located.[102,103]

For this exam, compression of the femoral vein is performed first, beginning superiorly at a level just below the inguinal ligament. The common femoral vein and artery should first be identified. Doppler flow can be used to differentiate arterial from venous structures. The vein should be located medially to the artery and fully compressible with probe pressure. Serial compressions of the vein in a short-axis, or side-to-side, orientation can then be performed every centimeter, moving the probe inferiorly past the confluence of the saphenous vein down to the bifurcation of the vein into the femoral vein of the thigh and the deep femoral vein. The femoral vein of the thigh (formerly the superficial femoral vein) then continues down the leg to become the popliteal vein behind the knee. From a posterior position behind the knee, the vein will generally be seen above or closer to the probe, in relation to the popliteal artery. The popliteal vein should be evaluated with serial compressions from high in the popliteal fossa down inferiorly to the level of trifurcation into the three calf veins. Failure to fully compress the femoral or popliteal vein with direct probe pressure is pathognomonic of thrombosis.

PUTTING RUSH INTO ACTION

The RUSH protocol—pump, tank, and pipes—was created as an easily remembered physiologic roadmap for use in the resuscitation of the critical patient. The RUSH protocol was designed to be performed expediently by specifically choosing those exam components most applicable to the patient's clinical context. While the entire protocol is extensive and incorporates multiple US elements, the clinician should generally begin with evaluation of the heart, IVC, and/or the IJ veins. The RUSH exam should then be tailored based on clinical suspicion, as many patients may be assessed with an abbreviated exam. Incorporation of other components, such as the lung, FAST, aorta, and DVT

TABLE 6.8 Using the RUSH Protocol to Diagnose the Type of Shock

RUSH Exam:	Hypovolemic Shock	Cardiogenic Shock	Obstructive Shock	Distributive Shock
Pump	Hypercontractile heart Small heart size	Hypocontractile heart Dilated heart size	Pericardial effusion RV strain Hypercontractile heart	Hypercontractile heart (early sepsis) Hypocontractile heart (late sepsis)
Tank	Flat IVC Flat IJV Peritoneal fluid Pleural fluid	Distended IVC Distended IJV B-lines Pleural effusions Ascites	Distended IVC Distended IJV Absent lung sliding (PTX)	Normal/small IVC Normal/small IJV Pleural fluid (Empyema) Peritoneal fluid (Peritonitis)
Pipes	AAA Aortic dissection	Normal	DVT	Normal

exams, can be determined as the clinical picture dictates. Table 6.8 demonstrates how using the RUSH exam at the bedside can assist in the diagnosis of the type of shock in the critically ill patient.

Response to therapy can also be evaluated by repeating the RUSH exam in the hypotensive patient. Specifically as mentioned above, the clinician can monitor the function of the heart and the size and respiratory variation of the IVC and IJ veins over time to assess for the response to fluid loading or for the need to initiate vasopressor agents in the patient in shock.

CONCLUSION

Focused bedside US has evolved to become a key assessment tool in the evaluation of the critically ill patient in shock. Clinical information that once necessitated invasive measures, such as placement of a central line or a Swan-Ganz catheter, can now be measured by US assessment. The RUSH exam represents one of a series of resuscitation US algorithms for use in the critically ill patient. The physiologic basis for the protocol, simplified to "the pump, tank, and pipes," allows for an easily remembered and rapidly performed protocol for shock assessment. While the RUSH protocol provides an extensive roadmap for shock evaluation, the exam should be adapted to best match the clinical presentation and not all elements may need to be performed in any given patient. Emergency physicians and critical care physicians caring for the sickest of patients should consider integrating US techniques, including the RUSH protocol, into their care.

ACKNOWLEDGMENT

Funding Sources: All authors disclose no funding sources.

Conflicts of Interest: Phillips Perera is an educational consultant for SonoSite Ultrasound. Diku Mandavia is the Chief Medical Officer for SonoSite Ultrasound, Bothell, WA. All other authors disclose no conflicts of interest.

LITERATURE TABLE

TRIAL	DESIGN	RESULT
Jones et al., *Shock.* 2005[34]	Single-center, prospective, randomized trial of 103 patients with nontraumatic shock. The goal was to assess left ventricular contractility as a predictor for septic shock	The finding of hyperdynamic left ventricular contractility had a positive likelihood ratio of 5.3 for diagnosis of sepsis
Moore et al., *Acad Emerg Med.* 2002[35]	Single-center, prospective, observational study included 51 adult patients with symptomatic hypotension. Echocardiography exams were performed by emergency physicians and then later assessed by a cardiologist blinded to the preliminary emergency physician assessment. The goal was to assess agreement between the final reading by emergency physicians and cardiologists	Comparison of emergency physician vs. cardiology evaluation of left ventricular contractility yielded a Pearson correlation coefficient of $r = 0.86$. This compared favorably to the interobserver correlation of the reading between cardiologists $r = 0.84$. The conclusion was that emergency physicians with focused echo training can accurately determine left ventricular contractility in hypotensive patients
Joseph et al., *Chest.* 2004[36]	Single-center prospective study included 100 ICU patients in shock	Transthoracic echocardiography was performed by cardiologists. 63% of patients had a cardiac cause of shock present, defined as pericardial effusion, left or right ventricular failure, or valve dysfunction
Tayal et al., *Resuscitation.* 2003[44]	Single-center observational study of 20 patients with nontraumatic hemodynamic collapse. All patients had bedside echocardiography performed by emergency physicians during the resuscitation	12 of the 20 patients had cardiac kinetic activity on US. 8 of these 12 patients had a pericardial effusion noted. 3 patients required immediate pericardiocentesis for cardiac tamponade
Mandavia et al., *Ann Emerg Med.* 2001[45]	Single-center, prospective study enrolled 515 patients at high risk for pericardial effusion. Emergency physicians initially performed the echocardiography exam. Cardiologists later reviewed all studies for the presence of pericardial effusion	103 of 515 patients were found to have a pericardial effusion. Emergency physician-performed echocardiography had a sensitivity of 96% (95% CI 90.4–98.9), specificity of 98% (95% CI 95.8–99.1), and overall accuracy of 97.5% (95% CI 95.7–98.7) for the detection of pericardial effusions

CI, confidence interval.

REFERENCES

1. Rivers E, Nguyen B, Havstad S, et al. Early goal-directed therapy in the treatment of severe sepsis and septic shock. *N Engl J Med.* 2001;345(19):1368–1377.
2. Sebat F, Musthafa AA, Johnson D, et al. Effect of a rapid response system for patients in shock on time to treatment and mortality during 5 years. *Crit Care Med.* 2007;35(11):2568–2575.
3. Atkinson PRT, McAuley DJ, Kendall RJ, et al. Abdominal and cardiac evaluation with sonography in shock (ACES): an approach by emergency physicians for use of ultrasound in patients with undifferentiated hypotension. *Emerg Med J.* 2009;26:87–91.
4. Gunst M, Gaemmaghami V, Sperry J. Accuracy of cardiac function and volume status estimates using the bedside echocardiographic assessment in trauma/critical care (BEAT). *J Trauma.* 2008;65:509–516.
5. Pershad J, Myers S, Plouman C, et al. Bedside limited echocardiography by the emergency physician is accurate during evaluation of the critically ill patient (BLEEP). *Pediatrics.* 2004;114:e667–e671.
6. Boyd JH, Walley KR. The role of echocardiography in hemodynamic monitoring. *Curr Opin Crit Care.* 2009;15:239–243.
7. Lanctot YF, Valois M, Bealieu Y. EGLS: echo guided life support. An algorithmic approach to undifferentiated shock. *Crit Ultrasound J.* 2011;3:123–129.
8. Elmer J, Noble VA. An evidence based approach for integrating bedside ultrasound into routine practice in the assessment of undifferentiated shock. *ICU Director.* 2010;1(3):163–174.
9. Lichtenstein DA, Karakitsos D. Integrating ultrasound in the hemodynamic evaluation of acute circulatory failure (FALLS-the fluid administration limited by lung sonography protocol). *J Crit Care.* 2012;27:533el–533el9.
10. Jensen MB, Sloth E, Larsen M, et al. Transthoracic echocardiography for cardiopulmonary monitoring in intensive care (FATE). *Eur J Anaesthesiol.* 2004;21:700–707.

11. Rozycki G, Oschner MG, Schmidt JA, et al. A prospective use of surgeon's performed ultrasound as the primary adjunct modality for injured patient assessment. *J Trauma.* 1995;39:879–885.
12. Kirkpatrick AW, Sirois M, Laupland KB, et al. Hand-held sonography for detecting post-traumatic pneumothoraces: the extended focused assessment of sonography for trauma (E-FAST). *J Trauma.* 2004;57:288–295.
13. Breitkreutz R, Price S, Steiger HV, et al. Focused echocardiographic examination in life support and peri-resuscitation of emergency patients (FEEL-Resus): a prospective trial. *Resuscitation.* 2010;81: 1527–1533.
14. Breitkreutz R, Walcher F, Seeger F. Focused echocardiographic evaluation in resuscitation management (FEER): concept of an advanced life support-conformed algorithm. *Crit Care Med.* 2007;35(5): S150–S161.
15. Ferrada P, Murthi S, Anand RJ, et al. Transthoracic focused rapid echocardiography examination: real-time evaluation of fluid status in critically ill trauma patients (FREE). *J Trauma.* 2010;70(1): 56–64.
16. Liteplo A, Noble V, Atkinson P. My patient has no blood pressure: point of care ultrasound in the hypotensive patient-FAST and RELIABLE. *Ultrasound.* 2012;20:64–68.
17. Weingart SD, Duque D, Nelson B. *Rapid Ultrasound for Shock and Hypotension (RUSH-HIMAPP).* EMedHome.com article; April, 2009.
18. Perera P, Mailhot T, Riley D, et al. The RUSH exam: Rapid Ultrasound in SHock in the evaluation of the critically ill. *Emerg Med Clin North Am.* 2010;28:29–56.
19. Perera P, Mailhot T, Riley D, et al. The RUSH exam: Rapid Ultrasound in SHock in the evaluation of the critically ill (2012 update). *Ultrasound Clin.* 2012;7(2):255–278.
20. Seif D, Perera P, Mailhot T, et al. Bedside ultrasound in resuscitation and the Rapid Ultrasound in SHock protocol. *Crit Care Res Pract.* 2012;2012:Article ID 503254.
21. Bahner DP. Trinity, a hypotensive ultrasound protocol. *J Diagn Med Sonography.* 2002;18:193–198.
22. Rose JS, Bair AE, Mandavia DP. The UHP ultrasound protocol: a novel ultrasound approach to the empiric evaluation of the undifferentiated hypotensive patient. *Am J Emerg Med.* 2001;19:299–302.
23. American College of Emergency Physicians. Emergency ultrasound guidelines. *Ann Emerg Med.* 2009;53:550–570.
24. Akhtar S, Theodoro D, Gaspari R, et al. Resident training in emergency ultrasound: consensus recommendations from the 2008 council of emergency medicine residency directors conference. *Acad Emerg Med.* 2009;16:S32–S36.
25. Society for Academic Emergency Medicine. *Ultrasound Position Statement.* Available at: http//www.saem.org. Accessed January 20, 2013.
26. Jang TB, Coates WC, Jiu YT. The competency based mandate for emergency bedside sonography and a tale of two residency programs. *J Ultrasound Med.* 2012;31:515–521.
27. Neri L, Storti E, Lichtenstein D. Toward an ultrasound curriculum for critical care. *Crit Care Med.* 2007;35(5 suppl):S290–S304.
28. Bealieu Y. Specific skill set and goals of focused echocardiography for critical care physicians. *Crit Care Med.* 2007;35:S144–S149.
29. Mayo PH, Beaulieu Y, Doelken P, et al. American College of Chest Physicians/La Societe de Reanimation de Langue Francaise statement on competence in critical care ultrasonography. *Chest.* 2009;135:1050–1060.
30. International expert statement on training standards for critical care ultrasonography. *Intensive Care Med.* 2011;37(7):1077–1083.
31. Labovitz AJ, Noble VE, Bierig M, et al. Focused cardiac ultrasound in the emergent setting: a consensus statement of the American Society of Echocardiography and the American College of Emergency Physicians. *J Am Soc Echocardiogr.* 2010;23:1225–1230.
32. Weekes AJ, Quirke DP. Emergency echocardiography. *Emerg Med Clin North Am.* 2011;29:759–787.
33. Chen RS, Bivens MJ, Grossman SA. Diagnosis and management of valvular heart disease in emergency medicine. *Emerg Med Clin Nort Am.* 2011;29:801–810.
34. Jones AE, Craddock PA, Tayal VS, et al. Diagnostic accuracy of identification of left ventricular function among emergency department patients with nontraumatic symptomatic undifferentiated hypotension. *Shock.* 2005;24:513–517.
35. Moore CL, Rose GA, Tayal VS, et al. Determination of left ventricular function by emergency physician echocardiography of hypotensive patients. *Acad Emerg Med.* 2002;9:186–193.
36. Joseph M, Disney P. Transthoracic echocardiography to identify or exclude cardiac cause of shock. *Chest.* 2004;126:1592–1597.

37. Lang RM, Bierig M, Devereux RB, et al. Recommendations for chamber quantification. *Eur J Echocardiogr.* 2006;7(2):79–108.
38. Weekes AJ, Tassone HM, Babcock A, et al. Comparison of serial qualitative and quantitative assessments of caval index and left ventricular systolic function during early fluid resuscitation of hypotensive emergency department patients. *Acad Emerg Med.* 2011;18:912–921.
39. Secko MA, Lazar JM, Salciccioli, L, et al. Can junior emergency physicians use E-point septal separation to accurately estimate left ventricular function in acutely dyspneic patients? *Acad Emerg Med.* 2011;18:1223–1226.
40. Ahmadpour H, Shah AA, Allen JW. Mitral E point septal separation: a reliable index of left ventricular performance in coronary artery disease. *Am Heart J.* 1983;106(1):21–28.
41. Silverstein JR, Laffely NH, Rifkin RD. Quantitative estimation of left ventricular ejection fraction from mitral valve E-point to septal separation and comparison to magnetic resonance imaging. *Am J Cardiol.* 2006;97(1):137–140.
42. Weekes AJ, Reddy A, Lewis MR, et al. E-point septal separation compared to fractional shortening measurements of systolic function in emergency department patients. *J Ultrasound Med.* 2012;31:1891–1897.
43. Blaivas M. Incidence of pericardial effusion in patients presenting to the emergency department with unexplained dyspnea. *Acad Emerg Med.* 2001;8(12):1143–1146.
44. Tayal VS, Kline JA. Emergency echocardiography to determine pericardial effusions in patients with PEA and near PEA states. *Resuscitation.* 2003;59:315–318.
45. Mandavia DP, Hoffner RJ, Mahaney K, et al. Bedside echocardiography by emergency physicians. *Ann Emerg Med.* 2001;38:377–382.
46. Grecu L. Cardiac tamponade. *Int Anesthesiol Clin.* 2012;50(2):59–77.
47. Shabetai R. Pericardial effusions: haemodynamic spectrum. *Heart.* 2004;90:255–256.
48. Ma OJ, Mateer JR, Blaivas M. *Emergency Ultrasound.* New York: McGraw Hill Publishers; 2008.
49. Russo AM, O'Connor WH, Waxman HL. Atypical presentations and echocardiographic findings in patients with cardiac tamponade occurring early and late after cardiac surgery. *Chest.* 1993;104:71–78.
50. Trojanos CA, Porembka DT. Assessment of left ventricular function and hemodynamics with transesophageal echocardiography. *Crit Care Clin.* 1996;12:253–272.
51. Goodman A, Perera P, Mailhot T, et al. The role of bedside ultrasound in the diagnosis of pericardial effusions and cardiac tamponade. *J Emerg Trauma Shock.* 2012;5:72–75.
52. Nabazivadeh SA, Meskshar A. Ultrasonic diagnosis of cardiac tamponade in trauma patients using the collapsibility index of the inferior vena cava. *Acad Radiol.* 2007;14:505–506.
53. Armstrong WF, Ryan T. *Feigenbaum's Echocardiography.* 7th ed. Philadelphia, PA: Lippincott, Williams and Wilkins; 2010.
54. Tsang T, Enriquez-Sarano M, Freeman WK. Consecutive 1127 therapeutic echocardiographically guided pericardiocenteses: clinical profile, practice patterns and outcomes spanning 21 years. *Mayo Clin Proc.* 2002;77:429–436.
55. Salazar M, Mohar D, Bhardwaj R, et al. Use of contrast echocardiography to detect displacement of the needle during pericardiocentesis. *Echocardiography.* 2012;29:E60–E61.
56. Ainsworth CD, Salehian O. Echo-guided pericardiocentesis: let the bubbles show the way. *Circulation.* 2011;123:e210–e211.
57. Gifroni S, Olivotto I, Cecchini P, et al. Short term clinical outcome of patients with acute pulmonary embolism, normal blood pressure and echocardiographic right ventricular dysfunction. *Circulation.* 2000;101:2817–2822.
58. Becattini C, Agnelli G. Acute pulmonary embolism: risk stratification in the emergency department. *Intern Emerg Med.* 2007;2:119–129.
59. Nazeyrollas D, Metz D, Jolly D, et al. Use of transthoracic Doppler echocardiography combined with clinical and electrographic data to predict acute pulmonary embolism. *Eur Heart J.* 1996;17:779–786.
60. Jardin F, Duborg O, Bourdarias JP. Echocardiographic pattern of acute cor pulmonale. *Chest.* 1997;111:209–217.
61. Jardin F, Dubourg O, Gueret P, et al. Quantitative two dimensional echocardiography in massive pulmonary embolism: emphasis on ventricular interdependence and leftward septal displacement. *J Am Coll Cardiol.* 1987;10:1201–1206.
62. Rudoni R, Jackson R. Use of two-dimensional echocardiography for the diagnosis of pulmonary embolus. *J Emerg Med.* 1998;16:5–8.
63. Jackson RE, Rudoni RR, Hauser AM, et al. Prospective evaluation of two-dimensional transthoracic echocardiography in emergency department patients with suspected pulmonary embolism. *Acad Emerg Med.* 2000;7:994–998.

64. Miniati M, Monti S, Pratali L, et al. Value of transthoracic echocardiography in the diagnosis of pulmonary embolism: results of a prospective study in unselected patients. *Am J Med.* 2001;110(7):528–535.
65. Stein J. Opinions regarding the diagnosis and management of venous thromboembolic disease. ACCP Consensus Committee on pulmonary embolism. *Chest.* 1996;109:233–237.
66. Konstantinides S, Geibel A, Heusel G, et al. Heparin plus alteplase compared with heparin alone in patients with submassive pulmonary embolus. *N Engl J Med.* 2002;347:1143–1150.
67. Kucher N, Goldhaber SZ. Management of massive pulmonary embolism. *Circulation.* 2005;112:e28–e32.
68. Jaff MR, McMurtry S, Archer S, et al. Management of massive and submassive pulmonary embolism, iliofemoral deep venous thrombosis and chronic thromboembolic pulmonary embolism: a scientific statement from the American Heart Association. *Circulation.* 2011;123:1788–1830.
69. Vieillard-Baron A, Page B, Augarde R, et al. Acute cor pulmonale in massive pulmonary embolism: incidence, echocardiographic pattern, clinical implications and recovery rate. *Intensive Care Med.* 2001;27(9):1481–1486.
70. Mookadam F, Jiamsripong P, Goel R, et al. Critical appraisal on the utility of echocardiography in the management of acute pulmonary embolism. *Cardiol Rev.* 2010;18(1):29–37.
71. Cosby KS, Kendall JL. *Practical Guide to Emergency Ultrasound.* Philadelphia, PA: Lippincott Williams and Wilkins; 2006.
72. Riley D, Hultgren A, Merino D, et al. Emergency department bedside echocardiographic diagnosis of massive pulmonary embolism with direct visualization of thrombus in the pulmonary artery. *Crit Ultrasound J.* 2011;3(3):155–160.
73. Madan A, Schwartz C. Echocardiographic visualization of acute pulmonary embolus and thrombolysis in the ED. *Am J Emerg Med.* 2004;22:294–300.
74. Wallace DJ, Allison M, Stone MB. Inferior vena cava percentage collapse during respiration is affected by the sampling location: an ultrasound study in healthy volunteers. *Acad Emerg Med.* 2010;17(1):96–99.
75. Kircher BJ, Himelman RB, Schiller NB. Noninvasive estimation of right atrial pressure from the inspiratory collapse of the inferior vena cava. *Am J Cardiol.* 1990;66(4):493–496.
76. Simonson JS, Schiller NB. Sonospirometry: a new method for noninvasive estimation of mean right atrial pressure based on two-dimensional echographic measurements of the inferior vena cava during measured inspiration. *J Am Coll Cardiol.* 1988;11(3):557–564.
77. Randazzo MR, Snoey ER, Levitt, MA, et al. Accuracy of emergency physician assessment of left ventricular ejection fraction and central venous pressure using echocardiography. *Acad Emerg Med.* 2003;10(9):973–977.
78. Jardin F, Vieillard-Baron A. Ultrasonographic examination of the venae cavae. *Intensive Care Med.* 2006;32(2):203–206.
79. Marik PA. Techniques for assessment of intravascular volume in critically ill patients. *J Intensive Care Med.* 2009;24(5):329–337.
80. Blehar DJ, Dickman E, Gaspari R. Identification of congestive heart failure via respiratory variation of inferior vena cava diameter. *Am J Emerg Med.* 2009;27(1):71–75.
81. Nagdev AD, Merchant RC, Tirado-Gonzalez A, et al. Emergency department bedside ultrasonographic measurement of the caval index for noninvasive determination of low central venous pressure. *Ann Emerg Med.* 2010;55(3):290–295.
82. Schefold JC, Storm C, Bercker S, et al. Inferior vena cava diameter correlates with invasive hemodynamic measures in mechanically ventilated intensive care unit patients with sepsis. *J Emerg Med.* 2010;38(5):652–637.
83. Seif D, Mailhot T, Perera P, et al. Caval sonography in shock: a noninvasive method for evaluating intravascular volume in critically ill patients. *J Ultrasound Med.* 2012;31:1885–1890.
84. Rudski LG, Lai WW, Afilalo J, et al. Guidelines for the echocardiographic assessment of the right heart in adults: a report from the American society of echocardiography. *J Am Soc Echocardiogr.* 2010;23(7):685–713.
85. Barbier C, Loubieres Y, Schmit C, et al. Respiratory changes in the inferior vena cava diameter are helpful in predicting fluid responsiveness in ventilated septic patients. *Intensive Care Med.* 2004;30(9): 1740–1746.
86. Simon MA, Kliner DE, Girod JP, et al. Jugular venous distention on ultrasound: sensitivity and specificity for heart failure in patients with dyspnea. *Am Heart J.* 2010;159:421–427.
87. Jang T, Aubin C, Naunheim R, et al. Ultrasonography of the internal jugular vein in patients with dyspnea without jugular venous distention on physical examination. *Ann Emerg Med.* 2004;44(2):160–168.
88. Jang T, Aubin C, Naunheim R, et al. Jugular venous distention on ultrasound: sensitivity and specificity for heart failure in patients with dyspnea. *Ann Emerg Med.* 2011;29:1198–1202.

89. Killu K, Coba V, Huang Y, et al. Internal jugular vein collapsibility index associated with hypovolemia in intensive care unit patients. *Crit Ultrasound J.* 2010;1:13–17.
90. Volpicelli G, Caramello V, Cardinale L, et al. Bedside ultrasound of the lung for the monitoring of acute decompensated heart failure. *Am J Emerg Med.* 2008;26:585–591.
91. Soldati G, Copetti R, Sher S. Sonographic interstitial syndrome: the sound of lung water. *J Ultrasound Med.* 2009;28:163–174.
92. Liteplo AS, Marrill KA, Villen T, et al. Emergency thoracic ultrasound in the differentiation of the etiology of shortness of breath (ETUDES): sonographic B-lines and N-terminal pro-brain-type natriuretic peptide in diagnosing heart failure. *Acad Emerg Med.* 2009;16:201–210.
93. Volpicelli G, Noble VE, Liteplo A, et al. Decreased sensitivity of lung ultrasound limited to the anterior chest in emergency department diagnosis of cardiogenic pulmonary edema: a retrospective analysis. *Crit Ultrasound J.* 2010;2:47–52.
94. Lichtenstein DA, Menu Y. A bedside ultrasound sign ruling out pneumothorax in the critically ill. Lung sliding. *Chest.* 1995;108:1345–1348.
95. Lichtenstein D, Meziere G, Biderman P, et al. The comet-tail artifact: an ultrasound sign ruling out pneumothorax. *Intensive Care Med.* 1999;25:383–388.
96. Lichtenstein DA, Meziere GA. Relevance of lung ultrasound in the diagnosis of acute respiratory failure: the BLUE protocol. *Chest.* 2008;134:117–125.
97. Manson W, Hafez NM. The rapid assessment of dyspnea with ultrasound: RADIUS. *Ultrasound Clin.* 2011;6:261–276.
98. Rubano E, Mehta N, Caputo W, et al. Systematic review: emergency department bedside ultrasonography for diagnosing suspected abdominal aortic aneurysm. *Acad Emerg Med.* 2013;20:128–138.
99. Taylor RA, Oliva I, Van Tonder R, et al. Point of care focused cardiac ultrasound for the assessment of thoracic aortic dimensions, dilation and aneurysmal disease. *Acad Emerg Med.* 2012;19:244–247.
100. Fojtik, JP, Costantino TG, Dean AJ. The diagnosis of aortic dissection by emergency medicine ultrasound. *J Emerg Med.* 2007;32:191–196.
101. Budhram G, Reardon R. Diagnosis of ascending aortic dissection using emergency department bedside echocardiogram. *Acad Emerg Med.* 2008;15(6):584.
102. Bernardi E, Camporese G, Buller H, et al. Serial 2 point ultrasonography plus d-dimer vs. whole leg color ceded Doppler ultrasonography for diagnosing suspected symptomatic deep vein thrombosis. *JAMA.* 2008;300:1653–1659.
103. Farahmand S, Farnia M, Shahriaran S, et al. The accuracy of limited B-mode compression technique in diagnosing deep venous thrombosis in lower extremities. *Am J Emerg Med.* 2011;29(6):687–690.

7

Pulmonary Ultrasonography

Feras Khan and Anne-Sophie Beraud

BACKGROUND

Over the past decade, bedside point-of-care ultrasonography, or ultrasound (US), has become an indispensable tool in critical care and emergency medicine. It is an efficient and effective diagnostic aid myriad conditions and has improved procedure safety in both the emergency department (ED) and intensive care units (ICUs).[1] The American College of Emergency Physicians (ACEP) recommends that all emergency medicine residents train to proficiency in emergency US.[2] Lung US the subject of this chapter, is fast becoming an integral component of point-of-care US for both intensivists and emergency physicians. First developed in European ICUs, lung US has proven to be highly useful in detecting disease processes including pneumonia, pneumothorax, pleural effusions, and pulmonary edema.[3] With recent advances in technology, point-of-care US can now be performed at bedside with relatively small devices. This allows physicians to make decisions quickly and safely—without having to transport the patient out of a monitored setting—and has helped minimize computed tomography (CT) use and associated patient exposure to ionizing radiation. In 2012, the first evidence-based guidelines for point-of-care lung US were published in order to standardize definitions for a variety of lung pathologies.[4]

PROBE SELECTION, TECHNICAL EQUIPMENT, AND SCANNING TECHNIQUE

Transducer Selection

Lung US can be performed with three types of US transducers: linear (usually used for vascular access or nerve blocks), phased array ("cardiac"), or convex ("abdominal"). Because of its high frequency (7.5 to 10 MHz), the linear probe is preferred for analyzing superficial anatomy such as the pleura as well as individual rib interspaces. The linear probe, however, does not allow deep penetration to visualize deeper structures, such as the lungs themselves; better suited for this are the phased-array (2 to 8 MHz) and the convex probes (3.5 MHz).

Imaging Modalities

The US transducer generates US waves that are reflected back to the transducer. These returning waves generate a signal that is determined by the difference in the acoustic

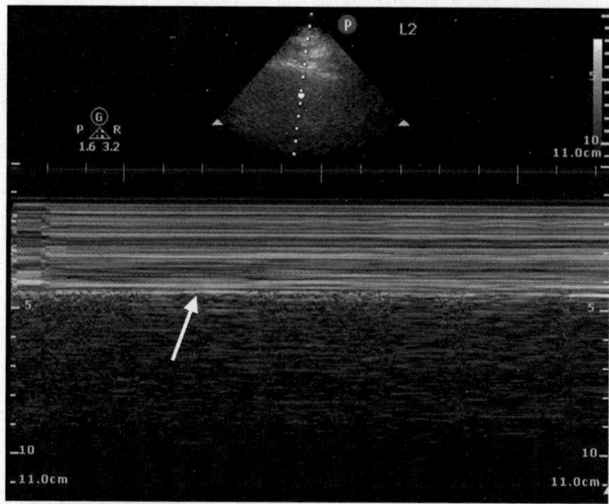

FIGURE 7.1 Seashore sign. This image is taken from the 3rd intercostal space in the midclavicular line using a convex probe in M-mode. The granular appearance of the lung creates the "seashore" sign. The arrow indicates the pleural line.

impedance of the tissues encountered.[5] There are two US modes commonly used for lung imaging. The first, B-mode (brightness mode), generates a 2D image. The second, M-mode (motion mode), displays images in relation to elapsed time (one axis showing the depth of the image-producing interface and the other showing time) (Fig. 7.1). M-mode allows recording of motion of the interface toward and away from the transducer. The use of each mode is discussed in detail in the sections below. When performing a bedside lung US exam, all preset filters should be turned off to allow lung artifacts to appear. The probe indicator points cephalad in all exams.

Imaging Technique

Prior to use, both machine and probe should be thoroughly cleaned with disinfectant to limit contamination and nosocomial infection spread.[6] The patient is typically imaged in the supine position. For patients in a critical care setting, it may be difficult to obtain true posterior views. In these patients, a protocol using the anterior and lateral chest walls has been described (Fig. 7.2) that images two interspaces (2nd and 5th) along the midclavicular line and at the midaxillary line.[7] This approach allows the clinician to quickly assess eight lung zones. For a more thorough examination in stable patients, the probe should be advanced longitudinally and transversely along the 2nd, 3rd, and 4th and 5th intercostal interspaces.

Training Requirements

No consensus exists regarding the number of supervised US exams needed for a clinician to achieve proficiency in lung US. The ACEP has proposed that 25 to 50 studies be reviewed by a qualified ultrasonographer in order to demonstrate competence in a specific exam (e.g., pulmonary, cardiac).

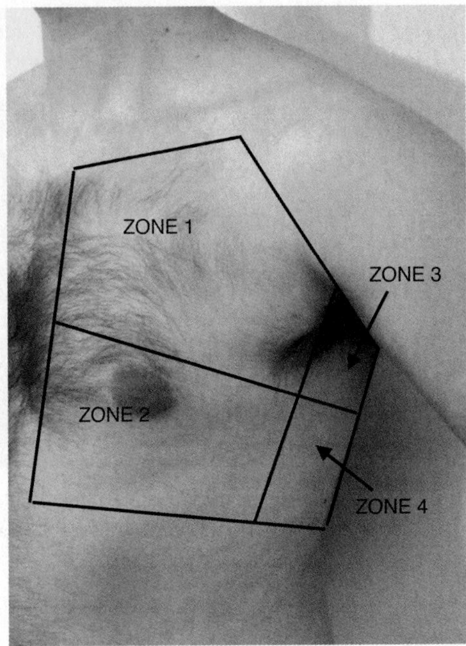

FIGURE 7.2 Lung zones. The four lung zones that are shown on this patient indicate areas that should be included when performing an ultrasound examination.

NORMAL SONOGRAPHIC THORACIC ANATOMY

The lung parenchyma is normally filled with air, which has very low acoustic impedance and is therefore not detected on ultrasonography. Pulmonary disease processes result in changes to the air–fluid interface in the lung. These changes generate unique US patterns, or artifacts, which can help identify a variety of conditions including pleural effusions, pneumothorax, pneumonia, and alveolar–interstitial syndrome (AIS).

Lung Sliding

The lung can be visualized in the intercostal spaces, which delineate US windows between each rib. The parietal pleura lines the thoracic wall, covers the superior surface of the diaphragm, and separates the pleural cavity from the mediastinum. The visceral pleura covers the surface of the lung. The pleural space is a virtual space between the parietal and the visceral pleura.

In the intercostal spaces, the pleural line is situated below the subcutaneous tissue, about 0.5 to 2 cm from the skin depending on chest wall thickness. It is a horizontal and thin structure that appears intensely hyperechoic on US imaging (Fig. 7.3). In normal healthy lungs, US imaging will demonstrate "lung sliding" of parietal pleura against the visceral pleura during the respiration.

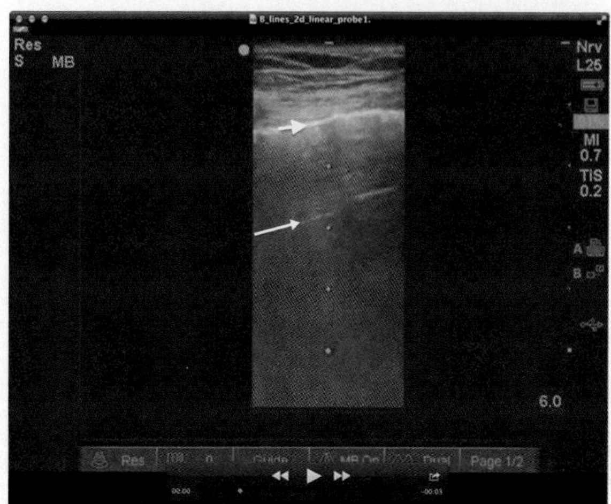

FIGURE 7.3 A-lines/pleural line. This image uses a vascular probe and shows a typical A-line (long arrow) as well as the pleural line (short arrow).

A-Lines

"A-lines" are hyperechoic horizontal artifacts seen in healthy lungs and represent repetition artifact generated by the pleural line (Fig. 7.3). Importantly, A-lines can also be seen in patients with pneumothorax as described below. In M-mode, healthy lungs will demonstrate a "seashore" sign (Fig. 7.1). This description captures the "wavelike" pattern produced by normal pleural line movement coupled with the "sandy beach" or granular appearance generated by lung parenchyma.

B-Lines

A "B-line" is a reverberation artifact with the following properties:[8]

1. A vertical comet-tail artifact
2. Arises from the pleural line
3. Well defined
4. Hyperechoic
5. Long (does not fade)
6. Erases A-lines
7. Moves with lung sliding

One or two B-lines may be seen in the dependent lung zones in the normal lungs.[9] A large number of B-lines are pathologic (Fig. 7.4A and B) and will be described below in the AIS section. These artifacts are also called "comet tails."

CLINICAL CONDITIONS

Pneumothorax

A pneumothorax can be traumatic or nontraumatic in etiology. A large pneumothorax, especially if causing hemodynamic compromise, may require emergent treatment.

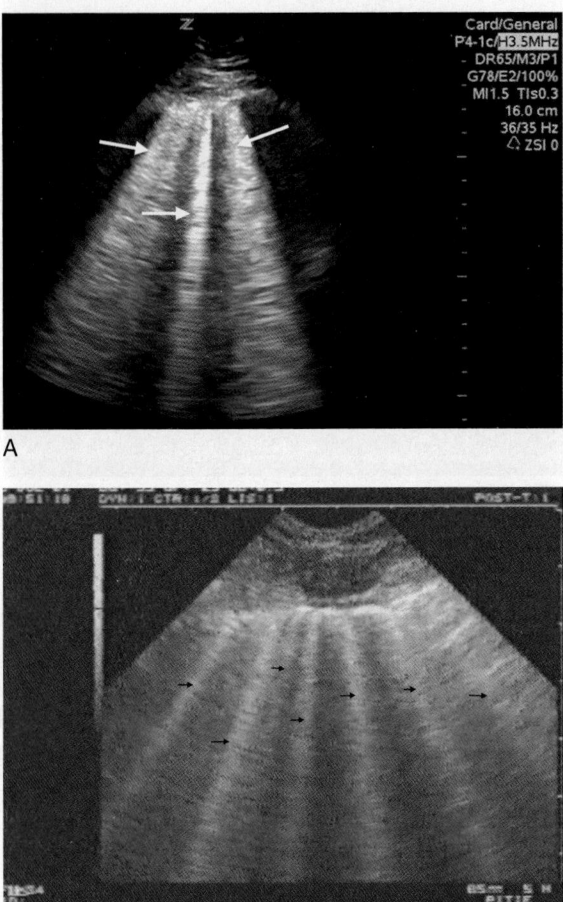

FIGURE 7.4 **A:** B-lines: alveolar–interstitial syndrome. This image shows three B-lines (arrows) in an interspace characteristic of AIS. There is a varying degree of thickness on each B-line. Image used courtesy of Dr. Darrell Sutijono. **B:** B-lines. This image shows 7 B-lines (arrows). Image used courtesy of Dr. Liz Turner.

Chest radiography (CXR) is the imaging modality most commonly used to evaluate pneumothorax; it has, however, been repeatedly demonstrated to be poorly sensitive (36% to 48%) for this condition.[10–13] CT remains the gold standard for the diagnosis of pneumothorax, but is time consuming and requires that the patient be transported out of the acute care setting.

Recent studies have demonstrated bedside lung US to have similar sensitivity to CT for the detection of pneumothorax,[10] making it ideal for the evaluation of hemodynamically unstable or ventilated patients in whom there is concern for lung collapse. A number of lung US findings exist that can help confirm or exclude pneumothorax. The presence of lung sliding has a negative predictive value for pneumothorax of close to 99%.[14] The lung sliding examination should be performed with the patient in a supine

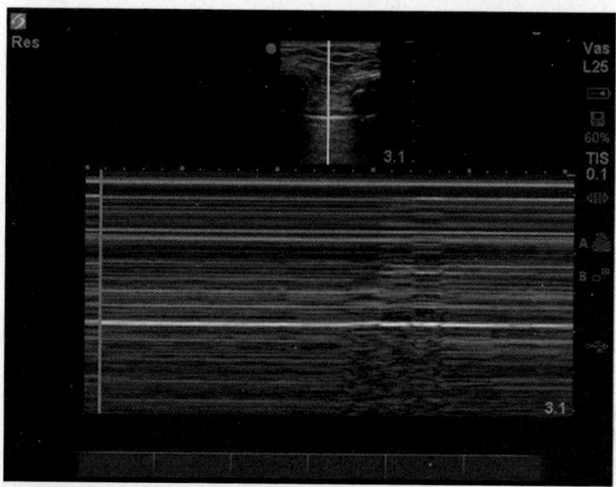

FIGURE 7.5 Stratosphere sign. This image uses a linear probe in M-mode and shows the "stratosphere sign," indicating a pneumothorax. Also known as the "bar-code sign."

position allowing air to rise to the most anterior part of the chest and should be evaluated at several points on the anterior and lateral chest wall. The presence of B-lines also rules out pneumothorax with a negative predictive value of 98% to 100%.[15–17] If a pneumothorax exists, a "stratosphere" or "bar-code" sign will replace the normal "seashore" sign seen using M-mode. The "stratosphere" sign is caused by air interrupting the normal pleural line reflection (Fig. 7.5). A "lung point," which represents the interface of normal lung next to an area of pneumothorax (Fig. 7.6A and B), may also be observed and is the most specific indicator for this condition.[18] Lung point is best visualized using M-mode with the probe held in the middle of the interspace transecting the lung—lung sliding will be seen on the part of the pleural line with intact lung and then will disappear in the area of pneumothorax. Finally, the absence of the "lung pulse" has also been described as a sign of pneumothorax.[18] The lung pulse refers to the rhythmic movement of the visceral and parietal pleural in step with the heart rate that is seen in normal healthy lungs. A combination of absent lung sliding and the presence of A-lines results in a sensitivity of 95% and a specificity of 94% for pneumothorax.[16] Guidelines recommend imaging at least four zones on each lung field to identify these findings.

In trauma, lung US has become a part of the Focused Assessment with Sonography for Trauma (FAST) as described in the extended FAST (E-FAST) protocol.[19] In this study of 225 trauma patients, a trained attending trauma surgeon using a 5- to 10-MHz linear transducer performed all US examinations. The protocol required imaging over the anteromedial chest at the second interspace at the midclavicular line and at the anterolateral chest wall near the 4th or 5th intercostal space at the midaxillary line. The absence of lung sliding and B-lines (comet tails) corresponded to an US diagnosis of pneumothorax. Lung US was found to be more sensitive than CXR alone (48.8% vs. 20.9%) with similar specificities (99.6% and 98.7% respectively). Compared with a composite standard (CXR, chest and abdomen CT, clinical course, and clinical interventions), the sensitivity of E-FAST was 58.9% with a specificity of 99.1%. The low

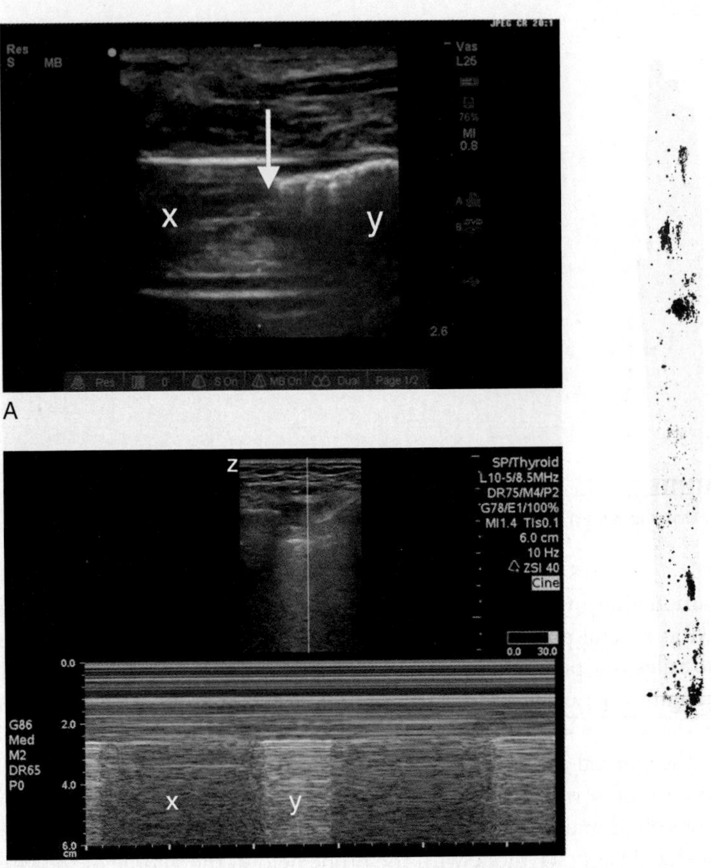

FIGURE 7.6 **A:** Lung point. This image uses a linear probe at the fourth right-sided intercostal space and shows the exact point at which a pneumothorax begins (arrow). Part (y) of the image shows normal sliding lung, while part (x) demonstrates absence of lung sliding consistent with a pneumothorax. Image used courtesy of Dr. Liz Turner. **B:** Lung point in M-mode. This image shows the alternating seashore (y) and stratosphere sign (x) in a patient with a pneumothorax demonstrating "lung point." Image used courtesy of Dr. Darrell Sutijono.

sensitivity of US in this study was attributed to the high rate of occult pneumothorax or partial pneumothorax. Nevertheless, the study highlights the importance of lung US as an integral part of trauma assessment and the need to incorporate lung US into the FAST protocol (E-FAST). In a 2012 systematic review of eight primarily trauma studies with a total of 1,048 patients, lung US was found to have superior sensitivity to CXR (90.9% vs. 50.2%) but similar specificity (98.2% vs. 99.4%) for detection of pneumothorax.[20]

Alveolar–Interstitial Syndrome

AIS describes a group of conditions—including pulmonary edema, interstitial pneumonia, and pulmonary fibrosis—that demonstrate similar findings on lung US.[9] Specifically,

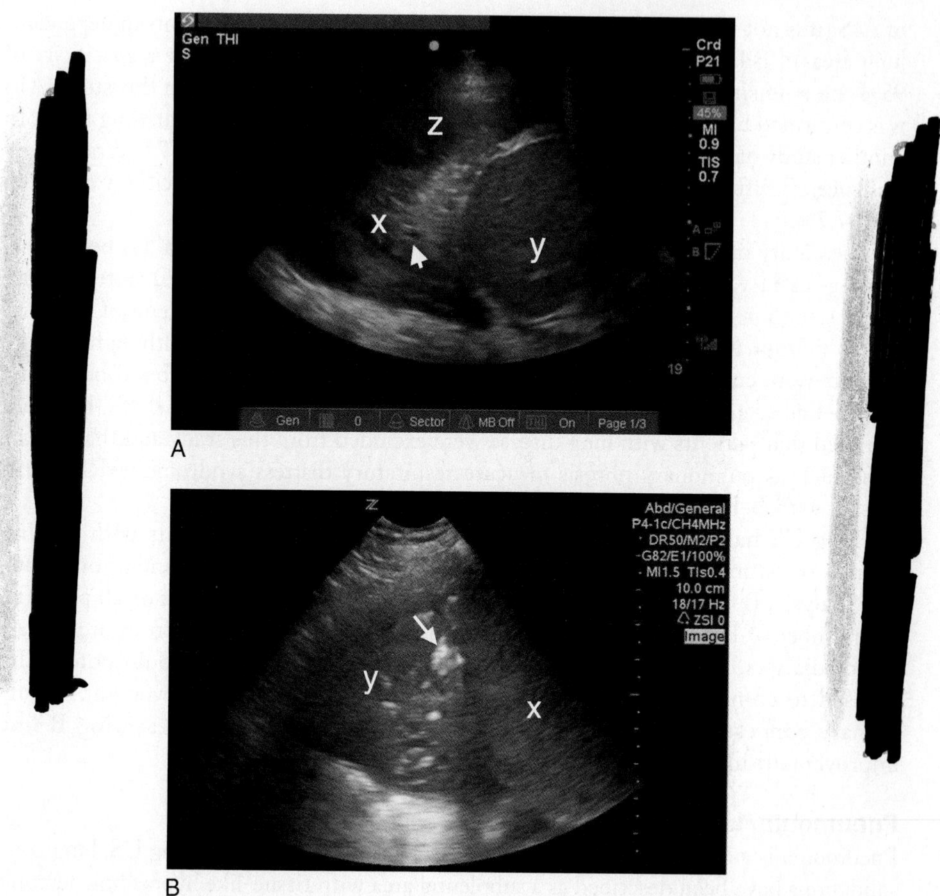

FIGURE 7.7 **A:** Pneumonia. This image shows a hyperechoic area (arrow) corresponding to an air bronchogram with pneumonia (x). The lung begins to resemble the liver (y) on US, a pattern termed "hepatization." There is also a pleural effusion (z). Image used courtesy of Dr. Liz Turner. **B:** Pneumonia. This image shows a hyperechoic area (arrow) that correlates to air bronchograms and pneumonia. The liver (x) and lung (y) are visible. Image used courtesy of Dr. Darrell Sutijono.

the normal air–fluid interface responsible for the artifacts seen on US imaging is shifted toward the fluid side. Cardiogenic pulmonary edema is the most common source of this change and is characterized on US by the presence of multiple B-lines (Fig. 7.4A and B). B-lines correspond to interlobular septal thickening on CT imaging, which denotes pulmonary vascular congestion.[9] B-lines are thought to be reverberation artifacts produced as the US beam strikes these congested areas.

To identify these findings, the US should be in B-mode, and at least eight lung zones should be imaged. A lung zone is considered "positive" when three or more B-lines are present.[4] Two or more positive zones bilaterally are required to meet the US definition of AIS (it is not uncommon to have one or two B-lines in normal patients in dependent lung areas).[4] Bilateral, diffuse B-lines have been demonstrated to have a specificity of 95% and a sensitivity of 97% for the diagnosis of pulmonary edema.[9] In this study, AIS was confirmed by CXR in 86 of 92 patients who had diffuse B-lines in all lung fields. In another study of 300 ED patients presenting with shortness of breath, 77 had radiologic evidence of diffuse AIS detected by lung US with a sensitivity and specificity of 85.7% and 97.7%.[21]

The ability of lung US to predict the presence of pulmonary edema has been compared to extra-vascular lung water (EVLW) calculations by the PiCCO system (Pulse index Contour Continuous Cardiac Output, Pulsion Medical Systems, Germany) and to pulmonary artery catheter (PAC)–derived wedge pressure.[22] Although only 20 patients were enrolled in this study, positive linear correlations were found between a total B-line score and EVLW ($r = 0.42$) and PAC wedge pressure ($r = 0.48$). It should be noted that patients with lung disease were excluded from this study and that conditions such as pulmonary fibrosis or acute respiratory distress syndrome (ARDS) can present with B-lines as well.

Lung US has also been used to monitor improvement in patients with varying degrees of pulmonary congestion/edema. In a study of 40 patients undergoing routine dialysis, B-lines were recorded pre- and postdialysis.[23] In 34 out of 40 patients, the number of B-lines underwent statistically significant reduction from predialysis to postdialysis. The study suggests that quantification of B-lines could potentially be used to complement daily patient weights in monitoring improvement in pulmonary congestion/edema. Lung US has also proven useful in measuring B-line improvement in acute decompensated heart failure.[22]

Pneumonia/Lung Consolidation

Pneumonia is a common diagnosis in both ED and ICU patients. Using US, lung consolidations have been described as a subpleural area with tissue-like hypoechoic texture[8] (Fig. 7.7A and B) and can resemble the US appearance of the liver, a pattern called "hepatization." Other US findings in patients with pneumonia include air bronchograms, comet-tail reverberation artifacts in a localized area, and a vascular pattern within the consolidation. Hyperechoic, linear, tubular artifacts within an isoechoic region suggest atelectasis.

In a prospective study of 65 ICU patients, US was found to have a sensitivity of 90% and a specificity of 98% for pneumonia when compared to alveolar consolidation on CT.[24] It should be noted that the ultrasonographers in this study were highly experienced and performed a thorough lung examination on each patient. In a separate study, lung US was used in 49 patients presenting to an ED with signs and symptoms of pneumonia.[25] All patients received both an US examination and a CXR. If the CXR was negative for pneumonia, and the US positive, a confirmatory CT was performed. Thirty-two out of 49 patients were confirmed to have pneumonia, with US outperforming CXR in diagnostic accuracy, 96.9% versus 75%, respectively. Limitations of the study included its nonblinded design, the small number of patients studied, and the variable experience of the ultrasonographers. Due to the design of the study, false negatives of US may have been missed.

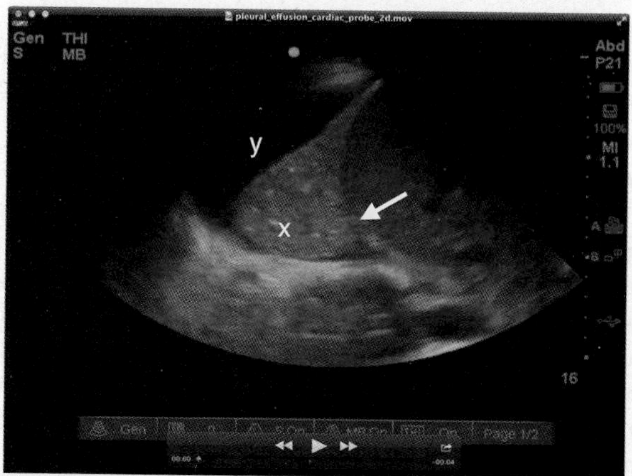

FIGURE 7.8 Pleural effusion. This image uses a convex probe in the midaxillary line and shows a pleural effusion (y). The collapsed lung is seen under the effusion (x) and the diaphragm can be seen (arrow) with the liver underneath.

Pleural Effusion

Detection of Pleural Effusion

Lung US is well validated as a tool for the detection of pleural fluid. Using B-mode, the probe is positioned along the mid- to posterior axillary line on the lateral aspect of the chest wall. The diaphragm should be identified as well as the liver (Fig. 7.8). Pleural fluid appears as an anechoic area superior to the diaphragm. The "sinusoid sign," which demonstrates variation in the interpleural distance with each respiratory cycle, has also been used as an indicator of pleural effusion.[26] A systematic review of four lung US studies, using chest CT as a gold standard, demonstrated US to have a mean sensitivity of 93% and specificity of 96% for detecting pleural effusion.[27]

In trauma patients, lung US has been used to rapidly detect hemothorax. In one study, 61 trauma patients underwent a standard FAST examination with two additional views used to evaluate the thoracic cavity laterally; the sensitivity and specificity of US for hemothorax were 92% and 100%, respectively.[28]

Quantification of Pleural Effusion

The amount of pleural fluid can also be quantified by US. A traditional posteroanterior CXR can identify effusions as small as 175 mL.[29] US has been able to detect as little as 20 mL of pleural fluid.[30] In a study of patients with known pleural effusions, 81 US examinations were performed to quantify amount of pleural fluid.[31] Patients were examined in a supine position with mild trunk elevation of 15 degrees and with the probe placed in the posterior axillary line perpendicular to the body axis. The maximal distance between the visceral and parietal pleural (Sep) in end-expiration was measured, which allowed calculation of the estimated volume (V). The volume estimated by US was compared to the volume of fluid obtained after thoracentesis:

$$V\,(\text{mL}) = 20 \times \text{Sep}\,(\text{mm})$$

A positive correlation was seen with both Sep and V ($r = 0.72$ and $r^2 = 0.52$, respectively). The mean prediction of error of V was 158.4 ± 160.5 mL. No complications were noted during US-guided thoracentesis in this study.

Characterization of Pleural Effusion

US may also be able to help identify subtypes of pleural effusion (transudate or exudate). Pleural fluid patterns are characterized as anechoic, complex nonseptated, and complex septated.[32] In a study of 320 patients undergoing both thoracentesis and lung US, transudates were anechoic in appearance (the type of effusion was determined by both chemical analysis of pleural fluid and clinical evaluation (i.e., evaluation of ascites, peripheral edema)).[33] Complex septated or nonseptated effusions were always found to be exudates. At this time, however, US should not be substituted for thoracentesis and definitive chemical evaluation of pleural fluid.

Ultrasound-Guided Thoracentesis

US-guided thoracentesis is both safe and efficient. A study of 67 patients with pleural effusion compared US-guided to blind thoracentesis; the use of US prevented organ puncture in 10% of cases and increased identification of accurate puncture sites by 26%.[34] When performing an US-guided thoracentesis, the clinician should place the patient in a supine position and use a convex probe in the midaxillary line to detect the effusion. Prior to insertion of a needle, relevant anatomic landmarks should also be identified, including the rib space, diaphragm, and depth of effusion. The needle should be directed superior to the rib to avoid the neurovascular bundle.

Acute Respiratory Distress Syndrome/Acute Lung Injury

Using traditional CXR, ARDS can appear similar to AIS, cardiogenic pulmonary edema, and pulmonary fibrosis. Recently, attempts have been made to identify a lung US pattern unique to ARDS. A recent study compared the lung US findings of 58 patients, in which 18 met criteria for acute lung injury (ALI)/ARDS (based on the American–European Consensus Conference diagnostic criteria) and 40 had acute pulmonary edema.[35] In ALI or ARDS, the lung examination showed areas that were spared of B-lines, while in cardiogenic pulmonary edema, the distribution of B-lines was more diffuse. ALI/ARDS patients also had more posterior lung consolidations with typical air bronchogram findings and a pleural line with reduced "sliding" and thickened and coarser appearance. A recently published guideline for lung US in ARDS lists the following associated findings[4]:

1. Anterior subpleural consolidation
2. Absence or reduced lung sliding
3. Sparred areas of normal parenchyma
4. Pleural line abnormalities
5. Nonhomogenous distribution of B-lines

To date, these findings have not been validated in a prospective study and should not replace the traditional diagnostic approach to APE or ARDS/ALI.

BEDSIDE LUNG ULTRASOUND IN EMERGENCY (BLUE) PROTOCOL

A recent major study used a lung US-based algorithm (Fig. 7.9) to categorize shortness of breath in patients presenting to the ICU and compared results to final ICU diagnosis.[7] Rare causes or uncertain diagnosis were excluded from the study (<2%). Six lung zones were analyzed for A- or B-lines, lung sliding, and alveolar consolidation. An US of both lower extremities was also performed for deep venous thrombosis.

A predominantly A-line pattern was seen in patients with chronic obstructive lung disease (89% sensitivity and 97% specificity). Multiple anterior diffuse B-lines with lung sliding were seen in patients with pulmonary edema (97% sensitivity and 95% specificity). A normal lung examination and deep venous thrombosis on lower extremity US indicated pulmonary embolism (81% sensitivity and 99% specificity). Lack of lung sliding plus A-lines and a lung point indicated pneumothorax (81% sensitivity and 100% specificity). Anterior and posterior consolidations, anterior asymmetric interstitial patterns, or anterior diffuse B-lines with abolished lung sliding indicated pneumonia (89% sensitivity and 94% specificity). The postero-lateral alveolar and/or pleural syndrome (PLAPs) is an entity seen on US that usually indicates pneumonia and was used in the BLUE protocol algorithm. The postero-lateral segment is found on the lower lateral part of the chest wall and is positive if there is evidence of effusion and areas of consolidation. These patterns correctly identified the final diagnosis in 90.5% of cases. It should be noted that 41 patients were excluded from the study for the following reasons: multiple diagnoses, no final diagnosis, and "rare" causes such as interstitial lung disease or massive pleural effusion.

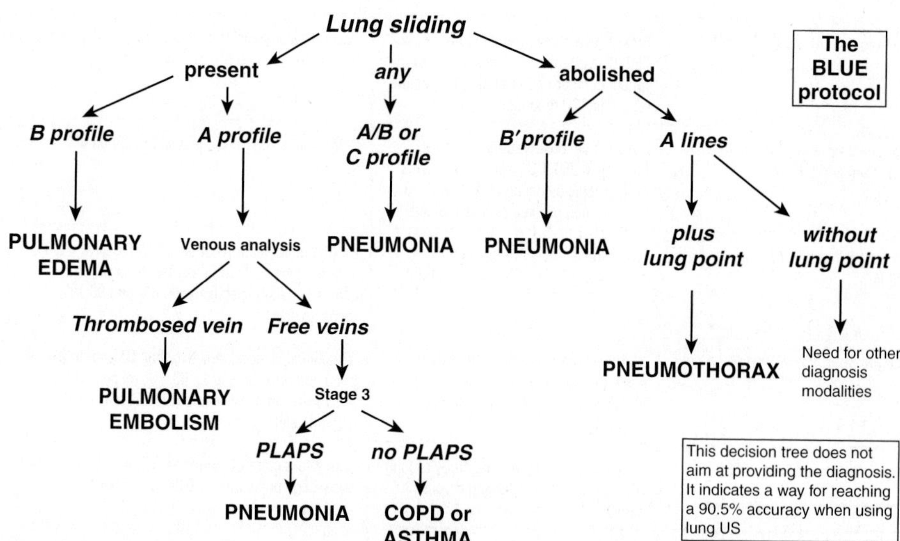

FIGURE 7.9 Blue Protocol Algorithm. PLAPS, posterior/lateral alveolar or pleural syndrome. From Lichtenstein D, Meziere G. Relevance of lung US in the diagnosis of acute respiratory failure: the BLUE protocol. *Chest.* 2008;134:117–125.

Limitations

Although bedside US is easy to perform in most patients, certain scenarios pose challenges. Obese patients with thick chest walls generate suboptimal images and limit artifact formation. Inadequate imaging may also occur in patients with subcutaneous emphysema or chest tubes and in trauma or postsurgical patients with large dressings in place. Adequate training is also essential in allowing a sonographer to recognize findings with confidence.[37]

CONCLUSION

The use of lung US has increased dramatically since its introduction in the 1980s. Portable US machines permit safe, cost-effective, and rapid detection of a variety of lung pathologies at bedside, while minimizing the need to transport patients away from the critical care setting. Lung US may help patients avoid harmful ionizing radiation exposure associated with repetitive CXR or CT.[36] Potential future uses of lung US include predicting successful extubation from the ventilator, evaluating recruitment maneuvers in mechanically ventilated patients, and differentiating ARDS from typical AIS patterns.

LITERATURE TABLE

TRIAL	DESIGN	RESULT
Volpicelli et al., *Intensive Care Med.* 2012[4]	Consensus recommendations	Definition of lung ultrasound findings
Lichtenstein et al., *Chest.* 2008[7]	Prospective observational study of 260 ICU patients with acute respiratory failure comparing initial lung US results with final ICU diagnosis	Accurate diagnosis of causes of respiratory failure by ultrasound in 90.5% of cases
Lichtenstein et al., *Am J Respir Crit Care Med.* 1997[9]	Prospective, observational study of lung US in 250 ICU patients, 121 with radiographic evidence of AIS and 129 without radiographic evidence of AIS	Comet-tail artifacts suggestive of AIS; 93.4% sensitivity
Kirkpatrick et al., *J Trauma.* 2004[19]	Prospective, observational cohort study of EFAST in 225 trauma patients	E-FAST more sensitive than CXR (48.8% vs. 20.9%) in detecting pneumothorax after trauma. Both exams had high specificity (99.6% and 98.7%, respectively)
Alrajhi et al., *Chest.* 2012[20]	Meta-analysis of 8 of 1,048 patients evaluated for pneumothorax, 864 of whom received with both CXR and lung US	Ultrasound is more sensitive than CXR to detect pneumothorax (90.9% vs. 50.2%, respectively). Both were similarly specific (98.2% and 99.4%, respectively)
Agricola et al., *Chest.* 2005[22]	Prospective, observational study of lung US in 20 patients following cardiac surgery	Comet tails correlate with EVLW ($r = 0.42$, $p = 0.001$) and wedge pressure ($r = 0.60$, $p = 0.0001$)
Noble et al., *Chest.* 2009[23]	Prospective, observational study of lung US in 40 patients undergoing hemodialysis	Significant B-line reduction as fluid is removed during dialysis ($p < 0.001$)
Mayo et al., *Chest.* 2009[37]	Consensus statement	Definition of competence in critical care ultrasonography

REFERENCES

1. National Institute of Clinical Excellence. *Final Appraisal Determination: Ultrasound Locating Devices for Placing Central Venous Catheters.* National Institute of Clinical Excellence; 2002.
2. American College of Emergency Physicians. Policy statement. Emergency ultrasound guidelines. *Ann Emerg Med.* 2009;53:550–570.
3. Lichtenstein D, Axler O. Intensive use of general ultrasound in the intensive care unit. Prospective study of 150 consecutive patients. *Intensive Care Med.* 1993;19(6):353–355.
4. Volpicelli G, Elbarbary M, Blaivas M, et al. International evidence-based recommendations for point-of-care lung ultrasound. *Intensive Care Med* 2012;38:577–591.
5. Chan VWS. *Ultrasound Imaging for Regional Anesthesia.* 2nd ed. Toronto, ON: Toronto Printing Company; 2009.
6. Fowler C, McCracken D. US Probes: risk of cross infection and ways to reduce it-comparison of cleaning methods. *Radiology.* 1999;213:299–300.
7. Lichtenstein D, Meziere G. Relevance of lung ultrasound in the diagnosis of acute respiratory failure: the BLUE protocol. *Chest.* 2008;134:117–125.
8. Lichtenstein DA. *Whole Body Ultrasonography in the Critically Ill.* Berlin, Germany: Springer-Verlag; 2010.
9. Lichtenstein D, Meziere G, Biderman P, et al. The comet-tail artifact. An ultrasound sign of alveolar-interstitial syndrome. *Am J Respir Crit Care Med.* 1997;156:1640–1646.
10. Rowan KR, Kirkpatrick AW, Liu D, et al. Traumatic pneumothorax detection with thoracic US: correlation with chest radiography and CT- initial experience. *Radiology.* 2002;225:210–214.
11. Neff MA, Monk JS, Peters K, et al. Detection of occult pneumothoraces on abdominal computed tomographic scans in trauma patients. *J Trauma.* 2000;49:281–285.
12. Tocino IM, Miller MH, Frederick PR, et al. CT detection of occult pneumothoraces in head trauma. *Am J Roentgenol.* 1984;143:987–990.
13. Rhea JT, Novelline RA, Lawrason J, et al. The frequency and significance of thoracic injuries detected on abdominal CT scans of multiple trauma patients. *J Trauma.* 1989;29:502–505.
14. Blaivas M, Lyon M, Duggal S. A prospective comparison of supine chest radiography and bedside ultrasound for the diagnosis of traumatic pneumothorax. *Acad Emerg Med.* 2005;12:844–849.
15. De Luca C, Valentino M, Rimondi M, et al. Use of chest sonography in acute-care radiology. *J Ultrasound.* 2008;11:125–134.
16. Lichtenstein DA, Meziere G, Lascols N, et al. Ultrasound diagnosis of occult pneumothorax. *Crit Care Med.* 2005;33:1231–1238.
17. Soldati G, Testa A, Pgnataro G, et al. The ultrasonographic deep sulcus sign in traumatic pneumothorax. *Ultrasound Med Biol.* 2006;32:1157–1163.
18. Lichtenstein D, Meziere G, Biderman P, et al. The "Lung Point": an ultrasound sign specific to pneumothorax. *Intensive Care Med.* 2000;26:1434–1440.
19. Kirkpatrick AW, Sirois M, Laupland KB, et al. Hand-held thoracic sonography for detecting post-traumatic pneumothoraces: the extended focused assessment with sonography for trauma (EFAST). *J Trauma.* 2004;57:288–295.
20. Alrajhi K, Woo MY, Vaillancourt C. Test characteristics of ultrasonography for the detection of pneumothorax: a systematic review and meta-analysis. *Chest.* 2012;141(3):703–708.
21. Volpicelli G, Caramello V, Cardinale L, et al. Bedside ultrasound of the lung for the monitoring of acute decompensated heart failure. *Am J Emerg Med.* 2008;26(5):585–591.
22. Agricola E, Bove T, Oppizzi M, et al. "Ultrasound comet-tail images": a marker of pulmonary edema: a comparative study with wedge pressure and extravascular lung water. *Chest.* 2005;127(5):1690–1695.
23. Noble V, Murray A, Capp R, et al. Ultrasound assessment for extravascular lung water in patients undergoing hemodialysis. *Chest.* 2009;135:1433–1439.
24. Lichtenstein DA, Lascols N, Meziere G, et al. Ultrasound diagnosis of alveolar consolidation in the critically ill. *Intensive Care Med.* 2004;30(2):276–281.
25. Parlamento S, Copetti R, Di Bartolomeo S. Evaluation of lung ultrasound for the diagnosis of pneumonia in the ED. *Am J Emerg Med.* 2009;27(4):379–384.
26. Lichtenstein D, Hulot JS, Rabiller A, et al. Feasibility and safety of ultrasound-aided thoracentesis in mechanically ventilated patients. *Intensive Care Med.* 1999;25:955–958.
27. Grimberg A, Shigueoka DC, Atallah AN, et al. Diagnostic accuracy of sonography for pleural effusion: systematic review. *Sao Paulo Med J.* 2010;128(2):90–95.

28. Brooks A, Davies B, Smethhurst M, et al. Emergency ultrasound in the acute assessment of haemothorax. *Emerg Med J.* 2004;21(1):44–46.
29. Webb WR, Higgins CB. *Thoracic Imaging: Pulmonary and Cardiovascular Radiology*. Philadelphia, PA: Lippincott Williams & Wilkins; 2004.
30. Rothlin MA, Nat R, Amgwerd M, et al. Ultrasound in blunt abdominal and thoracic trauma. *J Trauma.* 1993;34:488–495.
31. Balik M, Plasil P, Waldauf P et al. Usefulness of ultrasonography in predicting pleural fluid in mechanically ventilated patients. *Intensive Care Med.* 2006;32:318–321.
32. Marks WM, Filly RA, Callen PW. Real-time evaluation of pleural lesions: new observations regarding the probability of obtaining free fluid. *Radiology.* 1982;142:163–164.
33. Yang PC, Luh KT, Chang DB, et al. Value of sonography in determining the nature of pleural effusion: analysis of 320 cases. *AJR Am J Roentgenol.* 1992;159(1):29–33.
34. Diacon A, Brutsche M, Soler M. Accuracy of pleural puncture sites: a prospective comparison of clinical examination with ultrasound. *Chest.* 2003;123:436–441.
35. Copetti R, Soldati G, Copetti P. Chest sonography: a useful tool to differentiate acute cardiogenic pulmonary edema from acute respiratory distress syndrome. *Cardiovasc Ultrasound.* 2008;6:16.
36. Brenner D, Hall E. Computed tomography—an increasing source of radiation exposure. *N Engl J Med.* 2007;357:2277–2284.
37. Mayo PH, Beaulieu Y, Doelken P, et al. ACCP/La Societe de Reanimation de Langue Francaise statement on competence in critical care ultrasonography. *Chest.* 2009;135:1050–1060.

SECTION 4
Pulmonary Critical Care

8

Respiratory Failure and Mechanical Ventilation

Jon-Emile S. Kenny and Stephen Ruoss

BACKGROUND

Acute respiratory failure (ARF) is a life-threatening process that requires rapid identification and treatment by the emergency physician.[1] The causes of ARF are myriad, and its clinical presentation ranges from somnolence and hypopnea to profound tachypnea, tachycardia, and agitation. Appropriate diagnosis and treatment of ARF flow from a sound understanding of pulmonary pathophysiology.

Normal respiratory activity has been described as a functional chain, beginning with the central nervous system (CNS) and ending with the thoracic cage, muscles of respiration, pulmonary parenchyma, and the pulmonary vasculature.[3,4] A break in any of these links may result in ARF. ARF occurs when the respiratory system is unable to meet the metabolic needs of the tissues.[2] Classically, this clinical state is divided into hypoxemic and hypercapnic respiratory failure.

HYPOXEMIC RESPIRATORY FAILURE

Commonly cited causes of hypoxemia include global alveolar hypoventilation, diffusion impairment, ventilation–perfusion mismatch, and shunting.[2–4] Additionally, hypobaric (high-altitude) conditions, low inspired fraction of oxygen, and desaturated mixed venous blood can also cause hypoxemia.

Hypoventilation

Alveolar ventilation is the process by which the lungs deliver oxygen to the pulmonary capillaries and rid them of carbon dioxide. The alveolar gas equation describes the relationship between oxygen and carbon dioxide in the alveolus at a given atmospheric pressure and fraction of inspired oxygen:

$$PAO_2 = \left[P_{barometric} - P_{watervapor}\right] \times FiO_2 - \left[PaCO_2 / 0.8\right] \qquad \textbf{8.1}$$

(PAO_2 = alveolar partial pressure of oxygen, $PaCO_2$ = arterial partial pressure of carbon dioxide, FiO_2 = fraction of inspired oxygen)

This equation does not imply cause and effect; it is merely a description of the relationship between oxygen and carbon dioxide tensions in the alveolus. For instance, when the CNS is depressed as a result of a toxic or anatomical insult, normal alveolar ventilation may be impaired. In this context, the partial pressure of carbon dioxide in the alveolus will rise, and the partial pressure of oxygen in the alveolus will fall; the two processes however, are independent from one another—it is the alveolar hypoventilation that links both abnormalities.

The alveolar–arterial, or A–a, gradient is a calculation that provides a means of assessing how well oxygen is moving from the alveoli to the arterial blood:

$$\text{A-a gradient} = PAO_2 - PaO_2$$
$$\text{A-a gradient} = \left(\left[P_{\text{barometric}} - P_{\text{watervapor}}\right] \times FiO_2 - \left[PaCO_2 / 0.8\right]\right) - PaO_2 \quad \textbf{8.2}$$

An elevated A–a gradient (>10 mm Hg) is seen in patients with diffusion defects, ventilation–perfusion mismatch, or shunting. In the setting of hypoventilation, the difference between the alveolar oxygen concentration (as calculated from the alveolar gas equation above) and the measured arterial PaO_2 is minimal, and therefore the A–a gradient should be normal.

In practice, however, global alveolar hypoventilation is commonly complicated by states that also alter the pulmonary parenchyma (e.g., aspiration, compressive atelectasis). The administration of supplemental oxygen, a common intervention in these patients, can also cause ventilation–perfusion anomalies (See below) and nitrogen atelectasis.[2,3] These two factors can raise the A–a gradient, thereby diminishing the clinical utility of this calculation.

Diffusion Impairment

From the alveolus to the erythrocyte, a molecule of oxygen must pass through an alveolar epithelial cell, a small interstitial space, the pulmonary capillary endothelium and then into the erythrocyte. Any disease or disorder that disrupts this passive diffusion process is known as diffusion impairment. Diffusion impairment may contribute to—but rarely drives—hypoxemia. Normally, the concentration of oxygen in the alveolus and an erythrocyte equilibrate one-third of the way through the pulmonary capillary bed (carbon dioxide does so much more rapidly).[2,3] This rapid equilibration ensures that even when capillary transit time decreases substantially (e.g., during exercise) there will be no compromise of gas exchange. However, hypoxemia will be amplified when there is an effective decrease in alveolar–capillary surface area (e.g., severe emphysema or severe interstitial lung disease such as pulmonary fibrosis) in conjunction with increased pulmonary blood flow. When this pathologic state exists, the oxygen tension in the erythrocyte is unable to equilibrate with alveolar oxygen tension prior to the erythrocyte's passage through the pulmonary capillary bed.

Ventilation–Perfusion (V/Q) Mismatch

V/Q mismatch is the most common and important mechanism of hypoxemia encountered by the emergency physician.[1] Alveolar ventilation (Va) is determined by three variables: (1) respiratory rate (RR), (2) tidal volume (Vt), and (3) dead space fraction (Vd/Vt), as related in the following equation:

$$Va = [RR \times Vt] \times [1 - (Vd / Vt)] \quad \textbf{8.3}$$

(Va = alveolar ventilation, RR = respiratory rate, Vd = dead space ventilation, Vt = tidal volume)

The product of the RR and Vt is known as the minute ventilation (Mve). If alveolar ventilation to a unit of lung exceeds its blood flow (Q), the Va/Q ratio exceeds 1. Such Va/Q mismatch produces alveolar and capillary gas tensions similar to air (i.e., high oxygen and low carbon dioxide). While one would expect such lung units to be beneficial, they are, in fact, inefficient. Lung units with Va/Q ratios >1 yield a high partial pressure of oxygen in the pulmonary capillary; however, the arterial oxygen content draining from these units does not dramatically increase. Recall that the total oxygen content of blood is primarily determined by hemoglobin concentration and saturation, and that only a small portion of blood oxygen content is composed of dissolved oxygen. Because the oxyhemoglobin dissociation curve (Fig. 8.1) is largely flat once the PaO_2 is much >60 mm Hg, large increases in PaO_2 do not greatly increase oxygen saturation.

Unlike the oxyhemoglobin dissociation curve, the carbon dioxide dissociation curve is linear. Therefore, decrements in the partial pressure of carbon dioxide in high Va/Q lung units result in decreased carbon dioxide concentration, and therefore content, in pulmonary capillary blood. This is why normal, or low, carbon dioxide levels frequently accompany hypoxemia; the small increase in pH caused by carbon dioxide retention is a potent stimulus to augment alveolar ventilation and lower the $PaCO_2$.

Dead space is an area of the lung that is ventilated but not perfused. There is a normal amount of physiologic dead space in all lungs as the conducting airways do not participate in gas exchange. However, alveoli that are not perfused are considered pathologic dead space. These two types of dead space are referred to as anatomical and physiologic dead space, respectively. Dead space (both anatomical and physiologic)

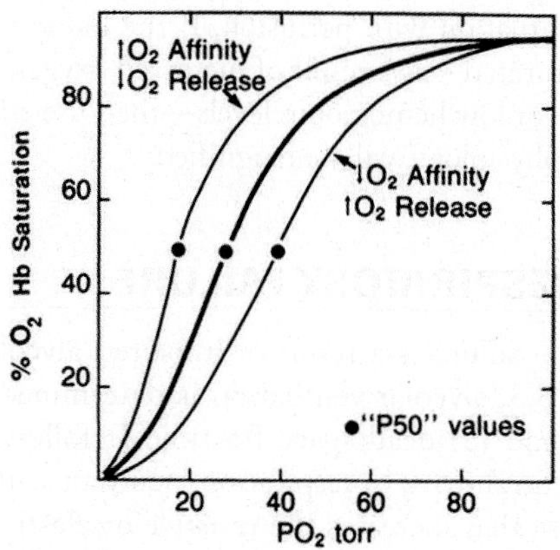

FIGURE 8.1 Oxyhemoglobin dissociation curve

is, by mathematical definition, a high Va/Q unit. However, rather than being a function of increased ventilation, dead space is the result of absent pulmonary blood flow (i.e., a Va/Q ratio of infinity). These portions of the lung behave differently from lung units with Va/Q ratios >1 (i.e., high Va/Q ratios). Examination of Equation 8.3 (above) reveals that dead space and alveolar ventilation (Va) are inversely proportional. Therefore, increased dead space results in a functionally low Va/Q physiology. As discussed below, the consequence of low Va/Q physiology is both hypoxemia and hypercapnia.

When alveolar ventilation (Va) falls in relation to perfusion (i.e., a low Va/Q), alveolar gas approaches the composition of mixed venous blood, resulting in a low partial pressure of oxygen and a high partial pressure of carbon dioxide. Consequently, these lung units result in low oxygen- and high carbon dioxide–containing blood. Because blood flow from low Va/Q lung units is by definition proportionately large relative to blood flow from normal or high Va/Q lung units, these lung units contribute disproportionately to the composite arterial blood gas values.

Shunt

Shunt is the most severe form of low Va/Q physiology (i.e., a Va/Q ratio of zero); shunt occurs when mixed venous blood passes into the left heart without participating in gas exchange. Shunt may have cardiac (e.g., patent foramen ovale) and/or pulmonary (e.g., severe pneumonia and acute respiratory distress syndrome [ARDS]) etiologies. The result of shunt is that mixed venous blood returns to the left heart without being exposed to alveolar gas. The more shunt a lung has, the more mixed venous blood oxygen content will contribute to arterial oxygen content. While it is commonly taught that shunt physiology does not respond to supplemental oxygen, this is only partly true. Oxygen-refractory hypoxemia due to shunt only begins to occur when the shunt fraction of the lung approaches 40% to 50%.[3] Notably, acute lung injury and ARDS typically occur when the shunt fraction approaches 20% to 30%.

Arterial oxygen saturation is determined by the mixed venous oxygen saturation—that is, the blood entering the lungs from the right ventricle—and the degree to which the lungs can match ventilation with perfusion. If the blood returning to the lungs is disproportionately desaturated—as a result of increased oxygen consumption in the tissues, low cardiac output, or low hemoglobin levels—then the effects of Va/Q mismatch, and in particular shunt physiology, will be magnified.

HYPERCAPNIC RESPIRATORY FAILURE

Hypercapnic respiratory failure is a result of impaired alveolar ventilation (Va). As described in Equation 8.3, alveolar ventilation is determined by three variables: (1) RR, (2) tidal volume, and (3) dead space fraction. It follows that hypercapnia can result from impaired central drive to respiration, neuromuscular weakness, chest wall deformities, lung disease that increases the resistive or elastic load on the lungs, and increased dead space. Many of the aforementioned disease states are also associated with Va/Q mismatch.

While it is intuitive how CNS depression and neuromuscular weakness lead to hypoventilation and hypercapnia, it is less obvious how diseases with increased pulmonary elastic and resistive loads like chronic obstructive pulmonary disease (COPD), asthma, and chronic heart failure (CHF) result in hypercapnia, as patients with these issues typically present with dramatically increased RRs. The important physiologic anomaly in these disease states is rapid shallow breathing. The shallow tidal volume (Vt) serves, despite the tachypnea, to both decrease minute ventilation (Mve) and increase the dead space fraction of ventilation. Because anatomical dead space (Vd) stays relatively constant, a precipitous drop in Vt acts to increase dead space fraction (Vd/Vt). As described above, true dead space ventilation prevents the lung from removing carbon dioxide, and while dead space is technically a high Va/Q ratio, its physiology mirrors that of low Va/Q units with hypoxemia and hypercapnia as a consequence.

The differential diagnosis of arterial hypercapnia should also include increased carbon dioxide production. Arterial carbon dioxide content is directly proportional to the tissue production of carbon dioxide and indirectly proportional to alveolar ventilation (Va).

$$PaCO_2 = VCO_2 / Va$$
$$\text{Or} \qquad (8.4)$$
$$PaCO_2 = VCO_2 / [RR \times Vt] \times [1 - (Vd / Vt)]$$

(VCO_2 = carbon dioxide production)

While increased production rarely is the sole cause of hypercapnia, it can be an important contributor, especially when work of breathing is high. With extremis, the muscles of respiration can increase total body carbon dioxide production by fourfold.[5] Fever also increases CO_2 production by approximately 10% per degree celsius.[6]

AN ALTERNATIVE DIAGNOSTIC APPROACH TO ARF

The traditional classification of respiratory failure as either hypoxemic or hypercapneic does provide some indication of underlying etiology of failure, and can help direct initial ventilator settings. Given the overlap between these etiologies discussed above, and the fact that Va/Q mismatch is by far the most common cause of ARF, a more physiologically intuitive and clinically useful approach to ARF may be to overlay the common insults to alveolar ventilation and perfusion onto the framework of the respiratory chain. To this end, a simplified scheme (Table 8.1) thus divides ARF into neuromuscular abnormalities and parenchymal abnormalities which include airway injury or dysfunction, alveolar injury, and pulmonary vascular injury.[2]

BASICS OF MECHANICAL VENTILATION

Mastering the basic nomenclature of mechanical ventilation is challenging, and is complicated by inconsistent naming among manufacturers and by novel ventilation modes available with newer devices. This section outlines the basics of mechanical ventilation. Ventilation strategies for specific disease entities are elaborated upon in following chapters.

TABLE 8.1 Causes of Acute Respiratory Failure

Neuromuscular Abnormalities	Pulmonary Parenchyma Abnormalities	
Hypoventilation	High Va/Q physiology and dead space	Low Va/Q physiology and Shunt
Typically hypoxemic and hypercapnic respiratory failure	Typically hypoxemic ± hypercapnic respiratory failure if dead space fraction high	Typically hypoxemic ± hypercapnic respiratory failure if dead space fraction high
Impaired central drive: brainstem lesions, toxicologic insults, nonconvulsive status epilepticus, myxedema, and CNS infection **Neuromuscular weakness:** C-spine injury, transverse myelitis, organophosphate toxicity, Guillain-Barré, phrenic nerve palsy, electrolyte disorders **Chest wall deformity:** kyphoscoliosis, thoracoplasty, obesity, massive ascites, flail chest	**Obstructive lung disease**: emphysema and bronchiectasis Acutely diminished cardiac output that lowers perfusion of the lungs relative to ventilation Pulmonary emboli Compromise of pulmonary perfusion due to high positive pressure ventilation and PEEP Rapid shallow breathing	**Diffuse bilateral lung lesions:** pulmonary edema, ARDS, alveolar hemorrhage **Unilateral lung lesion:** aspiration, atelectasis, edema, pneumothorax **Focal or multifocal lung lesions:** pneumonia, lung contusion, segmental atelectasis, infarction, effusion **Diffusion impairment:** interstitial lung disease, primary pulmonary hypertension

Modes of Invasive Mechanical Ventilation

Invasive ventilation entails the application of positive pressure via an endotracheal tube. The breath type delivered to the patient defines a mode of ventilation. Breath types, in turn, are defined by three variables: what triggers (initiates), limits (maintains), and cycles (terminates) a breath. While there are three variables, it is typically how a breath is cycled that categorizes the ventilation mode. Volume-cycled breaths are terminated when a preset volume has been achieved. Pressure-cycled breaths are terminated when a preset time has been reached (Fig. 8.2). While the later are technically time-cycled breaths, the common clinical parlance of 'pressure-cycled' is used here.

The choice between using volume-cycled and pressure-cycled modes of ventilation depends mostly on what the clinician desires to control. When a patient needs a guaranteed Mve (e.g., a patient with severe acid–base disturbances), it is prudent to choose a volume-cycled mode of ventilation because Mve is controlled directly. However, when airway pressure needs to be strictly managed (e.g., in a patient at risk of ventilator-induced lung injury and/or high airway pressures) then a pressure-cycled mode of mechanical ventilation should be instituted.

Importantly, when a clinician initiates and monitors ventilation that is volume cycled, there will be varying peak and plateau pressures depending on airway resistance and thoracic compliance, respectively. Conversely, Vt—and therefore Mve—will vary when pressure is the predetermined variable. A more detailed discussion of thoracic compliance and the relationship between airway pressure and Vt is presented below.

Volume-Cycled Ventilation

The two most common modes of volume-cycled ventilation are volume assist–control ventilation (AC; also known simply as assist–control), and synchronized

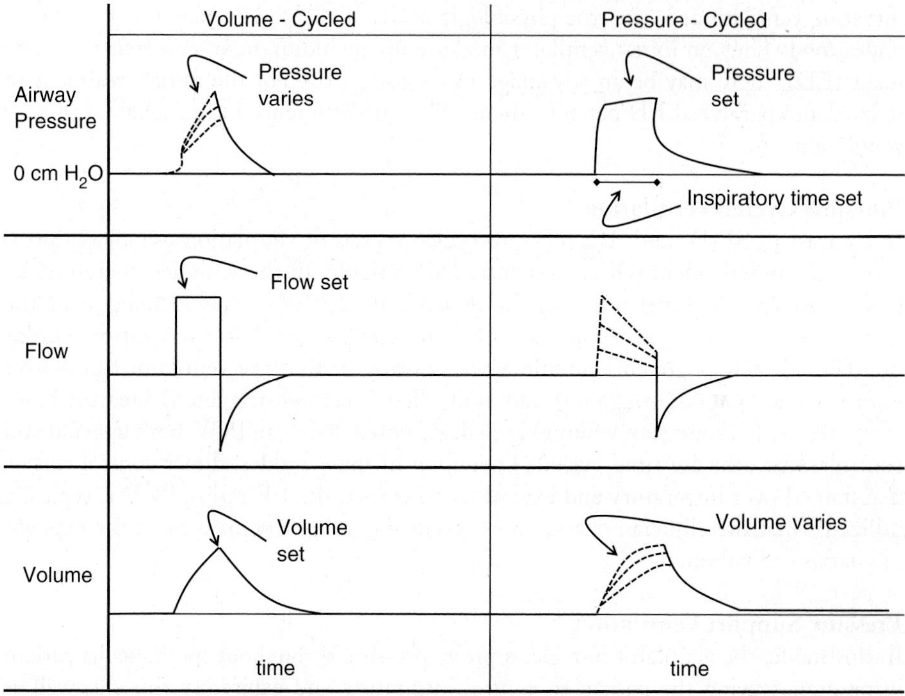

FIGURE 8.2 Volume-cycled versus pressure-cycled breaths

intermittent mandatory ventilation (SIMV). AC is defined by delivery of a set Vt for each breath, regardless of whether the breath is initiated by the ventilator or the patient. In AC mode, the patient receives, at a minimum, the ventilation rate and the tidal volume set on the ventilator. If a patient has an intrinsic respiratory drive to breathe at a rate faster than the one set on the mechanical ventilator in AC mode, the patient will still receive the full machine-delivered tidal volume for every breath initiated. Thus, AC ventilation mode involves assured delivery of a set and consistent Vt for any net RR, regardless of whether the patient or the machine is initiating the breath.

In contrast to AC, the central ventilation feature of SIMV is the delivery of the preset Vt to the patient only at the rate set on the ventilator. Breaths initiated by the patient over the set machine ventilation rate are not assisted with a preset Vt, but instead follow a Vt that is generated independently by the patient. Preset inspiratory pressure assistance—or pressure support—is an added feature that helps the patient to achieve a physiologically reasonable Vt in the absence of a set Vt for breaths initiated by the patient above and beyond the set RR.

Both AC and SIMV guarantee a minimum Mve, because the clinician directly sets both RR and Vt. An important operational difference between AC and SIMV is that AC will allow full Vt support for a patient breathing over the preset ventilation rate; in SIMV, if the preset ventilator rate is not sufficient for the patient's ventilator requirements, the patient will not receive an adequate Mve. This is particularly important when initiating ventilation, as the true physiologic needs of the patient may not yet be fully understood. Thus, in initial ventilator mode setup, including in an emergency department (ED), there may be an advantage in choosing AC. For the initial treatment of sedated and paralyzed ED patients, there will be no difference in the achieved minute ventilation.

Pressure-Cycled Ventilation

In contrast to SIMV and AC, pressure-cycled modes of ventilation use airway pressure as the independent (clinician-controlled) variable. In these modes, therefore, Vt (and consequently Mve) becomes the dependent variable and is a function of the preset pressure, airway resistance, and thoracic compliance. Pressure control ventilation (PCV) is analogous to volume assist–control, in that the ventilator can deliver both assisted (patient-triggered) and controlled (machine-triggered) breaths; however, they are pressure (not volume) cycled. As noted above, in PCV, both assisted and controlled breaths are time-cycled. Therefore, in these modes, direct control can be maintained over inspiratory and expiratory time (i.e., the I:E ratio). PCV is typically utilized when the clinician desires direct control over airway pressure at the expense of guaranteed volume.

Pressure Support Ventilation

In this mode, the ventilator provides a preset pressure throughout spontaneous patient inspiration, leaving the patient to control inspiratory and expiratory times as well as achieved Vt. Given the dependence of pressure support ventilation (PSV) on patient cooperation and effort, respiratory support provided by this mode can be altered substantially by patient sedation, respiratory muscular weakness, or clinical features such as pain or agitation. PSV is commonly used in the ICU prior to extubation (i.e., as a "weaning" mode), and so is unlikely to be encountered in the ED.

Noninvasive Positive Pressure Ventilation

Noninvasive positive pressure ventilation (NIPPV) entails the application of positive pressure to the patient via a tight-fitting mask over the nose or mouth and nose. Essentially, there are two modes of NIPPV—bilevel positive airway pressure (BiPAP) and continuous positive airway pressure (CPAP). As the name suggests, BiPAP requires that the clinician set two pressure variables: the inspiratory positive airway pressure (IPAP) and the expiratory positive airway pressure (EPAP). The change in pressure in BiPAP—referred to as the "delta"—is the IPAP minus the EPAP, because both pressures are referenced to zero (atmospheric) pressure. The difference between inspiratory and expiratory pressure is the driving pressure to support alveolar ventilation and CO2 clearance. Note that the EPAP is equivalent to the positive end-expiratory pressure, or PEEP, value used with invasive modes of ventilation, and is defined as the set pressure above atmospheric pressure that is delivered throughout expiration. BiPAP can be thought of as the noninvasive equivalent to PSV. One important difference between PSV and BiPAP is the terminology used to define the pressure parameters. In PSV, the inspiratory pressure is delivered above a baseline PEEP. In BiPAP, the IPAP is always delivered above atmospheric pressure, not above EPAP.

CPAP, by contrast, requires only one pressure preset. A single pressure is delivered throughout the respiratory cycle; that is, the IPAP and EPAP are the same. CPAP mainly benefits oxygenation by stenting open collapsed airways, thereby reducing the number of low Va/Q lung units. Because BiPAP has preset inspiratory and expiratory pressures, BiPAP increases the Vt and therefore aids in ventilation (CO2 elimination) as well as oxygenation.

AIRWAY PRESSURES DURING MECHANICAL VENTILATION

Two important physiologic aspects of mechanical ventilator support are airway pressures and PEEP. The peak airway pressure (also known as the peak inspiratory pressure or PIP) measured by the ventilator is the pressure required to overcome both the thoracic (lung and chest wall) compliance and the airway resistance (Equation 8.5). Compliance describes the change in volume with respect to a change in pressure in a deformable object. For example, a poorly compliant thorax has a small change in volume for a large change in pressure. Airway resistance, analogous to resistance in blood vessels, describes the mechanical factors that limit airflow. There are approximately 23 generations, or branching points, of airways from the trachea to the alveoli, and the resistance to airflow is highly dependent upon the cumulative cross-sectional area of each generation in parallel. While the trachea has a larger diameter than a single terminal bronchiole, the trachea has a much smaller diameter than the entire cross-sectional diameter of all the terminal bronchioles in parallel. Hence, the trachea contributes more to airway resistance than do the terminal bronchioles in the healthy lung.

$$\mathrm{PIP} = (\mathrm{Vt} / \mathrm{Ct}) + (\mathrm{Raw} \times \mathrm{Q}) \qquad \textbf{8.5}$$

(PIP = peak inspiratory pressure, Vt = tidal volume, Ct = thoracic compliance, Raw = airway resistance, Q = airflow)

Note that Equation 8.5 divides PIP into two components—a static component that is determined by the Vt and the compliance of the thorax, and a dynamic component that is determined by the flow of gas and the composite resistance of the lungs' airways. Consequently, an increase in airway resistance or a decrease in thoracic compliance will increase peak airway pressure. Distinguishing between the two requires a cessation of airflow at end-inspiration. In the absence of airflow (i.e., Q is zero), the resistive component is removed from the equation, and the pressure that remains is related only to the thoracic compliance; this pressure is referred to as the plateau pressure.

When evaluating a patient with high PIPs, a large pressure drop between the peak and plateau pressure suggests an excess of airway resistance. Conversely, if there is little difference between the peak and plateau pressures, there is likely a poorly compliant lung or chest wall (Fig. 8.3). Normal peak and plateau values are approximately 20 and 10 cm H_2O, respectively. An inspiratory hold maneuver is best carried out in a volume-cycled mode of ventilation rather than a pressure-cycled one. This is because in volume-cycled ventilation, pressure is the dependent variable.

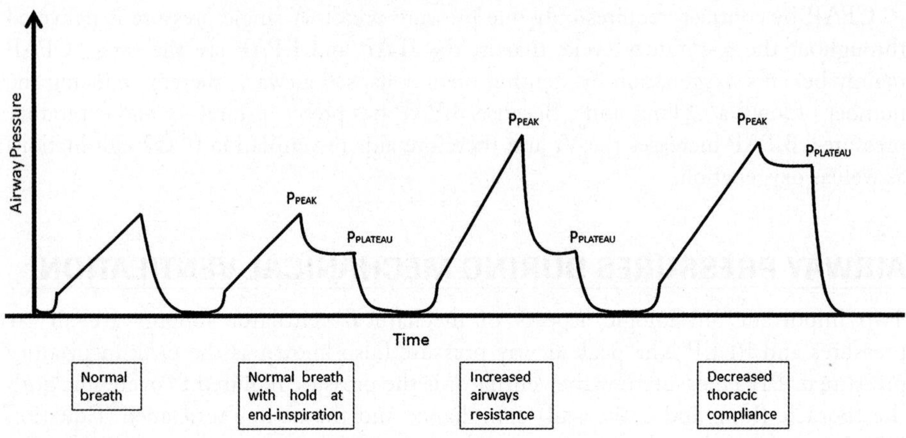

FIGURE 8.3 Peak and plateau pressures

PEEP may be applied to a patient supported with either invasive or noninvasive ventilation. It is often applied to some small degree under the guise of replacing the "physiologic PEEP," which is reportedly lost when the endotracheal tube separates the vocal cords.[7] While there is little evidence that physiologic PEEP exists, PEEP can be applied therapeutically to aid in oxygenation.[8] Typical PEEP levels range between 5 and 15 cm H_2O. PEEP promotes oxygenation by preventing alveolar and small airway closure at end-expiration. As previously noted, multiple mechanisms may result in low Va/Q lung units. For example, increased airway resistance due to inflammation, secretions and airway edema; physical compression secondary to habitus; and excessively compliant airways may all lead to low alveolar ventilation relative to perfusion. The judicious application of PEEP preserves patent airways and maintains the lung on a mechanically favorable portion of its compliance curve.

While PEEP has beneficial applications, it can be detrimental to both the heart and lungs. PEEP has a profound effect on mean airway pressure and can exert a multitude of effects on the right heart, pulmonary vasculature, and left heart. Specifically, excessive PEEP can impair venous return, which in turn has the potential to diminish cardiac output and compromise oxygen delivery to the tissues.[9] Excessive PEEP can also lead to alveolar rupture.[10]

The time constant of a lung unit describes the length of time required for inflation and deflation of a ventilated portion of the lung. The time constant is directly proportional to the resistance and compliance of the lung unit. Hence, if the resistance or the compliance of a lung unit increases, the time it takes to deflate increases. This is particularly important in patients with emphysema, as both resistance and compliance may be dramatically elevated. If lung units fail to deflate before a subsequent breath is taken (or delivered by a ventilator), retained volume—and consequently pressure—can build within portions of the lung. This phenomenon is called auto-PEEP or intrinsic PEEP. The risk of auto-PEEP becomes greatest in patients with airway obstruction and tachypnea. In order to detect auto-PEEP, the clinician must first anticipate its existence. On the ventilator, the presence of an expiratory

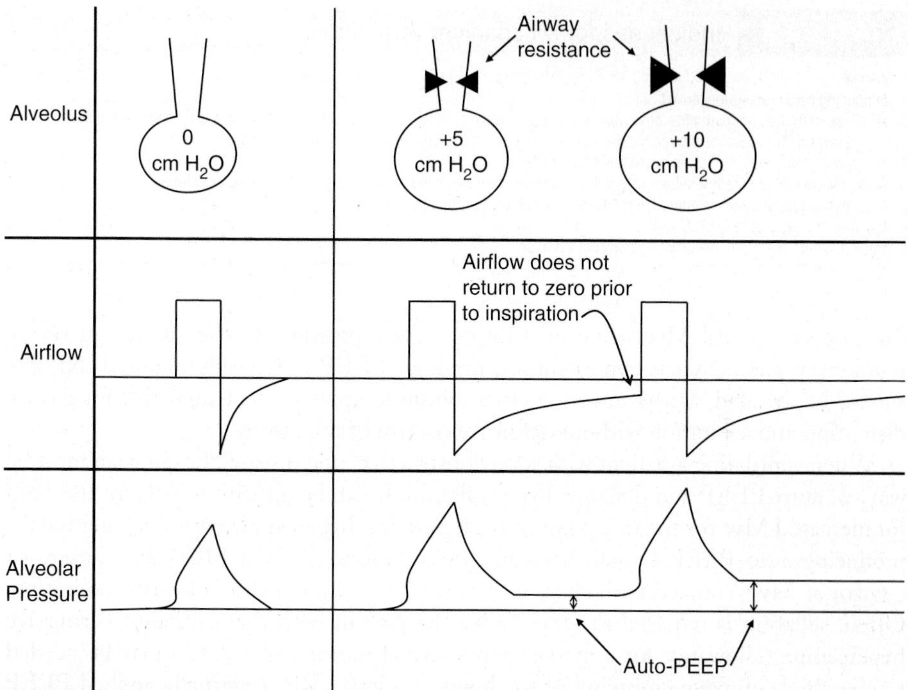

FIGURE 8.4 Auto-PEEP

flow curve that does not reach zero flow prior to a subsequent breath is suggestive of auto-PEEP (Fig. 8.4). Since the pressure at end-expiration is the sum total of both extrinsic (machine delivered) and intrinsic PEEP, an end-expiratory breath hold maneuver is another way to reveal pressure present in the airway. Just as with extrinsic PEEP, excessive auto-PEEP can diminish venous return to the right heart and negatively impact cardiac output. Treatment of auto-PEEP that results in hemodynamic compromise includes briefly removing the patient from the ventilator to allow for lung and chest decompression. For ongoing correction of intrinsic PEEP, sedating the patient and/or lowering the set RR and decreasing the inspiratory time (and thus prolonging the expiratory time at any given ventilation rate) will all help avoid or reverse intrinsic PEEP.

BASIC STRATEGIES OF MECHANICAL VENTILATION IN RESPIRATORY FAILURE

Indications for mechanical ventilation can be difficult to define for all clinical conditions. Often, it is a gestalt decision based upon the clinical status of the patient in combination with objective measures such as pulse oximetry and arterial blood gas sampling (Table 8.2). When neurologic insult impairs global alveolar ventilation, the resultant hypoxemia and hypercapnia are usually easily managed with invasive mechanical ventilation. A volume-cycled mode such as AC or SIMV is preferred, because the clinician

TABLE 8.2 Indications for Mechanical Ventilation

1. Apnea
2. Impending cardiorespiratory arrest
3. Acute exacerbation of obstructive airways disease with acute respiratory acidosis especially if any of the following are present: Cardiovascular instability, altered mental status, excessive secretions, inability to tolerate NIPPV, pH < 7.2
4. Acute ventilatory insufficiency in neuromuscular disease
5. Acute hypoxemic respiratory failure despite high supplemental FiO_2 especially if any of the following are present: Cardiovascular instability, altered mental status, inability to protect the airway
6. Inability to protect airway (GCS < 9)
7. Head and neck trauma or mass with airway compromise

can directly control Mve while monitoring airway pressure. In the absence of severe pulmonary parenchymal abnormalities, minimal PEEP is typically required. NIPPV should be avoided, as the unconscious or obtunded patient is at high risk for gastric distention and aspiration without definitive control of the airway.

When ventilating a patient with severe obstructive lung disease, the clinician must be wary of auto-PEEP and dynamic hyperinflation. It can be difficult to balance the need for increased Mve for the treatment of these patients' hypercapnia with the potential for producing auto-PEEP. Usually a volume-cycled mode (A/C or SIMV) is chosen for control of Mve, coupled with short inspiratory times to allow for adequate expiration. Often, sedation is required to synchronize the patient with the ventilator. Permissive hypercapnia (allowance for a modest supranormal increase in $PaCO_2$) may be needed to allow for complete emptying of the lungs at a lower RR. Externally applied PEEP can be useful in emphysema, a condition in which increased airway compliance makes the alveoli susceptible to collapse during positive pressure ventilation (See Chapter 9). Furthermore, when auto-PEEP exists, extrinsic PEEP may decrease the pressure gradient required to trigger the ventilator. While adding extrinsic PEEP to aid a patient with excessive intrinsic PEEP may seem counterintuitive, the rationale is that ventilators use small deflections in airway pressure as the signal to begin a subsequent breath (pressure triggered). Ventilators may also use changes in flow and time as other variables to trigger breaths. The drop in pressure that must be achieved to trigger a breath is referenced to the preset (extrinsic) PEEP. If there is superimposed intrinsic PEEP, then the patient must create a pressure drop that includes all of the intrinsic PEEP plus the trigger value below the extrinsic PEEP. Increasing the extrinsic PEEP will narrow this pressure differential and ease breath triggering.[11]

When managing alveolar and/or interstitial edema, it is recommended to adopt a low-lung-volume ventilation strategy, especially if ARDS is the presumed cause of ARF.[2] In this paradigm, plateau pressures of <30 cm H_2O are desirable. If a volume-cycled mode of ventilation is chosen, peak and plateau pressures should be closely monitored. This hazard can be avoided by placing the patient on a pressure-cycled mode (e.g., PCV), which allows the clinician to select the delivered pressure. The trade-off of selecting a pressure-cycled mode, however, is that close observation of Vt and Mve (the dependent variables) is required. As ventilators become more sophisticated, modes of ventilation that deliver safe levels of pressure to obtain a preset volume (e.g., pressure-regulated volume control) are being adopted. However, the only mode of ventilation known to improve mortality in ARDS is volume control, as this was used in the ARDSNet trial.[2]

The use of NIPPV for COPD exacerbations has been demonstrated to decrease mortality and intubation rates, and improved long-term outcomes.[13] Evidence for the application of NIPPV in acute asthma is less robust.[14] While there is evidence to support the use of NIPPV in cardiogenic pulmonary edema to improve dyspnea, gas exchange, and perhaps prevent intubation,[15,16] the data for ARDS are less definitive.[17,18]

CONCLUSION

Acute respiratory failure is a life-threatening process that requires rapid identification and treatment. The decision to initiate mechanical ventilation is always best made by the emergency physician at bedside, however a nuanced understanding of the different etiologies of respiratory failure and optimal corresponding modes of ventilatory support described in this chapter can help ensure patient safety and improve outcomes.

LITERATURE TABLE

TRIAL	DESIGN	RESULT
Acute Respiratory Distress Syndrome		
The ARDS Network, *N Engl J Med.* 2000[12]	861 patients with acute lung injury and ARDS in a multicenter, randomized controlled trials (RCT) comparing ventilation with Vt of 12 mL/kg and Pplat of 50 cm H_2O or less to ventilation with Vt of 6 mL/kg and Pplat of 30 cm H_2O or less	In patients with acute lung injury or ARDS ventilated with Vt targeted to 6 mL/kg and Pplat <30 cm H_2O, there was a 9% absolute risk reduction in mortality (31% vs. 39.8%, $p = 0.007$) compared to 12 mL/kg and Pplat of <50 cm H_2O
Agarwal et al., *Respir Care.* 2010[17]	Meta-analysis of 13 studies including 540 patients assessing the efficacy of NIPPV in patients with ALI/ARDS by means of measured intubation and mortality rates	The pooled intubation rate was 48% in patients treated with NIPPV, and the pooled mortality rate was 35%. There were no trials comparing NIPPV and standard mechanical ventilation
Zhan et al., *Crit Care Med.* 2012[18]	Multicenter prospective RCT that compared the use of high-concentration oxygen therapy to NIPPV in 40 patients with acute lung injury (P/F ratio <300, but >200)	NIPPV reduced intubation rate (1 in 21 in the NIPPV group vs. 4 in 19 in the control group, $p = 0.04$), and number of organ system failures (3 in NIPPV vs. 14 in control, $p < 0.001$); as well, there was a trend towards reduced in-hospital mortality in the NIPPV group
Exacerbations of Obstructive Airways Disease		
Ram et al., *Cochrane Database Syst Rev.* 2004[13]	Meta-analysis of 14 RCTs that compared NIPPV versus usual medical care in patients with respiratory failure due to COPD with a $PaCO_2$ >45 mm Hg	NIPPV compared to usual medical care resulted in decreased mortality (RR 0.52; 95% CI, 0.35, 0.76), decreased need for intubation (RR 0.41; 95% CI 0.33, 0.53), reduction in treatment failure (RR 0.48; 95% CI 0.37, 0.63), reduction in hospital stay (mean difference −3.24 days; 95% CI −4.42, −2.06) and improved physiologic parameters such as pH and vital signs
Soroksky et al., *Chest.* 2004[14]	Prospective, RCT comparing BiPAP to sham BiPAP in 30 patients with acute exacerbations of asthma in the emergency department	Patients who received treatment compared to sham were more likely to improve their FEV1 by at least 50% (80% vs. 20%, $p < 0.004$) and were less likely to require hospitalization (18% vs. 63%, $p = 0.013$)

(*Continued*)

LITERATURE TABLE (*Continued*)

TRIAL	DESIGN	RESULT
Cardiogenic Pulmonary Edema		
Gary et al., 3CPO Trial Group. *NEJM.* 2008[15]	Multicenter, prospective, RCT of nearly 1,100 patients with acute cardiogenic pulmonary edema assigned to standard O_2 therapy, CPAP (5–15 cm H_2O), or BiPAP (IPAP 8–20 cm H_2O; EPAP, 4–10 cm of water). The primary end point for the comparison between noninvasive ventilation and standard oxygen therapy was death within 7 d after the initiation of treatment, and the primary end point for the comparison between BiPAP and CPAP was death or intubation within 7 d	No significant difference in 7-d mortality between patients receiving standard therapy and those undergoing noninvasive ventilation. No significant difference in the combined end point of death or intubation between the two groups of patients undergoing noninvasive ventilation (11.7% for CPAP and 11.1% for BiPAP). As compared with standard oxygen therapy, NIPPV was associated with greater improvements at 1 h in patient-reported dyspnea, heart rate, acidosis, and hypercapnia. There were no treatment-related adverse events
Weng et al., *Ann Intern Med.* 2010[16]	Meta-analysis of randomized trials that compared CPAP and BiPAP with standard therapy or each other in patients with acute cardiogenic pulmonary edema. The outcomes were mortality, intubation rate, and new incidence of MI	Compared with standard therapy, CPAP reduced mortality (RR 0.64; 95% CI, 0.44–0.92) and need for intubation (RR 0.44; 95% CI, 0.32–0.60), but not new incidence of MI. BiPAP reduced the need for intubation (RR 0.54; 95% CI, 0.33–0.86) but did not reduce mortality or new MI. No differences were detected between CPAP and BiPAP on any clinical variables for which they were compared

CI, confidence interval; RR, relative risk.

REFERENCES

1. Stefan MS, Shieh MS, Pekow PS, et al. Epidemiology and outcomes of acute respiratory failure in the United States, 2001 to 2009: a national survey. *J Hosp Med.* 2013;8:76–82.
2. Greene KE, Peters JI. Pathophysiology of acute respiratory failure. *Clin Chest Med.* 1994;15:1–12.
3. D'Alonzo GE, Dantzger DR. Mechanisms of abnormal gas exchange. *Med Clin North Am.* 1983;67:557–571.
4. MacSweeney RM, McAuley DF, Matthay MA. Acute lung failure. *Semin Respir Crit Care Med.* 2011;32:607–625.
5. Roussos C, Koutsoukou A. Respiratory failure. *Eur Respir J.* 2003;22:3S–14S.
6. Manthous CA, Hall JB, et al. Effect of cooling on oxygen consumption in febrile critically ill patients. *Am J Respir Crit Care Med.* 1995;151:10–14.
7. Fernández-Mondéjar E. Prophylactic positive end-expiratory pressure: are good intentions enough? *Crit Care.* 2003;7:191.
8. Rimensberger PC, Cox PN, et al. The open lung during small tidal volume ventilation: concepts of recruitment and "optimal" positive end-expiratory pressure. *Crit Care Med.* 1999;27(9):1946–1952.
9. Lueke T, Pelosi P. Clinical review: positive end-expiratory pressure and cardiac output. *Crit Care.* 2005;9(6):607–621.
10. Dos Santos CC, Slutsky AS. Mechanisms of ventilator-induced lung injury: a perspective. *J Appl Physiol.* 2000;89:1645–1655.
11. MacIntyre NR, et al. Applied PEEP during pressure support reduces the inspiratory threshold load of intrinsic PEEP. *Chest.* 1997;111(1):188–193.
12. The Acute Respiratory Distress Network. Ventilation with lower tidal volumes as compared with traditional tidal volumes for acute lung injury and the acute respiratory distress syndrome. *N Engl J Med.* 2000;342(18):1301–1308.
13. Ram FS, Picot J, et al. Non-invasive positive pressure ventilation for treatment of respiratory failure due to exacerbations of chronic obstructive pulmonary disease. *Cochrane Database Syst Rev.* 2004;(3):CD004104.

14. Soroksky A, et al. A pilot prospective, randomized, placebo-controlled trial of bilevel positive airway pressure in acute asthmatic attack. *Chest.* 2003;123(4):1018.
15. Gray A, Goodacre S, et al. 3CPO Trialists. Noninvasive ventilation in acute cardiogenic pulmonary edema. *N Engl J Med.* 2008;359(2):142–151.
16. Weng CL, Zhao YT, et al. Meta-analysis: noninvasive ventilation in acute cardiogenic pulmonary edema. *Ann Intern Med.* 2010;152(9):590–600.
17. Agarwal R, Aggarwal AN, Gupta D. Role of noninvasive ventilation in acute lung injury/acute respiratory distress syndrome: a proportion meta-analysis. *Respir Care.* 2010;55(12):1653–1660.
18. Zhan Q, et al. Early use of noninvasive positive pressure ventilation for acute lung injury; a multicenter randomized controlled trial. *Crit Care Med.* 2012;40(2):455.

9

Ventilation Strategies in COPD, Asthma, and Pulmonary Arterial Hypertension

Jey K. Chung, Paul K. Mohabir, and Stephen Ruoss

BACKGROUND

Chronic obstructive pulmonary disease (COPD), asthma, and pulmonary arterial hypertension (PAH) are diseases that are commonly encountered in an emergency department (ED) setting. It is estimated that 1.5 million patients visit the ED in the United States each year for COPD exacerbations, 1.75 million for acute asthma, and 200,000 for PAH.[1–3] The appropriate initiation and management of emergent ventilatory support in these patients requires a nuanced understanding of the pathophysiology of these diseases.

DISEASE PATHOPHYSIOLOGY

Severe airflow obstruction is typically encountered in asthma and COPD, the latter of which includes both chronic bronchitis and emphysema. In both asthma and chronic bronchitis, the central pathologic events include inflammation, increased mucus (due to both hypersecretion and inflammation), and airway caliber reduction due to the combination of these processes. Airways in asthma and chronic bronchitis also suffer from decreased compliance, or compromised airway caliber expansion during spontaneous inspiration or positive pressure ventilation. The consequence of these pathologic effects is a limitation of airflow during both inspiration and expiration, both of which are important considerations when initiating mechanical ventilation in these patients.

The pathology of emphysema is different, even while the resulting expiratory airflow limitation can be similarly extreme. Emphysema is characterized by a loss of parenchymal lung elastic tissue, and thus a loss of the normal elastic recoil forces that hold open the smaller conducting airways. The result is that conducting airways tend to collapse with normal expiration; in marked contrast to airways in asthma, conducting airways in emphysema have greater compliance, and this airflow obstruction can magnify with increased expiratory effort during spontaneous breathing. Appreciating these distinct disease processes is critically important when considering mechanical ventilation for these patients.

Another important pathologic feature present in all patients with acute airflow obstruction is an increase in the work of breathing because of the greater airway resistance in these diseases; left untreated, a sustained increase in work of breathing can quickly lead to respiratory muscle fatigue and failure.

PAH has diverse pathologic causes, but a number of characteristics are common to all etiologies of this disease. These include an already-increased pulmonary arterial resistance and an associated increase in right ventricular afterload. Increases in pulmonary arterial resistance are seen with hypoxemia, hypercapnia (with magnified response to the combination of both), as well as with significant increases or decreases in lung volume because of lung parenchymal compression and overdistension of the pulmonary vascular beds, respectively.

VENTILATION STRATEGIES IN COPD AND ASTHMA

Patients who present with exacerbations of obstructive airway disease have an acute or chronic increase in airway resistance and an associated increase in work of breathing. This process heightens the risk of respiratory muscle fatigue and decompensation, which can compound already inadequate ventilation and increase the risk of respiratory failure. The application of assisted ventilation, by either noninvasive or invasive modes, can help reduce a patient's work of breathing. The underlying increased airway resistance persists, however, and can be challenging to manage. Comprehensive therapy therefore combines support of respiratory mechanics (assistance with ventilation as well as reduction of work of breathing) with administration of bronchodilator and anti-inflammatory medications.

Noninvasive Ventilation Support

Noninvasive positive pressure ventilation (NIPPV) can be an appropriate first-line adjunct to medical therapy in the management of obstructive airway disease. When properly applied, NIPPV can preclude the need for invasive mechanical ventilation and its associated risks of trauma (direct, mechanical trauma or barotrauma), infection, adverse effects of sedation, increased length of hospital stay, and difficulty or failure to wean from the ventilator.[4]

The benefits of NIPPV assistance in respiratory distress from COPD are significant and well documented. A 1995 multicenter randomized control trial (RCT) of 85 patients with COPD compared NIPPV with standard treatment and demonstrated a decreased rate of intubation (26% vs. 74%), frequency of complications (16% vs. 48%), length of hospital stay (23 vs. 35 days), and inpatient mortality rates (9% vs. 29%).[5] A MEDLINE and EMBASE review of similarly designed RCTs from 1968 to 2006 confirmed a consistent significant reduction in the risk of intubation (65%), in-hospital mortality (55%), and length of hospitalization (1.9 days) when NIPPV was used for acute exacerbation of COPD.[6] A 2003 Cochrane systemic review meta-analysis of eight RCTs evaluating the use of NIPPV as an adjunct to usual medical care in COPD exacerbations similarly demonstrated a lower mortality risk (RR 0.41), shorter hospital stays (−3.24 days), and greater improvements at 1 hour in pH (+0.03), $PaCO_2$ (−0.04 kPa), and respiratory rate (−3.08 breaths per minute).[7] While the benefits of noninvasive ventilation are well established in COPD, its efficacy is less well established, and its use more controversial, in the setting of status asthmaticus.[8]

The decision to undertake a trial of noninvasive ventilation rather than proceed directly to intubation and mechanical ventilation is largely based on clinical judgment. Studies show that the majority of patients with asthma, even those with some degree of hypercapnia, can be successfully managed noninvasively.[9,10] Similarly, in an RCT of 49 patients who failed standard ED medical therapy for COPD exacerbations, the use of NIPPV as a rescue therapy averted the need for intubation in 48%. Factors supporting the decision to initiate invasive ventilation in both COPD and asthma include refractory hypoxemia, severe hypercapnia ($PaCO_2$ > 60 mm Hg), significant acidosis (pH < 7.25), and the inability to tolerate noninvasive ventilation, whether due to unsustainable dyspnea with increased respiratory frequency or altered mental status. Certainly, failure of a noninvasive ventilation trial or cardiorespiratory arrest calls for immediate intubation.[11,12]

Mechanical Ventilation Support

If the decision is made to initiate invasive ventilatory support, either assist–control ventilation or synchronized intermittent mandatory ventilation, using volume or pressure cycling, may be used; no one mode of ventilation has been found consistently superior in the treatment of these conditions. There are, however, a number of ventilator parameters that should be carefully selected and continuously evaluated when managing these patients.

The initiation of mechanical ventilation involves a substantial shift in the physiology of ventilation, with multiple, immediately relevant effects. The principal physiologic differences for the clinician to remember are that:

- Positive pressure (with or without patient assistance) is now being used to achieve lung inflation.
- Inspiratory peak pressures from positive pressure ventilation will necessarily be increased in the context of the high airflow resistance caused by airway inflammation and narrowing and/or dynamic collapse.
- The time needed for complete exhalation will be substantially increased due to the marked airflow obstruction, and if adequate (prolonged) expiratory times are not allowed by the ventilator parameters, lung gas volumes will increase ("air trapping" and "hyperinflation") and intrapulmonary and intrathoracic pressures will rise ("induced, or intrinsic, positive end-expiratory pressure [PEEP]").

By far, the most potentially harmful of these adverse physiologic effects is the production of higher intrathoracic pressures and induced PEEP, which can result in both pulmonary and cardiac compromise. Pulmonary effects include barotrauma (i.e., pneumothorax, interstitial emphysema with pneumomediastinum) and parenchymal ventilator–induced lung injury. In addition, increased intrathoracic pressure increases thoracic volume, which results in chest wall distension (and a less compliant chest wall) and a greater ventilator workload for any patient assisting with mechanical ventilation (i.e., taking spontaneous breaths in addition to the set mechanical respiratory rate). This increased work of breathing can raise metabolic demand, further destabilizing an already compromised patient. Cardiac effects include reduced biventricular preload and increased pulmonary artery resistance (increased RV afterload), with resulting diminished cardiac output. Given this array of potential issues, the goal when initiating mechanical ventilation in patients with severe airflow obstruction is to employ techniques and parameters that avoid or at least limit pulmonary and cardiac compromise.

Minimization of induced intrathoracic air trapping and intrinsic PEEP is achieved by using either a shorter inspiratory time (which, for a fixed respiratory rate, will produce a lengthened I:E ratio) or a lower respiratory rate (which, with a fixed inspiratory time, will also produce a lengthened I:E ratio). As inspiratory time is shortened, ventilator inspiratory flow rate will necessarily be increased in volume-cycle ventilation modes to achieve the specified tidal volume, often into the range of 80–100 L/min.

As a working example of the adjustment of ventilator parameters to achieve a lengthened I:E ratio and lessened barotrauma risk, consider the following example in volume-cycled ventilation:

A. Initial ventilator settings:
- ○ Ventilator mode: volume cycle assist control ventilation
- ○ Ventilator rate: 20 (i.e., a 3-second breath cycle)
- ○ Inspiratory time: 1 second (with resulting I:E ratio of 1:2)

B. Adjusted ventilator settings to avoid air trapping:
- ○ Ventilator mode: volume cycle assist control ventilation
- ○ Ventilator rate: 20
- ○ Inspiratory time: 0.5 second (with resulting I:E ratio now increased to 1:5)

While different ventilator manufacturers use different default parameters to adjust the I:E ratio (i.e., either adjustment of the I:E ratio directly, or conversely, adjustment of inspiratory time to alter the dependent I:E ratio), the important points are the following: a) it is imperative to recognize the need for a lengthened I:E ratio for optimal control of ventilation in severe obstructive diseases, and b) careful monitoring and appropriate adjustment of the I:E ratio will help to avoid increments in intrinsic PEEP and resulting cardiopulmonary function compromise. Peak inspiratory pressures will necessarily increase with a shorter inspiration but will not contribute to patient injury.

It is important to understand the role of increased peak inspiratory pressures seen in severe airflow obstruction. While high inspiratory peak pressures have historically been thought to produce an increased risk for barotrauma, this has been proven false.[13] To avoid air trapping and hyperinflation—by far the more harmful consequences of mechanical ventilation in these patients—ventilator settings that are invariably associated with higher peak inspiratory pressures (e.g., shorter inspiratory times with higher ventilator inspiratory flow rates) are reasonable and should be tolerated by the treating physician. In addition, these same physiological considerations also underlie the strong recommendation to not use pressure-control ventilation modes in acute severe airflow obstruction. Using pressure-limited ventilation modes in severe obstruction will produce very small, and likely much more variable tidal volumes and resulting minute ventilation, and thus should be avoided, particularly when higher peak pressures of volume-cycle modes are known to be tolerated well.

In contrast to peak pressures, high plateau pressures are known to be harmful and to be associated with barotrauma. While few studies have looked specifically at patients with COPD or asthma, lower plateau pressures (<30 cm H_2O) have been shown to decrease the incidence of ALI and acute respiratory distress syndrome (ARDS) in mechanically ventilated patients.[14,15] As in circumstances of acute lung injury, the delivery of smaller tidal volumes may also be necessary to achieve target plateau pressures and avoid traumatic complications in patients with COPD or asthma.[16] A tidal volume of 6 to 8 mL/kg of ideal body weight, with further adjustments as needed, is a reasonable initial strategy. Lower tidal volumes, however, produce lower minute ventilation, which can be a physiologic confounder in the already hypercapnic patient. Increasing set ventilatory rates can counter the effect on MV of lower tidal volumes but will, in turn, accelerate air trapping. To minimize air trapping, a set respiratory rate of 10 to 14 breaths per minute is preferred. Significant air trapping is indicated by increasing levels of intrinsic PEEP and should be closely monitored and minimized where possible.[17] Careful consideration of physiology and available ventilator support options is necessary to balance acceptable ventilation with the associated risks of mechanical ventilation in these patients; some degree of "permissive hypercapnia"—that is, allowing for an abnormal rise in PCO_2 to enable minimization of delivered tidal volumes and breaths per minute—is often required to avoid exacerbation of lung injury and barotrauma.

While the addition of PEEP is known to contribute to lung hyperinflation in patients with obstructive airway disease, there are certain circumstances in which added PEEP can help relieve airflow obstruction. This is particularly true in patients in whom airflow obstruction and respiratory failure are associated with increased airway compliance (e.g., emphysema) as opposed to decreased compliance (e.g., acute asthma flare or bronchiolitis). When intrinsic PEEP is present in these patients, the application of added PEEP can provide a "stenting" effect to maintain airway caliber during exhalation, which can improve overall airflow obstruction, assist the patient's ability to trigger subsequent breaths, and minimize the associated hypercapnia, increased work of breathing, and hemodynamic compromise. If this technique is used, additional extrinsic PEEP should be set to a level that is approximately 75% of the intrinsic PEEP.[18–20]

The optimal fraction of inspired oxygen (FiO_2) provided to the mechanically ventilated patient with COPD or asthma has not been clearly determined. While low pO_2 (>60) and Hgb saturations (>90%) may be acceptable in ARDS, the avoidance of additional cardiopulmonary compromise from hypoxemia may require a higher FiO_2 in this setting.

Helium can be mixed with oxygen to form a gas with a lower density than ambient air or than ambient air mixed with oxygen. Termed "heliox," and generally available in helium:oxygen ratios of 80:20 or 70:30, this gas can decrease airway resistance by increasing the proportion of laminar to turbulent flow in the airways, thereby improving airflow and decreasing a patient's work of breathing. Heliox can be delivered either noninvasively or with mechanical ventilation. It should be noted, however, that there are limited data supporting the routine use of heliox in obstructive airway diseases.[21] While there are minimal adverse effects associated with the use of heliox, the physician should be aware that ventilator adjustments might be necessary to correct for changes in flow of this less dense gas. The use of heliox mixtures can produce erroneous volume delivery measurements in some mechanical ventilators, with a resulting need to use pressure-cycle rather than volume-cycle ventilation modes. It is important to determine the specific needs of the ventilators used and to make any necessary adjustments, before using heliox mixtures for ventilator support.

VENTILATION STRATEGIES IN PULMONARY ARTERIAL HYPERTENSION

PAH is a significant contributor to right ventricular dysfunction.[22–24] The challenges to mechanical ventilation in patients with PAH are significant, as positive pressure ventilation can exert a destabilizing hemodynamic impact on an already stressed right heart. Positive pressure ventilation increases intrathoracic pressures, including right atrial pressures, which in turn decreases venous return to the right ventricle. This drop in right ventricular preload decreases right ventricular output, contributing to ventricular dysfunction. Compounding this process, as lung volumes increase with positive pressure ventilation and larger tidal volumes, alveolar distention leads to compression of the associated vessels, including the inferior vena cava. The resultant increase in pulmonary vascular resistance (PVR) is reflected as an increase in right ventricular afterload, which exacerbates existing PAH and tricuspid regurgitation, and contributes to further right ventricular dysfunction.[25–27]

Both hypoxemia and hypercapnia/acidemia independently increase PVR, and the combination of the two has a greater effect on PVR than either alone. The choice of ventilation parameters thus needs to optimize oxygenation and ventilation as much as can be safely achieved without adding greater stress on RV function.

Initial ventilation management strategies for patients with PAH should focus on limiting intrathoracic pressures. High applied PEEP and large tidal volumes should be avoided if possible. Lower tidal volumes (4 to 6 mL/kg ideal body weight) will help limit plateau pressures while still allowing for adequate oxygenation and ventilation. Similarly, lower levels of applied PEEP, typically to remain <15 cm H_2O, will limit the detrimental effects of high plateau and intrathoracic pressures. Careful monitoring is required to avoid the problem of mechanical ventilation-induced increased intrinsic PEEP, as can be produced in severe airflow obstruction (e.g., asthma and COPD). Oxygen saturation should be maintained at or above 92%. When employing a low tidal volume ventilation approach, a higher set respiratory rate can help minimize hypercapnia and acidemia; this is unlikely to create physiologic problems so long as there is no concurrent severe airflow obstruction present. If airflow obstruction is present concurrently with PAH, then the ventilator management guidelines outlined earlier in this chapter will also need to be employed.[28]

CONCLUSION

Optimal support of severe COPD and asthma requires recognition of the central and critically important role of increased airway resistance in these diseases. NIPPV can assist significantly in reducing the work of breathing and helping to alleviate respiratory failure. Intubation and mechanical ventilation are typically necessary when progressive respiratory muscle fatigue and/or worsening airflow obstruction produce hypercapnic ventilatory decompensation. Critical parameters to consider for achieving optimal mechanical ventilation support in these patients include

- Shorter inspiratory times and prolonged expiratory times, with resulting longer I:E ratios
- Acceptance of higher peak inspiratory airway pressures to achieve shortened inspiratory times
- Reduced tidal volumes to avoid higher inspiratory plateau pressures

- Avoidance of increases in trapped gas, hyperinflation, and the induction of increased intrinsic PEEP
- Application of PEEP in select patients with emphysema to assist in the relief of airflow obstruction resulting from dynamic expiratory airway compression

Mechanical ventilator support of patients with significant PAH requires taking steps to minimize physiologic stressors that can increase pulmonary arterial resistance. These include

- Avoidance of hypercapnia and hypoxemia
- Avoidance of high tidal volumes, as these can contribute to increased PVR

While these diseases can be associated with complex clinical conditions, their optimal ventilatory management is based on well-understood pathophysiology. The considerations and approaches outlined in this chapter provide a basis for the initial aspects of ventilatory care, with the goal of improving outcomes in ED and ICU care (Table 9.1).

TABLE 9.1 Ventilation Strategies for COPD, Asthma, and Pulmonary Hypertension

NIPPV for COPD and Asthma	Mechanical Ventilation Strategies for COPD and Asthma	Mechanical Ventilation Strategies for Pulmonary Hypertension
• Appropriate for initial supportive therapy • Indications for immediate intubation include refractory hypoxemia, severe hypercapnia ($PaCO_2$ > 60 mm Hg), significant acidosis (pH < 7.25), inability to tolerate noninvasive ventilation, and cardiorespiratory arrest	• Initial tidal volumes 6–8 mL/kg ideal body weight • Limit plateau pressures (<30 cm H_2O) • Decrease I/E ratio to allow for complete exhalation • Increase inspiratory flow rates (80–100 L/min) to decrease inspiratory time • Monitor closely for air trapping with increased respiratory rates • Accept mild hypercapnia and acidemia (keep pH > 7.2) • Titrate FiO_2 to maintain PaO_2 > 60 mm Hg (SaO_2 > 90%) • In patients with emphysema, careful application of PEEP to ~75% of intrinsic PEEP	• Initial tidal volumes 6–6 mL/kg ideal body weight • Limit use of higher PEEP levels • Limit plateau pressures • Avoid hypoxemia, hypercapnia, and acidemia

LITERATURE TABLE

TRIAL	DESIGN	RESULT
Brochard et al., *N Engl J Med.* 1995[5]	Multicenter RCT of 85 patients with COPD comparing NIPPV with standard therapy	NIPPV significantly reduced the need for endotracheal intubation (26% vs. 74%, $p < 0.001$), frequency of complications (16% vs. 48%, $p = 0.001$), mean hospital stays (23 vs. 35 d, $p = 0.005$), and in-hospital mortality (9% vs. 29%, $p = 0.02$)
Quon et al., *Chest.* 2008[6]	MEDLINE and EMBASE search of RCT from 1968 to 2006 that evaluated the advantages of specific medical therapies as well as the use of NIPPV for acute exacerbations of COPD	Compared to standard therapy, NIPPV significantly reduced the risk of intubation by 65% (95% CI, 0.32–0.92), in-hospital mortality by 55% (95% CI, 0.08–0.62), and length of hospitalization by 1.9 d (95% CI, 0.0–3.9)

LITERATURE TABLE (*Continued*)

TRIAL	DESIGN	RESULT
Lightowler et al., *BMJ.* 2003[7]	Systematic review of eight RCTs comparing NIPPV plus usual medical care with medical care alone in patients with respiratory failure secondary COPD exacerbation	Using NIPPV as an adjunct to usual care was associated with a lower mortality (relative risk 0.41, 95% CI, 0.26–0.64), and greater improvements at 1 h in pH (mean difference 0.03), $PaCO_2$ (mean difference of –0.04 kPa), and respiratory rate (mean difference –3.08 breaths per minute). NIPPV was also associated with shorter hospital stays (mean difference –3.24 d)
Gupta et al., *Respir Care.* 2010[8]	RCT of 53 patients with asthma comparing NIPPV with standard treatment	NIPPV significantly reduced ICU length of stays (10 vs. 24 h, $p = 0.01$) and hospital length of stays (38 vs. 54 h, $p = 0.01$) as well as decreased doses of bronchodilator treatments; however, there were no significant differences in FEV1s, respiratory rates, pHs, P/F ratios, $PaCO_2$s, or mortality rates. A nonsignificant trend toward ≥ 50% improvement in FEV1 values at 1, 2, and 4 h after treatment initiation was noted in the NIPPV arm
Conti et al., *Intensive Care Med.* 2002[12]	RCT of 49 patients with COPD who failed standard medical treatment in the ED setting comparing NIPPV with conventional ventilation via endotracheal intubation	Forty-eight percent of patients in the NIPPV arm avoided intubation. Overall, the two groups had similar lengths of ICU stay, days on mechanical ventilation, and overall complications. 1-y follow-up showed significantly fewer hospital readmissions (65% vs. 100%) or need for de novo oxygen supplementation (0% vs. 36%) in the NIPPV arm. There was also a trend toward increased survival (54% vs. 74%) in the NIPPV arm

CI, confidence interval.

REFERENCES

1. Mannino DM, Homa DM, Akinbami LJ, et al. Chronic obstructive pulmonary disease surveillance—United States, 1971–2000. *MMWR Surveill Summ.* 2002;51:1–16.
2. Centers for Disease Control and Prevention. Hospital Ambulatory Medical Care Survey: 2010 Emergency Department Summary Table. http://www.cdc.gov/nchs/data/ahcd/nhamcs_emergency/2010_ed_web_tables.pdf
3. Hyduk A, Croft JB, Ayala C, et al. Pulmonary hypertension surveillance—United States, 1980–2002. *MMWR Surveill Summ.* 2005;54:1–28.
4. Esteban A, Anzueto A, Frutos F, et al. Characteristics and outcomes in adult patients receiving mechanical ventilation: a 28-day international study. *JAMA.* 2002;287(3):345–355.
5. Brochard L, Mancebo J, Wysocki M, et al. Noninvasive ventilation for acute exacerbations of chronic obstructive pulmonary disease. *N Engl J Med.* 1995;333(13):817–822.
6. Quon BS, Gan WQ, Sin DD. Contemporary management of acute exacerbations of COPD: a systematic review and metaanalysis. *Chest.* 2008;133(3):756–766.
7. Lightowler JV, Wedzicha JA, Elliott MW, et al. Non-invasive positive pressure ventilation to treat respiratory failure resulting from exacerbations of chronic obstructive pulmonary disease: Cochrane systematic review and meta-analysis. *BMJ.* 2003;326(7382):185.
8. Gupta D, Nath A, Agarwal R, et al. A prospective randomized controlled trial on the efficacy of noninvasive ventilation in severe acute asthma. *Respir Care.* 2010;55(5):536–543.
9. Braman SS, Kaemmerlen JT. Intensive care of status asthmaticus: a 10-year experience. *JAMA.* 1990;264:366–368.
10. Mountain RD, Sahn SA. Acid–base disturbances in acute asthma. *Chest.* 1990;98:651–655.

11. Rabe KF, Hurd S, Anzueto A, et al. Global strategy for the diagnosis, management, and prevention of chronic obstructive pulmonary disease: GOLD executive summary. *Am J Respir Crit Care Med.* 2007;176(6):532–555.
12. Conti G, Antonelli M, Navalesi P, et al. Noninvasive vs. conventional mechanical ventilation in patients with chronic obstructive pulmonary disease after failure of medical treatment in the ward: a randomized trial. *Intensive Care Med.* 2002;28(12):1701–1707.
13. Williams TJ, Tuxen DV, Scheinkestel CD, et al. Risk factors for morbidity in mechanically ventilated patients with acute severe asthma. *Am Rev Respir Dis.* 1992;607–615.
14. Jia X, Malhotra A, Saeed M, et al. Risk factors for ARDS in patients receiving mechanical ventilation for >48 h. *Chest.* 2008;133(4):853–861.
15. Yilmaz M, Keegan MT, Iscimen R, et al. Toward the prevention of acute lung injury: protocol-guided limitation of large tidal volume ventilation and inappropriate transfusion. *Crit Care Med.* 2007;35(7):1660–1666.
16. Brenner B, Corbridge T, Kazzi A. Intubation and mechanical ventilation of the asthmatic patient in respiratory failure. *J Emerg Med.* 2009;37(Suppl 2):S23–S34.
17. Reddy VG. Auto-PEEP: how to detect and how to prevent—a review. *Middle East J Anesthesiol.* 2005;18:293–312.
18. MacIntyre NR, Cheng KC, McConnell R. Applied PEEP during pressure support reduces the inspiratory threshold load of intrinsic PEEP. *Chest.* 1997;111(1):188–193.
19. Petrof BJ, Legaré M, Goldberg P, et al. Continuous positive airway pressure reduces work of breathing and dyspnea during weaning from mechanical ventilation in severe chronic obstructive pulmonary disease. *Am Rev Respir Dis.* 1990;141(2):281–289.
20. Smith TC, Marini JJ. Impact of PEEP on lung mechanics and work of breathing in severe airflow obstruction. *J Appl Physiol.* 1988;65(4):1488–1499.
21. Hurford WE, Cheifetz IM. Respiratory controversies in the critical care setting. Should heliox be used for mechanically ventilated patients? *Respir Care.* 2007;52(5):582–591.
22. Konstantinides S. Clinical practice. Acute pulmonary embolism. *N Engl J Med.* 2008;359(26):2804–2813.
23. Chan CM, Klinger JR. The right ventricle in sepsis. *Clin Chest Med.* 2008;29(4):661–676, ix.
24. Vieillard-Baron A, Jardin F. Why protect the right ventricle in patients with acute respiratory distress syndrome? *Curr Opin Crit Care.* 2003;9(1):15–21.
25. Jardin F, Vieillard-Baron A. Right ventricular function and positive pressure ventilation in clinical practice: from hemodynamic subsets to respirator settings. *Intensive Care Med.* 2003;29(9):1426–1434.
26. Zapol WM, Snider MT. Pulmonary hypertension in severe acute respiratory failure. *N Engl J Med.* 1977;296(9):476–480.
27. Zamanian RT, Haddad F, Doyle RL, et al. Management strategies for patients with pulmonary hypertension in the intensive care unit. *Crit Care Med.* 2007;35(9):2037–2050.
28. Bindslev L, Jolin-Carlsson A, Santesson J, et al. Hypoxic pulmonary vasoconstriction in man: effects of hyperventilation. *Acta Anaesthesiol Scand.* 1985;29(5):547–551.

10

Acute Pulmonary Edema

Nina Patel Shah and Margaret J. Neff

BACKGROUND

No single test can distinguish cardiogenic from non-cardiogenic pulmonary edema. A clear understanding of the physiology of each disease processes, however, enables the clinician to better integrate patient history, exam, and diagnostic tests into a cohesive management strategy. This chapter outlines a systematic approach to the identification of the most common etiologies of acute pulmonary edema. Management details are addressed separately (see Chapters 12 and 14).

ETIOLOGY OF PULMONARY EDEMA

Noncardiogenic pulmonary edema, often referred to as increased permeability pulmonary edema, is caused by an increase in the vascular permeability of the lung—specifically the epithelial barrier—with subsequent movement of protein-rich fluid into the lung intersitium.[1] Increased vascular permeability is commonly associated with acute respiratory distress syndrome (ARDS) and can be due to a myriad of pathologies including pneumonia, sepsis, ingestions, and trauma associated with large-volume transfusions. It is also the disease process associated with neurogenic and high-altitude pulmonary edema.

Cardiogenic pulmonary edema results when increased left ventricular end-diastolic and left atrial pressures elevate hydrostatic pressure in the pulmonary capillaries, leading to transmission of protein-poor edema fluid across the lung endothelium and into the alveoli.[2] Alveolar edema reduces diffusion capacity, leading to hypoxia and dyspnea. The physiologic stress of the dyspnea results in a catecholamine surge, which produces tachycardia and increased afterload that can, in turn, further augment left-sided pulmonary pressures and exacerbate the edema. Cardiogenic pulmonary edema can result from a variety of pathologies, including acute decompensated heart failure, mitral or aortic valve dysfunction, tachyarrhythmias, and renovascular hypertension.[3]

CARDIOGENIC PULMONARY EDEMA

Acute decompensated heart failure accounts for more than 650,000 emergency department (ED) visits in the United States per year.[4] By itself, acute heart failure is associated with a 5% mortality rate; this number rises to 12% to 15% when the failure produces pulmonary edema.[5] Acute decompensated heart failure can result from impaired systolic or diastolic function. Impaired left ventricle (LV) systolic function is associated with coronary artery disease, hypertension, valvular heart disease, viral myocarditis, and dilated cardiomyopathies, as well as with toxins and metabolic disorders such as hypo- and hyperthyroidism. Impaired LV systolic function results in decreased cardiac output, which increases pulmonary capillary pressure and activates the renin–angiotensin–aldosterone system; this, in turn, triggers sodium and fluid retention.[6] In diastolic heart failure, the LV becomes less compliant, leading to coronary ischemia (since the coronary arteries fill during diastole), arrhythmias (especially atrial fibrillation), reduced ventricular filling, and increased end-diastolic pressure.

Valvular abnormalities, particularly stenosis of the mitral and aortic valves, are common culprits in acute cardiogenic pulmonary edema. Mitral stenosis, a known complication of rheumatic heart disease, causes an atrial obstruction that leads to pulmonary capillary congestion. Although mitral stenosis generally develops in a chronic manner, stresses such as tachycardia and decreased diastolic filling can lead to acute increases in hydrostatic pressure. Aortic valve stenosis limits LV outflow, resulting in a similar upstream increase in hydrostatic pressure in the pulmonary capillaries.[7]

Renal artery stenosis is a less common etiology for cardiogenic pulmonary edema. It causes long-standing hypertension, leading to diastolic dysfunction as well as chronic physiologic activation of the renin–angiotensin system with resulting increases in sodium and water retention.[8]

Of the tachyarrhythmias associated with acute pulmonary edema, atrial fibrillation is the most common. In a study of more than 200 consecutive elderly patients presenting with acute cardiogenic pulmonary edema, approximately 36% had an arrhythmia; 24% were in rapid atrial fibrillation, causing an elevation in end-diastolic pressure and subsequent drop in cardiac output.[9] Ventricular arrhythmias can also account for acute cardiogenic pulmonary edema, especially when associated with myocardial ischemia.

NONCARDIOGENIC PULMONARY EDEMA

The functional definition of noncardiogenic edema is the presence of increased vascular permeability, resulting in protein-rich fluid leaking into the pulmonary interstitium and air spaces.[1] It is most commonly associated with ARDS, defined as acute bilateral pulmonary edema in the absence of heart failure or other causes of hydrostatic edema.[10] With the advent of a therapeutic strategy for ARDS—namely, low tidal volume ventilation—prompt recognition and treatment of this condition are essential.[11] A predisposing risk factor is not a diagnostic criterion for ARDS; in fact, 20% of diagnosed cases of ARDS have no identifiable risk factor.[12] The most commonly associated conditions are trauma and sepsis;[12] others include massive transfusion, aspiration, inhalation injury, and pancreatitis.

Other etiologies of noncardiogenic pulmonary edema likely to be encountered by the emergency physician include neurogenic edema, opiate toxicity, and high-altitude pulmonary edema.[13–15] Neurogenic pulmonary edema can be a consequence of seizures, blunt or penetrating head injuries, and cerebral, especially subarachnoid, hemorrhage. Treatment of neurogenic, nonhydrostatic pulmonary edema—thought to be due to catecholamine excess—consists of supportive treatment and management of the underlying brain injury. Opiate toxicity—from narcotics including street drugs (e.g., heroin), hospital-prescribed methadone, intravenous narcotics (e.g., a bolus of fentanyl), and even the narcotic antagonist naloxone—can also precipitate noncardiogenic pulmonary edema; the exact mechanism in this process is, however, unclear. Lastly, high-altitude pulmonary edema can result from rapid ascent to high altitudes. In this case, profound hypoxia leads to pulmonary vasoconstriction, causing capillary leak permeability edema; the primary treatment strategy is descent and supplemental oxygen (see Chapter 54).

DIAGNOSTIC EVALUATION

The diagnosis of pulmonary edema is achieved via patient history and physical exam, chest radiograph, ultrasound, chemistries, and biomarker tests. A cardiogenic etiology is suggested by a history of hypertension, heart failure, aortic or mitral valve disease, or coronary artery disease or its accompanying disease states (e.g., diabetes, hyperlipidemia, obesity). A patient with this history may exhibit findings suggestive of elevated left ventricular end-diastolic pressure, including an S3 gallop, which has a high specificity (90% to 97%) but low sensitivity (9% to 51%) for a reduced ejection fraction.[1,16] In addition, the patient may have cool extremities and preferential vasoconstriction resulting from compromised cardiac output. Other physical signs are less reliable indicators of etiology, as they can result from multiple noncardiogenic processes. For example, lower extremity edema can be due to chronic kidney or liver disease, and findings of inspiratory crackles and rhonchi on examination of the lung—while consistent with the finding of pulmonary edema—can also result from aspiration of gastric contents, sepsis, trauma, or recent blood transfusion.

Imaging modalities are useful in the workup of acute pulmonary edema, but often cannot be relied upon to establish etiology. The chest radiograph, almost universally used in the initial workup of dyspnea, can reveal findings highly specific for pulmonary edema—such as the characteristic patterns of cephalization (by which upper lobe vessels are recruited to carry more blood when lower lobe vessels are compressed by increased hydrostatic pressure), interstitial edema, and alveolar edema. However, these findings cannot be used to establish etiology.[3] Importantly, in almost 20% of patients with clinically significant heart failure, chest radiograph will show no evidence of pulmonary edema; this is likely because lung fluid must increase 30% before becoming evident radiographically.[3,17] Vascular pedicle width (VPW) has also been used to help distinguish between cardiogenic and noncardiogenic causes of pulmonary edema, but its sensitivity and specificity (71% and 66%, respectively) are inadequate for independent use.[18] The electrocardiogram (EKG) can also be useful in the initial workup; patients with clinically significant heart failure from various etiologies rarely present with a normal EKG. EKG findings commonly associated with heart failure, as discussed above, include tachycardia (the natural response of the heart to preserve cardiac output in the setting of impaired stroke volume), arrhythmias such as atrial fibrillation, and myocardial infarctions. Finally, a pulmonary artery wedge pressure of ≤18 mmHg—measured using a pulmonary artery catheter (PAC)—has traditionally been part of the definition of noncardiogenic pulmonary edema. Wedge pressure has since been disproved as a useful marker and has fallen out of favor as diagnostic tools less invasive than the PAC have become available.[19]

In the past decade, bedside, or point-of-care, ultrasound has increasingly been used to evaluate the lungs for various insults, including pulmonary edema, pneumothorax,

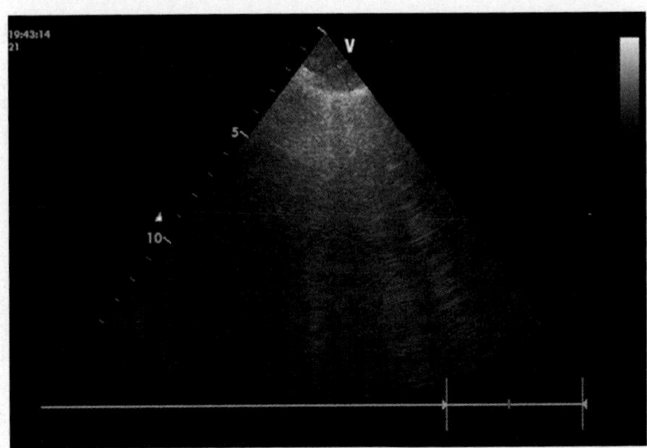

FIGURE 10.1 Three B-lines/comet tails in cardiogenic pulmonary edema. Image courtesy of Dr. Anne-Sophie Beraud, Stanford University Medical Center.

and pleural effusion. The finding of at least three to six bilateral "B-lines" (vertical lines that extend from the pleural surface and obliterate the A-lines that occur horizontally as reflections of the pleura) has been demonstrated to be up to 95% specific for pulmonary edema and correlates with the radiographic finding of alveolar–interstitial syndrome—a condition most commonly associated with cardiogenic pulmonary edema[20–22] (Fig. 10.1). Some caution is advised in the interpretation of these findings, however, as B-lines in clusters can be found in dependent lung zones in up to 28% of normal patients and may be limited or absent in patients with milder forms of pulmonary edema.[21–23] Bedside ultrasound to evaluate cardiac function and assess intravascular volume is also increasingly used by the critical care community.[24] The combination of LV and right ventricle (RV) assessment, when coupled with an assessment of inferior vena cava size and respiratory variation, can help include or exclude volume overload and heart failure as a likely cause of the pulmonary edema (see Chapters 6 and 7).

Biomarkers, such as B-type natriuretic peptide (BNP), are also useful in determining the etiology of acute pulmonary edema and can help prompt early implementation of targeted interventions, such as diuretics and vasodilators for cardiogenic edema or lung-protective ventilation strategy for nonhydrostatic ARDS.[25] A recent study evaluated the utility of BNP in distinguishing cardiogenic from noncardiogenic pulmonary edema and found that a BNP level of 100 pg/mL or less was highly specific for noncardiogenic pulmonary edema in ED patients, with a negative predictive value (NPV) for heart failure of >90%.[26] Similarly, a BNP level >500 pg/mL was strongly suggestive of heart failure ([positive predictive value] PPV > 90%).[27]

Direct analysis of pleural fluid using thoracentesis, although unlikely to be used in a busy ED, is another classic test for distinguishing cardiogenic and noncardiogenic etiology.[28] A pleural fluid/serum protein concentration ratio >0.65 has been shown to be over 80% sensitive and specific for noncardiogenic edema in intubated patients being evaluated for ARDS.

CONCLUSION

There is no one test that determines the cause or detects the presence of acute pulmonary edema. A detailed history and physical exam followed by diagnostic testing, including chest radiography, BNP, and ultrasound (cardiac and lung), can help differentiate the cause of acute edema and guide appropriate treatment.

LITERATURE TABLE

TRIAL	DESIGN	RESULT
Ware and Matthay. *N Engl J Med.* 2005[1]	Review of diagnostic strategies for pulmonary edema	Algorithm developed for the clinical differentiation of cardiogenic and non-cardiogenic pulmonary edema
Knudsen et al., *Am J Med.* 2004[17]	Cohort study of BNP and chest radiography interpretation	BNP (BNP levels ≥ 100 pg/mL, OR = 12.3; 95% CI: 7.4–20.4) and radiographic evaluation (cardiomegaly: OR = 2.3; 95% CI: 1.4–3.7, cephalization: OR = 6.4; 95% CI: 3.3–12.5, and interstitial edema: OR = 7.0; 95% CI: 2.9–17.0) can provide complementary information to the clinical exam in diagnosing the cause of pulmonary edema
Rice et al., *Crit Care.* 2011[18]	Retrospective cohort study comparing VPW to intravascular pressure measurements	VPW was neither sensitive nor specific enough to determine fluid status in patients with acute lung injury (ALI) (71% sensitivity and 68% specificity for a pulmonary artery opening pressure <8 mmHg)
Volpicelli et al., *Am J Emerg Med.* 2006[22]	Prospective evaluation of 300 emergency department patients with lung ultrasound	Comet tails/B-lines were highly associated with interstitial edema (sensitivity of 85.7% and a specificity of 97.7% in recognition of radiologic alveolar–interstitial syndrome)
Levitt et al., *Crit Care.* 2008[26]	Prospective, blinded cohort study of BNP in the ICU	BNP can help identify heart failure in the ED (<100 pg/mL consistent with noncardiogenic edema (NPV for cardiogenic edema 90%); >500 pg/mL consistent with heart failure). This marker is not as useful in the ICU setting
Ware et al., *Eur Respir J.* 2010[28]	Prospective study of edema fluid: plasma protein concentrations in intubated patients	An edema fluid: plasma protein concentration >0.65 was over 80% sensitive and specific for the diagnosis of ALI

CI, confidence interval; NPV, negative predictive value; OR, odds ratio.

REFERENCES

1. Ware LB, Matthay MA. Acute pulmonary edema. *N Engl J Med.* 2005;353:2788–2796.
2. Staub NC. Pulmonary edema. *Physiol Rev.* 1974;54:678–811.
3. Collins S, Storrow AB, Kirk JD, et al. Beyond pulmonary edema: diagnostic, risk stratification, and treatment challenges of acute heart failure management in the emergency department. *Ann Emerg Med.* 2008;51(1):45–57.
4. Schappert S, Rechtsteiner E. Ambulatory medical care utilization estimates for 2006. *Natl Health Stat Report.* 2008;(8):1–29.
5. Mac Sweeney R, McAuley DF, Matthay MA. Acute lung failure. *Semin Respir Crit Care Med.* 2011;32:607–625.
6. Francis GS, Goldsmith SR, Levine TB, et al. The neurohumoral axis in congestive heart failure. *Ann Intern Med.* 1984;101(3):370–377.
7. Gandhi SK, Powers JC, Nomeir AM, et al. The pathogenesis of acute pulmonary edema associated with hypertension. *N Engl J Med.* 2001;344:17–22.

8. Pickering TG. Recurrent pulmonary oedema in hypertension due to bilateral renal artery stenosis. *Lancet.* 1988;2(8610):551.
9. Bentancur AG, Rieck J, Koldanov R, et al. Acute pulmonary edema in the emergency department: clinical and echocardiographic survey in an aged population. *Am J Med Sci.* 2002;323(5):238–243.
10. Ranieri VM, et al. Acute respiratory distress syndrome: the Berlin definition. *JAMA.* 2012;307(23): 2526–2533.
11. The Acute Respiratory Distress Syndrome Network. Ventilation with lower tidal volumes as compared with traditional tidal volumes for acute lung injury and the acute respiratory distress syndrome. *N Engl J Med.* 2000;342:1301–1308.
12. Hudson LD, Milberg JA, Anardi D, et al. Clinical risks for development of the acute respiratory distress syndrome. *Am J Respir Crit Care Med.* 1995;151:293–301.
13. Muroi C, Keller M, Pangalu A, et al. Neurogenic pulmonary edema in patients with subarachnoid hemorrhage. *J Neurosurg Anesthesiol.* 2008;20(3):188.
14. Sporer KA, Dorn E. Heroin-related noncardiogenic pulmonary edema: a case series. *Chest.* 2001;120(5): 1628.
15. Stream JO, Grissom CK. Update on high-altitude pulmonary edema: pathogenesis, prevention, and treatment. *Wilderness Environ Med.* 2008;19(4):293–303.
16. Marcus GM, Gerber IL, McKeown BH, et al. Association between phonocardiographic third and fourth heart sounds and objective measures of left ventricular function. *JAMA.* 2005;293(18):2238–2244.
17. Knudsen CW, Omland T, Clopton P, et al. Diagnostic value of B-type natriuretic peptide and chest radiographic findings in patients with acute dyspnea. *Am J Med.* 2004;116:363–368.
18. Rice TW, Ware LB, Haponik EF, et al. Vascular pedicle width in acute lung injury: correlation with intravascular pressures and ability to discriminate fluid status. *Crit Care.* 2011;15(2):R86.
19. Bernard GR, Artigas A, Brigham KL, et al. The American-European Consensus Conference on ARDS. Definitions, mechanisms, relevant outcomes, and clinical trial coordination. *Am J Respir Crit Care Med.* 1994;149:818–824.
20. Turner JP, Dankoff J. Thoracic ultrasound. *Emerg Med Clin North Am.* 2012;30(2):451–473.
21. Lichtenstein D, Meziere G, Biderman P, et al. The comet-tail artifact. An ultrasound sign of alveolar-interstitial syndrome. *Am J Respir Crit Care Med.* 1997;156(5):1640–1646.
22. Volpicelli G, Mussa A, Garofalo G, et al. Bedside lung ultrasound in the assessment of alveolar-interstitial syndrome. *Am J Emerg Med.* 2006;24(6):689–696.
23. Volpicelli G, Caramello V, Cardinale L, et al. Detection of sonographic B-lines in patients with normal lung or radiographic alveolar consolidation. *Med Sci Monit.* 2008;14(3):CR122–CR128.
24. Duane PG, Colice GL. Impact of noninvasive studies to distinguish volume overload from ARDS in acutely ill patients with pulmonary edema: analysis of the medical literature from 1966 to 1998. *Chest.* 2000;118:1709–1717.
25. Noveanu M, Mebazaa A, Mueller C. Cardiovascular biomarkers in the ICU. *Curr Opin Crit Care.* 2009;15:377–383.
26. Levitt JE, Vinayak AG, Gehlbach BK, et al. Diagnostic utility of B-type natriuretic peptide in critically ill patients with pulmonary edema: a prospective cohort study. *Crit Care.* 2008;12:R3.
27. Silver MA, Maisel A, Yancy CW, et al. BNP consensus panel 2004: a clinical approach for the diagnostic, prognostic, screening, treatment monitoring, and therapeutic roles of natriuretic peptides in cardiovascular diseases. *Congest Heart Fail.* 2004;10(Suppl 3):1–30.
28. Ware LB, Fremont RD, Bastarache JA, et al. Determining the aetiology of pulmonary oedema by the oedema fluid-to-plasma protein ratio. *Eur Respir J.* 2010;35(2):331–337.

11

High Risk Pulmonary Embolism

Tsuyoshi Mitarai

BACKGROUND

In an autopsy series of hospital deaths, pulmonary embolism (PE) was found in approximately 15% of the cases and—after excluding incidental PE—to be a primary or contributing cause of death in 3.4% to 8.9% of cases.[1–5] In only 30% of this group had there been an antemortem suspicion or diagnosis of PE, a statistic that fueled the argument that PE is an underdiagnosed disease.[3–6] Conversely, another study, done after the introduction of multidetector row computed tomographic pulmonary angiography (MDCTPA) in 1998, pointed to the possible overdiagnosis of PE.[7] No significant change in the incidence of PE was reported between 1993 and 1998 (from 58.8 to 62.3 per 1,00,000; annual percentage change [APC] 0.5%). Between 1998 and 2006, when the use of MDCTPA increased 7- to 13-fold,[8–11] an 81% increase in incidence of PE was reported (from 62.1 to 112.3 per 1,00,000; APC 7.1%).[7] Despite this improved detection of PE, reduction in PE-associated mortality has been modest,[7] raising concern that we are diagnosing and treating (and sometimes overdiagnosing/overtreating) patients with low-risk PE and an intrinsically low mortality rate, while underdiagnosing and/or undertreating patients with high-risk PE. This hypothesis is supported by the findings in the Emergency Medicine Pulmonary Embolism in the Real World Registry (EMPEROR).[12] In the analysis of 1,880 emergency department (ED) patients with confirmed PE (88% diagnosed with CTPA), the all-cause mortality rate at 30 days was only 5.4%.[12] Although only 3% of the registry had a systolic blood pressure (SBP) <90 mm Hg at presentation, 30-day mortality of this subgroup was much higher than those with SBP >90 (14.0% vs. 1.8%).[13] Furthermore, only 15.5% (9/58) of this high-risk subgroup received reperfusion therapy (systemic thrombolytic therapy or embolectomy).[13] The review of data from the Nationwide Inpatient Sample also shows underutilization of reperfusion therapy among PE patients with shock or ventilator dependence (30%, 1.2%, and 0.3% for systemic thrombolytic therapy, surgical embolectomy, and catheter embolectomy, respectively). The review also reports higher case fatality rate attributable to PE not treated versus treated with systemic thrombolytic therapy (42% vs. 8.4%).[14] To improve the mortality outcome of this disease, there needs to be an improvement in the care of patients in the high-risk PE subgroups. This chapter focuses on the diagnostic approach and management of unstable patients with suspected and confirmed PE in the ED. A discussion of the diagnosis and management of PE in stable patients may be found elsewhere.[15–18]

CLASSIFICATION OF ACUTE PULMONARY EMBOLISM

One of the hallmarks of PE is its wide spectrum of clinical presentation. The mortality rate of PE ranges from approximately 1% for low-risk PE to 65% for massive PE with cardiac arrest.[19–22] Classification of PE into different risk subgroups is important for appropriate prognostication, treatment selection, and disposition. Classification of PE based solely on the degree of clot burden fails to account for the patient's underlying cardiopulmonary reserve or physiologic response against the clot. In fact, anatomically massive PE—defined by an angiographic obstruction of >50% or obstruction of two lobar arteries—is rarely associated with shock and accounts for only 50% of fatal PE[8]; in patients with saddle emboli, only 8% to 14% are reported to have sustained hypotension.[23,24] Right ventricular (RV) failure and associated hemodynamic compromise, on the other hand, reflect both embolism size as well as underlying cardiopulmonary status and serve as a better indicator of clinical outcome.[6,25–27] In 2011, the American Heart Association (AHA) proposed classifying PE into three groups based on the patient's physiologic response to the embolus: massive, submassive, and low-risk PE.[28] The European Society of Cardiology (ESC) guidelines use the terms high-risk, intermediate-risk, and low-risk PE.[15]

Massive PE is defined as an acute PE accompanied by any of the following:

- Systolic blood pressure < 90 mm Hg for at least 15 minutes or requiring inotropic support without alternative cause of hypotension, such as arrhythmia, hypovolemia, sepsis, or left ventricular dysfunction
- Pulselessness
- Persistent bradycardia with heart rate < 40 bpm with signs of shock

ESC guidelines include a drop of SBP > 40 mm Hg over 15 minutes in this category.[15,22]

Submassive PE is defined as an acute PE without hypotension with any of the following:

- Myocardial necrosis
    - Troponin I > 0.4 ng/mL or troponin T > 0.1 ng/mL
- RV dysfunction
    - RV systolic dysfunction or dilation (apical four-chamber RV diameter divided by LV diameter > 0.9) on echocardiography
    - RV dilation on CT (four-chamber RV diameter divided by LV diameter > 0.9)
    - Brain natriuretic peptide (BNP) > 90 pg/mL
    - N-terminal pro-BNP > 500 pg/mL
    - Electrocardiographic (ECG) changes (new complete or incomplete right bundle branch block, anteroseptal ST elevation or depression, or anteroseptal T-wave inversion)

Low-risk PE encompasses all other patients with PE not included in these first two categories.

In large registries, massive PE accounts for <5% of patients with acute PE,[12,29] but it is associated with a high mortality rate. The International Cooperative Pulmonary Embolism Registry (ICOPER) reported 90-day mortality rates of nonmassive and massive PE to be 15.1% and 58.3%, respectively.[29] The Management Strategy and

Prognosis of Pulmonary Embolism Registry (MAPPET) reported an in-hospital mortality rate of 8.1% for submassive PE, 15% for massive PE meeting hypotension criteria without signs of shock or vasopressor use, 25% for massive PE with signs of shock or requiring use of vasopressors, and 65% in patients requiring cardiopulmonary resuscitation (CPR).[22] A conceptual guide to the triage of PE patients by clinical severity subgroups is shown in Figure 11.1. The determination of which low-risk PE patients may be treated as an outpatient is outside the scope of this chapter.

MASSIVE PULMONARY EMBOLISM

Pathophysiology

The relative utility of various therapies for massive PE, including inotropic and vasopressor drugs, has yet to be assessed in a robust trial. However, a rational management strategy can be guided by an understanding of the pathophysiology of cardiovascular compromise in these patients (Fig. 11.2).

Acute PE produces an increase in pulmonary vascular resistance (PVR) through not only mechanical obstruction but also pulmonary artery vasoconstriction from hypoxia,[30] neural reflexes,[31] and humoral factors.[32] This sudden increase in PVR is poorly tolerated by the right ventricle (RV), which cannot generate mean pulmonary artery pressures (PAPs) of ≥40 mm Hg.[33] The increase in RV afterload results in a proportional decrease in RV stroke volume (RVSV) as well as RV dilation.[34,35] The decrease in

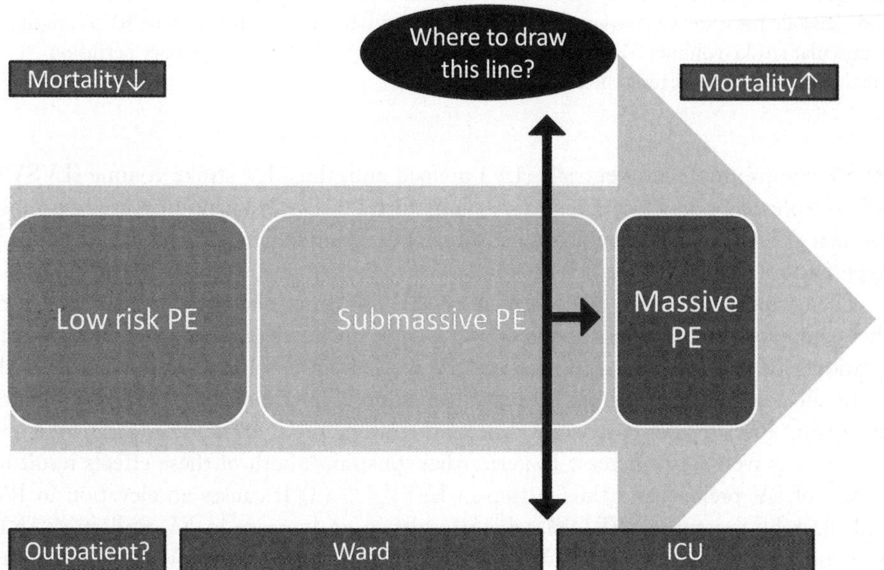

FIGURE 11.1 Triage concept of acute pulmonary embolism: Three PE risk subgroups and potential disposition site. PE, pulmonary embolism; ICU, Intensive Care Unit.

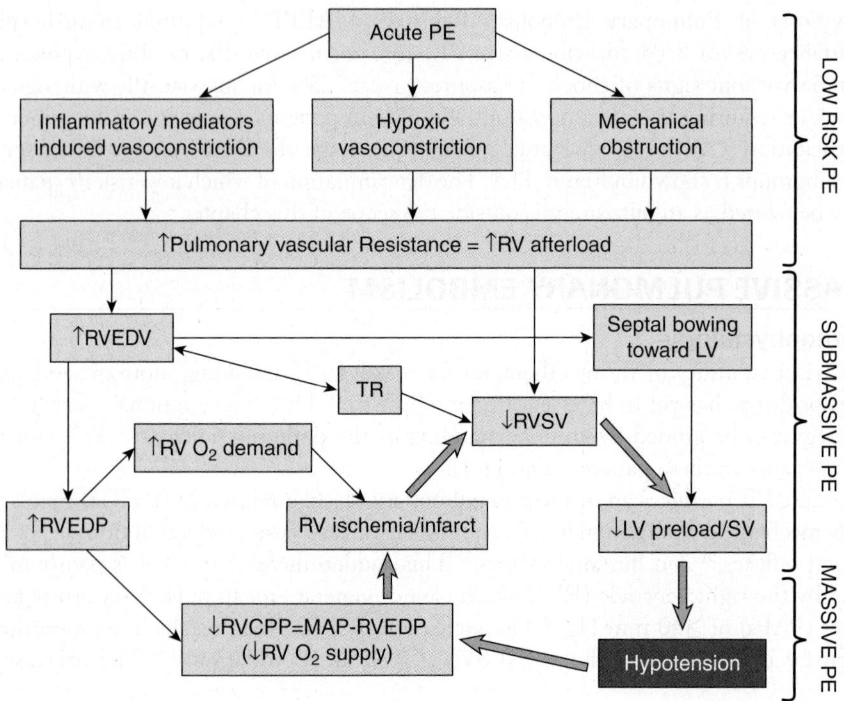

FIGURE 11.2 Pathophysiology of pulmonary embolism. Large arrows indicate how patients with massive PE can continue to deteriorate without a recurrent PE. PE, pulmonary embolism; RV, right ventricular; RVEDV, right ventricular end-diastolic volume; RVEDP, right ventricular end-diastolic pressure; O_2, oxygen; TR, tricuspid regurgitation; LV, left ventricle; RVSV, right ventricular stroke volume; SV, stroke volume; RVCPP, right ventricular coronary perfusion pressure; MAP, mean arterial pressure.

RVSV compromises left ventricle (LV) preload and, thus, LV stroke volume (LVSV), which—once a patient's compensatory sympathetic tachycardia and increased systemic vascular resistance (SVR) are no longer sufficient—eventually results in systemic arterial hypotension.

The accompanying RV dilation/increased RV end-diastolic volume (RVEDV) further complicates this process in several ways: (1) It produces significant tricuspid regurgitation (TR), which results in increased RV preload.[36] A volume-overloaded RV will eventually take residence on the descending portion of the Frank-Starling curve, further decreasing RVSV.[34] (2) It causes a shift of the interventricular septum toward the left ventricle, as well as an increase in pericardial constraint; both of these effects result in a drop of LV preload and thus a drop in LVSV.[36–39] (3) It causes an elevation in RV end-diastolic pressure (RVEDP), which results in an increase in RV wall stress (RV wall stress = RV radius × RVEDP) and an associated decrease in RV coronary perfusion pressure (RVCPP) (RVCPP = Mean arterial pressure - RVEDP).[6] This increase in RV wall stress and decrease in RVCPP will produce higher RV oxygen demand and lower oxygen supply, respectively. These changes—particularly in the context of systemic hypotension—can easily precipitate RV ischemia or infarction.[40–43] Figure 11.2 demonstrates this vicious cycle, which explains how patients with massive PE can continue to deteriorate without a recurrent PE.

Considerations during Patient Stabilization

Untreated patients with massive PE can further decompensate through a loss of physiologic compensation, recurrent PE, and/or in response to interventions. Two-thirds of patients with a fatal PE die within the first hour of presentation.[6] Careful stabilization, rapid diagnostic efforts, and appropriate treatment of suspected massive PE therefore need to take place simultaneously. The concept of a golden hour should be applied to these patients just as with patients with major trauma, ST elevation myocardial infarction (STEMI), and acute stroke.[6] Understanding the physiology of massive PE as described above illuminates several key points that are important in stabilization of such patients in the ED:

- Excessive intravenous (IV) fluid in patients with massive PE suffering from RV dilation and failure can further compromise cardiac output by worsening of RV ischemia and increasing septal bowing toward the LV.[44–46] An initial 500-mL IV fluid bolus is reasonable, but if hemodynamic improvement is not observed, use of vasopressors should not be delayed. This is in stark contrast to the majority of hypotensive patients in the ED who typically require aggressive fluid resuscitation, including those with nonmassive PE but hemodynamic instability caused by sepsis and/or hypovolemia. Clinical impression and early bedside transthoracic echocardiogram (TTE) (see Diagnostic Approach to Suspected Massive PE) are therefore important determinants of the early resuscitative pathway.
- Vasopressor therapy should be considered early in massive PE in order to maintain RVCPP and minimize RV ischemia and infarction. There are no human trials data to establish superiority of one vasopressor over another in massive PE. In a canine PE model with relative hypotension, both norepinephrine and phenylephrine showed restoration of hemodynamics, but only the norepinephrine group showed improved RV function, presumably through its beta-1 properties.[47] Dopamine is known to have a higher tachyarrhythmia risk compared to norepinephrine for the treatment of patients with shock,[48] and such arrhythmia is poorly tolerated in patients with acute right ventricular failure.[35,49] Epinephrine has a theoretical benefit for its combined property of positive inotropy and vasoconstriction, but clinical evidence on its use is limited.[50] Therefore, norepinephrine seems to be a reasonable vasopressor of choice for massive PE, with epinephrine as a possible alternative. The risk of vasopressor infusion through a peripheral IV should be weighed against the risks of delay in blood pressure restoration and of increased bleeding from a central line insertion site (if thrombolytic agents are to be used).
- The inotropic agent dobutamine has been shown to improve cardiac output in PE patients with evidence of cardiogenic shock without profound hypotension in a small ICU study.[51] However, in massive PE with significant hemodynamic compromise, dobutamine should be used cautiously, as it can worsen hypotension through systemic vasodilation and may necessitate the concurrent use of norepinephrine.[35]

- Providing adequate oxygen promptly reduces PAP and improves cardiac output in patients with pulmonary hypertension.[35,52] Orotracheal intubation, however, poses a threat to patients with massive PE, as it removes the compensatory sympathetic tone and can exacerbate systemic hypotension.[6] If intubation is necessary, vasopressor therapy should be titrated to maintain adequate mean arterial pressure (MAP) (i.e., ≥65 mm Hg), and induction agents known to cause systemic vasodilation, such as propofol, should be avoided. Care should be taken to minimize hypoxia, prolonged hypercarbia, and worsening of acidosis, all of which may increase PVR.[53–55] Unfortunately, despite these precautionary measures, a patient may still decompensate following intubation. A retrospective chart review of 52 normotensive and nonintubated patients requiring emergent pulmonary embolectomy showed 19% rate of hemodynamic collapse (refractory to fluid, inotrope, or vasopressor administration and requiring emergent cardiopulmonary bypass [CPB]) after receiving induction of general anesthesia for intubation.[56] The rate of hemodynamic collapse following emergency intubation for massive PE patients in the ED may be even higher. Although there are no data for the use of noninvasive positive-pressure ventilation (NIPPV) in massive PE, carefully selected patients may benefit from the use of short-term NIPPV as a bridge to definitive therapies, including administration of thrombolytic agents.
- Even after successful intubation, positive-pressure mechanical ventilation can produce substantial destabilizing cardiovascular effects, including a decrease in venous return and an increase in PVR, resulting in further RV decompensation and subsequent hypotension.[6] It is thought that lung hyperinflation along with excessive positive end-expiratory pressure (PEEP) can significantly reduce RV systolic function and cardiac output.[57] A low tidal volume (6 mL/kg ideal body weight) with plateau pressure goal below 30 cm H_2O should be used in massive PE,[15] since this strategy seems to provide both lung and RV protection in acute respiratory distress syndrome (ARDS)[58] with lower incidence of acute cor pulmonale.[59]

Diagnostic Evaluation

Massive PE poses unique challenges for the emergency physician: time constraints, physiology that is unforgiving in response to common stabilizing measures, and diagnostic uncertainty where clinical instability may preclude or delay confirmatory diagnostic studies. A step-by-step diagnostic approach to suspected massive PE is proposed below:

Step 1. Suspecting massive PE among hypotensive patients:

Massive PE should be considered in all hypotensive patients, especially with suggestive symptoms. In the MAPPET study, which included both massive and submassive PE, acute onset of symptoms (<48 hours), dyspnea, and syncope were reported in 70%, 96%, and 35% of patients, respectively.[22] In the subgroup analysis of massive PE patients in the ICOPER study, reported symptoms included dyspnea (81%), chest pain (40%), and syncope (39%).[60]

Step 2: Transthoracic echocardiogram:

TTE is a noninvasive and easily repeatable bedside procedure that can be performed by the emergency physician without interfering with ongoing stabilizing interventions.

In cases of massive PE, TTE may demonstrate RV dilation and hypokinesis, septal shift, and tricuspid regurgitation (TR). While the absence of these echocardiographic findings does not rule out PE (sensitivity 60% to 70%), it effectively eliminates PE as a cause of hemodynamic instability and encourages a search for alternative explanations of a patient's hypotension.[15] The presence of such TTE findings should change the urgency of a confirmatory PE study and justifies the initiation of stabilizing maneuvers discussed above. Finally, TTE will identify emboli in transit in 4% to 18% of patients with acute PE[61–64] and can help identify other causes of shock, including cardiac tamponade, aortic dissection, hypovolemia, LV dysfunction, and valvular insufficiency (see Chapter 6).[15]

Step 3: Confirmatory studies for massive PE:

Pending a confirmatory study, therapeutic anticoagulation with intravenous unfractionated heparin (UFH) should be started (in the absence of a drug contraindication) for all patients in whom there is high or intermediate suspicion of PE.[28] The standard dose of UFH for the treatment of PE is an 80 unit/kg IV bolus followed by 18 unit/kg/min.[65]

Given its widespread availability, diagnostic accuracy, and short study time, MDCTPA is the study of choice for confirmation of massive PE. Because of the frequent finding of proximal or central pulmonary circulation clot in massive PE, MDCTPA is usually able to confirm the diagnosis.[15,66] Even in patients with renal insufficiency, the risk of contrast-induced nephropathy is likely outweighed by the risk of delay in the diagnosis and treatment.

Although its availability in the ED may be limited, transesophageal echocardiogram (TEE) should be considered in cases in which a patient has an IV contrast allergy or is hemodynamically too unstable to be transported to CT. In patients with suspected PE noted to have RV dysfunction on TTE, TEE has been shown to have a sensitivity of 80% to 96.7% and specificity of 84% to 100% for massive PE (by detection of proximal clots).[67–70]

Ventilation/perfusion (V/Q) studies require a prolonged departure from the ED and have limited utility in a patient with massive PE. Similarly, lower extremity Doppler ultrasound, while increasing the likelihood of PE diagnosis if positive, neither confirms nor excludes a diagnosis of massive PE.

A confirmatory diagnosis of massive PE, while not required before initiating therapeutic anticoagulation, is preferred before initiating reperfusion therapy such as systemic thrombolytic therapy, surgical embolectomy, or catheter-directed therapy (CDT). However, if severe hemodynamic instability does not permit additional testing, aggressive measures may be warranted based on clinical suspicion and TTE findings alone.[15] One study tested an institution-specific algorithm for suspected PE in ED patients with the goal of implementing appropriate treatment, including reperfusion therapy, in a timely manner. Twenty-one of the 204 patients had a shock index (SI) (SI = HR/SBP, normal range 0.5 to 0.7) of $\geq$1; of these, 14 demonstrated RV dysfunction on TTE. All 14 patients with RV dysfunction received reperfusion treatment without a confirmatory study (systemic thrombolysis, 7; catheter fragmentation, 4; and surgical embolectomy, 3) with an averaged time interval between ED admission and start of reperfusion therapy of 32 $\pm$ 12 minutes. In all 14 patients, PE was confirmed after initiation of reperfusion therapy.[71]

Management Guidelines

Systemic Thrombolytic Therapy

The Food and Drug Administration (FDA) has approved the following three drugs in the treatment of massive PE[15,28]:

- *Streptokinase*: 250,000 IU IV bolus over 30 minutes followed by 100,000 IU/hour for 12 to 24 hours (or 1.5 million IU IV over 2 hours[72])
- *Urokinase*: 4,400 IU/kg IV bolus over 10 minutes followed by 4,400 IU/kg/h for 12 to 24 hours (or 1 million IU IV bolus over 10 minutes followed by 2 million IU IV over 110 minutes[73])
- *Alteplase*: 100-mg IV infusion over 2 hours (or 0.6 mg/kg IV over 15 minutes with maximum dose of 50 mg[74,75])

Systemic thrombolytic therapy is associated with more rapid clot lysis than heparin therapy alone.[76–81] In a study comparing a 2-hour infusion of 100 mg of alteplase (a recombinant tissue plasminogen activator [rt-PA]) combined with heparin versus heparin alone, at the 2-hour mark the alteplase group showed a 12% decrease in vascular obstruction, 30% reduction in mean PAP, and 15% increase in cardiac index. No changes were observed in the heparin group except for an 11% rise in mean PAP.[79] One week postintervention, however, the severity of vascular obstruction[79,82] and reversal of RV dysfunction[83] were similar in both groups.[6,15,28] Systemic thrombolytic therapy has been shown to have greatest benefit when started within 48 hours of symptom onset[80] but may still be useful for patients who have had symptoms for up to 14 days.[15,84]

A mortality benefit of thrombolysis has not been found in patients with nonmassive PE and remains speculative in patients with massive PE, since there exists no large randomized controlled trial in this subgroup. One meta-analysis failed to demonstrate a superiority of thrombolysis compared with heparin alone with regard to recurrent pulmonary embolism or death as a composite outcome. However, when the study restricted analysis to trials that included massive PE patients, the composite outcome was 9.4% with the thrombolysis group versus 19.0% with heparin alone (odds ratio 0.45; NNT = 10).[85] In a large retrospective study that analyzed patients with a diagnosis of PE and shock or ventilator dependence, the case fatality rate attributable to PE was higher among patients not receiving systemic thrombolytic therapy (42% vs. 8.4%).[14]

The three drugs listed above appear to be comparable in efficacy and bleeding risk, provided doses are equivalent and given over the same time period.[72,73] Shorter infusion regimens (i.e., $\leq$2 hours) are preferred as they are associated with lower bleeding risk and more rapid clot lysis.[86] Drug delivery via peripheral IV is preferred, as pulmonary artery catheters are associated with an increased bleeding risk at the insertion site without an increase in efficacy.[86,87] IV UFH should be discontinued during systemic thrombolytic therapy.[15,28] Activated partial thromboplastin time (aPTT) should be checked after the completion of alteplase, and maintenance IV heparin should be restarted without a bolus if aPTT is <80 seconds (if not, it should be checked again in 4 hours).[88]

An alteplase bolus regimen (0.6 mg/kg, maximum of 50 mg) given over 15 minutes appears to be comparable in both efficacy and bleeding risk to the more commonly used 100-mg infusion given over 2 hours.[74,75] Limited data exist for more rapid bolus infusions. In a study of a 2-minute alteplase infusion protocol (0.6 mg/kg ideal body weight, maximum dose not specified) versus heparin alone, a significant mean relative improvement in perfusion after 24 hours was reported (measured by perfusion lung scan, 37% vs. 18.8%, respectively) without an increase in major bleeding (minor bleeding was 45% vs. 4%).[81] In patients in extremis, including cardiac arrest from massive PE, a bolus dose should be given.[86] However, thrombolysis for undifferentiated cardiac arrest is not recommended.[28]

All thrombolytic drugs carry a risk of bleeding. The cumulative rate of major bleeding and intracranial/fatal hemorrhage in early trials was shown to be to be 13% and 1.8%, respectively.[73,74,79,81,82,87,89–92] Life-threatening hemorrhage is less common in more recent trials.[78,91] Thrombolysis-related major bleeding is also less frequent when noninvasive imaging methods are used for PE diagnosis.[93] Of note, massive PE patients have higher bleeding rates when compared to patients with nonmassive PE, regardless of whether they are receiving thrombolysis plus heparin or heparin alone.[85,88] A retrospective chart review of patients who received IV alteplase 100 mg for PE between 1996 and 2004 showed a significant increase in bleeding risk among patients with hemodynamic instability requiring vasopressors prior to treatment (multivariate analysis: odds ratio 115).[94] Systemic thrombolytic therapy is nevertheless recommended for patients with massive PE considered to have acceptably low bleeding risk.[15,28,86] Absolute contraindications to systemic thrombolytic therapy for PE (listed after this paragraph) are extrapolated from guidelines for ST-segment elevation MI[95]; clinicians are, however, encouraged to judge the relative merits of the therapy on a case-by-case basis.[28] Absolute contraindications to systemic thrombolytic therapy for MI might become relative in a patient with immediately life-threatening high-risk PE.[15] Despite the recommendations of current guidelines and evidence in favor of systemic thrombolytic therapy in massive PE, this therapy continues to be grossly underutilized.[13,14]

Absolute contraindications to systemic thrombolytic therapy in PE[28]:

- Any prior intracranial hemorrhage
- Known structural intracranial malignant neoplasm or cerebrovascular disease (e.g., arteriovenous malformation)
- Ischemic stroke within 3 months
- Suspected aortic dissection
- Active bleeding or bleeding diathesis
- Recent (i.e., within preceding 3 weeks[15]) surgery encroaching on the spinal canal or brain
- Recent (i.e., within preceding 3 weeks[15]) significant closed-head or facial trauma with radiographic evidence of bony fracture or brain injury

Surgical Embolectomy

Historically, surgical embolectomy for PE was considered an option of last resort, reserved for patients in cardiogenic shock or requiring CPR.[15,96,97] However, as mortality rates have improved from 57% in the 1960s[98] to 26% (16% to 46%) in the late 1980s/early 1990s,[99] this procedure has reemerged as a viable treatment option for massive PE. Certain authors have attributed this change not to surgical technique, but rather to a more expeditious diagnostic approach and to advances in the perioperative management of these patients, specifically the preoperative application of CPB in moribund patients.[99] A more rigorous and discriminating patient selection process has likely also contributed to the improved outcomes. For example, instead of undergoing surgical embolectomy, patients with acute PE superimposed on chronic thromboembolic pulmonary hypertension are now transferred to centers that specialize in pulmonary endarterectomy.[15,100] The wide range of mortality rates reported in various case series reflects the importance of presurgical clinical status on postsurgical outcome; patients with no preoperative CPR, intermittent CPR with stable hemodynamics on arrival to the OR, and continuous CPR on arrival to the OR were reported to have mortality rate of 10%, 40%, and 80%, respectively.[101]

A recent study, extended inclusion criteria for surgical embolectomy to include hemodynamically stable patients with large clot and RV dysfunction, demonstrated an even lower mortality rate of 6%.[96] Although extending the indications to include submassive PE remains controversial, this and another recent series (0% perioperative mortality, 8% 30-day mortality)[97] suggest that surgical embolectomy is not as futile as once believed, provided there is appropriate patient selection and consideration of technical factors.

If surgical expertise and resources are available, indications for surgical embolectomy for massive PE are the presence of a contraindication to systemic thrombolytic therapy, failed systemic thrombolytic therapy, or hemodynamic instability that is likely to cause death before systemic thrombolytic therapy can take effect.[86] A surgical approach may also be appropriate in the case of impending paradoxical embolism (thrombus entrapped within a patent foramen ovale [PFO]).[28] Absolute contraindications to systemic thrombolytic therapy are present in approximately one-third of massive PE[88] (although this number varies depending on what is considered to be an absolute vs. relative contraindications). Failure of systemic thrombolytic therapy is defined as persistent clinical instability and residual echocardiographic RV dysfunction at 36 hours and is reported to occur in 8.2% of cases.[102] In these cases, rescue embolectomy is recommended over repeat systemic thrombolytic therapy.[102]

Catheter Embolectomy

The goal of the CDT is rapid central clot debulking to relieve life-threatening heart strain and improve pulmonary perfusion.[103] Modern CDT for massive PE is defined as the use of low-profile catheters and devices (<10 F) for the purpose of catheter-directed mechanical fragmentation and/or aspiration of emboli, as well as optional intraclot thrombolytic agent injection.[103] To avoid the risk of perforation, CDT is recommended only for use on major branches of the pulmonary artery and should be terminated as soon as hemodynamics improves, regardless of angiographic result.[15,104] However, because successful clot fragmentation increases the surface area of thrombus, some authors advocate giving an extended intraclot infusion of low-dose thrombolytics, especially to patients with residual elevation of PA pressure with right heart strain.[103,105,106]

Large randomized controlled trials on CDT have been hindered by device variations, lack of well-established protocols, and feasibility issues. A meta-analysis of 35 studies conducted from January 1990 through September 2008 evaluated the safety and efficacy of CDT for massive PE.[107] Clinical success—defined as stabilization of hemodynamics, resolution of hypoxia, and survival to hospital discharge—was 86.5%.[103,107] In 96% of patients, systemic thrombolytic therapy was not given, and CDT was used as the first adjunct to heparin.[107] Approximately 30% of patients received mechanical fragmentation and/or aspiration of emboli only, and 60% of patients received an extended thrombolytic infusion through the catheter.[107] The pooled risk of major procedural complications (e.g., groin hematoma requiring transfusion) was 2.4%.[107]

CDT shares the same indications as surgical embolectomy and is a relatively safe and highly effective treatment option for massive PE in an experienced center. Knowledge of local expertise should guide the emergency physician's decision to pursue one or the other option,[28] and establishing a transfer protocol is encouraged in facilities that lack either option. A management algorithm for suspected massive PE in the ED is shown in Figure 11.3.

Adjunctive Therapies

Inferior Vena Cava (IVC) Filter Subgroup analysis of massive PE patients in the ICOPER showed reduced 90-day mortality among patients with IVC filters (hazard ratio 0.12). However, only 11 of 108 patients with massive PE in this registry received an IVC filter. Some authors of case series for surgical embolectomy and catheter embolectomy advocate the use of IVC filters for their patients with massive PE, given relatively the low procedural risk and potentially lethal nature of recurrent PE in this group.[96,99,106,108] In the absence of data from large randomized controlled

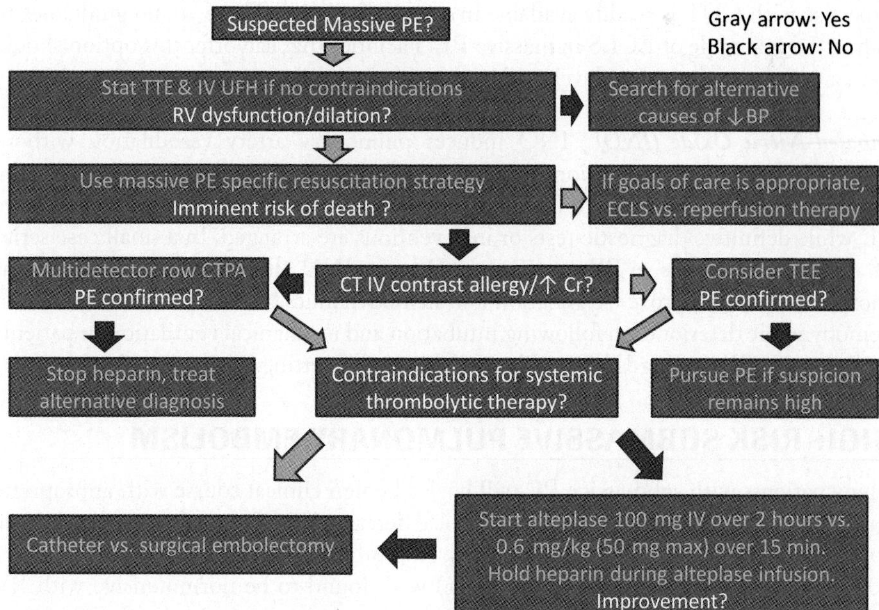

FIGURE 11.3 Management algorithm for suspected massive PE. PE, pulmonary embolism; TTE, transthoracic echocardiogram; IV, intravenous; UFH, unfractionated heparin; BP, blood pressure; RV, right ventricular; ECLS, extracorporeal life support; CTPA, computed tomographic pulmonary angiography; CT, computed tomography; Cr, creatinine; TEE, transesophageal echocardiogram; min., minutes.

trials, AHA guidelines state that placement of an IVC filter may be considered for patients with acute PE with very poor cardiopulmonary reserve, including those with massive PE.[28]

Extracorporeal Life Support (ECLS) ECLS can be lifesaving for massive PE patients who are too unstable to tolerate other interventions or have failed reperfusion therapy.[109] Bedside cannulation and placement on ECLS are possible during cardiac arrest, and patients can be transferred to institutions with higher levels of care while receiving ECLS.[109] A study of 21 patients with massive PE receiving ECLS (8 in cardiac arrest at ECLS initiation) demonstrated a mortality rate of 38% and mean ECLS bypass duration of 4.7 days.[109] Of note, 10/13 survivors in this study required no additional therapy other than anticoagulation. Excluding patients in hypercoagulable states, the study noted that these 10 patients had sufficient amount of emboli autolysis to allow recovery of RV function within 5 days.[109] A recent case series of patients with massive PE requiring ECLS (9/10 in cardiac arrest) reported a 30-day mortality of 30%.[110] Of note, 8 out of 10 patients had CDT while on ECLS, which improved hemodynamics and allowed early weaning of ECLS (mean ECLS bypass was 48 ± 44 hours).[110] Although this was a small study without a comparative group, it suggests that early CDT to shorten ECLS bypass time may have both clinical and financial benefit, given the complications associated with prolonged ECLS. However, it should also be noted that a small case series of successful CDT during cardiac arrest (6/7 survived) suggests less of a need for ECLS if expertise with CDT is readily available in a given facility.[111] There are no guidelines to define the exact role of ECLS in massive PE. Facilities that can offer this option should have a treatment algorithm developed by an interdisciplinary team.

Inhaled Nitric Oxide (INO) INO induces pulmonary artery vasodilation without generating systemic hypotension, making it a physiologically attractive adjunct in the management of massive PE. INO may help stabilize patients with suspected massive PE while definitive diagnostic tests or interventions are arranged. In a small case series of patients with massive PE requiring intubation, INO at a dose of 10–20 ppm was shown to rapidly improve oxygenation and hemodynamics.[112] Given the known risk of hemodynamic deterioration following intubation and mechanical ventilation in patients with massive PE, having INO readily available in this setting is a reasonable strategy.

HIGH-RISK SUBMASSIVE PULMONARY EMBOLISM

Many patients with submassive PE will have a benign clinical course with appropriate anticoagulation; others will experience clinical deterioration due to a loss of physiologic compensation or recurrent embolic events. In a prospective clinical outcome study of 209 patients with confirmed PE, 65 (31%) were found to be normotensive with RV dysfunction on initial TTE; of these, 10% developed shock within the first 24 hours despite initiation of heparin therapy; half of these 10% died.[113] Important issues that remain to be addressed include: (1) How to identify submassive PE patients with poor short-term prognosis who may benefit from ICU admission (Fig. 11.1), and (2) What treatment beyond anticoagulation can be provided to improve the outcome of this subgroup.

Research has assessed a variety of risk-stratification tools for normotensive patients with PE. Current risk stratification tools include clinical scores (e.g., the pulmonary embolism severity index [PESI],[114] simplified PESI[115]), biomarkers (e.g., troponin,[116,117] highly sensitive troponin T assay,[118] heart-type fatty acid–binding protein,[119] brain-type natriuretic peptides [BNP]/N-terminal–pro-BNP [NT-proBNP][120]), cardiopulmonary imaging (e.g., RV dysfunction in CT/TTE),[121] or combinations of these indicators.[122–124] Unfortunately, identification of a definitive risk assessment tool has been hampered by a paucity of studies focusing on short-term mortality/deterioration risk (i.e., within the first 48 hours) and lack of a universally accepted definition of RV dysfunction and threshold values for diagnostic biomarkers.

Even if such a high-risk subgroup can be successfully identified, it remains unclear what therapeutic interventions would prove safe and superior to the current approach of anticoagulation with the option of subsequent reperfusion therapy for patients who further deteriorate. In a trial comparing heparin plus alteplase versus heparin alone for submassive PE, the requirement for escalation of treatment was significantly lower in the first group (10.2% vs. 24.6%), but no difference in all-cause mortality was observed (3.4% vs. 2.2%).[91] The study showed that in the majority of submassive PE patients who experience subsequent deterioration, providers had sufficient time to intervene with reperfusion therapy. Preemptive reperfusion therapy with the goal of reducing short-term mortality therefore appears unjustified at this time.

The use of preemptive reperfusion therapy to prevent long-term RV dysfunction is also of questionable value. In patients with submassive PE who survive to receive 1 week of anticoagulation alone, the degree of pulmonary vascular obstruction and reversal of RV dysfunction appear similar to patients who receive systemic thrombolytic therapy.[6,15,28] Reperfusion therapy may possibly have benefit in preventing persistent or worsening RV systolic pressure (RVSP) in the long term (i.e., 6 months),[125] but the clinical significance of changes (or lack thereof) in RVSP have yet to be demonstrated in a large-scale study.

Four major interventions are being investigated in the treatment of the high-risk subgroup in submassive PE. The use of systemic rt-PA, soon to be addressed by the ongoing PEITHO trial (tenecteplase vs. placebo); surgical embolectomy, as described in more recent surgical case series[96]; CDT with extended catheter-based infusion of rt-PA[126]; and half-dose alteplase as described in the MOPETT trial.[127] Besides safety, clinically meaningful outcome benefits should be demonstrated before these strategies can routinely be recommended over anticoagulation alone in this subgroup of patients

CONCLUSION

Massive PE comprises a small fraction of PE, particularly now that we are detecting a greater number of lower-risk patients with the advent of MDCTPA; it remains, however, an undertreated, lethal, and challenging condition to manage. Optimal management requires a sophisticated understanding of the unique physiology of PE, an efficient and systemic approach to diagnosis and treatment, and an institution-based management algorithm based on available resources and expertise. If there are no contraindications, systemic thrombolytic therapy should be offered to patients with confirmed massive PE, as well as suspected massive PE with suggestive TTE findings when there is no time for confirmatory study due to imminent risk of death. A decision to withhold thrombolysis based on the risk of bleeding needs to be followed by an attempt to provide either surgical or catheter-directed embolectomy in massive PE. As for submassive PE, a large-scale study is needed to determine what risk factors predict short-term (i.e., <48 hours) deterioration. The challenge remains to identify the high-risk subgroup in patients with submassive PE who may benefit from more aggressive care, and it is still unknown what specific preemptive reperfusion therapy should be offered to them.

LITERATURE TABLE

TRIAL	DESIGN	RESULT
Torbicki et al., *Eur Heart J.* 2008[15]	Guidelines and expert consensus documents by the European Society of Cardiology on the diagnosis and management of acute PE	Extensive review of diagnostic and treatment strategy for acute PE with an emphasis on risk stratification into high-, intermediate-, and low-risk PE
Kasper et al., *J Am Coll Cardiol.* 1997[22] MAPPET	Prospective observational study of 1,001 patients with confirmed or suspected PE plus (1) acute right ventricular pressure overload/pulmonary hypertension without hypotension, (2) arterial hypotension, (3) cardiogenic shock, or (4) circulatory collapse requiring CPR	Associated in-hospital mortality rate for each group was (1) 8.1%, (2) 15%, (3) 25%, and (4) 65%. Groups with more hemodynamic instability received confirmatory imaging studies less often and early thrombolysis more often
Jaff et al., *Circulation.* 2011[28]	A scientific statement from the American Heart Association on the management of PE, proximal DVT, and chronic thromboembolic pulmonary hypertension	Acute PE is classified into massive, submassive, and low-risk PE. Management recommendations are provided using classifications of recommendations and level of evidence
Goldhaber et al., *Lancet.* 1999[29] ICOPER	Prospective observational study of 2,454 patients with acute PE; primary outcome was all-cause mortality at 3 mo. The prognostic effect of baseline factors on survival was also assessed using multivariate analyses	Mortality rate was 58.3% for massive PE and 15.1% for nonmassive PE. Age over 70 y (HR 1.6, 95% CI 1.1–2.3), cancer (HR 2.3, 95% CI 1.5–3.5), congestive heart failure (HR 2.4, 95% CI 1.5–3.7), chronic obstructive pulmonary disease (HR 1.8, 95% CI 1.5–3.7), systolic arterial hypotension (HR 2.4, 95% CI 1.2–2.7), tachypnea (HR 2.0, 95% CI 1.2–3.2), and RV hypokinesis on echocardiography (HR 2.0, 95% CI 1.3–2.9) were identified as significant prognostic factors
Wan et al., *Circulation.* 2004[85]	Meta-analysis of 11 randomized trials comparing heparin vs. thrombolytic therapy in treatment of PE; primary outcomes included rate of recurrent PE or death during hospitalization or within 30 d	No difference in the primary outcome. However, in a subgroup analysis of five trials that included massive PE, thrombolytic therapy was associated with lower rate of recurrent PE or death than heparin (9.4% vs. 19.0%; OR 0.45, 95% CI 0.22–0.92, NNT 10)
Kuo et al., *J Vasc Interv Radiol.* 2009[107]	Meta-analysis of modern catheter-directed thrombolysis (CDT) in massive PE. Successful outcome defined as stabilization of hemodynamics, resolution of hypoxia, and survival to hospital discharge	The pooled clinical success rate from CDT was 86.5% (95% CI 82.1%, 90.2%) and pooled risks of minor and major procedural complications were 7.9% (95% CI 5.0%, 11.3%) and 2.4% (95% CI 1.9%, 4.3%), respectively

CI, confidence interval; HR, hazard ratio; NNT, number needed to treat; OR, odds ratio.

REFERENCES

1. Stein PD, Henry JW. Prevalence of acute pulmonary embolism among patients in a general hospital and at autopsy. *Chest.* 1995;108(4):978–981.
2. Rubinstein I, Murray D, Hoffstein V. Fatal pulmonary emboli in hospitalized patients: an autopsy study. *Arch Intern Med.* 1988;148(6):1425–1426.
3. Goldhaber SZ, Hennekens CH, Evans DA, et al. Factors associated with correct antemortem diagnosis of major pulmonary embolism. *Am J Med.* 1982;73(6):822–826.
4. Clagett GP, Reisch JS. Prevention of venous thromboembolism in general surgical patients. Results of meta-analysis. *Ann Surg.* 1988;208(2):227–240.
5. Moser KM, Fedullo PF, LitteJohn JK, et al. Frequent asymptomatic pulmonary embolism in patients with deep venous thrombosis. *JAMA.* 1994;271(3):223–225.
6. Wood KE. Major pulmonary embolism: review of a pathophysiologic approach to the golden hour of hemodynamically significant pulmonary embolism. *Chest.* 2002;121(3):877–905.
7. Wiener RS, Schwartz LM, Woloshin S. Time trends in pulmonary embolism in the United States: evidence of overdiagnosis. *Arch Intern Med.* 2011;171(9):831–837.
8. Wittram C, Meehan MJ, Halpern EF, et al. Trends in thoracic radiology over a decade at a large academic medical center. *J Thorac Imaging.* 2004;19(3):164–170.
9. Donohoo JH, Mayo-Smith WW, Pezzullo JA, et al. Utilization patterns and diagnostic yield of 3421 consecutive multidetector row computed tomography pulmonary angiograms in a busy emergency department. *J Comput Assist Tomogr.* 2008;32(3):421–425.
10. Auer RC, Schulman AR, Tuorto S, et al. Use of helical CT is associated with an increased incidence of postoperative pulmonary emboli in cancer patients with no change in the number of fatal pulmonary emboli. *J Am Coll Surg.* 2009;208(5):871–878; discussion 878–880.
11. Weir ID, Drescher F, Cousin D, et al. Trends in use and yield of chest computed tomography with angiography for diagnosis of pulmonary embolism in a Connecticut hospital emergency department. *Conn Med.* 2010;74(1):5–9.
12. Pollack CV, Schreiber D, Goldhaber SZ, et al. Clinical characteristics, management, and outcomes of patients diagnosed with acute pulmonary embolism in the emergency department: initial report of EMPEROR (Multicenter Emergency Medicine Pulmonary Embolism in the Real World Registry). *J Am Coll Cardiol.* 2011;57(6):700–706.
13. Lin BW, Schreiber DH, Liu G, et al. Therapy and outcomes in massive pulmonary embolism from the emergency medicine pulmonary embolism in the real world registry. *Am J Emerg Med.* 2012;30(9):1774–1781.
14. Stein PD, Matta F. Thrombolytic therapy in unstable patients with acute pulmonary embolism: saves lives but underused. *Am J Med.* 2012;125(5):465–470.
15. Torbicki A, Perrier A, Konstantinides S, et al. Guidelines on the diagnosis and management of acute pulmonary embolism: the Task Force for the Diagnosis and Management of Acute Pulmonary Embolism of the European Society of Cardiology (ESC). *Eur Heart J.* 2008;29(18):2276–2315.
16. Fesmire FM, Brown MD, Espinosa JA, et al. Critical issues in the evaluation and management of adult patients presenting to the emergency department with suspected pulmonary embolism. *Ann Emerg Med. 2011*;57(6):628–652.e675.
17. Church A, Tichauer M. The emergency medicine approach to the evaluation and treatment of pulmonary embolism. *Emerg Med Pract.* 2012;14(12):1–22.
18. Aujesky D, Roy PM, Verschuren F, et al. Outpatient versus inpatient treatment for patients with acute pulmonary embolism: an international, open-label, randomised, non-inferiority trial. *Lancet.* 2011;378(9785):41–48.
19. Post F, Mertens D, Sinning C, et al. Decision for aggressive therapy in acute pulmonary embolism: implication of elevated troponin T. *Clin Res Cardiol.* 2009;98(6):401–408.
20. Palmieri V, Gallotta G, Rendina D, et al. Troponin I and right ventricular dysfunction for risk assessment in patients with nonmassive pulmonary embolism in the emergency department in combination with clinically based risk score. *Intern Emerg Med.* 2008;3(2):131–138.
21. Bova C, Pesavento R, Marchiori A, et al. Risk stratification and outcomes in hemodynamically stable patients with acute pulmonary embolism: a prospective, multicentre, cohort study with three months of follow-up. *J Thromb Haemost.* 2009;7(6):938–944.
22. Kasper W, Konstantinides S, Geibel A, et al. Management strategies and determinants of outcome in acute major pulmonary embolism: results of a multicenter registry. *J Am Coll Cardiol.* 1997;30(5):1165–1171.
23. Ryu JH, Pellikka PA, Froehling DA, et al. Saddle pulmonary embolism diagnosed by CT angiography: frequency, clinical features and outcome. *Respir Med.* 2007;101(7):1537–1542.

24. Sardi A, Gluskin J, Guttentag A, et al. Saddle pulmonary embolism: is it as bad as it looks? A community hospital experience. *Crit Care Med.* 2011;39(11):2413–2418.
25. McIntyre KM, Sasahara AA. Correlation of pulmonary photoscan and angiogram as measures of the severity of pulmonary embolic involvement. *J Nucl Med.* 1971;12(11):732–738.
26. McDonald IG, Hirsh J, Hale GS, et al. Major pulmonary embolism, a correlation of clinical findings, haemodynamics, pulmonary angiography, and pathological physiology. *Br Heart J.* 1972;34(4):356–364.
27. Alpert JS, Smith R, Carlson J, et al. Mortality in patients treated for pulmonary embolism. *JAMA.* 1976;236(13):1477–1480.
28. Jaff MR, McMurtry MS, Archer SL, et al. Management of massive and submassive pulmonary embolism, iliofemoral deep vein thrombosis, and chronic thromboembolic pulmonary hypertension: a scientific statement from the American Heart Association. *Circulation.* 2011;123(16):1788–1830.
29. Goldhaber SZ, Visani L, De Rosa M. Acute pulmonary embolism: clinical outcomes in the International Cooperative Pulmonary Embolism Registry (ICOPER). *Lancet.* 1999;353(9162):1386–1389.
30. Alpert JS, Godtfredsen J, Ockene IS, et al. Pulmonary hypertension secondary to minor pulmonary embolism. *Chest.* 1978;73(6):795–797.
31. Stein M, Levy SE. Reflex and humoral responses to pulmonary embolism. *Prog Cardiovasc Dis.* 1974;17(3):167–174.
32. Malik AB. Pulmonary microembolism. *Physiol Rev.* 1983;63(3):1114–1207.
33. McIntyre KM, Sasahara AA. The hemodynamic response to pulmonary embolism in patients without prior cardiopulmonary disease. *Am J Cardiol.* 1971;28(3):288–294.
34. Matthews JC, McLaughlin V. Acute right ventricular failure in the setting of acute pulmonary embolism or chronic pulmonary hypertension: a detailed review of the pathophysiology, diagnosis, and management. *Curr Cardiol Rev.* 2008;4(1):49–59.
35. Zamanian RT, Haddad F, Doyle RL, et al. Management strategies for patients with pulmonary hypertension in the intensive care unit. *Crit Care Med.* 2007;35(9):2037–2050.
36. Haddad F, Doyle R, Murphy DJ, et al. Right ventricular function in cardiovascular disease, part II: pathophysiology, clinical importance, and management of right ventricular failure. *Circulation.* 2008;117(13):1717–1731.
37. Taylor RR, Covell JW, Sonnenblick EH, et al. Dependence of ventricular distensibility on filling of the opposite ventricle. *Am J Physiol.* 1967;213(3):711–718.
38. Jardin F, Dubourg O, Gueret P, et al. Quantitative two-dimensional echocardiography in massive pulmonary embolism: emphasis on ventricular interdependence and leftward septal displacement. *J Am Coll Cardiol.* 1987;10(6):1201–1206.
39. Belenkie I, Dani R, Smith ER, et al. Ventricular interaction during experimental acute pulmonary embolism. *Circulation.* 1988;78(3):761–768.
40. Vlahakes GJ, Turley K, Hoffman JI. The pathophysiology of failure in acute right ventricular hypertension: hemodynamic and biochemical correlations. *Circulation.* 1981;63(1):87–95.
41. Coma-Canella I, Gamallo C, Martinez Onsurbe P, et al. Acute right ventricular infarction secondary to massive pulmonary embolism. *Eur Heart J.* 1988;9(5):534–540.
42. Adams JE III, Siegel BA, Goldstein JA, et al. Elevations of CK-MB following pulmonary embolism. A manifestation of occult right ventricular infarction. *Chest.* 1992;101(5):1203–1206.
43. Jerjes-Sanchez C, Ramirez-Rivera A, de Lourdes Garcia M, et al. Streptokinase and heparin versus heparin alone in massive pulmonary embolism: a randomized controlled trial. *J Thromb Thrombolysis.* 1995;2(3):227–229.
44. Ducas J, Prewitt RM. Pathophysiology and therapy of right ventricular dysfunction due to pulmonary embolism. *Cardiovasc Clin.* 1987;17(2):191–202.
45. Molloy WD, Lee KY, Girling L, et al. Treatment of shock in a canine model of pulmonary embolism. *Am Rev Respir Dis.* 1984;130(5):870–874.
46. Ghignone M, Girling L, Prewitt RM. Volume expansion versus norepinephrine in treatment of a low cardiac output complicating an acute increase in right ventricular afterload in dogs. *Anesthesiology.* 1984;60(2):132–135.
47. Hirsch LJ, Rooney MW, Wat SS, et al. Norepinephrine and phenylephrine effects on right ventricular function in experimental canine pulmonary embolism. *Chest.* 1991;100(3):796–801.
48. De Backer D, Biston P, Devriendt J, et al. Comparison of dopamine and norepinephrine in the treatment of shock. *N Engl J Med.* 2010;362(9):779–789.
49. Goldstein JA, Harada A, Yagi Y, et al. Hemodynamic importance of systolic ventricular interaction, augmented right atrial contractility and atrioventricular synchrony in acute right ventricular dysfunction. *J Am Coll Cardiol.* 1990;16(1):181–189.
50. Layish DT, Tapson VF. Pharmacologic hemodynamic support in massive pulmonary embolism. *Chest.* 1997;111(1):218–224.

51. Jardin F, Genevray B, Brun-Ney D, et al. Dobutamine: a hemodynamic evaluation in pulmonary embolism shock. *Crit Care Med.* 1985;13(12):1009–1012.
52. Roberts DH, Lepore JJ, Maroo A, et al. Oxygen therapy improves cardiac index and pulmonary vascular resistance in patients with pulmonary hypertension. *Chest.* 2001;120(5):1547–1555.
53. Moloney ED, Evans TW. Pathophysiology and pharmacological treatment of pulmonary hypertension in acute respiratory distress syndrome. *Eur Respir J.* 2003;21(4):720–727.
54. Viitanen A, Salmenpera M, Heinonen J. Right ventricular response to hypercarbia after cardiac surgery. *Anesthesiology.* 1990;73(3):393–400.
55. Balanos GM, Talbot NP, Dorrington KL, et al. Human pulmonary vascular response to 4 h of hypercapnia and hypocapnia measured using Doppler echocardiography. *J Appl Physiol (1985).* 2003;94(4):1543–1551.
56. Rosenberger P, Shernan SK, Shekar PS, et al. Acute hemodynamic collapse after induction of general anesthesia for emergent pulmonary embolectomy. *Anesth Analg.* 2006;102(5):1311–1315.
57. Tsapenko MV, Tsapenko AV, Comfere TB, et al. Arterial pulmonary hypertension in noncardiac intensive care unit. *Vasc Health Risk Manag.* 2008;4(5):1043–1060.
58. Vieillard-Baron A, Loubieres Y, Schmitt JM, et al. Cyclic changes in right ventricular output impedance during mechanical ventilation. *J Appl Physiol.* 1999;87(5):1644–1650.
59. Jardin F, Vieillard-Baron A. Is there a safe plateau pressure in ARDS? The right heart only knows. *Intensive Care Med.* 2007;33(3):444–447.
60. Kucher N, Rossi E, De Rosa M, et al. Massive pulmonary embolism. *Circulation.* 2006;113(4):577–582.
61. Casazza F, Bongarzoni A, Centonze F, et al. Prevalence and prognostic significance of right-sided cardiac mobile thrombi in acute massive pulmonary embolism. *Am J Cardiol.* 1997;79(10):1433–1435.
62. Ferrari E, Benhamou M, Berthier F, et al. Mobile thrombi of the right heart in pulmonary embolism: delayed disappearance after thrombolytic treatment. *Chest.* 2005;127(3):1051–1053.
63. Pierre-Justin G, Pierard LA. Management of mobile right heart thrombi: a prospective series. *Int J Cardiol.* 2005;99(3):381–388.
64. Torbicki A, Galie N, Covezzoli A, et al. Right heart thrombi in pulmonary embolism: results from the International Cooperative Pulmonary Embolism Registry. *J Am Coll Cardiol.* 2003;41(12):2245–2251.
65. Raschke RA, Gollihare B, Peirce JC. The effectiveness of implementing the weight-based heparin nomogram as a practice guideline. *Arch Intern Med.* 1996;156(15):1645–1649.
66. Agnelli G, Becattini C. Acute pulmonary embolism. *N Engl J Med.* 2010;363(3):266–274.
67. Pruszczyk P, Torbicki A, Pacho R, et al. Noninvasive diagnosis of suspected severe pulmonary embolism: transesophageal echocardiography vs spiral CT. *Chest.* 1997;112(3):722–728.
68. Steiner P, Lund GK, Debatin JF, et al. Acute pulmonary embolism: value of transthoracic and transesophageal echocardiography in comparison with helical CT. *AJR Am J Roentgenol.* 1996;167(4):931–936.
69. Wittlich N, Erbel R, Eichler A, et al. Detection of central pulmonary artery thromboemboli by transesophageal echocardiography in patients with severe pulmonary embolism. *J Am Soc Echocardiogr.* 1992;5(5):515–524.
70. Vieillard-Baron A, Qanadli SD, Antakly Y, et al. Transesophageal echocardiography for the diagnosis of pulmonary embolism with acute cor pulmonale: a comparison with radiological procedures. *Intensive Care Med.* 1998;24(5):429–433.
71. Kucher N, Luder CM, Dornhofer T, et al. Novel management strategy for patients with suspected pulmonary embolism. *Eur Heart J.* 2003;24(4):366–376.
72. Meneveau N, Schiele F, Metz D, et al. Comparative efficacy of a two-hour regimen of streptokinase versus alteplase in acute massive pulmonary embolism: immediate clinical and hemodynamic outcome and one-year follow-up. *J Am Coll Cardiol.* 1998;31(5):1057–1063.
73. Goldhaber SZ, Kessler CM, Heit JA, et al. Recombinant tissue-type plasminogen activator versus a novel dosing regimen of urokinase in acute pulmonary embolism: a randomized controlled multicenter trial. *J Am Coll Cardiol.* 1992;20(1):24–30.
74. Sors H, Pacouret G, Azarian R, et al. Hemodynamic effects of bolus vs 2-h infusion of alteplase in acute massive pulmonary embolism. A randomized controlled multicenter trial. *Chest.* 1994;106(3):712–717.
75. Goldhaber SZ, Agnelli G, Levine MN. Reduced dose bolus alteplase vs conventional alteplase infusion for pulmonary embolism thrombolysis. An international multicenter randomized trial. The Bolus Alteplase Pulmonary Embolism Group. *Chest.* 1994;106(3):718–724.
76. Tibbutt DA, Davies JA, Anderson JA, et al. Comparison by controlled clinical trial of streptokinase and heparin in treatment of life-threatening pulmonay embolism. *Br Med J.* 1974;1(5904):343–347.
77. Urokinase pulmonary embolism trial. Phase 1 results: a cooperative study. *JAMA.* 1970;214(12):2163–2172.
78. Goldhaber SZ, Haire WD, Feldstein ML, et al. Alteplase versus heparin in acute pulmonary embolism: randomised trial assessing right-ventricular function and pulmonary perfusion. *Lancet.* 1993;341(8844):507–511.

79. Dalla-Volta S, Palla A, Santolicandro A, et al. PAIMS 2: alteplase combined with heparin versus heparin in the treatment of acute pulmonary embolism. Plasminogen activator Italian multicenter study 2. *J Am Coll Cardiol.* 1992;20(3):520–526.
80. Ly B, Arnesen H, Eie H, et al. A controlled clinical trial of streptokinase and heparin in the treatment of major pulmonary embolism. *Acta Med Scand.* 1978;203(6):465–470.
81. Levine M, Hirsh J, Weitz J, et al. A randomized trial of a single bolus dosage regimen of recombinant tissue plasminogen activator in patients with acute pulmonary embolism. *Chest.* 1990;98(6):1473–1479.
82. The urokinase pulmonary embolism trial. A national cooperative study. *Circulation.* 1973;47(suppl 2): II1–II108.
83. Konstantinides S, Tiede N, Geibel A, et al. Comparison of alteplase versus heparin for resolution of major pulmonary embolism. *Am J Cardiol.* 1998;82(8):966–970.
84. Daniels LB, Parker JA, Patel SR, et al. Relation of duration of symptoms with response to thrombolytic therapy in pulmonary embolism. *Am J Cardiol.* 1997;80(2):184–188.
85. Wan S, Quinlan DJ, Agnelli G, et al. Thrombolysis compared with heparin for the initial treatment of pulmonary embolism: a meta-analysis of the randomized controlled trials. *Circulation.* 2004; 110(6):744–749.
86. Kearon C, Akl EA, Comerota AJ, et al. Antithrombotic therapy for VTE disease: Antithrombotic Therapy and Prevention of Thrombosis, 9th ed: American College of Chest Physicians Evidence-Based Clinical Practice Guidelines. *Chest.* 2012;141(suppl 2):e419S–e494S.
87. Verstraete M, Miller GA, Bounameaux H, et al. Intravenous and intrapulmonary recombinant tissue-type plasminogen activator in the treatment of acute massive pulmonary embolism. *Circulation.* 1988;77(2):353–360.
88. Kucher N, Goldhaber SZ. Management of massive pulmonary embolism. *Circulation.* 2005;112(2): e28–e32.
89. Meyer G, Sors H, Charbonnier B, et al. Effects of intravenous urokinase versus alteplase on total pulmonary resistance in acute massive pulmonary embolism: a European multicenter double-blind trial. The European Cooperative Study Group for Pulmonary Embolism. *J Am Coll Cardiol.* 1992;19(2):239–245.
90. Goldhaber SZ, Kessler CM, Heit J, et al. Randomised controlled trial of recombinant tissue plasminogen activator versus urokinase in the treatment of acute pulmonary embolism. *Lancet.* 1988;2(8606): 293–298.
91. Konstantinides S, Geibel A, Heusel G, et al. Heparin plus alteplase compared with heparin alone in patients with submassive pulmonary embolism. *N Engl J Med.* 2002;347(15):1143–1150.
92. Kanter DS, Mikkola KM, Patel SR, et al. Thrombolytic therapy for pulmonary embolism. Frequency of intracranial hemorrhage and associated risk factors. *Chest.* 1997;111(5):1241–1245.
93. Stein PD, Hull RD, Raskob G. Risks for major bleeding from thrombolytic therapy in patients with acute pulmonary embolism. Consideration of noninvasive management. *Ann Intern Med.* 1994; 121(5):313–317.
94. Fiumara K, Kucher N, Fanikos J, et al. Predictors of major hemorrhage following fibrinolysis for acute pulmonary embolism. *Am J Cardiol.* 2006;97(1):127–129.
95. Antman EM, Anbe DT, Armstrong PW, et al. ACC/AHA guidelines for the management of patients with ST-elevation myocardial infarction: a report of the American College of Cardiology/American Heart Association Task Force on Practice Guidelines (Committee to revise the 1999 Guidelines for the Management of Patients with Acute Myocardial Infarction). *Circulation.* 2004;110(9):e82–e292.
96. Leacche M, Unic D, Goldhaber SZ, et al. Modern surgical treatment of massive pulmonary embolism: results in 47 consecutive patients after rapid diagnosis and aggressive surgical approach. *J Thorac Cardiovasc Surg.* 2005;129(5):1018–1023.
97. Kadner A, Schmidli J, Schonhoff F, et al. Excellent outcome after surgical treatment of massive pulmonary embolism in critically ill patients. *J Thorac Cardiovasc Surg.* 2008;136(2):448–451.
98. Cross FS, Mowlem A. A survey of the current status of pulmonary embolectomy for massive pulmonary embolism. *Circulation.* 1967;35(suppl 4):I86–I91.
99. Stulz P, Schlapfer R, Feer R, et al. Decision making in the surgical treatment of massive pulmonary embolism. *Eur J Cardiothorac Surg.* 1994;8(4):188–193.
100. Hoeper MM, Mayer E, Simonneau G, et al. Chronic thromboembolic pulmonary hypertension. *Circulation.* 2006;113(16):2011–2020.
101. Ullmann M, Hemmer W, Hannekum A. The urgent pulmonary embolectomy: mechanical resuscitation in the operating theatre determines the outcome. *Thorac Cardiovasc Surg.* 1999;47(1):5–8.
102. Meneveau N, Seronde MF, Blonde MC, et al. Management of unsuccessful thrombolysis in acute massive pulmonary embolism. *Chest.* 2006;129(4):1043–1050.

103. Kuo WT. Endovascular therapy for acute pulmonary embolism. *Journal of vascular and interventional radiology: JVIR.* 2012;23(2):167–179 e164; quiz 179.
104. Uflacker R. Interventional therapy for pulmonary embolism. *J Vasc Interv Radiol.* 2001;12(2):147–164.
105. Schmitz-Rode T, Kilbinger M, Gunther RW. Simulated flow pattern in massive pulmonary embolism: significance for selective intrapulmonary thrombolysis. *Cardiovasc Intervent Radiol.* 1998;21(3):199–204.
106. de Gregorio MA, Laborda A, de Blas I, et al. Endovascular treatment of a haemodynamically unstable massive pulmonary embolism using fibrinolysis and fragmentation. Experience with 111 patients in a single centre. Why don't we follow ACCP recommendations? *Arch Bronconeumol.* 2011;47(1):17–24.
107. Kuo WT, Gould MK, Louie JD, et al. Catheter-directed therapy for the treatment of massive pulmonary embolism: systematic review and meta-analysis of modern techniques. *J Vasc Interv Radiol.* 2009;20(11):1431–1440.
108. Dauphine C, Omari B. Pulmonary embolectomy for acute massive pulmonary embolism. *Ann Thorac Surg.* 2005;79(4):1240–1244.
109. Maggio P, Hemmila M, Haft J, et al. Extracorporeal life support for massive pulmonary embolism. *J Trauma.* 2007;62(3):570–576.
110. Munakata R, Yamamoto T, Hosokawa Y, et al. Massive pulmonary embolism requiring extracorporeal life support treated with catheter-based interventions. *Int Heart J.* 2012;53(6):370–374.
111. Fava M, Loyola S, Bertoni H, et al. Massive pulmonary embolism: percutaneous mechanical thrombectomy during cardiopulmonary resuscitation. *J Vasc Interv Radiol.* 2005;16(1):119–123.
112. Summerfield DT, Desai H, Levitov A, et al. Inhaled nitric oxide as salvage therapy in massive pulmonary embolism: a case series. *Respir Care.* 2012;57(3):444–448.
113. Grifoni S, Olivotto I, Cecchini P, et al. Short-term clinical outcome of patients with acute pulmonary embolism, normal blood pressure, and echocardiographic right ventricular dysfunction. *Circulation.* 2000;101(24):2817–2822.
114. Aujesky D, Obrosky DS, Stone RA, et al. A prediction rule to identify low-risk patients with pulmonary embolism. *Arch Intern Med. 2006*;166(2):169–175.
115. Jimenez D, Aujesky D, Moores L, et al. Simplification of the pulmonary embolism severity index for prognostication in patients with acute symptomatic pulmonary embolism. *Arch Intern Med.* 2010;170(15):1383–1389.
116. Jimenez D, Uresandi F, Otero R, et al. Troponin-based risk stratification of patients with acute nonmassive pulmonary embolism: systematic review and metaanalysis. *Chest.* 2009;136(4):974–982.
117. Pruszczyk P, Bochowicz A, Torbicki A, et al. Cardiac troponin T monitoring identifies high-risk group of normotensive patients with acute pulmonary embolism. *Chest.* 2003;123(6):1947–1952.
118. Lankeit M, Friesen D, Aschoff J, et al. Highly sensitive troponin T assay in normotensive patients with acute pulmonary embolism. *Eur Heart J.* 2010;31(15):1836–1844.
119. Dellas C, Puls M, Lankeit M, et al. Elevated heart-type fatty acid-binding protein levels on admission predict an adverse outcome in normotensive patients with acute pulmonary embolism. *J Am Coll Cardiol.* 2010;55(19):2150–2157.
120. Klok FA, Mos IC, Huisman MV. Brain-type natriuretic peptide levels in the prediction of adverse outcome in patients with pulmonary embolism: a systematic review and meta-analysis. *Am J Respir Crit Care Med.* 2008;178(4):425–430.
121. Sanchez O, Trinquart L, Colombet I, et al. Prognostic value of right ventricular dysfunction in patients with haemodynamically stable pulmonary embolism: a systematic review. *Eur Heart J.* 2008;29(12):1569–1577.
122. Lankeit M, Jimenez D, Kostrubiec M, et al. Predictive value of the high-sensitivity troponin T assay and the simplified Pulmonary Embolism Severity Index in hemodynamically stable patients with acute pulmonary embolism: a prospective validation study. *Circulation.* 2011;124(24):2716–2724.
123. Kang DK, Sun JS, Park KJ, et al. Usefulness of combined assessment with computed tomographic signs of right ventricular dysfunction and cardiac troponin T for risk stratification of acute pulmonary embolism. *Am J Cardiol.* 2011;108(1):133–140.
124. Lankeit M, Gomez V, Wagner C, et al. A strategy combining imaging and laboratory biomarkers in comparison with a simplified clinical score for risk stratification of patients with acute pulmonary embolism. *Chest.* 2012;141(4):916–922.
125. Kline JA, Steuerwald MT, Marchick MR, et al. Prospective evaluation of right ventricular function and functional status 6 months after acute submassive pulmonary embolism: frequency of persistent or subsequent elevation in estimated pulmonary artery pressure. *Chest.* 2009;136(5):1202–1210.
126. Kucher N, Boekstegers P, Muller OJ, et al. Randomized, controlled trial of ultrasound-assisted catheter-directed thrombolysis for acute intermediate-risk pulmonary embolism. *Circulation.* 2014;129(4):479–486.

12

Acute Respiratory Distress Syndrome

Darryl Abrams and Daniel Brodie

BACKGROUND

Acute respiratory distress syndrome (ARDS) is characterized by the rapid onset of hypoxemia and bilateral pulmonary infiltrates consistent with pulmonary edema that cannot be fully attributed to cardiac failure or fluid overload.[1] The ARDS Definition Task Force has recently revised this definition, which uses the ratio of the partial pressure of arterial oxygen to the fraction of inspired oxygen (PaO_2 to FIO_2 ratio), to classify ARDS into mild ($200 < PaO_2/FIO_2 \leq 300$), moderate ($100 < PaO_2/FIO_2 \leq 200$), and severe ($PaO_2/FIO_2 \leq 100$), with a positive end-expiratory pressure (PEEP) of at least 5 cm of water.[2] By these criteria, there are estimated to be over 190,000 cases of ARDS in the United States annually.[3] In clinical trials involving patients with ARDS, mortality remains in the range of 22% to 45%, with lower PaO_2 to FIO_2 ratios correlating with worse survival rates.[2,4–9] The majority of ARDS cases are caused by bacterial or viral pneumonia, extrapulmonary sepsis, aspiration, and trauma. Less common causes include acute pancreatitis, transfusions, and drug reactions.[3,10,11] Pathologically, diffuse alveolar damage results from injury to both the capillary endothelium and the lung epithelium, increasing permeability and allowing protein-rich alveolar edema to form. Surfactant production and function are impaired, promoting alveolar collapse.[7,12] The result is abnormal gas exchange, with hypoxemia and impaired carbon dioxide excretion, as well as decreased lung compliance.[13] The distribution of ARDS is heterogeneous within the lung. Positive pressure ventilation, although potentially lifesaving in ARDS, may cause ventilator-associated lung injury (VALI) and exacerbate the inflammatory process by overdistending less affected regions of the lung and repeatedly collapsing and reopening small bronchioles and alveoli.[13,14] The use of a high fraction of inspired oxygen may also contribute to lung injury.[14,15] The cornerstone of management of ARDS is treatment of the precipitating illness and minimization of VALI.[4,12] This chapter discusses ARDS therapies available to the emergency physician and the rationale behind them.

MANAGEMENT GUIDELINES

Lung-Protective Ventilation

The only intervention that definitively demonstrates a survival benefit in ARDS is a volume- and pressure-limited ventilation strategy. In 2000, the ARDS Network published the results of a prospective randomized trial (ARMA) in which 861 intubated patients with ARDS were assigned to receive either (1) a tidal volume of 6 mL/kg predicted body weight (based on height) with a goal airway pressure measured after a 0.5-second pause at the end of inspiration (plateau pressure) of 30 cm of water or less or (2) a traditional tidal volume of 12 mL/kg with a goal plateau pressure of 50 cm of water or less.[4] Tidal volumes in each group were reduced stepwise by 1 mL/kg (minimum tidal volume 4 mL/kg) as needed to achieve the target plateau pressures, with an increase in respiratory rate as needed to maintain adequate minute ventilation up to a maximum set respiratory rate of 35 breaths/min. For the group treated with the volume- and pressure-limited strategy, results showed significantly lower mortality (31% vs. 39.8%), more ventilator-free days (12 ± 11 vs. 10 ± 11), and more days without nonpulmonary organ failure (15 ± 11 vs. 12 ± 11). Of note, the actual plateau pressures achieved in the low and traditional tidal volume groups were 25 ± 6 and 33 ± 8 cm of water, respectively. Additionally, oxygenation early in the trial was not a good predictor of outcome, as the low tidal volume group had lower PaO_2 to FIO_2 ratios on days 1 and 3, yet this group had better survival. The results of this and two other randomized trials with similar interventions have led to the adoption of a lung-protective strategy targeting low volume (6 mL/kg predicted body weight or less) and low pressure (plateau pressures of 30 cm of water or less) as the standard of care in ventilator management in ARDS.[4,16,17]

PEEP Strategy

Nonaerated portions of the lung in ARDS—those not adequately exchanging gas due to alveolar edema and collapse—may contribute significantly to shunt physiology and hypoxemia; in addition, the shear forces of cyclic opening and closing of alveolar units with positive pressure ventilation may precipitate worsening inflammation and VALI.[13,18] By applying PEEP via the ventilator, a portion of the collapsed alveoli may be reopened or "recruited." With this intervention, the proportion of nonaerated lung may be reduced and arterial oxygenation goals met, with lower levels of FIO_2 delivered by the ventilator. However, increased levels of PEEP may cause circulatory compromise by impeding venous return and may lead to increased regional airway pressures and lung volumes, further exacerbating VALI.

The effect of different levels of PEEP on clinical outcomes was investigated by the ARDS Clinical Trials Network in a prospective, randomized trial in which 549 intubated patients with ARDS were randomized to either a high or low PEEP strategy.[5] PEEP and FIO_2 were adjusted in discrete steps to maintain an arterial oxyhemoglobin saturation (measured by pulse oximetry, SpO_2) of 88% to 95% or a PaO_2 of 55 to 80 mm Hg. There was no difference in mortality, ventilator-free days, ICU-free days, or organ failure–free days between the two groups, despite higher PaO_2 to FIO_2 ratios and respiratory system compliance in the high PEEP group. A subsequent multicenter study randomized 767 subjects with ARDS to either a minimal distention strategy (moderate PEEP of 5 to 9 cm of water) or an increased recruitment strategy (a level of PEEP set to reach a plateau pressure of 28 to 30 cm of water).[8] Both groups were managed with low tidal volume ventilation (6 mL/kg of predicted body weight). Mean PEEP values in the minimal distention and increased recruitment strategy groups on day 1 were 8.4 cm of water and 15.8 cm of water, respectively. The increased recruitment strategy was associated with more ventilator-free days (7 vs. 3) and organ failure–free days

(6 vs. 2), but there was no difference in 28- or 60-day mortality. In meta-analyses of 2,299 individual subjects from three randomized trials of high versus low PEEP (including the two previously mentioned trials), there was no significant difference in overall mortality between PEEP strategies (adjusted relative risk 0.94), though subset analysis demonstrated a survival benefit in subjects with moderate to severe ARDS who received a higher PEEP strategy (34.1% vs. 39.1%, adjusted relative risk 0.90).[5,8,19–21]

Based on the above results, there may be a role for higher levels of PEEP in improving surrogate outcomes (ventilator-free days, ICU-free days, organ failure–free days) in ARDS, and a high PEEP strategy may confer a survival benefit in patients with more severe cases of ARDS. However, the potential benefits of higher levels of PEEP have to be balanced against the risk of hemodynamic compromise. In the acute care setting, regardless of the PEEP strategy utilized, it is essential to institute early and appropriate standard-of-care ventilator management, which requires careful attention to tidal volumes, plateau airway pressures, and acceptable combinations of PEEP and FIO_2.[22]

Fluid Management and Hemodynamic Monitoring

Noncardiogenic pulmonary edema in ARDS results from increased capillary permeability and is exacerbated by increased intravascular hydrostatic pressure and decreased oncotic pressure. This argues in favor of a strategy that minimizes fluid administration. However, given that mortality in ARDS is often the result of nonpulmonary organ failure, a conservative fluid strategy may worsen organ perfusion and outcomes. To help guide fluid management in ARDS, the ARDS Clinical Trials Network conducted the Fluid and Catheter Treatment Trial (FACTT), a randomized controlled trial of 1,001 patients assigned to receive either a liberal or conservative fluid strategy, guided by intravascular pressure monitoring.[6] The 7-day cumulative fluid balance in the conservative-strategy group was −136 ± 491 mL, compared to 6,992 ± 502 mL in the liberal-strategy group. There was no significant difference in in-hospital mortality between groups (25.5 ± 1.9% in the conservative-strategy group, 28.4 ± 2.0% in the liberal-strategy group). However, the conservative-strategy group had significantly more ventilator-free days (14.6 vs. 12.1) and ICU-free days (13.4 vs. 11.2) than did the liberal-strategy group, without increasing the rate of nonpulmonary organ failure. Based on these data, it is generally recommended to adhere to a conservative fluid strategy to help improve lung function and minimize the duration of mechanical ventilation and intensive care. Despite the recommendation to minimize intravascular pressure, this same trial found no benefit in guiding hemodynamic management using a pulmonary artery catheter (PAC) versus a central venous catheter. PACs were, however, associated with a higher rate of atrial and ventricular arrhythmias. Based on these results, PACs are not recommended for routine use in ARDS.

Corticosteroids

ARDS is characterized by diffuse lung inflammation, which is further exacerbated by positive pressure ventilation and resulting VALI. Corticosteroids, with their anti-inflammatory properties, have been hypothesized to have a role in treating ARDS; however, multiple randomized trials have not demonstrated a clear and consistent benefit from corticosteroids in either the early or late phases of ARDS.[23–26] One RCT found no difference in 45-day mortality, resolution of ARDS, or infectious complications among 99 patients with early ARDS (onset within 48 hours) who were randomized to either high-dose corticosteroids (methylprednisolone 30 mg/kg every 6 hours for 24 hours) or placebo.[23] Another randomized trial of 24 patients demonstrated a benefit in mortality when a prolonged course of corticosteroids was administered after 7 days of persistent ARDS[24]; however, a subsequent multicenter trial conducted by the ARDS Clinical Trials Network (Late Steroid Rescue Study, LaSRS), randomizing 180 patients with ARDS of 7 to 28 days' duration to methylprednisolone versus placebo, showed no difference in 60-day mortality (28.6% vs. 29.2%).[25] Corticosteroids were associated with increases in the number of ventilator-free days (11.2 vs. 6.8) and shock-free days (20.7 vs. 17.9), but they were also associated with significantly more episodes of neuromyopathy (9 vs. 0) and a higher mortality when steroids were started 14 or more days after ARDS onset (35% vs. 8%). Based on the existing evidence, the routine use of corticosteroids is not generally recommended for ARDS; however, this remains an area of controversy. Also, such recommendations do not apply to patients whose acute hypoxemic respiratory failure is due to an etiology for which corticosteroids are indicated, such as collagen vascular disease or acute eosinophilic pneumonia.

Neuromuscular Blocking Agents

Neuromuscular blocking agents (NMBAs) are often used in severe ARDS to decrease patient–ventilator dyssynchrony and improve oxygenation when sedation alone is insufficient. However, their use has also been associated with muscle weakness.[27,28] The ACURASYS trial, a recent multicenter study from France, was conducted to evaluate the effect of NMBAs in early, severe ARDS.[29] Three hundred and forty patients with ARDS for <48 hours, a PaO_2 to FIO_2 ratio of <150, and a Ramsey sedation score of 6 (no response on glabellar tap) were randomized to receive cisatracurium or placebo for 48 hours. Those who received cisatracurium had a significantly lower 90-day mortality (hazard ratio 0.68) after post hoc adjustments were made for the degree of hypoxemia, severity of illness, and plateau airway pressure; however, this difference did not become apparent until well after NMBAs were discontinued. There were also more ventilator-free and ICU-free days within the cisatracurium group, without a significant difference in ICU-acquired paresis. NMBAs remain an option early in the course of severe ARDS when severe gas exchange abnormalities persist despite deep sedation, but their use has yet to be widely accepted as standard of care.

Extracorporeal Membrane Oxygenation

Extracorporeal membrane oxygenation (ECMO) refers to an extracorporeal circuit that directly oxygenates and removes carbon dioxide from the blood. In most cases of ECMO for ARDS, a cannula is placed in a central vein. Blood is withdrawn into an extracorporeal circuit by a mechanical pump and passed through an oxygenator, where the blood passes along one side of a semipermeable membrane that allows for diffusion of gases. The oxygenated blood is then returned to a central vein. This technique is referred to as "venovenous" ECMO because blood is withdrawn from and returned to the venous system.[1] ECMO may be considered as a rescue therapy in patients whose gas exchange abnormalities are so severe that positive pressure ventilation alone is insufficient to maintain adequate gas exchange. Additionally, ECMO may be indicated in patients who can be maintained on positive pressure ventilation only at the expense of excessively high airway pressures or in patients who cannot tolerate a lung-protective ventilation strategy because of unacceptable levels of hypercapnia and acidemia.

The results of two early, randomized controlled trials with outdated ECMO technology failed to show a survival benefit with ECMO for ARDS.[30,31] However, in the interval since those trials, there have been significant advances in ECMO technology, with observational reports demonstrating higher rates of survival and fewer complications. The only controlled clinical trial using modern ECMO technology is Conventional Ventilation or ECMO for Severe Adult Respiratory Failure (CESAR), in which 180 subjects with severe but potentially reversible respiratory failure were randomized to conventional mechanical ventilation or referral to a specialized center for consideration of ECMO.[32] There was a significantly lower rate of death or severe disability at 6 months in the group referred for consideration of ECMO (37% vs. 53%, relative risk 0.69). The major limitation of the study was that only 70% of the conventionally managed patients received a lung-protective ventilation strategy at any time in the study because such a strategy was not mandated despite the fact that it is the widely accepted standard of care. Regardless, the results of this trial and other observational studies (particularly those published during the influenza A (H1N1) pandemic) have given momentum to the belief that there is a role for ECMO in ARDS when gas exchange is markedly abnormal or airway pressures are excessively high. A randomized controlled trial of ECMO versus standard-of-care mechanical ventilation is needed to better define the use of this therapy in severe cases of ARDS. The initiation of ECMO should be reserved for centers with extensive experience in its use. Early referral to such a center is recommended, since the benefits of ECMO may be lessened by prolonged mechanical ventilation with plateau pressures exceeding 30 cm of water for >7 days or prolonged exposure to high FIO_2.[33–37] Earlier initiation of ECMO has been associated with better outcomes in some, but not all, observational studies.[35,38–40]

ADDITIONAL RESCUE THERAPIES

Prone Positioning

ARDS affects the lung heterogeneously, with more consolidation and atelectasis occurring in the dependent portions of the lung and with alveolar inflation and ventilation distributing preferentially to the nondependent lung regions. Hypoxemia results from ventilation–perfusion mismatch and from the development of physiologic shunt as blood flow remains prominent in the dependent, atelectatic lung regions. Prone positioning has been proposed as a way of improving oxygenation by improving ventilation–perfusion matching. Prone positioning achieves this through redistribution of perfusion, recruitment of previously dependent lung regions, more homogeneous distribution of ventilation, and alterations in chest wall compliance.[41,42]

Despite demonstrating a consistent relationship between prone positioning and improved oxygenation, multiple randomized trials and meta-analyses initially failed to show any mortality benefit,[43–49] with prone positioning associated with a higher rate of complications, including hemodynamic instability, loss of venous access, and endotracheal tube displacement.[42] However, post hoc analyses of several trials and two meta-analyses have suggested a mortality benefit in patients with the most severe forms of ARDS,[50,51] leading to a multicenter randomized trial of prone versus supine positioning in 466 patients with ARDS with a PaO_2 to FIO_2 ratio <150.[52] Twenty-eight–day mortality was significantly lower in the prone group than the supine group (16.0% vs. 32.8%, hazard ratio 0.42), a difference that persisted at 90 days. Adverse event rates were comparable between the two groups, except for a higher rate of cardiac arrests in the supine group. Based on the results of this trial, the early institution of prone positioning is not recommended for routine use in ARDS, but may be considered in cases of severe hypoxemia at centers experienced in its use.

High-Frequency Oscillatory Ventilation

The principle of high-frequency oscillatory ventilation (HFOV) is to maintain alveolar patency while avoiding low end-expiratory pressure and high peak pressures. Ventilation is achieved with an oscillating piston that creates pressure cycles around a constant mean airway pressure at a very high frequency (180 to 900/min), resulting in low tidal volumes (<2.5 mL/kg).[53,54] Early randomized trials demonstrated a trend toward decreased mortality with HFOV compared to conventional mechanical ventilation.[55] Two multicenter randomized controlled trials comparing HFOV to standard-of-care lung-protective ventilation, the Oscillation for Acute Respiratory Distress Syndrome Treated Early Trial (OSCILLATE) and High-Frequency Oscillation in ARDS (OSCAR), have recently been conducted.[56,57] OSCAR failed to show a difference from HFOV in 30-day mortality (41.7% vs. 41.1%), and OSCILLATE was terminated early by the data monitoring committee due to increased in-hospital mortality in the HFOV group (47% vs. 35%, RR 1.33). Given the findings of these studies, HFOV is not recommended for routine use in ARDS.

Inhaled Vasodilators

Inhaled vasodilator therapy delivers aerosolized vasodilator medications to the alveoli by way of a ventilator. The effect of the vasodilators will not be significant in areas of the lung where edema and atelectasis are plentiful and delivery is hampered. However, in well-ventilated portions of the lung, inhaled vasodilators may improve oxygenation in ARDS by preferentially recruiting blood flow and simultaneously diverting it from areas with high levels of shunt.

Commonly used vasodilators include inhaled nitric oxide and inhaled epoprostenol. Despite demonstrating improvements in oxygenation, randomized trials have failed to show a survival benefit from vasodilator therapy, and concerns have been raised about side effects from prolonged nitric oxide administration, including cyanide toxicity, methemoglobinemia, and worsening renal function.[58–60] Side effects from epoprostenol may include flushing and hypotension if there is systemic absorption of the medication.[61] Both therapies may worsen hypoxemia by worsening ventilation–perfusion mismatch if systemic absorption results in vasodilation of the pulmonary vasculature in areas of the lung where ventilation is low. Inhaled vasodilators should not be used routinely in ARDS, but may be considered in cases of severe, refractory hypoxemia.

Recruitment Maneuvers

Recruitment maneuvers, often used in conjunction with high levels of PEEP, are intended to improve aeration to collapsed or fluid-filled alveoli, thus improving oxygenation, minimizing shear stress on alveoli, and increasing pulmonary compliance.[54,62] A recruitment maneuver involves increasing airway pressures to levels above tidal ventilation for a brief period of time. Risks of achieving these higher airway pressures include overinflation of unaffected alveoli, increased VALI, decreased alveolar fluid clearance, and hemodynamic compromise.[21,63–65] In a prospective trial of 983 patients with ARDS randomized to recruitment maneuvers and high levels of PEEP (40-second breath hold at 40 cm of water followed by a PEEP of 20 cm of water) or standard-of-care lung-protective ventilation, the intervention group had lower rates of refractory hypoxemia (4.6% vs. 10.2%) and death with refractory hypoxemia (4.2% vs. 8.9%), but there was no difference in all-cause mortality (36.4% vs. 40.4%, RR, 0.90).[21] Recruitment maneuvers were complicated by hypotension, worsening hypoxemia, arrhythmia, or barotrauma in 22% of the subjects in the intervention group. Similar to the results of trials evaluating high PEEP strategies, these results show that recruitment maneuvers may improve surrogate outcomes but do not demonstrate a definitive mortality benefit.[21,65,66] Recruitment maneuvers may be considered in severe ARDS with refractory hypoxemia, but should be avoided in patients in shock and those with pneumothoraces or focal disease. The maneuver should be aborted if hypotension or worsening hypoxemia develops and should not be repeated if there is no improvement after the initial maneuver.[54]

OTHER THERAPIES

The utility of noninvasive positive pressure ventilation (NIPPV), although well established in exacerbations of chronic obstructive pulmonary disease and cardiogenic pulmonary edema, is limited in ARDS and not recommended as routine therapy.[67] High failure rates have been reported in several studies of NIPPV in ARDS, with severe hypoxemia, shock, and metabolic acidosis identified as independent risk factors for NIPPV failure.[68] In patients with ARDS who have lower severity of illness scores and more mild hypoxemia, there may be a role for the cautious application of NIPPV.[67,69] However, such patients must be assessed frequently for signs of failure of NIPPV and for the need for prompt institution of invasive mechanical ventilation. Ventilatory strategies that have been used as rescue therapies for severe ARDS include airway pressure release ventilation, inverse-ratio ventilation, and open lung ventilation. These therapies may demonstrate a benefit in surrogate outcomes, but none has been shown to affect major clinical outcomes in ARDS favorably.[21,70–77]

CONCLUSION

Management of ARDS should focus on treatment of the underlying etiology and application of a volume- and pressure-limited ventilation strategy. A conservative fluid management strategy is recommended, and the administration of NMBAs may be associated with decreased mortality when used early in cases of severe ARDS. In patients with refractory gas exchange abnormalities despite these interventions, other therapies,

TABLE 12.1 Therapies for ARDS

Standard of Care	Therapies to Consider	Controversial Therapies
• Volume- and pressure-limited ventilation • Conservative fluid strategy	• High PEEP strategy • NMBAs • ECMO • Inhaled vasodilators • Recruitment maneuvers • Prone positioning	• Corticosteroids • HFOV

ARDS, acute respiratory distress syndrome; PEEP, positive end-expiratory pressure; NMBAs, neuromuscular blocking agents; ECMO, extracorporeal membrane oxygenation; HFOV, high-frequency oscillatory ventilation.

including ECMO, high levels of PEEP, prone positioning, inhaled vasodilators, and recruitment maneuvers, may be considered (Table 12.1). The use of HFOV, corticosteroids, and PACs for hemodynamic monitoring is generally not recommended. Whether to use alternative therapies depends on the preference of the treating clinician and the resources available at a given institution or in that institution's referral network, since there are no evidence-based algorithms to guide decision making.

LITERATURE TABLE

TRIAL	DESIGN	RESULT
Lung-protective ventilation		
The Acute Respiratory Distress Syndrome Network. *N Engl J Med.* 2000[4] ARMA	Multicenter RCT of 861 patients with ARDS, randomized to conventional (higher tidal volume) or lung-protective (lower tidal volume) ventilation	Lower mortality with tidal volume of 6 mL/kg and plateau pressure ≤30 cm H_2O than 12 mL/kg and plateau pressure ≤50 cm H_2O (31% vs. 39.8%, $p = 0.007$)
Amato et al., *N Engl J Med.* 1998[16]	RCT of 53 patients with ARDS in 2 ICUs, randomized to conventional or lung-protective ventilation	Lower 28-d mortality with low tidal volume (<6 mL/kg) than high tidal volume (12 mL/kg) (38% vs. 71%, $p < 0.001$)
Villar et al., *Crit Care Med.* 2006[17]	Multicenter RCT of 103 patients with ARDS in mixed ICUs, randomized to conventional or lung-protective ventilation	Lower hospital mortality with lower tidal volume (6–8 mL/kg) than higher tidal volume (9–11 mL/kg) (34% vs. 66%, $p = 0.041$)
Positive end-expiratory pressure (PEEP) and recruitment maneuvers		
Brower et al., *N Engl J Med.* 2004[5]	Multicenter RCT of 549 patients with ARDS, randomized to a high or low PEEP strategy	No difference in mortality between high and low PEEP strategies (27.5% vs. 24.9% $p = 0.48$)
Mercat et al., *JAMA.* 2008[8]	Multicenter RCT of 767 patients with ARDS, randomized to a high or low PEEP strategy	More ventilator-free days (7 vs. 3, $p = 0.04$) and organ failure–free days (6 vs. 2, $p = 0.04$) in high PEEP strategy, no difference in mortality
Briel et al., *JAMA.* 2010[19]	Meta-analysis of 2,299 patients from 3 RCTs of high vs. low PEEP in ARDS	Lower in-hospital mortality with high PEEP strategy in moderate to severe ARDS (34.1% vs. 39.1%, adjusted RR 0.90, 95% CI, 0.81–1.00, $p = 0.049$)
Putensen et al., *Ann Intern Med.* 2009[20]	Meta-analysis of 2,299 patients from 3 RCTs of high vs. low PEEP in ARDS	No difference in mortality between high and low PEEP strategies
Meade et al., *JAMA.* 2008[21]	Multicenter RCT of 983 patients with ARDS randomized to recruitment maneuvers and high PEEP or conventional ventilation	Lower rates of hypoxemia in intervention arm, but no difference in mortality (36.4% vs. 40.4%, RR, 0.90, 95% CI, 0.77–1.05, $p = 0.19$). High rate of complications in intervention arm (22%)

(Continued)

LITERATURE TABLE *(Continued)*

TRIAL	DESIGN	RESULT
Fluid management		
Wiedemann et al., *N Engl J Med.* 2006[6] FACTT	Multicenter RCT of 1,001 patients with ARDS, randomized to conservative or liberal fluid strategy	No difference in mortality in conservative vs. liberal fluid strategy (25.5% vs. 28.4%, $p = 0.30$), but significantly more ventilator-free days (14.6 vs. 12.1, $p < 0.001$) and ICU-free days (13.4 vs. 11.2, $p < 0.001$) with conservative strategy
Corticosteroids		
Bernard et al., *N Engl J Med.* 1987[23]	Multicenter RCT of 99 patients treated with high-dose steroids or placebo in early ARDS	No difference in mortality between high-dose steroids and placebo (60% vs. 63%, $p = 0.74$)
Meduri et al., *JAMA.* 1998[24]	RCT of 24 patients in 4 ICUs with ARDS for more than 7 d, randomized to steroids or placebo	Decreased hospital mortality in steroid group (12% vs. 62%, $p = 0.03$). Small study
Steinberg et al., *N Engl J Med.* 2006[25] LaSRS	Multicenter RCT of 180 patients with ARDS for more than 7 d, randomized to steroids or placebo	No difference in mortality between steroids and placebo (28.6% vs. 29.2%, $p = 1.0$), but higher mortality when steroids started 14 or more days after ARDS onset (35% vs. 8%, $p = 0.02$). Higher rate of neuromyopathy in the steroid group
Neuromuscular blocking agents (NMBAs)		
Papazian et al., *N Engl J Med.* 2010[29] ACURASYS	Multicenter RCT of 340 patients with ARDS, randomized to NMBA or placebo	Decreased risk of death in NMBA group (HR 0.68, 95% CI, 0.48–0.98, $p = 0.04$)
Extracorporeal membrane oxygenation (ECMO)		
Peek et al., *Lancet.* 2009[32] CESAR	RCT of 180 patients with ARDS randomized to conventional mechanical ventilation or referral for consideration of ECMO	Decreased rate of death or severe disability in ECMO referral group (37% vs. 53%, RR 0.69, 95% CI, 0.05–0.97; $p = 0.03$)
Prone positioning		
Taccone et al., *JAMA.* 2009[43]	Multicenter RCT of 342 patients with moderate to severe ARDS, randomized to prone or supine positioning	No difference in 28-d and 6-mo mortality. Higher rate of complications in prone group
Gattinoni et al., *N Engl J Med.* 2001[49]	Multicenter RCT of 304 patients with ARDS, randomized to prone or supine positioning	No difference in mortality at time of ICU discharge (RR 1.05; 95% CI, 0.84–1.32) or at 6 mo (RR 1.06; 95% CI, 0.88–1.28). Post hoc analysis suggested benefit of prone positioning in those with the most severe ARDS
Guerin et al., *N Engl J Med.* 2013[52]	Multicenter RCT of 466 patients with ARDS with $PaO_2/FIO_2 < 150$, randomized to prone or supine positioning	Decreased 28- and 90-d mortality in the prone group (16.0% vs. 32.8%, HR 0.42, 95% CI 0.26–0.66; $p < 0.001$)
High frequency oscillatory ventilation (HFOV)		
Ferguson et al., *N Engl J Med.* 2013[56] OSCILLATE	Multicenter RCT of HFOV vs. conventional lung-protective ventilation	Increased in-hospital mortality in the HFOV group (47% vs. 35%, RR 1.33, 95% CI 1.09–1.64, $p = 0.005$)
Young et al., *N Engl J Med.* 2013[57] OSCAR	Multicenter RCT of HFOV vs. conventional lung-protective ventilation	No difference in 30-d mortality (41.7% vs. 41.1%, $p = 0.85$)

CI, confidence interval; HR, hazard ratio; RR, relative risk; RCT, randomized controlled trial.

REFERENCES

1. Brodie D, Bacchetta M. Extracorporeal membrane oxygenation for ARDS in adults. *N Engl J Med.* 2011;365(20):1905–1914.
2. Ranieri VM, Rubenfeld GD, Thompson BT, et al. Acute respiratory distress syndrome: the Berlin Definition. *JAMA.* 2012;307(23):2526–2533.
3. Rubenfeld GD, Caldwell E, Peabody E, et al. Incidence and outcomes of acute lung injury. *N Engl J Med.* 2005;353(16):1685–1693.
4. The Acute Respiratory Distress Syndrome Network. Ventilation with lower tidal volumes as compared with traditional tidal volumes for acute lung injury and the acute respiratory distress syndrome. *N Engl J Med.* 2000;342(18):1301–1308.
5. Brower RG, Lanken PN, MacIntyre N, et al. Higher versus lower positive end-expiratory pressures in patients with the acute respiratory distress syndrome. *N Engl J Med.* 2004;351(4):327–336.
6. Wiedemann HP, Wheeler AP, Bernard GR, et al. Comparison of two fluid-management strategies in acute lung injury. *N Engl J Med.* 2006;354(24):2564–2575.
7. Spragg RG, Lewis JF, Walmrath HD, et al. Effect of recombinant surfactant protein C-based surfactant on the acute respiratory distress syndrome. *N Engl J Med.* 2004;351(9):884–892.
8. Mercat A, Richard JC, Vielle B, et al. Positive end-expiratory pressure setting in adults with acute lung injury and acute respiratory distress syndrome: a randomized controlled trial. *JAMA.* 2008;299(6):646–655.
9. Matthay MA, Brower RG, Carson S, et al. Randomized, placebo-controlled clinical trial of an aerosolized beta(2)-agonist for treatment of acute lung injury. *Am J Respir Crit Care Med.* 2011;184(5):561–568.
10. Ware LB, Matthay MA. The acute respiratory distress syndrome. *N Engl J Med.* 2000;342(18):1334–1349.
11. Rubenfeld GD, Herridge MS. Epidemiology and outcomes of acute lung injury. *Chest.* 2007;131(2):554–562.
12. Matthay MA, Ware LB, Zimmerman GA. The acute respiratory distress syndrome. *J Clin Invest.* 2012;122(8):2731–2740.
13. Piantadosi CA, Schwartz DA. The acute respiratory distress syndrome. *Ann Intern Med.* 2004;141(6):460–470.
14. International consensus conferences in intensive care medicine: Ventilator-associated Lung Injury in ARDS. This official conference report was cosponsored by the American Thoracic Society, The European Society of Intensive Care Medicine, and The Societe de Reanimation de Langue Francaise, and was approved by the ATS Board of Directors, July 1999. *Am J Respir Crit Care Med.* 1999;160(6):2118–2124.
15. Lodato R. Oxygen toxicity. In: Tobin MJ, ed. *Principles and Practice of Mechanical Ventilation.* 2nd ed. New York, NY: McGraw-Hill; 2006:965–989.
16. Amato MB, Barbas CS, Medeiros DM, et al. Effect of a protective-ventilation strategy on mortality in the acute respiratory distress syndrome. *N Engl J Med.* 1998;338(6):347–354.
17. Villar J, Kacmarek RM, Pérez-Méndez L, et al. A high positive end-expiratory pressure, low tidal volume ventilatory strategy improves outcome in persistent acute respiratory distress syndrome: a randomized, controlled trial. *Crit Care Med.* 2006;34(5):1311–1318.
18. Muscedere JG, Mullen JB, Gan K, et al. Tidal ventilation at low airway pressures can augment lung injury. *Am J Respir Crit Care Med.* 1994;149(5):1327–1334.
19. Briel M, Meade M, Mercat A, et al. Higher vs lower positive end-expiratory pressure in patients with acute lung injury and acute respiratory distress syndrome: systematic review and meta-analysis. *JAMA.* 2010;303(9):865–873.
20. Putensen C, Theuerkauf N, Zinserling J, et al. Meta-analysis: ventilation strategies and outcomes of the acute respiratory distress syndrome and acute lung injury. *Ann Intern Med.* 2009;151(8):566–576.
21. Meade MO, Cook DJ, Guyatt GH, et al. Ventilation strategy using low tidal volumes, recruitment maneuvers, and high positive end-expiratory pressure for acute lung injury and acute respiratory distress syndrome: a randomized controlled trial. *JAMA.* 2008;299(6):637–645.
22. Checkley W, Brower R, Korpak A, et al. Effects of a clinical trial on mechanical ventilation practices in patients with acute lung injury. *Am J Respir Crit Care Med.* 2008;177(11):1215–1222.
23. Bernard GR, Luce JM, Sprung CL, et al. High-dose corticosteroids in patients with the adult respiratory distress syndrome. *N Engl J Med.* 1987;317(25):1565–1570.
24. Meduri GU, Headley AS, Golden E, et al. Effect of prolonged methylprednisolone therapy in unresolving acute respiratory distress syndrome: a randomized controlled trial. *JAMA.* 1998;280(2):159–165.
25. Steinberg KP, Hudson LD, Goodman RB, et al. Efficacy and safety of corticosteroids for persistent acute respiratory distress syndrome. *N Engl J Med.* 2006;354(16):1671–1684.
26. Meduri GU, Golden E, Freire AX, et al. Methylprednisolone infusion in early severe ARDS: results of a randomized controlled trial. *Chest.* 2007;131(4):954–963.

27. Segredo V, Caldwell JE, Matthay MA, et al. Persistent paralysis in critically ill patients after long-term administration of vecuronium. *N Engl J Med.* 1992;327(8):524–528.
28. Murray MJ, Coursin DB, Scuderi PE, et al. Double-blind, randomized, multicenter study of doxacurium vs. pancuronium in intensive care unit patients who require neuromuscular-blocking agents. *Crit Care Med.* 1995;23(3):450–458.
29. Papazian L, Forel JM, Gacouin A, et al. Neuromuscular blockers in early acute respiratory distress syndrome. *N Engl J Med.* 2010;363(12):1107–1116.
30. Zapol WM, Snider MT, Hill JD, et al. Extracorporeal membrane oxygenation in severe acute respiratory failure. A randomized prospective study. *JAMA.* 1979;242(20):2193–216.
31. Morris AH, Wallace CJ, Menlove RL, et al. Randomized clinical trial of pressure-controlled inverse ratio ventilation and extracorporeal CO_2 removal for adult respiratory distress syndrome. *Am J Respir Crit Care Med.* 1994;149(2 Pt 1):295–305.
32. Peek GJ, Mugford M, Tiruvoipati R, et al. Efficacy and economic assessment of conventional ventilatory support versus extracorporeal membrane oxygenation for severe adult respiratory failure (CESAR): a multicentre randomised controlled trial. *Lancet.* 2009;374(9698):1351–1363.
33. Rouby JJ, Brochard L. Tidal recruitment and overinflation in acute respiratory distress syndrome: yin and yang. *Am J Respir Crit Care Med.* 2007;175(2):104–106.
34. Pugin J, Verghese G, Widmer MC, et al. The alveolar space is the site of intense inflammatory and profibrotic reactions in the early phase of acute respiratory distress syndrome. *Crit Care Med.* 1999;27(2):304–312.
35. Pranikoff T, Hirschl RB, Steimle CN, et al. Mortality is directly related to the duration of mechanical ventilation before the initiation of extracorporeal life support for severe respiratory failure. *Crit Care Med.* 1997;25(1):28–32.
36. Jackson RM. Pulmonary oxygen toxicity. *Chest.* 1985;88(6):900–905.
37. Davis WB, Rennard SI, Bitterman PB, et al. Pulmonary oxygen toxicity. Early reversible changes in human alveolar structures induced by hyperoxia. *N Engl J Med.* 1983;309(15):878–883.
38. Beiderlinden M, Eikermann M, Boes T, et al. Treatment of severe acute respiratory distress syndrome: role of extracorporeal gas exchange. *Intensive Care Med.* 2006;32(10):1627–1631.
39. Mols G, Loop T, Geiger K, et al. Extracorporeal membrane oxygenation: a ten-year experience. *Am J Surg.* 2000;180(2):144–154.
40. Lewandowski K, Rossaint R, Pappert D, et al. High survival rate in 122 ARDS patients managed according to a clinical algorithm including extracorporeal membrane oxygenation. *Intensive Care Med.* 1997;23(8):819–835.
41. Pelosi P, Brazzi L, Gattinoni L. Prone position in acute respiratory distress syndrome. *Eur Respir J.* 2002;20(4):1017–1028.
42. Gattinoni L, Caironi P. Prone positioning: beyond physiology. *Anesthesiology.* 2010;113(6):262–264.
43. Taccone P, Pesenti A, Latini R, et al. Prone positioning in patients with moderate and severe acute respiratory distress syndrome: a randomized controlled trial. *JAMA.* 2009;302(18):1977–1984.
44. Piehl MA, Brown RS. Use of extreme position changes in acute respiratory failure. *Crit Care Med.* 1976;4(1):13–14.
45. Slutsky AS. The acute respiratory distress syndrome, mechanical ventilation, and the prone position. *N Engl J Med.* 2001;345(8):610–612.
46. Abroug F, Ouanes-Besbes L, Elatrous S, et al. The effect of prone positioning in acute respiratory distress syndrome or acute lung injury: a meta-analysis. Areas of uncertainty and recommendations for research. *Intensive Care Med.* 2008;34(6):1002–1011.
47. Alsaghir AH, Martin CM. Effect of prone positioning in patients with acute respiratory distress syndrome: a meta-analysis. *Crit Care Med.* 2008;36(2):603–609.
48. Sud S, Sud M, Friedrich JO, et al. Effect of mechanical ventilation in the prone position on clinical outcomes in patients with acute hypoxemic respiratory failure: a systematic review and meta-analysis. *CMAJ.* 2008;178(9):1153–1161.
49. Gattinoni L, Tognoni G, Pesenti A, et al. Effect of prone positioning on the survival of patients with acute respiratory failure. *N Engl J Med.* 2001;345(8):568–573.
50. Gattinoni L, Carlesso E, Taccone P, et al. Prone positioning improves survival in severe ARDS: a pathophysiologic review and individual patient meta-analysis. *Minerva Anestesiol.* 2010;76(6):448–454.
51. Sud S, Friedrich JO, Taccone P, et al. Prone ventilation reduces mortality in patients with acute respiratory failure and severe hypoxemia: systematic review and meta-analysis. *Intensive Care Med.* 2010;36(4):585–599.

52. Guerin C, et al. Prone Positioning in Severe Acute Respiratory Distress Syndrome. *N Engl J Med.* 2013;368(23):2159–2168.
53. Derdak S, Mehta S, Stewart TE, et al. High-frequency oscillatory ventilation for acute respiratory distress syndrome in adults: a randomized, controlled trial. *Am J Respir Crit Care Med.* 2002;166(6):801–808.
54. Diaz JV, Brower R, Calfee CS, et al. Therapeutic strategies for severe acute lung injury. *Crit Care Med.* 2010;38(8):1644–1650.
55. Ip T, Mehta S. The role of high-frequency oscillatory ventilation in the treatment of acute respiratory failure in adults. *Curr Opin Crit Care.* 2012;18(1):70–79.
56. Ferguson ND, Cook DJ, Guyatt GH, et al. High-Frequency Oscillation in Early Acute Respiratory Distress Syndrome. *N Engl J Med.* 2013;368(9):795–805.
57. Young D, Lamb SE, Shah S, et al. High-frequency oscillation for acute respiratory distress syndrome. *N Engl J Med.* 2013;368(9):795–805.
58. Taylor RW, Zimmerman JL, Dellinger RP, et al. Low-dose inhaled nitric oxide in patients with acute lung injury: a randomized controlled trial. *JAMA.* 2004;291(13):1603–1609.
59. Walmrath D, Schneider T, Schermuly R, et al. Direct comparison of inhaled nitric oxide and aerosolized prostacyclin in acute respiratory distress syndrome. *Am J Respir Crit Care Med.* 1996;153(3):991–996.
60. Adhikari NK, et al. Effect of nitric oxide on oxygenation and mortality in acute lung injury: systematic review and meta-analysis. *BMJ.* 2007;334(7597):779.
61. Barst RJ, et al. A comparison of continuous intravenous epoprostenol (prostacyclin) with conventional therapy for primary pulmonary hypertension. *N Engl J Med.* 1996;334(5):296–301.
62. Barbas CS, et al. Lung recruitment maneuvers in acute respiratory distress syndrome. *Respir Care Clin N Am.* 2003;9(4):401–418, vii.
63. Constantin JM, et al. Response to recruitment maneuver influences net alveolar fluid clearance in acute respiratory distress syndrome. *Anesthesiology.* 2007;106(5):944–951.
64. Kacmarek RM, Kallet RH. Respiratory controversies in the critical care setting. Should recruitment maneuvers be used in the management of ALI and ARDS? *Respir Care.* 2007;52(5):622–631; discussion 631– 635.
65. Grasso S, et al. Effects of recruiting maneuvers in patients with acute respiratory distress syndrome ventilated with protective ventilatory strategy. *Anesthesiology.* 2002;96(4):795–802.
66. Gattinoni L, et al. Lung recruitment in patients with the acute respiratory distress syndrome. *N Engl J Med.* 2006;354(17):1775–1786.
67. Hill NS, et al. Noninvasive ventilation in acute respiratory failure. *Crit Care Med.* 2007;35(10):2402–2407.
68. Rana S, et al. Failure of non-invasive ventilation in patients with acute lung injury: observational cohort study. *Crit Care.* 2006;10(3):R79.
69. Antonelli M, et al. A multiple-center survey on the use in clinical practice of noninvasive ventilation as a first-line intervention for acute respiratory distress syndrome. *Crit Care Med.* 2007;35(1):18–25.
70. Burchardi H. New strategies in mechanical ventilation for acute lung injury. *Eur Respir J.* 1996;9(5):1063–1072.
71. Maung AA, Kaplan LJ. Airway pressure release ventilation in acute respiratory distress syndrome. *Crit Care Clin.* 2011;27(3):501–509.
72. Daoud EG, Farag HL, Chatburn RL. Airway pressure release ventilation: what do we know? *Respir Care.* 2012;57(2):282–292.
73. Stawicki SP, Goyal M, Sarani B. High-frequency oscillatory ventilation (HFOV) and airway pressure release ventilation (APRV): a practical guide. *J Intensive Care Med.* 2009;24(4):215–229.
74. Zavala E, et al. Effect of inverse I:E ratio ventilation on pulmonary gas exchange in acute respiratory distress syndrome. *Anesthesiology.* 1998;88(1):35–42.
75. Marcy T. In: Tobin MJ, ed. *Principles and Practice of Mechanical Ventilation.* 2nd ed. New York, NY: McGraw-Hill; 2006:319–332.
76. Rasanen J. In: Tobin MJ, ed. *Principles and Practice of Mechanical Ventilation.* 2nd ed. New York, NY: McGraw-Hill; 2006:341–348.
77. Hodgson CL, et al. A randomised controlled trial of an open lung strategy with staircase recruitment, titrated PEEP and targeted low airway pressures in patients with acute respiratory distress syndrome. *Crit Care.* 2011;15(3):R133.

13

Extracorporeal Membrane Oxygenation

Vidya K. Rao, Darryl Abrams, Cara Agerstrand, and Daniel Brodie

BACKGROUND

Extracorporeal membrane oxygenation (ECMO) is a term often used broadly to describe an extracorporeal circuit that provides short-term support of respiratory or cardiac function. In this chapter, we use the acronym ECMO in this expansive way, although ECMO is most accurately used to describe an extracorporeal circuit in which the primary goal is to provide oxygenation. Extracorporeal carbon dioxide removal ($ECCO_2R$, pronounced ee-kor) is the more appropriate terminology when the primary function of the circuit is correction of hypercapnia. Extracorporeal cardiopulmonary resuscitation (ECPR) is used to describe the initiation of ECMO for resuscitation during cardiac arrest when conventional resuscitative efforts have failed.

The appropriate use of ECMO in the emergency department or intensive care unit requires an understanding of the principles behind extracorporeal support and an ability to identify circumstances in which its use would provide sufficient benefit to justify its associated risk. While ECMO is used in the neonatal, pediatric, and adult populations, this chapter only focuses on the use of ECMO in the adult population.

BRIEF HISTORY

In 1971, Dr. J.D. Hill documented the first successful case of ECMO for severe, post-traumatic hypoxemic respiratory failure.[1] A subsequent multicenter, randomized, controlled trial published in 1979 evaluated conventional mechanical ventilation with and without venoarterial ECMO support for severe hypoxemic respiratory failure.[2] This study failed to demonstrate a survival benefit from ECMO (9.5% in the ECMO group vs. 8.3% in the control group). Despite these findings, and inspired by the success of others in using $ECCO_2R$ to minimize respiratory rates and airway pressures in patients with severe hypoxemic respiratory failure,[3–6] a subsequent randomized trial of $ECCO_2R$ was conducted in 1994, but again failed to demonstrate survival benefit (33% in the $ECCO_2R$ group, 42% in the control group).[7] Both trials, however, had significant limitations, especially with regard to extracorporeal technology and mechanical ventilation practices, making their relevance in the era of modern-day ECMO and ventilation strategies questionable at best.

Enthusiasm for ECMO in the adult population was initially tempered by the lack of survival benefit in these early studies, but multiple subsequent observational reports, particularly during the influenza A (H1N1) pandemic in 2009, demonstrated high rates of survival with ECMO for the acute respiratory distress syndrome (ARDS).[8–11] In an attempt to investigate the effect of ECMO on ARDS in the era of more advanced technology, the Conventional Ventilation or ECMO for Severe Adult Respiratory Failure (CESAR) trial was performed.[12] One hundred eighty subjects with severe but potentially reversible respiratory failure were randomized to conventional mechanical ventilation or transfer to a single ECMO center for consideration of ECMO. Death or severe disability at 6 months occurred in 37% of the subjects in the ECMO-referred group, compared with 53% in the control group (relative risk 0.69). However, the lack of a standardized ventilation strategy in the control group; the differences in adherence to a low-volume, low-pressure strategy between the groups; and the fact that only 76% of patients referred for ECMO actually received ECMO limit the conclusions that can be drawn from this study. Nonetheless, the results of the CESAR study suggest there may be a benefit in referring patients with severe ARDS to a center capable of conducting ECMO as part of a larger management protocol.

INDICATIONS AND TECHNIQUE

ECMO may be initiated as salvage therapy in patients with life-threatening cardiac or respiratory failure that is refractory to conventional therapy. Regardless of the specific indication, it is important to note that extracorporeal support does not treat a patient's underlying disease. Rather, it provides supportive care while the cause of cardiac or respiratory failure is addressed. In patients with end-stage respiratory failure, ECMO may be used, where appropriate, as a bridge to lung transplantation. In patients with end-stage cardiac failure, ECMO may be used as a bridge to either heart transplantation or a ventricular assist device (or total artificial heart), which itself may be used as destination therapy or as a bridge to transplantation.

If life-threatening respiratory or cardiac failure persists despite conventional management therapies, emergency medicine physicians should consider prompt ECMO consultation in appropriate patients. In centers where there is limited ECMO experience, early referral to a regional ECMO center is advised.

Respiratory Failure

ECMO and $ECCO_2R$ may be considered in cases of severe hypoxemic or hypercapnic respiratory failure. Etiologies of respiratory failure for which these modalities have been initiated include, but are not limited to, ARDS, refractory status asthmaticus, acute pulmonary embolism, pulmonary hypertensive crisis, end-stage respiratory failure pretransplant, and primary graft dysfunction in the posttransplant period. Uncommonly, ECMO has been instituted in cases of severe air leak syndromes.[13,14]

There is no universally accepted set of criteria for initiating ECMO in severe hypoxemic respiratory failure. However, reasonable proposed criteria include a partial pressure of oxygen to fraction of inspired oxygen ratio (PaO_2/FIO_2) <80 despite the use of high levels of positive end-expiratory pressure (PEEP) for several hours, uncompensated hypercapnia with acidemia ($pH < 7.15$), or excessively high end-inspiratory plateau airway pressures despite standard-of-care lung protective ventilation strategies.[15]

ECMO is considered a rescue strategy and should not be initiated, either in the medical intensive care unit or from the emergency department (ED), until conventional strategies to optimize oxygenation and ventilation have proven inadequate.

Cardiac Failure

ECMO can be used to provide hemodynamic support in cardiogenic shock that is refractory to aggressive inotropic support. Although it is an application that requires continued study, ECMO may also be employed in cases of respiratory failure with concomitant hemodynamic instability, including sepsis-induced cardiomyopathy or severe septic shock.[16]

With advances in extracorporeal technology that allow for rapid cannulation, there has been increasing interest in the use of ECPR for in-hospital cardiac arrest, typically in cases where return of spontaneous circulation has not occurred within 10 minutes or more of maximal resuscitative efforts.[17,18] This application requires availability of an on-site ECMO team, which in some institutions may include emergency medicine physicians. Recent data show that patients with in-hospital cardiac arrest, who received conventional cardiopulmonary resuscitation (CPR) that was escalated to ECPR or to ECPR combined with intraarrest percutaneous coronary intervention, had better survival than patients receiving conventional CPR alone.[19–21]

Contraindications

While ECMO may benefit select critically ill patients, there are situations in which extracorporeal support has an unacceptable risk to benefit ratio. Relative contraindications include limitations in vascular access that would preclude cannulation and comorbid conditions or concomitant organ dysfunction for which aggressive management would not provide meaningful benefit (e.g., advanced metastatic cancer or devastating neurologic injury). Finally, since the use of systemic anticoagulation is strongly recommended to maintain the integrity of the ECMO circuit, a contraindication to the use anticoagulation is also a relative contraindication for ECMO.

Technique

The initiation and management of ECMO requires a trained, multidisciplinary team, typically consisting of surgeons, intensivists, ECMO specialists, and nurses. ECMO circuits most often require insertion of a drainage cannula into a central vein. Deoxygenated blood is withdrawn by a pump and passes through an oxygenator, where gas exchange occurs. The blood passes along one side of a semipermeable membrane, and "sweep gas," typically 100% oxygen, is delivered to the other side. Oxygen is taken up by the blood, and carbon dioxide is removed. The oxygenated blood may be heated or cooled as necessary and is returned to the patient via a reinfusion cannula. The reinfusion cannula can be inserted into either a central vein (venovenous ECMO) or artery (venoarterial ECMO) (Fig. 13.1).[15]

Venovenous ECMO is indicated in patients with hypoxemic or hypercapnic respiratory failure but preserved cardiac function. The configuration may consist of either single-site or multisite cannulation. In single-site cannulation, a dual-lumen cannula is inserted into the internal jugular vein and advanced through the superior vena cava and right atrium into the inferior vena cava under transthoracic echocardiographic or fluoroscopic

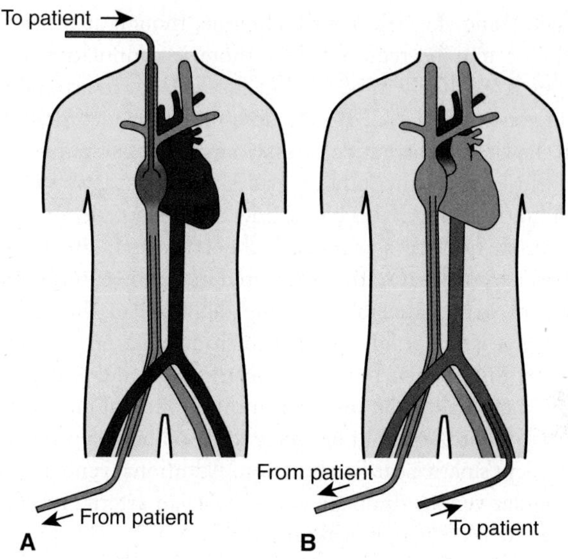

FIGURE 13.1 **A:** Venovenous extracorporeal cannulation; deoxygenated blood is drained from the femoral vein with oxygenated blood being returned to the right atrium. **B:** Venoarterial cannulation; deoxygenated blood is drained from the femoral vein and returned to the femoral artery where oxygenated blood flows in a retrograde direction up along the aorta. When some residual cardiac function remains, oxygenated ECLS blood mixes with deoxygenated blood ejected from the left ventricle. ECLS, extracorporeal life support. Adapted from Gaffney AM, Wildhirt SM, Griffin MJ, et al. Extracorporeal life support. *BMJ.* 2010;341:982–986. Copyright ©2010, *British Medical Journal*, with permission from BMJ publishing group.

guidance.[22,23] Drainage ports of one lumen are positioned in the superior and inferior vena cavae, and the port of the second lumen is positioned such that the reinfusion jet is directed across the tricuspid valve. Multisite (typically dual-site) venovenous cannulation is commonly performed using the internal jugular and femoral veins and requires less sophisticated radiographic guidance and technical expertise radiographic guidance than single-site cannulation. While more expedient in emergent situations, this cannulation strategy is more prone to recirculation, which occurs when reinfused oxygenated blood is drawn back into the extracorporeal circuit by the venous drainage cannula instead of flowing across the tricuspid valve and contributing to systemic oxygenation. Single-site cannulation, when properly positioned, is less prone to recirculation. In venovenous ECMO, blood pressure and heart rate are managed in standard fashion, as they would be for any patient not receiving extracorporeal support. Because oxygenation in ECMO is dependent on the amount of blood passing through the oxygenator, some cases of severe hypoxemia may require a second venous drainage cannula to maximize the rate of blood flow through the circuit (veno–venovenous ECMO) (see Fig. 13.1).

Venoarterial ECMO is indicated in cases of severe cardiac failure refractory to conventional therapy, combined respiratory and cardiac failure, and ECPR. Femoral venous and arterial cannulation is the most common configuration and is the approach of choice in unstable patients and in the ED, as it can be performed rapidly and with minimal interference of ongoing resuscitative efforts in cases of ECPR. Vascular access is typically obtained using the Seldinger technique, though at times surgical cutdown or a hybrid technique may be required. Intrathoracic cannulation may be performed intraoperatively, but is less likely to be used in the ED. Mean arterial pressure and systemic perfusion in venoarterial ECMO are determined by a combination of the blood flow rate through the circuit, the native cardiac output, and systemic vascular resistance. Because blood reinfused from the femoral arterial cannula flows in a retrograde direction in the descending aorta, ECMO blood flow can be impeded by the patient's native cardiac output and may not necessarily reach the aortic arch, great vessels, or coronary arteries. Furthermore, oxygen saturation measured in the lower limbs may not accurately reflect the amount of oxygenated blood being delivered to the brain and heart, and because of this, oxygen is preferably monitored from a site on the upper body, such as the right upper extremity. When there is concern for adequate upper body perfusion, a second reinfusion cannula can be inserted into the internal jugular vein (venoarterial venous ECMO), with that portion of oxygenated blood being pumped into the ascending aorta via the patient's native cardiac function. Additional venoarterial configurations include internal jugular venous drainage and subclavian arterial reinfusion, though the latter requires placement in the operating room.[24]

MANAGEMENT GUIDELINES

Circuit-Related Factors

A trained ECMO team manages the extracorporeal circuit. A brief description of these management principles is provided here in order to highlight the possible complications and concerns associated with extracorporeal circuitry.

Anticoagulation

In preparation for vascular cannulation, patients are given a bolus of unfractionated heparin, followed by a continuous heparin infusion. To assess the adequacy of anticoagulation, activated clotting time (ACT) or activated partial thromboplastin time (aPTT) is followed; other evaluations, such as anti–factor Xa assays and thromboelastography, have also been employed.[25–27] When heparin is contraindicated, direct thrombin inhibitors may be used.[28,29] Platelet counts typically decrease with ECMO and should also be monitored. Although platelet transfusion thresholds vary by center, 20,000 platelets/cm^3 is a reasonable trigger for transfusion in the absence of bleeding. The ECMO circuit should be periodically inspected for thrombi, whose presence may indicate a need to increase anticoagulation or change circuit components.

Gas Exchange

The sweep gas is the source of oxygen for the circuit and also provides a gradient for carbon dioxide diffusion out of the blood. The fraction of oxygen delivered in the sweep gas (FDO_2) is adjusted by a blender, but is typically maintained at 1.0. Goal arterial oxygen saturation is generally ≥88%, although this may vary by patient and institution. The amount of oxygen supplied by ECMO is determined primarily by the blood flow rate through the circuit, since oxygen transfer across the membrane is highly efficient. A higher blood flow rate means that a greater proportion of the patient's cardiac output passes through the oxygenator and, therefore, makes a greater contribution to systemic oxygenation. It is important to note that the proportion of cardiac output that passes through the circuit depends not only on the circuit blood flow rate but also on the total cardiac output of the patient. Any increase in a patient's cardiac output, for a given extracorporeal blood flow rate, will translate to a lower proportion of blood flowing through the circuit and a decrease in ECMO's contribution to systemic oxygenation. Oxygen delivery is also affected by hemoglobin concentration; however, there is no universally accepted transfusion threshold for packed red blood cells. Current recommendations for transfusion during ECMO are the same as for all critically ill patients.

Carbon dioxide removal is primarily dependent on the sweep gas flow rate, as carbon dioxide diffusion across the oxygenator is extremely efficient. The sweep gas flow rate should be adjusted as needed to achieve appropriate pH and $PaCO_2$ goals.

Blood Flow

Blood flow through the ECMO circuit is determined by the revolutions per minute (RPMs) of the pump (although newer pumps allow the blood flow rate to be set with variability in RPMs), the sizes of the drainage and reinfusion cannulae, the intravascular volume of the patient, and the resistance to reinfusion flow. Increasing the RPMs on the pump will usually increase blood flow, but close attention must be paid to the pressure within the venous drainage cannula. As the RPMs are increased, pressure will become more negative in the venous limb; excessively negative pressures (typically more negative than minus 50 to 100 mm Hg) may cause trauma to red blood cells. High positive pressures (typically >300 to 400 mm Hg) in the reinfusion cannula are also potentially problematic. Adequacy of blood flow is monitored by levels of oxygen saturation and markers of end-organ perfusion.

Patient-Related Factors

Sedation, Analgesia, and Neuromuscular Blockade

During cannulation, sedation, analgesia, and neuromuscular blockade may be required to provide comfort and minimize patient movement. Following stabilization on ECMO, sedation and analgesia should be titrated as they would in other critically ill patients. Select patients, once in the ICU, will be able to tolerate decreased sedation. In such patients, sedation is minimized in favor of allowing the patient to be awake and potentially participate in physical rehabilitation.

Occasionally, ongoing neuromuscular blockade may be required in order to optimize cardiac or respiratory function. When neuromuscular blocking agents are administered, the patient must be adequately sedated, and the degree of neuromuscular blockade should be monitored with "train of four" sequences by a peripheral nerve stimulator.

Adequate dosing of sedatives can be challenging due to pharmacokinetic alterations in the ECMO circuit. The circuit provides an additional volume of distribution and may adsorb certain, especially lipophilic, medications onto the surfaces of the tubing and oxygenator, reducing their bioavailability. This is an area of active investigation, and the behavior of many medications in the setting of ECMO is not known. Frequent reassessment is recommended to ensure that the desired effect of a given medication is being achieved.

Hemodynamics

In patients receiving venovenous ECMO, manifestations of hemodynamic instability, including hypotension, tachycardia, dysrhythmias, and inadequate perfusion, are managed as they would be in any other critically ill patient. In venoarterial ECMO, blood flow rate may be adjusted to increase mean arterial pressure and enhance perfusion.

Ventilator Management

Ventilator management practices vary based on the underlying condition necessitating the use of ECMO. In patients with ARDS, once stabilized on ECMO, the goal of mechanical ventilation is to minimize the deleterious effects of positive pressure ventilation, using a low-volume, low-pressure strategy. The ARDS Clinical Trials Network ARMA trial demonstrated mortality benefit when using goal tidal volume and plateau airway pressure ≤6 mL/kg predicted body weight and 30 cm of water, respectively.[30] Lower tidal volumes and plateau airway pressures than those used in the ARMA trial, a target often referred to as "lung rest," may provide additional benefit for patients receiving ECMO for ARDS, although this remains an area of continued study.[31–33] FIO_2 should also be minimized as tolerated, though it is prudent to continue moderate to high levels of PEEP to maintain alveolar patency and minimize atelectasis. In patients with severe air leak syndromes, extracorporeal support could allow complete discontinuation of the ventilator to allow sealing of the leak.[13] In patients requiring venoarterial ECMO for the treatment of cardiac failure, lung rest setting should be avoided to prevent the development of atelectasis.

Volume Status and Electrolyte Management

Patients are often volume overloaded at the time of ECMO initiation as a result of resuscitative efforts related to their critical illness. In patients with ARDS, additional volume infusions should be minimized, and aggressive diuresis should be instituted, as tolerated, to minimize extravascular lung water. If diuresis is limited by renal dysfunction, or if it alone does not achieve adequate euvolemia, ultrafiltration should be considered.

In patients without ARDS who are receiving venoarterial ECMO, optimal volume status should be determined clinically. Patients receiving ECPR and therapeutic hypothermia may experience cold diuresis; their volume status must be closely assessed in order to avoid hypovolemia. Electrolyte derangements may also occur following resuscitation or during diuresis and should be managed as in other critically ill patients.

Infection

In ECMO, as with any vascular access, precautions must be taken to minimize infection. Antibiotic prophylaxis is not specifically required, but patients should continue to receive any antibiotic therapy clinically indicated prior to ECMO initiation as well as standard monitoring for general infection. Cannula maintenance and dressing changes require strict aseptic techniques, and access points within the circuit should be kept to a minimum. It is important to note that the pharmacokinetics of antibiotics, much like sedative agents, may be altered with the use of the extracorporeal circuit, and antibiotic drug levels should be monitored to ensure adequate dosing.

Temperature Regulation

Temperature regulation can be achieved within the ECMO circuit. In most cases of venovenous and venoarterial ECMO, normothermia is the goal; warming of the blood within the oxygenator counteracts the effect of the extracorporeal blood cooling.

In cases of ECPR or other neurologic injury, therapeutic hypothermia may be induced following the initiation of ECMO and stabilization of the patient. Counterregulatory mechanisms, such as shivering, electrolyte derangements, insulin resistance, platelet dysfunction, and hemodynamic changes associated with cutaneous vasoconstriction, must be recognized and appropriately managed.

Procedures

Procedures should be minimized while a patient is receiving ECMO. If an intervention is necessary, anticoagulation may be temporarily discontinued; however, prolonged periods without anticoagulation should be avoided. Close attention must be paid to cannula positioning if the patient requires repositioning for a procedure. Ideally, patients should not be moved without the assistance or approval of the ECMO team.

Complications

Despite close monitoring, life-threatening complications do occur during all stages of ECMO, from initiation to weaning and decannulation. Therefore, ECMO should be instituted only when its benefits are believed to outweigh its risks. Bleeding complications may occur due to anticoagulation or as a result of vascular injury during cannulation. Additionally, cellular destruction and factor consumption by the circuit may lead to a clinical picture consistent with disseminated intravascular coagulation. ECMO cannulae are a nidus for thrombus formation, and inadequate anticoagulation may lead to thromboembolic complications. Air embolism has also been reported during cannulation. Adverse events related to the circuit and oxygenator, including oxygenator failure from thrombosis, have also been reported and require the vigilance of a trained ECMO specialist.[34] Fortunately, complications have become considerably less frequent with recent improvements in ECMO technology.

CONCLUSION

The availability of extracorporeal support enables an ED to initiate early escalation of care in patients with severe respiratory or cardiac failure for whom the expectation of survival without such intervention is low. Emergency physicians have an opportunity to identify both patients who might benefit from ECMO support and those for whom it is inappropriate. At certain institutions, they may be responsible for initiating early consultation or regional referral to an ECMO center as well as providing essential ongoing management while the patient awaits transfer.

It should be emphasized that the initiation and management of ECMO is an involved process that requires a trained team and that inexperienced providers should never attempt extracorporeal cannulation or management without involvement from clinicians with ECMO expertise. That said, the ED's role in providing extracorporeal support is likely to continue to expand as more centers include emergency physicians on ECMO teams to enable more efficient initiation of therapy.

LITERATURE TABLE

TRIAL	DESIGN	RESULT
ECMO for Respiratory Failure		
Zapol et al. *JAMA. 1979*[2]	Multicenter RCT of 90 patients with severe hypoxemic respiratory failure randomized to either conventional mechanical ventilation (MV) or conventional MV and venoarterial ECMO	No difference in survival (8.3% conventional MV vs. 9.5% conventional MV and venoarterial ECMO)
Gattinoni et al. *JAMA. 1986*[6]	Prospective cohort study of 43 patients receiving venovenous ECMO for CO_2 removal ($ECCO_2R$)	Patients underwent venovenous ECMO for CO_2 removal and low-frequency rest ventilation with 49% surviving to hospital discharge
Morris et al. *Am J Resp Crit Care Med. 1994*[7]	Single-center RCT of 43 patients with ARDS randomized to either $ECCO_2R$ or pressure controlled inverse ratio ventilation	No difference in survival (33% $ECCO_2R$ vs. 42% non-$ECCO_2R$, $p = 0.8$)
Peek et al. *Lancet. 2009 CESAR Trial*[12]	Multicenter RCT of 180 patients with severe respiratory failure randomized to either conventional treatment or transfer to regional ECMO center for consideration for ECMO.	There was a significant survival without disability benefit in the ECMO referral group (63% vs. 47%, $p = 0.03$)
ECMO for Cardiac Failure		
Chen et al. *Lancet. 2008*[17]	Prospective observational study of 172 patients with in-hospital cardiac arrests. Patients received either extracorporeal support after 10 minutes of CPR (ECPR) or CPR alone.	Patients who underwent ECPR had a higher survival rate to discharge ($p < 0.001$) and greater 1-y survival ($p = 0.007$)
Thiagarajan et al. *Ann Thorac Surg. 2009*[18]	Multicenter retrospective cohort study of 295 patients who received ECPR following cardiac arrest	The use of ECPR in initial resuscitation of cardiac arrest was associated with a 27% survival rate
Kagawa et al. *Circulation. 2012*[20]	Multicenter cohort study of 86 patients with cardiac arrest from acute coronary syndrome who received rapid response ECMO	Emergency coronary angiography was performed in 81 patients (94%) and intraarrest percutaneous coronary intervention in 61 (71%). Rates of return of spontaneous circulation, 30-d survival, and favorable neurologic outcomes were 88%, 29%, and 24%, respectively

RCT, randomized controlled trial.

REFERENCES

1. Hill JD, O'Brien TG, Murray JJ, et al. Prolonged extracorporeal oxygenation for acute post-traumatic respiratory failure (shock-lung syndrome). Use of the Bramson membrane lung. *N Engl J Med.* 1972;286:629–634.
2. Zapol WM, Snider MT, Hill JD, et al. Extracorporeal membrane oxygenation in severe acute respiratory failure. A randomized prospective study. *JAMA.* 1979;242:2193–2196.
3. Gattinoni L, Kolobow T, Damia G, et al. Extracorporeal carbon dioxide removal (ECCO2R): a new form of respiratory assistance. *Int J Artif Organs.* 1979;2:183–185.
4. Gattinoni L, Kolobow T, Agostoni A, et al. Clinical application of low frequency positive pressure ventilation with extracorporeal CO2 removal (LFPPV-ECCO2R) in treatment of adult respiratory distress syndrome (ARDS). *Int J Artif Organs.* 1979;2:282–283.
5. Gattinoni L, Pesenti A, Caspani ML, et al. The role of total static lung compliance in the management of severe ARDS unresponsive to conventional treatment. *Intensive Care Med.* 1984;10:121–126.
6. Gattinoni L, Pesenti A, Mascheroni D, et al. Low-frequency positive-pressure ventilation with extracorporeal CO_2 removal in severe acute respiratory failure. *JAMA.* 1986;256:881–886.
7. Morris AH, Wallace CJ, Menlove RL, et al. Randomized clinical trial of pressure-controlled inverse ratio ventilation and extracorporeal CO2 removal for adult respiratory distress syndrome. *Am J Respir Crit Care Med.* 1994;149:295–305.
8. Davies A, Jones D, Bailey M, et al. Extracorporeal membrane oxygenation for 2009 influenza A(H1N1) acute respiratory distress syndrome. *JAMA.* 2009;302:1888–1895.

9. Roch A, Lepaul-Ercole R, Grisoli D, et al. Extracorporeal membrane oxygenation for severe influenza A (H1N1) acute respiratory distress syndrome: a prospective observational comparative study. *Intensive Care Med.* 2010;36:1899–1905.
10. Freed DH, Henzler D, White CW, et al. Extracorporeal lung support for patients who had severe respiratory failure secondary to influenza A (H1N1) 2009 infection in Canada. *Can J Anaesth.* 2010;57:240–247.
11. Noah MA, Peek GJ, Finney SJ, et al. Referral to an extracorporeal membrane oxygenation center and mortality among patients with severe 2009 influenza A(H1N1). *JAMA.* 2011;306:1659–1668.
12. Peek GJ, Mugford M, Tiruvoipati R, et al. Efficacy and economic assessment of conventional ventilatory support versus extracorporeal membrane oxygenation for severe adult respiratory failure (CESAR): a multicentre randomised controlled trial. *Lancet.* 2009;374:1351–1363.
13. Fica M, Suarez F, Aparicio R, et al. Single site venovenous extracorporeal membrane oxygenation as an alternative to invasive ventilation in post-pneumonectomy fistula with acute respiratory failure. *Eur J Cardiothorac Surg.* 2012;41:950–952.
14. Daoud O, Augustin P, Mordant P, et al. Extracorporeal membrane oxygenation in 5 patients with bronchial fistula with severe acute lung injury. *Ann Thorac Surg.* 2011;92:327–330.
15. Brodie D, Bacchetta M. Extracorporeal membrane oxygenation for ARDS in adults. *N Engl J Med.* 2011;365:1905–1914.
16. Brechot N, Luyt CE, Schmidt M, et al. Venoarterial extracorporeal membrane oxygenation support for refractory cardiovascular dysfunction during severe bacterial septic shock. *Crit Care Med.* 2013;41:1616–1626.
17. Chen YS, Lin JW, Yu HY, et al. Cardiopulmonary resuscitation with assisted extracorporeal life-support versus conventional cardiopulmonary resuscitation in adults with in-hospital cardiac arrest: an observational study and propensity analysis. *Lancet.* 2008;372:554–561.
18. Thiagarajan RR, Brogan TV, Scheurer MA, et al. Extracorporeal membrane oxygenation to support cardiopulmonary resuscitation in adults. *Ann Thorac Surg.* 2009;87:778–785.
19. Shin TG, Choi JH, Jo IJ, et al. Extracorporeal cardiopulmonary resuscitation in patients with inhospital cardiac arrest: a comparison with conventional cardiopulmonary resuscitation. *Crit Care Med.* 2011;39:1–7.
20. Kagawa E, Dote K, Kato M, et al. Should we emergently revascularize occluded coronaries for cardiac arrest?: rapid-response extracorporeal membrane oxygenation and intra-arrest percutaneous coronary intervention. *Circulation.* 2012;126:1605–1613.
21. Megarbane B, Leprince P, Deye N, et al. Emergency feasibility in medical intensive care unit of extracorporeal life support for refractory cardiac arrest. *Intensive Care Med.* 2007;33:758–764.
22. Wang D, Zhou X, Liu X, et al. Wang-Zwische double lumen cannula-toward a percutaneous and ambulatory paracorporeal artificial lung. *ASAIO J.* 2008;54:606–611.
23. Javidfar J, Brodie D, Wang D, et al. Use of bicaval dual-lumen catheter for adult venovenous extracorporeal membrane oxygenation. *Ann Thorac Surg.* 2011;91:1763–1768; discussion 9.
24. Javidfar J, Brodie D, Costa J, et al. Subclavian artery cannulation for venoarterial extracorporeal membrane oxygenation. *ASAIO J.* 2012;58:494–498.
25. Bembea MM, Schwartz JM, Shah N, et al. Anticoagulation monitoring during pediatric extracorporeal membrane oxygenation. *ASAIO J.* 2013;59:63–68.
26. Chen A, Teruya J. Global hemostasis testing thromboelastography: old technology, new applications. *Clin Lab Med.* 2009;29:391–407.
27. Bembea MM, Annich G, Rycus P, et al. Variability in anticoagulation management of patients on extracorporeal membrane oxygenation: an international survey. *Pediatr Crit Care Med.* 2013;14:e77–e84.
28. Young G, Yonekawa KE, Nakagawa P, et al. Argatroban as an alternative to heparin in extracorporeal membrane oxygenation circuits. *Perfusion.* 2004;19:283–288.
29. Ranucci M, Ballotta A, Kandil H, et al. Bivalirudin-based versus conventional heparin anticoagulation for postcardiotomy extracorporeal membrane oxygenation. *Crit Care.* 2011;15:R275.
30. The Acute Respiratory Distress Syndrome Network. Ventilation with lower tidal volumes as compared with traditional tidal volumes for acute lung injury and the acute respiratory distress syndrome. *N Engl J Med.* 2000;342:1301–1308.
31. Terragni PP, Del Sorbo L, Mascia L, et al. Tidal volume lower than 6 ml/kg enhances lung protection: role of extracorporeal carbon dioxide removal. *Anesthesiology.* 2009;111:826–835.
32. Frank JA, Gutierrez JA, Jones KD, et al. Low tidal volume reduces epithelial and endothelial injury in acid-injured rat lungs. *Am J Respir Crit Care Med.* 2002;165:242–249.
33. Hager DN, Krishnan JA, Hayden DL, et al. Tidal volume reduction in patients with acute lung injury when plateau pressures are not high. *Am J Respir Crit Care Med.* 2005;172:1241–1245.
34. Wendel HP, Philipp A, Weber N, et al. Oxygenator thrombosis: worst case after development of an abnormal pressure gradient—incidence and pathway. *Perfusion.* 2001;16:271–278.

SECTION 5
Cardiac Critical Care

14

Heart Failure and Cardiogenic Shock

Daniel Sedehi and Venu Menon

ACUTE HEART FAILURE SYNDROME

Background

Acute heart failure syndrome (AHFS) is a term intended to capture pathologic changes in cardiac function that are new or that destabilize an already vulnerable cardiac substrate. These alterations in myocardial, valvular, pericardial, or electrical function frequently result in admission to the emergency department (ED), where rapid recognition and correction of the destabilizing change are essential to successful therapy.[1,2] AHFS now accounts for over 3 million ED visits annually—a number that has increased dramatically over the last several decades as a result of an aging population as well as significant advances in acute reperfusion therapy, neurohumoral modulation for heart failure (HF), preventive strategies for sudden cardiac death, and primary prevention strategies that limit and attenuate the consequences of cardiac injury.[2–9] Nearly 80% of AHFS patients have an established diagnosis of HF; 20% of AHFS patients will present with new-onset HF. Common comorbid conditions in these patients include coronary artery disease, hypertension (HTN), diabetes mellitus, atrial fibrillation, and chronic renal dysfunction.

The 2009 American College of Cardiology/American Heart Association (ACC/AHA) guidelines define three classes of AHFS:

Class 1—volume overload: pulmonary congestion, systemic congestion
Class 2—impaired cardiac output: hypotension, organ failure, shock
Class 3—combination of classes 1 and 2

This classification of AHFS echoes a diagnostic approach developed in 1999[10] (Fig. 14.1). The figure, which shows fluid status on one axis and cardiac output on the other, provides a useful description of four hemodynamic profiles based on evidence of resting congestion and hypoperfusion. As the majority of AHFS presenting to the ED will fall into class 1, or "B" in Figure 14.1, this chapter focuses on the diagnostic and therapeutic strategies involved in the care of this patient population. Cardiogenic shock (CS) is addressed in the second part of the chapter.

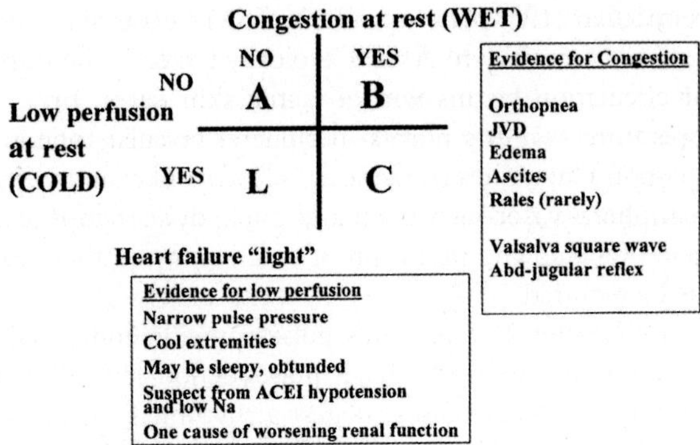

FIGURE 14.1 Four hemodynamic profiles describing cardiac function based on evidence of resting congestion and/or hypoperfusion. *A*: normal cardiac function. *B* (wet and warm): require only diuresis in addition to their regular regimen of ACE inhibitors and digoxin. *C* (cold and wet): in general cannot be effectively "dried out" until they have "warmed up," usually with monitored vasodilation, rarely requiring inotropic therapy as well. *L* (cold and dry): comfortable at rest but have no cardiac reserve or exercise capacity. Adjustment of the oral regimen for L patients is unlikely to yield direct improvement, and most will require increased doses of vasodilators or imitation of IV vasodilators or inotropes. Na, serum sodium level. Adapted from: Stevenson LW. Tailored therapy to hemodynamic goals for advanced heart failure. *Eur J Heart Fail.* 1999;1:251–257.

History and Physical Exam

An essential component of the AHFS patient history is identification of possible triggers of cardiac decompensation, including dietary indiscretion, physician-prescribed adjustments in medication dosage, medication nonadherence, and usage of new medications, including over-the-counter medications such as NSAIDs. Infections, particularly of the respiratory or genitourinary tract, may also trigger decompensation.

AHFS patients with pulmonary congestion will commonly report dyspnea, orthopnea, and postural nocturnal dyspnea. Patients will often deny an inability to sleep but will admit to sleeping in a reclining chair or even upright. Many of these patients also complain of lower extremity edema, a sign of underlying right HF. Right HF can also present with nausea, vomiting, anorexia, and gradually increasing abdominal girth.

Most cases of acute HF originate in the left ventricle and result in shortness of breath, exercise intolerance, and clinical signs of pulmonary congestion. In the ED, initial assessment should focus on respiratory status and adequacy of circulation.

Observation of the patient's presenting position (e.g., sitting, recumbent) can provide important information regarding the severity of pulmonary edema; patients sitting erect or leaning on their knees in a "tripod" position are typically the most dyspneic and congested. Attention should also be paid to a patient's respiratory rate and the ability to speak in full sentences; aberrations in either of these may suggest an urgent need for ventilatory support and/or rapid correction of volume overload. The pulmonary exam should evaluate for signs of congestion, including inspiratory crackles suggestive of elevated left ventricular (LV) pressures. Percussion of posterior chest walls may also reveal pleural effusions secondary to AHFS, typically larger in the right lung.

Assessment of circulation begins with a tactile skin exam. In a "warm and wet" patient, skin temperature suggests normal peripheral vascular tone and implies there will be a positive response to a diuretic alone. In a "cold and clammy" patient, skin findings result from peripheral vasoconstriction and the body's attempt to maintain central vascular tone, blood pressure, and perfusion of vital organs; in these cases, vasodilators and inotropes may be required.

The quality and character of a patient's pulses provide additional information on circulatory adequacy. Diminished and thready pulses denote low pulse pressure and suggest low cardiac output. Irregular pulses suggest arrhythmias such as atrial fibrillation, while frequent ectopic beats may accompany electrolyte imbalances. Pulsus alternans, a clinical feature seen almost exclusively in severe LV dysfunction, is characterized by alternating forceful and weak peripheral pulses at regular beat intervals.

Jugular venous distension (JVD), a marker of fluid status, is often pronounced in patients presenting with AHFS.[11] Careful examination of the neck veins—starting with the patient sitting upright and then with the bed lowered—can provide vital information about a patient's intravascular volume status. As a marker for right atrial pressure, and thereby right-sided preload, jugular venous pressure (JVP) should also be measured, using the technique described in Chapter 15. JVP also may also be assessed using the hepatojugular reflex; continued abdominal compression will result in sustained (>3 seconds) elevation of the JVP in patients with volume overload or a failing right ventricle. Assessment of inspiratory change in JVP is important as well; Kussmaul sign (a failure to decrease or even an increase in the mean JVP during inspiration) can be seen in constrictive and restrictive processes, as well as in the setting of an acute right ventricular (RV) infarction.[12,13]

Precordial palpation should be performed for determination of displaced cardiac apex, parasternal heaves, and thrills. A displaced apex with sustained impulse suggests either long-standing HTN or LV cavity enlargement in a dilated cardiomyopathy. Parasternal heave can accompany this in the setting of RV hypertrophy or enlargement. Any palpable murmur is abnormal and classified as a thrill or an 4/6 murmur on the Levine grading scale.

Auscultation of the heart should focus on extra heart sounds; in patients with volume overload, for example, a postsystolic sound (the S3) is a very specific marker for reduced ejection fraction.[14] Murmurs and their characteristics are important to note, as a patient with 3/6 or greater holosystolic murmur over the apex radiating to the axilla may have hemodynamically significant mitral regurgitation.[15] Finally, irregular heart rhythms may suggest a new destabilizing arrhythmia.

Bilateral lower extremity pitting edema may be seen in patients with AHFS and elevated JVP. Lower extremity edema may be present in other conditions (such as liver failure and nephrotic syndrome) and is not specific to HF. As the location of edema is gravity dependent, patients who are not upright (e.g., bedbound) must be examined for edema in the dependent parts of their body, such as the sacrum.

Ascites can also be seen in AHFS and is often associated with severe right-sided HF. Palpation of the liver will reveal enlargement and sometimes tenderness, both signs of hepatic congestion. Pulsatility of the liver may be observed in patients with severe tricuspid insufficiency.

Diagnostic Evaluation

Electrocardiogram

Sinus tachycardia is the most common finding on an electrocardiogram (ECG) in AHFS. This reflects compensatory response to preserve cardiac output in the setting of impaired stroke volume. Arrhythmias such as atrial fibrillation are present in approximately 20% of patients with AHFS who present to the ED. Acute coronary syndromes (ACS)—as an ST-segment elevation myocardial infarction (STEMI), a non–ST-segment elevation myocardial infarction (NSTEMI), or an unstable angina—can cause an acute decompensation in patients with underlying structural heart disease or even severe dysfunction in a previously normal heart.[27]

Laboratory Testing

Hyponatremia is a common finding in AHFS; up to 25% of patients will have a serum sodium of <135 mEq/L. Patients with baseline serum sodium of <137 mEq/L have been shown to have significantly shorter life expectancy than patients with a normal baseline serum sodium, and patients with a baseline serum sodium <130 mEq/L have a 15% 12-month survival rate.[16] While potassium is within the normal range for most AHFS patients, potassium levels can be elevated by typical AHFS medications, including angiotensin-converting enzyme (ACE) inhibitors, angiotensin receptor blockers, or aldosterone antagonist diuretics such as spironolactone. Concomitant renal dysfunction—the result of impaired perfusion due to diminished cardiac output or venous renal congestion—can exacerbate this hyperkalemia, sometimes to dangerous levels.[17,18] In patients with severe right HF, a hepatic transaminitis may also be observed.[19]

Natriuretic peptides (BNP, NT-proBNP) are normally secreted in response to ventricular distension and stretch and may be of particular use to the emergency physician (EP). Brain natriuretic peptide (BNP) and N-terminal pro–brain natriuretic peptide (NT-proBNP) act as endogenous diuretics, cardiac myocyte relaxants (lusitropic agents), and vasodilators. In the clinical setting, they have been shown to aid in the differentiation of the causes of acute dyspnea in patients with concomitant COPD and HF.[20–24] Natriuretic peptides have a high negative predictive value for cardiac failure–induced dyspnea in the patient with AHFS. In a recent prospective cohort study of 1,586 patients, the diagnostic accuracy of BNP at a cutoff of 100 pg/mm was 83.4 % and the negative predictive value at levels of <50 pg/mm was 96%.[21] Importantly, natriuretic peptides are insensitive in patients with marked obesity and may be elevated in patients with chronic renal failure or long-standing HF.[22,23,25] In these cases, knowledge of the patient's baseline (dry weight) BNP level aids in decision making.

Chest Radiograph

Obtaining a chest radiograph (CXR) is considered standard of care in the evaluation of dyspnea, and approximately 80% of patients with AHFS will have radiographic evidence of pulmonary edema. Attention should be paid to the cardiac silhouette, as well. Enlargement can indicate chronic LV dysfunction; a globular appearance, pericardial effusion; and pericardial calcification, constriction.[26] Significant pleural effusions (typically left greater than right) are often present in patients with congestive HF.

Differential Diagnosis

The differential diagnosis for causes of AHFS is extensive but may be broadly divided into ischemic and nonischemic (Table 14.1).

Management Guidelines

The initial assessment of the patient with AHFS begins with an assessment of respiratory status and the need for immediate respiratory support with either invasive or noninvasive positive pressure ventilation (NIPPV). In patients with intact mental status but severe respiratory distress, NIPPV has been shown to improve ventilation and reduce cardiac strain. A recent RCT of 2,096 patients with acute cardiogenic pulmonary edema compared standard O_2 supplementation and NIPPV and showed significant reductions in breathlessness, heart rate, acidosis, and hypercapnia at 1 hour with NIPPV use.[28] In patients with altered sensorium who are unable to adequately protect their airway, rapid sequence intubation should be performed immediately. In patients who are not hypoxemic, supplemental oxygen therapy is still effective at relieving dyspnea and should be provided.

TABLE 14.1 Causes of AHFS

Ischemic	Nonischemic
ACS ○ Large anterior wall MI ○ RV infarction ○ Acute ischemic mitral regurgitation *Mechanical complications* ○ Ventricular septal rupture ○ Papillary muscle rupture ○ Free wall rupture/tamponade	*End-stage cardiomyopathy* *Medication/Toxin induced* ○ Calcium channel blocker induced ○ β-Blocker induced *Stress cardiomyopathy* ○ Takotsubo *Myocarditis* ○ Infectious ○ Inflammatory *Myocardial stunning after fatal arrhythmia and ICD discharge* *Cardiomyopathy of sepsis* *Hypertrophic cardiomyopathy* *Acute valvular pathology* ○ Acute aortic insufficiency • Infectious endocarditis • Type A aortic dissection ○ Acute mitral regurgitation • Infectious endocarditis *Acute tamponade*

In the severely hypertensive patient, sublingual nitroglycerin can favorably alter hemodynamics by decreasing afterload and preload. Sublingual administration is preferred as it rapidly increases blood levels in a bolus fashion, after which a nitroglycerin drip can be initiated.

Morphine is commonly administered for patient comfort but may produce undesirable effects, including a higher incidence of need for mechanical ventilation, intensive care unit admission, and prolonged hospital stay. Morphine has also been associated with increased mortality in patients presenting with NSTEMI.[28]

Most AHFS patients will benefit from diuretic therapy instituted in the ED, with the notable exception of patients with hypertrophic obstructive cardiomyopathy, whose cardiac output is dependent on adequate preload. Intravenous (IV) furosemide is the safest and most effective initial therapy, resulting in rapid diuresis. A recent RCT of patients with AHFS demonstrated IV bolus dosing of furosemide—preferred in the ED for ease of administration—to be equivalent to continuous infusion, with no significant difference in patients' assessment of symptoms or in the change in renal function.[29]

Arrhythmias can be the precipitating event in AHFS.[30] For the AHFS patient presenting with a tachyarrhythmia—such as atrial fibrillation with rapid ventricular response—IV calcium channel and β-blocking agents should be avoided, as their negative inotropic effect may produce further hemodynamic deterioration. The COMMIT trial demonstrated that routine use of IV β blockade in patients with STEMI reduced the risks of reinfarction and ventricular fibrillation, but these gains were offset by increased rates of CS.[31] In the absence of STEMI, consideration can be given to IV β blockade in low dosages, such as 5 to 15 mg total of IV metoprolol. In a state of volume overload, diuresis can sometimes be a more effective modality for rate control. In the patient with hemodynamic instability, immediate electrical cardioversion should be performed.

CARDIOGENIC SHOCK

Background

CS is defined as severely depressed cardiac output leading to life-threatening tissue hypoperfusion. In-hospital mortality from CS is approximately 60%, a number that has not changed dramatically over the last 20 years.[32] Approximately 3% to 5% of patients with AHFS and 5% to 8% of patients with STEMI will present in CS. Of patients with CS in the setting of STEMI, the majority will have left anterior descending artery occlusions.[33,34] Other risk factors for CS in the setting of myocardial infarction (MI) include advanced age, diabetes, a history of peripheral arterial disease, stroke, transient ischemic attack, coronary artery bypass grafting, and prior STEMI.[35,36] The remainder of this chapter discusses the management of CS due to acute MI.

LV failure is the most common cause of CS. LV failure may result from one significant ischemic event or from a series of smaller ischemic insults over time. Subjects who are not reperfused, or who present late in the course of their MI, are particularly vulnerable. Importantly, when the degree of hemodynamic compromise is disproportionate to the area of myocardium at risk (i.e., as seen on ECG), alternate etiologies for the patient's hemodynamic instability should be sought. These include

TABLE 14.2 Causes of Cardiogenic Shock

Cause of Cardiogenic Shock	Diagnostic Tests	Management
Acute ischemia	ECG, echocardiogram for wall motion abnormalities	Proceed with left heart catheterization with possible percutaneous coronary intervention
Papillary muscle rupture	Cardiac auscultation for holosystolic murmur at apex with radiation to the axilla, echocardiogram	IABP, vasodilator therapy (nitroprusside) to decrease afterload and improve forward flow, early surgical intervention
Ventricular septal rupture	ECG with new Q-waves, auscultation for holosystolic murmur, echocardiogram, right heart catheterization for shunt fraction	Afterload reduction with IABP, nitroprusside, and possible mechanical support (ECMO, Tandem Heart, Impella 5.0), early surgical correction
β-Blocker or calcium channel blocker overdose	Historical use, ECG looking for bradycardia	Calcium gluconate or chloride
Ventricular tachycardia storm	ECG looking for long QT_c, Brugada syndrome, or other proarrhythmic substrate, interrogation of ICD (if possible)	Amiodarone bolus and infusion, lidocaine bolus and infusion, possible electrophysiology mapping and ablation
Takotsubo cardiomyopathy	History of recent emotionally traumatic event, ECG, echocardiogram for apical ballooning and hinge-point, cardiac catheterization with normal coronary arteries	Support of blood pressure acutely, β blockade to decrease catecholamine surge
Acute myocarditis	History of recent viral illness, ECG with possible low voltage, echocardiogram with global hypokinesis	Supportive measures (vasopressors and inotropes as needed), possible IABP or mechanical circulatory support, possible high-dose steroids
Tamponade	Physical exam notable for Beck triad (elevated JVD, hypotension, distant heart sounds), pulsus paradoxus, echocardiogram with pericardial effusion	Rapid infusion of IV fluids, percutaneous drainage or surgical pericardial window procedure

mechanical complications such as ventricular septal rupture and papillary muscle rupture—which can occur as early as the first day of infarction—as well as tamponade, acute aortic dissection, pulmonary embolism, medication effect, and occult blood loss (Table 14.2).

Physical Exam

Cold and clammy extremities are common in patients with an inadequate cardiac output and are due to the compensatory release of endogenous catecholamines that cause peripheral vasoconstriction and shunting of blood to vital organs. Diminished stroke volume may also result in a thready pulse, low pulse pressure, and a compensatory tachycardia.[37,38] Importantly, attenuation of this tachycardic response may be noted in patients with chronic β-blocker use or conduction abnormalities.

Determination of volume status is a challenging but important step in the management of CS. As with any patient with HF, measurement of JVP, lung and thoracic auscultation, and assessment of extremity and dependent edema should be performed. CS remains one of the few clinical entities in which use of a pulmonary artery catheter (PAC) continues to be recommended. PAC monitoring can help confirm adequate intravascular status and enables the clinician to differentiate true CS from a mixed cardiogenic and vasodilatory process. Only experienced clinicians should perform PAC insertion, preferably in a medical or cardiac ICU.

The cardiac examination in a patient in CS should focus on the auscultation of cardiac murmurs. Holosystolic murmurs can suggest either a ventricular septal rupture or acute mitral regurgitation secondary to papillary muscle rupture. Distant heart sounds suggest a pericardial effusion and possibly tamponade secondary to free wall rupture.

Diagnostic Evaluation

Electrocardiogram

ST elevation consistent with acute ischemic injury is an indication for prompt reperfusion.[32] Care must be taken to look for new arrhythmias, such as atrial fibrillation, ventricular tachycardia, or heart blocks, that can result in severe bradycardia.[39]

Laboratory Testing

New-onset end-organ dysfunction is a defining feature of shock. Newly elevated creatinine or hepatic enzymes suggest poor delivery of blood to the kidneys and liver. Elevated lactate levels, seen with any tissue hypoperfusion, are a quantitative measure of shock severity. Cardiac enzyme levels, as well, may be useful in helping elucidate the magnitude and timing of the ischemic event.[40]

Chest Radiograph

In patients with difficult physical exams, a CXR is useful in assessing for pulmonary edema and pleural effusions.[27] Although not specific, a bulbous cardiac silhouette may suggest pericardial fluid or tamponade from a free wall rupture, while unilateral pulmonary edema may be seen in the setting of acute mitral regurgitation due to papillary muscle rupture.[41]

Echocardiogram

Echocardiography is an invaluable diagnostic tool in CS and can help identify the precipitating pathology. Acute valvular pathology, tamponade, RV infarction, takotsubo cardiomyopathy, LV wall motion abnormalities, and ventricular septal rupture—to name a few—can be ruled in or out by echocardiography.[42]

Management Guidelines

Primary reperfusion therapy is the mainstay of treatment in patients presenting with CS secondary to acute myocardial ischemia. The SHOCK trial demonstrated an initial early revascularization strategy—using either percutaneous coronary intervention or coronary artery bypass grafting—to be associated with a 13% decrease in mortality when compared to medical stabilization strategy (50.3% vs. 63.1%).[32] In the absence of contraindications, these patients should be taken for mechanical revascularization as urgently as possible. Pharmacologic lytic therapy is ineffective in this population, as poor blood flow leads to low drug concentration in the target coronary arteries.

Mechanical complications of MIs, such as ventricular septal rupture or papillary muscle rupture, are surgical emergencies minimally amenable to medical management. Adjunctive mechanical support devices, such as an Impella, Tandem Hearts, or intra-aortic balloon pumps (IABPs), may be considered as a bridge to surgical intervention but are not definitive therapies. Although IABPs and Impellas have often been used to provide adjunctive hemodynamic support in the setting of CS, they have yet to be proven to improve clinical outcomes or decrease mortality. In the IABP SHOCK-2 trial, patients with CS due to MI in whom an early invasive strategy was planned were randomized to either IABP or medical therapy alone. No difference was seen between the patient groups in terms of mortality (relative risk with IABP, 0.96).[43] As an alternative therapy for the same clinical scenario, Impella 2.5 L/min was compared with IABP in the ISAR-Shock 2 trial. Both therapies were shown to have similar effects on 30-day mortality (30-day mortality 46% in both groups).[44]

Vasopressors and Inotropes

In an ED setting, temporary stabilization of the patient with vasopressors or inotropes may be necessary. The use of vasopressors in CS should be limited to patients with hypotension (systolic blood pressure <80 mm Hg or mean arterial pressure <65 mm Hg). Increasing afterload provides a temporizing solution for a failing heart but will also increase cardiac oxygen consumption. An understanding of the appropriate application of these agents is important.

Norepinephrine is a synthetic catecholamine with vasoconstrictive as well as positive chronotropic (heart rate) and inotropic (contractility) effects. Its primary effect is stimulation of α receptors, which raises systemic vascular resistance (SVR) leading to an increase in blood pressure. Norepinephrine also increases heart rate and contractility through a weak but present agonism of β receptors. As with any α receptor agonist, or vasopressor, long-term use or sustained high doses can result in peripheral tissue ischemia.

Phenylephrine is pure α receptor agonist and vasoconstrictor; like norepinephrine, it raises blood pressure by increasing SVR. It has no direct effect on the heart but will increase blood pressure. Phenylephrine should be limited to use in patients with hypertrophic obstructive cardiomyopathy.

Epinephrine is a powerful vasoconstrictor and inotrope and acts directly on both α and β receptors. The result is a more dramatic increase in inotropy and chronotropy with a similar, or even more powerful, degree of vasoconstriction than norepinephrine. As a potent chronotropic agent, the drug is capable of inducing cardiac arrhythmias, including atrial fibrillation and ventricular fibrillation. For this reason, it is considered a second- or third-line agent in CS.

Vasopressin is an analog of antidiuretic hormone and acts on the vasopressin receptor. A powerful vasoconstrictor, it works best at a fixed dose in concert with another vasoconstrictor such as norepinephrine or phenylephrine. There is limited data for the use of vasopressin in CS, and for this reason, it is recommended only as a third- or fourth-line agent.

Dopamine is weaker version of epinephrine and has effects on the α, β, and Dopamine (D) receptors. Traditional teaching is that at increasing doses, dopamine affects different receptors; in practice, dopamine can be used simultaneously as a vasoconstrictor, inotrope, and chronotrope. Data from the SOAP II trial suggested dopamine and norepinephrine to have similar efficacy in CS but found dopamine to be associated with more adverse events, specifically arrhythmias[43] (Table 14.3).

TABLE 14.3 Vasopressors and Inotropes in Cardiogenic Shock

Agent	Action	Benefits	Toxicity	Notes/Recs
Norepinephrine	Increase BP through vasoconstriction, mild increase inotropy and chronotropy	Increased BP without significant increase in HR or arrhythmias	Increase afterload	Typical first agent of choice in CS
Epinephrine	Powerful inotropy, chronotropy, vasoconstriction	Can increase cardiac output and improve vasoconstriction	Greater arrythmogenicity, tachycardia	Can be a second-line agent, particularly in setting of bradycardia
Dopamine	Mild to moderate inotropy, chronotropy, vasoconstriction	Weaker than epinephrine	Mild to moderate level of arrythmogenicity	No longer first-line agent, except in setting of bradycardia
Phenylephrine	Potent vasoconstrictor without effect on inotropy or chronotropy	Pure afterload agent, useful in hypotension with takotsubo or hypertrophic cardiomyopathy	Potent increase in afterload can lead to decrease cardiac output	Use as adjunctive therapy in CS, second or third line
Vasopressin	Potent vasoconstrictor without effect on inotropy or chronotropy	Pure afterload agent, helpful as adjunctive therapy	Potent increase in afterload can lead to decrease cardiac output	Use as adjunctive therapy in CS, second or third line No ability to titrate

CONCLUSION

In patients with HF and CS, early and accurate assessment of volume status and cardiac function improves outcome. Close hemodynamic monitoring is vital, and the use of intra-arterial blood pressure monitoring is strongly recommended. Early involvement of a cardiology intensivist is recommended for any unstable patient with AHFS.

LITERATURE TABLE

TRIAL	DESIGN	RESULT
Acute Heart Failure Syndrome		
Maisel et al., *New Engl J Med.* 2002[21] BNP	Prospective cohort study of 1,586 patients adding bedside B-type natriuretic peptide (BNP) to improve diagnosis of cardiac cause of dyspnea	In addition to other clinical findings, the addition of BNP improved diagnostic accuracy regarding cause of dyspnea in ER setting. The diagnostic accuracy of BNP at a cutoff of 100 pg/mL was 83.4%. The negative predictive value of BNP at levels of <50 pg/mL was 96%
Gray et al., *Health Technol Assess.* 2009[28] 3CPO	RCT of 1,096 patients comparing standard O_2 supplementation, continuous positive airway pressure (CPAP) or bi-level positive airway pressure (BiPAP) for acute cardiogenic pulmonary edema and effects on mortality	No different in mortality or need for intubation with CPAP or BiPAP (11.7% vs. 11.1%; $p = 0.81$) but was associated with reductions in breathlessness (visual analogue scale score 0.7, 95% CI 0.2–1.3; $p = 0.008$), heart rate (4/min, 95% CI 1–6; $p = 0.004$), improvement in acidosis (pH 0.03, 95% CI 0.02–0.04; $p < 0.001$), and hypercapnia (0.7 kPa, 95% CI 0.4–0.9; $p < 0.001$) at 1 h
Felker et al., *New Engl J Med* 2011[29]	RCT of 308 patients comparing IV furosemide in bolus dose (q12h) or continuous infusion and high vs. low dose	No difference in symptoms or renal function at 72 h in either bolus or continuous, high or low dose

(*Continued*)

LITERATURE TABLE (*Continued*)

TRIAL	DESIGN	RESULT
Chen et al., *Lancet* 2005[31] COMMIT	RCT of 45,852 patients admitted within 24 h of suspected acute MI assigned to either metoprolol (up to 15 mg IV then 200 mg oral daily) or matching placebo	Early β-blocker therapy in acute MI reduced the risks of reinfarction (464 [2.0%] metoprolol vs. 568 [2.5%] placebo; OR 0.82, 0.72–0.92; $p = 0.001$) and ventricular fibrillation (581 [2.5%] vs. 698 [3.0%]; OR 0.83, 0.75–0.93; $p = 0.001$) but increased the risk of CS (1,141 [5.0%] vs. 885 [3.9%]; OR 1.30, 1.19–1.41; $p < 0.00001$), especially when given during the first days following admission. The study recommended starting β-blocker therapy only once a patient's hemodynamic condition after MI has stabilized
Cardiogenic Shock		
Hochman et al., *New Engl J Med* 1999[32] SHOCK	RCT of 302 patients comparing initial revascularization strategy vs. initial medical stabilization in patients with CS complicating MI	No difference in 30-d mortality, but at 6 mo, reperfusion strategy had a 50.3% mortality compared with a 63.1% mortality for medical stabilization strategy ($p = 0.027$). Reperfusion is the standard of care for CS complicating acute coronary intervention
Seyfarth et al., *JACC.* 2008[45] ISAR-SHOCK	Trial of 26 patients comparing IABP to percutaneous left ventricular assist device (LVAD, Impella 2.5) in MI and LV failure	No difference in mortality between the Impella 2.5 device and traditional IABP
Thiele et al., *New Engl J Med* 2012[46] IABP-SHOCK 2	Randomized trial of 598 patients with CS and acute ischemia, undergoing percutaneous coronary intervention, with or without placement of IABP	No difference in 30-d mortality in patients who had IABP placed for LV dysfunction secondary to acute ischemia (relative risk of death with IABP, 0.96; 95% CI, 0.79–1.17; $p = 0.69$)

CI, confidence interval; OR, odds ratio.

REFERENCES

1. Gheorghiade M, Zannad F, Sopko G, et al; International Working Group on Acute Heart Failure Syndromes. Acute heart failure syndromes: current state and framework for future research. *Circulation.* 2005;112:3958–3968.
2. Hunt SA, Abraham WT, Chin MH, et al. 2009 Focused Update Incorporated into the ACC/AHA 2005 Guidelines for the diagnosis and management of heart failure in adults. *J Am Coll Cardiol.* 2009;53:e1–e90.
3. Tracy CM, Epstein AE, Darbar D, et al. 2012 ACCF/AHA/HRS focused update incorporated into the ACCF/AHA/HRS 2008 guidelines for device-based therapy of cardiac rhythm abnormalities. *J Am Coll Cardiol.* 2013;61:e6–e75.
4. Moss AJ, Hall WJ, Cannom DS, et al. Improved survival with an implanted defibrillator in patients with coronary disease at high risk for ventricular arrhythmia. Multicenter Automatic Defibrillator Implantation Trial Investigators. *N Engl J Med.* 1996;335:1933–1940.
5. The effects of tissue plasminogen activator, streptokinase, or both on coronary-artery patency, ventricular function, and survival after acute myocardial infarction. The GUSTO Angiographic Investigators. *N Engl J Med.* 1993;329:1615–1622.
6. A clinical trial comparing primary coronary angioplasty with tissue plasminogen activator for acute myocardial infarction. The Global Use of Strategies to Open Occluded Coronary Arteries in Acute Coronary Syndromes (GUSTO IIb) Angioplasty Substudy Investigators. *N Engl J Med.* 1997;336:1621–1628.
7. Van de Werf F, Ross A, Armstrong P, et al. Primary versus tenecteplase-facilitated percutaneous coronary intervention in patients with ST-segment elevation acute myocardial infarction (ASSENT-4 PCI): randomised trial. *Lancet.* 2006;367:569–578.

8. Bigger JT. Prophylactic use of implanted cardiac defibrillators in patients at high risk for ventricular arrhythmias after coronary-artery bypass graft surgery. Coronary Artery Bypass Graft (CABG) Patch Trial Investigators. *N Engl J Med.* 1997;337:1569–1575.
9. Buxton AE, Fisher JD, Josephson ME, et al. Prevention of sudden death in patients with coronary artery disease: the Multicenter Unsustained Tachycardia Trial (MUSTT). *Prog Cardiovasc Dis.* 1993;36:215–226.
10. Stevenson LW. Tailored therapy to hemodynamic goals for advanced heart failure. *Eur J Heart Fail.* 1999;1:251–257.
11. Drazner MH, Rame JE, Stevenson LW, et al. Prognostic importance of elevated jugular venous pressure and a third heart sound in patients with heart failure. *N Engl J Med.* 2001;345:574–581.
12. Cintron GB, Hernandez E, Linares E. Bedside recognition, incidence and clinical course of right ventricular infarction. *Am J Cardiol.* 1981;47:224–227.
13. Vaitkus PT, Kussmaul WG. Constrictive pericarditis versus restrictive cardiomyopathy: a reappraisal and update of diagnostic criteria. *Am Heart J.* 1991;122:1431–1441.
14. Johnston M, Collins SP, Storrow AB. The third heart sound for diagnosis of acute heart failure. *Curr Heart Fail Rep.* 2007; 4:164–168.
15. Bonow RO, Carabello BA, Chatterjee K, et al. 2008 focused update incorporated into the ACC/AHA 2006 guidelines for the management of patients with valvular heart disease. *J Am Coll Cardiol.* 2008;52:e1–e142.
16. Lee WH, Packer M. Prognostic importance of serum sodium concentration and its modification by converting-enzyme inhibition in patients with severe chronic heart failure. *Circulation.* 1986;73:257–267.
17. Juurlink DN, Mamdani MM, Lee DS, et al. Rates of hyperkalemia after publication of the randomized aldactone evaluation study. *N Engl J Med.* 2004;351:543–551.
18. Pitt B, Zannad F, Remme WJ, et al. The effect of spironolactone on morbidity and mortality in patients with severe heart failure. Randomized aldactone evaluation study investigators. *N Engl J Med.* 2000;341:709–717.
19. Matthews JC, Dardas TF, Dorsch MP. Right-sided heart failure: diagnosis and treatment strategies. *Curr Treat Options Cardiovasc Med.* 2008;10:329–341.
20. McCullough PA, Nowak RM, McCord J, et al. B-Type natriuretic peptide and clinical judgment in emergency diagnosis of heart failure. *Circulation.* 2002;106:416–422.
21. Maisel AS, Krishnaswamy P, Nowak RM, et al; Breathing Not Properly Multinational Study Investigators. Rapid measurement of B-type natriuretic peptide in the emergency diagnosis of heart failure. *N Engl J Med.* 2002;347:161–167.
22. Daniels LB, Clopton P, Bhalla V, et al. How obesity affects the cut-points for B-type natriuretic peptide in the diagnosis of acute heart failure. *Am Heart J.* 2006;151:999–1005.
23. McCullough PA, Duc P, Omland T, et al. B-type natriuretic peptide and renal function in the diagnosis of heart failure: an analysis from the breathing not properly multinational study. *Am J Kidney Dis.* 2003;41:571–579.
24. Januzzi JL Jr, Camargo CA, Anwaruddin S, et al. The N-terminal Pro-BNP Investigation of Dyspnea in the Emergency department (PRIDE) study. *Am J Cardiol.* 2005;95:948–954.
25. Tsutamoto T, Wada A, Maeda K, et al. Attenuation of compensation of endogenous cardiac natriuretic peptide system in chronic heart failure: prognostic role of plasma brain natriuretic peptide concentration in patients with chronic symptomatic left ventricular dysfunction. *Circulation.* 1997;96:509–516.
26. Gimlette T. Constrictive pericarditis. *Br Heart J.* 1959;21:9–16.
27. Killip T III, Kimball JT. Treatment of myocardial infarction in a coronary care unit. *Am J Cardiol.* 1967;20:457–464.
28. Gray AJ, Goodacre S, Newby DE, et al; 3CPO Study Investigators. A multicentre randomised controlled trial of the use of continuous positive airway pressure and non-invasive positive pressure ventilation in the early treatment of patients presenting to the emergency department with severe acute cardiogenic pulmonary oedema: the 3CPO trial. *Health Technol Assess.* 2009;13:1–106.
29. Felker GM, Lee KL, Bull DA, et al. Diuretic strategies in patients with acute decompensated heart failure. *N Engl J Med.* 2011;364:797–805.
30. Karasek J, Widimsky P, Ostadal P, et al. Acute heart failure registry from high-volume university hospital ED: comparing European and US data. *Am J Emerg Med.* 2012;30:695–705.
31. Chen ZM, Pan HC, Chen YP, et al; COMMIT (Clopidogrel and Metoprolol in Myocardial Infarction Trial) collaborative Group. Early intravenous then oral metoprolol in 45,852 patients with acute myocardial infarction: randomised placebo-controlled trial. *Lancet.* 2005;366:1622–1632.
32. Hochman JS, Sleeper LA, Webb JG, et al. Early revascularization in acute myocardial infarction complicated by cardiogenic shock. SHOCK Investigators. Should we emergently revascularize occluded coronaries for cardiogenic shock. *N Engl J Med.* 1999;341:625–634.

33. Bengtson JR, Kaplan AJ, Pieper KS, et al. Prognosis in cardiogenic shock after acute myocardial infarction in the intervencional era. *J Am Coll Cardiol.* 1992;20:1482–1489.
34. Webb JG, Sleeper LA, Buller CE, et al. Implications of the timing of onset of cardiogenic shock after acute myocardial infarction: a report from the SHOCK Trial Registry. *J Am Coll Cardiol.* 2000;36:1084–1090.
35. Zeymer U. Predictors of in-hospital mortality in 1333 patients with acute myocardial infarction complicated by cardiogenic shock treated with primary percutaneous coronary intervention (PCI) Results of the primary PCI registry of the Arbeitsgemeinschaft Leitende Kardiologische Krankenhausärzte (ALKK). *Eur Heart J.* 2004;25:322–328.
36. Hasdai D, Holmes DR Jr, Califf RM, et al. Cardiogenic shock complicating acute myocardial infarction: predictors of death. *Am Heart J.* 1999;138:21–31.
37. Menon V, Hochman JS. Management of cardiogenic shock complicating acute myocardial infarction. *Heart.* 2002;88(5):531–537.
38. Reynolds HR, Hochman JS. Cardiogenic shock: current concepts and improving outcomes. *Circulation.* 2008;117:686–697.
39. Berger PB, Ryan TJ. Inferior myocardial infarction. High-risk subgroups. *Circulation.* 1990;81:401–411.
40. Katus HA, Remppis A, Neumann FJ, et al. Diagnostic efficiency of troponin T measurements in acute myocardial infarction. *Circulation.* 1991;83:902–912.
41. Stout KK, Verrier ED. Acute valvular regurgitation. *Circulation.* 2009;119:3232–3241.
42. Gianni M. Apical ballooning syndrome or takotsubo cardiomyopathy: a systematic review. *Eur Heart J.* 2006;27:1523–1529.
43. De Backer D, Biston P, Devriendt J, et al. Comparison of dopamine and norepinephrine in the treatment of shock. *N Engl J Med.* 2010;362:779–789.
44. Pfeffer MA, Braunwald E, Moyé LA, et al. Effect of captopril on mortality and morbidity in patients with left ventricular dysfunction after myocardial infarction. Results of the survival and ventricular enlargement trial. The SAVE Investigators. *N Engl J Med.* 1992;327:669–677.
45. Seyfarth M, Sibbing D, Bauer I, et al. A randomized clinical trial to evaluate the safety and efficacy of a percutaneous left ventricular assist device versus intra-aortic balloon pumping for treatment of cardiogenic shock caused by myocardial infarction. *J Am Coll Cardiol.* 2008;52:1584–1588.
46. Thiele H, Zeymer U, Neumann F-J, et al. Intraaortic balloon support for myocardial infarction with cardiogenic shock. *N Engl J Med.* 2012;367:1287–1296.

15

Right Ventricular Failure

Joshua Sternbach, Francois Haddad, John E. Arbo, and Anne-Sophie Beraud

BACKGROUND

Accurate and rapid assessment of right ventricular failure (RVF) is challenging. The thin-walled right ventricle (RV), which serves as a conduit to the typically high-flow low-pressure pulmonary circulation, is less tolerant of increases in afterload and wall stress. Right ventricular hemodynamic compromise can occur as a result of a variety of clinical insults and can benefit from an equally diverse group of therapies. This chapter presents the clinical approach to the evaluation of the failing right heart, while providing evidence-based strategies for effective therapeutic intervention.

CLASSIFICATION AND EPIDEMIOLOGY

RVF is a complex clinical process defined by the inability to provide adequate blood flow through the pulmonary circulation at a normal central venous pressure (CVP).[1,2] Although heart failure is often ascribed to either the left or the right ventricle, the interdependence of these structures renders this division somewhat artificial. Isolated left ventricular failure can create an unhealthy milieu for an otherwise well-functioning RV, just as a struggling RV can hinder the performance of a normal LV. In the latter case, RV distension and diminished contractility may lead to paradoxical interventricular septal motion, producing an acute deficit in LV filling and therefore decreased cardiac output and oxygen delivery.

PATHOPHYSIOLOGY

RV dysfunction or failure occurs as the result of one or more of three pathophysiologic processes: RV pressure overload, volume overload, or reduced contractility (see Fig. 15.1). RV pressure overload may occur in conditions such as pulmonary embolism (PE), pulmonary arterial hypertension (PAH) (with or without associated lung disease), and positive pressure ventilation. RV volume overload occurs in the setting of valvular (tricuspid or pulmonic) regurgitation and has particularly deleterious effects on LV systolic function. Finally, depressed RV contractility may manifest as a result of myocardial ischemia, arrhythmia, or sepsis.

Specific etiologies of RV dysfunction include intrinsic pulmonary or pulmonary vascular conditions (also termed cor pulmonale) or cardiac disease. Data regarding the

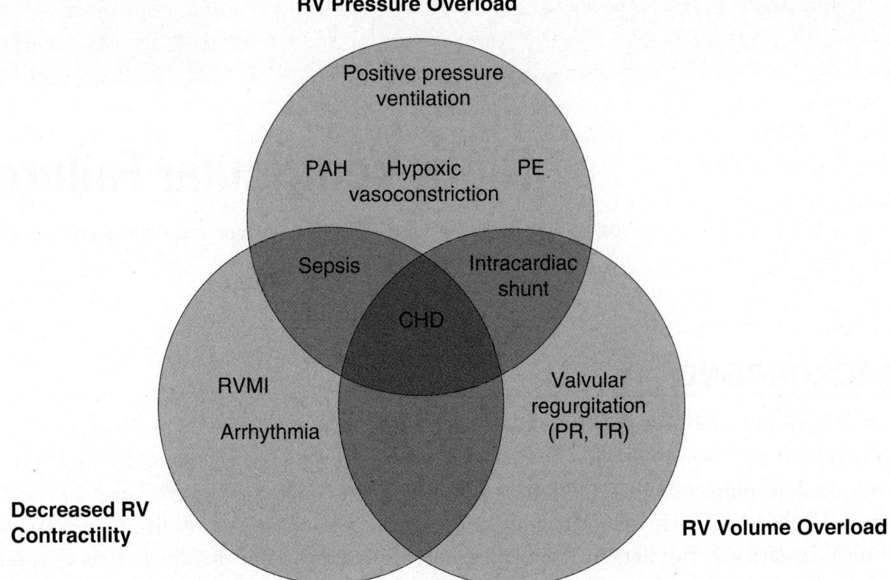

FIGURE 15.1 Pathophysiologic contributors in acute right heart failure. (RVMI, right ventricular myocardial infarction; PAH, pulmonary arterial hypertension; PE, pulmonary embolism; CHD, congenital heart disease; PR, pulmonic regurgitation; TR, tricuspid regurgitation). Adapted from Piazza G, Goldhaber SZ. The acutely decompensated right ventricle, pathways for diagnosis and management. *Chest.* 2005;128:1836–1852.[3] Reproduced with permission from Stanford University School of Medicine.

incidence and associated morbidity and mortality of various causes are presented in Table 15.1. Patients requiring ICU admission for RV failure frequently experience high mortality rates and require prolonged medical intensive care.[31,32] Other conditions not mentioned in Table 15.1 that can result in RV failure include adult congenital heart disease, sleep-disordered breathing, any disorder associated with pulmonary hypertension (PH)—including chronic thromboembolic disease—and connective tissue disorders such as scleroderma (Table 15.2).

HISTORY AND PHYSICAL EXAM

In patients with mild to moderate chronic right heart disease, reports of dyspnea, fatigue, lethargy, light-headedness, angina, and exertional syncope or presyncope will predominate.[3] Patients with a more severe disease may initially present with lower extremity edema or ascites, prompting complaints of abdominal pain or fullness due to hepatic congestion.

In a patient with established RV dysfunction, a careful review of medications is an essential part of the initial patient history, as any missed doses or lapses in compliance can result in a dramatic clinical decline. Patients with chronic PH treated with vasodilatory agents—or patients with chronic lung diseases treated with daily inhalers or immunomodulators—may develop advanced symptoms, despite seemingly minimal changes

TABLE 15.1 Epidemiology and Associated Morbidity and Mortality of RV Dysfunction

Disease Process	Epidemiology	Associated Morbidity and Mortality
PE	40%–70% of PEs present with RV dysfunction.[a,4] 8% of PEs present with circulatory collapse.[b,5] Overall PE incidence: 112.3 per 100,000 US adults,[6] 600,000 cases per year, >50,000 deaths per year[2]	15.3% mortality rate for all acute pulmonary emboli at 3 mo The presence of right ventricular hypokinesis on the baseline echocardiogram confers twofold mortality risk at 3 mo[7]
Right ventricular myocardial infarction (RVMI)	43% of inferior MIs present with RV involvement.[c,8] 6.9% of RV infarcts result in cardiogenic shock.[9] 85% of RV infarcts resulting in shock have an inferior location on ECG[10]	In-hospital mortality of 31% in patients with inferior MI and RVMI (vs. 6% in those with no RV involvement) In-hospital mortality 53% in patients with RVMI when shock present[10]
Acute respiratory distress syndrome (ARDS)	Acute cor pulmonale present in 25% of ARDS patients on transesophageal echocardiography (TEE)[d,11]	Longer duration of mechanical ventilation, no apparent difference in mortality[11]
PAH	A rare disease: 26–52 cases per million of total population.[12] 1% of all causes of cor pulmonale.[13] A higher incidence of PAH exists in certain at-risk groups: HIV: 0.5%[14] Systemic sclerosis: 7%–12%[15,16] Sickle cell disease: 2%–3.75%[17,18]	RV failure is the leading cause of hospitalization in PAH patients (56%). Mortality is 40%–48% for those PAH patients admitted to the ICU with RV failure.[19,20] 29% with PAH and RV failure die or require urgent transplantation within 90 d of admission[21]
Chronic obstructive pulmonary disease (COPD)	Most common cause of cor pulmonale in North America.[12] Cor pulmonale present in 40% of those with FEV1 <1.0 L; 70% when FEV1 falls to 0.6 L[22]	4-y mortality rate of 73% when cor pulmonale[e] present[23]
Interstitial pulmonary fibrosis (IPF)	65% with RV dysfunction[f] in end-stage disease patients being evaluated for transplant.[24] The prevalence of PH[g] ranges from 20% to 32%[25–27]	1-y survival: 45% when pulmonary artery systolic (PAS) pressure >50 mm Hg on echocardiogram, 83% when PAS <50[28]
Sepsis	30%–40% have evidence of nonisolated RV dysfunction.[h] Isolated RV dysfunction ~10%[29,30]	Lower overall cardiac output. Higher vasopressor requirements. Higher median troponin and lactate levels. No difference in 30-d or 1-y mortality rates when compared to patients with normal myocardial function[30]

[a]No uniform criteria exists to assess the presence of right ventricular dysfunction. In the majority of studies included in this meta-analysis, right ventricular dysfunction was defined as right ventricular hypokinesis as assessed by a qualitative evaluation of the right ventricular wall motion.
[b]Circulatory collapse defined as loss of consciousness or systolic blood pressure ≤80 mm Hg.
[c]Technetium-99m pyrophosphate scintigraphy and a dynamic flow study performed to detect right ventricular involvement.
[d]Acute cor pulmonale defined as RV dilation (a right ventricular end-diastolic area to left ventricular end-diastolic area ratio >0.6 on long-axis view) associated with septal dyskinesia on the short-axis view.
[e]Presence of RHF with no demonstrable cause other than COPD.
[f]RV dysfunction defined as a right ventricular ejection fraction (RVEF) <45% as determined by radionuclide ventriculography.
[g]Defined as a mean pulmonary artery pressure of >25 mm Hg on cardiac catheterization.
[h]RV function evaluated with a multimodal approach (lateral tricuspid annulus peak systolic velocity was used in association with the relative RV to LV size, motion of the RV wall, and expert evaluation).

in their prescribed routine. Likewise, recreational or illicit drug use may trigger new, or exacerbate chronic, RV dysfunction. In particular, amphetamines, cocaine, and dietary supplements containing fenfluramine constitute a common cohort of agents known to cause PH and subsequent cor pulmonale.[34,46]

TABLE 15.2 World Health Organization Classification of PH

WHO Group	Characteristic Disease(s)
I	Disease inherent to the pulmonary arterial system (not a manifestation of L-sided heart disease). This includes the so-called idiopathic or primary PH as well as PH secondary to connective tissues disorders (scleroderma, rheumatoid arthritis, etc.) and drugs/toxins (methamphetamines, dietary supplements)
II	PH secondary to L-sided heart disease (left ventricular systolic or diastolic dysfunction or valvular disease)
III	PH arising from pulmonary disorders (COPD, interstitial lung disease, or sleep-disordered breathing)
IV	Chronic thromboembolic PH—a result of chronic inflammatory and constrictive changes in the pulmonary vascular bed following an initial thromboembolic insult or recurrent embolic events
V	Miscellaneous or multifactorial PH (myeloproliferative disorders, glycogen storage disease, sickle cell anemia, etc.)

Adapted from Simonneau G, Robbins IM, Beghetti M, et al. Updated clinical classifications of pulmonary hypertension. *J Am Coll Cardiol.* 2009;54:S43.[33]

The initial physical exam centers on a determination of CVP and signs of low cardiac output or hemodynamic compromise. In the absence of significant tricuspid valve stenosis, CVP provides a reasonable estimate of the filling pressure of the RV, in much the same way that the pulmonary capillary wedge pressure can estimate LV diastolic pressure.[1] Jugular venous pressure (JVP) is a surrogate for CVP, but it can be measured by direct visualization of the internal jugular vein. To perform the exam, position the patient at a 45-degree angle and measure at the vertical height of the jugular vein, just above the sternal angle (or angle of Louis).[36] Calculate the JVP by adding 5 cm to this height (the distance from the middle of the right atrium to the sternal angle). CVP can also be estimated using ultrasound and examining the inferior vena cava (IVC) diameter (see Echocardiography below). A JVP >8 cm is suggestive of elevated right-sided filling pressures.

Additional physical exam signs suggestive of RV failure include an increase in intensity of the pulmonic component of S2, a narrowly split S2, a holosystolic murmur at the left lower sternal border (usually compatible with tricuspid regurgitation), a prominence of the "A" wave in the jugular venous pulse (corresponding to atrial contraction), and either a left parasternal heave or a downward subxiphoid thrust. In the patient presenting with severe decompensated disease, systemic signs of cardiogenic shock may manifest as cool extremities, diminished peripheral pulses, and decreased urine output.[37]

DIFFERENTIAL DIAGNOSIS

Identifying conditions that mimic RV failure requires consideration of disease processes that cause either a real or perceived elevation in CVP. For example, constrictive pericarditis produces elevated right-sided filling pressures with elevations in CVP as well as signs and symptoms of acute heart failure. Superior vena cava syndrome, as might be seen in patients with a history of central venous catheters, device placement, or known malignancies, can present with an increase in jugular venous distension, or height, without a true elevation in right atrial pressure.

Because lower extremity edema, abdominal ascites, and even hepatic engorgement can result from RVF, other syndromes marked by anasarca—or total body fluid excess—must also be excluded. Cirrhosis, nephrotic syndrome, or disorders disruptive of the hepatic circulation (such as Budd-Chiari or hepatic venoocclusive disease) may produce a pattern of edema identical to that found in states of RVF.

DIAGNOSTIC EVALUATION

Electrocardiogram

The initial evaluation of a patient with suspected RV dysfunction should begin with an assessment using simple and noninvasive diagnostic modalities. An electrocardiogram (ECG) can offer significant insight into the presence or absence of RV strain. Significant ECG findings include an S1Q3T3 pattern, right axis deviation, or signs of RV hypertrophy such as a dominant R wave in V1 and V2 with a prominent S wave in V5 and V6.[38] A low threshold for performing a right-sided ECG (providing the additional leads of V3R to V6R) can improve the detection of RV infarction and inferior wall ischemia.[8] In a prospective study of patients with acute inferior myocardial infarction (MI) complicated by RV involvement (evidenced by ST-segment elevation in V4R), in-hospital mortality rate was significantly higher when compared to those with inferior MI in the absence of RV ischemia (31% vs. 6%, respectively).[39] Posterior MI, especially in patients with a right dominant coronary circulation, represents another potential insult to RV perfusion. This can manifest with subtle ECG findings, including prominent R wave amplitude and ST depressions in V1 to V3. However, more demonstrative ST-segment elevations can become evident with the use of posterior or the so-called esophageal ECG leads (V7 to V9).[40]

Chest Radiography

Appreciating signs of RV enlargement on a single- or two-view chest x-ray (CXR) requires close attention to subtle findings. PH and RV hypertrophy may produce enlargement of the proximal pulmonary arteries or a reduction in retrosternal air space (Fig. 15.2). Classic CXR findings in PE include Westermark sign (focal oligemia) and Hampton hump (peripheral area of opacification representing pulmonary infarction); note that these findings lack in sensitivity and specificity.[41] The absence of pulmonary edema in the setting of elevated JVP is considered to be the most specific sign for isolated RVF.[1,2]

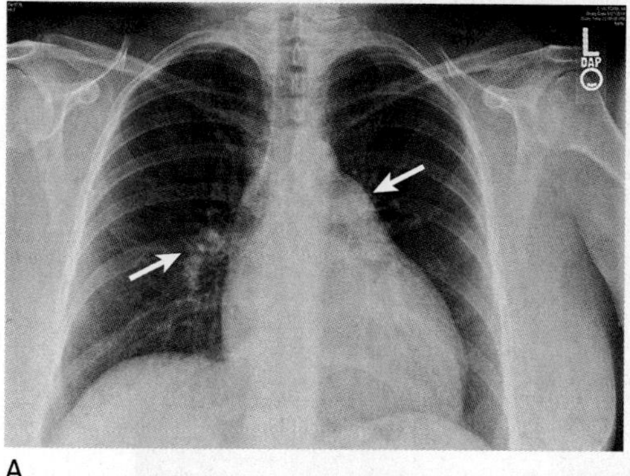

A

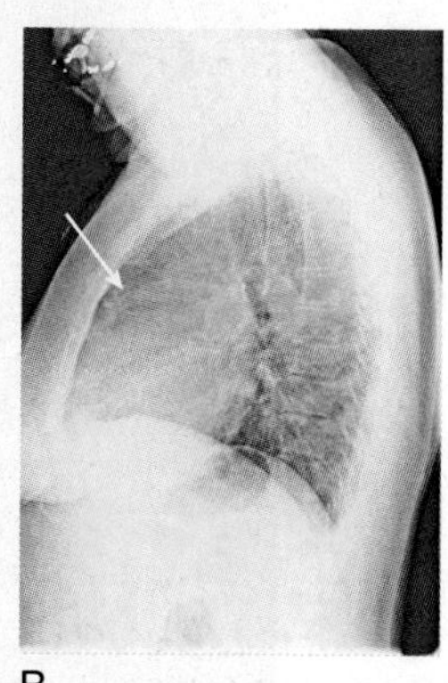

B

FIGURE 15.2 Signs of right ventricular hypertrophy/pulmonary hypertension. **A:** Enlarged pulmonary arteries and **(B)** loss of retrosternal airspace in a patient with chronic PAH.

Once conventional imaging studies such as CXR and computed tomography demonstrate evidence for RV dysfunction, however, the disease process is likely already advanced.

Echocardiography

Bedside portable ultrasound and echocardiography has gained widespread popularity and can provide direct assessment of cardiac function. Findings indicative of RV dysfunction include tricuspid regurgitation, RV hypokinesis or dilatation (Fig. 15.3), right atrial enlargement, and paradoxical septal motion.[12,37] CVP can be evaluated echocardiographically by measurement of the degree of IVC collapse with inspiration.[42] RV failure due to acute PE—or occasionally MI—may present with diffuse hypokinesis of the RV free wall sparing the apex (McConnell sign).[3] Echocardiographic findings in RV failure are discussed in further detail in Chapter 6.

Laboratory Investigation

Poor end-organ perfusion as a result of diminished right heart function may be suggested by elevations in serum lactate or evidenced by markers of organ-specific injury such as serum creatinine (kidney) or hepatic function tests and bilirubin (liver).[37] Troponin and brain natriuretic peptide (BNP)—two biomarkers of cardiac injury—also have predictive value in the setting of RV dysfunction due to PE or acute exacerbations of PH. In acute PE, an elevated troponin T was found to be associated with in-hospital and 30-day mortality, prolonged hypotension, cardiogenic shock, and need for resuscitation.[43,44] BNP has also been shown to have significant predictive value for outcomes in PE. In one study of 79 patients with acute PE, those who had an uncomplicated clinical course (16.5%) all had normal BNP values, whereas all in-hospital deaths and serious events occurred in the group with elevated measures. BNP also serves as a reliable marker of RV strain and correlates well with echocardiographic measurements of RV/LV ratio and IVC dimension.[45] In patients with PAH requiring hospitalization for ICU management of acute right heart failure, elevations in admission BNP, C-reactive protein, and creatinine were found to negatively correlate with survival.[20]

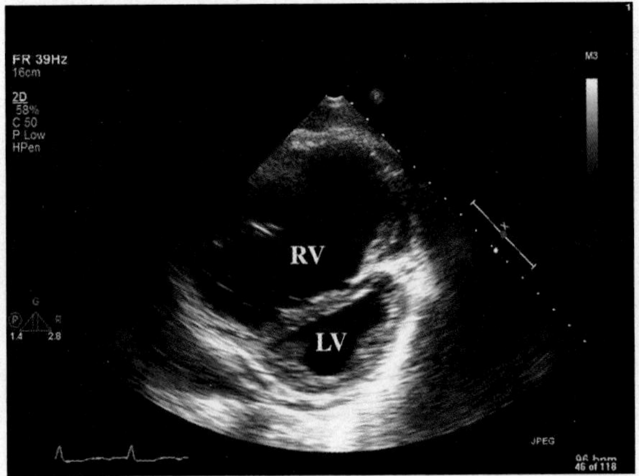

FIGURE 15.3 Bedside echocardiogram in short-axis view demonstrating sizeable RV dilatation in a patient with PH. (RV, right ventricle; LV, Left ventricle.)

MONITORING AND SUPPORTIVE CARE

Initial treatment of RVF requires the basic supportive care necessary for all critically ill patients. Monitoring of blood pressure, heart rate, and pulse oximetry—whether performed noninvasively or with the assistance of an intra-arterial catheter—is essential. Central venous access, in addition to enabling complex pharmacotherapy, offers the additional benefit of regular CVP measurement and central venous oxygen saturation ($ScvO_2$), data that can assist in the assessment of response to vasoactive medications and fluid therapy.

Supplemental oxygen administration to maintain oxygen saturation >92% can reverse one of the more injurious influences on RV afterload, namely, hypoxic vasoconstriction (see below). Basic lab work, including a complete blood count, coagulation studies, and a comprehensive metabolic panel, permits identification of easily correctable disorders such as anemia, electrolyte or acid/base abnormalities, as well as renal or hepatic dysfunction.

Once advanced monitoring is in place, and initial diagnostic studies performed, targeted interventions should be implemented to relieve RV strain. Prior to initiating medical therapy, however, consideration of the following unique characteristics of RV failure can help avoid unintentional exacerbation of cardiopulmonary function.

Afterload Reduction

Administration of RV afterload-reducing agents such as inhaled nitric oxide can precipitate acute pulmonary edema if the RV failure is secondary to a left-sided cardiac process (e.g., LV systolic or diastolic failure, mitral stenosis). This occurs as a result of decreased pulmonary vascular resistance in the face of a relatively fixed left-sided obstruction or defect.[46]

Inotropic Support

In the case of RV failure presenting with systemic hypotension, initiation of certain vasopressor therapies may become necessary. There is no evidence to suggest that one inotrope or vasopressor has greater success than another at maintaining circulatory support in RVF. However, careful consideration should precede the use of strong alpha-1 agonists as they can increase pulmonary vascular tone and further impinge on RV function.

Volume Resuscitation

Although a trial of intravenous volume administration may be appropriate in hypotensive patients without an increased CVP or evidence of pulmonary edema (as in the case of right ventricular MI), signs of RV volume overload including a CVP of >12 to 15 mm Hg should preclude this therapy. In these instances, initiation of vasopressors or inotropes may be preferable; if uncertainty exists, aggressive fluid therapy should be avoided. A trial bolus of 500 cc of crystalloid, with careful monitoring of clinical response, should be used instead.[3,47]

MANAGEMENT GUIDELINES

Oxygen

Hypoxic pulmonary vasoconstriction—although normally a protective physiologic response against V/Q mismatching when pO_2 levels drop below 50 to 60 mm Hg—requires a reversal in instances of life-threatening RV failure. Application of supplemental oxygen via nasal cannula, Venturi mask, simple face mask, nonrebreathing face mask, or other device depending on the degree of hypoxia can reduce pulmonary vascular resistance.[48] Additionally, systemic acidosis, if present, can worsen hypoxic vasoconstriction and should be corrected.[49]

Nitric Oxide

Available in the inhaled form (iNO), nitric oxide can diffuse rapidly across the alveolo-capillary membrane into adjacent smooth muscle of pulmonary vessels to increase cyclic guanosine monophosphate, leading to vasodilatation. In right heart failure (RHF), iNO is an attractive therapeutic option given its ability to preferentially improve perfusion to well-ventilated pulmonary segments while avoiding unwanted systemic hypotension (prevented by the scavenging of NO by native hemoglobin). Initial dosing begins at 20 parts per million or less; higher concentrations provide little additional hemodynamic benefit.[50] Disadvantages of iNO include the risk of developing methemoglobinemia as well as rebound PH upon discontinuation.[51,52]

Vasopressors and Inotropes

Improvement of a poorly contractile RV requires augmentation of ventricular perfusion, RV ejection fraction, and ultimately stroke volume. Various agents have been employed for this purpose, and each agent comes with different risks and benefits depending on the underlying etiology of the dysfunction (Table 15.3). Definitive evidence to guide choice of vasopressor or inotrope in patients with acute RHF is lacking. Experimental studies suggest that dobutamine may be more beneficial than norepinephrine.[47,54] A recent extensive literature review gave weak evidence-based recommendations for the use of norepinephrine, vasopressin, dobutamine, and levosimendan. Strong recommendations were made for the use of PDE3 inhibitors (e.g., milrinone) for improvement in RV performance and reduction in pulmonary vascular resistance (PVR). A strong recommendation advised against the use of dopamine in cardiogenic shock secondary to an increase in tachyarrhythmias.[55]

Diuretics

Although a key therapy for the volume-overloaded RV, achieving clinically meaningful diuresis in the emergency department may be impractical and, at times, detrimental depending upon the patient's hemodynamic stability. Inpatient therapy in the intensive care unit may include salt and fluid restriction, intermittent or continuous administration of loop diuretics, or more rigorous approaches such as continuous or intermittent renal replacement therapy.[56] In the emergency setting, however, a more reasonable approach may be to pursue diuresis or natriuresis by augmenting RV contractility, cardiac output, and, by extension, renal perfusion.

Antiarrhythmics

The importance of maintaining sinus rhythm and heart rate control during an episode of acute right heart failure cannot be overstated. Atrial tachyarrhythmias, such as atrial fibrillation or flutter, are the most common ectopic rhythms observed in RV failure and can increase morbidity and mortality.[47] Although no randomized, controlled data exist to guide the management of unstable atrial arrhythmias, consensus guidelines characterize unstable patients as those with ventricular rates >150 accompanied by ongoing chest pain or poor perfusion (a systolic blood pressure <90, heart failure, or reduced level of consciousness).[57,58] Patients with hemodynamic instability due to a tachyarrhythmia,

TABLE 15.3 Common Agents Used in the Treatment of RV Failure

Agent/Class	Receptor	Ideal Use	Infusion Rate	Notes
Catecholamines				
Epinephrine	α1 > β1 > β2	Hypotension, unresponsiveness	0.01–0.1 μg/kg/min	Caution if arrhythmia present
Norepinephrine	α1 > β1 > β2	Hypotension, unresponsiveness	0.01–3 μg/kg/min	Increases RV perfusion pressure and CO Caution if arrhythmia present
Phenylephrine	α1	Tachycardia (as may produce a reflex bradycardia)	0.4–9.1 μg/kg/min	May increase PVR
Dobutamine	β1 > β2 (3:1 ratio)	Normotension	2–20 μg/kg/min	At doses of 2–5 μg/kg/min increases cardiac output while decreasing pulmonary vascular resistance Increased cardiac contractility without affecting peripheral resistance Increased myocardial oxygen consumption
Dopamine	DA > β1 > α1 (as dosing escalates)	Hypotension, nontachycardic	2–20 μg/kg/min (max 50 μg/kg/min)	Caution if arrhythmia present
Phosphodiesterase inhibitors (e.g., milrinone)	N/A	Normotension, chronic beta-blocker use (where adrenergic receptors may be desensitized)	0.375–0.75 μg/kg/min	Caution in hypotension given vasodilator properties
Vasopressin	V_1, V_2	Hypotension, tachycardia	Fixed dose of 0.04 units/min	Produces less coronary, cerebral, and pulmonary vascular vasoconstriction
Calcium-sensitizing agents (e.g., levosimendan)	N/A	Need for increase in CO with decrease in PVR	Loading dose: 12–24 μg/kg over 10 min Infusion: 0.05–0.2 μg/kg/min	Approved in Europe, not in the United States

Adapted from Overgaard CB, Dzavík V. Inotropes and vasopressors: review of physiology and clinical use in cardiovascular disease. *Circulation.* 2008;118(10):1047–1056.[53]

regardless of the presence of RV strain, should receive direct current cardioversion for restoration of sinus rhythm. For those deemed appropriate for rate control or pharmacologic therapy, evidence for specific treatment in RVF is once again sparse. Digoxin, although not a first-line agent in those who can tolerate calcium channel blockers or beta-blockers, may be useful in decompensated heart failure given its modest inotropic properties and ability to slow conduction velocity. PH patients with evidence of RV dysfunction in sinus rhythm have demonstrated improvements in cardiac output following the administration of this agent.[59] Figure 15.4 summarizes a therapeutic approach to the patient with RV failure.

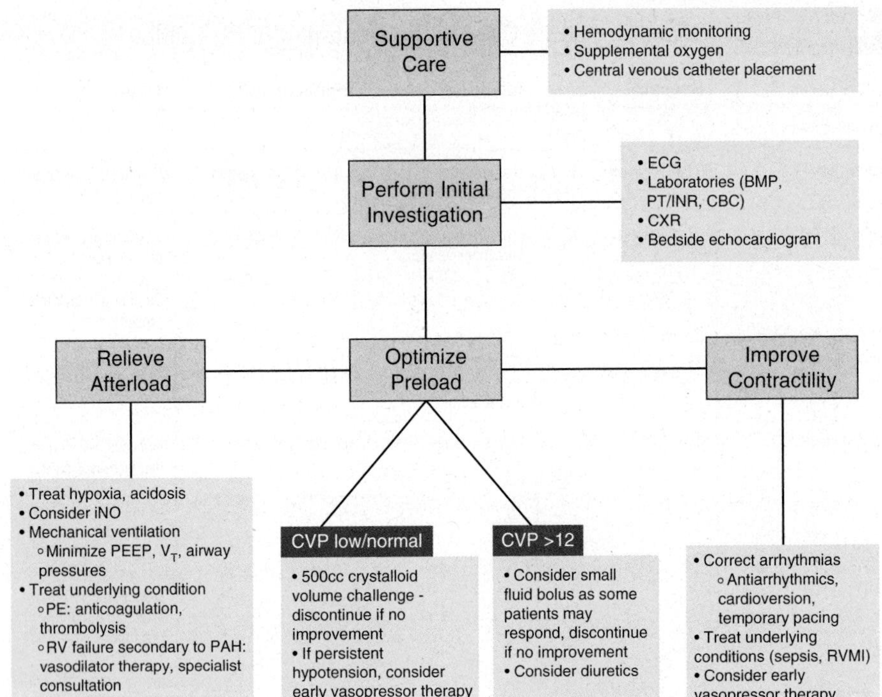

FIGURE 15.4 Therapeutic approach to RV failure. (ECG, electrocardiogram; BMP, basic metabolic panel; PT, prothrombin time; INR, international normalized ratio; CBC, complete blood count; CXR, chest x-ray; iNO, inhaled nitric oxide; PEEP, positive end-expiratory pressure; V_T, tidal volume; PE, pulmonary embolism; RV, right ventricle; PAH, pulmonary arterial hypertension; CVP, central venous pressure; RVMI, right ventricular myocardial infarction.)

SPECIAL CONSIDERATIONS

Sepsis

The current accepted definition of sepsis-induced myocardial dysfunction requires only a reduced LV ejection fraction—in the absence of cardiac disease—that demonstrates reversibility on the correction of the septic state.[30] Sepsis-induced cardiomyopathy affects both ventricles and causes dilation, diminished ejection fraction, and poor response to fluid resuscitation and catecholamines. The underlying pathophysiologic mechanisms are myriad; however, increased concentrations of myocardial suppressant substances such as bacterial toxins, cytokines, tumor necrosis factor–alpha, interleukin-1, and nitric oxide have been implicated. Key treatment strategies involve correction of the underlying infectious disease while providing adequate fluid resuscitation and vasopressor support so as to optimize mean arterial pressure and organ perfusion.[60]

Severe Pulmonary Hypertension

Whether idiopathic or originating from a known cause, this disease group may require consideration of specialized therapies such as prostacyclin derivatives (e.g., epoprostenol, iloprost), endothelin receptor antagonists (e.g., bosentan), and phosphodiesterase inhibitors (e.g., sildenafil) due to marked elevations in pulmonary vascular resistance. However, such advanced pharmacologic interventions can usually be delayed until clinical stability and transfer to an intensive care setting has occurred. Enlisting specialist consultation early in the clinical course should always be considered.

Massive Pulmonary Embolism

The defining characteristics of massive PE include arterial hypotension (systolic arterial pressure <90 mm Hg or a drop in systolic arterial pressure of at least 40 mm Hg for at least 15 minutes) and cardiogenic shock.[61] Diagnosis is suggested by RV strain demonstrated on ECG as well as RV dilation on echocardiogram. Following diagnosis, aggressive interventions such as thrombolysis or thrombectomy (performed via surgical or interventional radiologic methods) in addition to systemic anticoagulation may become necessary. A detailed discussion of massive PE is provided in Chapter 11.

Mechanical Ventilation

In the event that intubation and mechanical ventilation become necessary, the physiologic characteristics of RV dysfunction should be carefully considered. High tidal volumes (V_T) and positive end-expiratory pressures (PEEP) can increase pulmonary arterial and right atrial pressures, worsen tricuspid regurgitation, increase RV afterload, and decrease preload.[55] This contrasts with the influence of positive pressure ventilation on the failing left ventricle, where reductions in preload and afterload can be a welcome effect.[62] As such, the lowest V_T and PEEP settings should be sought in order to help preserve adequate oxygenation and ventilation. It is equally important to avoid excessive hypercapnia, which can exacerbate pulmonary vasoconstriction and lead to an increase in RV afterload. This can be attenuated with some measure of hyperventilation, although care must be taken to avoid air trapping (especially in those with a history of obstructive lung disease) that can lead to elevated pleural and pericardial pressures and impaired diastolic filling.[3]

Pregnancy

Maternal and fetal mortality risk is increased in the presence of cardiac disease. Pregnancy in the setting of PH, for example, is associated with a combined mortality rate that approaches 50%.[63] In general, the goals of treatment in pregnant patients are similar to those in nonpregnant patients. Periods of greatest risk include the second trimester and active labor and delivery.[47] Consultation with a cardiologist, and if available, a maternal–fetal medicine specialist, is warranted early in the clinical course.

Advanced Mechanical Support

In more severe cases of circulatory collapse, advanced mechanical support devices, including ventricular assist devices or extracorporeal membrane oxygenation, may have clinical utility. These interventions as well as measures such as intraaortic balloon counterpulsation and atrial septostomy have been implemented successfully in cases of severe PH and massive PE and as a bridge to lung transplantation.[64–66] Although only low-grade evidence exists for their use, such salvage therapies merit consideration, especially in centers with advanced cardiothoracic surgical capability.

CONCLUSION

Recognizing and successfully treating acute right heart failure require the consideration of a unique collection of illnesses and thoughtful integration of critical care resources. Although some of the available strategies and pharmacotherapies differ from those used in left ventricular disease, the underlying treatment principles are much the same. All clinical efforts should be aimed at preserving and aiding myocardial function, while maintaining focus on correction of precipitating illness and contributing systemic comorbidities. Historically, right ventricular dysfunction has been the subject of less academic study than left ventricular disorders. Future investigation, from both the clinical and basic science realms, will be needed to delineate the optimal therapeutic approach. At present, clinicians faced with the acutely failing RV may still draw upon a broad armamentarium to achieve hemodynamic and respiratory stability.

LITERATURE TABLE

TRIAL	DESIGN	RESULT
Piazza et al., *Chest.* 2005[3]	Review article	Excellent summary of pathophysiology of RV failure and mechanisms of successful treatment
Simonneau et al., *J Am Coll Cardiol.* 2009[33]	The classification of PAH as developed at the World Conference on PH in Dana Point, CA, in 2008	PH classification has undergone a number of revisions since the initial WHO-endorsed meeting in 1973. This latest symposium addressed changes to the definitions of familial PAH, schistosomiasis, hemolytic anemia, and chronic thromboembolic pulmonary hypertension (CTEPH)
Zehender et al., *N Engl J Med.* 1993[39]	Prospective 5-y study of 200 patients with acute inferior MIs	ST-segment elevation in V4R found to be a reliable indicator of RV involvement during acute inferior MI. Patients with ST-segment elevations in V4R had higher in-hospital mortality (31% vs. 6%, $p < 0.001$), and a higher incidence of major complications (64% vs. 28%, $p < 0.001$) than those without ST-segment elevation in V4R
Giannitsis et al., *Circulation.* 2000[43]	Single-center, prospective study of troponin T levels in 56 patients with confirmed PE	Elevated troponin found in 32%. In-hospital death (OR 29.6, 95% CI, 3.3–265.3), prolonged hypotension and cardiogenic shock (OR 11.4, 95% CI, 2.1–63.4), and need for resuscitation (OR 18.0, 95% CI, 2.6–124.3) were more prevalent in patients with elevated troponin T. The presence of troponin elevation, in the absence of coronary artery disease, underscored the hypothesis of ischemic injury to the RV in acute PE
Pruszczyk et al., *Eur Respir J.* 2003[45]	Single-center, prospective study of 79 patients with acute PE. Compared NT-proBNP to echocardiography for assessment of severity of RV overload	16.5% of patients had normal NT-proBNP values and had an uncomplicated clinical course, whereas all in-hospital deaths and serious events occurred in the group with elevated levels. Additionally, RV to left ventricular ratio and IVC dimension correlated with NT-proBNP
Price et al., *Crit Care.* 2010[55]	Systematic literature review from 1980 to 2010 of over 200 studies regarding intensive care management of pulmonary vascular dysfunction	Evidence level recommendations made regarding management of volume use, specific vasopressors/inotropes, pulmonary vasodilators, and mechanical therapies

CI, confidence interval; OR, odds ratio.

REFERENCES

1. Greyson CR. Pathophysiology of right ventricular failure. *Crit Care Med.* 2008;36(suppl 1):S57–S65.
2. Greyson CR. Right heart failure in the intensive care unit. *Curr Opin Crit Care.* 2012;18(5):424–431.
3. Piazza G, Goldhaber SZ. The acutely decompensated right ventricle, pathways for diagnosis and management. *Chest.* 2005;128:1836–1852.
4. ten Wolde M, Söhne M, Quak E, et al. Prognostic value of echocardiographically assessed right ventricular dysfunction in patients with pulmonary embolism. *Arch Intern Med.* 2004;164(15):1685–1689.
5. Stein PD, Beemath A, Matta F, et al. Clinical characteristics of patients with acute pulmonary embolism: data from PIOPED II. *Am J Med.* 2007;120(10):871–879.
6. Wiener RS, Schwartz LM, Woloshin S. Time trends in pulmonary embolism in the United States: evidence of overdiagnosis. *Arch Intern Med.* 2011;171(9):831.
7. Goldhaber SZ, Visani L, De Rosa M. Acute pulmonary embolism: clinical outcomes in the International Cooperative Pulmonary Embolism Registry (ICOPER). *Lancet.* 1999;353(9162):1386–1389.
8. Braat SH, Brugada P, de Zwaan C, et al. Value of electrocardiogram in diagnosing right ventricular involvement in patients with an acute inferior wall myocardial infarction. *Br Heart J.* 1983;49(4):368.
9. Mehta SR, Eikelboom JW, Natarajan MK, et al. Impact of right ventricular involvement on mortality and morbidity in patients with inferior myocardial infarction. *J Am Coll Cardiol.* 2001;37:37–43.
10. Jacobs AK, Leopold JA, et al. Cardiogenic shock caused by right ventricular infarction: a report from the SHOCK registry. *J Am Coll Cardiol.* 2003;41:1273–1279.
11. Vieillard-Baron A, et al. Acute cor pulmonale in acute respiratory distress syndrome submitted to protective ventilation: incidence, clinical implications, and prognosis. *Crit Care Med.* 2001;29(8):1551–1555.
12. Peacock AJ, Murphy NF, McMurray JJV, et al. An epidemiological study of pulmonary arterial hypertension. *Eur Respir J.* 2007;30:104–109.
13. Budev MM, Arroliga AC, Wiedemann HP, et al. Cor Pulmonale: an overview. *Semin Respir Crit Care Med.* 2003;24(3):233–244.
14. Sitbon O, Lascoux-Combe C, Delfraissy JF, et al. Prevalence of HIV-related pulmonary arterial hypertension in the current antiretroviral therapy era. *Am J Respir Crit Care Med.* 2008;177:108–113.
15. Hachulla E, Gressin V, Guillevin L, et al. Early detection of pulmonary arterial hypertension in systemic sclerosis: a french nationwide prospective multicenter study. *Arthritis Rheum.* 2005;52:3792–3800.
16. Mukerjee D, St George D, Coleiro B, et al. Prevalence and outcome in systemic sclerosis associated pulmonary arterial hypertension: application of a registry approach. *Ann Rheum Dis.* 2003;62:1088–1093.
17. Machado RF, Gladwin MT. Pulmonary hypertension in hemolytic disorders: pulmonary vascular disease: the global perspective. *Chest.* 2010;137:30S–38S.
18. Fonseca GH, Souza R, Salemi VM, et al. Pulmonary hypertension diagnosed by right heart catheterization in sickle cell disease. *Eur Respir J.* 2012;39(1):112–118.
19. Campo A, Mathai SC, Le Pavec J, et al. Outcomes of hospitalisation for right heart failure in pulmonary arterial hypertension. *Eur Respir J.* 2011;38(2):359–367.
20. Sztrymf B, Souza R, Bertoletti L, et al. Prognostic factors of acute heart failure in patients with pulmonary arterial hypertension. *Eur Respir J.* 2010;35:1286–1293.
21. Haddad F, Peterson T, Fuh E, et al. Characteristics and outcome after hospitalization for acute right heart failure in patients with pulmonary arterial hypertension. *Circ Heart Fail.* 2011;4(6):692–699.
22. Macnee W. Pathophysiology of cor pulmonale in chronic obstructive pulmonary disease. *Am J Respir Crit Care Med.* 1994;150(3):833–852.
23. Renzetti AD, McClement JG, Litt BD. The Veterans administration cooperative study of pulmonary function. *Am J Med.* 1966;41:115–129.
24. Vizza CD, Lynch JP, Ochoa LL, et al. Right and left ventricular dysfunction in patients with severe pulmonary disease. *Chest.* 1998;113:576–583.
25. Lettieri CJ, Nathan SD, Barnett SD, et al. Prevalence and outcomes of pulmonary arterial hypertension in advanced idiopathic pulmonary fibrosis. *Chest.* 2006;129:746–752.
26. Patel NM, Lederer DJ, Borczuk AC, et al. Pulmonary hypertension in idiopathic pulmonary fibrosis. *Chest.* 2007;132(3):998.
27. Shorr AF, Davies DB, Nathan SD. Outcomes for patients with sarcoidosis awaiting lung transplantation. *Chest.* 2002;122:233–238.
28. Strange C, Highland KB. Pulmonary hypertension in interstitial lung disease. *Curr Opin Pulm Med.* 2005;11(5):452–455.
29. Redl G, Germann P, Plattner H, et al. Right ventricular function in early septic shock states. *Intensive Care Med.* 1993;19(1):3–7.

30. Pulido JN, Afessa B, Masaki M, et al. Clinical spectrum, frequency, and significance of myocardial dysfunction in severe sepsis and septic shock. *Mayo Clin Proc.* 2012;87(7):620–628.
31. Green EM, Givertz MM. Management of acute right ventricular failure in the intensive care unit. *Curr Heart Fail Rep.* 2012;9(3):228–235.
32. Nieminen MS, Brutsaert D, Dickstein K, et al. EuroHeart Failure Survey II (EHFS II): a survey on hospitalized acute heart failure patients: description of population. *Eur Heart J.* 2006;27:2725–2736.
33. Simonneau G, Robbins IM, Beghetti M, et al. Updated clinical classification of pulmonary hypertension. *J Am Coll Cardiol.* 2009;54:S43.
34. Brenot F, Herve P, Petitpretz P, et al. Primary pulmonary hypertension and fenfluramine use. *Br Heart J.* 1993;70(6):537.
35. Albertson TE, Walby WF, Derlet RW. Stimulant-induced pulmonary toxicity. *Chest.* 1995;108(4):1140.
36. Cook DJ, Simel DL. The rational clinical examination. Does this patient have abnormal central venous pressure? *JAMA.* 1996;275(8):630–637.
37. Matthews JC, McLaughlin V. Acute right ventricular failure in the setting of acute pulmonary embolism or chronic pulmonary hypertension: a detailed review of the pathophysiology, diagnosis, and management. *Curr Cardiol Rev.* 2008;4(1):49–59.
38. Harrigan RA, Jones K. ABC of clinical electrocardiography. Conditions affecting the right side of the heart. *BMJ.* 2002;324(7347):1201–1204.
39. Zehender M, Kasper W, Kauder E, et al. Right ventricular infarction as an independent predictor of prognosis after acute inferior myocardial infarction. *N Engl J Med.* 1993;328(14):981–988.
40. Casas RE, Marriott HJ, Glancy DL. Value of leads V7-V9 in diagnosing posterior wall acute myocardial infarction and other causes of tall R waves in V1-V2. *Am J Cardiol.* 1997;80(4):508.
41. Stein PD, Terrin ML, Hales CA, et al. Clinical, laboratory, roentgenographic, and electrocardiographic findings in patients with acute pulmonary embolism and no pre-existing cardiac or pulmonary disease. *Chest.* 1991;100(3):598.
42. Blehar DJ, Dickman E, Gaspari R. Identification of congestive heart failure via respiratory variation of inferior vena cava diameter. *Am J Emerg Med.* 2009;27:71–75.
43. Giannitsis E, Müller-Bardorff M, Kurowski V, et al. Independent prognostic value of cardiac troponin T in patients with confirmed pulmonary embolism. *Circulation.* 2000;102(2):211–217.
44. Becattini C, Vedovati MC, Agnelli G. Prognostic value of troponins in acute pulmonary embolism: a meta-analysis. *Circulation.* 2007;116:427–433.
45. Pruszczyk P, Kostrubiec M, Bochowicz A, et al. N-terminal pro-brain natriuretic peptide in patients with acute pulmonary embolism. *Eur Respir J.* 2003;22(4):649–653.
46. Bocchi EA, Bacal F, Auler JO Jr, et al. Inhaled nitric oxide leading to pulmonary edema in stable severe heart failure. *Am J Cardiol.* 1994;74:70–72.
47. Haddad F, Doyle R, Murphy DJ, et al. Right ventricular function in cardiovascular disease, part II: pathophysiology, clinical importance, and management of right ventricular failure. *Circulation.* 2008;117(13):1717–1731.
48. Forfia PR, Vaidya A, Wiegers SE. Pulmonary heart disease: the heart-lung interaction and its impact on patient phenotypes. *Pulm Circ.* 2013;3(1):5–19.
49. Lejeune P, Brimioulle S, Leeman M, et al. Enhancement of hypoxic pulmonary vasoconstriction by metabolic acidosis in dogs. *Anesthesiology.* 1990;73(2):256–264.
50. Ichinose F, Roberts JD, Zapol WM. Inhaled nitric oxide: a selective pulmonary vasodilator current uses and therapeutic potential. *Circulation.* 2004;109(25):3106–3111.
51. Weinberger B, Laskin DL, Heck DE, et al. The toxicology of inhaled nitric oxide. *Toxicol Sci.* 2001;59(1):5–16.
52. Christenson J, Lavoie A, O'Connor M, et al. The incidence and pathogenesis of cardiopulmonary deterioration after abrupt withdrawal of inhaled nitric oxide. *Am J Respir Crit Care Med.* 2000;161(5):1443.
53. Overgaard CB, Dzavík V. Inotropes and vasopressors: review of physiology and clinical use in cardiovascular disease. *Circulation.* 2008;118(10):1047–1056.
54. Kerbaul F, Rondelet B, Motte S, et al. Effects of norepinephrine and dobutamine on pressure load-induced right ventricular failure. *Crit Care Med.* 2004;32:1035–1040.
55. Price, LC, Wort SJ, et al. Pulmonary vascular and right ventricular dysfunction in adult critical care: current and emerging options for management: a systemic literature review. *Crit Care.* 2010;14:R169.
56. Lahm T, McCaslin CA, Wozniak TC, et al. Medical and surgical treatment of acute right ventricular failure. *J Am Coll Cardiol.* 2010;56(18):1435–1446.

57. Khoo CW, Lip GY. Acute management of atrial fibrillation. *Chest.* 2009;135(3):849–859.
58. Fuster V, Ryden LE, Cannom DS, et al. ACC/AHA/ESC 2006 guidelines for the management of patients with atrial fibrillation: full text: a report of the American College of Cardiology/American Heart Association Task Force on practice guidelines and the European Society of Cardiology Committee for Practice Guidelines (Writing Committee to Revise the 2001 guidelines for the management of patients with atrial fibrillation) developed in collaboration with the European Heart Rhythm Association and the Heart Rhythm Society. *Europace.* 2006;8:651–745.
59. Rich S, Seidlitz M, Dodin E, et al. The short-term effects of digoxin in patients with right ventricular dysfunction from pulmonary hypertension. *Chest.* 1998;114(3):787–792.
60. Romero-Bermejo FJ, Ruiz-Bailen M, Gil-Cebrian J, et al. Sepsis-induced cardiomyopathy. *Curr Cardiol Rev.* 2011;7(3):163–183.
61. Kucher N, Goldhaber SZ. Management of massive pulmonary embolism. *Circulation.* 2005;112(2):e28.
62. Pinsky MR. Cardiovascular issues in respiratory care. *Chest.* 2005;128(5 suppl 2):592S–597S.
63. Franklin WJ, Benton MK, Parekh DR. Cardiac disease in pregnancy. *Tex Heart Inst J.* 2011;38(2):151–153.
64. Chan CY, Chen YS, Ko WJ, et al. Extracorporeal membrane oxygenation support for single lung transplantation in a patient with primary pulmonary hypertension. *J Heart Lung Transplant.* 1998;17:325–327.
65. Gregoric ID, Chandra D, Myers TJ, et al. Extracorporeal membrane oxygenation as a bridge to emergency heart-lung transplantation in a patient with idiopathic pulmonary arterial hypertension. *J Heart Lung Transplant.* 2008;27:466–468.
66. Deehring R, Kiss AB, Garrett A, et al. Extracorporeal membrane oxygenation as a bridge to surgical embolectomy in acute fulminant pulmonary embolism. *Am J Emerg Med.* 2006;24:879–880.

16

Hypertensive Crises

Anand Swaminathan and Michael P. Jones

BACKGROUND

Hypertension affects an estimated 50 million individuals in the United States.[1] Management of this largely preventable disease focuses on chronic reduction of blood pressure through dietary and lifestyle modifications and, when necessary, pharmacologic management. Patients with hypertension frequently seek emergency care, and hypertension is one of the most common primary diagnoses of patients admitted with critical illness.

Hypertensive emergency refers to the presence of end-organ damage directly attributable to uncontrolled elevations in blood pressure and requires immediate administration of antihypertensive medications to prevent irreversible injury. Hypertensive urgency, a more benign diagnosis, is defined as symptomatic (e.g., headache, shortness of breath, anxiety) hypertension without evidence of end-organ damage. The most common presentations of hypertensive emergency include cerebral infarction or hemorrhage (24.5%), acute pulmonary edema (APE) (22.5%), and hypertensive encephalopathy (16.3%). Other complications include acute coronary syndrome (ACS), aortic dissection (AD), preeclampsia and eclampsia, acute renal failure, microangiopathic hemolytic anemia, and hypertensive retinopathy.

This chapter presents an approach to the management of severe hypertension in the setting of four important emergency department (ED) diagnostic concerns: APE, hypertensive encephalopathy, ACS, and AD. Stroke—the most common of all hypertensive emergencies—is addressed in detail in Chapter 20. A review of antihypertensive agents used in the management of these four conditions is provided in Tables 16.1 and 16.2.

ACUTE PULMONARY EDEMA

History and Physical Exam

Cardiogenic APE is a relatively common clinical entity in the ED and carries a mortality rate of 15% to 20%. The most common presenting complaints are dyspnea, tachypnea, and, in severe cases, cough productive of frothy sputum.

The history and physical exam in patients with APE should focus on determining the etiology of the heart failure causing the edema. Potential etiologies include myocardial infarction (MI), exacerbation of chronic CHF, mitral/aortic valve dysfunction, and infection. Eliciting a history of chronic renal failure is also important, as these patients, if volume overloaded, will often require hemodialysis to remove excess fluid. Physical exam will reveal findings—such as tachypnea and abnormal lung sounds—common to other disease processes such as pneumonia. Findings more specific to APE include elevated jugular venous pressure and an S_3 gallop.[2,3] New murmurs are also important to note as these may suggest rupture of a valve leaflet—a critical finding that can require surgical management.

Diagnostic Evaluation

There is no single test that confirms the diagnosis of APE. Diagnostic evaluation commonly employs laboratory testing, electrocardiogram (ECG), chest radiography (CXR), and bedside ultrasound (US). Serum B-type natriuretic peptide is a relatively sensitive marker for APE (90%), but lacks specificity (76%).[4] Cardiac-specific troponin (cTnT) assays can be helpful in establishing myocardial ischemia or infarction as the underlying cause of APE, but troponin levels may also be elevated secondary to increased right ventricular wall stress, rate-related or stress ischemia, or underlying end-stage renal disease (ESRD).[5] As a result, many patients with CHF will have chronically mild troponin elevations. A number of trials have found a correlation between an elevated cTnT and increased mortality in acute heart failure patients.[6,7]

The ECG is an essential diagnostic test in APE, as it can reveal precipitating ischemia or dysrhythmias that require additional interventions (cardiac catheterization or rate/rhythm control, respectively). The CXR is equally important; in diagnosing APE, its findings of cephalization, interstitial edema, and alveolar edema are highly specific (96%, 98%, and 99%, respectively) but have low sensitivity (41%, 27%, and 6%, respectively). Up to 18% of CXRs in patients with APE will demonstrate no vascular congestion.[8,9] Finally, bedside ultrasonography is a relatively new but valuable tool for evaluation of patients with suspected APE. Bedside transthoracic echocardiography (TTE) can be used to estimate left ventricular (LV) function and diagnose valvular rupture; it can also reveal B-lines, a highly sensitive and specific finding (97% and 95%, respectively) for interstitial edema. In trained hands, lung ultrasonography is more accurate than plain radiography for the diagnosis of APE.[10,11]

Management Guidelines

In patients with APE, treatment focuses on reducing the work of breathing (and thus the risk of respiratory failure) and shifting fluid out of the interstitial and alveolar spaces through reduction of preload and afterload. Respiratory support for patients with APE traditionally necessitated intubation and mechanical ventilation. In the last 10 years, the use of noninvasive positive pressure ventilation (NIPPV) using continuous positive airway pressure (CPAP) and bilevel positive airway pressure (BiPAP) has become increasingly common. NIPPV, by increasing intrathoracic pressure, effects a reduction in preload, thereby decreasing blood flow into the pulmonary vasculature and reducing pulmonary capillary pressures. Although not shown to reduce mortality, NIPPV has been associated with decreased need for intubation, fewer critical care unit admissions, and fewer overall treatment failures.[12–16]

Pharmacologic treatment of increased preload emphasizes use of nitrates (specifically nitroglycerin), morphine sulfate, and loop diuretics (furosemide).

Nitroglycerin (sublingual, topical, or intravenous) is a potent vasodilator, and small studies have shown it to be capable of producing rapid, significant decreases in LV pressure.[17] Sublingual nitroglycerin (SLNTG) should be started immediately upon recognition of APE and followed by a continuous IV infusion. A 400-mcg tab of SLNTG provides a dose equivalent to an intravenous infusion of 80 mcg/min for 5 minutes, so the IV infusion should be started at this or a similar infusion rate and rapidly titrated to effect. Morphine and loop diuretics have been used for decades in the treatment of APE, but the physiologic rationale for their efficacy is flawed, and there is little evidence to support their use. The ADHERE study group found that APE patients receiving morphine had increased rates of mechanical ventilation (15.4% vs. 2.8%), ICU admissions (38.7% vs. 14.4%), and mortality (13.0% vs. 2.4%).[6] These results have also been reproduced in ED-based studies.[17] Loop diuretics for the treatment of APE historically were recommended based on the cardiorenal pathogenesis model, which hypothesized that edema and decreased cardiac function result from decreased kidney function and subsequent volume overload. However, more recent studies have shown that less than half of patients with APE have total body increased volume.[18,19] Furosemide was shown to initially increase PCWP in patients in the ICU with APE and did not lead to significant drops in preload until 20 minutes after administration.[20] Additionally, loop diuretics activate the renin–angiotensin–aldosterone system (RAAS) and the sympathetic nervous system, leading to increased vasoconstriction and impaired cardiac function.[21] Finally, many patients with APE also have ESRD and will not benefit from loop diuretics regardless of volume status.

Correction of elevated afterload—the result of activation of the RAAS and an increase in sympathetic drive—is equally important in the management of APE; afterload reduction improves LV function and helps restore adequate circulation. Bilevel positive airway pressure (BPAP), in addition to its ability to reduce preload and support respiratory function, produces afterload reduction; however, the mechanism of this response is not fully understood.[12–16] High-dose IV nitroglycerin (>100 mcg/min) also results in arterial vasodilation and afterload reduction. The use of angiotensin-converting enzyme inhibitors (ACEI) for afterload reduction in the treatment of cardiogenic APE is supported by a number of small studies. One of these demonstrated a reduced need for mechanical ventilation in patients receiving ACEI, while a second demonstrated a lower ICU admission rate (OR = 0.29) and lower intubation rates (OR = 0.16) with its use.[22,23] Nicardipine is another alternative for achieving afterload reduction; it can be rapidly titrated and effects a coronary blood flow increase, which may be beneficial in systolic heart failure.[24,25]

Finally, emphasis should be placed on identifying reversible causes of APE and involving subspecialty consultation—cardiac catheterization for AMI, cardiac surgery for valvular rupture, and hemodialysis for ESRD—as appropriate.

HYPERTENSIVE ENCEPHALOPATHY

History and Physical Exam

Hypertensive encephalopathy is one of the more insidious consequences of uncontrolled hypertension. It is classically defined as the triad of hypertension, altered mental status, and papilledema.[26] Hypertensive encephalopathy must be treated immediately to prevent further end-organ damage. First described in 1928, hypertensive encephalopathy is a rare disease that leads to death if untreated.[27]

A patient history may be difficult to obtain, as these patients may in fact be obtunded; in this case, evaluation for other life-threatening causes of altered mental status—such as hypoglycemia, hypoxia, and intracranial injury—should take precedence. Once these causes have been ruled out, hypertensive encephalopathy should be considered. Symptoms will commonly include headache, irritability and nausea. Seizures may also be reported. Physical exam should center on accurate measurement of blood pressure (using an appropriately sized cuff or arterial blood pressure monitoring) and a detailed neurologic examination looking for focal deficits. Papilledema and retinal hemorrhages may be observed. There is no set value of measured blood pressure required for hypertensive encephalopathy; a patient with long-standing hypertension may tolerate blood pressures greater than 200 mm Hg systolic and 150 mm Hg diastolic, while a pregnant woman or child can develop symptoms at diastolic blood pressures greater than 100 mm Hg.[28]

Diagnostic Evaluation

Hypertensive encephalopathy is a diagnosis of exclusion. Its workup includes a noncontrast CT head to rule out mass lesion or hemorrhagic or ischemic stroke as well as laboratory examinations to exclude metabolic causes of altered mental status. Suggestive findings on CT include signs of edema, particularly in the posterior regions. Brain MRI will show edema of a vasogenic origin, but obtaining this degree of imaging is often neither feasible nor necessary in the ED, unless there is concern for a more subtle focal insult not visualized on CT.

Electroencephalographic (EEG) examination will show evidence of generalized slowing and epileptiform discharges as well as loss of alpha-wave rhythms, signifying an impaired consciousness. The utility of continuous EEG monitoring in the ED, however, is not well established; this is in part due to the typically rapid improvement in symptoms following initiation of aggressive therapy, and in part to the practical challenges of obtaining an EEG in the ED.

Management Guidelines

Hypertensive encephalopathy is a fully reversible condition if appropriate treatment is instituted in a timely manner. The mainstay of treatment is a rapid, but controlled, decline in blood pressure, with adequate maintenance of cerebral perfusion pressure. Most experts recommend a reduction in mean arterial pressure of no more than 20% to 25% in the first hour of therapy guided by an arterial blood pressure monitor for more timely and accurate monitoring. In a busy emergency department, at a minimum, the blood pressure should be noninvasively monitored every 3 to 5 minutes until more invasive monitoring can be made available. Preferred antihypertensive agents include sodium nitroprusside, labetalol, and nicardipine.

Literature suggests that labetalol, in particular, has minimal impact on cerebral perfusion pressure—making it optimal for treating hypertensive encephalopathy. Unlike pure beta-blocking agents (e.g., esmolol) that reduce cardiac output, labetalol reduces systemic vascular resistance (SVR) without reducing total peripheral blood flow, which is essential in maintaining cerebral, renal, and cardiac perfusion.[29–32]

ACUTE CORONARY SYNDROME

History and Physical Exam

Hypertension is a known risk factor for the development of coronary artery disease.[1,33] Acute elevations in blood pressure can lead to increased LV demand without a proportionate increase in myocardial perfusion, resulting in ischemia. In all patients with elevated blood pressure who complain of chest pain or chest pain equivalents (e.g., shortness of breath), ACS should be considered.

The physical exam in the patient with ACS is nonspecific but plays an important role in ruling out the alternative diagnoses of AD and APE. The presence, in particular, of pulse deficits, aortic insufficiency murmurs, and neurologic deficits points to AD.[26] The presence of jugular venous distension, lower extremity edema, severe dyspnea, and crackles on pulmonary exam points to APE.

Diagnostic Evaluation

ECG, CXR, bedside echocardiography, and serum cardiac enzyme testing are essential to the evaluation of ACS in the setting of hypertensive emergency. An ECG should be performed immediately and evaluated for the presence of an ST-segment elevation myocardial infarction (STEMI) necessitating emergent cardiac catheterization. While CXR rarely establishes a diagnosis of ACS on its own, it is helpful in identifying alternative hypertensive emergencies (e.g., AD or APE). Similarly, echocardiography may reveal LV wall motion abnormalities consistent with MI, but may also show findings consistent with AD (pericardial effusion, proximal dissection flap) or APE (B-lines, flail leaflet). An elevated serum cardiac troponin (cTn) supports a diagnosis of ACS; however, it is important to note that cTn may be elevated in a number of disease processes including pericarditis/myocarditis, pulmonary embolism, tachydysrhythmias, takotsubo cardiomyopathy, ESRD, sepsis, stroke, and rhabdomyolysis.[5]

Management Guidelines

The treatment of ACS in the setting of hypertensive emergency requires the use of pharmacologic agents directed both at blood pressure control—to reduce shear forces, LV strain, and ischemia and platelet activation—and platelet inhibition. Antiplatelet agent recommendations can be found in the American College of Cardiology/American Heart Association (ACC/AHA) guidelines.[34,35] For rapid reduction in blood pressure, nitroglycerin and beta-blockers are the most commonly recommended agents.[34,35] Nitroglycerin (sublingual or intravenous) reduces both LV filling pressure and SVR, thereby decreasing both myocardial oxygen demand and the likelihood of further ischemia.[36] At higher doses, nitroglycerin produces coronary artery vasodilation.[36] These factors, along with its short half-life and ease in titration, make it an ideal therapeutic agent in hypertension-associated ACS.

Beta-blockers are beneficial both for blood pressure reduction and for prevention of ventricular dysrhythmias in ACS. The ACC/AHA recommends beta-blockers be given within 24 hours of presentation, with a goal of 20% to 30% blood pressure reduction.[35,37–39] Although both labetalol and esmolol are commonly recommended, esmolol has a more favorable profile with rapid onset, short half-life, and ease of titration.[28] Beta-blocking agents should, however, be used with caution in the setting of ACS, as these agents can exacerbate LV failure. The COMMIT trial found that patients with acute MI given beta-blockers early in their clinical course had higher rates of cardiogenic shock and recommended beta-blocker therapy be considered only after a patient's hemodynamic condition had stabilized.[40] In patients at risk for cardiogenic shock, it is advisable to obtain an echocardiogram to further assess cardiac function prior to the administration of intravenous beta-blockers.

AORTIC DISSECTION

History and Physical Exam

AD represents one of the most challenging diagnoses to make in the emergency department. The disease carries a high mortality rate (Stanford type A, 34.9%, and Stanford type B, 14.9%) and should be considered in any patient with hypertension and a complaint of chest or back pain. The majority of patients with AD complain of chest pain (72.7%), abrupt onset of pain (84.8%), and severe pain at onset (90.6%).[41] The classic presentation—sudden onset of sharp or tearing chest pain radiating to the back—is, however, rarely observed.[41] Patients with Stanford type B dissections (descending aorta only) can present with isolated back pain.

Commonly described physical exam findings are equally unreliable in ruling out AD. While the majority of patients (72.1%) have a history of hypertension, only 50% will be hypertensive on presentation (in the patient in whom an ascending dissection has resulted in a pericardial effusion, hypotension may actually be observed).[41] Other exam findings, including a murmur of aortic insufficiency (31.6%) and pulse deficit (15.1%), are equally unlikely to be found. However, in a patient with chest pain that has one of these findings, the diagnosis of AD should be more seriously considered.

Diagnostic Evaluation

The most important diagnostic modalities in AD are the ECG, CXR, and chest CT with IV contrast. An ECG will frequently demonstrate either no abnormal findings or nonspecific findings (31.3% and 41.4%, respectively); about 3.2%, however, will show findings consistent with an STEMI. An STEMI can be observed in the setting of an ascending AD when the dissection extends into either the right or left coronary ostium, leading to occlusion of any of the major coronary arteries. The most common coronary artery involvement occurs via extension into the right coronary artery leading to an inferior wall infarction. In patients with evidence of STEMI on ECG, a diagnosis of AD should be considered if the patient's symptoms or presentation are atypical for ACS.

Chest radiography may reveal a widened mediastinum (61.6%) or abnormal aortic contour (49.6%), but is normal in up to 15% of patients. Chest CT with IV contrast, which has a high sensitivity (95%) and specificity (87% to 100%) and can be performed rapidly, is the primary diagnostic modality for AD in the ED.[42] Transesophageal echocardiography is an effective alternative imaging modality (sensitivity of 98%, specificity of 95%) for patients that cannot tolerate CT, but may not be available in the ED and/or may delay diagnosis. Although TTE is rarely adequate to make a definitive diagnosis of AD, it can help identify pericardial effusions or tamponade that provide indirect evidence of AD.

Management Guidelines

Once AD is diagnosed, all efforts should be made to obtain emergent cardiothoracic surgery consultation for operative repair. Mortality increases by 1% to 2% for every hour from symptom onset to definitive treatment.[8] ED management should focus on "anti-impulse therapy," that is, control of blood pressure and heart rate in order to reduce the shear forces of LV ejection (dP/dT). Elevated shear forces result in a forceful flow of blood against the dissection flap that can cause the flap to extend.[42] AD is the only hypertensive emergency in which rapid lowering of blood pressure (ideally within 5 to 10 minutes) is indicated. The recommended target systolic blood pressure is 100 to 110 mm Hg, with some experts advocating lowering to subnormal numbers (SBP = 90 to 100).[28,42] Heart rate should be lowered to less than 60 bpm.[28,42]

First-line agents for anti-impulse therapy are beta-blockers, as they have the ability to lower heart rate and blood pressure simultaneously. Although there is no consensus on a preferred beta blocker, esmolol's rapid onset and ease of titration make it an ideal agent.[28,39,42,43] Labetalol can be used, but has a slower onset of action and a longer half-life and is more difficult to titrate. If beta-blockers are contraindicated, calcium channel blockers (CCBs) (e.g., diltiazem) are acceptable alternatives.

Once goal heart rate is achieved, an arterial vasodilator should be added to achieve an SBP <110 mm Hg. Historically, sodium nitroprusside was the vasodilator of choice, but this agent has multiple limitations, including labile blood pressure and reflex tachycardia.[28,39,42,43] Clevidipine and nicardipine offer more reliable effects on blood pressure. Both agents are dihydropyridine CCBs and pure afterload reducers that have a rapid onset and a short half-life, are easily titratable, and have been demonstrated safe to use concurrently with intravenous beta-1–selective agents.[44] An ED-based study found that 89% of patients with hypertensive emergencies who received clevidipine reached goal BP targets within 30 minutes.[44] If neither of these agents is available, intravenous nitroglycerin at higher doses may provide adequate blood pressure control, however use as a solo agent can produce a reflex tachycardia.

Finally, bedside US should be performed in all patients with AD to determine whether the patient has cardiac tamponade and requires immediate pericardiocentesis.

CONCLUSION

Hypertensive crisis requires prompt intervention. Recognition of the common complications of severe hypertension and appreciation of optimal antihypertensive agents enable the emergency physician to respond to these emergencies in a timely and effective manner.

TABLE 16.1 Common Antihypertensive Agents—Preferred Use, Starting Dose, Side Effects, and Contraindications

Antihypertensive Agent	Preferred Use	Starting Dose	Side Effects and Contraindications
Sodium nitroprusside	Hypertensive encephalopathy, AD[a]	0.25–10 mcg/kg/min IV gtt	Reflex tachycardia, coronary steal, methemoglobinemia. Is metabolized to cyanide
Nitroglycerin	MI, CHF, LV dysfunction	5–100 mcg/min IV gtt	Hypotension Contraindicated in severe aortic stenosis, LV outflow obstruction, and inferior wall MI
Nicardipine	Hypertensive encephalopathy, MI, CHF, cerebral infarction/hemorrhage	5 mg/h IV gtt, increasing by 2.5 mg/h IV every 5 min to a maximum of 30 mg/h IV gtt	Hypotension Contraindicated in severe aortic stenosis Reflex tachycardia
Labetalol	Hypertensive encephalopathy, MI, preeclampsia/eclampsia, cerebral infarction/hemorrhage	20–80 mg IV bolus every 10 min, 0.5–2 mg/min IV gtt	Hypotension Contraindicated in acute asthma, COPD, acute CHF, heart block, and sympathomimetic intoxication (e.g., cocaine)
Esmolol	Hypertensive encephalopathy, MI, eclampsia, cerebral infarction/hemorrhage	Loading dose 500 mcg/kg IV over 1 min, 25–50 mcg/kg/min IV gtt	See labetalol
Fenoldopam	Acute renal failure, CHF	0.1–0.6 mcg/kg/min IV gtt	Contraindicated in increased intraocular pressure
Enalaprilat	CHF, active renin–angiotensin system	1.25–5 mg IV every 6 h	Contraindicated in pregnancy and ACEI-related angioedema
Hydralazine	Preeclampsia/eclampsia	5–10 mg IV bolus can be repeated every 10–15 min	Reflex tachycardia, CNS, and myocardial ischemia

[a]Should be administered with a beta-blocker to avoid reflex tachycardia.

TABLE 16.2 Common Antihypertensive Agents—Pharmacology

Sodium Nitroprusside	An arterial and venous vasodilator that decreases both afterload and preload. It results in decreased cerebral blood flow while increasing intracranial pressure, making it a poor agent for patients with acute neurological conditions (e.g., hypertensive encephalopathy). Nitroprusside has a quick onset of action (seconds) and a short half life of 3–4 minutes. Coronary steal can occur in patients with coronary artery disease leading to reduction in regional blood flow
Nitroglycerin	A potent vasodilator that acts mainly on the venous system. It decreases preload and also increases coronary blood flow to the subendocardium. Nitroglycerin can be administered as a paste, sublingual spray, dissolvable tablet, or an infusion. It has a rapid onset and is considered the drug of choice in hypertensive emergencies in patients with cardiac ischemia, LV dysfunction, and pulmonary edema. It is not recommended in patients with severe aortic stenosis, LV outflow obstruction, or inferior wall MI because of the potential to precipitate cardiovascular collapse

(*Continued*)

TABLE 16.2	Common Antihypertensive Agents–Pharmacology (*Continued*)
Nicardipine	A dihydropyridine CCB. It may have unique benefits in hypertensive encephalopathy as it crosses the blood–brain barrier to vasorelax the cerebrovascular smooth muscle and minimize vasospasm, especially in subarachnoid hemorrhage. Nicardipine is contraindicated in patients with advanced aortic stenosis. The principal adverse effect is abrupt reduction in blood pressure and reflex tachycardia, which can be harmful in patients with coronary heart disease
Labetolol	A combined selective alpha-1 and nonselective beta-adrenergic receptor blocker. Its alpha:beta blocking ratio is 1:7. Labetalol begins to act in lowering blood pressure 2–5 minutes after administration and reaches it's peak within 5–15 minutes. It reduces systemic vascular resistance without compromising cardiac output or decreasing cerebral, renal or coronary artery blood flow
Esmolol	A short-acting selective beta-1–adrenergic blocker. It has a rapid onset and short duration of action. These properties make it easy to titrate. Esmolol is effective in blunting the reflex tachycardia induced by nitroprusside. It carries the same contraindications as other beta-blockers (see Labetalol)
Fenoldopam	A selective peripheral dopamine type 1 (D_1) agonist that has recently been added to the list of medications used in the treatment of hypertensive emergencies. It causes both vasodilation and natriuresis. It has the advantage of increasing renal blood flow and improving creatinine clearance. As a result, fenoldopam may be the drug of choice in treating hypertensive emergencies in the setting of impaired renal function. It is contraindicated in patients with increased intraocular pressure
Enalaprilat	It is the active IV form of enalapril, an angiotensin-converting enzyme (ACE) inhibitor. Enalaprilat lowers SVR, pulmonary capillary pressure, and heart rate while increasing coronary vasodilation. It has minimal effect on cerebral perfusion pressure. Some studies have found enalaprilat to be particularly useful in hypertensive emergency with APE. ACE inhibitors are contraindicated in pregnancy.
Hydralazine	Lowers blood pressure by a direct vasodilatory effect on arteriolar smooth muscle. The exact mechanism of this effect is unknown. It is the preferred agent for treatment of preeclampsia/eclampsia, but has fallen out of favor for treatment of hypertension in other conditions. Hydralazine can cause reflex tachycardia as well as CNS and myocardial ischemia. An additional downside of hydralazine is that while its half-life is 3–6 h, the total duration of effect is unpredictable and extend to 36 h.

LITERATURE TABLE

TRIAL	DESIGN	RESULT
Mehta and Jay. *Crit Care Med.* 1997[14]	27 patients presenting with APE, characterized by dyspnea, tachypnea, tachycardia, accessory muscle use, bilateral rales, and typical findings of congestion on a CXR. Randomized to receive nasal CPAP vs. nasal BiPAP	After 30 min, significant reductions in breathing frequency, heart rate, blood pressure, and $PaCo_2$ were observed in the BiPAP group, as were significant improvements in arterial pH and dyspnea scores. BiPAP improves ventilation and vital signs more rapidly than does CPAP in patients with APE
Bussmann and Schupp. *Am J Card.* 1978[17]	22 patients with the classical clinical signs of pulmonary edema (orthopnea, cyanosis, sweating, and rales heard at a distance) were divided into those observed clinically and those given 0.8–2.4 mg nitroglycerin sublingually one to six times at 5–10 min intervals	This early study showed qualitatively that the use of nitroglycerin leads to marked improvement in dyspnea
COMMIT collaborative group. *Lancet.* 2005[40]	Randomized placebo-controlled trial of early intravenous followed by oral metoprolol in 45,852 patients with acute MI. Prespecified co-primary outcomes were (1) composite of death, reinfarction, or cardiac arrest; and (2) death from any cause during the treatment period	Use of early beta-blocker therapy in acute MI reduces the risk of reinfarction (2.0% metoprolol vs. 2.5% placebo; OR 0.82, 0.72–0.92; $p = 0.001$) and ventricular fibrillation (2.5% vs. 3.0%; OR 0.83, 0.75–0.93; $p = 0.001$), but increases the risk of cardiogenic shock (5.0% vs. 3.9%; OR 1.30, 1.19–1.41; $p < 0.00001$), especially during days 0–1 after admission. No difference in mortality

LITERATURE TABLE (*Continued*)		
TRIAL	DESIGN	RESULT
Hagan et al., *JAMA.* 2000[41]	Case series of 464 patients with aortic dissection. Data were collected at presentation and by physician review of hospital records. Of the 464 patients (mean age, 63 years; 65.3% male), 62.3% had type A dissection	Sudden onset of severe sharp pain was the single most common presenting complaint. Classic physical findings such as aortic regurgitation and pulse deficit were noted in only 31.6% and 15.1% of patients, respectively, and initial CXR and ECG were frequently not helpful (no abnormalities were noted in 12.4% and 31.3% of patients, respectively). Computed tomography was the initial imaging modality used in 61.1%. Overall in-hospital mortality was 27.4%

OR, odds ratio.

REFERENCES

1. Chobanian AV, Bakris GL, Black HR, et al. The Seventh Report of the Joint National Committee on Prevention, Detection and Evaluation, and Treatment of High Blood Pressure. *Hypertension.* 2003;42(6):1206–1252. Epub 2003 Dec 1.
2. Allen LA, O'Conor CM. Management of acute decompensated heart failure. *CMAJ.* 2007;176(6):797–805.
3. Ware LB, Matthay MA. Acute pulmonary edema. *NEJM.* 2005;353(26):2788–2796.
4. Maisel AS, Krishnaswamy P, Nowak RM, et al. Breathing not properly multinational study investigators. Rapid measurement of B-type natriuretic peptide in the emergency diagnosis of heart failure. *NEJM.* 2002;347:161–167.
5. Agewall S, Giannitsis E, Jernberg T, et al. Troponin elevation in coronary vs. non-coronary disease. *Eur Heart J.* 2011;32:404–411.
6. Peacock WF IV, De Marco T, Fonarow GC, et al.; ADHERE Investigators. Cardiac troponin and outcome in acute heart failure. *NEJM.* 2008;358:2117–2126.
7. Januzzi JL, van Kimmenade R, Lainchbury J, et al. NT-proBNP testing for diagnosis and short-term prognosis in acute destabilized heart failure: an international pooled analysis of 1256 patients: the International Collaborative of NT-proBNP Study. *Eur Heart J.* 2006;27:330–337.
8. Knudsen CW, Omland T, Clopton P, et al. Diagnostic value of B-type natriuretic peptide and chest radiographic findings in patients with acute dyspnea. *Am J Med.* 2004;116:363–368.
9. Collins S, Lindsell CJ, Storrow AB, et al. Prevalence of negative chest radiography in the emergency department patient with decompensated heart failure. *Ann Emerg Med.* 2006;47:13–18.
10. Lichtenstein DA, Meziere GA. Relevance of lung ultrasound in the diagnosis of acute respiratory failure: the BLUE protocol. *Chest.* 2008;134:117–125.
11. Martindale JL, Noble VE, Liteplo A. Diagnosing pulmonary edema: lung ultrasound versus chest radiography. *Eur J Emerg Med.* 2013;20:356–360.
12. Bersten AD, et al. Treatment of severe cardiogenic pulmonary edema with continuous positive airway pressure delivered by face mask. *NEJM.* 1991;325(36):825–830.
13. Gray A, et al. Noninvasive ventilation in acute cardiogenic pulmonary edema. *NEJM.* 2008;359:142–151.
14. Mehta S, Jay G. Randomized, prospective trial of bilevel versus CPAP in acute pulmonary edema. *Crit Care Med.* 1997;25(4):620–628.
15. Nava S, et al. Noninvasive ventilation in cardiogenic pulmonary edema: a multicenter randomized trial. *Am J Respir Crit Care Med.* 2003;168:1432–1437.
16. Rasanen J, et al. CPAP by facemask in acute cardiogenic pulmonary edema. *Am J Cardiol.* 1985;55:296–300.
17. Bussmann W, Schupp D. Effect of sublingual nitroglycerin in emergency treatment of severe pulmonary edema. *Am J Cardiol.* 1978;41:931–936.
18. Zile MR, Bennett TD, Sutton MSJ, et al. Transition from chronic compensated to acute decompensated heart failure: pathophysiological insights obtained from continuous monitoring of intracardiac pressures. *Circulation.* 2008;118:1433–1441.
19. Chaudhry SI, Wang Y, Concato J, et al. Patterns of weight change preceding hospitalization for heart failure. *Circulation.* 2007;116:1549–1554.
20. Kraus PA, Lipman J, Becker PJ. Acute preload effects of furosemide. *Chest.* 1990;98:124–128.

21. Felker GM, et al. Loop diuretics in acute decompensated heart failure. Necessary? Evil? A Necessary Evil? *Circulation.* 2009;2:56–62.
22. Sacchetti A, Ramoska E, Moakes ME, et al. Effect of ED management on ICU use in acute pulmonary edema. *Am J Emerg Med.* 1999;17(6):571–574.
23. Hamilton RJ, Carter WA, Gallagher JE. Rapid improvement of acute pulmonary edema with sublingual captopril. *Acad Emerg Med.* 1996;3:205–212.
24. Schillinger D. Nifedipine in hypertensive emergencies: a prospective study. *J Emerg Med.* 1987;5:463–473.
25. Lambert CR, Hill JA, Feldman RL, et al. Effects of nicardipine on left ventricular function and energetics in man. *Int J Cardiol.* 1986;10:237–250.
26. Amraoui F, van Montfrans GA, van den Born BJ. Value of retinal examination in hypertensive encephalopathy. *J Hum Hypertens.* 2010;24(4):274–279.
27. Oppenheimer BS, Fishberg AM. Hypertensive encephalopathy. *Arch Intern Med.* 1928;41(2):264–278.
28. Marik PE, Rivera R. Hypertensive emergencies: an update. *Curr Opin Crit Care.* 2011;17:569–580.
29. Olsen KS, Svendsen LB, Larsen FS, et al. Effect of labetalol on cerebral blood flow, oxygen metabolism and autoregulation in healthy humans. *Br J Anaesth.* 1995;75(1):51–54.
30. Pearce CJ, Wallin JD. Labetalol and other agents that block both alpha- and beta-adrenergic receptors. *Cleve Clin J Med.* 1994;61(1):59–69; quiz 80–82.
31. Varon J, Marik PE. Clinical review: the management of hypertensive crises. *Crit Care.* 2003;7(5):374–384.
32. van Beek AH, Claassen JA, Rikkert MG, et al. Cerebral autoregulation: an overview of current concepts and methodology with special focus on the elderly. *J Cereb Blood Flow Metab.* 2008;28(6):1071–1085.
33. Hajjar I, Kotchen TA. Trends in prevalence, awareness, treatment, and control of hypertension in the United States, 1988–2000. *JAMA.* 2003;290:199–206.
34. Anders JL, Adams CD, Antman EM, et al. 2011 ACCF/AHA focused updated incorporated into the ACC/AHA guidelines for the management of patients with unstable angina/non-ST-elevation myocardial infarction. *Circulation.* 2011;123:e426–e579.
35. Kushner FG, Hand M, Smith SC, et al. 2009 focused updates: ACC/AHA guidelines for the management of patients with ST-elevation myocardial infarction and ACC/AHA/SCAI guidelines on percutaneous coronary intervention. *Circulation.* 2009;120:2271–2306.
36. Flaherty JT. Role of nitroglycerin in acute myocardial infarction. *Cardiology.* 1989;76(2):122–131.
37. Nadar SK, Tayebjee MH, Messerli F, et al. Target organ damage in hypertension: pathophysiology and implications for drug therapy. *Curr Pharm Des.* 2006;12:1581–1592.
38. Amin A. Parenteral medication for hypertension with symptoms. *Ann Emerg Med.* 2008;51(3):S9–S15.
39. Marik PE, Varon J. Hypertensive crises—challenges and management. *Chest.* 2007;131:1949–1962.
40. COMMIT collaborative group. Early intravenous then oral metoprolol in 45,852 patients with acute myocardial infarction: randomized placebo-controlled trial. *Lancet.* 2005;366:1622–1632.
41. Hagan PG, et al. The International Registry of Acute Aortic Dissection (IRAD). *JAMA.* 2000;283(7): 897–903.
42. Tsai TT, Nienaber CA, Eagle KA. Acute aortic syndromes. *Circulation.* 2005;112(24):3802–3813.
43. Wittels K. Aortic emergencies. *Emerg Med Clin North Am.* 2011;29:789–800.
44. Pollack CV, Varon J, Garrison NA, et al. Clevidipine, an intravenous dihydropyridine calcium channel blocker, is safe and effective for the treatment of patients with acute severe hypertension. *Ann Emerg Med.* 2009;53:329–338.

17

Controversies in Arrhythmia Management

Sam Senturia

BACKGROUND

Emergency physicians are tasked with managing a wide range of arrhythmias. Rather than reviewing the management of all common arrhythmias, this chapter addresses three controversies of arrhythmia management encountered by emergency and critical care physicians: (1) rate control versus rhythm control in atrial fibrillation (AF), (2) the use of adenosine for the diagnosis and treatment of undifferentiated wide complex tachycardia (WCT), and (3) the use of procainamide versus amiodarone for the treatment of ventricular tachycardia (VT). A review of the evidence relevant to these topics will help physicians make informed evidence-based decisions when these dilemmas arise.

There are no evidence-based guidelines to help the emergency physician decide when to involve critical care services in the management of arrhythmias. It is reasonable to do so when there is concern that an arrhythmia may cause hemodynamic deterioration. Whether an arrhythmia will cause hemodynamic deterioration will depend on both the electrical properties of the arrhythmia and the physiologic reserve of the patient. Many patients, for example, tolerate supraventricular tachyarrhythmias with minimal symptoms, whereas in others with compromised cardiac function, the addition of a supraventricular arrhythmia may lead to life-threatening deterioration. Ventricular arrhythmias always are considered capable of producing hemodynamic deterioration because of the risk of degenerating into pulseless VT or ventricular fibrillation. For example, AF with a wide QRS complex and a ventricular rate exceeding 200 beats per minute may represent atrioventricular (AV) conduction over an accessory pathway, which can precipitate ventricular fibrillation. A commonsense approach to arrhythmia management should involve critical care services in the following situations:

1. Patients with any arrhythmia for which there is concern about the possibility of associated hemodynamic deterioration
2. Patients with ventricular arrhythmias
3. Patients with AF, a wide QRS complex, and a ventricular rate exceeding 200 beats per minute
4. Patients with high-grade AV block, complete heart block, or bradyarrhythmias that require transvenous pacing
5. Patients successfully resuscitated from cardiac arrest

RATE CONTROL VERSUS RHYTHM CONTROL FOR RECENT-ONSET ATRIAL FIBRILLATION

Controversy exists regarding whether rate control or rhythm control is the best management strategy for recent-onset atrial fibrillation (ROAF), a condition commonly defined as AF of <48 hours' duration. Rate control is defined as ventricular rate control without an attempt to convert the patient to sinus rhythm. Rhythm control requires either pharmacologic or electrical cardioversion to sinus rhythm. In a recent survey of members of national emergency medicine associations, 94% (234/249) of American emergency physician respondents indicated that they use rate control, and 26% (65/249) indicated that they use rhythm control.[1] In Canada, 71% of respondents indicated that they use rate control, and 66% indicated that they use rhythm control. In the United Kingdom and Australasia, 50% of respondents indicated that they use rhythm control. The American College of Cardiology (ACC)/American Heart Association (AHA)/European Society of Cardiology (ESC) Guidelines for the Management of Patients with AF do not provide recommendations for management in the emergency department (ED).[2,3]

Large Multicenter Randomized Trials

Several multicenter randomized controlled trials (AFFIRM,[4] RACE,[5] PIAF,[6] STAF,[7] HOT CAFÉ[8]) have compared rate and rhythm control in the general population of patients with AF and have demonstrated equivalent outcomes, including rates of death and thromboembolism. The largest of these was the AFFIRM trial,[4] which compared outcomes in 4,060 patients aged 65 or older with AF and risk factors for stroke who were randomized to rate control (RaC) or rhythm control (RhC). After a mean follow-up of 3.5 years, the rhythm control group had an almost significant trend toward increase in the primary endpoint of death (25.9% RaC vs. 26.7% RhC). There was no significant difference between the groups in a composite secondary endpoint composed of death, disabling stroke, disabling anoxic encephalopathy, major bleeding, and cardiac arrest (32.7% RaC vs. 32.0% RhC). There also was no difference in overall frequency of central nervous system events (7.4% RaC vs. 8.9% RhC) or ischemic strokes (5.5% RaC vs. 7.1% RhC). In both groups, the majority of strokes occurred in patients who had discontinued warfarin or had a subtherapeutic international normalized ratio (INR). The rhythm control group had higher hospitalization rates during follow-up (73.0% RaC vs. 80.1% RhC). A subsequent analysis suggested that adverse effects of antiarrhythmic drugs could explain the trend toward increased mortality in the rhythm control group.[9] In this analysis, the use of antiarrhythmic drugs was associated with increased mortality (hazard ratio 1.49), and the presence of sinus rhythm was associated with reduced mortality (hazard ratio 0.53).

The AFFIRM trial and the other large trials comparing rate control and rhythm control included very few patients with ROAF. As a result, these studies may have limited applicability to the management of ROAF in the ED. In the AFFIRM trial, the qualifying episode of AF had a duration >48 hours in more than 69% of patients and was the first episode of AF in only 36% of patients.[10] The RACE trial included only patients who had persistent AF after a previous cardioversion.[5] The median duration of the qualifying episode of AF was >30 days, and the median duration of AF was >300 days. An *Annals of Emergency Medicine* systematic review abstract reported on a

Cochrane review of the RACE, STAF, and HOT CAFÉ trials and found that the mean age in these studies was more than 60 years and the mean duration of AF was more than 200 days. The report concluded that the Cochrane review provided little evidence on which to base decisions in the ED.[11]

ED Studies Comparing Rate Control with Rhythm Control

Although the large RCTs have provided only limited information relevant to ED management, several studies of ED patients with ROAF support the efficacy and safety of rhythm control. A 2004 multicenter retrospective cohort study reported on 388 stable patients with ROAF who were electrically cardioverted in the ED.[12] Eighty-six percent (332/388) were successfully converted to sinus rhythm; of these, 91% (301/332) were discharged from the ED. All patients received IV procedural sedation before cardioversion. Chemical cardioversion was attempted before electrical cardioversion in 29%. Twenty-five cardioversion attempts (6%) were associated with 28 complications: 22 complications from procedural sedation (oxygen desaturation below 90% in 12 patients, use of bag-valve-mask device in 6 patients, and emesis, hypotension, bradycardia, and agitation each in 1 patient) and 6 complications from the cardioversion itself (three minor burns, two episodes of VT, and one episode of bradycardia). Ten percent (39/388) of patients returned to the ED within 7 days, including 6% (25/388) for relapse of AF.

A 2008 prospective controlled study from the Mayo Clinic reported on 153 patients with ROAF who were randomly assigned to either protocolized treatment in an ED observation unit or hospital admission with usual care.[13] The ED observation unit protocol consisted of administration of a calcium channel blocker or beta blocker for rate control followed by procedural sedation and electrical cardioversion if AF persisted at 6 hours, followed by observation for an additional 2 hours. Among the ED observation unit cohort, 32% (24/75) reverted to sinus rhythm after rate control, and 51% (38/75) required electrical cardioversion, creating an 85% (64/75) conversion rate. Nine patients (12%) of the ED cohort were admitted. The median length of stay was 10 hours for the ED observation unit group versus 25 hours for the inpatient group. During 6 months of follow-up, there were no differences between the two groups in rates of recurrent AF (10%) or MI, congestive heart failure, stroke, or death (zero patients with each diagnosis except for one MI in the inpatient group).

A recent review considered five ED studies that specifically examined the outcome of patients discharged after cardioversion in the ED.[14] No patient in any of the studies suffered a thromboembolic event. Among all five studies, there were only three cardioversion-related complications that resulted in a disposition change, and each of these was an arrhythmia that resolved in the ED.

In Ontario, Canada, emergency physicians have long followed a protocolized management of ROAF called the Ottawa Aggressive Protocol.[15] The protocol consists of chemical cardioversion followed, in case of failure, by electrical cardioversion and discharge from the ED (see Table 17.1). A 2010 retrospective cohort study at a university hospital in Ontario evaluated the effectiveness and safety of this protocol. Of 660 ED visits in which the protocol was applied, 40% (261/660) received rate control drugs, 100% (660/660) received IV procainamide, and 37% (243/660) subsequently underwent electrical cardioversion. The rate of conversion to sinus rhythm was 58% (385/660)

TABLE 17.1 The Ottawa Aggressive Protocol

1. Assessment: The patient must be stable, without ischemia, hypotension, or acute congestive heart failure (CHF). Onset must be clear and <48 h, unless the patient is on warfarin and has had a therapeutic INR for at least 3 wk
2. Rate control: If highly symptomatic or not planning to convert. Often omitted because of lack of compelling evidence that it facilitates cardioversion. Typical agents used: diltiazem or metoprolol
3. Pharmacologic cardioversion: Procainamide (1 g IV over 60 min; hold if BP < 100 mm Hg; if 250 mL normal saline bolus corrects hypotension, the infusion is resumed). Not attempted if patient deemed unstable (cardiac ischemia, severe CHF, or hypotension) or if failure of this approach on a previous visit
4. Electrical cardioversion: If chemical cardioversion fails. Consider keeping patient NPO × 6 h. Procedural sedation given by EP (propofol and fentanyl). Start at 150–200 J biphasic synchronized. Use anterior–posterior pads
5. Anticoagulation: Usually no heparin or warfarin if onset clearly <48 h or INR therapeutic for >3 wk
6. Disposition: Home within 1 h after cardioversion. Usually no antiarrhythmic prophylaxis or anticoagulation given. Arrange outpatient echocardiography if first episode. Cardiology follow-up if first episode or frequent episodes
7. Patients not treated with cardioversion: Achieve rate control with diltiazem IV (target heart rate < 100 beats per minute). Discharge home on diltiazem (or metoprolol) and warfarin. Arrange INR monitoring and outpatient echocardiography. Follow-up with cardiology at 4 wk for elective cardioversion
8. Recommended additions to the protocol: If onset unclear, consider transesophageal echocardiography (TEE). If TEE-guided cardioversion >48 h, start warfarin. If $CHADS_2$ score ≥ 1,[53] consider warfarin, and arrange early follow-up

CHF, congestive heart failure; INR, international normalized ratio; IV, intravenously; NPO, nothing by mouth.
Modified from Stiell IG, Clement CM, Perry JJ, et al. Association of the Ottawa Aggressive Protocol with rapid discharge of emergency department patients with recent-onset atrial fibrillation or flutter. *CJEM.* 2010;12:181–191. Box 1, with permission.

for procainamide and 92% (223/243) for electrical cardioversion. 97% (639/660) were discharged from the ED, and 90% (595/660) were discharged in normal sinus rhythm. The median lengths of stay from ED arrival to discharge were 4.9 hours (all patients), 3.9 hours (cardioversion with procainamide), and 6.5 hours (electrical cardioversion). Adverse ED events occurred in 7.6% (50/660): 6.6% (44/660) experienced transient hypotension, and 1% (7/66) experienced either bradycardia, AV block, or atrial or ventricular tachyarrhythmia. 3.2% (21/660) required admission. During the 7 day follow-up period, 8.6% (57/660) had relapse of AF. There was no stroke or death.

Arguments for Rate Control

Arguments for rate control include the following. The large, randomized controlled trials (AFFIRM, RACE, etc.) have shown that—over the long term—outcomes with rate control are as good as (or better than) outcomes with rhythm control.[4–8] In the AFFIRM trial, rhythm control was associated with a higher mortality than rate control among older patients.[4] Achieving rate control in the ED may be faster and less operationally complicated than cardioversion.[16] Rate control does not expose the patient to the risk of procedural sedation associated with electrical cardioversion. Finally, many patients will spontaneously convert to sinus rhythm. In one study, 32% (24/75) of patients spontaneously converted in the ED within 6 hours of arrival.[13] In another study, 29% (59/206) of patients spontaneously converted in the ED, and an additional 11/16 patients discharged in AF returned the next day having converted to sinus rhythm.[17]

Arguments for Rhythm Control

Arguments for rhythm control include the following. The mean age in the AFFIRM trial was 70 years.[4] Younger, more physically active patients would be expected to show benefit from conversion to sinus rhythm. It seems reasonable to offer rhythm control to those patients having a first episode of AF and no known cardiac structural abnormality. There is mounting evidence that AF itself leads to electrical and structural remodeling of the atria that, in turn, make the arrhythmia intractable.[18] Current theory suggests that rhythm control should be established as soon as possible to improve the chances of remaining in sinus rhythm.[19] Rhythm control strategies allow for high rates of discharge from the ED, usually without warfarin or rate control medication.[20] In contrast, patients treated with rate control usually require rate control medications and often warfarin; this frequently requires hospital admission and chronic INR monitoring and carries a risk of serious bleeding.

ADENOSINE IN THE MANAGEMENT OF WIDE-COMPLEX TACHYCARDIA

The 2010 AHA Guidelines for Advanced Cardiovascular Life Support (ACLS) recommend adenosine for the diagnosis and treatment of stable undifferentiated regular WCT.[21] The principal effect of adenosine is transient AV nodal blockade. Thus, if a WCT is caused by a supraventricular tachycardia (SVT), administration of adenosine will do one of two things: (1) Terminate the arrhythmia if the AV node is part of a reentry loop, or (2) block AV nodal conduction and reveal the previously hidden atrial activity. If the WCT is VT, administration of adenosine is expected to have no effect on the rhythm (in most cases) and no adverse hemodynamic effect. The AHA executive summary emphasizes that this dual diagnostic/treatment capability is an important change for the 2010 guidelines.[22]

Early Studies of Adenosine for WCT

Several small studies in the late 1980s and 1990s attempted to clarify the efficacy and safety of adenosine administration for WCT. In a 1994 prospective study of ED patients, adenosine was administered (maximum dose 18 mg) to 12 patients during 29 episodes of WCT.[23] Adenosine terminated 59% (17/29) of episodes, all of which were identified as atrioventricular reentry tachycardia (AVRT). Transient AV block occurred in 10% (3/29) of episodes, revealing atrial flutter or AF. No response occurred in 31% (9/29) of episodes, which were identified as AVRT (5) and VT (4). In a second, prospective, study in 2001—also of emergency patients—adenosine was administered (maximum dose 18 mg) to 26 patients with WCT.[24] Adenosine terminated 27% (7/26) of episodes. Transient AV block occurred in 42% (11/26) allowing diagnosis of the underlying arrhythmia. No response occurred in 31% (8/26), all of which were VT. No patient suffered serious hemodynamic deterioration in either study.

Two electrophysiology studies, performed in a more controlled lab setting, supported the findings of the ED-based studies. In a 1988 study, adenosine was administered to 26 consecutive patients with WCT.[25] Of these, 35% (9/26) were SVT, and 65% (17/26) were VT. Adenosine terminated 67% (6/9) of SVTs and 6% (1/17) of VTs. As a diagnostic test for supraventricular origin of a regular WCT, the investigators calculated that adenosine administration had 89% (8/9) sensitivity and 94% (16/17) specificity. In a 1990 electrophysiology study, adenosine was administered to 34 consecutive patients with WCT.[26] Adenosine terminated 7/10 arrhythmias using reentry mechanisms involving the AV node, 1/10 atrial arrhythmias, and 1/14 VTs. As with the ED studies, no patients in the electrophysiology studies experienced adverse hemodynamic effects after adenosine administration.

Studies Demonstrating Adenosine Terminates VT

The studies noted above demonstrate that adenosine can terminate VT. Additional studies have clarified that the episodes of VT terminated by adenosine are predominately exercise-induced VT caused by triggered automaticity in patients with structurally normal hearts and not reentry-related VT in patients with structural (including ischemic) heart disease.[27–30] The only known mechanism of adenosine activity on ventricular conduction is antagonism of catecholamine-induced stimulation of intracellular cAMP production. Based on these findings, the authors of one study postulated that the mechanism underlying this form of exercised-induced VT is mediated by cyclic adenosine monophosphate (cAMP).[27] Since then, this form of VT has been documented in multiple studies, where it manifests with left bundle branch block (LBBB) pattern in most cases.[27–30] In a subsequent retrospective study of patients with WCT who received adenosine, 10/18 patients had VT, and 50% of these (5/10) were terminated with adenosine.[30] Four of the five patients whose VT was terminated by adenosine had structurally normal hearts, exercise-induced VT, and LBBB VT pattern consistent with the group of patients described in the initial study.

Concerns About Safety of Adenosine

Concerns have been raised about the safety of adenosine administration because of case reports of persistent bradycardia or asystole, induction of AF, ventricular fibrillation, torsades de pointes, and accelerated ventricular response in patients with AF or atrial flutter with and without preexcitation.[31,32] In the 2001 study discussed above, 160 consecutive ED patients were treated with adenosine for narrow complex tachycardia and WCT in order to determine the prevalence of arrhythmogenic effects.[24] Of these, 84% (134/160) had narrow complex tachycardia, and 16% (26/160) had WCT. In the narrow complex group, the adenosine-related arrhythmias observed included the following: prolonged AV block (>4 seconds) in 6% (8/134), AF in 1.5% (2/134), and nonsustained VT in 6% (8/134). In the wide complex group, the only adenosine-related arrhythmia observed was prolonged AV block (>4 seconds) in 11% (3/26). All arrhythmias were transient and resolved spontaneously; none required treatment. In a 2001 retrospective study of 187 episodes of tachycardia treated with adenosine in 127 ED patients, VT occurred following successful termination of an arrhythmia of supraventricular origin in 19% (31/160) of episodes.[33] All adenosine-related episodes of VT were brief (mean duration 6.0 beats, range 3 to 26 beats) and spontaneously resolved. AF was induced in 5% (8/160) of episodes. There is only one case report of degeneration of VT to ventricular fibrillation (VF) after administration of adenosine for WCT.[34]

Perhaps the greatest safety concern is that adenosine will accelerate conduction over an accessory pathway in patients with AF or atrial flutter, leading to hemodynamic deterioration or ventricular fibrillation. Neither of the two electrophysiology studies of adenosine use in WCT discussed above reported any adverse hemodynamic effects on patients with AF and preexcitation.[25,26] In the first of these two studies, there was also no effect on the mean RR interval.[25] In the second of these studies, antegrade accessory pathway conduction was transiently enhanced in all nine patients, and the average RR interval and the shortest RR interval shortened but again without hemodynamic consequence.[26] Similarly, in a study of 30 patients with Wolff-Parkinson-White syndrome (WPW), adenosine administration was shown to lead to shortened antegrade refractoriness of the accessory pathway, but again, the effects were brief and no patient suffered clinical deterioration.[35]

There have been, however, isolated case reports of VF after administration of adenosine to patients with AF and preexcitation.[36–38] In one study, four patients who presented to the ED with preexcited AF degenerated to VF after administration of adenosine.[38] These four patients were compared to five control patients with preexcitation who underwent induction of AF and administration of adenosine in the electrophysiology lab and did not develop VF. The four patients who developed VF in response to adenosine demonstrated a shorter RR interval during AF and a shorter antegrade effective refractory period of the accessory tract than the five who did not develop VF.

A recently published investigation has attempted to clarify the efficacy and safety of adenosine administered for WCT in ED patients.[39] This was a retrospective observational study at nine hospitals in five cities of 197 patients with WCT who received adenosine. Adenosine terminated 15% (29/197) of the WCTs. Overall, 59% (116/197) of the WCTs were diagnosed as SVT, and 41% (81/197) were diagnosed as VT. There was a positive response to adenosine, defined as termination of the WCT or temporary AV block or any other change in rhythm except for retrograde ventriculoatrial block, in 90% (104/116) of patients with SVT and in 2% (2/81) of patients with VT. The investigators calculated that a positive response to adenosine increased the odds of SVT by a factor of 36. A negative response to adenosine, defined as no apparent change in rhythm or transient retrograde ventriculoatrial block, increased the odds of VT by a factor of 9. The rate of primary adverse events, defined as need for emergent electrical or medical intervention in response to adenosine administration, was 0% (0/116) of patients with SVT and 0% (0/81) of patients with VT. In 48% (56/116) of patients diagnosed as SVT, the diagnosis was determined by a positive response to adenosine. As a result, there may have been cases of VT terminated by adenosine that were misdiagnosed as SVT. Therefore, a positive response to adenosine may increase the odds of SVT by less than the factor of 36 calculated by the investigators. Since the calculation that adenosine distinguishes SVT from VT was itself determined by the response to adenosine, this limits the validity of the odds calculation.

Administration of adenosine to patients with stable undifferentiated regular WCT appears to be relatively safe. Except for isolated case reports, no patients in the above studies developed significant arrhythmic or hemodynamic deterioration or required electrical or pharmacologic resuscitation after administration of adenosine. Adenosine is not recommended for irregular WCT, but it is worth noting that none of the 15 patients with WPW and AF in the two electrophysiology studies discussed developed VF or hemodynamic deterioration after administration of adenosine. Some caution needs to be exercised as these observations were based on a very small number of subjects. Because of the possibility of arrhythmic deterioration, defibrillator pads should be attached to patients receiving adenosine for undifferentiated WCT. According to the AHA 2010 guidelines, when faced with a stable WCT, if the mechanism cannot be determined and the rate is regular and the QRS is monomorphic, adenosine is recommended for both diagnosis and treatment.[21]

The diagnostic use of adenosine to distinguish SVT from VT does have one notable drawback. As a diagnostic test for supraventricular origin of a regular WCT, studies have calculated that adenosine administration has 89% to 90% sensitivity and 93% to 94% specificity.[25,40] The less-than-perfect specificity reflects the false-positive VTs that terminated with adenosine. If termination of a WCT by adenosine is accepted as proof of supraventricular origin, some patients with VT will be mislabeled as SVT, with the consequence of not receiving the appropriate workup and treatment for VT (e.g., electrophysiology studies, ablation, implantable cardioverter defibrillator placement). The best approach for the emergency physician probably is to avoid labeling WCTs that terminate with adenosine as SVT and to have these patients receive consultation by a cardiologist. Although SVT is the most likely explanation, a definitive electrophysiologic explanation is warranted.

PROCAINAMIDE VERSUS AMIODARONE FOR TERMINATION OF VENTRICULAR TACHYCARDIA

In the 2010 AHA Guidelines for ACLS, procainamide is the preferred drug for the treatment of stable monomorphic VT.[21] Procainamide is rated class IIa (administration is reasonable), whereas amiodarone is now rated class IIb (administration may be considered). Arguments against procainamide have included a long administration time, QT prolongation and hypotension, and a contraindication for use in patients with depressed left ventricular function. Thus, situational variables often dictate pharmacologic choice. Additional agents that have been used in VT include lidocaine and sotalol. The latter agents will be reviewed briefly, followed by a more extensive consideration of evidence surrounding procainamide and amiodarone.

Lidocaine and Sotalol

Lidocaine is mentioned in the 2010 ACLS guidelines as a second-line agent for treatment of VT.[21] In multiple studies, lidocaine had poor efficacy in terminating VT, with success ranging between 19% and 29%.[41–44] This termination rate is inferior to that seen with sotalol,[42] procainamide,[44] and amiodarone.[45] Sotalol was shown in a single randomized double-blind crossover study of 33 conscious patients with sustained VT to terminate VT in 69% of patients.[42] Hypotension required electrical cardioversion in 10% of patients. Since this 1994 study, there appears to be no high-quality evidence addressing the efficacy and safety of IV sotalol for termination of acute hemodynamically stable VT. Until recently, sotalol had little use in the emergency management of VT in the United States because it was not available in intravenous form. The FDA approved an intravenous form of sotalol in July 2009. Sotalol received a class IIb recommendation in the 2010 ACLS guidelines.

Early Studies of Procainamide

Studies of procainamide in the 1990s reported rates of termination of VT as high as 80% to 90%. A 2002 randomized crossover study compared procainamide (10 mg/kg at 100 mg/min) and lidocaine (1.5 mg/kg over 2 minutes) in 29 consecutive patients with hemodynamically stable monomorphic VT.[44] The investigators excluded patients with severe heart failure or hypotension during VT (mean LV ejection fraction (LVEF) = 30%; mean systolic BP during VT = 115 mm Hg). When VT did not terminate within 15 minutes of the first drug, the crossover drug was administered. Initial treatment was successful in 80% (12/15) of patients receiving procainamide and in 21% (3/14) of patients receiving lidocaine. After 25 episodes of recurrent VT and 24 episodes that crossed over to the second agent, a total of 79 drug infusions for VT were given; procainamide terminated 79% (38/48), and lidocaine terminated 19% (6/31).

Administration of procainamide was associated with prolongation of the QRS width and QT interval, whereas administration of lidocaine was not. Adverse events requiring termination of the protocol occurred in 13% (2/15) of patients receiving procainamide (hypotension in one patient and acceleration of VT in one patient) and were quickly reversible. The procainamide infusion rate of 100 mg/min in this study is at least double the current 2010 AHA ACLS recommended 20 to 50 mg/min. In this study, a 70-kg patient received the total infusion in 7 minutes, and termination of VT occurred within 15 minutes of finishing the infusion. While this study is limited by the small sample size, the crossover design allowed the testing of the second drug during the same episode when the first was not effective. Procainamide still terminated 70% to 80% of episodes after lidocaine was ineffective. When administered sequentially, a carryover effect of one drug to the other cannot be excluded because only 15 minutes elapsed between the first and second drugs. The authors considered the likelihood of significant crossover effect to be small because lidocaine remained less effective after procainamide. If there had been an interaction between the two drugs, a greater effect would be expected for lidocaine after procainamide than the reverse because of the longer half-life of procainamide.

In a 1992 electrophysiology study, VT was induced by programmed electrical stimulation in 15 patients with prior myocardial infarction (12 with recurrent hemodynamically tolerated VT, 1 with syncope, 2 with history of cardiac arrest and inducible VT).[46] Infusion of procainamide at 50 mg/min terminated VT in 93% (14/15) of patients. The total dose of procainamide required to terminate the tachycardia ranged from 100 to 1,080 mg (median 600 mg). The systolic BP during VT was >100 mm Hg in all patients and remained >80 mm Hg in all patients during and after infusion of procainamide. No patients had symptoms related to hypotension.

Early Studies of Amiodarone

The benefit of IV amiodarone in terminating acute hemodynamically stable VT has been extrapolated from studies of prolonged infusions to suppress recurrent unstable ventricular tachyarrhythmias. In a 1996 randomized controlled double-blind dose-range study of amiodarone by continuous infusion in 273 patients with recurrent hypotensive ventricular tachyarrhythmias refractory to lidocaine, procainamide, and bretylium, subjects received 525, 1,050, or 2,100 mg of amiodarone by continuous infusion over 24 hours.[47] During VT, all patients had systolic BP < 80 mm Hg with clinical signs or symptoms of shock. All patients had had at least two episodes (mean 5.9) of hypotensive tachyarrhythmias in the 24 hours before admission to the study or were in incessant VT despite attempts at cardioversion. While on continuous amiodarone infusion, 40% (110/273) of patients survived 24 hours without another episode of hypotensive ventricular arrhythmia. There was no clear dose–response relationship with respect to success rate. In a second study that administered prolonged amiodarone infusions to 46 patients with recurrent life-threatening VT or VF that had failed to respond to at least two other antiarrhythmic agents, amiodarone was administered as 5 mg/kg over 30 minutes followed by continuous infusion of 1 g/24 hours for 72 hours, followed by oral amiodarone.[48] This protocol led to resolution of recurrent VT or VF in 33% (15/46) of patients within 2 hours and 58.5% (27/46) of patients within 84 hours.

Until recently, few studies examined the use of IV amiodarone to terminate discrete episodes of hemodynamically stable VT. One study in 1989 examined the efficacy of

IV amiodarone to terminate sustained VT in 19 patients with depressed LV function (mean EF = 30.1%) who had suffered recurrent sustained VT and VF.[49] All patients were hemodynamically stable during VT. Amiodarone was administered as 5 mg/kg over 20 minutes followed by continuous infusion of 1,050 mg over 24 hours. Amiodarone terminated sustained VT in 42% (8/19) of patients within a mean effect time of 31 (±20) minutes.

Recent Studies of Amiodarone and Procainamide

In the past several years, two important studies have provided evidence that neither amiodarone nor procainamide is effective for termination of VT. A retrospective review in 2008 evaluated 41 consecutive patients with hemodynamically tolerated sustained monomorphic VT who were administered bolus dose amiodarone 300 mg IV.[50] Amiodarone was administered over <30 minutes in 36 patients and over 30 to 60 minutes in 5 patients. The mean LVEF was 31%, and the mean systolic BP was 112 mm Hg. The median VT duration was 70 min (range 15 to 6,000). VT termination occurred within 20 minutes of the start of the amiodarone infusion in 15% (6/41) and within 1 hour in 29% (12/41). Hemodynamic deterioration requiring emergency cardioversion occurred in 17% (7/41).

A 2010 multicenter historical cohort study evaluated consecutive patients with stable VT treated with IV amiodarone or procainamide.[51] Response to the medication was defined as termination of VT within 20 minutes of initiation of the infusion. Rates of termination of VT were 25% (13/53) and 30% (9/30) for amiodarone and procainamide, respectively. The adjusted odds of termination with procainamide compared with amiodarone was 1.2. Eventually, electrical therapy was required to terminate VT in 53% (35/66) of patients receiving amiodarone and 42% (13/31) of patients receiving procainamide. Hypotension requiring cessation of infusion or immediate electrical cardioversion occurred in 6% (4/66) of amiodarone patients and in 19% (6/31) of procainamide patients. The investigators note that the retrospective design of the study, limited data set, and potential for confounders limit the ability to draw firm conclusions about the relative effectiveness of amiodarone and procainamide. The 21-mg/min mean rate of infusion of procainamide is also lower than the 50- to 100-mg/min rate used in other studies and may have limited both the efficacy and the adverse effects of procainamide.

Based on these more recent studies, it appears that neither procainamide nor amiodarone is highly effective or safe in terminating hemodynamically stable VT. The authors of the 2010 study note several limitations that highlight the difficulty of performing their retrospective study, including limited use of procainamide by the physicians at the study hospitals, potential bias in the choice of medicine, and the 20-minute treatment interval allowed for successful termination of VT, which might bias against procainamide since it is often infused over 1 hour. The current 2010 AHA Guidelines for ACLS cite the 2008 study, but not the 2010 study, which was likely unavailable at time of publication.[21] Given the unclear effectiveness and risk of significant hypotension associated with procainamide administration, procedural sedation and electrical cardioversion remain the currently recommended approach to hemodynamically stable VT. An early study published in 1973 demonstrated a 98% success rate of electrical cardioversion of 116 episodes of VT in 39 patients, and the incidence of significant complications of electrical cardioversion was low.[52]

CONCLUSION

Among American emergency physicians, the most common strategy for managing ROAF is rate control. Several studies have, however, demonstrated the efficacy and safety of rhythm control, which offers the advantage of high rates of discharge from the ED, usually without warfarin or rate control medication. No patient in any of the rhythm control studies reviewed suffered a thromboembolic event. The use of adenosine for the diagnosis and treatment of stable undifferentiated regular WCT appears to be safe. Termination of a WCT by adenosine should not be accepted as proof of supraventricular origin because adenosine also can terminate VT. The optimal approach is to consult an electrophysiologist for all episodes of undifferentiated WCT terminated by adenosine. Recent studies have provided evidence that neither amiodarone nor procainamide is highly effective or safe in terminating hemodynamically stable VT. Procedural sedation and electrical cardioversion appears to be the safest and most effective approach.

LITERATURE TABLE

TRIAL	DESIGN	RESULT
AF: Rate control vs. rhythm control		
Wyse et al. *N Engl J Med. 2002*[4] AFFIRM	Multicenter RCT of rhythm control vs. rate control in 4,060 patients >65 years old with risk factors for stroke	No significant difference in death or stroke (mean follow-up 3.5 y) Mortality at five years, 23.8% and 21.3%, for rhythm control vs. rate control respectively, (HR, 1.15, 95% CI, 0.99 to 1.34, $p = 0.08$)
Van Gelder et al. *N Engl J Med. 2002*[5] RACE	Multicenter RCT of rhythm control vs. rate control in 522 patients, with recurrent persistent AF after at least one cardioversion	No significant difference in death. Near significant trend toward lower incidence of composite endpoint (death, CHF, thromboembolism, bleeding, implantation of pacemaker, adverse effects of drugs) with rate control (17.2%) vs. rhythm control (22.6%)
Burton et al. *Ann Emerg Med.* 2004[12]	Multicenter retrospective cohort, 388 patients with atrial fibrillation who received electrical cardioversion	Cardioversion successful in 86%. Complications in 6% (mostly from procedural sedation). 6% returned to ED within 7 days for recurrent AF
Decker et al. *Ann Emerg Med.* 2008[13]	Prospective controlled study of 153 patients randomized to ED observation unit protocol (calcium channel blocker or beta blocker followed by electrical cardioversion if still in AF at 6 hours) vs. routine inpatient care	ED observation unit vs. inpatient: conversion to sinus rhythm, 85% vs. 73% (not statistically significant); median length of stay, 10 h vs. 25 h (difference 15.1 hours; 95% CI 11.2 to 19.6; $P < 0.001$). No difference in rate of recurrent AF (10%) or adverse events in 6-mo follow-up
Stiell et al. *CJEM.* 2010[15]	Retrospective review of 660 consecutive patient visits treated with Ottawa Aggressive Protocol	All patients initially received procainamide, with 58% (385/660) conversion to sinus. 243 pts received subsequent electrical cardioversion, with 92% conversion rate. Median length of stay <5 h. Adverse ED events in 7.6% (mostly transient hypotension). 97% discharged. 8.6% relapse of AF in 7-d follow-up
Adenosine for regular wide complex tachycardia (WCT)		
Domanovits et al. *Eur Heart J.* 1994[23]	Prospective study, 29 episodes of WCT in 12 ED patients. Diagnosis based on ECG and/or EP study	Effect of adenosine on WCT: terminated WCT in 59% (17/29). Transient AVB in 10% (3/29). No response in 31% (9/29)

(*Continued*)

LITERATURE TABLE (*Continued*)

TRIAL	DESIGN	RESULT
Camaiti et al. *Eur J Emerg Med.* 2001[24]	Prospective study, 26 ED patients with WCT. Diagnosis based on 12-lead ECG and esophageal ECG	Effect of adenosine on WCT: terminated WCT in 27% (7/26). Transient AVB in 42% (11/26). No response in 31% (8/26)
Griffith et al. *Lancet.* 1988[25]	EP study of 26 patients with WCT	Adenosine terminated 67% (6/9) of SVTs and 6% (1/17) of VTs. VT terminated by adenosine in one pt. In six patients with AF and preexcitation: no adverse effect of adenosine. Adenosine as diagnostic test for supraventricular origin of WCT: 89% sensitivity, 94% specificity
Hina et al. *Jpn Heart J.* 1996[30]	Retrospective EP study of 18 patients with WCT	Adenosine terminated 50% (5/10) of VTs
Marill et al. *Crit Care Med.* 2009[39]	Retrospective observational study of 197 patients with WCT	Effect of adenosine on WCT: positive response (termination of WCT or transient AVB) in 90% (104/116) of SVTs and in 2% (2/81) of VTs. Positive response increased odds of SVT by factor of 36. Negative response increased odds of VT by factor of 9
Procainamide vs. amiodarone for VT		
Gorgels et al. *Am J Cardiol.* 1996[44]	Randomized crossover study of procainamide vs. lidocaine in 29 patients with stable VT resulting in 79 drug infusions. Procainamide infusion rate 100 mg/min	Procainamide terminated 79% (38/48); lidocaine terminated 19% (6/31) ($p < 0.001$). Procainamide adverse events in 13% (2/15: hypotension in 1 patient, acceleration of VT in 1 patient)
Schutzenberger et al. *Br Heart J.* 1989[49]	19 patients with stable VT, given amiodarone 5 mg/kg over 20 min followed by 1,050-mg infusion over 24 h	Amiodarone terminated VT in 42% (8/19) within a mean of 31 min
Tomlinson et al. *Emerg Med J.* 2008[50]	Retrospective case series of 41 patients with stable VT given amiodarone 300 mg IV	Amiodarone terminated 15% (6/41) within 20 min and 29% (12/41) within 1 h. Hypotension requiring cardioversion in 17% (7/41)
Marill et al. *Acad Emerg Med.* 2010[51]	Multicenter historical cohort study comparing amiodarone and procainamide in 90 patients with stable VT. Amiodarone mean dose 166 mg. Procainamide mean infusion rate 21 mg/min	Amiodarone terminated 25% (13/53) within 20 min. Procainamide terminated 30% (9/30) within 20 min. Hypotension required cessation of infusion or immediate cardioversion in 6% (4/66) of amiodarone patients and in 19% (6/31) of procainamide pts

RCT, randomized controlled trial; pts, patients; AF, atrial fibrillation; CHF, congestive heart failure; ED, emergency department; WCT, wide-complex tachycardia; EP, electrophysiology; AVB, atrioventricular block; sens, sensitivity; spec, specificity; VT, ventricular tachycardia; SVT, supraventricular tachycardia; CI, confidence interval; HR, hazard ratio.

REFERENCES

1. Rogenstein C, Kelly AM, Mason S, et al. An international view of how recent-onset atrial fibrillation is treated in the emergency department. *Acad Emerg Med.* 2012;19:1255–1260.
2. Fuster V, Ryden LE, Cannom DS, et al. ACC/AHA/ESC 2006 Guidelines for the management of patients with atrial fibrillation: a report of the American College of Cardiology/American Heart Association Task Force on Practice Guidelines and the European Society of Cardiology Committee for practice guidelines (writing committee to revise the 2001 guidelines for the management of patients with atrial fibrillation): developed in collaboration with the European Heart Rhythm Association and the Heart Rhythm Society. *Circulation.* 2006;114:e257–e354.

3. Wann LS, Curtis AB, January CT, et al. 2011 ACCF/AHA/HRS focused update on the management of patients with atrial fibrillation (updating the 2006 guideline): a report of the American College of Cardiology Foundation/American Heart Association Task Force on Practice Guidelines. *J Am Coll Cardiol.* 2011;57:223–242.
4. Wyse DG, Waldo AL, DiMarco JP, et al. A comparison of rate control and rhythm control in patients with atrial fibrillation. *N Engl J Med.* 2002;347(23):1825–1833.
5. Van Gelder IC, Hagens VE, Bosker HA, et al. A comparison of rate control and rhythm control in patients with recurrent persistent atrial fibrillation. *N Engl J Med.* 2002;347(23):1834–1840.
6. Hohnloser SH, Kuck KH, Lilienthal J. Rhythm or rate control in atrial fibrillation—Pharmacological Intervention in Atrial Fibrillation (PIAF): a randomised trial. *Lancet.* 2000;356(9244):1789–1794.
7. Carlsson J, Miketic S, Windeler J, et al. Randomized trial of rate-control versus rhythm-control in persistent atrial fibrillation: the Strategies of Treatment of Atrial Fibrillation (STAF) study. *J Am Coll Cardiol.* 2003;41(10):1690–1696.
8. Opolski G, Torbicki A, Kosior DA, et al. Rate control vs rhythm control in patients with nonvalvular persistent atrial fibrillation: the results of the Polish How to Treat Chronic Atrial Fibrillation (HOT CAFE) Study. *Chest.* 2004;126(2):476–486.
9. Corley SD, Epstein AE, DiMarco JP, et al. Relationships between sinus rhythm, treatment, and survival in the Atrial Fibrillation Follow-Up Investigation of Rhythm Management (AFFIRM) Study. *Circulation.* 2004;109:1509–1513.
10. AFFIRM Investigators. Baseline characteristics of patients with atrial fibrillation: the AFFIRM Study. *Am Heart J.* 2002;143(6):991–1001.
11. Stead LG, Vaidyanathan L. Rhythm control with electrical cardioversion for atrial fibrillation and flutter. *Ann Emerg Med.* 2009;54:745–747.
12. Burton JH, Vinson DR, Drummond K, et al. Electrical cardioversion of emergence department patients with atrial fibrillation. *Ann Emerg Med.* 2004;44:20–30.
13. Decker WW, Smars PA, Vaidyanathan L, et al. A prospective, randomized trial of an emergency department observation unit for acute onset atrial fibrillation. *Ann Emerg Med.* 2008;52:322–328.
14. von Besser K, Mills AM. Is discharge to home after emergency department cardioversion safe for the treatment of recent-onset atrial fibrillation? *Ann Emerg Med.* 2011;58:517–520.
15. Stiell IG, Clement CM, Perry JJ, et al. Association of the Ottawa Aggressive Protocol with rapid discharge of emergency department patients with recent-onset atrial fibrillation or flutter. *CJEM.* 2010;12:181–191.
16. Decker WW, Stead LG. Selecting rate control for recent-onset atrial fibrillation. *Ann Emerg Med.* 2011;57:32–33.
17. Vinson DR, Hoehn T, et al. Managing emergency department patients with recent-onset atrial fibrillation. *J Emerg Med.* 2012;42:139–148.
18. Van Gelder IC, Haegeli LM, Brandes A, et al. Rationale and current perspective for early rhythm control therapy in atrial fibrillation. *Europace.* 2011;13:1517–1525.
19. Cosio FG, Aliot E, Botto GL, et al. Delayed rhythm control of atrial fibrillation may be a cause of failure to prevent recurrences: reasons for change to active antiarrhythmic treatment at the time of the first detected episode. *Europace.* 2008;10:21–27.
20. Stiell IG, Birnie D. Managing recent-onset atrial fibrillation in the emergency department. *Ann Emerg Med.* 2011;57:31–32.
21. Neumar RW, et al. Part 8: Adult Advanced Cardiovascular Life Support: 2010 American Heart Association Guidelines for Cardiopulmonary Resuscitation and Emergency Cardiovascular Care. *Circulation.* 2010;122:S729–S767.
22. Field JM, Hazinski MF, Sayre MR, et al. Part 1: Executive Summary : 2010 American Heart Association Guidelines for Cardiopulmonary Resuscitation and Emergency Cardiovascular Care. *Circulation.* 2010;122:S640–S656.
23. Domanovits H, Laske H, Stark G, et al. Adenosine for the management of patients with tachycardias—A new protocol. *Eur Heart J.* 1994;15:589–593.
24. Camaiti A, Pieralli F, Olivotto I, et al. Prospective evaluation of adenosine-induced proarrhythmia in the emergency room. *Eur J Emerg Med.* 2001;8:99–105.
25. Griffith MJ, Linker NJ, Ward DE, et al. Adenosine in the diagnosis of broad complex tachycardia. *Lancet.* 1988;1:672–675.
26. Sharma AD, Klein GJ, Yee R. Intravenous adenosine triphosphate during wide QRS complex tachycardia: safety, therapeutic efficacy, and diagnostic utility. *Am J Med.* 1990;88:337–343.
27. Lerman BB, Belardinelli L, West A, et al. Adenosine-sensitive ventricular tachycardia: evidence suggesting cyclic AMP-mediated triggered activity. *Circulation.* 1986;74:270–280.

28. Wilber DJ, Baerman J, Olshansky B, et al. Adenosine-sensitive ventricular tachycardia. Clinical characteristics and response to catheter ablation. *Circulation.* 1993;87:126–134.
29. Ng KS, Wen MS, Yeh SJ, et al. The effects of adenosine on idiopathic ventricular tachycardia. *Am J Cardiol.* 1994;74:195–197.
30. Hina K, Kusachi S, Takaishi A, et al. Effects of adenosine triphosphate on wide QRS tachycardia. Analysis in 18 patients. *Jpn Heart J.* 1996;37:463–470.
31. Mallet ML. Proarrhythmic effects of adenosine: a review of the literature. *Emerg Med J.* 2004;21:408–410.
32. Pelleg A, Pennock RS, Kutalek SP. Proarrhythmic effects of adenosine: one decade of clinical data. *Am J Ther.* 2002;9:141–147.
33. Tan HL, Spekhorst HHM, Peters RJG, et al. Adenosine induced ventricular arrhythmias in the emergency room. *Pacing Clin Electrophysiol.* 2001;24:450–455.
34. Parham WA, Mehdirad AA, Biermann KM, et al. Case report: adenosine induced ventricular fibrillation in a patient with stable ventricular tachycardia. *J Interv Card Electrophysiol.* 2001;5:71–74.
35. Garratt CJ, Griffith MJ, O'Nunain S, et al. Effects of intravenous adenosine on antegrade refractoriness of accessory atrioventricular connections. *Circulation.* 1991;84:1962–1968.
36. Exner DV, Muzyka T, Gillis AM. Proarrhythmia in patients with the Wolff-Parkinson-White syndrome after standard doses of intravenous adenosine. *Ann Intern Med.* 1995;122:351–352.
37. Shah CP, Gupta AK, Thakur RK, et al. Adenosine-induced ventricular fibrillation. *Indian Heart J.* 2001;53:208–210.
38. Gupta AK, Shah CP, Maheshwari A, et al. Adenosine induced ventricular fibrillation in Wolff-Parkinson-White syndrome. *Pacing Clin Electrophysiol.* 2002;25:477–480.
39. Marill KA, Wolfram S, Desouza IS, et al. Adenosine for wide-complex tachycardia: efficacy and safety. *Crit Care Med.* 2009;37:2512–2518.
40. Rankin AC, Oldroyd KG, Chong E, et al. Value and limitations of adenosine in the diagnosis and treatment of narrow and broad complex tachycardias. *Br Heart J.* 1989;62:195–203.
41. Armengol RE, Graff J, Baerman JM, et al. Lack of effectiveness of lidocaine for sustained, wide QRS complex tachycardia. *Ann Emerg Med.* 1989;18:254–257.
42. Ho DS, Zecchin RP, Richards DA, et al. Double-blind trial of lignocaine versus sotalol for acute termination of spontaneous sustained ventricular tachycardia. *Lancet.* 1994;344:18–23.
43. Marill KA, Greenberg GM, Kay D, et al. Analysis of the treatment of spontaneous sustained stable ventricular tachycardia. *Acad Emerg Med.* 1997;4:1122–1128.
44. Gorgels AP, van den Dool A, Hofs A, et al. Comparison of procainamide and lidocaine in terminating sustained monomorphic ventricular tachycardia. *Am J Cardiol.* 1996;78:43–46.
45. Somberg JC, Bailin SJ, Haffajee CI, et al. Intravenous lidocaine versus intravenous amiodarone (in a new aqueous formulation) for incessant ventricular tachycardia. *Am J Cardiol.* 2002;90:853–859.
46. Callans DJ, Marchlinski FE. Dissociation of termination and prevention of inducibility of sustained ventricular tachycardia with infusion of procainamide: evidence for distinct mechanisms. *J Am Coll Cardiol.* 1992;19:111–117.
47. Levine JH, Massumi A, Scheinman MM, et al. Intravenous amiodarone for recurrent sustained hypotensive ventricular tachyarrhythmias. *J Am Coll Cardiol.* 1996;27:67–75.
48. Helmy I, Herre JM, Gee G, et al. Use of intravenous amiodarone for emergency treatment of life-threatening ventricular arrhythmias. *J Am Coll Cardiol.* 1988;12:1015–1022.
49. Schutzenberger W, Leisch F, Kerschner K, et al. Clinical efficacy of intravenous amiodarone in the short term treatment of recurrent sustained ventricular tachycardia and ventricular fibrillation. *Br Heart J.* 1989;62:367–371.
50. Tomlinson DR, Cherian P, Betts TR, et al. Intravenous amiodarone for the pharmacological termination of haemodynamically-tolerated sustained ventricular tachycardia: is bolus dose amiodarone an appropriate first-line treatment? *Emerg Med J.* 2008;25:15–18.
51. Marill KA, deSouza IS, Nishijima DK, et al. Amiodarone or procainamide for the termination of sustained stable ventricular tachycardia: an historical multicenter comparison. *Acad Emerg Med.* 2010;17:297–306.
52. Lown B, Temte JV, Arter WJ. Ventricular tachyarrhythmias. Clinical aspects. *Circulation.* 1973;47:1364–1381.
53. Gage BF, Waterman AD, Shannon W, et al. Validation of clinical classification schemes for predicting stroke: results from the National Registry of Atrial Fibrillation. *JAMA.* 2001;285(22):2864–2870.

18

Left Ventricular Assist Devices

Joe L. Hsu and Rachel H. Dotson

BACKGROUND

Heart failure affects over 6 million people in the United States and accounts for 1 million hospital admissions annually.[1,2] Despite this prevalence, the number of hearts transplanted annually in the United States has remained fixed over the past decade at approximately 2,000 per year.[3] In response to the disparity between need for transplantation and organ availability, in 1994, the U.S. Food and Drug Administration approved the use of left ventricular assist devices (LVADs) for patients awaiting heart transplantation and more recently for long-term support (i.e., destination therapy) in 2010. Although left ventricular (LV) assist technology to provide mechanical circulatory assistance for the failing heart has existed since 1963, it has only been in the last decade, with the advent of a continuous-flow pump, that these devices have become capable of providing reliable long-term support.[4,5] Based on data from the Interagency Registry for Mechanically Assisted Circulatory Support (INTERMACS), the number of LVADs implanted increased nearly sixfold from 276 in 2006 to an estimated 1,600 patients in 2011.[6] Among the 5,407 patients with LVADs registered in INTERMACS, approximately ¾ had devices placed as a bridge to transplant, and ¼ had them placed as a destination therapy.[6] As the number of patients with LVADs continues to rise and as their survival improves, the emergency physician will increasingly be tasked with their acute care. This review focuses on a single LVAD system, the HeartMate II (Thoratec, Pleasanton, CA); this is the most commonly-installed assist device worldwide, and knowledge of this system is applicable to the management of other continuous-flow systems. This chapter addresses (1) the evolution of the LVAD, (2) the management of LVAD-associated complications, and (3) the use of radiographic imaging in diagnosing these complications.

EVOLUTION AND GENERAL FUNCTION OF LEFT VENTRICULAR ASSIST DEVICES

The two main groups of LVADs are distinguished by pump type: pulsatile and continuous flow (Fig. 18.1). Pulsatile pumps are analogous to the heart: a pumping chamber, once filled, activates a pusher plate technology.[7] Newer continuous-flow pumps utilize a valveless system, in which centrifugal or axial pumping propels blood forward (Fig. 18.1B). Compared to the pulsatile system, continuous-flow pumps are smaller, lighter (0.75 vs. 2.6 pounds), and quieter. The Randomized

Evaluation of Mechanical Assistance for Congestive Heart Failure (REMATCH) trial demonstrated the pulsatile LVAD HeartMate XVE superior to medical therapy.[8] Patients with the HeartMate XVE had a 1-year survival rate of 52% and a 2-year survival rate of 23%; patients with medical therapy had a 1-year survival of 25% and a 2-year survival rate of 8%.[8] A follow-up trial compared the HeartMate XVE to the continuous-flow HeartMate II for use as destination therapy.[5] Patients with the pulsatile-flow pump had a 1-year survival rate of 55% and a 2-year survival rate of 24%; patients with the continuous-flow pump had a 1-year survival rate of 68% and a 2-year survival rate of 58%. Continuous-flow devices outperformed pulsatile pumps in rates of rehospitalization, pump replacement, and LVAD- and non-LVAD–related infections.[5] Adverse events associated with continuous-flow devices included hemorrhagic stroke (9%), right heart failure (5%), sepsis (4%), and bleeding (3%); the rate of these complications was, however, not significantly different from that of pulsatile-flow devices.[5] This trial highlighted the primary advantages of continuous-flow over pulsatile devices, namely, improved reliability and decreased pump wear, a lighter weight and less cumbersome design, and lower infection risk.[9] Newer second-generation LVADs include the HeartWare system (HeartWare, Framingham, MA, approved for bridge to transplant); this smaller "wearless" device is implantable within the pericardium, suspended by a passive magnet and a hydrodynamic thrust-bearing system.[10]

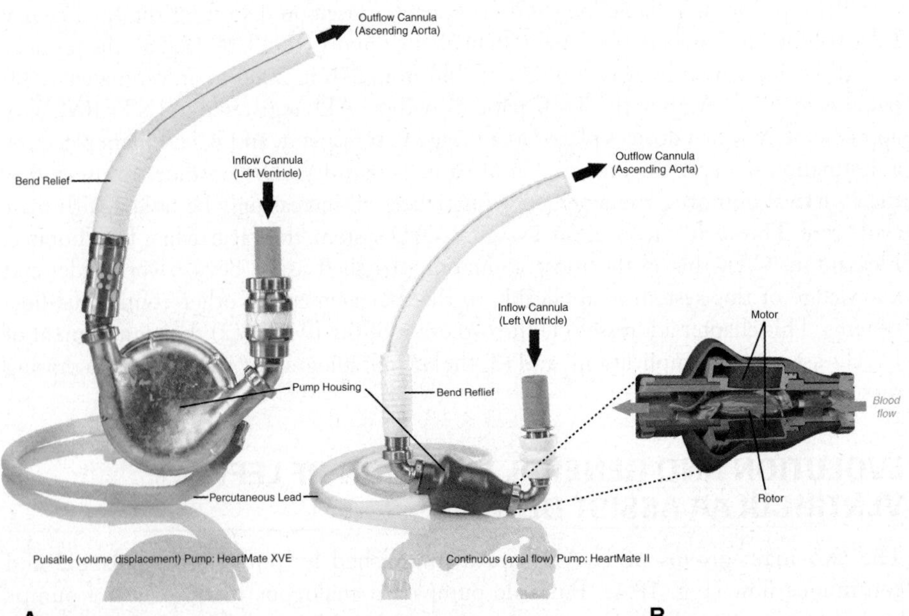

FIGURE 18.1 Pulsatile pump and continuous-flow pump. **A:** Pulsatile (HeartMate XVE, **left**) and continuous flow (HeartMate II, right). **B:** Internal mechanics of HeartMate II. Reprinted with the permission of Thoratec Corporation.

PUMP PARAMETERS

General Considerations

All LVAD flow parameters are set at the time of implantation; for the emergency physician needing to diagnose and manage acute illness and device-related complications in LVAD users, understanding the parameters displayed and their significance is essential. The HeartMate II control monitor displays the following parameters: pump speed (revolutions per minute [RPM]), pump power (watts [W]), flow estimate (liters per minute [LPM]), and pulse index (dimensionless value). Commonly, clinicians inexperienced with LVAD management will make decisions based on single parameters (e.g., decreased flow), failing to understand the significance of this parameter in the context of an acute change in condition. Instead, when troubleshooting a patient with an LVAD, clinicians should gather data from the whole patient, assessing volume status, presence of arrhythmias, mean arterial pressure (MAP), date of LVAD placement, recent echocardiography results, pump parameters, and history of LVAD alarms (e.g., suction events). Deviation from a functional baseline is more significant than the specific value of each parameter. Acquisition of additional hemodynamic data often requires use of echocardiography and pulmonary artery catheters (PACs).

Pump Speed

Pump speed is a fixed value set intraoperatively and often reassessed prior to hospital discharge in a process known as a "ramp study." This involves empirically adjusting pump speed under echocardiographic guidance to determine the patient's optimal LV cavity size and output at a given speed. Pump speed governs flow through the device and is a measure of assistance provided to the patient. Only an experienced VAD clinician should adjust pump speed, and always under echocardiographic guidance. Excessive pump speeds may be associated with ventricular arrhythmias.

Pump Power

The HeartMate II controller directly measures the amount of power delivered to maintain pump speed. This parameter is analogous to myocardial workload in normal individuals. An increase in speed, preload, or afterload will increase power consumption. In the absence of these conditions, a gradual increase in power use may indicate the formation of clot on the rotor (see Thrombotic Complications). Conversely, a decrease in afterload, preload, or speed as well as a blockage of inflow or outflow cannula will decrease power consumption. There is no generalizable power level, as it can vary from patient to patient; rather, it is the change (>2 W) from a previous level that may indicate a change in device or patient status.

Flow Estimate

The flow on the HeartMate II is derived from power and speed. Flow is not directly measured but rather is an estimate of the amount of fluid passing through the pump, assuming normal pump function. Using an ultrasonic probe, one study evaluated the differences between the "flow estimate," as reported on the HeartMate II control monitor, and the "absolute flow" measured by the probe. The study showed that at a flow of 4 to 6 LPM, there was a variable 15% to 20% difference between the estimated and absolute flow values.[11] Several factors affect "absolute flow" for continuous pumps; these include preload (LV preload and right ventricular [RV] function), speed, and afterload (the difference between outlet cannula and inlet cannula pressure).[9] Thus, hypervolemia, increased LV contractility, increased speed, and decreased pressure difference across the pump will increase flow. As mentioned, situations such as a clot on the rotor will cause power to increase, resulting in an erroneously high flow displayed as "+++." Flows displayed as "+++" or "−−−" (for high and low flows, respectively) are considered outside the range of the expected physiologic limits based on speed.[9] The HeartMate II low-flow alarm will signal when flow is <2.5 LPM. It is important to recognize that "flow estimate" is not analogous to cardiac output or "absolute flow" through the LVAD and thus should be used as a trended, directional value rather than a diagnostic tool to be used alone and without other patient and LVAD values.[11]

Pulse Index

Pulse index refers to the amount of flow that passes through the pump during a cardiac cycle as averaged over 15 seconds. It is calculated as [(flow max − flow minimum)/flow average] × 10.[9] It is a dimensionless value that is derived from the LVAD estimated flow. The degree of LVAD support is the primary variable that correlates with pulse index, and the two are inversely related. During LV systole, the flow through the pump increases due to an increased pressure at the pump inlet approximating the pressure at the outlet cannula (aortic pressure). During cardiac diastole, this inlet pressure drops, while the outlet pressure remains high (increased pressure difference) and, consequently, flow decreases. Therefore, pulse index is directly proportional to LV contractility (increases in which are due to preload, inotropic support, and myocardial recovery) and inversely proportional to the assistance provided by the pump.

ADVERSE EVENTS AND COMPLICATIONS

Common LVAD-related complications include hemorrhage, arrhythmias, infections, hemodynamic instability, and thrombosis (Table 18.1).[5,13] When any of these are encountered in an LVAD-supported patient, a multidisciplinary approach to management is required; the patient's cardiologist and/or VAD coordinator should be contacted to discuss the plan of care. If hospitalization is indicated, then the patient should be transferred to a VAD center when stable for transport.

Infections

Infections are common in LVAD patients and are a leading cause of hospital readmission and mortality.[5,13–17] Based on an analysis of 2,006 patients registered in the INTERMACS database, nearly 19% of patients will develop a percutaneous site infection within 1 year.[14] The percutaneous lead acts as a portal of entry for pathogens, which can progress to the subcutaneous tunnel, pump pocket, device, heart (i.e., endocarditis), and bloodstream (Figs. 18.2 and 18.3). Recommendations for the evaluation of an LVAD patient with suspected infection are outlined in Table 18.1. Patients with suspected LVAD-related infections should be treated with empiric broad-spectrum antimicrobials to cover nosocomial pathogens, including Methicillin-resistant Staphylococcus aureus (MRSA) and *Pseudomonas aeruginosa*.[16,18] Fungemia has also been reported in LVAD-supported patients.[19] Surgical consultation should be obtained, as incision and drainage, debridement, and/or percutaneous lead revision may be required.[16] The ongoing development of LVADs that do not require a percutaneous lead should reduce the risk of these infections.

TABLE 18.1 Diagnosis and Management of Adverse Events and Complications

Complication	Clinical Features	LVAD Parameters	Diagnosis: Diagnostic Studies	Diagnosis: CT Findings[7]	Management Strategies
Inflow cannula complications					
Kinking of inflow cannula	↑ Cardiac pulse pressure, hypotension	↓ Flow, power, variable flow	Coagulation parameters (INR 1.5–2.5), CT	Kinking of inflow cannula Cannula malposition (Fig. 18.4)	Surgical consultation Anticoagulation Maintain adequate volume status.
Thrombus in cannula	↑ Cardiac pulse pressure, acute anemia (due to hemolysis), hypotension	↓ Flow, power	Evaluate for hemolysis: ↑ cell-free plasma Hgb, indirect bilirubin, LDH; ↓ haptoglobin, CT	Low-attenuation lesion in inflow/outflow cannula	Surgical consultation Anticoagulation
Outflow cannula complications					
Tearing of aortic anastomosis	Hypotension, hemorrhage	No specific change	Serial Hgb, TEE, CT	Extravasation of contrast material at anastomosis	Emergent surgical consultation Can occur over time
Kinking of outflow cannula	↑ Cardiac pulse pressure, hypotension	↓ Flow, power, variable flow (positional)	Coagulation parameters (INR 1.5–2.5), CT	Kinking of outflow cannula Disruption of cannula patency	Surgical consultation Anticoagulation
Hemodynamic complications					
Arrhythmia	±Hemodynamic instability, symptoms of ↓ perfusion	↓ Flow, power	ECG, electrolyte panel, TTE/TEE (to assess LV geometry, fluid status, and cannula position)	None	Control arrhythmia and defibrillation Evaluate for suction events-VT Watch for RVF External chest compression only if in extremis
Right ventricular failure	Hypotension, ↑ CVP, PVR	↓ Flow, power, suction events	TTE, TEE, CT CVC ± PAC	Intraventricular septum bowed leftward RV dilated Dilation of IVC	RV contractility: inotropes (milrinone) Decrease PVR: Avoid hypercapnia, hypoxemia, and pulmonary vasodilators (iNO) Avoid overfilling Control arrhythmias
Pericardial tamponade	↑ CVP, hypotension, preload dependent	↓ Flow, power, suction events	TTE, TEE (pericardial effusion may not be visualized on TTE), CT	Dilation of IVC Compression of RV or atrium, flattening of heart border Pericardial effusion	Pericardiocentesis

(*Continued*)

TABLE 18.1 Diagnosis and Management of Adverse Events and Complications (*Continued*)

Complication	Clinical Features	LVAD Parameters	Diagnosis: Diagnostic Studies	Diagnosis: CT Findings[7]	Management Strategies
Aortic valve insufficiency	Decompensated heart failure, ↓ systemic perfusion, cardiogenic shock	↑ High flow	TTE ramp study to evaluate speed, ECG-gated CT	Presence of valvular thickening Aortic valve visualized on ECG-gated CT	May develop over time Consult cardiology and cardiac surgery Diuretics, afterload reduction AI may improve with decreased pump speed
Coagulation-related complications					
Thrombus on rotor	Acute anemia (due to hemolysis) ↑ Cardiac pulse pressure	"+++" flow, ↑ Power (>10–12 W) — hours to days	Evaluate for hemolysis: ↑ cell-free plasma Hgb, indirect bilirubin, LDH; ↓ haptoglobin, CT	Low-attenuation lesion near inflow	Surgical consultation Anticoagulation
Hemorrhage	Primarily GI also: epistaxis, hematuria, mediastinal, thoracic, ICH	↓ Flow, power, suction events	TTE, TEE, EGD, serial CBC, coagulation parameters, CT Evaluate for acquired vWD: vWF antigen, vWF activity, and factor VIII activity. Evaluate for hemolysis: ↓ cell-free plasma Hgb, indirect bilirubin, LDH; ↓ haptoglobin.	Evidence of bleed (e.g., ICH on CT head)	PRBC and procoagulant factors and vWF as indicated Avoid excessive transfusions in: • Bridge to transplant • History of RVF
Infectious complications					
LVAD specific[12] • Pump/cannula infections • Pocket infections • Percutaneous driveline infections *LVAD related*[12] • Endocarditis • Bacteremia • Mediastinitis	Fever, chills, hypotension 2/2 sepsis, sequelae of embolic events	Variable effect on LVAD	CBC with differential, lactate Exit site wound Cx, plus fungal Cx if risk factors TEE, if TTE negative Blood cultures, if + CVC obtain "time to positivity" Cx Imaging: ultrasound, CT (c/a/p)	Gas or fluid collection around pump components, percutaneous lead Figure 18.2, pocket infection Figure 18.3, percutaneous lead infection	Broad-spectrum antimicrobials for nosocomial pathogens ± fungal coverage based on risk factors EGDT Surgical consultation for incision and drainage, debridement, device exchange

CVC, central venous catheter; CVP, central venous pressure; Cx, culture; EGDT, early goal-directed therapy; GI, gastrointestinal; Hgb, hemoglobin; ICH, intracranial hemorrhage; LDH, lactate dehydrogenase; PAC, pulmonary artery catheter; PVR, pulmonary vascular resistance; RV, right ventricle; RVF, right ventricular failure; TEE, transesophageal echocardiogram; TTE, transthoracic echocardiogram; vWD, von Willebrand disease; vWF, von Willebrand factor; W, watts.

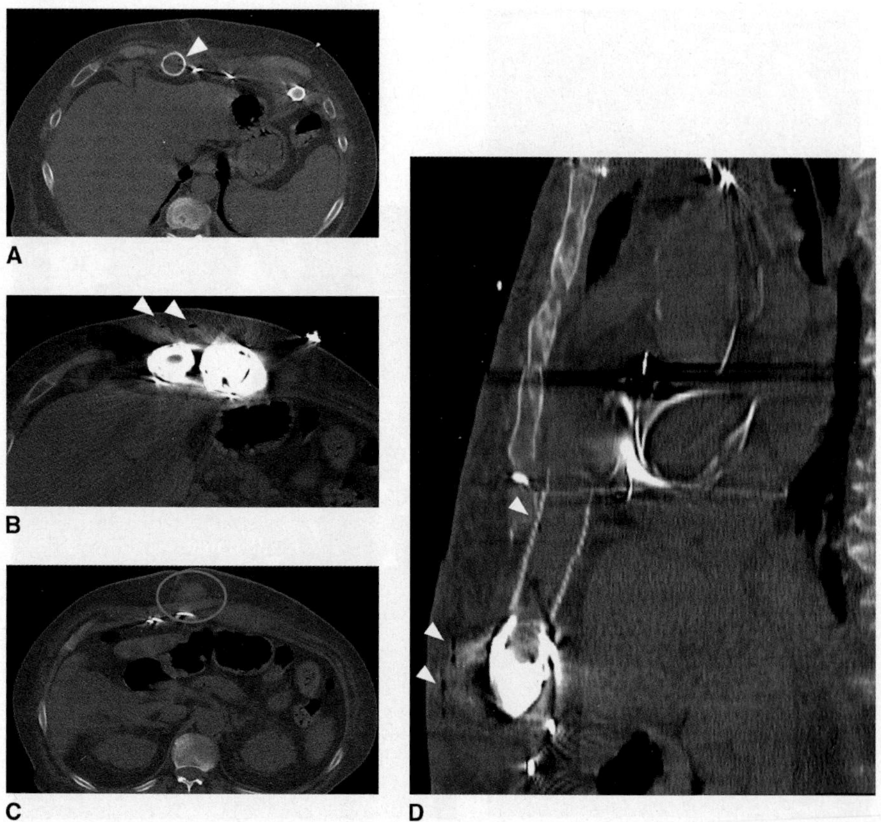

FIGURE 18.2 Computed tomography images of pump pocket infection. **A:** Gas bubble (arrows) in outflow cannula. **B:** Gas bubbles in pocket space surrounding LVAD pump. **C:** Hyperdense area inferior to pump pocket (oval). **D:** Sagittal view of pump pocket infection; gas bubbles can be seen in outflow cannula and pump pocket.

Hypotension and Hemodynamic Instability

Continuous-flow pumps unload the LV throughout the cardiac cycle, resulting in a diminished or absent pulse pressure.[20] Thus, noninvasive measurement of blood pressure and pulse oximetry are often unreliable.[9] Blood pressure is best measured as a mean arterial pressure (MAP) obtained by Doppler and sphygmomanometer or, alternatively, by placement of an arterial catheter. Goal MAP in most LVAD patients is 70 to 80 mm Hg. In general, MAP should not exceed 90 mm Hg; LVAD patients are sensitive to increases in afterload, and higher blood pressures increase their risk for adverse neurological events.[9] For the hypertensive LVAD patient, beta-blockers and angiotensin-converting enzyme inhibitors are generally used for blood pressure control. For the hypotensive patient, the etiology should be identified (hypovolemic, vasodilatory, or cardiogenic shock due to RV or LV failure) and treated accordingly with volume repletion, vasopressor, and/or inotropic medications. Echocardiography and pulmonary artery catheterization may provide valuable data for diagnosis and management. Additionally,

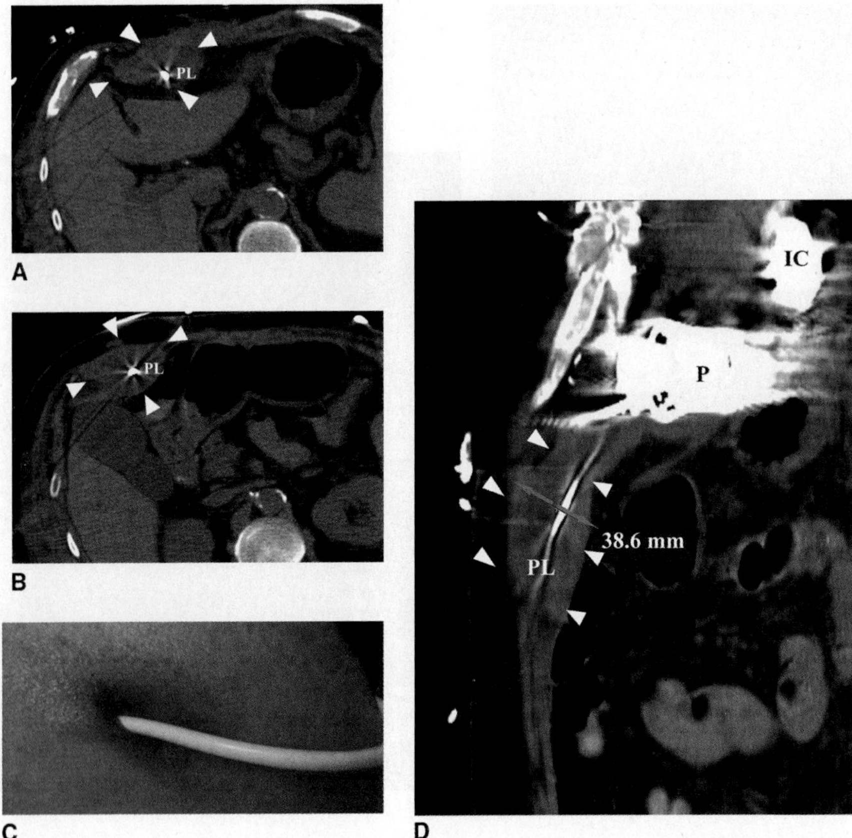

FIGURE 18.3 Computed tomography images of percutaneous lead infection. **A, B:** Hyperattenuated area surrounding percutaneous lead (PL), borders marked by arrows. **C:** Local erythema at exit site of PL. **D:** Sagittal view of hyperattenuated area surrounding PL (diameter: 38.6 mm). IC, inflow cannula; P, pump; PL, percutaneous lead.

problems intrinsic to the device, such as oversuctioning, may contribute to diminished blood flow and should be considered when evaluating the hypotensive LVAD patient.

Right Ventricular Failure

Right ventricular failure (RVF) is one of the more dreaded etiologies of hypotension after LVAD placement. RVF is estimated to occur in up to 20% of LVAD patients[21] and is associated with a 1-year mortality of 83%.[22] While this condition is usually recognized in the immediate perioperative period, the emergency physician may have to contend with the management of LVAD patients with RV dysfunction. Because of the complexity of managing an LVAD patient with RVF, early consultation with a VAD specialist or a cardiologist is recommended, as the patient may require more advanced mechanical circulatory assistance. Causes of RVF specific to LVADs include (1) leftward bowing of the intraventricular septum due to LVAD-related LV emptying, reducing its capacity to participate in RV contractility, and (2) increased venous return from the LVAD, outmatching the capacity of a failing right heart.[23] Table 18.1 details the management strategy for patients with RVF, including transfer to a critical care unit for placement of a pulmonary artery catheter (PAC) and/or transesophageal echocardiography. Among inotropes, milrinone is particularly beneficial because it decreases pulmonary vascular resistance (PVR) and improves RV contractility and matching of RV and LVAD outputs.[24] Additional therapies for RVF include pulmonary vasodilators, such as inhaled nitric oxide (iNO) and/or aerosolized prostacyclin, that lower PVR. Avoidance of conditions that aggravate pulmonary vasoconstriction, such as hypercapnia and hypoxemia, is also essential. In a randomized trial of 11 patients with increased PVR after LVAD placement, iNO significantly reduced PVR and increased LVAD flow in patients with pulmonary hypertension.[25] Avoidance of excessive preload is also important in the management of patients with RVF; thus, particular caution should be paid to the LVAD patient with a history of RVF who presents to the emergency department with hemorrhagic shock and who may require large-volume blood and factor transfusions. Patients who do not respond to these medical therapies for RVF (e.g., iNO, inotropes) may require more advanced mechanical circulatory support including the placement of a right ventricular assist device (RVAD). Risk factors that predict the need for an RVAD placement include female gender, low right ventricular stroke work index, history of pulmonary hypertension, and intraoperative high central venous pressure.[21,22,26,27]

Suction Events

A suction event occurs when there is excessive LV unloading due to a pump speed that is too high relative to LV volume. Suction events may manifest as a decrease in pump flow, arrhythmias, or transient and intermittent decreases in the pump speed to the low-speed limit (a result of LVAD auto-correction). During a suction event, echocardiography will demonstrate a leftward shift of the intraventricular septum with an underfilled LV. Other potential causes of poor LV filling include hypovolemia, RVF, pulmonary hypertension, and malposition of the inflow cannula toward the intraventricular septum or the lateral wall (Fig. 18.4). Suction events can be alleviated by volume repletion or by decreasing the pump speed, tasks best performed by an LVAD specialist using echocardiographic guidance.

Arrhythmias

Patients with advanced heart failure have a high prevalence of cardiac arrhythmias both prior to and following LVAD placement.[28] When patients develop new arrhythmias postimplantation, an underlying etiology, such as ischemia, suction events, or electrolyte imbalances, should be excluded. Although the LVAD continues to unload the LV during arrhythmic events, the right heart is unsupported and is at risk of acute dysfunction. The management of most arrhythmias in LVAD patients is similar to that of patients with advanced heart failure.

Atrial Fibrillation

Medications used for rate and rhythm control in patients with advanced heart failure are also appropriate for LVAD-supported patients. In addition to impairing right heart function (resulting in decreased LVAD preload), atrial fibrillation increases the risk of thromboembolism. Due to the risk of embolic events, which may occur peripherally or within the LVAD pump itself, warfarin is typically dosed to achieve a target INR of 2 to 2.5.[29]

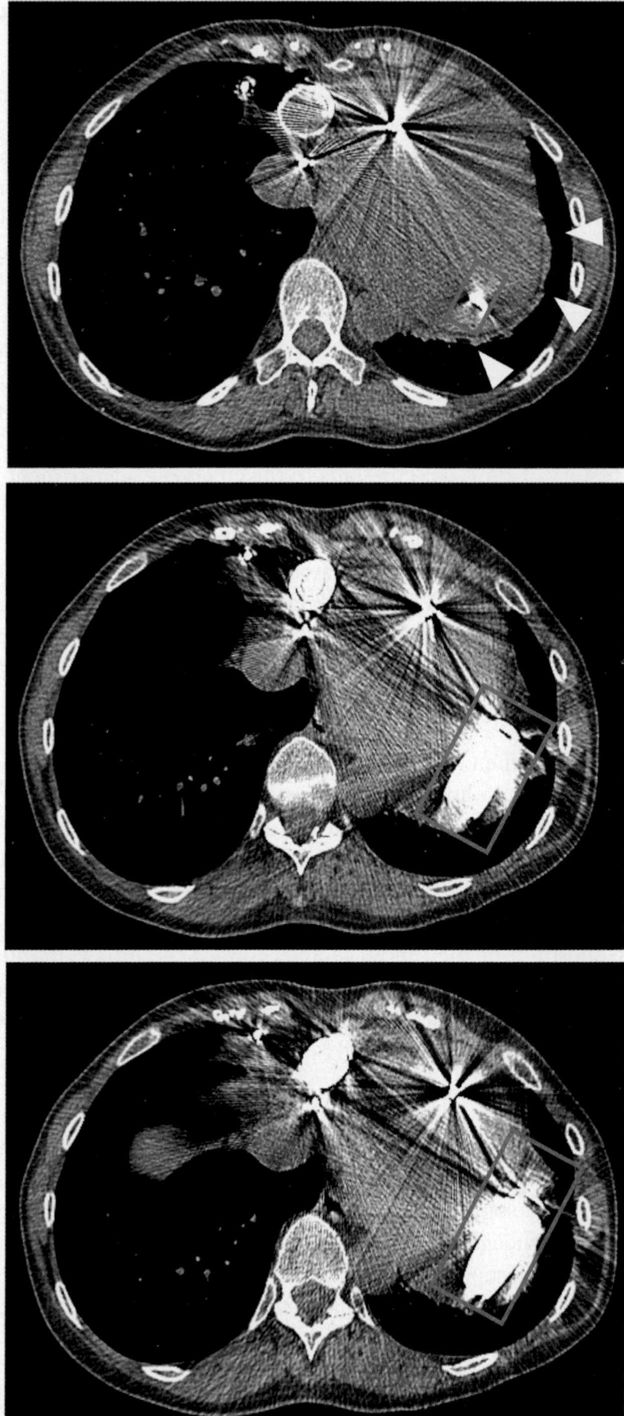

FIGURE 18.4 Inflow cannula malposition. CT images depicting malposition of the inflow cannula toward the posterior–lateral cardiac wall (arrows). Cannula orientation depicted by rectangle.

Ventricular Arrhythmias

Because the LVAD continues to function during otherwise life-threatening arrhythmias, patients with these arrhythmias may present with hemodynamic stability. However, the unsupported RV is at high risk of failure, placing the patient at risk of cardiogenic shock or sudden cardiac death. All ventricular arrhythmias require immediate treatment. Beta-blockers and other antiarrhythmic medications may be beneficial; however, defibrillation is indicated in patients with persistent ventricular arrhythmias or arrhythmia-induced hypotension. Given the high prevalence of ventricular arrhythmias in end-stage heart failure patients, the majority of LVAD patients will have implanted cardiac defibrillators (ICDs). Patients who do not have ICDs should be considered for this intervention.

Cardiac Arrest

External chest compressions may disrupt the aortic anastomosis or LVAD inflow tract and are generally contraindicated, particularly shortly after implant when the sternum has not healed; however, they may be helpful in patients in extremis. Prior to mediastinal wound healing, direct cardiac massage by a qualified surgeon may be effective in patients with recent device implantation. External defibrillation should be performed with the pump running and the system controller connected to the percutaneous lead. The system controller should be disconnected only if open-chest defibrillation is required. All drugs routinely given per advanced cardiac life support (ACLS) protocols may be administered.

Thrombotic Complications

The routine use of systemic anticoagulation and antiplatelet therapy has resulted in a low incidence of device thrombosis and thromboembolism.[30–33] Current guidelines recommend administering warfarin with a target INR of 1.5 to 2.5 alongside daily aspirin. In a study of 331 HeartMate II patients treated with warfarin and antiplatelet therapy, ischemic strokes occurred in 2.4% of patients and pump thrombosis in 0.9%.[30] The risk of thrombosis was highest when the INR was <1.5. Hemorrhagic complications, including hemorrhagic stroke or blood loss requiring transfusions of ≥2 units PRBC or surgical intervention, were more common than thrombotic events (2.1%, 15.4%, and 1.2%, respectively) particularly in patients with an INR >2.5. Pump thrombus is a rare but serious complication, as it may result in obstruction of blood flow. Gradual increases in pump power (often >10 to 12 W) occurring over hours to days may herald a thrombus in contact with the rotor or bearings.[9] Thrombus may be initially noted as unexplained hemolysis (see Hemolysis).

Blood Loss and Coagulopathy

Acute anemia in an LVAD patient may be due to hemorrhage caused by anticoagulation and/or acquired coagulopathies and hemolysis. In some cases, hemorrhage may be severe enough to require blood transfusions or surgery.[5] The gastrointestinal (GI) tract is a particularly common source of bleeding, and in a retrospective study of 154 LVAD patients, GI bleeds were most often due to peptic ulcer disease and vascular malformations.[34] Esophagogastroduodenoscopy (EGD) is a reasonable first diagnostic study in most LVAD patients with a suspected upper GI bleed, as it is well tolerated, diagnostic, and therapeutic. Bleeding may also manifest as epistaxis, hematuria, or mediastinal, thoracic, or intracranial hemorrhage. Depending on the severity and location of the hemorrhage, anticoagulants should be reduced or withheld. Patients should be transfused as clinically indicated with packed red blood cells and procoagulant factors. Unnecessary or excessive transfusions in candidates for heart transplantation should be avoided, as there is an increased risk of graft rejection due to transfusion-related allosensitization. As previously discussed, invasive monitoring (e.g., PAC) may be useful to avoid exacerbating RV dysfunction in patients requiring large-volume transfusions.

Acquired von Willebrand Disease

In addition to bleeding due to therapeutic anticoagulation, other derangements in hemostasis are associated with LVADs. Acquired von Willebrand disease (vWD) may occur following continuous-flow LVAD placement.[35] A postulated mechanism involves excessive cleavage of high molecular weight von Willebrand factor (vWF) multimers by continuous-flow, pump–related shear stress forces,[36] a process analogous to the acquired vWD associated with severe aortic stenosis.[37] At this time, no studies have clarified the potential benefits of vWF replacement therapy for LVAD patients with active hemorrhage. Generally, empiric use of desmopressin is both appropriate and efficacious in reducing hemorrhage with acquired vWD.

Hemolysis

Acute anemia in the LVAD patient may also be the result of hemolysis. Hemolysis may be diagnosed by laboratory findings, including increased cell-free plasma hemoglobin, indirect bilirubin, and lactate dehydrogenase, and decreased haptoglobin. Although the incidence of hemolysis due to mechanical shearing from the pump is low (3%), it may be observed with pump-related thrombus.[33,38] Thus, the observation of hemolysis should prompt a workup for a pump or cannula-related thrombus.

Aortic Insufficiency

Aortic insufficiency (AI) adversely affects pump function by causing rapid LV filling and high pump flow.[9] Studies have demonstrated the development of de novo AI, as well as the progression of AI to at least moderate severity, in up to 64% of patients within 18 months after HeartMate II implantation.[39,40] The patient with clinically significant AI may present with decompensated heart failure, decreased systemic perfusion, cardiogenic shock, and high pump flow. Mild AI can often be managed with diuretics and afterload reduction. As long as systemic perfusion is not compromised, decreasing pump speed may reduce regurgitant flow across the valve. Moderate or severe symptomatic AI after LVAD implantation requires surgical repair, including bioprosthetic aortic valve replacement, coaptation of the aortic valve leaflets, or complete oversewing of the aortic valve outflow tract.[41]

RADIOGRAPHIC EVALUATION OF THE HEARTMATE II

For the emergency physician, radiographic imaging is one of the most accessible and useful tools for diagnosing potential problems in an LVAD patient (Figs. 18.5 and 18.6). Figure 18.6 depicts the typical contrast computed tomography (CT) appearance

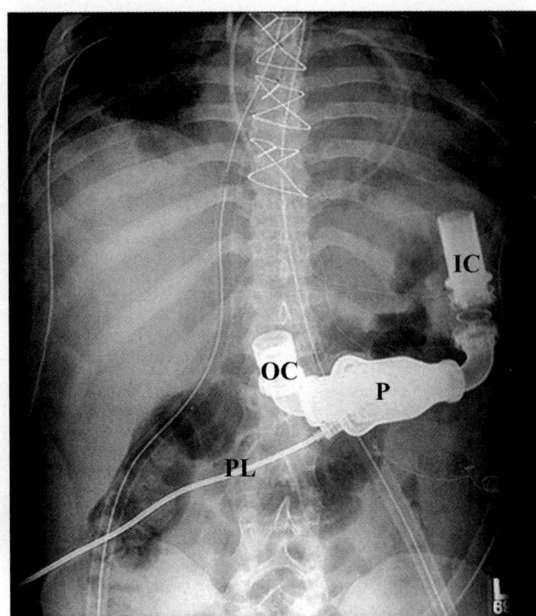

FIGURE 18.5 Plain radiograph of HeartMate II. IC, inflow cannula; OC, outflow cannula; P, pump; PL, percutaneous lead. Reprinted with the permission of Thoratec Corporation.

of the LVAD in situ. CT imaging can inform diagnoses both anatomic (e.g., pocket and percutaneous lead infections, Figs. 18.2 and 18.3, respectively) and, with ECG gating, dynamic (e.g., AI). The HeartMate II is implanted anterior to the rectus sheath, preperitoneally.[9] The distal end is attached via an end-to-side anastomosis to the ascending aorta (Fig. 18.6A). Both the inflow and outflow cannula can be visualized using CT with intravenous contrast and should be patent without evidence of kinking or obstruction (Fig. 18.6B and C). The inflow cannula attaches to the LV apex (Fig. 18.6C). A bend relief allows the inflow cannula to attach to the pump in the upper abdomen pocket without kinking. Similarly, the outflow cannula attaches to the pump with a bend relief. The pump itself cannot be visualized on CT (Fig. 18.6D). Table 18.1 lists potential complications and their characteristic CT findings.

CONCLUSION

As the prevalence of LVADs increases, more of these patients will present to the emergency department, challenging the emergency physician to recognize and manage the complications that can arise in this complex group of patients. An emergency medical service (EMS) LVAD guide, produced by the Mechanical Circulatory Support Organization, provides instructions and important facts for the emergency personnel (www.mylvad.com). For the HeartMate II, 24-hour clinical and technical support and manuals with information pertaining to routine operating procedures, alarms, and emergencies are available to clinicians via the Thoratec website (www.thoratec.com). A multidisciplinary approach including the patient's cardiologist, VAD coordinator, and, when indicated, cardiothoracic surgeon and/or infectious disease specialist, is necessary for successful clinical outcomes in this patient population.

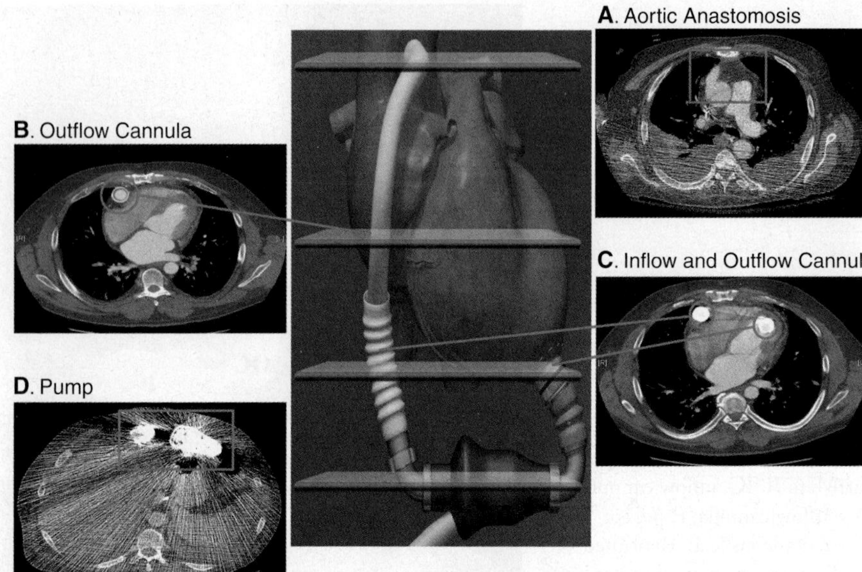

FIGURE 18.6 Computed tomography images of HeartMate II pump. Cross-sectional CT images of HeartMate II pump, in situ. **A:** Aortic anastomosis: end-to-side anastomosis of outflow cannula to ascending aorta. **B:** Outflow cannula: Cannula is patent without evidence of obstruction or kinking. **C:** Outflow and inflow cannula: Note position at ventricular apex oriented toward mitral valve. **D:** Pump itself cannot be visualized. HeartMate II graphic images reprinted with the permission of Thoratec Corporation.

LITERATURE TABLE

TRIAL	DESIGN	RESULT
Slaughter et al., *NEJM.* 2009[5]	Multicenter randomized trial of 200 patients with advanced heart failure compared continuous-flow vs. pulsatile-flow LVADs for destination therapy.	2-year survival continuous- vs. pulsatile-flow LVADs (58% and 24%, respectively, $p = 0.008$). Both devices improved quality of life and functional capacity
Rose et al., *NEJM.* 2001[8]	Multicenter RCT of 129 NYHA class IV heart failure patients for destination therapy	Pulsatile LVAD compared to optimal medical management resulted in improved survival and quality of life. The study demonstrated a 48% reduction in risk of death from any cause for the device group vs. the medical therapy group (relative risk 0.52; 95% CI 0.34–0.78, $p = 0.001$). One- and two-year survival rates in the device group vs. medical therapy group were 52% vs. 25% ($p = 0.002$) and 23% vs. 8% ($p = 0.09$), respectively
Topkara et al., *Ann Thoracic Surg.* 2010[16]	Retrospective, single-center study of 81 patients with continuous-flow LVADs	51.9% of patients diagnosed with ≥1 infection. Mean follow-up period of 9.2 mo
Boyle et al., *J Heart Lung Transplant.* 2009[30]	Cohort study of 331 patients with HeartMate II LVADs	Low rate of thromboembolism in anticoagulated patients. Increased bleeding if INR > 2.5
Miller et al., *NEJM.* 2007[31]	Prospective, multicenter study of 133 patients with end-stage heart failure after implantation of continuous-flow LVADs for bridge to transplant	LVADs survival: 75% at 6 mo, 68% at 12 mo. Improved quality of life and functional status

CI, confidence interval.

ACKNOWLEDGMENTS

We would like to thank Dipanjan Banerjee, MD, MS; Greg Rosselini, MD; and Robert Smith, CCP, RN, for their careful review of the manuscript. We would also like to thank Dominik Fleischmann, MD for providing radiographic images used in the figures.

REFERENCES

1. Hall MJ, Levant S, DeFrances CJ. Hospitalization for congestive heart failure: United States, 2000–2010. *NCHS Data Brief.* 2012;108:1–8.
2. Rathi S, Deedwania PC. The epidemiology and pathophysiology of heart failure. *Med Clin North Am.* 2012;96:881–890.
3. Organ Procurement and Transplantation Network and Scientific Registry of Transplant Recipients 2010 data report. *Am J Transplant.* 2012;12 (suppl 1):1–156.
4. DeBakey ME. Left ventricular bypass pump for cardiac assistance. Clinical experience. *Am J Cardiol.* 1971;27:3–11.
5. Slaughter MS, Rogers JG, Milano CA, et al. Advanced heart failure treated with continuous-flow left ventricular assist device. *N Engl J Med.* 2009;361:2241–2251.
6. Kirklin J, Naftel DC, Myers SL, et al. INTERMACS Interagency Registry for Mechanically Assisted Circulatory Support Quarterly Statistical Report Implant dates: June 23, 2006–December 31, 2011. 2012:15.
7. Carr CM, Jacob J, Park SJ, et al. CT of left ventricular assist devices. *Radiographics.* 2010;30:429–444.
8. Rose EA, Gelijns AC, Moskowitz AJ, et al. Long-term use of a left ventricular assist device for end-stage heart failure. *N Engl J Med.* 2001;345:1435–1443.
9. Slaughter MS, Pagani FD, Rogers JG, et al. Clinical management of continuous-flow left ventricular assist devices in advanced heart failure. *J Heart Lung Transplant.* 2010;29:S1–S39.
10. Slaughter MS, Sobieski MA II, Tamez D, et al. HeartWare miniature axial-flow ventricular assist device: design and initial feasibility test. *Tex Heart Inst J.* 2009;36:12–16.
11. Slaughter MS, Bartoli CR, Sobieski MA, et al. Intraoperative evaluation of the HeartMate II flow estimator. *J Heart Lung Transplant.* 2009;28:39–43.
12. Hannan MM, Husain S, Mattner F, et al. Working formulation for the standardization of definitions of infections in patients using ventricular assist devices. *J Heart Lung Transplant.* 2011;30:375–384.
13. Hasin T, Marmor Y, Kremers W, et al. Readmissions after implantation of axial flow left ventricular assist device. *J Am Coll Cardiol.* 2013;61:153–163.
14. Goldstein DJ, Naftel D, Holman W, et al. Continuous-flow devices and percutaneous site infections: clinical outcomes. *J Heart Lung Transplant.* 2012;31:1151–1157.
15. Gordon RJ, Weinberg AD, Pagani FD, et al. Prospective, multicenter study of ventricular assist device infections. *Circulation.* 2013;127:691–702.
16. Topkara VK, Kondareddy S, Malik F, et al. Infectious complications in patients with left ventricular assist device: etiology and outcomes in the continuous-flow era. *Ann Thorac Surg.* 2010;90:1270–1277.
17. Kirklin JK, Naftel DC, Kormos RL, et al. Second INTERMACS annual report: more than 1,000 primary left ventricular assist device implants. *J Heart Lung Transplant.* 2010;29:1–10.
18. Maniar S, Kondareddy S, Topkara VK. Left ventricular assist device-related infections: past, present and future. *Expert Rev Med Devices.* 2011;8:627–634.
19. Bagdasarian NG, Malani AN, Pagani FD, et al. Fungemia associated with left ventricular assist device support. *J Card Surg.* 2009;24:763–765.
20. Myers TJ, Bolmers M, Gregoric ID, et al. Assessment of arterial blood pressure during support with an axial flow left ventricular assist device. *J Heart Lung Transplant.* 2009;28:423–427.
21. Dang NC, Topkara VK, Mercando M, et al. Right heart failure after left ventricular assist device implantation in patients with chronic congestive heart failure. *J Heart Lung Transplant.* 2006;25:1–6.
22. Drakos SG, Janicki L, Horne BD, et al. Risk factors predictive of right ventricular failure after left ventricular assist device implantation. *Am J Cardiol.* 2010;105:1030–1035.
23. Haddad F, Couture P, Tousignant C, et al. The right ventricle in cardiac surgery, a perioperative perspective: II. Pathophysiology, clinical importance, and management. *Anesth Analg.* 2009;108:422–433.
24. Kihara S, Kawai A, Fukuda T, et al. Effects of milrinone for right ventricular failure after left ventricular assist device implantation. *Heart Vessels.* 2002;16:69–71.

25. Argenziano M, Choudhri AF, Moazami N, et al. Randomized, double-blind trial of inhaled nitric oxide in LVAD recipients with pulmonary hypertension. *Ann Thorac Surg.* 1998;65:340–345.
26. Fukamachi K, McCarthy PM, Smedira NG, et al. Preoperative risk factors for right ventricular failure after implantable left ventricular assist device insertion. *Ann Thorac Surg.* 1999;68:2181–2184.
27. Ochiai Y, McCarthy PM, Smedira NG, et al. Predictors of severe right ventricular failure after implantable left ventricular assist device insertion: analysis of 245 patients. *Circulation.* 2002;106:I198–I202.
28. Raasch H, Jensen BC, Chang PP, et al. Epidemiology, management, and outcomes of sustained ventricular arrhythmias after continuous-flow left ventricular assist device implantation. *Am Heart J.* 2012;164:373–378.
29. Boyle A. Arrhythmias in patients with ventricular assist devices. *Curr Opin Cardiol.* 2012;27:13–18.
30. Boyle AJ, Russell SD, Teuteberg JJ, et al. Low thromboembolism and pump thrombosis with the HeartMate II left ventricular assist device: analysis of outpatient anti-coagulation. *J Heart Lung Transplant.* 2009;28:881–887.
31. Miller LW, Pagani FD, Russell SD, et al. Use of a continuous-flow device in patients awaiting heart transplantation. *N Engl J Med.* 2007;357:885–896.
32. Struber M, Sander K, Lahpor J, et al. HeartMate II left ventricular assist device; early European experience. *Eur J Cardiothorac Surg.* 2008;34:289–294.
33. John R, Kamdar F, Liao K, et al. Improved survival and decreasing incidence of adverse events with the HeartMate II left ventricular assist device as bridge-to-transplant therapy. *Ann Thorac Surg.* 2008;86:1227–1234; discussion 1234–1225.
34. Kushnir VM, Sharma S, Ewald GA, et al. Evaluation of GI bleeding after implantation of left ventricular assist device. *Gastrointest Endosc.* 2012;75:973–979.
35. Crow S, Chen D, Milano C, et al. Acquired von Willebrand syndrome in continuous-flow ventricular assist device recipients. *Ann Thorac Surg.* 2010;90:1263–1269; discussion 1269.
36. Uriel N, Pak SW, Jorde UP, et al. Acquired von Willebrand syndrome after continuous-flow mechanical device support contributes to a high prevalence of bleeding during long-term support and at the time of transplantation. *J Am Coll Cardiol.* 2010;56:1207–1213.
37. Vincentelli A, Susen S, Le Tourneau T, et al. Acquired von Willebrand syndrome in aortic stenosis. *N Engl J Med.* 2003;349:343–349.
38. Bhamidipati CM, Ailawadi G, Bergin J, et al. Early thrombus in a HeartMate II left ventricular assist device: a potential cause of hemolysis and diagnostic dilemma. *J Thorac Cardiovasc Surg.* 2010;140:e7–e8.
39. Aggarwal A, Raghuvir R, Eryazici P, et al. The development of aortic insufficiency in continuous-flow left ventricular assist device-supported patients. *Ann Thorac Surg.* 2013;95:493–498.
40. Cowger J, Pagani FD, Haft JW, et al. The development of aortic insufficiency in left ventricular assist device-supported patients. *Circ Heart Fail.* 2010;3:668–674.
41. Park SJ, Liao KK, Segurola R, et al. Management of aortic insufficiency in patients with left ventricular assist devices: a simple coaptation stitch method (Park's stitch). *J Thorac Cardiovasc Surg.* 2004;127:264–266.

19

Management of the Post–Cardiac Arrest Patient

Cappi Lay

BACKGROUND

In the United States, out-of-hospital cardiac arrest (OHCA) affects roughly 300,000 people each year.[1] Despite herculean efforts in improving outcome, mortality from cardiac arrest remains high, with only 8% to 10% of these patients surviving to hospital discharge.[1,2] Between 35% and 61% of OHCA victims will have return of spontaneous circulation (ROSC) either in the prehospital setting or in the emergency department (ED),[3–5]; of those, between 36% and 79% will rearrest in the acute care setting.[6]

Anoxic brain injury is the leading cause of morbidity in patients with cardiac arrest who survive to hospital admission. Over the last decade, the development and use of therapeutic hypothermia has made neuroprotection the cornerstone of therapy for hemodynamically stable survivors of cardiac arrest. Sustained reperfusion is also fundamental to neurologic salvage, and identifying and addressing the initial cause of cardiac failure is essential if further episodes of hemodynamic instability are to be prevented.

ACUTE CARE AND DIAGNOSTIC EVALUATION

A sense of relief often comes over ED staff in the aftermath of successful ROSC, once the flurry of CPR activity has subsided and the patient has regained a pulse. However, a continued sense of urgency is required for the phases of evaluation and treatment that follow. As with all critically injured patients, the first priorities of management for a post–cardiac arrest patient are to secure and confirm the placement of a definitive airway and obtain intravenous access for the delivery of fluid and vasoactive medications. Although multiple large-bore peripheral IVs are acceptable initially, a central venous catheter (CVC) is preferred, in order to accommodate potential vasopressor administration. The goals of post–cardiac arrest management in the ED are subsequently organized along two parallel paths: identifying and treating the primary cause of the arrest; and initiating therapeutic cooling in appropriate candidates.

Understanding the context of the arrest can be critical in determining its cause. Witnesses—whether emergency medical services (EMS), family members, or bystanders—should be questioned about symptoms that preceded the collapse, such as chest pain, shortness of breath, dizziness, or severe headache. It is equally important to identify preexisting conditions that predispose to cardiac events, including coronary artery disease (CAD), congestive heart failure (CHF), deep venous thrombosis (DVT), or renal disease.

A twelve-lead electrocardiogram (ECG) should be obtained as early as possible to look for evidence of cardiac ischemia. Multiple studies have shown that acute coronary thrombosis is the single most common cause of sudden atraumatic cardiac arrest. Other potential causes include primary arrhythmia, electrolyte disturbances, dilated cardiomyopathy, pulmonary embolus, hypoglycemia, accidental hypothermia, tension pneumothorax, cardiac tamponade, toxic overdose, and subarachnoid hemorrhage. Of these, several can be eliminated based on history and physical exam. A basic metabolic panel or an arterial blood gas can be used to identify dangerous electrolyte abnormalities, while pneumothorax and tamponade, although uncommon in the absence of trauma, can be identified with chest radiography and bedside cardiac ultrasound.

Given the diagnostic uncertainty that can be present after ROSC, the International Liaison Committee On Resuscitation (ILCOR) has emphasized the importance of a comprehensive search for reversible causes of OHCA.[7] A recent study retrospectively reviewed 896 cases of OHCA in PROCAT, a cardiac arrest registry in Paris, France, in which all patients received a diagnostic procedure to identify the cause of arrest.[1] The authors describe an algorithm in which, following ROSC, patients suspected of underlying cardiac etiology were taken for immediate cardiac catheterization regardless of initial rhythm and ECG changes. For patients suspected of having a noncardiac etiology, brain computed tomography (CT) and chest CT angiography (CTA) could be performed to assess for intracranial hemorrhage or pulmonary embolism (PE), respectively. When cardiac catheterization did not reveal a culprit lesion, the patient could then be taken for CT; similarly, if an initial CT did not reveal a cause of arrest, the patient could be taken for cardiac catheterization. Out of 896 patients without an obvious cause of OHCA, 729 (81%) received an immediate diagnostic coronary angiogram. In approximately 39% of patients taken to the catheterization lab initially, no culprit lesion could be identified. Following a negative coronary angiogram, 188 patients underwent CT, which revealed a diagnosis in 33 cases (17.6%). Conversely, 167 patients underwent initial CT at the time of hospital admission that demonstrated a cause of arrest in 39 cases (23.4%). Sixteen of the patients whose initial CT was negative went on to receive a cardiac catheterization, which revealed a cause of arrest in 5 cases. Overall, using this approach, physicians were able to identify a cause of cardiac arrest in 524 of 896 cases based on the results of 452 cardiac catheterizations and 72 CT studies. The most common extracardiac cause of OHCA identified by CT was stroke, followed by PE.

The routine use of head CT is not endorsed in established guidelines on the management of cardiac arrest after ROSC; however, CT effectively rules out brain hemorrhage, which, if detected, would affect the decision to treat the patient with anticoagulants fundamental to therapy for both coronary and pulmonary thrombosis.

CARDIAC CATHETERIZATION

The single most common cause of OHCA is myocardial infarction due to acute coronary artery occlusion. Because of neurologic injury, survivors of OHCA are often unresponsive after CPR and/or are heavily sedated and paralyzed. Few physicians would disagree that in the presence of true ST-segment elevation >0.5 mm in two or more contiguous leads, patients should be taken emergently for cardiac catheterization and percutaneous coronary intervention (PCI) regardless of the patient's mental status. Considerably more controversy exists regarding the proper course of action for the comatose patient for whom a twelve-lead ECG is nondiagnostic following ROSC. In one study, among survivors of OHCA without a history of chest pain or diagnostic ECG changes, 26% had evidence of recent coronary occlusion on angiography.[8] Similar rates of significant coronary occlusion have been demonstrated in other cohorts of patients lacking diagnostic ECG findings. In a study of OHCA patients with angiographic evidence of acute myocardial infarction (MI), 12% were without evidence of ST-segment elevation on their postresuscitation ECG.[9]

The high rate of electrographically silent myocardial ischemia in cardiac arrest patients has led some authors to suggest that all survivors of OHCA should be taken for coronary angiography, regardless of ECG findings. Others reason that such aggressive screening has not been shown to improve outcomes in this group of patients; not only is their prognosis frequently dictated by the degree of neurologic damage rather than that of myocardial necrosis, but also, unselected angiography of all OHCA patients is economically wasteful. Proponents counter by pointing out that neurologic prognosis based on clinical exam and imaging is unreliable immediately after ROSC, and that the potential for lethal, untreated coronary artery occlusion necessitates immediate investigation and treatment in patients with amenable lesions, in order to limit myocardial damage.

A 2012 study of 240 patients after resuscitation from cardiac arrest found improved survival to discharge among the 25% of patients who were taken for coronary angiography within 6 hours of reaching the hospital compared to patients who were taken later or not at all (72% vs. 49% discharged alive).[10] In another report of 72 angiograms performed on survivors of OHCA (at an institution that performed cardiac catheterization on all OHCA patients with successful ROSC), the diagnosis of acute MI was made in 37.5% of all patients. ST-segment elevation on admission ECG yielded a positive predictive value (PPV) for a final diagnosis of acute MI of 82.6% and a negative predictive value (NPV) of 83.7%. In this study, the roughly 16% of missed MI in patients with a normal ECG strongly suggests that ECG alone is not a sufficiently sensitive test to rely on in a potentially lethal disease process.[11]

Another recent study attempted to analyze the impact of emergency cardiac catheterization on in-hospital outcome among unconscious survivors of OHCA. The study reviewed the outcomes of 93 patients with OHCA and ROSC after <20 minutes; of these, 66 received a cardiac catheterization, and of those, 52% were found to have an acute or recent culprit lesion. Forty-two percent of those with an acute or recent culprit lesion identified did not demonstrate ST-segment elevation on their post-ROSC ECG. Sixty percent of patients who received emergency coronary angiography were discharged from the hospital alive compared to 54% overall.[12]

A large prospective cohort study completed in 2012 analyzed the 1- and 5-year outcomes of 5,958 patients with OHCA who were admitted alive to the hospital. One thousand and one (16.8%) were discharged alive; of these, 384 (38.4%) received cardiac catheterization, 80% of whom had PCI performed. Therapeutic hypothermia (TH) was performed in 241 of 941 (25.6%) patients comatose at hospital admission. Patient outcomes were analyzed in groups according to whether they received PCI, therapeutic hypothermia, both therapies, or neither. At 1 and 5 years after discharge, survival was highest in those patients who had received both PCI and TH.[13]

CARDIAC ARREST WITH MASSIVE PULMONARY EMBOLISM

The percentage of OHCA caused by PE is estimated to be between 0.2% and 13.3%.[14–16] Differentiating between PE and other causes of cardiac arrest has profound implications for patient treatment, since PE may be amenable to treatment with thrombolytics and catheter or surgical embolectomy. In a 2008 study, patients with OHCA and a suspected cardiac etiology (without a confirmed ST segment elevation myocardial infarction [STEMI]) were randomized to empiric intravenous tissue plasminogen activator (tPA) or placebo; there was no demonstrable benefit from tPA, effectively limiting this therapy to cardiac arrest cases with a strong suspicion of PE etiology.[17] Making this distinction, however, is challenging and complicated by considerable overlap of symptoms among arrest-inducing etiologies. In the ED, CTA of the chest is the optimal diagnostic test for PE, and should be considered in all patients without an obvious etiology for their arrest.[7] Echocardiography is another useful diagnostic modality in massive PE (discussed in detail in Chapter 11), and will typically demonstrate right ventricular dysfunction, including RV/LV end-diastolic diameter ratio ≥1 in four-chamber view, paradoxical septal motion, and pulmonary hypertension with RV/atrial gradient ≥30 mm Hg.

Intravenous tPA is the standard of care for a massive PE that results in hemodynamic instability or cardiac arrest, and is given in a dose of 100 mg, with 10 mg given as a bolus and the remaining 90 mg infused over a period of 2 hours.[18] Catheter-directed embolectomy and open thoracotomy are other, albeit less well-researched, interventions for massive PE. Catheter-directed embolectomy is performed using a combination of aspiration, clot fragmentation, rheolysis, and direct administered thrombolysis at the site of the clot. In a cohort of patients with persistent hemodynamic instability after receiving thrombolytics for PE, one study observed that patients who received a rescue embolectomy with a catheter-based approach had lower mortality (7% vs. 38%) and lower risk of recurrent PE (0% versus 35%).[19] Catheter-directed embolectomy is still rarely performed in most medical centers and should be considered only when cardiothoracic surgical services exist to manage the potential vascular complications. ED staff who suspect PE as the cause of cardiac arrest or hemodynamic instability should involve interventional radiology and cardiothoracic surgery early in the decision-making process.

THERAPEUTIC HYPOTHERMIA

As already noted, mortality and long-term disability resulting from cardiac arrest are frequently due to severe neurologic injury during and after the ischemic period of the arrest. To date, most experiments with neuroprotective strategies aimed at improving clinical outcome after cardiac arrest have failed, with the notable exception of therapeutic hypothermia (TH). The benefit of postarrest hypothermia is likely mediated though multiple pathways. Neuronal injury after cardiac arrest is the result of disrupted calcium homeostasis, inflammatory cell migration, excitatory neurotransmission, and the activation of proteolytic and apoptotic pathways.[20] Several investigators have shown that for every 1°C drop in body temperature, the cerebral metabolic rate decreases by approximately 7%, effectively blunting the effects of neuronal injury.[21] Hypothermia is also thought to protect the integrity of the blood–brain barrier, which may attenuate ischemia-related cerebral edema.

Two randomized trials of therapeutic hypothermia after OHCA were published in 2002; both demonstrated benefits in neurologic outcome and survival. Both sets of investigators randomly assigned survivors of OHCA to a target temperature of between 32°C and 34°C after ROSC, for a duration of 12 to 24 hours. The first study showed a significant reduction in neurological morbidity in patients receiving TH; this finding was confirmed by the second study, performed by the Hypothermia After Cardiac Arrest (HACA) investigators.[22,23] In addition, HACA also found a significant reduction in 30-day mortality associated with TH. Although it has been more than a decade since these and many confirmatory follow-up studies have been published, recent surveys show that TH is still underutilized. Based on the initial two studies, six patients need to be treated (NNT) to prevent one poor neurologic outcome, and seven treated to prevent one death. To put this statistic into perspective, the NNT to prevent one poor neurologic outcome using tissue plasminogen activator in stroke is eight. For thrombolytics in acute myocardial infarction, the NNT to save one life is between 20 and 33.

Current recommendations that guide which patient groups should receive therapeutic hypothermia are based on the populations included in the original two studies, and include those comatose patients with successful ROSC following ventricular fibrillation (VF) and pulseless ventricular tachycardia (VT).[22,23] Patients with an initial rhythm of pulseless electrical activity have a poorer prognosis than do those with rhythms responsive to defibrillation; however, it is likely that once ROSC is established, these patients will benefit from the neuroprotective effect of TH as well. Treatment should thus be initiated as soon as possible in all nontraumatic cardiac arrest patients with significantly altered mental status or coma. TH should probably be withheld in those patients with significant ongoing hemorrhage or sepsis. Although the original trials demonstrating benefit for TH excluded patients with cardiogenic shock, more recent studies have confirmed that these patients also derive a mortality benefit from TH, and that cooling in fact decreases vasopressor requirements.[24]

In the setting of STEMI, immediate PCI or thrombolysis can be lifesaving; several reports have shown that both procedures are compatible with cooling. Early TH should be instituted prior to hospital transfer and continued throughout the catheterization procedure. Several published reports have demonstrated the compatibility of TH with anticoagulation, thrombolytics, and PCI without a significant increase in complications.[25,26] When compared with historical controls that were not cooled, rates of bleeding complications in patients receiving TH were identical, even in those patients receiving clopidogrel, GPIIA/IIIB inhibitors, and heparin. Studies have also reported that TH can be initiated prior to cardiac catheterization with no impact on door-to-balloon time.[25] To effectively implement early TH in cardiac arrest patients who need immediate PCI, the ED and the catheterization team must collaboratively create standing protocols on TH indications and method of use, and discern how best to achieve rapid goal temperature without sacrificing door-to-balloon time.

Therapeutic hypothermia should be initiated as soon as possible after ROSC is achieved. Animal models of VF arrest have shown that even a 15-minute delay in the initiation of cooling results in markedly worse neurologic outcome and more severe histologic damage of brain tissue.[27,28] If ROSC is achieved in the field, induction of hypothermia should begin with EMS providers and continue through transfer to the ED. The application of therapeutic hypothermia consists of three phases: (1) The induction phase, during which core body temperature is actively decreased; (2) the maintenance phase; and (3) the rewarming phase, when body temperature is allowed to return to its physiologic baseline.

At the end of 2013, a randomized controlled trial of patients with OHCA compared therapeutic hypothermia with a standard target temperature of 33° Celsius to that with a target temperature of 36°.[29] This multi-center trial enrolled 939 patients and demonstrated no significant difference in mortality or neurological outcome between management strategies, raising questions about the optimal target temperature for TH after OSCA. Patients in both arms of the study received bystander CPR roughly 73% of the time and had a median ROSC time of 25 minutes. The trail leaves unanswered whether patients surviving arrest under different circumstances would still benefit from more aggressive temperature lowering. Patients were eligible for inclusion in the trial if they were screened within 4 hours of their arrest. It is at least possible that more aggressive cooling has a larger beneficial impact when initiated earlier in the course, after reperfusion has occurred. The study has also been criticized for failing to test for subtle differences in cognitive ability between the groups and for failing to control for differing sedation strategies that may have influenced outcomes. Further research is warranted to determine which subgroups of cardiac arrest patient can safely be treated with therapeutic hypothermia using this less aggressive strategy.

Cooling Methods

Therapeutic hypothermia may be initiated via several methods, including surface cooling, endovascular cooling, and infusions of iced saline. Surface cooling employs ice packs, evaporative sprays, cooling blankets, or fitted pads with circulating cold water to lower temperature. Both of the original TH studies demonstrated profound clinical benefit using surface cooling alone, often only with the use of ice packs. Cold intravenous saline, which is easy to apply and provides for rapid induction of TH at low cost, is being utilized with increasing frequency. In healthy anesthetized volunteers, one study found that rapid infusion of 40 mL/kg of 4°C normal saline via a CVC resulted in a drop in core temperature of 2.5°C in 30 minutes.[30] This drop was greater than expected due to peripheral vasoconstriction, which caused relative isolation of the core and peripheral body compartments. Conversely, peripheral vasoconstriction decreases the efficacy of cooling when surface techniques are used. In another study, OHCA victims were randomized to cold saline infusion of up to 2 L upon ROSC while still in the care of EMS providers. Field cooling was associated with a mean drop in temperature of 1.2°C from initiation of infusion to arrival in the ED.[31] No significant differences were found between groups in the PaO_2, vasopressor requirements, or pulmonary edema on initial chest radiograph. In a study examining the effects of large-volume cold saline infusion on respiratory function after cardiac arrest, 52 patients who received an average of 3 L of cold saline experienced only a small decrease in their PaO_2 to FiO_2 ratio—from 290 at admission to the intensive care unit (ICU) to 247.5—while maintaining oxygen saturation in the normal range.[32]

A 2005 prospective study reported on 134 cardiac arrest patients, including those with cardiogenic shock, who received 4°C saline in addition to surface cooling for the induction of hypothermia. On average, patients without shock received approximately 2 L of cold fluid in 60 minutes and experienced a drop in temperature from 36.9°C to 32.9°C.[33] In the patients with cardiogenic shock, a more conservative protocol with slower fluid administration was used, but still resulted in a change in core temperature from 36.8°C to 33.1°C over 120 minutes. Only 8 of 134 patients in the study required modest increases in positive end-expiratory pressure (PEEP) to maintain PaO_2 during fluid administration, of which 5 demonstrated evidence of cardiogenic shock prior to fluid infusion. Overall, the data support the routine use of large volume (30 mL/kg) of ice-cold (4°C) saline for the induction of HACA.

Physiologic Effects of Hypothermia

Induction of mild hypothermia alters normal cardiac, pulmonary, endocrine, and renal functions and carries a risk of adverse effects. At temperatures between 32°C and 34°C, myocardial contractility increases and heart rate declines as a result of decreased spontaneous depolarization of pacemaker cells.[34] Peripheral vasoconstriction causes an increase in systemic vascular resistance that may manifest as an increased blood pressure during induction. Metabolic rate decreases by 7% to 8% for every 1°C decrease in core body temperature, so decreases in cardiac output as a result of induced bradycardia do not usually result in unmet oxygen demand or tissue ischemia. A brisk diuresis occurs in response to an expansion of central blood volume and may require aggressive fluid repletion to maintain cardiac filling pressures.[35] Below 30°C, the risk of clinically relevant arrhythmias increases steeply, with atrial fibrillation occurring most commonly, and ventricular tachycardia and fibrillation becoming more likely as temperature drops further.[35] Careful observation of body temperature during induction is important to avoid overcooling and the associated risk of malignant arrhythmia.

As core body temperature drops, observed changes in serum electrolytes are due to intracellular shifts in potassium, magnesium, calcium, and phosphate.[36,37] Hourly monitoring of electrolytes, with repletion as needed, is recommended during the induction phase of cooling to maintain normal levels. Later on, as rewarming is started, potassium that shifted into cells during the induction phase may suddenly exit the cells, creating a risk of rebound hyperkalemia. Ensuring slow rates of rewarming—no faster than 0.25°C per hour—helps minimize this complication, as well the risk of rebound cerebral edema.[21]

Mild hypothermia causes decreased insulin secretion and insulin resistance, which may result in hyperglycemia and increased insulin requirements during the induction and maintenance phases of cooling.[21] In brain-injured patients, the optimal serum glucose level has not been determined, but maintaining levels between 100 and 180 mg/dL is reasonable.

Platelet function is impaired and clotting times are increased with TH. These effects however, have not been associated with increased rates of clinically significant bleeding after OHCA, even when TH is used in conjunction with antiplatelet drugs, anticoagulants, and thrombolytics.[38]

Hypothermia also impairs leukocyte migration and the production of inflammatory mediators, thereby reducing the body's ability to fight off infection. The HACA trial demonstrated a trend toward increased risk of pneumonia and sepsis with cooling, and other studies have confirmed the association between TH and increased rates of infection.[23,39] Close observation for signs of evolving infection should be maintained throughout the cooling process. During active cooling, fever may not reliably be observed, but the work required to achieve cooling goals—a measure indicated on multiple newer devices—can be used as a surrogate for the development of fever.

Shivering

The normal shivering response is the greatest obstacle to rapid cooling; if not aggressively controlled, shivering can contribute to increased metabolic demand and undermine the beneficial effects of TH. Management follows a stepwise protocol that begins with measures to decrease the shivering threshold, and proceeds to include nonvolatile anesthetics such as propofol and, rarely, paralytics for severe refractory shivering. Initial agents used for shivering control include buspirone, meperidine, magnesium sulfate, and alpha-2 agonists. Buspirone, a serotonin (5HT)-1A partial agonist, is thought to lower the shivering threshold by activating hypothalamic heat loss mechanisms. Meperidine, which acts synergistically with buspirone, is a unique opiate agonist of both *kappa* and *mu* receptors shown to be effective in decreasing shivering. Magnesium sulfate, when targeted to a serum level of between 3 and 4 mg/dL, reduces shivering by promoting peripheral vasodilation and muscle relaxation. Alpha-2 agonists, such as clonidine and dexmedetomidine, are thought to inhibit neuronal firing related to thermosensitivity. Finally, skin surface rewarming, although counterintuitive, has also been shown to decrease the core temperature shivering threshold by 1°C for every 4°C rise in skin temperature.[40]

When the above therapies fail, fentanyl and propofol infusions can be employed to suppress refractory shivering. During the rapid induction phase of cooling, a bolus dose of a long acting paralytic such as rocuronium or vecuronium is encouraged; however, because of the concern for critical illness myopathy, ongoing infusions of paralytic medications to suppress shivering are discouraged for all but the most refractory cases.

Continuous EEG

Seizure activity is common in victims of anoxic brain injury but may be easily missed in the setting of therapeutic hypothermia where deep sedation or paralysis is required. Nonconvulsive status epilepticus (NCSE), defined as unremitting epileptiform activity in the absence of clinical seizures, has been reported in 8% to 9% of patients in undifferentiated coma.[41–43] The presence of NCSE has been associated with increased risk of mortality and severe disability at hospital discharge. In one study, 10% of comatose patients in the ICU had continuous seizure activity on cEEG, 68% of which was not detected clinically. Seizure activity was associated with a 19-fold increase in the odds of death or severe disability.[44] It is not clear whether seizures are the direct cause of poor outcome or merely a marker of severe brain injury; nevertheless, in those patients for whom aggressive care is appropriate, it is reasonable to monitor and treat seizures in the immediate postarrest period under the assumption that unceasing epileptiform discharges inhibit neurologic recovery.

PERCUTANEOUS HEMODYNAMIC SUPPORT

Following resuscitation from cardiac arrest, many patients will experience significant hemodynamic instability requiring varying degrees of vasopressor and inotropic support. In patients with cardiogenic shock from acute myocardial infarction or other cardiac insult, high-dose vasopressors and inotropes may be required. By augmenting cardiac contractility and afterload, however, these medications can increase myocardial oxygen consumption and exacerbate cardiac ischemia. In patients requiring cardiac catheterization, extracorporeal membrane oxygenation (ECMO) and intra-aortic balloon pump (IABP) are two temporizing percutaneous interventions that may be used to maintain hemodynamic stability.

As percutaneous hemodynamic support devices have become smaller, they have begun to gain wider use in the management of acute cardiogenic shock. Unlike veno–veno ECMO that can only be used to support oxygenation, venoarterial (VA) ECMO can be used to provide hemodynamic support. These devices typically consist of two 18-gauge French catheters that are inserted into the femoral artery and vein, essentially creating a right atrial-to-aortic shunt. Blood is removed through the femoral vein catheter where it enters the ECMO circuit for oxygenation and is returned via pump in retrograde fashion to the aorta. A side-port is inserted into the distal femoral artery to prevent limb ischemia.

A 2011 study described the creation of an Extracorporeal life support (ECLS) team capable of quickly establishing a VA ECMO circuit to provide rapid hemodynamic support, and demonstrated that ECLS could be used to facilitate CT imaging and PCI in survivors of cardiac arrest.[45] Over the course of 6 years, the ECLS team was activated for 144 patients, 58 of whom had ECLS established. Overall survival in the ECLS group was 38%. A 2012 study described initiating percutaneous hemodynamic support with a VA ECMO circuit in a combination of 28 patients with cardiac arrest from acute myocardial infarction (AMI) or PE. In all AMI patients, hemodynamic support was initiated while the patient was still in arrest; in the patients with PE, 10 of 12 survived, 70% with good neurologic outcome.[46] A similar study of 22 patients who received VA ECMO initiated during cardiac arrest reported that 41% were discharged home from the hospital with no disability.[47] In the last two studies, an IABP was frequently used in conjunction with VA ECMO to reduce LV afterload.

Percutaneous hemodynamic support of the type described above requires a cardiothoracic surgeon or interventional cardiologist to establish the perfusion circuit, and is only being used in a minority of academic medical centers. To date, no randomized trials of this technology in selected cardiac arrest patients have been performed.

CONCLUSION

OHCA remains a catastrophic event that continues to claim tens of thousands of lives each year in the U.S. alone. Rapidly identifying the etiology of the arrest is essential to initiating the correct treatment. Myocardial infarction is the single most common cause of OHCA and may present in approximately 10% of patients without characteristic ECG changes. Diagnostic algorithms that combine CT imaging and cardiac catheterization will increase accurate diagnosis of the etiology of cardiac arrest and may improve outcomes by prompting early identification and treatment. Therapeutic hypothermia is still the only therapy proven to have a mortality benefit after cardiac arrest and should be initiated as soon as possible in all eligible patients. Therapeutic hypothermia has been shown to be compatible with anticoagulants, thrombolytics, and cardiac catheterization, and should not be delayed for any of these treatments.

LITERATURE TABLE

TRIAL	DESIGN	RESULT
Spaulding et al., *N Engl J Med.* 1997[8]	Prospective cohort study of 84 consecutive cardiac arrest survivors taken for immediate coronary angiography	Coronary occlusion the most common (48%) etiology of OHCA. 15% of patients with recent coronary occlusions had no STE on admission ECG
Bottiger et al., *N Engl J Med.* 2008[17]	RCT of OHCA patients randomized to empiric IV thrombolysis vs. placebo during cardiopulmonary resuscitation	No difference between IV thrombolysis and placebo in 30-d mortality (14.7% vs. 17% $p = 0.36$), hospital admission (53.5% vs. 55% $p = 0.67$), ROSC (55% vs. 54.6% $p = 0.96$), 24-h survival (30.6% vs. 33.3% $p = 0.39$), survival to hospital discharge (15.1% vs. 17.5% $p = 0.33$), or neurologic outcome ($p = 0.69$)
Bernard et al., *N Engl J Med.* 2002[22]	RCT of 77 OHCA survivors randomized to mild TH vs. normothermia × 12 h	Significant improvement in neurologic outcome in treatment group (OR 5.25, 95% CI, 1.47–18.76; $p = 0.011$)
Hypothermia after Cardiac Arrest Study (HACA) group. *N Engl J Med.* 2002[23]	Multicenter RCT of 136 OHCA survivors randomized to mild TH vs. normothermia × 24 h	TH resulted in significant improvement in neurologic outcome (55% vs. 39%, RR 1.40; 95% CI, 1.08–1.81) and 6-mo mortality (41% vs. 55%, RR 0.74; 95% CI, 0.58–0.95) in treatment group
Nielsen et al., *N Engl J Med.* 2013[29]	RCT of 950 survivors of OHCA assigned to either 33°C or 36°C targeted temperature management	All cause mortality 50% in the 33°C group and 48% in the 36°C (HR with a temperature of 33°C, 1.06; 95% CI, 0.89–1.28; $p = 0.51$). Study concluded that hypothermia at a targeted temperature of 33°C did not confer a benefit as compared with a targeted temperature of 36°C
Polderman et al., *Crit Care Med.* 2005[33]	Prospective cohort study of 134 OHCA patients given iced cold saline for induction of TH	Iced saline infusion achieved ~4°C drop in temperature within 60 min. Minimal effects on respiratory function, even in patient group with cardiogenic shock

CI, confidence interval; HR, hazard ratio; OR, odds ratio; RR, relative risk.

REFERENCES

1. Roger VL, et al. Heart Disease and Stroke Statistics–2011 Update: a report from the American Heart Association. *Circulation.* 2011;123:e18–e209.
2. Centers for Disease Control and Prevention. Out-of-hospital Cardiac Arrest Surveillance—Cardiac Arrest Registry to Enhance Survival (CARES), United States, October 1, 2005–December 31, 2010. *MMWR.* 2011;60(8):1–19.
3. Grasner JT, et al. A national resuscitation registry of out of hospital cardiac arrest in Germany: a pilot study. *Resuscitation.* 2009;80:199–203.
4. Grmec S, et al. Utstein style analysis of out of hospital cardiac arrest—bystander CPR and end expired CO2. *Resuscitation.* 2007;72:404–14.
5. Nichol G, Thomas E, Callaway C, et al. Regional variation in out of hospital cardiac arrest incidence and outcome. *JAMA.* 2008;300:1423–31.
6. Salcido DD, et al. Incidence of re-arrest after return of spontaneous circulation in out of hospital cardiac arrest. *Prehosp Emerg Care.* 2010;14(4):413–18.
7. Chelly J, Mongardon N, Dumas F, et al. Benefit of an early and systematic imaging procedure after cardiac arrest: insights from the PROCAT registry. *Resuscitation.* 2012;83:1444–50.
8. Spaulding C, Joly LM, Rosenberg A, et al. Immediate coronary angiography in survivors of out-of-hospital cardiac arrest. *N Engl J Med.* 1997;336(23):1629–1633.
9. Sideris G, et al. Value of post resuscitation electrocardiogram in the diagnosis of acute myocardial infarction in out of hospital cardiac arrest patients. *Resuscitation.* 2011;82:1148–1153.
10. Strote JA, et al. Comparison of role of early to later or no cardiac catheterization after resuscitation from out-of-hospital cardiac arrest. *Am J Cardiol.* 2012;109:451–454.

11. Anyfantakis ZA, et al. Acute coronary angiographic findings in survivors of out-of-hospital cardiac arrest. *Am Heart J.* 2009;157(2):312–8.
12. Zanuttini D, et al. Impact of emergency coronary angiography on in-hospital outcome of unconscious survivors after out of hospital cardiac arrest. *Am J Cardiol.* 2012;110:1723–1728.
13. Dumas F, et al. Long term prognosis following resuscitation from out of hospital cardiac arrest. *J Am Coll Cardiol.* 2012;60:21–7.
14. Pell JP, Sivel JM, et al. Presentation, management and outcome of out-of-hospital-cardiac arrest: comparison by underlying aetiology. *Heart.* 2003;89:839–42.
15. Hess EP, Campbell RL, White RD, et al. Epidemiology, trends, and outcome of out-of-hospital-cardiac arrest of non-cardiogenic origin. *Resuscitation.* 2007;72:200–6.
16. Deasy C, Bray JE, et al. Out-of-hospital cardiac arrest in young adults in melbourne, australia: adding coronial data to a cardiac arrest registry. *Resuscitation.* 2011;82:1302–6.
17. Bottiger BW, Arntz HR, Chamberlain DA, et al. Thrombolysis during resuscitation for out-of-hospital cardiac arrest. *N Engl J Med.* 2008;359(25):2651–62.
18. Konstantinides SV. Massive pulmonary embolism: what level of aggression? *Semin Respir Crit Care Med.* 2008;29:47–55.
19. Meneveau N, et al. Management of unsuccessful thrombolysis in acute massive pulmonary embolism. *Chest.* 2006;129:1043–50.
20. Schneider A, Bottiger BW, Popp E. Cerebral resuscitation after cardiocirculatory arrest. *Anesth Analg.* 2009;108(3):971–979.
21. Polderman KH. Mechanisms of action, physiological effects, and complications of hypothermia. *Crit Care Med.* 2009;37(suppl 7):S186–S202.
22. Bernard SA, Gray TW, Buist MD, et al. Treatment of comatose survivors of out-of-hospital cardiac arrest with induced hypothermia. *N Engl J Med.* 2002;346:557–563.
23. HACA Group. Mild therapeutic hypothermia to improve the neurologic outcome after cardiac arrest. *N Engl J Med.* 2002;346:549–556.
24. Zobel C, Adler C, et al. Mild therapeutic hypothermia in cardiogenic shock syndrome. *Crit Care Med.* 2012;40:1715–1723.
25. Hovdeness J, Laake JH, Aaberge L, et al. Therapeutic hypothermia after out-of-hospital cardiac arrest: experiences with patients treated with percutaneous coronary intervention and cardiogenic shock. *Acta Anaesthesiol Scand.* 2007;51:137–142.
26. Wolfrum S, Pierau C, Radke PW, et al. Mild therapeutic hypothermia in patients after out-of-hospital cardiac arrest due to acute ST-segment elevation myocardial infarction undergoing immediate percutaneous coronary intervention. *Crit Care Med.* 2008;36:1780–1786.
27. Kuboyama K, Safar P, Radovsky A, et al. Delay in cooling negates the beneficial effect of mild resuscitative cerebral hypothermia after cardiac arrest in dogs: a prospective, randomized study. *Crit Care Med.* 1993;21:1348–1358.
28. Nozari A, Safar P, Stezoski SW, et al. Critical time window for intra-arrest cooling with cold saline flush in a dog model of cardiopulmonary resuscitation. *Circulation.* 2006;113:2690–2696.
29. Nielsen N, Wetterslev J, Cronberg T, et al. Targeted Temperature Management at 33°C versus 36°C after Cardiac Arrest. *New England Journal of Medicine* 2013;369:2197–2206.
30. Rajek A, Greif R, Sessler DI, et al. Core cooling by central venous infusion of ice-cold (4 degrees C and 20 degrees C) fluid: isolation of core and peripheral thermal compartments. *Anesthesiology.* 2000;93:629–637.
31. Kim F, Olsufka M, Longstreth WT Jr, et al. Pilot randomized clinical trial of prehospoital induction of mild hypothermia in out-of-hospital cardiac arrest patients with a rapid infusion of 4 degrees C normal saline. *Circulation.* 2007;115:3064–3070.
32. Jacobshagen C, Pax A, Unsold BW, et al. Effects of large volume, ice-cold intravenous fluid infusion on respiratory function in cardiac arrest survivors. *Resuscitation.* 2009;80:1223–1228.
33. Polderman KH, Rijnsburger ER, Peerdeman SM, et al. Induction of hypothermia in patients with various types of neurologic injury with use of large volumes of ice-cold intravenous fluid. *Crit Care Med.* 2005;33:2744–2751.
34. Weisser J, Martin J, Bisping E, et al. Influence of mild hypothermia on myocardial contractility and circulatory function. *Basic Res Cardiol.* 2001;96:198–205.
35. Polderman KH, Peerdeman SM, Girbes AR. Hypophosphatemia and hypomagnesemia induced by cooling in patients with severe head injury. *J Neurosurg.* 2001;94:697–705.
36. Schaller B, Graf R. Hypothermia and stroke: the pathophysiological background. *Pathophysiology.* 2003;10:7–35.

37. Soliman HM, Mercan D, Lobo SS, et al. Development of ionized hypomagnesemia is associated with higher mortality rates. *Crit Care Med.* 2003;31:1082–1087.
38. Schefold JC, Storm C, Joerres A, et al. Mild therapeutic hypothermia after cardiac arrest and the risk of bleeding in patients with acute myocardial infarction. *Int J Cardiol.* 2009;132:387–391.
39. Nielsen N, Hovdenes J, Nilsson F, et al. Outcome, timing and adverse events in therapeutic hypothermia after out-of-hospital cardiac arrest. *Acta Anaesthesiol Scand.* 2009;53:926–934.
40. Badjatia N, Strongilis E, Gordon E, et al. Metabolic impact of shivering during therapeutic temperature modulation: the Bedside Shivering Assessment Scale. *Stroke.* 2008;39:3242–3247.
41. Alroughani R, Javidan M, Qasem A, et al. Non-convulsive status epilepticus; the rate of occurrence in a general hospital. *Seizure.* 2009;18:38–42.
42. Legriel S, Bruneel F, Sediri H, et al. Early EEG monitoring for detecting post-anoxic status epilepticus during therapeutic hypothermia: a pilot study. *Neurocrit Care.* 2009;11:338–344.
43. Towne AR, Waterhouse EJ, Boggs JG, et al. Prevalence of nonconvulsive status epilepticus in comatose patients. *Neurology.* 2000;54:340–345.
44. Oddo M, Carrera E, Claassen J, et al. Continuous electroencephalography in the medical intensive care unit. *Crit Care Med.* 2009;37:2051–2056.
45. Kjaergaard B, et al. Extra-corporeal life support makes advanced radiologic examination and cardiac interventions possible in patients with cardiac arrest. *Resuscitation.* 2011;82:623–626.
46. Hashiba K, et al. Percutaneous cardiopulmonary support (PCPS) in pulmonary embolism with cardiac arrest. *Resuscitation.* 2012;83;183–187.
47. Sung K, et al. Improved survival after cardiac arrest using emergent autopriming percutaneous cardiopulmonary support. *Ann Thorac Surg.* 2006;82:651–656.

SECTION 6
Neurological Critical Care

20

Ischemic Stroke

Mohamed Teleb and Paul Singh

BACKGROUND

Stroke is the fourth leading cause of mortality in the United States and incurs an estimated cost of 38.6 billion dollars anually.[1] Although the overall mortality from this disease has declined over the last decade, 50% of individuals who suffer a stroke at an age of >65 will die within 5 years.[1] Traditionally a clinical diagnosis, evaluation of stroke is now highly reliant on imaging. While new multimodality radiologic technologies are being developed to determine brain ischemia and penumbral tissue, the most important imaging for acute care remains the noncontrast computed tomography (CT) of the head. With this in mind, this chapter reviews both the pathogenesis and clinical manifestation of stroke as well as a basic approach to its image interpretation in the acute setting.

HISTORY AND PHYSICAL EXAM

Patient History

Obtaining a quick and accurate history in patients with stroke facilitates optimal clinical care. It is essential to determine the exact time at which brain ischemia started. Because this can be a difficult task unless bystanders are present at the onset of symptoms, the practitioner should rely on the time of "last seen normal," as opposed to when the patient was first witnessed having symptoms. For example, if a patient were to wake up with symptoms of a stroke, his or her time last seen normal would be the night before when he went to sleep. This information is required to determine a patient's eligibility to receive specific interventions, including intravenous tissue plasminogen activator (IV tPA) or endovascular intra-arterial (IA) thrombolysis/thrombectomy. In addition to the time of onset and duration of symptoms, delineating the progression of neurologic findings is also important. Most vascular events result in immediate deficits; exceptions to this include stuttering transient ischemic attacks and flow related symptoms caused by an intracranial or extracranial stenosis.

The emergency provider should also attempt to identify nonstroke conditions, referred to as "stroke mimics" that can produce focal neurologic deficits (Table 20.1).

TABLE 20.1 Stroke Mimics and Their Features

Stroke Mimics	Comment/Features of Mimics
Seizure	Postictal Todd paralysis or generalized tonic–clonic can be confused with a basilar stroke
Migraine headache	Headaches may come after onset of focal neurologic symptoms (e.g., hemiparesis, aphasia, visual field cuts)
Syncope	Usually associated with hypotension or cardiac arrhythmia. Other brainstem findings, such as focal cranial nerve deficits, can help with identification of possible vertebral basilar insufficiency
Hypoglycemia	May produce a focal weakness. History of diabetes mellitus should raise concern. A glucose level should always be obtained in any patient with stroke-like symptoms
Metabolic encephalopathy	Confusion, slurred speech, or aphasia. The onset of symptoms may be more gradual when compared to an actual stroke
Drug overdose	Obtundation related to drug toxicity can be confused for posterior circulation strokes or a catastrophic intracranial bleed. Physical exam—especially pupillary size and reactivity and deep painful stimuli—and vital signs may be helpful. Pinpoint pupils can represent opioid intoxication, whereas asymmetric, nonreactive pupils raise suspicion for elevated ICP/cerebral herniation. Bradycardia in the setting of hypertension (Cushing response) also suggests elevated ICPs
Herpes encephalitis	HSV encephalitis affects the temporal lobes, leading to confusion, aphasia, and visual field cuts. The presence of other signs of CNS infection, including fever and progression of symptoms, should help distinguish from stroke
Subdural hematoma	May present with confusion and focal neurologic symptoms corresponding to the compressed hemisphere. Seen in elderly with minor trauma. Imaging rules this out
PNC	PNC is usually not sudden in onset unless witnessed postsurgically (OR positioning), or noted following awaking with symptoms (slept on an arm). Weakness and/or numbness are in a particular peripheral nerve distribution
Bell palsy	Patients may have sudden weakness in eye closure and in their forehead muscles, for example, raising the eyebrow (peripheral CN 7 features), although this can appear slowly in some Bell palsy patients. Recent infection/trauma can be the etiology of a peripheral CN 7 deficit. A peripheral CN 7 palsy can also occur with pontine stroke, but other CNs are usually involved (e.g., CN 6)
BPPV	Symptoms include vertigo, nausea, vomiting, and a sense of imbalance, usually with turning of the head in one direction. In a brainstem stroke, other focal CN deficits such as diplopia, facial palsies, or hemifacial sensory deficits should be present
Conversion disorder	Patients will often present with unilateral weakness, sensory deficits, or speech difficulties. Whether these symptoms are organic or psychiatric is often difficult to determine. Inquire about psychiatric history and recent drug use. Once stroke has been ruled out, treat the symptoms as if they are organic with positive reinforcement (PT/OT evaluations)
Reactivation of old stroke	Sudden onset of a focal neurologic deficit. The patient will have a clinical or radiographic history of stroke. Can occur with fatigue or any metabolic derangement

BPPV, benign paroxysmal positional vertigo; PNC, peripheral nerve compression; CN, cranial nerves ; HSV, herpes simplex virus; ICP, intracranial pressure; CPP, cerebral perfusion pressure.

A thorough history and exam can help distinguish brain infarction from stroke mimics, and, in the event of a true central ischemic process, help pinpoint the specific etiology of the neurologic insult. Stroke symptoms accompanied by severe chest pain radiating to neck are suggestive of a myocardial infarction with associated cardiac emboli. Stroke symptoms accompanied by severe chest and back pain can suggest an aortic dissection with extension into the carotid or the vertebral arteries. Such combinations

TABLE 20.2 Pertinent History in Stroke Patients

HPI	Time of onset, accompanying symptoms (headache, seizures), evolution of symptoms (sudden, gradual), accompanying chest pain, back pain, rhythmic movements, and eye deviation
PMH	Prior intracerebral hemorrhage, ischemic stroke, head trauma, myocardial infarction, or atrial fibrillation
PSH	Recent or major surgeries, arterial punctures in noncompressible sites
Allergies	Contrast, aspirin, heparin, anticoagulants
Medications	Anticoagulant, antiplatelet, antihypertensive

HPI, history of present illness; PMH, past medical history; PSH, past surgical history.

of findings not only help identify a specific pathologic process but also may dramatically alter patient management by avoiding hemorrhagic complications of thrombolytic therapy in patients with specific contraindications, for example, an intracerebral tumor.

The diagnosis of stroke mimics can often be difficult during the acute phase. Studies show anywhere between 3% and 16% of patients treated with tPA are stroke mimics.[2,3] Fortunately, multiple studies have reported stroke mimics treated with tPA to have no increased rate of symptomatic intracranial bleeds.[3] The pathogenesis of intracranial hemorrhage after tPA is secondary to reperfusion hemorrhage into a region of infarcted brain tissue. Because stroke mimics do not have actual brain ischemia, they are less likely to have hemorrhage after tPA. The exception to this is patients with intracranial tumors, but these are typically visualized on a CT scan prior to IV tPA administration.

In addition to accompanying symptoms, the patient's past medical and surgical history needs to be quickly established, focusing on exclusion and inclusion criteria for administration of IV tPA. IV tPA is the current standard of care for patients who present within 3 hours of symptoms and is recommended in patients up to 4.5 hours if they meet the criteria (Table 20.2).[4]

Physical Exam

Assessment of the ABCs (airway, breathing, circulation) and vital signs may also provide clues as to the nature and cause of the stroke (whether hemorrhagic or ischemic). Tachycardia with an irregular heartbeat may support a cardioembolic ischemic stroke. Elevated blood pressure in the setting of headache, nausea/vomiting, and obtundation is more likely to be indicative of a hemorrhagic stroke, although posterior circulation strokes (e.g., a basilar artery occlusion) can present similarly. Once the ABCs are stabilized, a rapid neurologic examination using the National Institutes of Health Stroke Scale (NIHSS) should be obtained (Table 20.3).[5,6]

The NIHSS is easy to perform, helps predict short-term and long-term outcomes, and can help identify large-vessel occlusion (LVO) strokes.[7,8] The scale has been demonstrated to be reliable and reproducible, but proper use requires training and certification, which can be obtained through the American Stroke Association's Web site (www.strokeassociation.org).[9,10]

Common clinical syndromes ascribed to specific subtypes of stroke are listed in Table 20.4.[11–13] While not an exhaustive list, familiarity with these signs and symptoms

TABLE 20.3 NIHSS (National Institutes of Health Stroke Scale)

1a. Level of consciousness	0 = Alert 1 = Not alert, arousable 2 = Not alert, obtunded 3 = Unresponsive
1b. Questions	0 = Answers both correctly 1 = Answers one correctly 2 = Answers neither correctly
1c. Commands	0 = Performs both tasks correctly 1 = Performs one task correctly 2 = Performs neither task
2. Gaze	0 = Normal 1 = Partial gaze palsy 2 = Total gaze palsy
3. Visual fields	0 = No visual loss 1 = Partial hemianopsia 2 = Complete hemianopsia 3 = Bilateral hemianopsia
4. Facial palsy	0 = Normal 1 = Minor paralysis 2 = Partial paralysis 3 = Complete paralysis
5a. Left motor arm	0 = No drift 1 = Drift before 10 s 2 = Falls before 10 s 3 = No effort against gravity 4 = No movement
5b. Right motor arm	Scored in same fashion as left arm
6a. Left motor leg	0 = No drift 1 = Drift before 5 s 2 = Falls before 5 s 3 = No effort against gravity 4 = No movement
6b. Right motor leg	Scored in same fashion as right arm
7. Ataxia	0 = Absent 1 = One limb 2 = Two limbs
8. Sensory	0 = Normal 1 = Mild loss 2 = Severe loss
9. Language	0 = Normal 1 = Mild aphasia 2 = Severe aphasia 3 = Mute or global aphasia
10. Dysarthria	0 = Normal 1 = Mild 2 = Severe
11. Extinction/inattention	0 = Normal 1 = Mild 2 = Severe

Available at www.ninds.nih.gov/doctors/NIH_Stroke_Scale.pdf

TABLE 20.4 Common Signs and Symptoms by Type of Stroke

Vessel/Type of Stroke	Signs and Symptoms
MCA	Contralateral loss of strength and sensation in the face, arm, and, to a lesser extent, leg. Aphasia if dominant hemisphere; neglect if nondominant
ACA	Contralateral loss of strength and sensation in the leg and, to a lesser extent, arm
PCA	Contralateral visual field deficit. Possibly confusion and aphasia if dominant hemisphere. Left-sided gives alexia without agraphia
Basilar	Various combinations of limb ataxia, dysarthria, dysphagia, facial and limb weakness and sensory loss (may be bilateral), pupillary asymmetry, disconjugate gaze, visual field loss, decreased responsiveness. Also visual hallucinations, dreamlike behavior, agitated behavior, and amnesia
SCA	Dysarthria and limb ataxia
AICA	Gait and limb ataxia, dysfunction of ipsilateral CN-5, 7, and 8. Acute hearing loss with ataxia
PICA	Vertigo, nausea, vomiting, gait ataxia
Vertebral	Ipsilateral limb ataxia and Horner syndrome, crossed sensory loss, vertigo, dysphagia, hoarseness (lateral medullary/Wallenberg syndrome)
Penetrating arteries (lacunar syndromes) MCA penetrators (internal capsule/corona radiata) Basilar penetrators (ventral pons)	Contralateral hemiparesis alone (pure motor stroke) or contralateral hemiparesis + ataxia out of proportion to weakness (ataxic–hemiparesis); no cortical signs
PCA penetrators (thalamus)	Contralateral sensory loss alone (pure sensory stroke); no cortical signs

MCA, middle cerebral artery; ACA, anterior cerebral artery; PCA, posterior cerebral artery; SCA, superior cerebellar artery; AICA, anterior inferior cerebellar artery; PICA, posterior inferior cerebellar artery.
From Levine J, Johnston K. Diagnosis of stroke and stroke mimics in the emergency setting. *Continuum Lifelong Learning Neurol.* 2008; Jones HR, Srinivasan J, Allam GJ, et al. *Netter's Neurology.* W. B. Saunders Co; 2011; Uchino K, Pary J, Grotta J. *Acute Stroke Care.* 2011.

can help providers localize the region of ischemia. Stroke patients often present with dramatic findings, such as hemiparesis; in isolation, however, weakness can be representative of both large- and small-territory strokes. The presence of cortical signs, such as aphasia, visual field deficits, or a gradient in weakness (face and arm greater than leg involvement), suggests a LVO that may eventually require endovascular therapy. The presence of cranial nerve deficits or cerebellar findings, such as ataxia or dysmetria, may help localize a stroke to the brainstem or posterior fossa.[14]

PATHOGENESIS

Ischemic stroke is commonly classified according to the following subtypes: small-vessel atherosclerosis, large-artery atherosclerosis, cardioembolic, cryptogenic, or other.[15] Other known causes include arterial dissections, infections, trauma, sickle cell disease, and hypercoagulable states. A patient's particular diagnostic course will depend in part on his or her history of illness and clinical presentation. For example, a patient who presents with heart palpitations followed by stroke symptoms will require a cardiac evaluation for arrhythmias; whereas a patient with stroke symptoms who has sustained neck trauma would need vascular imaging of the chest, neck, and head to identify potential arterial dissections.

DIAGNOSTIC EVALUATION

The initial ED diagnostic workup should consist of a focused history, exam, labs, and imaging. Per the American Heart Association/American Stroke Association (AHA/ASA) guidelines, only a noncontrast CT of the head is required, even though advanced imaging, if available, may help delineate the stroke.[4] The rationale for this recommendation is that a noncontrast head CT is sufficient to determine a patient's eligibility for IV tPA, provided that clinical criteria are already met. Although other imaging such as CT angiogram or MRI may ultimately be required, the decision to give tPA should be made immediately following noncontrast CT so as to avoid delays that can lessen benefit from IV tPA (Table 20.5).

Recommended initial orders and labs include (per AHA/ASA guidelines)

- Vital Signs
- ECG and cardiac enzymes
- INR, PT, PTT, BMP, CBC, troponin, urinalysis, and toxicology (urine studies help in identification of stroke mimics such as hypo/hyperglycemia, DKA, infection, metabolic encephalopathy)
- Noncontrast CT of the head

The noncontrast CT allows a radiologist to distinguish hemorrhagic from ischemic stroke; the relative acuity of an ischemic stroke; the presence of mass effect or imminent midline shift that would necessitate more aggressive treatment; and the degree of brain parenchyma that is unsalvageable. In patients with stroke onset >3 hours, a hypodensity of greater than or equal to one-third of middle cerebral artery (MCA) territory excludes use of tPA. For ischemic stroke, the emergency physician should be aware of the following radiographic findings indicative of a stroke (Fig. 20.1); these findings may sway the decision to administer IV tPA based on the presumed degree of infarcted brain tissue:

- A hyperdense MCA
- Blurring of the insular ribbon
- Sulcal effacement
- Blurring of the gray–white junction, especially of the deep structures of the caudate, internal capsule, and putamen

TABLE 20.5 Diagnostic Approach by Time Line

Time[a]	Action
0–10 min	Check vital signs Get history: symptoms, time of onset, recent surgeries Draw labs: Glucose, INR/PTT, BMP, CBC, troponin
10–20 min	Review vital signs again Conduct neurologic exam and record the NIHSS score
20–40 min	Acute imaging—noncontrast CT, CTA, CTP, or MRI[b]
40–60 min	Decide on treatment course in consultation with neurology service

[a]This is a relative time scale and defines the maximum allotted time to complete each step.
[b]Imaging will differ depending on the institution. Only CT of the head is required.

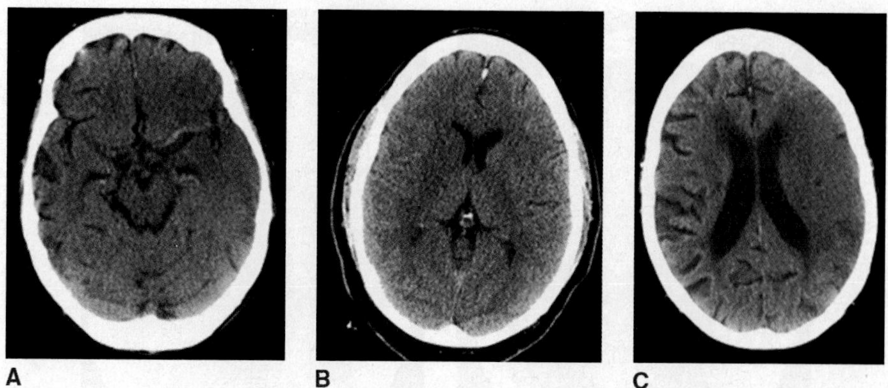

FIGURE 20.1 **A:** A hyperdense left MCA with blurring of the insular ribbon and sulcal effacement of the left temporal lobe. **B:** Blurring of the gray–white junction involving the right caudate, internal capsule, and putamen. **C:** Sulcal effacement and blurring of the gray–white junction over the entire left MCA territory.

In addition to the subtle findings above, one should evaluate for midline shift, masses/mass effect, blood (in the brain or at the base of the skull), cerebral edema, or herniation. A frequently used tool for the evaluation of ischemic stroke on a head CT is the Alberta Stroke Program Early CT Score (ASPECTS).[16] The ASPECTS tool evaluates 10 commonly viewed areas of the MCA territory. Every area of hypodensity is subtracted from 10; a lower composite score indicates more areas of infarcted brain. This tool can be used to evaluate functional outcome (a score of 7 or less associated with poor functional outcome) as well as to estimate the size of any MCA stroke (Fig. 20.2).

MANAGEMENT GUIDELINES

The treatment of acute ischemic stroke centers on urgent revascularization of occluded vessels or augmentation of collateral cerebral blood flow in order to minimize brain infarct size and salvage penumbra. Equally important is the provision of supportive care to minimize stroke complications, including intracerebral hemorrhage, increasing stroke size, and brain herniation, as well as identification of concomitant disease processes such as myocardial infarction, aortic dissection, aspiration pneumonia, or drug intoxication. Management aims to provide appropriate treatment, and to proceed as rapidly as possible to improve neurologic outcome with an acceptably low risk of complications. A decision tree for the management of ischemic stroke is provided in Figure 20.3. Guidelines for standard medical management are detailed in Table 20.6. Potential complications of stroke therapy and their management are reviewed in Table 20.7. Additional standard ischemic stroke protocols, criteria, and order sets are provided in Table 20.8.[4,17–19] Indications and contraindications to IV tPA are listed in Table 20.9.

Intravenous Tissue Plasminogen Activator (IV t-PA)

The most commonly asked questions regarding the acute management of ischemic stroke relate to the risks and benefits of IV tPA. Major clinical trials evaluating the efficacy of IV tPA include ECASS 3, NINDS 2, and IST 3.[20,21,32,33] In order to better

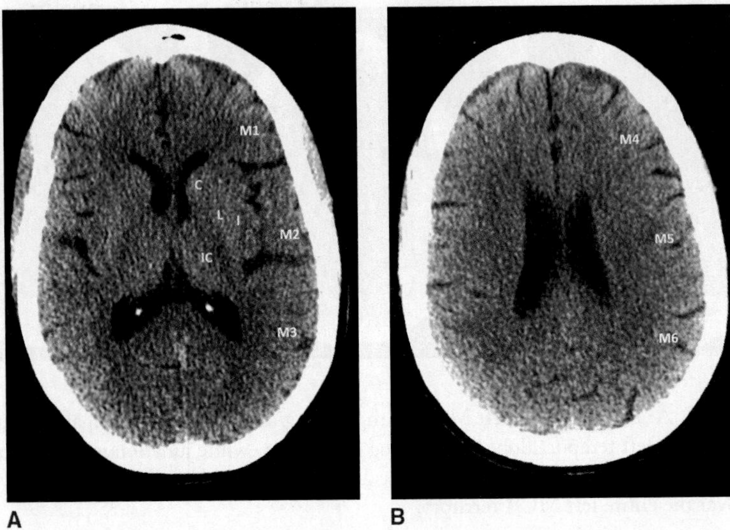

FIGURE 20.2 ASPECTS stroke regions (10 regions assessed). **(A)** Lower cross-sectional region of interest with deep structures. **(B)** Higher cross-sectional region of interest for cortex evaluation. C, caudate; L, lentiform nucleus; IC, internal capsule; I, insula; M1–6, corresponding regions of the MCA territory.

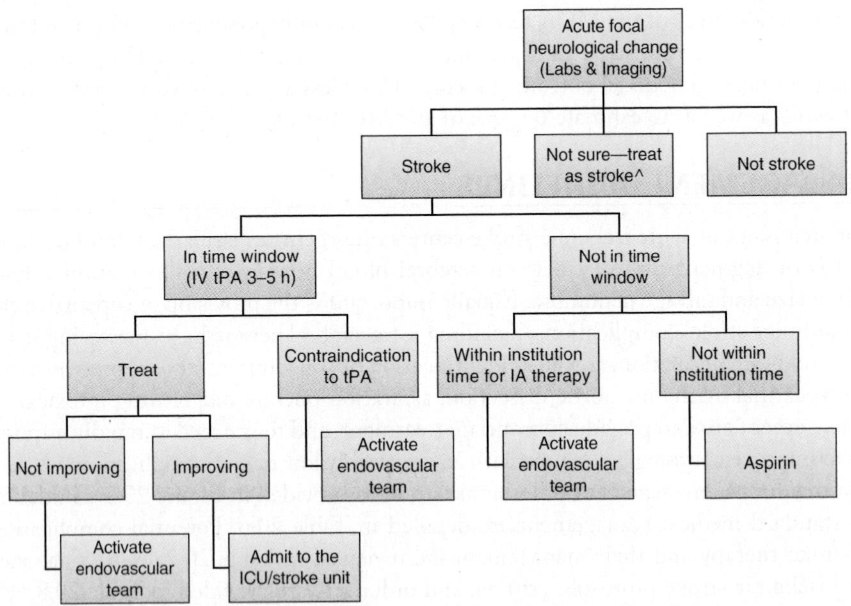

FIGURE 20.3 Acute-Stroke Flow Chart. ^Meta-analysis of stroke mimics treated with IV tPA revealed no adverse events (involve stroke team in decision). From Chang J, Teleb M, Yang JP, et al. A model to prevent fibrinolysis in patients with stroke mimics. *J Stroke Cerebrovasc Dis.* 2011;21(8):839–843. doi:10.1016/j.jstrokecerebrovasdis.2011.04.018; Tsivgoulis G, Alexandrov AV, Chang J, et al. Safety and outcomes of intravenous thrombolysis in stroke mimics: a 6-year, single-care center study and a pooled analysis of reported series. *Stroke.* 2011;42(6):1771–1774. doi:10.1161/STROKEAHA.110.609339

TABLE 20.6 Medical Management of Ischemic Stroke

Management	Indication	Guidelines/Recommendations
Intravenous (IV) tPA	Ischemic stroke within 3 or 4.5 h if meets ECASS 3 criteria.[a] Given as 0.9 mg/kg, maximum dose 90 mg, 10% as bolus and rest over 1 h	Class I, Level of Evidence A and B[a]
Intra-arterial (IA) tPA	Major stroke of <6h duration due to occlusions of the MCA and are not otherwise candidates for IV tPA	Class I, Level of Evidence B
IA mechanical thrombectomy	Large MCA stroke <8 h	Class IIb, Level of Evidence B
Antiplatelet	All ischemic stroke unless otherwise contraindicated. Oral administration of aspirin (initial dose 325 mg) within 24–48 h	Class I, Level of Evidence A
Anticoagulation	Not indicated. More bleeds in all trials	Class III, Level of Evidence A
Acute blood pressure/ maintain CPP	If the patient does not receive tPA, BP goal should be <220/120 in order to maintain brain perfusion and to reverse and preserve hypoxic brain tissue If the patient receives tPA, BP goal should be <185/110 to decrease the risk of intracranial hemorrhage	Class I, Level of Evidence C Class I, Level of Evidence B
Hyper/hypoglycemia	Treat BG > 140 mg/dL consistently (goal 140–185). Nonrandomized studies showed worse recovery in patients with hyperglycemia Expert consensus, hypoglycemia should be treated when <60 mg/dL	Class IIa, Level of Evidence C Class I, Level of Evidence C
Airway/oxygenation/and aspiration precautions	Use supplemental oxygen if SpO_2 < 94%. Consider early intubation if the patient is not protecting his or her airway	Class I, Level of Evidence C
Cardiac monitoring for 24 h	Screen for atrial fibrillation and other potential cardiac arrhythmias that would necessitate urgent cardiac interventions, that is, rate/rhythm control and prompt anticoagulation	Class I, Level of Evidence B
Antipyretics	Fever. Attempt to identify and treat the source	Class I, Level of Evidence C

From Jauch EC, Saver JL, Adams HP, et al. Guidelines for the early management of patients with acute ischemic stroke: a guideline for healthcare professionals from the American Heart Association/American Stroke Association. *Stroke.* 2013;44(3):870–947. doi: 10.1161/STR.0b013e318284056a
[a]Age >80, combination of previous stroke and diabetes, NIHSS >25, >1/3 MCA infarct on CT are the exclusions for 3–4.5 h as these patients were not in trial. From Hacke W, Kaste M, Bluhmki E, et al. Thrombolysis with alteplase 3 to 4.5 hours after acute ischemic stroke. *N Engl J Med.* 2008;359(13):1317–1329. doi:10.1056/NEJMoa0804656.

TABLE 20.7 Potential Complications and Treatment of Stroke Therapy

Complication	To do	Guidelines/Recommendations
Post-tPA: headache, worsening exam, acute hypertension, nausea/vomiting	Stop tPA and obtain immediate CT of the head. If hemorrhagic conversion, proceed with your institution's tPA reversal protocol	Class I, Level of Evidence C
Angioedema	Occurs in 1.3%–5.1% of patients who receive IV tPA. Stabilize the airway and initiate treatment with ranitidine, diphenhydramine, methylprednisolone, and epinephrine as needed	Class I, Level of Evidence B
Cerebellar reperfusion hemorrhage/brainstem compression	Neurosurgical consult for occipital craniectomy or EVD. Life-saving technique with good outcomes	Class I, Level of Evidence B

TABLE 20.7 Potential Complications and Treatment of Stroke Therapy (*Continued*)

Complication	To do	Guidelines/Recommendations
Large MCA stroke with midline shift	Institute medical ICP reduction techniques if obtunded (head of bed at 30°, 1 g/kg of IV mannitol ±30-mL bolus of 23.4% hypertonic saline) Neurosurgical consult for possible hemicraniectomy. Hemicraniectomy can be a life-saving procedure when performed within 48 h of stroke in patients who are <60 y of age and present with an NIHSS < 25 Do not use steroids for edema	Class IIb, Level of Evidence C Class I, Level of Evidence B Class III, Level of Evidence A
Seizures	Treat rapidly with IV antiepileptic agents to prevent brain injury from prolonged seizures (e.g., IV phenytoin, levetiracetam, lacosamide)	Class I, Level of Evidence B
Acute hydrocephalus	Neurosurgical consult for placement of EVD	Class I, Level of Evidence C

From Jauch EC, Saver JL, Adams HP, et al. Guidelines for the early management of patients with acute ischemic stroke: a guideline for healthcare professionals from the American Heart Association/American Stroke Association. *Stroke.* 2013;44(3):870–947. doi: 10.1161/STR.0b013e318284056a
EVD, extraventricular drain.

TABLE 20.8 Important Ischemic Stroke Protocols, Criteria, and Order Sets

tPA Reversal Protocol[a]	Hemicraniectomy Inclusion Criteria[b]	Post-tPA Orders
• Stop tPA • Goal: fibrinogen level >100 mg/dL with cryoprecipitate • Type and cross • Check fibrinogen level immediately and every 6 h • Give 10–20 units cryoprecipitate before level returns (1 unit raises fibrinogen by 5–10 mg/dL; assume there is no fibrinogen and adjust dose when level is back) • Repeat cryoprecipitate if needed • May use fresh frozen plasma (FFP) if cryoprecipitate unavailable (1 unit of cryoprecipitate is made from one bag of FFP) • Maintain platelets > 50,000/μL • Activated factor VII is untested in this situation and should not be used • Neurosurgery consult	• Age 18–60 y • Clinical deficits suggestive of the MCA with an NIHSS > 15 • Decrease in the level of consciousness to a score of 1 or greater on item 1a of the NIHSS • CT with infarct of >50% of the MCA, with or without additional infarction in the ACA or PCA on the same side, or infarct volume >145 cm³ as shown on diffusion-weighted MRI • Inclusion within 45 h after onset • Written informed consent by the patient or a legal representative	• Neurologic checks and blood pressure q 15 min × 2 h, then q 30 min × 6 h, and then hourly for first 24 h. • Defer NG, Foley, arterial line for 24 h • CT scan at 24 h **Angioedema Treatment** • Epinephrine 0.5 mL via nebulizer or 0.3 mL of 0.1% solution subcutaneously (may repeat 2) • Diphenhydramine (Benadryl) 50 mg IV followed by 25 mg every 6 h × 4 • Methylprednisolone (Solumedrol) 100 mg IV; may follow with 20–80 mg IV daily for 3–5 d depending on the degree and course of angioedema • Famotidine 20 mg IV followed by 20 mg IV every 12 h × 2

[a]Consensus recommendations based on the AHA/ASA 2007 Guidelines. From Broderick J, Connolly S, Feldmann E, et al. Guidelines for the Management of Spontaneous Intracerebral Hemorrhage in Adults: 2007 Update: a guideline from the American Heart Association/American Stroke Association Stroke Council, High Blood Pressure Research Council, and the Quality of Care and Outcomes in Research Interdisciplinary Working Group: the American Academy of Neurology affirms the value of this guideline as an educational tool for neurologists. *Stroke.* 2007;38(6):2001–2023. doi:10.1161/STROKEAHA.107.183689; Morgenstern LB, Hemphill JC, Anderson C, et al. Guidelines for the Management of Spontaneous Intracerebral Hemorrhage: a guideline for healthcare professionals from the American Heart Association/American Stroke Association. *Stroke.* 2010;41(9):2108–2129. doi:10.1161/STR.0b013e3181ec611b
[b]Evidence from Pooled Analysis of Hemicraniectomy Trials. From Vahedi K, Hofmeijer J, Juettler E, et al. Early decompressive surgery in malignant infarction of the middle cerebral artery: a pooled analysis of three randomised controlled trials. *Lancet Neurol.* 2007;6(3):215–222. doi:10.1016/S1474-4422(07)70036-4.
MCA, middle cerebral artery, ACA, anterior cerebral artery, PCA, posterior cerebral artery, hours (hours), tPA, tissue plasminogen activator.

TABLE 20.9 Indications and Contraindications for IV tPA

Indications	Contraindications
• Diagnosis of ischemic stroke causing measurable neurologic deficit • Onset of symptoms <3 h before beginning treatment • Aged ≥18 y **Relative Contraindications[a]** • Only minor or rapidly improving stroke symptoms (clearing spontaneously) • Pregnancy • Seizure at onset with postictal residual neurologic impairments • Major surgery or serious trauma within previous 14 d • Recent gastrointestinal or urinary tract hemorrhage (within previous 21 d) • Recent acute myocardial infarction (within previous 3 mo)	• Significant head trauma or prior stroke in previous 3 mo • Symptoms suggest subarachnoid hemorrhage • Arterial puncture at a noncompressible site in previous 7 d • History of previous intracranial hemorrhage • Intracranial neoplasm, arteriovenous malformation, or aneurysm • Recent intracranial or intraspinal surgery • Elevated blood pressure (systolic >185 mm Hg or diastolic >110 mm Hg) • Active internal bleeding • Acute bleeding diathesis, including but not limited 1. To Platelet count <100 000/mm³ 2. Heparin received within 48 h, resulting in abnormally elevated aPTT greater than the upper limit of normal 3. Current use of anticoagulant with INR > 1.7 or PT > 15 s 4. Current use of direct thrombin inhibitors or direct factor Xa inhibitors with elevated sensitive laboratory tests (such as aPTT, INR, platelet count, ECT, TT, or appropriate factor Xa activity assays) • Blood glucose concentration <50 mg/dL (2.7 mmol/L) • CT demonstrates multilobar infarction (hypodensity >1/3 cerebral hemisphere) **Additional Exclusions 3–4.5 h** • Age > 80 y • Combined history of diabetes and prior stroke • Any use of anticoagulation regardless of INR • NIHSS > 25 or CT with >1/3 MCA territory hypodensity

[a]Under some circumstances, patients may receive fibrinolytic therapy despite one or more relative contraindications. Consider risk to benefit of IV tPA carefully if any the relative contraindications are present. Based on the 2013 AHA/ASA Guidelines. From Jauch EC, Saver JL, Adams HP, et al. Guidelines for the early management of patients with acute ischemic stroke: a guideline for healthcare professionals from the American Heart Association/American Stroke Association. *Stroke.* 2013;44(3):870–947. doi: 10.1161/STR.0b013e318284056a

understand the results of these trials, it is important to recognize the outcome parameters being measured. The modified Rankin Scale (mRS) is a 6-point functional outcome parameter that ranges from no disability (0) to death (6). It is typically obtained 90 days after a patient has a stroke. The NIHSS, which is not a functional outcome scale but rather a 42-point measure of neurologic deficit, is more valuable during the initial evaluation. There is some controversy regarding these IV tPA trials, because in none of them were NIHSS scores at 24 hours different following IV tPA. At 3 months, however, the NIHSS and mRS demonstrated a significant benefit in patients treated within the 3-hour time window. These benefits were replicated in the 3- to 4.5-hour time window in the ECASS 3 trial. Importantly, earlier trials that extended IV tPA therapy to 6 hours revealed no difference in outcome and potential harm, and a 2010 meta-analysis of the ECASS, ATLANTIS, NINDS 2, and EPITHET trials demonstrated the same findings (no difference/potential harm) for IV tPA given after 4.5 hours.[33] Because of this, it is imperative to determine the time of onset of a patient's symptoms as well as to abide by the contraindications to therapy. The following is a summary of IV tPA outcome data:

- In patients receiving IV tPA within a 3-hour window, there is an absolute increase of 13% (39% vs. 26%) and a relative increase of 50% in an excellent outcome (mRS 0 to 1) versus placebo. In patients receiving IV tPA at the 3- to 4.5-hour mark, there is an absolute increase of 7% and a relative increase of 12% for this same outcome. The percentage of

individuals with a bad outcome (mRS 4 to 5) or dead (mRS 6) is also reduced for patients in both windows, even if patients with hemorrhagic conversion are included.[20,34,35]
- The odds ratio of a good outcome is 1.7 (95% confidence interval [CI] 1.2 to 2.6) when treated with IV tPA within 3 hours and is 1.3 (95% CI 1.0 to 1.7) when treated from 3 to 4.5 hours.[20]
- For IV tPA given within the 3-hour window, the number needed to treat (NNT) is 3; for IV tPA given with within the 3- to 4.5-hour window, the NNT is 6.[34,35]
- For IV tPA given within the 3-hour window, the number needed to harm (NNH) is 33; for IV tPA given with within the 3- to 4.5-hour window, the NNH is 37.[34,35]
- The risk of hemorrhagic conversion after IV tPA is 6%.[20]

Endovascular Therapy

Intra-arterial tPA (IA-tPA) and mechanical thrombectomy (IA-thrombectomy) are two endovascular therapeutic options that may be considered in patients with large vessel occlusions and NIHSS ≥ 8. The latest trial of endovascular therapy, in which patients within the IV tPA time window received either IV tPA alone or IV tPA and an endovascular intervention, did not show a significant difference in the outcome.[31] This study, however, did not use advanced perfusion imaging to confirm a large vessel clot, and nearly 20% of cases proved to have no large vessel occlusion. In addition, the majority of devices used in this trial are no longer used because of their inferior recanalization rates compared to newer models. Improved recanalization rates with the Trevo and Solitaire devices[24,25] have lead to continued research—not available at the time of this publication—regarding the benefits of endovascular therapy in large vessel occlusion (SWIFT PRIME and POSITIVE Trials). At this time, IA-tPA and IA--thrombectomy cannot be considered standard of care, but may be considered for patients with an NIHSS ≥ 8 who are either not candidates for IV tPA or who show no improvement following IV tPA.

Large MCA Stroke

For patients with a large MCA stroke seen on CT (>1/3 of MCA), admission to the ICU and neurosurgical consultation for consideration of hemicraniectomy may be considered, provided family members favor aggressive care. Hemicraniectomy trials have universally shown a significant mortality benefit, but have not demonstrated consistent improvement in functional status.[19] In patients with large MCA strokes, if signs or symptoms of herniation are encountered in the ED, ICP management should be implemented (see Table 20.7), including definitive airway management. Other potential complications that can arise in this setting include seizures and acute hydrocephalus.

CONCLUSION

Ischemic stroke continues to increase in prevalence, and is the cause of considerable morbidity in the United States. Fortunately, advances in diagnosis and in the armamentarium of therapeutic options, such as IV tPA and endovascular therapy, make stroke a highly treatable disease in the acute care setting. The protocols reviewed in this chapter can help guide a rapid diagnostic workup and facilitate the time-sensitive interventions necessary to minimize death and disability from to this devastating disease.

LITERATURE TABLE

TRIAL	DESIGN	RESULT
IV tPA		
The National Institute of Neurological Disorders and Stroke rt-PA Stroke Study Group. *NEJM.* 1995[20] NINDS 2	Randomized, double-blind trial (RCT) of 333 patients comparing IV tPA vs. placebo	Ninety-day functional outcome significantly better for all four outcome measures (OR 1.7, 95% CI, 1.2–2.6; $p = 0.008$) despite symptomatic bleed (SB) rate of 6.4% vs. 0.6% ($p < 0.001$)
Hacke et al., *NEJM.* 2008[21] ECASS 3	RCT of 821 patients comparing IV tPA vs. placebo 3 to 4.5 h	More patients with favorable outcome in the tPA group (52.4% vs. 45.2%; OR 1.34; 95% CI, 1.02–1.76; $p = 0.04$). SB, 2.4% treatment vs. 0.2% control; ($p = 0.008$). No mortality difference
Sandercock et al., *Lancet.* 2012[32] IST 3	RCT of 3,035 patients comparing IV tPA vs. placebo 0–6 h	Alive and favorable outcome (Oxford Handicap Scale (0–1)) at 6 mo 24% in the intervention group vs. 21% in controls ($p = 0.018$). More deaths occurred between 7 d and 6 mo in tPA group, but both groups had the same mortality at 6 mo (27%)
Endovascular Therapy: IA-tPA and IA-Thrombectomy		
Furlan et al., *JAMA.* 1999[22] PROACT 2	Randomized, controlled, open-label trial with blinded follow-up of 180 patients comparing IA tPA vs. no treatment at 3 to 6 h	Forty percent in treatment group vs. 25% in control group had a mRS of 2 or less ($p = 0.04$). Recanalization occured in 66% of treatment group vs. 18% of control group ($p = 0.001$). SB 10% in treatment group vs. 2% in control ($p = 0.06$). No difference in mortality
Saver et al., *Lancet.* 2012[24] SWIFT	RCT of 113 patients comparing Solitaire Stent vs. Merci device for large stroke	Recanalization rate, neurologic outcome, and mortality at 3 mo all statistically better then Merci device by a landslide
Nogueira et al., *Lancet.* 2012[25] TREVO	RCT of 178 patients comparingTrevo Stent vs. Merci device for large clot stroke	Recanalization rate of 86% in Trevo vs. 60% in Merci group (OR 4.22, 95% CI 1·92–9·69; p superiority <0·0001)
Broderick et al., *NEJM.* 2013[31] IMS 3	RCT of 656 patients who received either IV tPA alone or IV tPA and endovascular therapy (IA-tPA or IA-thrombectomy) within 3 h of stroke onset	No difference in 90-day mRS. No difference in SB or mortality
Hemicraniectomy		
Vahedi et al., *Lancet Neurol.* 2007[19]	Pooled analysis of three RCT of medical treatment vs. craniectomy for large MCA strokes with in 48 h	Surgery improved survival with mRS ≤ 4 (NNT= 2) and survival with mRS ≤ 3 (NNT = 4), and survival irrespective of functional outcome (NNT = 2)
Vahedi et al., *Stroke.* 2007[29] DECIMAL	RCT of 38 patients comparing medical therapy vs. hemicraniectomy for MCA stroke with shift	Early decompressive craniectomy increased by more than half the number of patients with moderate disability and significantly reduced the mortality rate compared with medical therapy (absolute mortality reduction of 52.8% in surgical group compared to medical therapy, $p < 0.0001$).
Jüttler et al., *N Eng J Med.* 2014[30] DESTINY 2	Medical therapy vs. craniectomy for malignant MCA stroke in patients 60 y of age or older	Hemicraniectomy increased survival without severe disability among patients 61 y of age or older with a malignant middle-cerebral-artery infarction (38% surgery vs. 18% control, OR, 2.91; 95% CI, 1.06–7.49; $p = 0.04$)

CI, confidence interval; OR, odds ratio SB, symptomatic bleed NNT, number needed to treat.

REFERENCES

1. Go AS, Mozaffarian D, Roger VL, et al. Heart disease and stroke statistics—2013 update: a report from the American Heart Association. *Circulation.* 2013;127(1):e6–e245. doi: 10.1161/CIR.0b013e31828124ad
2. Chang J, Teleb M, Yang JP, et al. A model to prevent fibrinolysis in patients with stroke mimics. *J Stroke Cerebrovasc Dis.* 2011;21(8):839–843. doi: 10.1016/j.jstrokecerebrovasdis.2011.04.018
3. Tsivgoulis G, Alexandrov AV, Chang J, et al. Safety and outcomes of intravenous thrombolysis in stroke mimics: a 6-year, single-care center study and a pooled analysis of reported series. *Stroke.* 2011;42(6):1771–1774. doi: 10.1161/STROKEAHA.110.609339
4. Jauch EC, Saver JL, Adams HP, et al. Guidelines for the early management of patients with acute ischemic stroke: a guideline for healthcare professionals from the American Heart Association/American Stroke Association. *Stroke.* 2013;44(3):870–947. doi: 10.1161/STR.0b013e318284056a
5. Brott T, Adams HP, Olinger CP, et al. Measurements of acute cerebral infarction: a clinical examination scale. *Stroke.* 1989;20(7):864–870.
6. Lyden PD, Lu M, Levine SR, et al. A modified National Institutes of Health Stroke Scale for use in stroke clinical trials: preliminary reliability and validity. editorial comment: The NIH stroke scale: is simpler better? *Stroke.* 2001;32(6):1310–1317.
7. Adams H Jr, Davis PH, Leira EC, et al. Baseline NIH Stroke Scale score strongly predicts outcome after stroke. *Neurology.* 1999;53(1):126–131.
8. Fischer U, Arnold M, Nedeltchev K, et al. NIHSS score and arteriographic findings in acute ischemic stroke. *Stroke.* 2005;36(10):2121–2125.
9. Lyden P, Raman R, Liu L, et al. NIHSS training and certification using a new digital video disk is reliable. *Stroke.* 2005;36(11):2446–2449. doi: 10.1161/01.STR.0000185725.42768.92
10. Goldstein LB, Bertels C, Davis JN. Interrater reliability of the NIH stroke scale. *Arch Neurol.* 1989;46(6):660. doi: 10.1001/archneur.1989.00520420080026
11. Levine J, Johnston K. Diagnosis of stroke and stroke mimics in the emergency setting. *Continuum Lifelong Learning Neurol*; 2008:13–20.
12. Jones HR, Srinivasan J, Allam GJ, et al. *Netter's Neurology.* W. B. Saunders Co; 2011:496–517.
13. Uchino K, Pary J, Grotta J. *Acute Stroke Care.* 2011:3–6.
14. Searls DE, Pazdera L, Korbel E, et al. Symptoms and signs of posterior circulation ischemia in the New England Medical Center Posterior Circulation registry. *Arch Neurol.* 2012;69(3):346–351. doi: 10.1001/archneurol.2011.2083
15. The Publications Committee for the Trial of ORG 10172 in Acute Stroke Treatment (TOAST) Investigators. Low molecular weight heparinoid, ORG 10172 (danaparoid), and outcome after acute ischemic stroke: a randomized controlled trial. *JAMA.* 1998;279(16):1265–1272.
16. Pexman JH, Barber PA, Hill MD, et al. Use of the Alberta Stroke Program Early CT Score (ASPECTS) for assessing CT scans in patients with acute stroke. *AJNR Am J Neuroradiol.* 2001;22(8):1534–1542.
17. Broderick J, Connolly S, Feldmann E, et al. Guidelines for the Management of Spontaneous Intracerebral Hemorrhage in Adults: 2007 Update: a guideline from the American Heart Association/American Stroke Association Stroke Council, High Blood Pressure Research Council, and the Quality of Care and Outcomes in Research Interdisciplinary Working Group: the American Academy of Neurology affirms the value of this guideline as an educational tool for neurologists. *Stroke.* 2007;38(6):2001–2023. doi:10.1161/STROKEAHA.107.183689
18. Morgenstern LB, Hemphill JC, Anderson C, et al. Guidelines for the Management of Spontaneous Intracerebral Hemorrhage: a guideline for healthcare professionals from the American Heart Association/American Stroke Association. *Stroke.* 2010;41(9):2108–2129. doi:10.1161/STR.0b013e3181ec611b
19. Vahedi K, Hofmeijer J, Juettler E, et al. Early decompressive surgery in malignant infarction of the middle cerebral artery: a pooled analysis of three randomised controlled trials. *Lancet Neurol.* 2007;6(3):215–222. doi:10.1016/S1474-4422(07)70036-4
20. The National Institute of Neurological Disorders and Stroke rt-PA Stroke Study Group. Tissue plasminogen activator for acute ischemic stroke. *N Engl J Med.* 1995;333(24):1581–1588. doi:10.1056/NEJM199512143332401
21. Hacke W, Kaste M, Bluhmki E, et al. Thrombolysis with alteplase 3 to 4.5 hours after acute ischemic stroke. *N Engl J Med.* 2008;359(13):1317–1329. doi:10.1056/NEJMoa0804656
22. Furlan A, Higashida R, Wechsler L, et al. Intra-arterial prourokinase for acute ischemic stroke. The PROACT II study: a randomized controlled trial. Prolyse in Acute Cerebral Thromboembolism. *JAMA.* 1999;282(21):2003–2011

23. Smith WS, Sung G, Saver J, et al. Mechanical thrombectomy for acute ischemic stroke: final results of the Multi MERCI trial. *Stroke.* 2008;39(4):1205–1212. doi:10.1161/STROKEAHA.107.497115
24. Saver JL, Jahan R, Levy EI, et al. Solitaire flow restoration device versus the Merci Retriever in patients with acute ischaemic stroke (SWIFT): a randomised, parallel-group, non-inferiority trial. *Lancet.* 2012;380(9849):1241–1249. doi:10.1016/S0140-6736(12)61384-1
25. Nogueira RG, Lutsep HL, Gupta R, et al. Trevo versus Merci retrievers for thrombectomy revascularisation of large vessel occlusions in acute ischaemic stroke (TREVO 2): a randomised trial. *Lancet.* 2012;380(9849):1231–1240. doi:10.1016/S0140-6736(12)61299-9
26. Bath PM, Lindenstrom E, Boysen G, et al. Tinzaparin in acute ischaemic stroke (TAIST): a randomised aspirin-controlled trial. *Lancet.* 2001;358(9283):702–710
27. International Stroke Trial Collaborative Group. The International Stroke Trial (IST): a randomised trial of aspirin, subcutaneous heparin, both, or neither among 19435 patients with acute ischaemic stroke. *Lancet.* 1997;349(9065):1569–1581. doi:10.1016/S0140-6736(97)04011-7
28. Berge E, Abdelnoor M, Nakstad PH, et al. Low molecular-weight heparin versus aspirin in patients with acute ischaemic stroke and atrial fibrillation: a double-blind randomised study. HAEST Study Group. Heparin in acute embolic stroke trial. *Lancet.* 2000;355(9211):1205–1210.
29. Vahedi K, Vicaut E, Mateo J, et al. Sequential-design, multicenter, randomized, controlled trial of early decompressive craniectomy in malignant middle cerebral artery infarction (DECIMAL Trial). *Stroke.* 2007;38(9):2506–2517. doi:10.1161/STROKEAHA.107.485235
30. Jüttler E, Unterberg A, Woitzik J, et al. Hemicraniectomy in older patients with extensive middle-cerebral artery stroke. *N Engl J Med.* 2014;370(12):1091–100.
31. Broderick JP, Palesch YY, Demchuk AM, et al. Endovascular therapy after intravenous t-PA versus t-PA alone for stroke. *N Engl J Med.* 2013;368(10):893–903. doi:10.1056/NEJMoa1214300.
32. IST-3 Collaborative Group, Sandercock P, Wardlaw JM, Lindley RI, et al. The benefits and harms of intravenous thrombolysis with recombinant tissue plasminogen activator within 6 h of acute ischaemic stroke (the third international stroke trial [IST-3]): a randomised controlled trial. *Lancet.* 2012;379(9834):2352–2363. doi:10.1016/S0140-6736(12)60768-5
33. Lees KR, Bluhmki E, Kummer von R, et al. Time to treatment with intravenous alteplase and outcome in stroke: an updated pooled analysis of ECASS, ATLANTIS, NINDS, and EPITHET trials. *Lancet.* 2010;375(9727):1695–1703. doi:10.1016/S0140-6736(10)60491-6.
34. Saver JL. Number needed to treat estimates incorporating effects over the entire range of clinical outcomes: novel derivation method and application to thrombolytic therapy for acute stroke. *Arch Neurol.* 2004;61(7):1066–1070. doi:10.1001/archneur.61.7.1066
35. Saver JL, Gornbein J, Grotta J, et al. Number needed to treat to benefit and to harm for intravenous tissue plasminogen activator therapy in the 3- to 4.5-hour window: joint outcome table analysis of the ECASS 3 Trial. *Stroke.* 2009;40(7):2433–2437. doi:10.1161/STROKEAHA.108.543561

21

Subarachnoid and Intracerebral Hemorrhage

A.L.O. Manoel, Cappy Lay, D. Turkel-Parrella, Joshua Stillman, and Alberto Goffi

BACKGROUND

Cerebrovascular disease is the fourth leading cause of death in North America and accounts for approximately 130,000 deaths per year. Eighty percent of strokes are ischemic; the remaining 20% are hemorrhagic. Hemorrhagic stroke is subdivided into spontaneous intracranial hemorrhage (ICH) (15%) and subarachnoid hemorrhage (5%). Although less common, hemorrhagic stroke has markedly worse outcomes than ischemic stroke, including higher mortality and poorer functional outcomes. This chapter reviews the management of both spontaneous ICH and aneurysmal subarachnoid hemorrhage.

SPONTANEOUS INTRACEREBRAL HEMORRHAGE

The estimated incidence of spontaneous ICH worldwide is 24.6/100,000 person-years; 67,000 cases are reported annually in the United States.[1] Among strokes, ICH carries the poorest prognosis for survival and functional recovery, with high rates of early mortality (median 30-day mortality 40.4%, with 50% of these deaths occurring within the first 2 days); poor long-term survival[2]; and moderate to severe persistent deficits among survivors (<40% ever achieve independent function).[1] Recent population-based studies, however, suggest that more than half of all patients present with small ICHs, where excellent and timely medical care can have a powerful, positive impact on morbidity and mortality.[3] In fact, observational reports suggest that misguided prognostic pessimism has led to withdrawal of life support in patients who would have had acceptable clinical outcomes if properly managed.[4–6] ICH must therefore be considered an acute neurologic emergency with potential interventions that may significantly mitigate primary and subsequent secondary brain injury. The following discussion focuses exclusively on spontaneous (i.e., not traumatic) ICH.

Etiology and Risk Factors for ICH

An increased incidence of spontaneous ICH is associated with many underlying conditions, including hypertension, advanced age, and male gender. Other conditions associated with a poorer prognosis—after controlling for age and gender—include

TABLE 21.1 Etiology and Risk Factors for ICH

- Hypertensive vasculopathy (leading cause for ICH; >50% of all ICHs)
- Cerebral amyloid angiopathy (most common cause of lobar ICH, especially in the elderly)
- Coagulopathy (bleeding disorders, antithrombotic agents, thrombolytic therapy)
- Underlying structural lesions
  - Brain tumor
  - Vascular malformations
  - Hemorrhagic transformation of ischemic stroke
  - Infections (especially "mycotic" aneurysms, endocarditis-related septic cerebral emboli, aspergillosis, and herpes simplex encephalitis)
  - Primary or secondary CNS vasculitis (rare cause)
  - Moyamoya disease (rare cause)
- Dural venous sinus thrombosis (hemorrhagic venous infarction)
- Post-reperfusion (e.g., post–carotid endoarterectomy)
- Drugs (e.g., cocaine, amphetamines)

diabetes mellitus and a posterior fossa location (Table 21.1). The most common risk factor associated with spontaneous ICH is chronic arterial hypertension, which is present in approximately 75% of all patients with ICH and is associated with deep hemorrhage. The most common sites for hypertensive bleeds are deep perforator arteries in the pons, midbrain, thalamus, basal ganglia, and the deep cerebellar nuclei.[7] The lobar region is the second most common location for ICH (45%). It is more common in the elderly and is associated with cerebral amyloid angiopathy. Posterior fossa hemorrhage accounts for the remaining 10% of ICH and carries the worst prognosis.

Important risk factors for secondary ICH are myriad: coagulopathies (resulting from the use of antithrombotic or thrombolytic agents or from congenital or acquired factor deficiencies); systemic diseases such as thrombocytopenia; lymphoproliferative disorders; and hepatic and renal failure. The increasing use of oral anticoagulants, especially vitamin K inhibitors (such as warfarin) and newer oral anticoagulants (such as dabigatran), has resulted in a surge of coagulopathy-associated ICH in recent years and now accounts for more than 15% of all cases of ICH.[8] Other identified risk factors for ICH are advanced age, high alcohol intake, low cholesterol, and low triglyceride levels.[9,10] Socioeconomic and ethnic factors also appear to play a role in the prevalence of cerebral hemorrhage. ICH is twice as common in low-income and middle-income countries when compared with high-income countries; Asians, African Americans, and Hispanics are at higher risk than Caucasians.[11,12]

Causes of ICH include intracranial aneurysms and arteriovenous malformations (AVMs). Aneurysms most commonly rupture into the subarachnoid space but may also cause intraparenchymal hematomas. AVMs typically remain asymptomatic; however, ICH is their most common presentation (60% of AVMs present with intraparenchymal hemorrhage).[13] Hemorrhage due to an AVM may occur at any location within the cerebrum, brainstem, or cerebellum.

Brain tumors are a rare cause of intracerebral hemorrhage and account for <5% of all cases.[14] These may be primary tumors, most commonly glioblastoma multiforme (GBM) or oligodendrogliomas, or they may be metastatic brain tumors. Lung cancer, because of its high prevalence, is the most common source for brain metastases causing ICH. Other sources of brain metastasis causing ICH include melanoma, renal cell carcinoma, thyroid carcinoma, and choriocarcinoma.[15]

Less frequent causes of secondary ICH include infections, vasculitis, sinus venous thrombosis, carotid endarterectomy, Moyamoya disease, and drug use (e.g., cocaine). Finally, it should be noted that hemorrhagic transformation of acute ischemic stroke is relatively common, but in the absence of anticoagulation or thrombolytic therapy, is most often asymptomatic.

Mechanisms of Brain Injury

Acute neurologic injuries cause immediate damage (primary brain injury) and delayed damage (secondary brain injury). In ICH, primary injury is defined by local tissue destruction, which results from the rupture of a blood vessel into the brain parenchyma and ensuing ischemia and elevated intracranial pressure (ICP). In more than one-third of patients, substantial expansion of the hemorrhage is observed during the first few hours, resulting in further mechanical injury and early clinical deterioration.[16] It is thought that much of this initial damage cannot be reversed.

Primary brain injury initiates a cascade of biochemical events at the cellular level, including ischemic and apoptotic cell injury cascades, edema, and excitotoxicity, resulting in delayed and often progressive secondary brain injury. Unlike primary injury, secondary brain injury is considered preventable or reversible in the first hours to days following the initial hemorrhagic event. If present, conditions that decrease cerebral oxygen and glucose delivery (e.g., hypotension, hypoxia, anemia, and hypoglycemia) or increase cerebral metabolic demand (e.g., fever, seizures, and hyperglycemia) exacerbate secondary brain injury.[17] Minimization of secondary brain injury requires an early, aggressive, and well-structured approach to patient care and may result in improved long-term functional outcomes.

History and Physical Exam

Classically, ICH presents as a sudden onset of a focal neurologic deficit that evolves over minutes to hours. Clinical assessment, however, cannot reliably distinguish intracerebral hemorrhage from ischemic stroke.[18] Neurologic signs and symptoms can help indicate the location of the hemorrhage: (1) hemiplegia/hemiparesis, hemisensory loss, or homonymous hemianopsia suggest putaminal and thalamic ICH; (2) ataxia, vomiting, headache, and coma indicate brainstem compression in cerebellar bleeding; (3) deep coma, total paralysis, and pinpoint pupils suggest pontine bleeding.

Common symptoms for all types of ICH include headache (~40%), nausea and vomiting (~40% to 50%), and alteration in level of consciousness (LOC) (~50%), particularly for large ICH. Seizures occur in up to one-third of patients and often reflect an expanding hemorrhage, an underlying vascular or neoplastic etiology, or a lobar hemorrhage affecting cortical tissue.[19]

Blood pressure (BP) is typically elevated in ICH. Nonspecific EKG abnormalities are common (e.g., prolonged QT interval, depressed ST segments, flat or inverted T waves) and are thought to result from a centrally mediated release of catecholamines. Ventricular arrhythmias have also been described with brainstem compression.

Progression of neurologic deficits with deterioration of LOC during the first 48 hours after hospital admission has been described in 22% to 50% of patients with ICH.[20,21]

Diagnostic Evaluation

Recently published Emergency Neurological Life Support (ENLS) protocols[22] emphasize the following aspects of emergent clinical assessment for patients presenting with suspicion of ICH: (1) a concise and targeted assessment of the patient's clinical condition and (2) rapid and accurate diagnosis using neuroimaging to define ICH characteristics (i.e., location, volume, and possible etiology). Clinical assessment proceeds as follows:

1. *ABCs.* Immediate assessment and stabilization of airway, breathing, and circulation.
2. *Evaluate all vital signs, oxygen saturation, and blood glucose.* Almost any alteration in vital signs can contribute to secondary brain injury.
3. *Perform and document a standardized neurologic stroke severity scale during the initial encounter.* This allows for easy communication about the initial level of disability and for comparison over time. The most common rating scales include the National Institutes of Health Stroke Scale (NIHSS)—appropriate for patients who are awake or drowsy—and the Glasgow Coma Scale (GCS)—for the obtunded or comatose patient. Often, both scales are used.
4. *Evaluate for bleeding disorders.* Investigate current anticoagulant use and any history of coagulopathy. Determine when the last dose of antithrombotic medication was taken. Measure the platelets count, partial thromboplastin time (PTT), and international normalized ratio (INR).
5. *Perform frequent neurologic assessments.* Ideally every 15 to 30 minutes, for rapid detection of clinical deterioration and signs of increased ICP.

The clinical presentation of ICH is indistinguishable from ischemic stroke, but its management can be very different; therefore, rapid neuroimaging is essential. Noncontrast computed tomography (CT) is the most commonly used imaging modality for emergency diagnosis and characterization of ICH (location and extent of the hematoma). Noncontrast CT is highly sensitive and specific for acute bleeding, which will appear hyperdense, then, over weeks, become isodense, and may have a ring-enhancing appearance. In addition to the location of the primary hematoma, the degree of bleeding (including volume, the presence of intraventricular hemorrhage [IVH], and signs of increased ICP or herniation) is among the strongest predictors of long-term outcome.

A rapid estimate of ICH volume helps determine stroke severity and delineate treatment options. A simple and validated method that can be used in the emergency department (ED) is the ABC/2 formula,[23] where A is the greatest hemorrhage diameter on the CT slice with the largest area of ICH, B is the largest perpendicular diameter on the same CT slice, and C is the approximate number of CT slices with hemorrhage multiplied by the slice thickness in centimeters, which is often 0.5 cm. For calculation of C, a slice is counted as 1 if the hemorrhage area is >75% of the largest hematoma area on the reference slice; as 0.5 if the hemorrhage area is approximately 25% to 75%; and not counted if the area is <25%. ABC/2 gives the ICH volume in cm^3. In children, the ABC/XYZ has been proposed, where X, Y, and Z are perpendicular measures of the supratentorial intracranial space (% of total brain volume).[24]

Recently, it has been suggested that identification of active extravasation of intravenous contrast into the hematoma, called the "spot sign," during contrast-enhanced CT and/or CT angiography (CTA) may predict hematoma expansion.[25,26]

In patients with confirmed acute ICH, CT or MR angiography, or catheter angiography is recommended to exclude an underlying lesion such as an aneurysm, AVM, or tumor. However, in hypertensive patients with a well-circumscribed hematoma in a typical location for hypertensive bleeding (thalamus, basal ganglia, pons, and cerebellum), the yield of such studies is extremely low, and a decision not to proceed with these additional diagnostic tests is reasonable.[27] At the other extreme, young, nonhypertensive patients with isolated intraventricular hemorrhage (IVH) deserve aggressive workup.

Risk Stratification and Prognostication

Several clinical grading scales have been developed to assist with risk stratification and prognostication. An easy-to-use and well-validated model is the ICH score[28] (Table 21.2), which is based on patient demographics (age), clinical condition (GCS), and neuroimaging findings (ICH volume, presence of IVH, and supratentorial or infratentorial origin of ICH). The ICH score has been validated for stratification of 30-day mortality[28] and 12-month functional outcome[29]; each point increase is associated with increased mortality risk and poorer functional outcome. However,

TABLE 21.2 ICH Score

Component	Points
Glasgow coma scale	
3–4	2
5–12	1
13–15	0
Age (years)	
≥80	1
<80	0
ICH volume (mL)	
≥30	1
<30	0
Presence of intraventricular hemorrhage	
Yes	1
No	0
Infratentorial origin of ICH	
Yes	1
No	0
Total ICH score	0–6
30 day-mortality at total points	
4	97%
3	72%
2	26%
1	13%

From Hemphill JC III, Bonovich DC, Besmertis L, et al. The ICH score: a simple, reliable grading scale for intracerebral hemorrhage. *Stroke.* 2001;32(4):891–897.

it has been shown that withdrawal of life support in patients likely to have a poor outcome may significantly bias these predictive models. In the ED, clinical grading scales should be used only for communication about a patient's condition, or for research purposes, and not to limit interventions in the initial management of patients with ICH.[22]

Management Guidelines

Emergency Department management of patients with acute ICH entails (1) initial stabilization of airway and hemodynamics, (2) minimization of primary injury and (3) prevention of secondary brain injury. The most recent American Heart Association/American Stroke Association guidelines[30] and the recently published ENLS protocols[22] are reviewed in the following sections.

Initial Stabilization

Management of ICH begins by ensuring adequate patient airway, breathing, and circulation. Early endotracheal intubation is essential for patients with a depressed LOC who are unable to protect their airway. Classically, a GCS $\leq$ 8, rapidly deteriorating LOC, and uncontrolled seizures are indications for intubation. Stable patients requiring transfer to another medical facility should be carefully assessed for the possibility of airway compromise in the the near term, and, if the risk is deemed high, be intubated prior to leaving the referring center. Whenever possible, a rapid and concise neurologic assessment should precede intubation in order to document the patient's baseline functioning before the exam is confounded by use of sedative or paralytic drugs.

Maintenance of both brain perfusion and oxygenation is critical for prevention of secondary brain injury. To this end, steps should be taken to prevent elevations in ICP, including minimization of airway manipulation and use of ICP lowering medications. Oxygen saturation should be maintained >94% and carbon dioxide ($PaCO_2$) levels should be kept in the normal range (35–45 mm Hg). In mechanically ventilated patients, use of lung-protective ventilation strategies (pressure- and volume-limited mechanical ventilation) is appropriate. In a setting of increased ICP and/or signs of acute brain herniation, hyperventilation to a goal $PaCO_2$ of 28 to 32 mm Hg may be used. Hyperventilation is not a definitive treatment for elevated ICP because of the risk of increased brain ischemia and rebound elevations in ICP; a normal $PaCO_2$ should be reinstituted as soon as definitive treatments to control ICP are in place.[31]

Minimization of Primary Injury

Blood Pressure Management Arterial blood pressure is elevated in the majority of patients who present with ICH. Mean arterial pressure (MAP) is >120 mm Hg in over two-thirds of ICH patients and >140 mm Hg in over one-third.[32] Such acute elevations in BP have been implicated as a cause of bleeding and as a normal physiologic response to maintain cerebral perfusion pressure (CPP). Although there is general agreement that low BP levels are associated with poorer outcome and must be corrected, it is not clear at this time whether this observation simply reflects the fact that low BP levels occur more often in severe cases.[30]

Current guidelines[30] recommend the following BP targets in patients with spontaneous ICH:

- SBP > 200 mm Hg or MAP > 150 mm Hg: Aggressive reduction of BP with target MAP of 110 mm Hg or BP 160/90 mm Hg
- SBP > 180 mm Hg or MAP > 130 mm Hg and no clinical evidence of elevated ICP: Target MAP of 110 mm Hg or BP 160/90 mm Hg
- SBP > 180 mm Hg or MAP > 130 mm Hg with clinical evidence of ICP elevation on exam, CT, or ICP monitor; If ICP monitoring is available, target a CPP of ≥ 60 mm Hg (50 to 70 mm Hg); if ICP monitoring is not available, target a MAP of 80 to 90 mm Hg (assuming an ICP of 20 to 30 mm Hg)

The evidence underlying these guidelines is controversial. In the recent, large multicenter trial "Intracerebral Hemorrhage Acutely Decreasing Arterial Pressure Trial 2" (INTERACT 2), 2,839 patients with spontaneous ICH were randomized to rapid blood pressure lowering with a target SBP = 140 mm Hg within 1 hour; or to the standard guideline-recommended target SBP of 180 mm Hg. Analysis of a composite outcome of death and severe disability on the modified Rankin scale (mRS = 3 to 6) showed an 8% benefit in the more aggressive treatment group; however, the result was not statistically significant. Although the safety of this lower-BP target has been demonstrated, an evidence-based benefit in clinical outcome has yet to be confirmed. More answers are expected from the Antihypertensive Treatment of Acute Cerebral Hemorrhage (ATACH) II trial.

If a decision is made to lower blood pressure, management should be started immediately. A short-acting, titratable, intravenous agent should be used to achieve the target quickly and with minimal risk for overshoot. Labetalol (initial bolus dose 5 to 20 mg titrated every 10 minutes to effect) is a reasonable agent if there are no contraindications. Nicardipine is another excellent option (initial dose 5 mg/hour, with titration by 2.5 mg/hour every 15 minutes as needed; maximum dose 15 mg/hour). Angiotensin-converting enzyme inhibitors (e.g., enalapril) and hydralazine may be used. Sodium nitroprusside and nitroglycerin increase ICP and lower cerebral blood flow and should be avoided.

Twenty-four to forty-eight hours following brain injury, oral/enteral antihypertensive medications should be initiated to help achieve individualized blood pressure targets for secondary stroke prevention.

Correction of Coagulopathy Coagulopathy in patients with ICH is most commonly due to use of therapeutic anticoagulation; other risk factors include acquired or congenital coagulation factor deficiencies and qualitative or quantitative platelet abnormalities. Coagulopathies in ICH are associated with poor prognosis because of prolonged bleeding and hematoma expansion; whenever possible, these deficits should be immediately corrected.

Specific Anticoagulants

1. Vitamin K antagonists (VKAs, e.g., warfarin) are currently the most commonly prescribed oral anticoagulants. ICH occurs 8 to 10 times more frequently in VKA anticoagulated patients than in non–anticoagulated patients, with a twofold

higher mortality rate. Therapy includes withholding anticoagulants and treating to rapidly normalize the INR with IV vitamin K (5 to 10 mg) and replacement of vitamin K–dependent factors. Debate continues over the optimal strategy for replacing vitamin K–dependent factors; currently both fresh frozen plasma (FFP; 10 to 15 mL/kg) and prothrombin complex concentrates (PCCs—25 to 50 IU/kg) are used. AHA/ASA guidelines recommend PCCs because of their smaller infusion volume and subsequently lower risk of volume overload and pulmonary edema.[30] PCCs have the added advantages of rapid reconstitution and administration and result in the correction of INR within minutes. The most recent American College of Chest Physicians (ACCP) Evidence-Based Clinical Practice Guidelines recommend using PCCs rather than FFP[33] to reverse significant warfarin-associated ICH.

2. Novel oral anticoagulants (direct thrombin inhibitors, e.g., dabigatran, and Xa inhibitors, e.g., rivaroxaban) have also been associated with ICH. Clinical experience in reversing coagulopathy from these agents is limited, and no specific reversal protocols or agents currently exist; inhibitors for dabigatran and rivaroxaban are under development, but not yet commercially available. There is some evidence that hemodialysis may be effective in dabigatran-associated bleeding, and, within 2 hours of ingestion, there may be a role for oral activated charcoal (also suggested for rivaroxaban).[34] PCCs may have a role in treating ICH related to rivaroxaban, but not to dabigatran. In the case of patients treated with one of these newer oral anticoagulants, urgent hematologic consultation is recommended.
3. For patients receiving unfractionated heparin (UFH), protamine sulfate is the reversal agent of choice. Standard dosing is 1 mg of protamine for every 100 units of heparin administered (maximum dose 50 mg). When UFH is given as continuous infusion, only the UFH given in the preceding 2 hours should be considered when estimating the quantity of heparin to be reversed. If more than 4 hours have elapsed since the last dose of UFH, reversal is unlikely to be necessary (PTT should still be documented). With low molecular weight heparin (LMWH), full reversal is not possible, although protamine may still be used in an attempt at partial reversal (provides a maximum of 60% to 75% inhibition of the anti-Xa activity).

Antiplatelet Agents Conflicting results have been published regarding the impact of antiplatelet agents on hematoma expansion and clinical outcomes. There is a small increased risk of ICH with the use of antiplatelet agents (0.2 events per 1,000 patient-years).[35,36] Some centers support empiric use of platelet transfusion, while others discourage this practice, or suggest assaying for platelet function to guide transfusion.[22] Current guidelines highlight a lack of evidence and consider platelet transfusion in ICH patients with a history of antiplatelet use as experimental.[30] Additionally, some authors suggest the use of desmopressin (DDAVP, 0.3 mcg/kg), as has been used in the treatment of uremia-associated bleeding.[22]

Fibrinolytic Agents Symptomatic ICH is one of the most life-threatening complications of thrombolytic therapy. The incidence of symptomatic ICH following recombinant tissue plasminogen activator (rt-PA) therapy for ischemic stroke is approximately 6%; of interest, symptomatic ICH following thrombolysis for myocardial infarction (MI), for which a higher dose of rt-PA is used than in stroke (1.1 mg/kg in MI vs. 0.9 mg/kg in stroke), is quite rare (0.4% to 1.3%). The difference is thought to reflect the fact that healthy cerebral vessels do not readily bleed from thrombolysis. Management of suspected ICH during or after fibrinolytic infusion begins with immediate cessation of the infusion, clinical stabilization (ABCs), and emergent noncontrast CT head. The NINDS rt-PA study[37] protocol recommends empiric treatment in these cases with 6 to 8 units of cryoprecipitate or FFP and 6 to 8 units of platelets; however, evidence on the most effective treatment in this situation is lacking.

Even patients without evidence of coagulopathy may experience hematoma expansion, especially in the first 24 hours. Because hematoma expansion is one of the major risk factors for poor outcome, it has been hypothesized that use of procoagulant agents could improve outcomes after ICH. Five randomized trials tested this hypothesis using recombinant factor VIIa (rFVIIa) (NovoSeven® RT) in non-coagulopathic patients with ICH (spontaneous and traumatic ICH). A meta-analysis[38] of these studies showed significant reduction in hematoma growth, but an increased rate of thromboembolic events and no overall net difference in mortality or long-term disability. Current guidelines do not recommend the use of rFVIIa in the treatment of ICH.[30] However, rFVIIa might benefit specific subsets of patients in whom the risk of hematoma expansion outweighs the risk of thromboembolic events. Two ongoing trials address this question in patients thought to be at high risk for hematoma expansion. The SPOTLIGHT trial (Spot Sign Selection of Intracerebral Hemorrhage to Guide Hemostatic Therapy) and the STOP-IT trial (Spot Sign for Predicting and Treating ICH Growth Study) are both addressing the role of rFVIIa in patients identified on CTA as having a positive "spot sign," a finding indicative of extravasation of contrast into the hematoma and suggestive of significant risk for imminent hematoma expansion.[39]

Surgical Interventions Based on current evidence and guidelines, surgical intervention may be considered in the following conditions.

Infratentorial ICH Although no randomized controlled trials (RCTs) of cerebellar hematoma evacuation have been undertaken, several case series suggest that surgical evacuation with cerebellar decompression is associated with improved outcomes in patients with ICH > 3 cm in diameter and clinical deterioration, or radiographic evidence of either brainstem compression or hydrocephalus. Treatment with external ventricular drainage (EVD) alone without posterior fossa decompression is not recommended because of the theoretical risk of upward herniation. Patients with cerebellar hemorrhage should be always referred for urgent neurosurgical consultation.

Supratentorial ICH Current guidelines suggest that surgical evacuation of supratentorial ICH should be considered only in patients presenting with lobar clots >30 mL that are within 1 cm of the surface.[30,40,41] The recently published Surgical Trial in Intracerebral Hemorrhage (STICH) II[41] did not show any difference in unfavorable outcomes at 6 months when comparing early surgery to conservative treatment in this specific subgroup of patients. The trial showed a slight survival advantage (OR = 0.86) for surgery within a few hours of the onset of hemorrhage in conscious patients with a modestly decreased

GCS (9 to 12) and with lobar hematomas, but the survival advantage was far from achieving statistical significance.[42] Expert consensus is that surgery should be considered as a life-saving procedure for treatment of refractory increased ICP, especially in patients with ongoing clinical deterioration, recent onset of hemorrhage, involvement of the nondominant hemisphere, and relatively accessible hematomas.

Intraventricular Hemorrhage and Hydrocephalus IVH is quite common in spontaneous ICH (45% of patients), especially in patients with hypertensive hemorrhages involving the basal ganglia and the thalamus.[43] Acute hydrocephalus may develop after ICH, either in association with IVH or because of direct mass effect on ventricles. Patients with acute hydrocephalus require urgent neurosurgical consultation for possible EVD placement. Unfortunately, ventriculostomy in the setting of IVH is difficult to manage because of frequent obstruction secondary to blood clots. Flushing the catheter helps remove the thrombus but may cause ventriculitis. Recently, use of intraventricular thrombolytic agents has been suggested as adjunct to EVD for accelerating blood clearance and clot lysis. The safety phase 2 trial of the CLEAR-IVH trial (Clot Lysis: Evaluating Accelerated Resolution of IVH) prospectively evaluated the safety of intraventricular use of 3 mg rt-PA versus placebo in 48 patients. Results from this study suggest that intraventricular rt-PA is safe and can have a significant benefit on clot clearance. However, pending results of the ongoing phase III CLEAR-IVH trial, current guidelines consider this treatment experimental.[30]

Prevention of Secondary Injury

Although this chapter focuses on the initial evaluation and management of patients with ICH, it is reasonable for the emergency physician to implement early intrventions that can help minimize secondary injury in the ensuing 24 to 72 hours.[22]

Intracranial Pressure Monitoring Few studies have addressed the incidence, management, and impact of elevated ICP on outcomes of ICH patients. Current guidelines are based on the principles and goals of traumatic brain injury (TBI) management.[22,30,44]

- *Indications for ICP monitoring*: GCS $\leq$ 8, large hematoma with mass effect suggestive of elevated ICP, or hydrocephalus
- *Goals*: ICP < 20 mm Hg, CPP 50 to 70 mm Hg (if possible, adjustments based on the patient's cerebral autoregulatory status)
- *Interventions*: Initial measures: elevate the patient's head (30 to 45 degrees), drain cerebral spinal fluid (CSF) using an EVD; provide analgesia and sedation to achieve a motionless state, and maintain normal body temperature
- *Advanced measures:* hypertonic solutions (e.g., mannitol and hypertonic saline); hyperventilation (as bridge to further management); neuromuscular blockade; hematoma evacuation/decompressive craniectomy; mild hypothermia; barbiturate coma

Seizure Prophylaxis Seizures frequently complicate ICH; however, their incidence varies widely depending on diagnostic criteria, duration of follow-up, and the population studied. The estimated incidence of clinical seizures in patients with ICH is 4.2% to 20%, subclinical seizures 29% to 31%, and status epilepticus 0.3% to 21.4%. About 50% to 70% of seizures will occur within the first 24 hours, and 90% in the first 3 days.[39] Predisposing factors include ICH with a lobar location (typically nonoccipital and subcortical hemorrhages), large hematoma size, hydrocephalus, midline shift, and low GCS. Although seizures theoretically may exacerbate brain injury, conflicting results have been reported on seizure association with clinical outcome and mortality. No RCTs exist to guide decision making for seizure prophylaxis or treatment specifically in patients with ICH.

As in traumatic brain injury, prophylactic anticonvulsants in patients with lobar ICH may reduce the risk of early seizures but do not affect long-term risk of developing epilepsy. In addition, two recent studies found their use to be associated with worse functional outcomes.[45,46] Based on available data, current guidelines do not recommend routine use of prophylactic anticonvulsants.[30]

However, if a patient with ICH develops clinical seizures, or there is a change in mental status associated with EEG evidence of seizures, experts recommend initiation of treatment with antiepileptic agents. The choice of initial drug should depend on individual patient characteristics (i.e., medical comorbidities, concurrent drugs, and contraindications). Initial treatment typically begins with an intravenous benzodiazepine (e.g., lorazepam 0.05 to 0.10 mg/kg), followed by a loading dose of an IV agent (e.g., phenytoin 15 to 20 mg/kg, valproic acid 15 to 45 mg/kg, levetiracetam 500 to 1,500 mg, or phenobarbital 10 to 20 mg/kg).

Glycemic Control A high proportion of patients with ICH (~60%) will develop stress hyperglycemia in the first 72 hours, even in the absence of a previous history of diabetes mellitus.[40] Multiple studies have associated increased serum glucose in the acute phase of ICH with higher risk of poor outcome (hematoma expansion, increased edema, and death or severe disability).[41] However, clear causality between hyperglycemia and poor outcome and, more interestingly, evidence of improved outcome with glycemic control have not been proven. Recent microdialysis studies have demonstrated increased cerebral hypoglycemic events in patients treated with tight glucose control strategy, and a large multicenter RCT in a general ICU population found increased mortality with intensive glucose control.[47] Current guidelines recommend close glucose monitoring and avoidance of both hypoglycemia (<70 mg/dL) and hyperglycemia (>180 mg/dL); most experts agree that an insulin infusion should aim for a serum glucose of 140 to 180 mg/dL.[39] By contrast, tight control (80 to 110 mg/dL) has been shown to increase mortality.[47]

Temperature Control Fever is relatively common in patients with ICH (up to 40%), and it has been independently associated with poor outcome. However, no RCT has yet demonstrated improved clinical outcome with induced normothermia.[39] Despite a lack of evidence, there is general agreement that the presence of fever should prompt an appropriately broad workup; infectious sources should be identified and treated, and hyperthermia should be corrected (target core temperature below 38°C–37.5°C).

Venous Thromboembolism Prophylaxis Patients with ICH are at high risk of venous thromboembolism (VTE). Independent risk factors for thromboembolic disease in patients with ICH include greater severity of stroke, prolonged immobilization, advanced age, female gender, African–American ethnicity, and thrombophilia. Discontinuation of antithrombotic agents is itself, of course, associated with an increased risk of deep vein thrombosis (DVT).[39] Guidelines suggest the use of intermittent pneumatic compression (IPC) devices in addition to elastic stockings in patients admitted for ICH, based on an RCT showing a reduced occurrence of asymptomatic DVT (4.7% vs. 15.9%).[48] Evidence regarding use of prophylactic UFH or LMWH is less definitive. Based on small studies showing safety of pharmacologic prophylaxis (no increased risk of hematoma expansion or further bleeding), current guidelines suggest consideration of LMWH starting 1 to 4 days after ICH, provided follow-up imaging has documented cessation of bleeding.[30]

Disposition

Patients with ICH are frequently medically and neurologically unstable and are at significant risk for sudden clinical deterioration, particularly in the immediate poststroke period. Care of ICH patients in highly specialized stroke or neurointensive intensive care units has been associated with lower mortality and better functional outcome,[49] and admission to such a unit is considered standard of care.[30] An institutional algorithm for referral protocol and/or transfer to centers with higher levels of care is recommended.

ANEURYSMAL SUBARACHNOID HEMORRHAGE

The challenge of emergency medicine lies in identifying those patients who can be treated and released and those patients whose complaints represent a life-threatening process requiring urgent intervention. Among the diseases with the greatest potential for catastrophic consequence when undiagnosed is subarachnoid hemorrhage from a ruptured cerebral aneurysm. When an emergency department patient presents with headache due to aneurysmal rupture, timely diagnosis by the emergency physician is the best chance for avoiding the devastating effects of rebleeding that so often result in severe disability or death.

Aneurysmal subarachnoid hemorrhage (aSAH) accounts for only a small proportion of patients who present to the ED with a complaint of headache. Unfortunately, despite our awareness of the severity of this disease, 12% of aSAH patients are misdiagnosed on initial presentation. Misdiagnosed patients are more likely to have normal mental status, to present more than a day after the onset of symptoms, be unmarried, less educated, and speak English as a second language.[50]

Epidemiology

Subarachnoid hemorrhage (SAH) is classified as either traumatic or spontaneous. Ruptured intracranial aneurysms are the leading cause of spontaneous SAH, followed by AVMs and nonaneurysmal "perimesencephalic" bleeding (characterized by a typical CT pattern and a benign clinical course). Cerebral aneurysms are vascular outpouchings that occur most frequently in the circle of Willis, where they typically form at branch points of the major cerebral arteries. Although cerebral aneurysms may be found at any arterial location in the cerebral circulation, the most common sites are the anterior communicating artery (30%), the posterior communicating artery (25%), the middle cerebral artery (20%), internal carotid bifurcation (7.5%), basilar tip (7%), and the posterior–inferior cerebellar artery (3%).[51]

Autopsy studies have shown that 6% to 8% of the general population harbors a cerebral aneurysm. The risk of rupture depends on many factors, including aneurysm location, size, and previous history of rupture.[52] In the United States, aSAH affects 30,000 persons per year and is twice as common in women (average age of 55 years old).[53–57] Although aSAH accounts for only 5% of all types of stroke, it is responsible for 27% of productive years of life lost from cerebrovascular diseases.[58]

Hypertension and smoking have a causative role in both aneurysm formation and rupture.[59] A recent study reported that smoking increased the odds of aneurysm rupture threefold.[60] Several heritable conditions are associated with the development of cerebral artery aneurysms, including a first-degree relative with aSAH, autosomal dominant polycystic kidney disease (PKD), neurofibromatosis type I, Marfan syndrome, multiple endocrine neoplasia (MEN) type I, pseudoxanthoma elasticum, hereditary hemorrhagic telangiectasia, and Ehlers-Danlos syndrome type II and IV.[61] Family history and PKD account for 10% and 1% of all cases of aSAH, respectively.

History and Physical Exam

Aneurysmal SAH patients typically present with a sudden onset of severe headache. It is commonly described as the "worst headache of life," but unfortunately, this description is given by more than 78% of all patients with headache of any etiology who present to the ED.[62] The development of pain from aSAH is almost always rapid, though not instantaneous, and will usually reach peak intensity within 30 minutes of onset. Pain can be accompanied by loss of consciousness, vomiting, and neck pain or stiffness. Clinical grading scales have been developed to classify the severity and to predict the long-term outcome of aSAH (Table 21.3).[63,64]

Although SAH represents only 2% of acute headaches in the ED, its potential for devastating outcomes makes accurate diagnosis essential.[65–67] A clinical decision rule was recently developed to rule out aSAH in patients with acute headache (Ottawa SAH rule).[68] In patients presenting to the ED with an acute headache and normal neurologic exam, any of the following factors raises the likelihood of aSAH and mandates additional workup (Table 21.4): age $\geq$ 40 years, neck pain or stiffness, witnessed loss of consciousness, onset during exertion, thunderclap headache (instantly peaking pain), and limited neck flexion on examination. This rule showed a sensitivity of 100% for detecting spontaneous SAH.

Diagnostic Evaluation

In a series of 482 patients with aSAH admitted to a tertiary hospital between 1996 and 2001, 56 patients (12%) of cases were initially misdiagnosed.[50] In 43% of cases, the misdiagnosis occurred in the ED. Most commonly, these patients received the diagnosis of tension headache or migraine (36%). The most common diagnostic error was the failure to acquire a head CT prior to discharge (73%). Three factors that were independently associated with misdiagnosis were normal mental status, small aSAH volume, and right-sided aneurysm location. Patients presenting with a normal mental status had higher rates of misdiagnosis (19%) than those with altered mental status.

TABLE 21.3 Clinical Grading Scales

	Hunt and Hess[63]	WFNS[64]
1	Asymptomatic or mild headache and slight nuchal rigidity	GCS 15 without hemiparesis
2	Moderate to severe headache, nuchal rigidity, no focal neurologic deficit other than cranial nerve palsy	GCS 14–13 without hemiparesis
3	Confusion, lethargy, or mild focal neurologic deficit other than cranial nerve palsy	GCS 14–13 with hemiparesis
4	Stupor or moderate to severe hemiparesis	GCS 12–7 with or without hemiparesis
5	Coma, extensor posturing, moribund appearance	GCS 6–3 with or without hemiparesis

WFNS, World Federation of Neurosurgical Societies.

The diagnostic workup for aSAH has traditionally included emergent noncontrast CT imaging followed by a lumbar puncture (LP) to evaluate for red blood cells or xanthochromia in the CSF if CT imaging is negative.[69]

Early studies of CT for detection of SAH demonstrated a sensitivity of 93% to 95% in the first 24 hours following onset of symptoms, dropping to 85% 3 days after, and 50% a week after symptom onset.[70] More recent studies have reported sensitivities close to 100% in the first 72 hours using more advanced CT technology, raising question of whether lumbar puncture is always required to rule out the diagnosis.[71,72] A recent prospective study of 3,132 patients with nontraumatic acute headache reported the sensitivity and negative predictive value of CT for the detection of SAH in the first 6 hours after symptom onset to be 100%.[73] All studies were performed on third-generation CT scanners and were interpreted by a trained radiologist. These results suggest that lumbar puncture may not be necessary to rule out the diagnosis of aSAH when a patient presents to an ED within 6 hours of ictus. Another less invasive diagnostic approach that has been proposed is noncontrast CT followed by CTA. The CT/CTA approach excludes aSAH with a >99% post-test probability.[74,75] The disadvantages of this last approach lie in the radiation dose and the need for iodinated contrast.

TABLE 21.4 Ottawa SAH Rule

Patients presenting with acute nontraumatic headache that reaches maximum intensity within 1 h and normal neurologic examination should undergo further workup, if one of the following is present:

1. Age ≥ 40 y
2. Neck pain or stiffness
3. Witnessed loss of consciousness
4. Onset during exertion
5. Thunderclap headache (instantly peaking pain)
6. Limited neck flexion on examination

Rule not applicable for the patient with neurologic deficits, previous aneurysms/SAH, brain tumors, or history of recurrent headaches (≥3 episodes over the course of ≥ 6 months)

SAH, Subarachnoid Hemorrhage.

From Perry JJ, Stiell IG, Sivilotti ML, et al. Clinical decision rules to rule out subarachnoid hemorrhage for acute headache. *JAMA*. 2013;310(12):1248–1255.

On CT, acute SAH appears as hyperdense material, most often filling the suprasellar, ambient, quadrigeminal, and prepontine cisterns, with extension into the sylvian fissures and interhemispheric fissure. IVH is common and is a risk for the development of communicating hydrocephalus. Thicker cisternal clots and IVH have been associated with the development of delayed cerebral ischemia (DCI) in the course of aSAH (Table 21.5).

Less frequently, aneurysmal rupture can occur directly into brain parenchyma, resulting in intracerebral hemorrhage in addition to SAH and IVH. Depending on the location of the ICH, this is often accompanied by clinical hemiplegia or hemiparesis. Global cerebral edema may also be present on initial head CT and is more commonly seen in patients with Hunt and Hess scores of 4 or 5.

Management Guidelines

Approximately 12% of aSAH patients will die immediately.[78] For patients who survive to reach medical attention, rebleeding is the most life-threatening entity, with mortality rates close to 70%.[79,80] Traditionally, the risk of rebleeding after SAH has been quoted as 4% in the first 24 hours, 1% to 2% per day for the next 14 days, 50% risk during the initial 6 months after ictus, and 3% yearly thereafter. This is now believed to be an underestimate,[81] with ultra-early rebleeding occurring in up to 17% of cases.[79] Proper initial management therefore includes taking steps to prevent rebleeding and to ensure transfer of patients to high-volume centers for definitive treatment. Other key interventions include implementation of strategies to prevent secondary complications, such as DCI. The following sections reference the most recent American Heart Association/American Stroke Association guidelines,[82] the recommendations from the Neurocritical Care Society's Multidisciplinary Consensus Conference,[83] and the recently published ENLS protocols.[84]

Initial Stabilization

As with any medical emergency, initial management focuses on the ABCs. Cardiopulmonary complications are not uncommon following aSAH and are likely

TABLE 21.5 CT Grading Scales

	Fisher Scale[76]	Modified Fisher Scale[77]
0		No SAH or IVH
1	No SAH or IVH	Minimum or thin SAH, and no IVH
2	Diffuse deposition of thin layer; all vertical layers of blood (interhemispheric fissure, insular cistern, or ambient cistern) <1 mm thick	Minimum or thin SAH, with IVH in both lateral ventricles
3	Vertical layers of blood ≥1 mm in thickness and/or localized clots (defined as >3 × 5 mm)	Thick SAH (completely filling one or more cistern or fissure), and no bilateral IVH
4	Intracerebral or intraventricular clots with diffuse or no subarachnoid blood	Thick SAH (completely filling one or more cistern or fissure) with IVH in both lateral ventricles

SAH, subarachnoid hemorrhage; IVH, intraventricular hemorrhage.

related to catecholamine discharge. Troponin elevation, arrhythmias (prolonged QT, ventricular arrhythmias, ST-segment changes), and wall motion abnormalities on echocardiography (stress-induced cardiomyopathy) are observed in 25% to 35% of patients. Severe cardiac compromise can occur and results in sudden death, cardiogenic shock, and pulmonary edema. Neurogenic pulmonary edema has also been described. These manifestations are usually transient and tend to resolve during the first week after hospitalization.[85]

Prevention of Rebleeding

Blood Pressure Management Blood pressure control is one of the most important early interventions in patients with aSAH. However, unlike for ICH, limited data exist to guide BP management in acute aSAH patients with an unsecured aneurysm (i.e., prior to either neurosurgical clipping or endovascular coiling). Lowering BP may decrease the risk of rebleeding but increases the risk of cerebral infarction in patients with impaired autoregulation. In a series of 134 patients with aSAH, a lower incidence of rebleeding (15% vs. 33%) but a higher incidence of infarction (43% vs. 22%) was reported in patients given antihypertensive therapy.[86] Randomized controlled studies are lacking. Current guidelines acknowledge the paucity of data and recommend balancing the risk of hypertensive-induced rebleeding with the risk of ischemia from reduced CPP. Maintaining an SBP below 160 mm Hg or a MAP below 110 mm Hg is considered reasonable.[82,84] Labetalol and nicardipine, both fast-acting and titratable drugs, are the preferred agents; as in ICH patients, the use of nitroprusside or nitroglycerine should be avoided because of the risk of increased ICP secondary to increased cerebral blood volume.[87]

Pain and Anxiety Management Pain (especially headache) and anxiety are common complaints after aSAH. Management of pain or anxiety in this population is challenging because of the difficult balance between effective management and avoidance of oversedation. There is no medication of choice; acetaminophen (1 g orally every 6 hours) along with an opioid agent (e.g., fentanyl, morphine, or hydromorphone) is a common strategy. Prior to the aneurysm being secured, NSAIDS should be avoided given their anti-platelet activity. Once the aneurysm is secured, the use of nonsteroid anti-inflammatory drugs (NSAIDs) as adjunctive opioid-sparing therapy may be considered. However, NSAID use has to be carefully considered because of potential detrimental effect on CPP and brain tissue hypoxia.[88] Small doses of benzodiazepines may help in a significantly anxious patient. However, agitation, confusion, and delirium can be insidious signs of symptomatic DCI and have to be carefully addressed in this population.[89]

Antifibrinolytic Agents Definitive aneurysm treatment often requires transfer to specialized centers (see Transfer to High-Volume Center); this strategy, however, can be associated with delay and potential increased risk of rebleeding. Antifibrinolytic therapy (e.g., tranexamic acid, aminocaproic acid) has therefore gained interest for its potential role in this group of patients at risk of ultraearly rebleeding. In one randomized trial, 254 patients with ruptured aneurysms received tranexamic acid (1 g IV immediately after CT diagnosis, followed by 1 g IV every 6 hours until aneurysm obliteration—for a maximum of 72 hours); 251 patients served as controls. Patients receiving tranexamic acid—70% of whom had the aneurysm secured within 24 hours—showed a reduction in the rebleeding rate from 10.8% to 2.4% and an inferred 80% reduction in the mortality rate due to early rebleeding.[90] Current recommendations suggest consideration of early (at diagnosis) and short (<72 hours) course of antifibrinolytic therapy (tranexamic acid or aminocaproic acid) for prevention of early rebleeding when definitive treatment of the aneurysm is unavoidably delayed and no risk factors for VTE are identified.[82,83] Delayed (>48 hours after the ictus) or prolonged (>72 hours) treatment with these agents is not recommended because of the associated risk of complications (VTE and cerebral ischemia).[83]

Correction of Coagulopathy The same principles of coagulopathy management discussed in the ICH section apply to spontaneous SAH. Although there are limited data available to support this guideline, most experts recommend reversal of all antithrombotic agents in patients with aSAH until definitive obliteration of the aneurysm has been achieved.[84]

Monitoring of Neurologic Status

Acute Hydrocephalus Acute hydrocephalus is one of the most common complications of aSAH (seen in 9% to 67% of patients), causing increased ICP and rapid neurologic deterioration.[91] Hydrocephalus in aSAH develops as a result of accumulation of subarachnoid blood on the arachnoid granulations, preventing the reabsorption of CSF. In addition, blood can obstruct the ventricular system, causing obstructive or noncommunicating hydrocephalus. Patients with aSAH and good neurologic grade (e.g., a WFNS of 1 to 3) require only frequent neurologic assessments. If clinical deterioration occurs (usually within 72 hours), an emergent noncontrast CT should be performed and, if hydrocephalus is confirmed, an EVD should be inserted. Patients with poor-grade (WFNS 4 and 5) and CT evidence of hydrocephalus require immediate EVD placement. Approximately 30% of these patients will demonstrate clinical improvement after EVD insertion.[92] While EVD insertion theoretically can cause rebleeding in unsecured ruptured aneurysms, observational studies have not confirmed this concern.[91]

Elevated ICP Elevated ICP secondary to acute hydrocephalus and reactive hyperemia/cerebral edema is common in patients suffering from high-grade aSAH, and is associated with poor outcomes. Definitive evidence is lacking in this population, and most of strategies, as in ICH, are derived from TBI management (see ICH section).[93]

Seizure Seizures are uncommon after aSAH (<20%), usually follow aneurysm re-rupture and are associated with poor outcome. Risk factors for seizures at onset are presence of intraparenchymal clot, middle cerebral artery aneurysm, and surgical clipping. There is, however, disagreement among experts regarding the routine use of anticonvulsants, and observational studies have shown worse cognitive and functional outcomes with prophylactic use of phenytoin.[82,83,89,94] If a decision to use seizure prophylaxis is undertaken, a very short course (3 to 7 days) with an agent other than phenytoin is advised.[83] For patients with documented clinical or electrographic seizures, treatment with an anticonvulsant is advised.

Transfer to High-Volume Center

Once a patient has been stabilized, transfer to a specialized high-volume center (>35 aSAH/year), with experienced neurovascular surgeons, endovascular specialists, and multidisciplinary neurointensive care services, is recommended.[82] Unfortunately, despite evidence of improved outcome, only a minority of aSAH patients are managed in these centers.[95]

Definitive Treatment of a Ruptured Aneurysm

Definitive treatment of a ruptured aneurysm involves either neurosurgical clipping or endovascular coiling to mechanically secure the lesion and isolate it from the intracranial circulation. The International Subarachnoid Aneurysm Trial (ISAT)[96] compared these two interventions in patients with aSAH, and showed that endovascular coiling resulted in significantly better disability-free survival at 1 year. However, debate still persists as to the superiority of one treatment over another.[97] There is general agreement that, regardless of modality, early treatment confers a clinical benefit.[82]

Postobliteration Management

Prevention of Delayed Cerebral Ischemia In the first 2 weeks following bleeding, patients with aSAH are at risk of deterioration as a result of cerebral vasospasm and DCI. The use of nimodipine (60 mg orally every 4 hours), started on ICU admission and continued for 21 days, is the only strategy currently available to decrease the risk of DCI and to improve functional outcomes.[98] Interestingly, oral nimodipine does not decrease the incidence of angiographic vasospasm, traditionally considered the primary cause of DCI. The most common complication of nimodipine use is hypotension, considered detrimental in aSAH patients because of the risk of cerebral hypoperfusion. In case of hypotension related to nimodipine, the dose can be changed to 30 mg every 2 hours.

Maintenance of euvolemia and normonatremia is fundamental in the management of patients suffering from aSAH. Typically, after aSAH, patients experience increased natriuresis and urine output, with subsequent hyponatremia and hypovolemia, respectively. Both entities are associated with increased risk of DCI and worse functional outcomes.[99] Unfortunately, routine fluid balance and vital signs are poor markers of intravascular fluid status in this population, and advanced hemodynamic monitoring may be required.[100] Strategies currently advocated are avoidance of hypotonic solutions; the use of isotonic (e.g., normal saline) or hypertonic solutions (e.g., 3% saline—especially if hyponatremia is present); and consideration of fludrocortisone in patients with persistent negative fluid balance. Finally, once the ruptured aneurysm has been secured, BP should not be reduced in the subsequent weeks.

Monitoring and Management of Symptomatic Vasospasm/Delayed Cerebral Ischemia

More than 60% of patients with aSAH will demonstrate vasospasm on CT or ultrasound, but only about 30% will become symptomatic.[89,101] Many monitoring techniques, including frequent neurologic examinations, daily transcranial Doppler, CTA and CT perfusion, and multimodal physiologic monitoring (brain tissue oxygenation, microdialysis, jugular oximetry, continuous EEG), are currently available and should be implemented during the first 2 weeks after aSAH.[89]

In case of acute neurologic deterioration (decrease in two or more GCS points or increase in two or more NIHSS points), confounding factors—such as fever, hyponatremia, infection, or seizures—should be immediately ruled out, and the patient should be promptly treated for presumptive DCI. Historically, triple-H therapy (hypertension, hypervolemia, and hemodilution) was considered standard of care for these patients; recent studies, however, have shown no additional benefit, and an increased complication rate, with hypervolemia when compared to euvolemia. Therefore, current guidelines suggest maintenance of euvolemia followed by induced hypertension with vasopressors (hemodynamic augmentation). No specific BP level has been defined; each patient should be managed in a stepwise approach with assessment of neurologic function at each SBP or MAP level. If the neurologic deficit does not reverse with aggressive hemodynamic augmentation, urgent angiography should be considered for angioplasty and/or intra-arterial infusion of vasodilators.

Identification and Management of Medical Complications

Finally, systemic complications are very common in the aSAH population, including fever (54%), anemia (36%), hyperglycemia (30%), pneumonia (20%), and pulmonary edema (14%). Hyperglycemia, fever, and anemia are significantly associated with higher mortality and worse functional outcome.[102] Interestingly, there is considerable uncertainty regarding anemia management in aSAH. Some studies suggest a risk of worsened outcomes with packed RBC transfusion, and there is no agreement on optimal transfusion threshold. Transfusion criteria for general medical patients (Hgb < 7 g/dL) are, however, considered inadequate, and guidelines support packed RBC transfusion to maintain hemoglobin concentration above 8 g/dL.[112]

CONCLUSION

ICH and SAH are diseases that both result in a high rate of morbidity and mortality. In the case of ICH, early, aggressive, and structured management of factors that cause secondary brain injury is essential for optimizing outcomes. Although there is much that is unknown, optimal outcomes result from management in experienced ICUs and, in particular, ICUs dedicated to neurocritical care. In the case of aSAH, the greatest challenges are avoiding misdiagnosis and preventing complications of vasospasm. Accurate diagnosis has improved with advanced imaging (CTA and MRI) but still requires a low threshold for lumbar puncture. Perhaps, someday there will be a "troponin" for SAH, but until then, vigilance and aggressive pursuit of the diagnosis are essential.

LITERATURE TABLE

TRIAL	DESIGN	RESULT
ICH-Blood Pressure Management		
Anderson et al., *Lancet Neurol.* 2008[103] INTERACT	RCT of 203 patients with ICH and elevated BP (150–220 mm Hg). Patients assigned either to an early intensive BP-lowering strategy (target SBP = 140 mm Hg) or to a standard approach (target SBP = 180 mm Hg). Primary end point: proportional change in hematoma volume at 24 h	Trend toward lower growth in hematoma volumes at 24 h in the intensive treatment group (difference 22.6%, 95% CI 0.6%–44.5%; $p = 0.04$; absolute difference in volume 1.7 mL, 95% CI 0.5–3.9 mL; $p = 0.13$)
Antihypertensive Treatment of Acute Cerebral Hemorrhage (ATACH) investigators. *Crit Care Med.* 2010[104] ATACH	Multicenter prospective study of 60 patients with spontaneous ICH and elevated SBP (>170 mm Hg) presenting to the ED within 6 h of symptom onset. Patients assigned to one of three levels of antihypertensive treatment goals (tier 1, SBP ≥ 170 and <200 mm Hg; tier 2, SBP ≥ 140 and <170 mm Hg, tier 3, SBP ≥ 110 and <140 mm Hg). Primary outcomes: (1) treatment feasibility (achieving and maintaining the SBP goals for 18–24 h); (2) neurologic deterioration within 24 h; and (3) serious adverse events within 72 h	9 patients in tier 3 had treatment failure. A total of 7 patients had neurologic deterioration (1, 2, and 4 in tier 1, 2, and 3, respectively). One subject in tier 2 and three in tier 3 had serious adverse events; however, the safety-stopping rule was not activated in any of the tiers. Results confirmed the feasibility and safety of early rapid lowering of BP in ICH and formed the based for the larger randomized ATACH II trial (ongoing)
Butcher et al., *Stroke.* 2013[105] ICHADAPT	Multicenter, prospective, RCT of 75 patients with spontaneous ICH diagnosed <24 h after onset and SBP ≥ 150 mm Hg. Patients randomized to an SBP target of <150 mm Hg or <180 mm Hg to be achieved within 1 h of randomization. Primary end point: difference in perihematoma cerebral blood flow (CBF) between treatment groups as assessed by CT perfusion imaging 2 h postrandomization	After adjustment for baseline intraparenchymal hematoma volume and time to randomization, perihematoma CBF not significantly lower in patients randomized to SBP < 150 mm Hg compared with <180 mm Hg (absolute difference, 0.03; 95% CI, −0.018–0.078, $p = 0.18$)
Anderson et al., *N Engl J Med.* 2013[106] INTERACT-2	Multicenter, prospective, RCT of 2,839 patients with spontaneous ICH and elevated BP (150–220 mm Hg) Patients assigned to either an early intensive BP-lowering strategy (target SBP = 140) or a standard approach (target SBP = 180 mm Hg). Primary outcome: death or major disability (defined as a modified Rankin scale score of 3–6 at 90 d)	No statistically significant difference in primary outcome between the two groups (52% vs. 55.6%; OR with intensive treatment 0.87; 95% CI, 0.75–1.01; $p = 0.06$)
ICH-Coagulopathy		
Mayer et al., *N Engl J Med.* 2008[107] FAST	Multicenter, RCT of 841 patients with spontaneous ICH documented by CT within 3 h after onset of symptoms. Patients randomized to single intravenous dose of rFVIIa (20 or 80 μg/kg) or placebo within 4 h from onset of symptoms. Primary outcome: death or severe disability (modified Rankin scale 5–6 at 90 d)	80 μg/kg of rFVIIa associated with significant reduction in ICH expansion (mean estimated increase in volume of ICH: 26% placebo; 18% 20 μg/kg; 11% 80 μg/kg). Despite reduction in bleeding, there was no significant difference in the proportion of patients with poor outcome (24% placebo; 26% 20 μg/kg; 29% 80 μg/kg). More arterial thromboembolic events occurred in the group receiving rFVII 80 μg/kg vs. placebo (9% vs. 4%, $p = 0.04$)

(Continued)

LITERATURE TABLE *(Continued)*

TRIAL	DESIGN	RESULT
ICH–Surgical Treatment		
Mendelow et al., *Lancet.* 2013[42] STICH II	Multicenter, prospective, RCT of 601 patients with spontaneous lobar ICH ≤ 1 cm from the cortical surface of the brain, blood volume between 10 and 100 mL; admitted within 48 of onset of ictus. Patients randomized to early surgery (evacuation of hematoma within 12 h of randomization) or initial conservative treatment (delayed evacuation permitted if judged clinically appropriate). Primary outcome: prognosis-based favorable or unfavorable outcome dichotomized from the Extended Glasgow Outcome Scale at 6 mo after randomization	No difference in the primary outcome (absolute difference 3.7%; 95% CI, –4.3 to 11.6%; (OR) 0.86, CI 95%, 0.62–1.20; $p = 0.37$). In the subgroup of patients with a poor expected prognosis at enrollment (lower GCS, greater age, and larger ICH volume), early surgical intervention was associated with more favorable outcome (OR, 0.49, CI 95%, 0.26–0.92; $p = 0.02$). No advantage for surgery in the good prognosis group (OR 1.2, 95% CI, 0.75–1.68; $p = 0.57$)
Mendelow et al., *Lancet.* 2005[108] STICH	Multicenter, prospective, RCT of 1,033 patients with spontaneous supratentorial ICH randomized to early surgery (hematoma evacuated within 24 h of randomization by the method of choice of the responsible neurosurgeon, combined with the best medical treatment) or to initial conservative management (best medical treatment; later surgical evacuation allowed in case of neurologic deterioration). Primary outcome: death or disability using the extended Glasgow Outcome Scale 6 mo after ictus	Of the 468 patients randomized to early surgery analyzed at 6 mo, 122 (26%) had a favorable outcome compared with 118 (24%) of 496 patients randomized to initial conservative treatment (OR 0.89; 95% CI, 0.66–1.19; $p = 0.414$; absolute benefit 2.3%; relative benefit 10%) suggesting no benefit from early surgery compared with initial conservative treatment Subjects with lobar ICH within 1 cm of the cortical surface who underwent surgery had a statistically significant increase in good outcomes compared with similar subjects in the medical arm (8% absolute increase; $p = 0.02$)
SAH–Detection		
Perry et al., *JAMA.* 2013[68]	Multicenter cohort study of 2,131 ED patients with acute onset of nontraumatic headache peaking within 1 h, with no neurologic deficits (Table 21.4). Study tested clinical decision rules for detection of SAH	132 patients (6.2%) had subarachnoid hemorrhage. Ottawa SAH decision rule had 100% sensitivity (95% CI, 97.2%–100.0%) and 15.3% specificity (95% CI, 13.8%–16.9%) for SAH
SAH–Prevention of Rebleeding		
Hillman et al., *J Neurosurg.* 2002[90]	Multicenter, RCT of 596 patients with aSAH. Patients received tranexamic acid 1 g, given in the referring hospital, followed by 1 g every 6 h, until aneurysm treatment or for a maximum of 72 h. Control group did not receive any intervention. Primary end point: early rebleeding	Reduction from 10.8% to 2.4% in rebleeding rate in the tranexamic group (80% reduction in the mortality from early rebleeding). No difference in DCI or favorable functional outcomes
SAH–Aneurysm Treatment		
Molyneux et al., *Lancet.* 2002[96] ISAT	Multicenter, RCT of 2,143 patients with SAH and an intracranial aneurysm assigned to either endovascular coiling or surgical clipping. Primary end point: dependency (modified Rankin scale) or death at 1 y	23.7% of patients allocated to the endovascular clipping group were dependent or dead at 1 y vs. 30.6% of patients who underwent neurosurgical clipping ($p = 0.0019$). Relative risk reduction 22.6% (95% CI, 8.9–34.2)

LITERATURE TABLE (*Continued*)

TRIAL	DESIGN	RESULT
SAH–DCI Prophylaxis		
Pickard et al., *BMJ*. 1989[109]	Multicenter, prospective, RCT of 554 patients with aSAH admitted within 96 h of symptoms onset. Patients assigned to either nimodipine 60 mg orally every 4 h for 21 d, or placebo. Primary outcomes: (1) incidence of cerebral infarction and DCI; and (2) functional outcome at 3 mo	22% of patients in the nimodipine group had cerebral infarction vs. 33% in the placebo (relative risk reduction, 34%; 95% CI, 13%–50%). Poor functional outcomes significantly reduced in the nimodipine group as well (20% in patients given nimodipine vs. 33% for placebo)
SAH–Triple-H Therapy		
Lennihan et al., *Stroke*. 2000[110]	Prospective, RCT of 82 patients with surgical clipping on or before SAH day 6 and no symptomatic vasospasm. Patients given 80 mL/h of isotonic crystalloid + 250 mL of 5% albumin solution every 2 h to maintain normovolemia or hypervolemia	No difference between groups in mean global cerebral blood flow or in symptomatic vasospasm
Egge et al., *Neurosurgery*. 2001[111]	Prospective, RCT of 32 patients with aSAH surgically treated within 72 h of hemorrhage. Patients assigned to either normovolemia or hypervolemia	No difference between groups in vasospasm, regional cerebral blood flow, or functional outcome. Patients in the hypervolemia group experienced more complications ($p < 0.001$), including congestive heart failure (CHF), bleeding, and extradural hematomas

CI, confidence interval; OR, odds ratio.

REFERENCES

1. van Asch CJ, Luitse MJ, Rinkel GJ, et al. Incidence, case fatality, and functional outcome of intracerebral haemorrhage over time, according to age, sex, and ethnic origin: a systematic review and meta-analysis. *Lancet Neurol.* 2010;9(2):167–176.
2. Saloheimo P, Lapp TM, Juvela S, et al. The impact of functional status at three months on long-term survival after spontaneous intracerebral hemorrhage. *Stroke.* 2006;37(2):487–491.
3. Zahuranec DB, Gonzales NR, Brown DL, et al. Presentation of intracerebral haemorrhage in a community. *J Neurol Neurosurg Psychiatry.* 2006;77(3):340–344.
4. Zahuranec DB, Morgenstern LB, Sánchez BN, et al. Do-not-resuscitate orders and predictive models after intracerebral hemorrhage. *Neurology.* 2010;75(7):626–633.
5. Becker KJ, Baxter AB, Cohen WA, et al. Withdrawal of support in intracerebral hemorrhage may lead to self-fulfilling prophecies. *Neurology.* 2001;56(6):766–772.
6. Tirschwell DL, Becker KJ, Creutzfeldt CJ, et al. Propensity score matching to estimate supported outcomes in intracerebral hemorrhage patients with withdrawal of life support. In: AHA, ed. International Stroke Conference; Honolulu, Hawaii. *Stroke.* 2013;44:ATMP83.
7. Rordorf G, McDonald C. Spontaneous intracerebral hemorrhage: pathogenesis, clinical features, and diagnosis. In: Kasner SE, ed. Waltham, MA: UpToDate; 2013.
8. Flaherty ML, Kissela B, Woo D, et al. The increasing incidence of anticoagulant-associated intracerebral hemorrhage. *Neurology.* 2007;68(2):116–121.
9. Ariesen MJ, Claus SP, Rinkel GJ, et al. Risk factors for intracerebral hemorrhage in the general population: a systematic review. *Stroke.* 2003;34(8):2060–2065.
10. Sturgeon JD, Folsom AR, Longstreth WT Jr, et al. Risk factors for intracerebral hemorrhage in a pooled prospective study. *Stroke.* 2007;38(10):2718–2725.
11. Labovitz DL, Halim A, Boden-Albala B, et al. The incidence of deep and lobar intracerebral hemorrhage in whites, blacks, and Hispanics. *Neurology.* 2005;65(4):518–522.
12. Feigin VL, Lawes CM, Bennett DA, et al. Worldwide stroke incidence and early case fatality reported in 56 population-based studies: a systematic review. *Lancet Neurol.* 2009;8(4):355–369.

13. Brown RD Jr, Wiebers DO, Torner JC, et al. Frequency of intracranial hemorrhage as a presenting symptom and subtype analysis: a population-based study of intracranial vascular malformations in Olmsted Country, Minnesota. *J Neurosurg.* 1996;85(1):29–32.
14. Licata B, Turazzi S. Bleeding cerebral neoplasms with symptomatic hematoma. *J Neurosurg Sci.* 2003;47(4):201–210; discussion 210.
15. Katz JM, Segal AZ. Incidence and etiology of cerebrovascular disease in patients with malignancy. *Curr Atheroscler Rep.* 2005;7(4):280–288.
16. Brott T, Broderick J, Kothari R, et al. Early hemorrhage growth in patients with intracerebral hemorrhage. *Stroke.* 1997;28(1):1–5.
17. Hemphill JC, Andrews P, De Georgia M. Multimodal monitoring and neurocritical care bioinformatics. *Nat Rev Neurol.* 2011;7(8):451–460.
18. Vincent JL. *Textbook of Critical Care.* 6th ed. Philadelphia, PA: Elsevier/Saunders; 2011: xli, 1698.
19. Claassen J, Jette N, Chum F, et al. Electrographic seizures and periodic discharges after intracerebral hemorrhage. *Neurology.* 2007;69(13):1356–1365.
20. Sahni R, Weinberger J. Management of intracerebral hemorrhage. *Vasc Health Risk Manag.* 2007;3(5):701–709.
21. Leira R, Davalos A, Silva Y, et al. Early neurologic deterioration in intracerebral hemorrhage: predictors and associated factors. *Neurology.* 2004;63(3):461–467.
22. Andrews CM, Jauch EC, Hemphill JC III, et al. Emergency neurological life support: intracerebral hemorrhage. *Neurocrit Care.* 2012;17(suppl 1):S37–S46.
23. Kothari RU, Brott T, Broderick JP, et al. The ABCs of measuring intracerebral hemorrhage volumes. *Stroke.* 1996;27(8):1304–1305.
24. Beslow LA, Ichord RN, Kasner SE, et al. ABC/XYZ estimates intracerebral hemorrhage volume as a percent of total brain volume in children. *Stroke.* 2010;41(4):691–694.
25. Goldstein JN, Fazen LE, Snider R, et al. Contrast extravasation on CT angiography predicts hematoma expansion in intracerebral hemorrhage. *Neurology.* 2007;68(12):889–894.
26. Wada R, Aviv RI, Fox AJ, et al. CT angiography "spot sign" predicts hematoma expansion in acute intracerebral hemorrhage. *Stroke.* 2007;38(4):1257–1262.
27. Zhu XL, Chan MS, Poon WS. Spontaneous intracranial hemorrhage: which patients need diagnostic cerebral angiography? A prospective study of 206 cases and review of the literature. *Stroke.* 1997;28(7):1406–1409.
28. Hemphill JC III, Bonovich DC, Besmertis L, et al. The ICH score: a simple, reliable grading scale for intracerebral hemorrhage. *Stroke.* 2001;32(4):891–897.
29. Hemphill JC III, Farrant M, Neill TA Jr. Prospective validation of the ICH Score for 12-month functional outcome. *Neurology.* 2009;73(14):1088–1094.
30. Morgenstern LB, Hemphill JC III, Anderson C, et al. Guidelines for the management of spontaneous intracerebral hemorrhage: a guideline for healthcare professionals from the American Heart Association/American Stroke Association. *Stroke.* 2010;41(9):2108–2129.
31. Seder DB, Riker RR, Jagoda A, et al. Emergency neurological life support: airway, ventilation, and sedation. *Neurocrit Care.* 2012;17(suppl 1):S4–S20.
32. Carlberg B, Asplund K, Hagg E. The prognostic value of admission blood pressure in patients with acute stroke. *Stroke.* 1993;24(9):1372–1375.
33. Guyatt GH, Akl EA, Crowther M, et al. Executive summary: Antithrombotic Therapy and Prevention of Thrombosis, 9th ed: American College of Chest Physicians Evidence-Based Clinical Practice Guidelines. *Chest.* 2012;141(Suppl 2):7S–47S.
34. Degos V, Westbroek EM, Lawton MT, et al. Perioperative management of coagulation in nontraumatic intracerebral hemorrhage. *Anesthesiology.* 2013;119(1):218–227.
35. He J, Whelton PK, Vu B, et al. Aspirin and risk of hemorrhagic stroke: a meta-analysis of randomized controlled trials. *JAMA.* 1998;280(22):1930–1935.
36. Gorelick PB, Weisman SM. Risk of hemorrhagic stroke with aspirin use: an update. *Stroke.* 2005;36(8):1801–1807.
37. Tissue plasminogen activator for acute ischemic stroke. The National Institute of Neurological Disorders and Stroke rt-PA Stroke Study Group. *N Engl J Med.* 1995;333(24):1581–1587.
38. Yuan ZH, Jiang JK, Huang WD, et al. A meta-analysis of the efficacy and safety of recombinant activated factor VII for patients with acute intracerebral hemorrhage without hemophilia. *J Clin Neurosci.* 2010;17(6):685–693.
39. Balami JS, Buchan AM. Complications of intracerebral haemorrhage. *Lancet Neurol.* 2012;11(1):101–118.

40. Godoy DA, Pinero GR, Svampa S, et al. Hyperglycemia and short-term outcome in patients with spontaneous intracerebral hemorrhage. *Neurocrit Care.* 2008;9(2):217–229.
41. Qureshi AI, Palesch YY, Martin R, et al. Association of serum glucose concentrations during acute hospitalization with hematoma expansion, perihematomal edema, and three month outcome among patients with intracerebral hemorrhage. *Neurocrit Care.* 2011;15(3):428–435.
42. Mendelow AD, Gregson BA, Rowan EN, et al. Early surgery versus initial conservative treatment in patients with spontaneous supratentorial lobar intracerebral haematomas (STICH II): a randomised trial. *Lancet.* 2013;382(9890):397–408.
43. Hallevi H, Albright KC, Aronowski J, et al. Intraventricular hemorrhage: anatomic relationships and clinical implications. *Neurology.* 2008;70(11):848–852.
44. Brain Trauma Foundation; American Association of Neurological Surgeons; Congress of Neurological Surgeons. Guidelines for the management of severe traumatic brain injury. *J Neurotrauma* 2007;24(suppl 1): S1–S106.
45. Messe SR, Sansing LH, Cucchiara BL, et al. Prophylactic antiepileptic drug use is associated with poor outcome following ICH. *Neurocrit Care.* 2009;11(1):38–44.
46. Naidech AM, Garg RK, Liebling S, et al. Anticonvulsant use and outcomes after intracerebral hemorrhage. *Stroke.* 2009;40(12):3810–3815.
47. Finfer S, Chittock DR, Su SY, et al. Intensive versus conventional glucose control in critically ill patients. *N Engl J Med.* 2009;360(13):1283–1297.
48. Lacut K, Bressollette L, Le Gal G, et al. Prevention of venous thrombosis in patients with acute intracerebral hemorrhage. *Neurology.* 2005;65(6):865–869.
49. Diringer MN, Edwards DF. Admission to a neurologic/neurosurgical intensive care unit is associated with reduced mortality rate after intracerebral hemorrhage. *Crit Care Med.* 2001;29(3):635–640.
50. Kowalski RG, Claassen J, Kreiter KT, et al. Initial misdiagnosis and outcome after subarachnoid hemorrhage. *JAMA.* 2004;291(7):866–869.
51. Brisman JL, Song JK, Newell DW. Cerebral aneurysms. *N Engl J Med.* 2006;355(9):928–939.
52. Morita A, Kirino T, Hashi K, et al. The natural course of unruptured cerebral aneurysms in a Japanese cohort. *N Engl J Med.* 2012;366(26):2474–2482.
53. Juvela S. Prehemorrhage risk factors for fatal intracranial aneurysm rupture. *Stroke.* 2003;34(8): 1852–1857.
54. Frontera JA, Fernandez A, Claassen J, et al. Hyperglycemia after SAH: predictors, associated complications, and impact on outcome. *Stroke.* 2006;37(1):199–203.
55. Ohkuma H, Tsurutani H, Suzuki S. Incidence and significance of early aneurysmal rebleeding before neurosurgical or neurological management. *Stroke.* 2001;32(5):1176–1180.
56. Kim HC, Nam CM, Jee SH, et al. Comparison of blood pressure-associated risk of intracerebral hemorrhage and subarachnoid hemorrhage: Korea Medical Insurance Corporation study. *Hypertension.* 2005;46(2):393–397.
57. Wijdicks EF, Kallmes DF, Manno EM, et al. Subarachnoid hemorrhage: neurointensive care and aneurysm repair. *Mayo Clin Proc.* 2005;80(4):550–559.
58. Johnston SC, Selvin S, Gress DR. The burden, trends, and demographics of mortality from subarachnoid hemorrhage. *Neurology.* 1998;50(5):1413–1418.
59. Juvela S, Porras M, Poussa K. Natural history of unruptured intracranial aneurysms: probability of and risk factors for aneurysm rupture. *J Neurosurg.* 2008;108(5):1052–1060.
60. Vlak MH, Rinkel GJ, Greebe P, et al. Independent risk factors for intracranial aneurysms and their joint effect: a case–control study. *Stroke.* 2013;44(4):984–987.
61. Caranci F, Briganti F, Cirillo L, et al. Epidemiology and genetics of intracranial aneurysms. *Eur J Radiol.* 2013;82(10):1598–1605.
62. Perry JJ, Stiell IG, Sivilotti ML, et al. High risk clinical characteristics for subarachnoid haemorrhage in patients with acute headache: prospective cohort study. *BMJ.* 2010;341:c5204.
63. Hunt WE, Hess RM. Surgical risk as related to time of intervention in the repair of intracranial aneurysms. *J Neurosurg.* 1968;28(1):14–20.
64. Report of World Federation of Neurological Surgeons Committee on a Universal Subarachnoid Hemorrhage Grading Scale. *J Neurosurg.* 1988;68(6):985–986.
65. Edlow JA, Panagos PD, Godwin SA, et al. Clinical policy: critical issues in the evaluation and management of adult patients presenting to the emergency department with acute headache. *Ann Emerg Med.* 2008;52(4):407–436.
66. Perry JJ, Stiell I, Wells G, et al. Diagnostic test utilization in the emergency department for alert headache patients with possible subarachnoid hemorrhage. *CJEM.* 2002;4(5):333–337.

67. Morgenstern LB, Huber JC, Luna-Gonzales H, et al. Headache in the emergency department. *Headache.* 2001;41(6):537–541.
68. Perry JJ, Stiell IG, Sivilotti ML, et al. Clinical decision rules to rule out subarachnoid hemorrhage for acute headache. *JAMA.* 2013;310(12):1248–1255.
69. Perry JJ, Spacek A, Forbes M, et al. Is the combination of negative computed tomography result and negative lumbar puncture result sufficient to rule out subarachnoid hemorrhage? *Ann Emerg Med.* 2008; 51(6):707–713.
70. van Gijn J, Kerr RS, Rinkel GJ. Subarachnoid haemorrhage. *Lancet.* 2007;369(9558):306–318.
71. Cortnum S, Sorensen P, Jorgensen J. Determining the sensitivity of computed tomography scanning in early detection of subarachnoid hemorrhage. *Neurosurgery.* 2010;66(5):900–902; discussion 903.
72. Byyny RL, Mower WR, Shum N, et al. Sensitivity of noncontrast cranial computed tomography for the emergency department diagnosis of subarachnoid hemorrhage. *Ann Emerg Med.* 2008; 51(6):697–703.
73. Perry JJ, Stiell IG, Sivilotti ML, et al. Sensitivity of computed tomography performed within six hours of onset of headache for diagnosis of subarachnoid haemorrhage: prospective cohort study. *BMJ.* 2011;343:d4277.
74. McCormack RF, Hutson A. Can computed tomography angiography of the brain replace lumbar puncture in the evaluation of acute-onset headache after a negative noncontrast cranial computed tomography scan? *Acad Emerg Med.* 2010;17(4):444–451.
75. Agid R, Andersson T, Almqvist H, et al. Negative CT angiography findings in patients with spontaneous subarachnoid hemorrhage: when is digital subtraction angiography still needed? *AJNR Am J Neuroradiol.* 2010;31(4):696–705.
76. Fisher CM, Kistler JP, Davis JM. Relation of cerebral vasospasm to subarachnoid hemorrhage visualized by computerized tomographic scanning. *Neurosurgery.* 1980;6(1):1–9.
77. Claassen J, Bernardini GL, Kreiter K, et al. Effect of cisternal and ventricular blood on risk of delayed cerebral ischemia after subarachnoid hemorrhage: the Fisher scale revisited. *Stroke.* 2001; 32(9):2012–2020.
78. Huang J, van Gelder JM. The probability of sudden death from rupture of intracranial aneurysms: a meta-analysis. *Neurosurgery.* 2002;51(5):1101–1105; discussion 1105–1107.
79. Fujii Y, Takeuchi S, Sasaki O, et al. Ultra-early rebleeding in spontaneous subarachnoid hemorrhage. *J Neurosurg.* 1996;84(1):35–42.
80. Naidech AM, Janjua N, Kreiter KT, et al. Predictors and impact of aneurysm rebleeding after subarachnoid hemorrhage. *Arch Neurol.* 2005;62(3):410–416.
81. Starke RM, Connolly ES Jr. Rebleeding after aneurysmal subarachnoid hemorrhage. *Neurocrit Care.* 2011;15(2):241–246.
82. Connolly ES Jr, Rabinstein AA, Carhuapoma JR, et al. Guidelines for the management of aneurysmal subarachnoid hemorrhage: a guideline for healthcare professionals from the American Heart Association/ American Stroke Association. *Stroke.* 2012;43(6):1711–1737.
83. Diringer MN, Bleck TP, Claude Hemphill J, et al. Critical care management of patients following aneurysmal subarachnoid hemorrhage: recommendations from the Neurocritical Care Society's Multidisciplinary Consensus Conference. *Neurocrit Care.* 2011;15(2):211–240.
84. Edlow JA, Samuels O, Smith WS, et al. Emergency neurological life support: subarachnoid hemorrhage. *Neurocrit Care.* 2012;17(suppl 1):S47–S53.
85. Bruder N, Rabinstein A. Cardiovascular and pulmonary complications of aneurysmal subarachnoid hemorrhage. *Neurocrit Care.* 2011;15(2):257–269.
86. Wijdicks EF, Vermeulen M, Murray GD, et al. The effects of treating hypertension following aneurysmal subarachnoid hemorrhage. *Clin Neurol Neurosurg.* 1990;92(2):111–117.
87. Suarez JI, Tarr RW, Selman WR. Aneurysmal subarachnoid hemorrhage. *N Engl J Med.* 2006;354(4):387–396.
88. Schiefecker AJ, Pfausler B, Beer R, et al. Parenteral diclofenac infusion significantly decreases brain-tissue oxygen tension in patients with poor-grade aneurysmal subarachnoid hemorrhage. *Crit Care.* 2013;17(3):R88.
89. Rabinstein AA, Lanzino G, Wijdicks EF. Multidisciplinary management and emerging therapeutic strategies in aneurysmal subarachnoid haemorrhage. *Lancet Neurol.* 2010;9(5):504–519.
90. Hillman J, Fridriksson S, Nilsson O, et al. Immediate administration of tranexamic acid and reduced incidence of early rebleeding after aneurysmal subarachnoid hemorrhage: a prospective randomized study. *J Neurosurg.* 2002;97(4):771–778.

91. Hellingman CA, van den Bergh WM, Beijer IS, et al. Risk of rebleeding after treatment of acute hydrocephalus in patients with aneurysmal subarachnoid hemorrhage. *Stroke.* 2007;38(1):96–99.
92. Ransom ER, Mocco J, Komotar RJ, et al. External ventricular drainage response in poor grade aneurysmal subarachnoid hemorrhage: effect on preoperative grading and prognosis. *Neurocrit Care.* 2007;6(3):174–180.
93. Mak CH, Lu YY, Wong GK. Review and recommendations on management of refractory raised intracranial pressure in aneurysmal subarachnoid hemorrhage. *Vasc Health Risk Manag.* 2013;9:353–359.
94. Naidech AM, Kreiter KT, Janjua N, et al. Phenytoin exposure is associated with functional and cognitive disability after subarachnoid hemorrhage. *Stroke.* 2005;36(3):583–587.
95. Vespa P, Diringer MN. High-volume centers. *Neurocrit Care.* 2011;15(2):369–372.
96. Molyneux A, Kerr R, Stratton I, et al. International Subarachnoid Aneurysm Trial (ISAT) of neurosurgical clipping versus endovascular coiling in 2143 patients with ruptured intracranial aneurysms: a randomised trial. *Lancet.* 2002;360(9342):1267–1274.
97. Spetzler RF, McDougall CG, Albuquerque FC, et al. The Barrow Ruptured Aneurysm Trial: 3-year results. *J Neurosurg.* 2013;119(1):146–157.
98. Dorhout Mees SM, Rinkel GJ, Feigin VL, et al. Calcium antagonists for aneurysmal subarachnoid haemorrhage. *Cochrane Database Syst Rev.* 2007(3):CD000277.
99. Rabinstein AA, Bruder N. Management of hyponatremia and volume contraction. *Neurocrit Care.* 2011;15(2):354–360.
100. Gress DR. Monitoring of volume status after subarachnoid hemorrhage. *Neurocrit Care.* 2011; 15(2):270–274.
101. Rowland MJ, Hadjipavlou G, Kelly M, et al. Delayed cerebral ischaemia after subarachnoid haemorrhage: looking beyond vasospasm. *Br J Anaesth.* 2012;109(3):315–329.
102. Wartenberg KE, Schmidt JM, Claassen J, et al. Impact of medical complications on outcome after subarachnoid hemorrhage. *Crit Care Med.* 2006;34(3):617–623; quiz 624.
103. Anderson CS, Huang Y, Wang JG, et al. Intensive blood pressure reduction in acute cerebral haemorrhage trial (INTERACT): a randomised pilot trial. *Lancet Neurol.* 2008;7(5):391–399.
104. Antihypertensive Treatment of Acute Cerebral Hemorrhage (ATACH) investigators. Antihypertensive treatment of acute cerebral hemorrhage. *Crit Care Med.* 2010;38(2):637–648.
105. Butcher KS, Jeerakathil T, Hill M, et al. The intracerebral hemorrhage acutely decreasing arterial pressure trial. *Stroke.* 2013;44(3):620–626.
106. Anderson CS, Heeley E, Huang Y, et al. Rapid blood-pressure lowering in patients with acute intracerebral hemorrhage. *N Engl J Med.* 2013;368(25):2355–2365.
107. Mayer SA, Brun NC, Begtrup K, et al. Efficacy and safety of recombinant activated factor VII for acute intracerebral hemorrhage. *N Engl J Med.* 2008;358(20):2127–2137.
108. Mendelow AD, Gregson BA, Fernandes HM, et al. Early surgery versus initial conservative treatment in patients with spontaneous supratentorial intracerebral haematomas in the International Surgical Trial in Intracerebral Haemorrhage (STICH): a randomised trial. *Lancet.* 2005;365(9457):387–397.
109. Pickard JD, Murray GD, Illingworth R, et al. Effect of oral nimodipine on cerebral infarction and outcome after subarachnoid haemorrhage: British aneurysm nimodipine trial. *BMJ.* 1989;298(6674):636–642.
110. Lennihan L, Mayer SA, Fink ME, et al. Effect of hypervolemic therapy on cerebral blood flow after subarachnoid hemorrhage: a randomized controlled trial. *Stroke.* 2000;31(2):383–391.
111. Egge A, Waterloo K, Sjoholm H, et al. Prophylactic hyperdynamic postoperative fluid therapy after aneurysmal subarachnoid hemorrhage: a clinical, prospective, randomized, controlled study. *Neurosurgery.* 2001;49(3):593–605; discussion 605–596.
112. Le Roux PD. Anemia and transfusion after subarachnoid hemorrhage. *Neurocrit Care.* 2011; 15(2):342–353.

22

Seizure and Status Epilepticus

Brandon Foreman and Anil Mendiratta

BACKGROUND

Seizure is a common emergency department (ED) presentation. Seizing patients may arrive actively convulsing, with a depressed level of consciousness, or comatose. In these patients, the emergency physician's challenges are to provide immediate and appropriate treatment, to evaluate for ongoing seizures or status epilepticus (SE), and to assess for seizure cause. The adage "time is brain" is as relevant to the treatment of seizure as it is in stroke therapy; early identification and control of ongoing seizures minimizes neurologic injury, reduces complications, and improves patient outcomes.

EPIDEMIOLOGY

Based on a nationwide sample, seizures account for an estimated 1.1 million visits to US EDs each year.[1] Just over 11% of the population will experience a seizure in the course of a lifetime, and approximately 1% of the population carries a diagnosis of epilepsy or recurrent unprovoked seizures.[2,3] Worldwide, the age-adjusted incidence of unprovoked seizures is around 60/100,000 person-years.[3,4] Approximately one-third of these are first-time seizures occurring in patients who otherwise will not develop epilepsy. Acute symptomatic seizures (also called provoked seizures) result from a clear underlying acute cause such as trauma, stroke, or hypoglycemia and have an age-adjusted incidence between 20 and 40/100,000 person-years.[4]

The majority of patients evaluated in the ED for seizures arrive by ambulance[5]; one-quarter of these patients require advanced life support (ALS) management by paramedics.[6] Over 25% of patients who present with seizures will be admitted to the hospital, and 1% will require endotracheal intubation for mechanical ventilation.[1] Mortality varies based on etiology, and while seizure patients rarely die in the ED,[1] the short-term 30-day mortality following an acute symptomatic seizure is reported to be as high as 19%.[7]

SE occurs when seizures are prolonged (>5 minutes) or recur before the patient fully recovers. Any patient who arrives to the ED seizing should be considered in SE. SE is diagnosed in up to 6% of all ED seizure presentations,[5] and has been estimated to occur in up to 152,000 patients annually in the United States alone.[8]

Nonconvulsive seizures are those in which the patient has only subtle or no overt clinical signs of ongoing seizures (other than depressed level of consciousness), but electroencephalography (EEG) demonstrates ongoing electrographic seizure activity. Nonconvulsive SE is seen in nearly half of patients who remain comatose after apparent control of initial convulsive SE.[9] While the incidence of nonconvulsive SE is reported to occur in one-quarter of all SE, this is likely an underestimate because continuous EEG monitoring is not immediately available in many medical centers.[10]

SE is associated with significant morbidity and mortality. Overall mortality is estimated to be 20%,[8] and this number climbs substantially when SE is associated with an acute symptomatic cause, advanced age, concurrent medical illness, and/or prolonged time to achieve seizure control.[11,12] Of these factors, only the duration of SE is modifiable, and it correlates with outcome: when SE resolves within 30 minutes, the reported mortality is 3%, compared to 19% with resolution after 30 minutes,[13] and 32% with resolution after 60 minutes.[11] Of those patients that survive SE, 41% will develop epilepsy.[14]

PREHOSPITAL EVALUATION AND MANAGEMENT

In the vast majority of cases, seizures will have resolved by the time paramedics arrive on the scene. Once in the ED, timely gathering of patient information—including a history of prior epilepsy or neurologic injury/disorder, an accurate medication list, and a point-of-care glucose—will facilitate appropriate care.

Patients in whom seizures have resolved may be safely transported to the ED by emergency medical services (EMS) for further evaluation without advanced life support (ALS) monitoring (i.e., a basic life support, or BLS unit).[6] However, one-quarter of patients with a chief complaint of seizure will have evidence of a serious concurrent illness/injury or neurologic/cardiopulmonary instability, often due to ongoing seizures or SE.[6] Given the delays associated with the resuscitation of the patient, transportation, and triage upon arrival,[15] it is essential to initiate early and adequate treatment of seizures prior to arrival to the ED. In addition to providing basic support, evidence supports the prompt administration of benzodiazepines (e.g., lorazepam, midazolam, or diazepam) in the prehospital setting by ALS providers, as these agents have been shown to terminate seizures and SE more effectively than placebo[16] or phenytoin alone.[17] Adequate benzodiazepine dosing in the field also results in significantly fewer seizure-related complications including respiratory failure requiring intubation[16] (Table 22.1).

Because intravenous (IV) lorazepam requires IV access and must be refrigerated in order to maintain stability in solution, rectal diazepam—despite its inferiority in a prospective, population-based study—has long been used in the home and acute care settings for children or adults with epilepsy who experience recurrent seizures.[18–20] In 2010, a meta-analysis of seizure control in children and young adults demonstrated intramuscular (IM), intranasal, or buccal midazolam also provides faster and more efficacious treatment when compared to diazepam by any route.[21] In 2012, a randomized controlled trial of IM midazolam versus IV lorazepam (the RAMPART trial) demonstrated IM midazolam to be more rapidly administered and at least as effective as IV lorazepam in terminating seizures and SE in adults, making IM midazolam an ideal choice for EMS or ED providers.[22] Evidence for the use of buccal and intranasal forms of midazolam in the adult population is lacking[23,24] (Fig. 22.1).

TABLE 22.1 Prehospital Evaluation of Seizures or SE

Prehospital Evaluation	
Vital signs	Heart rate, blood pressure, and oxygen saturation
Positioning	Left lateral decubitus; avoid placing objects inside mouth. If uncomplicated by other injury, no cervical stabilization is necessary
History of prior epilepsy or neurologic injury/disorder	If available, should include the name or contact information for the patient's neurologist
Concurrent illnesses or injuries	
Active medications	Including any available pill bottles (both full and empty)
Secondary injury screening	Fractures, hematoma, or burns may be seen
Point-of-care glucose testing	Low glucose should be treated with 100 mg IV thiamine prior to administration of 50% dextrose to prevent acute thiamine deficiency
IV access	Should not delay treatment in the case of ongoing seizures or status epilepticus. IM midazolam should be given if an IV site cannot be established immediately
ED activation by EMS	For any patient in status epilepticus, notification to prepare for incoming emergency by the ED is appropriate

ED, emergency department; EMS, emergency medical service; IM, intramuscular; IV, intravenous.

EMERGENCY DEPARTMENT DIAGNOSTIC EVALUATION

Seizures and SE resolve in approximately 70% of patients who are promptly treated with adequately dosed benzodiazepines, either en route to or upon arrival to the ED.[16,17,22,25] Once a patient demonstrates an improving level of consciousness, further treatment for the initial seizure may not be required. The emergency physician should continue the initial prehospital investigation into the cause of the seizures or SE and concurrently manage any recurrent seizures and associated illnesses (Table 22.2).

Patients with History of Epilepsy

If the patient takes antiepileptic drugs (AEDs) and/or has a known history of epilepsy, a careful history and evaluation should assess for a reason that the patient's seizure threshold might be reduced (e.g., missed medications, excessive sleep deprivation or alcohol intake, concurrent illness). The patient's neurologist should be contacted for further information and recommendations. If the patient has fully recovered, a safe discharge plan often can be made in conjunction with the patient's outpatient neurologist. If there is a history of missed medication doses, the neurologist may advise a partial "loading" dose in the ED. If there is no history of noncompliance, an increase in the standing AED dose may be advised. A brief low-dose benzodiazepine taper, such as lorazepam 0.5 to 1 mg once or twice daily for 1 to 3 days, may also be recommended in order to minimize the risk of seizure recurrence over the next few days as AED dosage adjustments are made. It is important to ensure that while the patient is being observed in the ED, he or she is administered all of his/her regularly scheduled AED doses. Of note, some of the newer AEDs are nonformulary in many hospitals; AEDs cannot be substituted for one

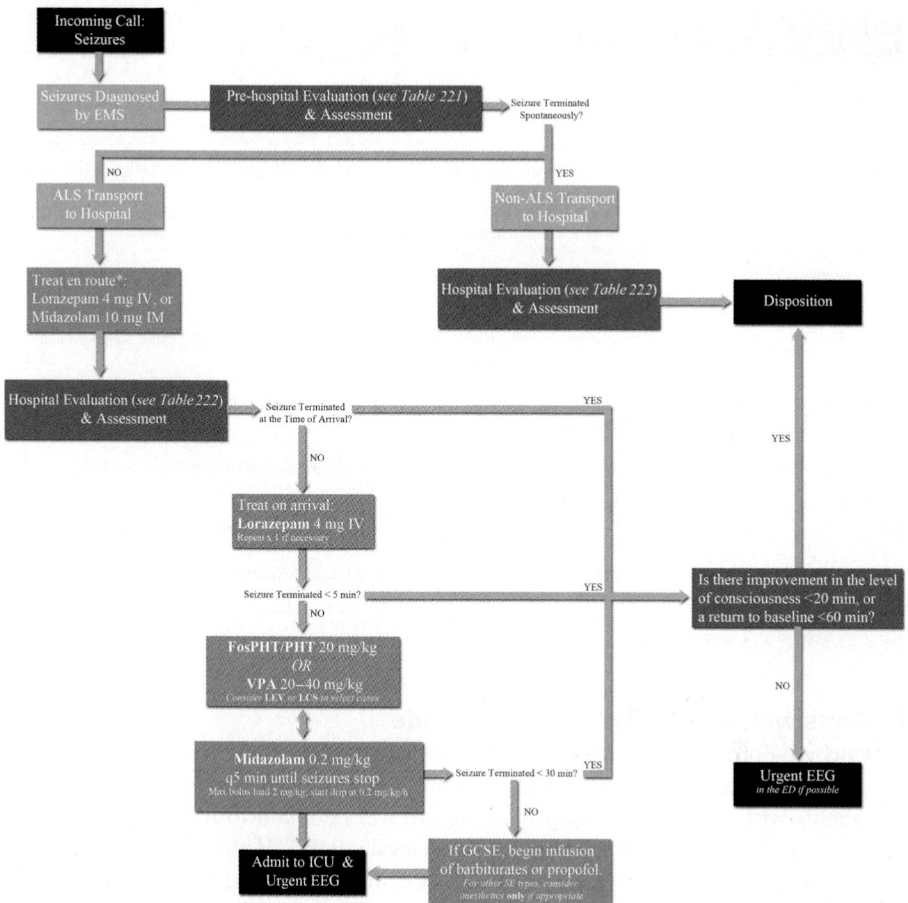

FIGURE 22.1 A sample protocol for the comprehensive evaluation and management of seizures and status epilepticus. *Treatment dosing recommendations are for adult patients >40 kg. ALS, advanced life support; EEG, electroencephalography; ED, emergency department; EMS, emergency medical services; GCSE, generalized convulsive status epilepticus; ICU, intensive care unit; IM, intramuscular; IV, intravenous; LCS, lacosamide; LEV, levetiracetam; FosPHT/PHT, fosphenytoin/phenytoin; SE, status epilepticus; VPA, valproic acid.

another (e.g., the patient who is taking lacosamide [LCS] should not be given phenytoin or carbamazepine because LCS is unavailable).

As emergency physicians often function as the default primary physician for many community patients, they should be alert for patients who repeatedly visit the ED for seizures. Patients with recurrent unprovoked seizures despite compliance with AEDs have refractory or pharmacoresistant epilepsy.[26] Refractory epilepsy patients should be referred to a comprehensive epilepsy center, where optimal management of AEDs may improve seizure control; these patients may also be evaluated for potentially curative epilepsy surgery, which has been shown to be more effective than medication in many patients.[27]

TABLE 22.2 ED Evaluation of Seizures or SE

Hospital Evaluation	
Vital signs	Continuous telemetry and pulse oximetry; intermittent blood pressure monitoring
Neurologic exam	Focal deficits may indicate underlying cause and/or help identify anatomic origin of the seizure
Contact outpatient physician	Obtain a history of prior hospitalizations, neurologic disorders/epilepsy, and current medications; involvement should help to facilitate management planning and safe disposition
Laboratory studies	Basic metabolic panel including calcium, magnesium, and glucose; complete blood count; liver function tests. A urinalysis and urine toxicology screen may be considered
AED levels	For patients already on AEDs, appropriate serum levels should be requested even if available assays are not run locally by the hospital
Lumbar puncture	In specific situations such as patients with fever, meningismus, acute headache, or a history of immunosuppression
Imaging (CT or MRI)	Not necessary in patients with a history of epilepsy in whom a clear cause for seizure exacerbation is identified (e.g., missed AEDs)
EEG	For first unprovoked seizures: Arrange as outpatient within shortest time possible
	For patients who remain comatose or do not return to baseline: Arrange emergently in the ED or immediately upon admission

AED, antiepileptic drug; CT, computed tomography; EEG, electroencephalogram; MRI, magnetic resonance imaging.

Patients with a Resolved Seizure Episode

Patients who present after a first-time unprovoked seizure should have a complete ED evaluation as outlined in Table 22.2. Prompt imaging is important, as approximately 10% of patients with a first-time unprovoked seizure will be found to have abnormality on head CT or brain MRI that warrants further evaluation.[28] If the patient has no risk factors for epilepsy (i.e., no history of neurologic injury, significant head trauma, CNS infection, or family history of epilepsy), and the neurologic examination and brain imaging (noncontrast head CT or brain MRI) are normal, an AED does not need to be started in the ED. These patients have a risk of seizure recurrence of approximately 40% over the next 2 years,[29] and consequently, many opt to defer AED treatment until a second definite unprovoked seizure occurs. However, an outpatient EEG should be arranged, as approximately one-third will have an EEG with epileptiform discharges, effectively doubling the risk for seizure recurrence.[28] Because of the risk of seizure recurrence, patients with a first-time unprovoked seizure should be advised against driving, and both patients and their families should be educated about seizure precautions and seizure first aid. An outpatient neurology consultation can help guide further diagnostic evaluation and discussions about prognosis with regard to risk of seizure recurrence, AEDs, and activity restrictions.

Importantly, the patient who has recovered to baseline following an isolated seizure does not require administration of IV/IM benzodiazepines, or the rapid IV loading dose of an AED, such as phenytoin. These may needlessly sedate the patient or cause unwarranted complications such as respiratory depression or hemodynamic instability.

Patients with acute symptomatic seizures (seizures provoked by systemic illness or brain injury, as opposed to seizures without a clear underlying cause) are typically admitted for evaluation and management of the underlying etiology (e.g., intracranial hemorrhage,

CNS infection) uncovered during their evaluation, as well as for observation for seizure recurrence. Depending upon the cause of the seizure, treatment with an AED may be indicated in order to minimize the risk of recurrent seizures and their associated complications. Consultation with a neurologist is always warranted in these cases.

MANAGEMENT GUIDELINES

First-Time or Resolved Seizure

Patients with a first-time seizure found to be at risk for seizure recurrence based on diagnostic evaluation (e.g., abnormal neuroimaging or epileptiform abnormalities on EEG) warrant treatment initiation with an AED. Consultation with a neurologist is advisable in order to guide the selection of the AED. However, if a neurologist is not available, the emergency physician should consider both the adverse effects and drug–drug interactions of the AED that is chosen. Although phenytoin (PHT) has traditionally been considered a default AED, current consensus recommends against PHT as a first-line agent because of its relatively unfavorable adverse effect profile, pharmacokinetics, and prominent drug–drug interactions. Newer-generation AEDs, such as levetiracetam (LEV), may be more appropriate for several reasons: broad-spectrum action (e.g., effective for both partial and generalized-onset seizures), renal excretion, lack of hepatic induction, and absence of drug–drug interactions. Importantly, the emergency physician should also consider individual medical and psychiatric comorbidities. Patients should be educated on potential adverse medication effects, such as allergic reactions, and arrangements should be made for neurology follow-up evaluation within a few weeks.

Status Epilepticus

For the patients who arrive to the ED seizing, or those who develop recurrent, ongoing seizures while in the ED, rapid and aggressive treatment to stop seizures is critical. Current laboratory evidence suggests that within minutes, seizure activity produces changes in the synaptic membrane receptors, altering the balance between inhibitory and excitatory neurotransmission, followed by changes in neuropeptide expression. The excitotoxicity that results culminates in neuronal death, which may be widespread after prolonged (or self-sustaining) SE.[30] Human data are limited, but seminal primate studies have clearly shown that even in the absence of the systemic effects of SE (e.g., hyperthermia, hypoxia), prolonged SE can cause ischemic neuronal loss, likely related to cerebral metabolic supply–demand mismatch.[31] In humans, even very focal seizures visible only using intracranial electrodes but lasting longer than 5 minutes create clear changes in brain and systemic physiology,[32] suggesting that seizures create a dangerous environment for sensitive neurons.

Response to medication can drop by as much as 50% when medications are either underdosed or given in a delayed manner such that SE is prolonged beyond 120 minutes.[33,34] Reducing the time to initial adequate treatment is challenging, as EMS run times average between 20 and 40 minutes,[6,16] and patients may experience subsequent delays to hospital triage and treatment of up to 50 minutes.[15,25] If SE continues from the ambulance to the hospital, adherence to an established ED clinical protocol may be the most important factor in shortening the duration of SE, minimizing the likelihood of conversion to refractory SE, and reducing the intensive care unit (ICU) length of stay[25] (Fig. 22.2).

Unfortunately, studies to date have demonstrated poor adherence to established ED protocols, including both dosage and timing of medications.[15,25,35] In one study, no patient received an adequate dose of phenytoin.[16] In another, more than 50% of patients received initial treatment more than 1 hour after the onset of SE.[35] The inclusion of both prehospital- and ED-based management as part of a unified treatment protocol for SE has not yet been studied adequately. A recently proposed Emergency Neurological Life Support protocol builds upon data showing improved outcomes with reduced treatment time in patients with acute myocardial infarction and highlights the importance of continuity in care from the ambulance to the hospital bed.[36]

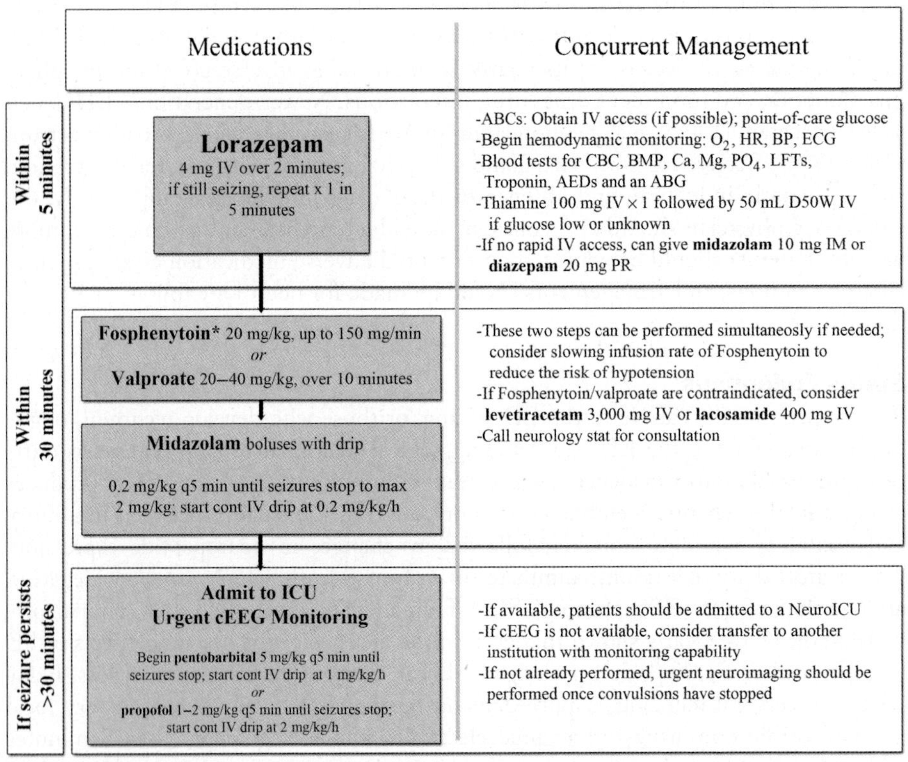

Medications
Concurrent Management
Within 5 minutes
Lorazepam
4 mg IV over 2 minutes; if still seizing, repeat x 1 in 5 minutes
-ABCs: Obtain IV access (if possible); point-of-care glucose
-Begin hemodynamic monitoring: O2, HR, BP, ECG
-Blood tests for CBC, BMP, Ca, Mg, PO4, LFTs, Troponin, AEDs and an ABG
-Thiamine 100 mg IV × 1 followed by 50 mL D50W IV if glucose low or unknown
-If no rapid IV access, can give midazolam 10 mg IM or diazepam 20 mg PR
Within 30 minutes
Fosphenytoin* 20 mg/kg, up to 150 mg/min
or
Valproate 20–40 mg/kg, over 10 minutes
Midazolam boluses with drip
0.2 mg/kg q5 min until seizures stop to max 2 mg/kg; start cont IV drip at 0.2 mg/kg/h
-These two steps can be performed simultaneosly if needed; consider slowing infusion rate of Fosphenytoin to reduce the risk of hypotension
-If Fosphenytoin/valproate are contraindicated, consider levetiracetam 3,000 mg IV or lacosamide 400 mg IV
-Call neurology stat for consultation
If seizure persists >30 minutes
Admit to ICU
Urgent cEEG Monitoring
Begin pentobarbital 5 mg/kg q5 min until seizures stop; start cont IV drip at 1 mg/kg/h
or
propofol 1–2 mg/kg q5 min until seizures stop; start cont IV drip at 2 mg/kg/h
-If available, patients should be admitted to a NeuroICU
-If cEEG is not available, consider transfer to another institution with monitoring capability
-If not already performed, urgent neuroimaging should be performed once convulsions have stopped
*Phenytoin may be used if Fosphenytoin is not available. Ensure quality IV access and reduce infusion rates to to 50 mg/min to reduce hypotension and cardiac dysrhyhtmias.

FIGURE 22.2 A sample protocol for the ED management of generalized convulsive SE. ABCs, airway, breathing, and circulation; ABG, arterial blood gas; AEDs, antiepileptic drugs; BMP, basic metabolic panel; BP, blood pressure; Ca, calcium; CBC, complete blood count; cEEG, continuous electroencephalographic monitoring; ECG electrocardiogram; HR, heart rate; ICU, intensive care unit; LFTs, liver function tests; Mg, magnesium; PO_4, phosphorous. Modified from Foreman B, Hirsch LJ. Epilepsy emergencies: diagnosis and management. *Neurol Clin.* 2012;30:11–41.

Medical Therapy

For the patient in SE (i.e., arrived to the ED seizing or with recurrent ongoing seizure in the ED), IV benzodiazepines are the first line of treatment. If IV access is available, lorazepam 4 mg IV over 2 minutes should be administered immediately. If IV access cannot be obtained rapidly, midazolam 10 mg IM should instead be administered. Rectal diazepam 15 to 20 mg is an alternative if IM midazolam is not immediately available. If the patient continues to have clinical seizures, benzodiazepine dosing may be repeated; at this point, the patient will likely require airway support. If not already done in the prehospital setting, point-of-care glucose testing should be performed immediately. Low or borderline low serum glucose should be treated with thiamine 100 mg IV followed by 50 mL D50W (given together to prevent acute thiamine deficiency).

Second-Line Agents

All patients presenting with SE should be started on a second-line AED following the administration of initial benzodiazepines—even if seizure activity is terminated—in order to prevent seizure recurrence as the effect of the benzodiazepines wanes over the next several hours. For patients who continue to seize, or who do not regain consciousness despite adequate benzodiazepine dosing (in the field and/or in the ED), rapid initiation of a second-line agent is critical. If benzodiazepines were given in the prehospital setting, second-line agents should be initiated at the same time as the first-line ED benzodiazepine therapy.

Phenytoin (PHT) is the traditional second-line agent. PHT is frequently underdosed (the usual 1,000 mg IV load is only adequate for a 50-kg person)[15]; the appropriate dosing is 20 mg/kg at a rate of 50 mg/min. For this dose, cardiac monitoring is required; hypotension is a common side effect requiring slower infusion rates.[17] Of note, PHT solvent extravasation from a peripheral IV can cause significant tissue injury. A rare idiosyncratic reaction causing digital ischemia, known as the "purple glove syndrome," has also been reported with IV PHT.

Fosphenytoin, a water-soluble PHT prodrug, avoids these complications, is associated with fever hypotensive episodes, and may be infused more rapidly (up to 150 mg/min). However, fosphenytoin is substantially more expensive, costing nearly eight times as much as PHT.[37] Cardiac arrhythmias and respiratory depression can occur with both medications. PHT is highly protein bound, induces the hepatic cytochrome P450 enzymatic system (specifically CYP3A and CYP2C), and may interact with other medications or AEDs. As such, PHT may cause problematic drug–drug interactions in patients with HIV, cancer, or solid organ transplants.

Valproic acid (VPA) has been studied in five randomized controlled trials recently included in a meta-analysis and appears to be at least as effective as PHT with fewer overall adverse effects.[38] VPA loading doses range between 20 and 40 mg/kg over 10 minutes. Side effects include hyperammonemia and pancreatitis and an increased risk of bleeding due to diminished platelet activation, prolonged thrombin time, and dose-dependent thrombocytopenia.[39,40] Importantly, cardiac arrhythmias and hypotension are rare, even among the elderly or critically ill.[41] VPA is protein bound like PHT, but acts as an inhibitor of CYP2C9, increasing the bioavailability of medications such as warfarin, amitriptyline, and clopidogrel. For both PHT and VPA, free and total serum drug levels should be drawn for the initial monitoring of these medications given their protein binding and pharmacokinetics.

Other Second-Line Agents

LEV, LCS, and phenobarbital are three additional second-line agents that may be considered in special circumstances. Intravenous LEV is negligibly protein bound and does not interact with hepatically cleared medications. Loading doses of 1,000 to 3,000 mg infused over 15 minutes are associated with minimal side effects.[42] However, studies of LEV as a second-line agent are lacking: Only one prospective study randomized patients to LEV either as a first-line or a second-line agent, and most were treated without benzodiazepines.[43] In a prospective observational study comparing LEV to phenobarbital and VPA as second-line agents in the treatment of SE, LEV demonstrated a higher risk for treatment failure compared to VPA when controlled for the severity of SE and potentially fatal underlying causes (odds ratio 2.69).[44] LCS is a relatively new IV agent with limited data available regarding efficacy. Like LEV, LCS has limited drug–drug interactions, and safety has been demonstrated with IV loading doses up to 400 mg over 15 minutes. Adverse effects include dizziness, nausea, and a dose-dependent prolongation of the PR interval on electrocardiography of unclear clinical significance.[45] Because of the lack of drug interactions, LCS and LEV may be considered as options in patients being treated for HIV, cancer, or solid organ transplants, although studies regarding this are lacking. Phenobarbital, an early antiepileptic agent limited by adverse effects, is administered as a 20 mg/kg load at 50 mg/min (similar to phenobarbital). Although its use in SE was comparable to lorazepam in a randomized clinical trial,[17] it requires a slow load time to avoid well-documented side effects including hypotension and respiratory depression. Airway support and possibly mechanical ventilation should be instituted prior to administration of an IV phenobarbital load. Phenobarbital should be considered only if other agents are unavailable, or if a patient on phenobarbital as an outpatient presents with subtherapeutic levels.

Refractory Status Epilepticus

SE usually stops after adequate dosages of first- and second-line medications. If not responsive to first- and second-line agents, SE is considered refractory.[46,47] When SE has truly stopped, a postictal state frequently develops, characterized by alterations in consciousness or cognition, behavior, or motor function. The postictal state is related to the type and duration of seizures: After focal seizures lasting a mean of 128 seconds recorded on video-EEG, one study documented postictal periods consisting of confusion, aphasia, or subtle nonpurposeful movements that lasted on average for 89 seconds.[48] In another study, following generalized convulsions captured on video, patients appeared unresponsive for up to 20 minutes (mean time of ~4 minutes) prior to first nonrespiratory movement.[49] Therefore, if seizures have stopped and the patient has not begun to improve neurologically within 20 minutes, or has not returned to baseline by 60 minutes, nonconvulsive SE should be considered.

Aggressive treatment for refractory generalized convulsive SE should begin in the ED. Close cardiopulmonary monitoring and support is crucial to reduce the risk for complications and ensure safe transition to the ICU. Endotracheal intubation and mechanical ventilation is frequently required.[46] Paralytics often given for intubation mask motor symptoms of generalized convulsive SE, and once paralysis has occurred, treatment decisions should be made with the assumption that the patient is very likely still seizing electrographically. Reviews of treatment for refractory SE are myriad[50];

however, available high-level evidence is currently limited to one randomized controlled trial that compared propofol and thiopental in a heterogeneous group of patients with refractory SE.[51] Questions remain regarding optimal approaches to treatment, and available evidence does not support any preference between midazolam, propofol, and pentobarbital.[52] Use of these medications, particularly if paralytics have been used for intubation, requires continuous EEG monitoring to guide therapy.

In patients with suspected nonconvulsive SE, the decision to intubate and/or begin anesthetic medications in the ED is complicated and requires consideration of underlying etiology, the risks of aggressive treatment, and the efficacy of nonaggressive treatment.[53] Similarly difficult situations include elderly patients with do-not-resuscitate/intubate orders and patients with focal motor SE and a preserved level of consciousness. In both of these groups, further treatment with second-line non-anesthetic agents (or even oral administration of AEDs) while avoiding associated hypotension or respiratory failure is preferred. Early consultation with a neurologist experienced in treating SE is required, and all patients with refractory SE or nonconvulsive SE should be admitted to an ICU for initiation of continuous EEG monitoring (or promptly transferred to an EEG-capable center).[9]

CONCLUSION

Patients with seizures and SE are commonly encountered in the ED. As a frontline provider, emergency physicians play a crucial role in the management of these patients. Most seizure patients present in noncritical condition following isolated seizures; in these patients, cautious management and avoidance of overly aggressive treatment can minimize complications, such as medication toxicity and sedation. A minority of patients will present in SE, and in these patients, early and aggressive protocol-based treatment is critical to terminating seizures and improving overall outcome.

LITERATURE TABLE

TRIAL	DESIGN	RESULT
Epidemiology		
Hauser et al., *Epilepsia.* 1993[3]	Population-based observational study of 880 patients that described the incidence of epilepsy or first-time unprovoked seizures over a 50-y period in Rochester, Minnesota	Age-adjusted incidence of epilepsy 44:100,000, cumulative incidence through 74 y of age 3.1%
DeLorenzo et al., *Neurology.* 1996[8]	Population-based observational study of 166 patients that described the incidence of SE over a 2-year period in Richmond, Virginia	Estimated incidence of SE was 61:100,000. Mortality was estimated at 17:100,000 patient-years
DeLorenzo et al., *Epilepsia.* 1998[9]	Population-based observational study of 164 patients that described frequency of nonconvulsive seizures and SE after control of convulsive SE over a 2-year period in Richmond, Virginia	48% with persistent electrographic seizures; 14% nonconvulsive SE
Hesdorffer et al., *Ann Neurol.* 1998[14]	Population-based observational study of 416 patients that assessed the risk of unprovoked seizure following acute symptomatic SE over a 30-y period in Rochester, Minnesota	The risk of unprovoked seizures following acute symptomatic SE was 41% compared to 13% following an acute symptomatic seizure

LITERATURE TABLE *(Continued)*

TRIAL	DESIGN	RESULT
Kwan and Brodie, *N Engl J Med.* 2000[26]	Single-center, prospective observational study of 525 patients that described the likelihood of seizure freedom in patients who do not respond to initial treatment	47% of previously untreated patients will respond with first epilepsy medicine compared to 14% who respond to second or third medication
Wiebe et al., *N Engl J Med.* 2001[27]	Randomized controlled trial of epilepsy surgery vs. medical treatment in 80 patients with temporal lobe epilepsy	58% of the surgery arm was free from seizures compared with 8% with epilepsy medication ($p < 0.001$)
Novy et al., *Epilepsia.* 2010[47]	Prospective observational study of 525 patients that described the frequency of refractory SE over a 2-y period in Lausanne, Switzerland	22.6% of all SE is refractory to first- and second-line therapy
Treatment		
Alldredge et al., *N Engl J Med.* 2001[16]	A randomized, double-blind controlled trial of 205 patients that compared lorazepam, diazepam, or placebo in the prehospital setting for SE	SE was aborted in 59.1% of the patients who received lorazepam compared with 21.1% of those who received placebo ($p = 0.001$). Rates of respiratory failure were significantly lower in the benzodiazepine groups: 10.6% for lorazepam, 10.3% for diazepam, and 22.5% for placebo ($p = 0.08$)
Treiman et al., *N Engl J Med.* 1998[17]	A randomized, double-blind controlled trial of 384 patients that compared diazepam, lorazepam, PHT, and phenobarbital as first-line treatment for SE	Lorazepam was superior to PHT in overt generalized convulsive SE. There was no difference in seizure cessation overall between drugs; lorazepam was noted to be easier to administer
Silbergleit et al., *N Engl J Med.* 2012[22] RAMPART	A randomized, double-blind controlled noninferiority trial of 448 patients that compared IM midazolam to IV lorazepam	IM midazolam aborted seizures in 73.4% compared to 63.4% in the IV lorazepam group (95% CI, 4.0–16.1; $p < 0.001$ for both noninferiority and superiority). Study concluded IM midazolam to be at least as safe and effective as IV lorazepam for prehospital seizure cessation
Alvarez et al., *Epilepsia.* 2011[44]	A prospective, observational study of 167 patients that compared PHT, VPA, and LEV as second-line agents in SE	LEV controlled SE less effectively than VPA when controlling for etiology and SE severity (OR 2.69; 95% CI 1.19–6.08). PHT was not statistically different from the other two compounds
Rossetti et al., *Neurocrit Care.* 2011[51]	A randomized, single-blind controlled trial of 24 patients that compared propofol to barbiturates for refractory SE	Although no differences were observed, the study was stopped early due to underenrollment

CI, confidence interval; OR, odds ratio.

REFERENCES

1. Pallin DJ, Goldstein JN, Moussally JS, et al. Seizure visits in US emergency departments: epidemiology and potential disparities in care. *Int J Emerg Med.* 2008;1:97–105.
2. Neligan A, Hauser WA, Sander JW. The epidemiology of the epilepsies. In: Stefan H, Theodore WH, eds. *Handbook of Clinical Neurology*. Philadelphia, PA: Elsevier B.V.; 2012:113–133.
3. Hauser WA, Annegers JF, Kurland LT. Incidence of epilepsy and unprovoked seizures in Rochester, Minnesota: 1935–1984. *Epilepsia.* 1993;34:453–468.
4. Hauser WA, Beghi E. First seizure definitions and worldwide incidence and mortality. *Epilepsia.* 2008;49(suppl 1):8–12.

5. Martindale JL, Goldstein JN, Pallin DJ. Emergency department seizure epidemiology. *Emerg Med Clin North Am.* 2011;29:15–27.
6. Abarbanell NR. Prehospital seizure management: triage criteria for the advanced life support rescue team. *Am J Emerg Med.* 1993;11:210–212.
7. Hesdorffer DC, D'Amelio M. Mortality in the first 30 days following incident acute symptomatic seizures. *Epilepsia.* 2005;46(suppl 11):43–45.
8. DeLorenzo RJ, Hauser WA, Towne AR, et al. A prospective, population-based epidemiologic study of status epilepticus in Richmond, Virginia. *Neurology.* 1996;46:1029–1035.
9. DeLorenzo RJ, Waterhouse EJ, Towne AR, et al. Persistent nonconvulsive status epilepticus after the control of convulsive status epilepticus. *Epilepsia.* 1998;39:833–840.
10. Shorvon S. The definition, classification and frequency of NCSE. In: Walker M, Cross H, Smith S, et al., eds. *Nonconvulsive status epilepticus: Epilepsy Research Foundation Workshop Reports: Epileptic Disorders.* Montrouge, France: John Libbey Eurotext Limited; 2005:255–258.
11. Towne AR, Pellock JM, Ko D, et al. Determinants of mortality in status epilepticus. *Epilepsia.* 1994;35:27–34.
12. Oddo M, Carrera E, Claassen J, et al. Continuous electroencephalography in the medical intensive care unit. *Crit Care Med.* 2009;37:2051–2056.
13. DeLorenzo RJ, Garnett LK, Towne AR, et al. Comparison of status epilepticus with prolonged seizure episodes lasting from 10 to 29 minutes. *Epilepsia.* 1999;40:164–169.
14. Hesdorffer DC, Logroscino G, Cascino G, et al. Risk of unprovoked seizure after acute symptomatic seizure: effect of status epilepticus. *Ann Neurol.* 1998;44:908–912.
15. Muayqil T, Rowe BH, Ahmed SN. Treatment adherence and outcomes in the management of convulsive status epilepticus in the emergency room. *Epileptic Disord.* 2007;9:43–50.
16. Alldredge BK, Gelb AM, Isaacs SM, et al. A comparison of lorazepam, diazepam, and placebo for the treatment of out-of-hospital status epilepticus. *N Engl J Med.* 2001;345:631–637.
17. Treiman DM, Meyers PD, Walton NY, et al. A comparison of four treatments for generalized convulsive status epilepticus. Veterans Affairs Status Epilepticus Cooperative Study Group. *N Engl J Med.* 1998;339:792–798.
18. Cereghino JJ, Mitchell WG, Murphy J, et al. Treating repetitive seizures with a rectal diazepam formulation: a randomized study. The North American Diastat Study Group. *Neurology.* 1998;51:1274–1282.
19. Cereghino JJ, Cloyd JC, Kuzniecky RI. Rectal diazepam gel for treatment of acute repetitive seizures in adults. *Arch Neurol.* 2002;59:1915–1920.
20. Chin RF, Neville BG, Peckham C, et al. Treatment of community-onset, childhood convulsive status epilepticus: a prospective, population-based study. *Lancet Neurol.* 2008;7:696–703.
21. McMullan J, Sasson C, Pancioli A, et al. Midazolam versus diazepam for the treatment of status epilepticus in children and young adults: a meta-analysis. *Acad Emerg Med.* 2010;17:575–582.
22. Silbergleit R, Durkalski V, Lowenstein D, et al. Intramuscular versus intravenous therapy for prehospital status epilepticus. *N Engl J Med.* 2012;366:591–600.
23. McIntyre J, Robertson S, Norris E, et al. Safety and efficacy of buccal midazolam versus rectal diazepam for emergency treatment of seizures in children: a randomised controlled trial. *Lancet.* 2005;366:205–210.
24. Holsti M, Dudley N, Schunk J, et al. Intranasal midazolam vs rectal diazepam for the home treatment of acute seizures in pediatric patients with epilepsy. *Arch Pediatr Adolesc Med.* 2010;164:747–753.
25. Aranda A, Foucart G, Ducasse JL, et al. Generalized convulsive status epilepticus management in adults: a cohort study with evaluation of professional practice. *Epilepsia.* 2010;51:2159–2167.
26. Kwan P, Brodie MJ. Early identification of refractory epilepsy. *N Engl J Med.* 2000;342:314–319.
27. Wiebe S, Blume WT, Girvin JP, et al. A randomized, controlled trial of surgery for temporal-lobe epilepsy. *N Engl J Med.* 2001;345:311–318.
28. Krumholz A, Wiebe S, Gronseth G, et al. Practice Parameter: evaluating an apparent unprovoked first seizure in adults (an evidence-based review): report of the Quality Standards Subcommittee of the American Academy of Neurology and the American Epilepsy Society. *Neurology.* 2007;69:1996–2007.
29. Berg AT. Risk of recurrence after a first unprovoked seizure. *Epilepsia.* 2008;49(suppl 1):13–18.
30. Chen JW, Wasterlain CG. Status epilepticus: pathophysiology and management in adults. *Lancet Neurol.* 2006;5:246–256.
31. Meldrum BS, Vigouroux RA, Brierley JB. Systemic factors and epileptic brain damage. Prolonged seizures in paralyzed, artificially ventilated baboons. *Arch Neurol.* 1973;29:82–87.
32. Claassen J, Perotte A, Albers D, et al. Nonconvulsive seizures after subarachnoid hemorrhage: multimodal detection and outcomes. *Ann Neurol.* 2013;74:53–64.

33. Cascino GD, Hesdorffer D, Logroscino G, et al. Treatment of nonfebrile status epilepticus in Rochester, Minn, from 1965 through 1984. *Mayo Clin Proc.* 2001;76:39–41.
34. Lowenstein DH, Alldredge BK. Status epilepticus at an urban public hospital in the 1980s. *Neurology.* 1993;43:483–488.
35. Rossetti AO, Alvarez V, Januel JM, et al. Treatment deviating from guidelines does not influence status epilepticus prognosis. *J Neurol.* 2013;260:421–428.
36. Claassen J, Silbergleit R, Weingart SD, et al. Emergency neurological life support: status epilepticus. *Neurocrit Care.* 2012;17(suppl 1):S73–S78.
37. Rudis MI, Touchette DR, Swadron SP, et al. Cost-effectiveness of oral phenytoin, intravenous phenytoin, and intravenous fosphenytoin in the emergency department. *Ann Emerg Med.* 2004;43:386–397.
38. Brigo F, Storti M, Del Felice A, et al. IV Valproate in generalized convulsive status epilepticus: a systematic review. *Eur J Neurol.* 2012;19:1180–1191.
39. Abou Khaled KJ, Hirsch LJ. Updates in the management of seizures and status epilepticus in critically ill patients. *Neurol Clin.* 2008;26:385–408, viii.
40. Zeller JA, Schlesinger S, Runge U, et al. Influence of valproate monotherapy on platelet activation and hematologic values. *Epilepsia.* 1999;40:186–189.
41. Sinha S, Naritoku DK. Intravenous valproate is well tolerated in unstable patients with status epilepticus. *Neurology.* 2000;55:722–724.
42. Zelano J, Kumlien E. Levetiracetam as alternative stage two antiepileptic drug in status epilepticus: a systematic review. *Seizure.* 2012;21:233–236.
43. Misra UK, Kalita J, Maurya PK. Levetiracetam versus lorazepam in status epilepticus: a randomized, open labeled pilot study. *J Neurol.* 2012;259:645–648.
44. Alvarez V, Januel JM, Burnand B, et al. Second-line status epilepticus treatment: comparison of phenytoin, valproate, and levetiracetam. *Epilepsia.* 2011;52:1292–1296.
45. Fountain NB, Krauss G, Isojarvi J, et al. Safety and tolerability of adjunctive lacosamide intravenous loading dose in lacosamide-naive patients with partial-onset seizures. *Epilepsia.* 2013;54:58–65.
46. Hocker SE, Britton JW, Mandrekar JN, et al. Predictors of outcome in refractory status epilepticus. *JAMA Neurol.* 2013;70:72–77.
47. Novy J, Logroscino G, Rossetti AO. Refractory status epilepticus: a prospective observational study. *Epilepsia.* 2010;51:251–256.
48. Theodore WH, Porter RJ, Penry JK. Complex partial seizures: clinical characteristics and differential diagnosis. *Neurology.* 1983;33:1115–1121.
49. Seyal M, Bateman LM, Li CS. Impact of periictal interventions on respiratory dysfunction, postictal EEG suppression, and postictal immobility. *Epilepsia.* 2013;54:377–382.
50. Fernandez A, Claassen J. Refractory status epilepticus. *Curr Opin Crit Care.* 2012;18:127–131.
51. Rossetti AO, Milligan TA, Vulliemoz S, et al. A randomized trial for the treatment of refractory status epilepticus. *Neurocrit Care.* 2011;14:4–10.
52. Brophy GM, Bell R, Claassen J, et al. Guidelines for the evaluation and management of status epilepticus. *Neurocrit Care.* 2012;17:3–23.
53. Ferguson M, Bianchi MT, Sutter R, et al. Calculating the risk benefit equation for aggressive treatment of non-convulsive status epilepticus. *Neurocrit Care.* 2013;18:216–227.

23

Myasthenic Crisis and Peripheral Neuromuscular Disorders

Christina Ulane

BACKGROUND

The diagnosis and management of peripheral neuromuscular disorders are generally the purview of neurologists in the outpatient setting. However, when these disorders present acutely, they can require the expertise of the emergency physician. This chapter discusses the clinical features, diagnosis, and treatment of the two peripheral neuromuscular disorders most commonly encountered in the emergency department (ED) setting: myasthenia gravis (MG) and Guillain-Barre syndrome (GBS), also known as acute inflammatory demyelinating polyradiculoneuropathy, or AIDP.

The incidence of MG is approximately 20 per 100,000; it is equally prevalent in men and women over age 40, but under the age of 40 is three times more common in women. The incidence of GBS is approximately 0.6 to 1.9 per 100,000; it is equally prevalent in men and women, with people over age 50 at greatest risk. Both MG and GBS are immune-mediated diseases. In MG, autoantibodies against the acetylcholine receptor (AchR) compete with acetylcholine at the neuromuscular junction. This blocks synaptic transmission and causes fluctuating motor weakness, the hallmark clinical feature of MG. MG may also result from antibodies acting against muscle-specific kinase; and finally, MG may be seronegative (lacking an antibody). GBS is an immune-mediated, often postinfectious polyradiculoneuropathy that produces both cellular and humoral responses. The exact pathophysiologic mechanisms of GBS are not completely understood, but it is thought that an antecedent infection or other stimulus activates an immune response, which, through molecular mimicry, cross-reacts with epitopes (the part of an antigen to which the antibody attaches) on the myelin and/or axon of peripheral nerves and nerve roots. Immune reaction to myelin components results in multifocal inflammatory demyelination that starts at the level of the nerve roots. Antibodies against gangliosides (which share antigens with *Campylobacter jejuni*, a commonly associated preceding infection) and complement deposition along axons are found in patients with acute axonal neuropathy variants.

CLINICAL PRESENTATION AND DIAGNOSTIC EVALUATION

Myasthenia Gravis

Patients with MG may present to the ED for different reasons. They may (1) have stable MG but have an unrelated acute problem, (2) have an MG exacerbation or crisis,

(3) present with new symptom onset for yet undiagnosed MG, and (4) present with cholinergic crisis as a result of acetylcholinesterase inhibitor use (this problem has lessened as the use of acetylcholinesterase inhibitor therapy has been replaced by immunosuppressive therapy). The classic clinical features of MG include:

- Weakness: proximal, fluctuating, usually worse after activity and at night, and improved after sleep and rest
- Ptosis (often asymmetric)
- Diplopia (with any combination of extraocular muscle palsies), fatigable upgaze
- Bulbar weakness (nasal speech, dysarthria, dysphagia)
- Respiratory muscle weakness (dyspnea, hypoxia, hypercapnia)
- Absence of any sensory deficits, normal reflexes

The diagnosis of MG is generally accomplished in the outpatient setting with laboratory and electrodiagnostic tests, such as repetitive nerve stimulation (demonstrating decrement in motor response) and single-fiber electromyography (demonstrating increased muscle fiber jitter). Myasthenic crisis—myasthenic weakness sufficient to cause respiratory failure requiring mechanical ventilation—is a true emergency that requires rapid assessment, diagnosis, and treatment. Myasthenic crisis and exacerbations can be triggered by infections, surgery, and medications (see Table 23.1). In the past 60 to 70 years, advances in pulmonary critical care and in the diagnosis of MG have reduced mortality rates for myasthenic crisis from 70% to 80% to approximately 4%.

In the ED, for a patient without established MG, making a clinical diagnosis is most practical; two easily administered tests—the ice test and the edrophonium, or Tensilon, test—can help confirm a diagnosis. The ice test is performed at bedside on patients with ptosis: A pack of ice is placed over the ptotic eye for 1 to 2 minutes; resolution or improvement in the ptosis is considered a positive result and is highly specific for MG.[1] In the Tensilon test, the short-acting acetylcholinesterase inhibitor edrophonium is administered in an intravenous (IV) dose of 2 mg, followed by up to 8 mg. Muscles

TABLE 23.1 Medications Exacerbating Myasthenia Gravis

Contraindicated	Alpha-interferon Penicillamine Telithromycin Botulinum toxin
Use with caution (may worsen MG)	Cardiac medications • Beta-blockers (propranolol, timolol maleate eye drops) • Calcium channel blockers • Quinine, quinidine, procainamide Neuromuscular blocking agents • Succinylcholine • D-Tubocurarine Antibiotics • Aminoglycosides (gentamicin, kanamycin, streptomycin, neomycin) • Macrolides (erythromycin, azithromycin) • Quinolones (ciprofloxacin, levofloxacin, norfloxacin, ofloxacin) • Magnesium salts (laxatives, antacids)

weak from MG will respond within 30 to 45 seconds, with a response lasting up to 5 minutes; an objective improvement in muscle strength is considered a positive result. The sensitivity of the Tensilon test, however, is only 60%, and false positives can occur in motor neuron and other diseases. The Tensilon test carries a low risk of serious cardiac complication, but life-threatening bradyrhythmias and ventricular fibrillation can occur, so the test should be done in a monitored setting with atropine at the bedside. Patients are also at risk for acute decompensation due to edrophonium-induced cholinergic crisis, which may result in excessive secretions and worsening neuromuscular weakness.

Guillain-Barre Syndrome

Guillain-Barre Syndrome and its variants (Miller Fisher syndrome, acute motor axonal neuropathy, acute motor and sensory axonal neuropathy) most often present with a subacute onset of progressive weakness, ascending sensory loss, and areflexia. Many patients will also have dysautonomia (with resultant fluctuations in heart rate and blood pressure), pain (often in the mid-back), and respiratory insufficiency. In the ED, the diagnosis of GBS is primarily made clinically; however, a cerebrospinal fluid analysis showing cytoalbuminologic dissociation (elevated protein in the absence of white blood cells) strongly supports the diagnosis and is recommended in patients with suspected GBS.

Differential Diagnosis

The primary alternative diagnostic considerations for MG and GBS are summarized in Table 23.2. While the differential diagnosis for acute weakness of unclear etiology is broad, alternative peripheral neuromuscular disorders such as amyotrophic lateral sclerosis are rarely encountered in the ED setting. Myopathies, which are slowly progressive, also rarely present to the ED, although fulminant cases with bulbar weakness and respiratory failure do occur.

Neuromuscular Respiratory Failure

In the ED, MG and GBS are the most common causes for neuromuscular respiratory failure. Twenty-five to fifty percent of GBS patients and 15% to 27% of MG patients will ultimately require intubation[19–22] though not necessarily upon arrival in the ED. Neuromuscular respiratory failure in both conditions is due to the following:

- Facial, laryngeal, and oropharyngeal muscle weakness (resulting in mechanical obstruction, especially when patient is supine, and increasing aspiration risk)
- Inspiratory muscle weakness (resulting in insufficient lung expansion and hypoxemia)
- Expiratory muscle weakness (resulting in hypoventilation, inadequate cough, and impaired secretion clearance)

MANAGEMENT GUIDELINES

Assessment and Monitoring of Pulmonary Function

Because neuromuscular weakness can result in respiratory muscle fatigue and rapid progression to respiratory failure, early identification of MG or GBS patients who will require intubation is important. Complicating this, however, are two factors: First, overt signs of respiratory distress may be absent; second, patients with known MG who are

TABLE 23.2 Differential Diagnosis for Peripheral Neuromuscular Weakness

Localization	Differential Diagnoses
Motor neuron	Upper motor neuron Primary lateral sclerosis Upper and lower motor neuron Amyotrophic lateral sclerosis Lower motor neuron Poliomyelitis Spinal muscular atrophy
Peripheral nerve	Motor Multifocal motor neuropathy Sensorimotor Peripheral neuropathy (toxic, metabolic, etc.) Vasculitis Acute intermittent porphyria Polyradiculoneuropathy GBS Chronic inflammatory demyelinating polyradiculoneuropathy Diabetic radiculoplexus neuropathy
Neuromuscular junction	Presynaptic Lambert-Eaton myasthenic syndrome Botulism Synaptic Organophosphate poisoning Cholinergic crisis Postsynaptic Myasthenia gravis
Muscle	Inflammatory Polymyositis Dermatomyositis Inclusion body myositis Toxic Metabolic Periodic paralyses Dystrophic Nondystrophic channelopathies

experiencing an exacerbation or crisis may be taking higher doses of acetylcholinesterase inhibitors as symptomatic treatment for increasing weakness, the cholinergic side effects of which can lead to increased oral secretions. Clinical assessment should focus on identifying clear indications for intubation, such as an inability to protect the airway, failure of ventilation or oxygenation, expected rapid deterioration, and paradoxical breathing, whereby the abdomen contracts and moves inward (rather than outward) with respiration, due to diaphragmatic weakness. Hypoxia, measured by pulse oximetry, is a late finding.

Tests of respiratory muscle strength (pulmonary function tests, or PFTs) and gas exchange (arterial blood gas, or ABG) are predictive of outcome in patients with neuromuscular weakness and are necessary to complement the clinical assessment and monitoring of respiratory function. Note that while the ABG is often abnormal in patients with MG, it can be normal even when respiratory fatigue and failure are imminent. Bedside PFTs include negative inspiratory force (NIF) or the similar measure maximal inspiratory pressure (MIP), vital capacity (VC), maximal expiratory pressure (MEP), and maximal single-breath count (normal ~50, impaired <30, very impaired <15). MIP and NIF reflect diaphragmatic and other inspiratory muscle strength, while MEP reflects the strength of expiratory muscles (intercostal and abdominal muscles) and indirectly the ability to cough and clear secretions. A normal MIP is > −100 cm H_2O in men and > −70 cm H_2O in women, with a critical cutoff value for all patients of −25 cm H_2O. A normal MEP is >200 cm H_2O in men and >140 cm H_2O in women, with a critical value of 40 cm H_2O. Depending on the particular manometer utilized, MIP, NIF, and MEP values are reported as either negative or positive pressures, but it is the absolute value in cm H_2O that is most significant. Normal VC is 40 to 70 mL/kg, with a critical cutoff value of 15 to 20 mL/kg. In a normal person, the VC decreases by <10% in the supine position; decreases >10% suggest diaphragmatic weakness (a 25% decrease is 79% sensitive and 90% specific for diaphragmatic weakness).[2] MIP and VC demonstrate a linear relationship in both acute and chronic neuromuscular respiratory failure.[3] In ED patients with suspected MG or GBS, a respiratory technician should be called to document respiratory function including PFTs. If a technician is not available, maximal single-breath count is an effective semiquantitative bedside test for VC and expiratory flow rate, with normal values in the range of 30 to 50.

A retrospective review of mechanically ventilated patients with neuromuscular diseases (of all types) found that (a) pre–mechanical ventilation ABGs with lower pH and pO_2 and higher pCO_2 were associated with poor functional outcome, (b) mechanical ventilation was required for more than 7 days if MIP was > −28 cm H_2O and/or MEP was ≤30 cm H_2O, and (c) death during hospitalization was predicted by pH < 7.30, serum bicarbonate >30 mg/dL, and pCO_2 >50 mm Hg.[4]

Predicting the Need for Intubation

Several studies have attempted to identify predictors of the need for intubation and mechanical ventilation in patients with MG or GBS. A retrospective review of 55 patients admitted to the intensive care unit (ICU) for MG identified three respiratory function parameters in patients unlikely to require mechanical ventilation: VC >20 mL/kg, MEP >40 cm H_2O, or MIP <−40 cm H_2O. Patients with a >30% decline in MIP and hypercapnia (pCO_2 >50 mm Hg) were more likely to require mechanical ventilation.[5]

A number of retrospective and prospective studies have evaluated the factors predicting the need for mechanical ventilation in patients with GBS and report similar findings. The most reliable bedside PFT predictors of the need for intubation are VC <20 mL/kg and an MIP >−30 cm H_2O. Other suggestive predictors include VC <60% of predicted and reduction of PFT values by >30% from baseline, inability to lift the head from the bed (a surrogate marker for neck flexor and extensor weakness), rapid disease progression (defined as reaching clinical nadir or worst neurologic status before clinical stabilization, within 7 days), bulbar dysfunction (identified by impaired gag reflex, dysarthria,

TABLE 23.3 Signs of Impending Neuromuscular Respiratory Failure

	Myasthenia Gravis	Guillain-Barre Syndrome
Clinical features	Prominent bulbar dysfunction Dysarthria, dysphagia Impaired gag reflex Tachypnea, dyspnea Use of accessory muscles Paradoxical breathing Single-breath count <15 Poor cough, secretion clearance	Prominent bulbar dysfunction Dysarthria, dysphagia Impaired gag reflex Bifacial weakness Dysautonomia Unexplained dysrhythmias Blood pressure fluctuations Rapid disease progression Inability to stand or cough
Laboratory signs	VC < 15–20 mL/kg (or VC < 1 L) NIF > −20 cm H_2O MEP < 40 cm H_2O $pCO_2 \geq 50$ mm Hg Tidal volume < 4–5 mL/kg	VC < 20 mL/kg MIP < 30 cm H_2O EP < 40 cm H_2O Elevated liver enzymes

VC, vital capacity; NIF, negative inspiratory force; MEP, maximal expiratory pressure; MIP, maximal inspiratory pressure.

and/or dysphagia), and dysautonomia (identified by unexplained dysrhythmias, blood pressure fluctuations, and/or bowel and bladder dysfunction). Elevated liver enzymes and inability to stand or cough are also predictive, but are considered less regularly in practice.[6–8] Indicators of impending respiratory failure in neuromuscular respiratory weakness are summarized in Table 23.3.

Unfortunately, no single clinical or laboratory finding adequately predicts the need for intubation in GBS and MG. The efficacy of bedside PFTs can be limited due to oropharyngeal weakness, and the usual signs of impending respiratory failure—such as distress, hypoxia, and ABG abnormalities—may not be present in patients with neuromuscular weakness. Finally, onset of respiratory muscle fatigue is unpredictable in patients with neuromuscular weakness. Because of this, serial functional and laboratory testing is essential to the management of these patients.

Noninvasive Ventilation

Because mechanical ventilation is, in general, associated with increased morbidity, mortality, and hospital length of stay, several studies have explored the benefits of noninvasive positive pressure ventilation (NIPPV) for patients with MG and GBS. NIPPV delivers continuous positive pressure in adjustable degrees: higher during inspiration (to overcome upper airway resistance and reduce the work of breathing) and lower during expiration (to prevent airway collapse and atelectasis). Two retrospective studies of myasthenic crisis found that more than half of patients placed on NIPPV avoided eventual intubation and that hypercapnia (pCO_2 >50 mm Hg) was the only predictor of NIPPV failure.[9–12] There are less robust data regarding NIPPV for GBS, but one case report suggests it may not be sufficient to prevent intubation.[13]

Intubation and Neuromuscular Blockade

Neuromuscular blocking agents should be avoided, if possible, in patients with MG who require intubation and mechanical ventilation. Depolarizing agents such as succinylcholine can be used safely, but because MG patients have reduced functional AchRs, more than twice the normal dose may be required. Nondepolarizing agents such as rocuronium should be avoided; they act as competitive inhibitors of postsynaptic AchR and may cause prolonged neuromuscular blockade because they imitate and thus enhance the effects of existing pathogenic antibodies.

In patients with GBS, because dysautonomia carries the risk of blood pressure and heart rate instability and arrhythmia, succinylcholine should not be used, as it increases the risk of life-threatening hyperkalemia. Succinylcholine should also be avoided in patients with myopathies or with hyperkalemia susceptibility (such as those with periodic paralyses). Only nondepolarizing agents such as rocuronium should be used in GBS, and even these with caution.[14]

Immunomodulatory Treatment

It is beyond the scope of this chapter to discuss immunomodulatory treatment of peripheral neuromuscular disorders in detail; however, certain general principles relevant to the emergency physician are worth mentioning. The treatment of acute MG exacerbations or crises entails the use of corticosteroids, intravenous immunoglobulin (IVIg), and plasma exchange (PE). If the exacerbation is mild, corticosteroids can be started in the ambulatory setting. It is important to note, however, that corticosteroids are known to cause an acute worsening of myasthenic symptoms within the first 2 weeks of initiating treatment. Thus, they should be administered with caution in the ambulatory setting, especially if the patient exhibits any bulbar weakness or respiratory symptoms. If the patient is in a closely monitored setting or already intubated and receiving mechanical ventilation, high-dose corticosteroids may be initiated, and doses of 60 to 80 mg of oral prednisone are commonly used. After remission is achieved (usually in 1 to 2 months), prednisone is slowly tapered over several months.

Numerous studies demonstrate the efficacy of IVIg and PE for treatment of myasthenic crisis.[15,16] These therapies are often given in conjunction with high-dose prednisone to achieve successful remission. As discussed, high-dose prednisone can cause an initial worsening of myasthenic weakness and thus should be initiated only after respiratory status is stabilized. Similarly, while IVIg or PE should begin as soon as possible, stable respiratory status is the first priority, and these definitive treatments can be initiated after admission to the hospital rather than in the ED. Long-term management of MG usually involves maintaining remission with low-dose prednisone and/or steroid-sparing immunosuppressants, such as azathioprine and mycophenolate mofetil.

Treatment of GBS also involves IVIg or PE[17] and may require more than one treatment in the acute setting, but long-term therapy is unnecessary as it is a monophasic illness. Similar to MG, IVIg or PE should be initiated after patient stabilization and admission to the hospital. Corticosteroids are not beneficial for GBS and should not be used.[18]

CONCLUSION

MG and GBS are the peripheral neuromuscular disorders most commonly encountered in the ED setting. Both diseases are associated with rapid respiratory muscle fatigue and respiratory failure. Early identification of these patients and accurate assessment of their need for ventilatory support are essential steps in optimizing patient outcomes.

LITERATURE TABLE

TRIAL	DESIGN	RESULT
Thieben et al., *Muscle Nerve.* 2005[5]	Retrospective review of utility of PFTs and ABGs in predicting need for mechanical ventilation in patients with MG	Patients unlikely to require mechanical ventilation if: • VC > 20 mL/kg • MEP > 40 cm H_2O or • MIP < −40 cm H_2O Higher risk for mechanical ventilation if: • >30% decline in MIP and • Hypercapnia (pCO_2 > 50 mm Hg)
Walgaard et al., *Ann Neurol.* 2010[6]	Prospective study of predictors of respiratory insufficiency in GBS	MV within 1 wk of hospital admission predicted by: • Rapid disease progression • Bulbar dysfunction • Bilateral facial weakness • Dysautonomia
Lawn et al., *Arch Neurol.* 2001[7]	Retrospective review of features associated with progression to respiratory failure patients with severe GBS	Progression to respiratory failure associated with: *Clinical features* • Rapid disease progression • Bulbar dysfunction • Bilateral facial weakness • Dysautonomia *PFTs* • VC < 20 mL/kg • MIP < 30 cm H_2O • MEP < 40 cm H_2O • PFT values reduced by >30%
Sharshar et al., *Crit Care Med.* 2003[8]	RCT of 722 patients to assess early predictors of need for mechanical ventilation in GBS	MV predicted by: • Symptom onset to hospital admission <7 d (OR 2.51) • Inability to lift head above the bed (OR 4.34) • Inability to stand or cough (OR 2.53 and 9.09 respectively) • Elevated liver enzymes (OR 2.09) • VC < 60% predicted (OR 2.86)
Seneviratne et al., *Arch Neurol.* 2008[9]	Retrospective review of predictors of need for mechanical ventilation and utility of NIPPV in patients with myasthenic crisis	More than half of patients placed on NIPPV avoided eventual intubation. Only hypercapnia (pCO_2 > 45 mm Hg, $p = 0.04$) predicted intubation
Wu et al., *Neurocrit Care.* 2009[11]	Retrospective review of utility of NIPPV in patients with myasthenic crisis	More than half of patients placed on NIPPV avoided eventual intubation
Zinman et al., *Neurology.* 2007[15]	RCT of 51 patients to determine effectiveness of IVIg in MG	Clinically meaningful and statistically significant improvement in patients with moderate to severe exacerbations of MG treated with IVIg over 2 d
Barth et al., *Neurology.* 2011[16]	RCT of 84 patients comparing IVIg vs. PE for treatment of MG	Both IVIg and PE are effective for treating patients with worsening MG with similar duration of benefit and safety profile
Plasma Exchange/Sandoglobulin Guillain-Barré Syndrome Trial Group. *Lancet.* 1997[17]	RCT of 383 patients comparing PE, IVIg, or PE followed by IVIg for treatment of GBS	Both PE and IVIg are effective for treating patients with GBS in the first 2 wk of symptoms. The combination of PE with IVIg did not confer significant benefit
Hughes et al., 2006[18]	Meta-analysis of utility of corticosteroids for treatment of GBS	Steroids should not be used for GBS; there is no significant difference in disability outcome compared to control

RCT, randomized controlled trial; OR, odds ratio.

REFERENCES

1. Browning J, Wallace M, Chana J, et al. Bedside testing for myasthenia gravis: the ice-test. *Emerg Med J.* 2011;28:709–711.
2. Prigent H, Orlikowski D, Letilly N, et al. Vital capacity versus maximal inspiratory pressure in patients with Guillain-Barre syndrome and myasthenia gravis. *Neurocrit Care.* 2012;17:236–239.
3. Perrin C, Unterborn JN, Ambrosio CD, et al. Pulmonary complications of chronic neuromuscular diseases and their management. *Muscle Nerve.* 2004;29:5–27.
4. Cabrera Serrano M, Rabinstein AA. Usefulness of pulmonary function tests and blood gases in acute neuromuscular respiratory failure. *Eur J Neurol.* 2012;19:452–456.
5. Thieben MJ, Blacker DJ, Liu PY, et al. Pulmonary function tests and blood gases in worsening myasthenia gravis. *Muscle Nerve.* 2005;32:664–667.
6. Walgaard C, Lingsma HF, Ruts L, et al. Prediction of respiratory insufficiency in Guillain-Barre syndrome. *Ann Neurol.* 2010;67:781–787.
7. Lawn ND, Fletcher DD, Henderson RD, et al. Anticipating mechanical ventilation in Guillain-Barre syndrome. *Arch Neurol.* 2001;58:893–898.
8. Sharshar T, Chevret S, Bourdain F, et al.; French Cooperative Group on Plasma Exchange in Guillain-Barre Syndrome. Early predictors of mechanical ventilation in Guillain-Barre syndrome. *Crit Care Med.* 2003;31:278–283.
9. Seneviratne J, Mandrekar J, Wijdicks EF, et al. Noninvasive ventilation in myasthenic crisis. *Arch Neurol.* 2008;65:54–58.
10. Rabinstein A, Wijdicks EF. Bipap in acute respiratory failure due to myasthenic crisis may prevent intubation. *Neurology.* 2002;59:1647–1649.
11. Wu JY, Kuo PH, Fan PC, et al. The role of non-invasive ventilation and factors predicting extubation outcome in myasthenic crisis. *Neurocrit Care.* 2009;10:35–42.
12. Chadda K, Clair B, Orlikowski D, et al. Pressure support versus assisted controlled noninvasive ventilation in neuromuscular disease. *Neurocrit Care.* 2004;1:429–434.
13. Wijdicks EF, Roy TK. Bipap in early Guillain-Barre syndrome may fail. *Can J Neurol Sci.* 2006;33:105–106.
14. Seder DB, Riker RR, Jagoda A, et al. Emergency neurological life support: airway, ventilation, and sedation. *Neurocrit Care.* 2012;17(suppl 1):S4–S20.
15. Zinman L, Ng E, Bril V. IV immunoglobulin in patients with myasthenia gravis: a randomized controlled trial. *Neurology.* 2007;68:837–841.
16. Barth D, Nabavi Nouri M, Ng E, et al. Comparison of IVIg and plex in patients with myasthenia gravis. *Neurology.* 2011;76:2017–2023.
17. Randomised trial of plasma exchange, intravenous immunoglobulin, and combined treatments in Guillain-Barre syndrome. Plasma exchange/sandoglobulin Guillain-Barre syndrome trial group. *Lancet.* 1997;349:225–230.
18. Hughes RA, Swan AV, van Koningsveld R, et al. Corticosteroids for Guillain-Barre syndrome. *Cochrane Database Syst Rev.* 2006:CD001446.
19. Nobuhiro Y, Hartung H-P. Guillain-Barre Syndrome. *N Engl J Med.* 2012;366:2294–2304.
20. Orlikowski, et al. Respiratory dysfunction in Guillain-Barre syndrome. *Neurocrit Care.* 2004;1(4):415–422.
21. Marinelli WA, Leatherman JW. Neuromuscular disorders in the intensive care unit. *Crit Care Clin.* 2002;18(4):915–929.
22. Murthy JM, et al. Myasthenic crisis: clinical features, complications, and mortality. *Neurol India.* 2005;53(1):37–40.

SECTION 7
Gastrointestinal and Hematological Critical Care

24

Gastrointestinal Hemorrhage

Parvathi A. Myer and Shai Friedland

LOWER GASTROINTESTINAL BLEEDING

Background

Lower gastrointestinal bleeding (LGIB), defined as bleeding below the ligament of Treitz, accounts for 20% of all acute GI bleeding.[1] In the United States, the incidence of LGIB ranges from 20.5 to 27 cases per 100,000 adults.[2] Compared to acute upper GI bleeding, patients with acute LGIB experience less shock, require fewer blood transfusions, and have a significantly higher hemoglobin level.[3] The mortality rate of acute LGIB is 2% to 4%, and bleeding stops spontaneously in 80% to 85% of patients.[3]

Epidemiology

The causes of hemodynamically significant hematochezia include diverticular bleeding (17% to 40%), angiodysplasia (9% to 21%), colitis (including ischemic, infectious, chronic inflammatory bowel disease [IBD], or radiation injury) (2% to 30%), neoplasia and postpolypectomy bleeding (11% to 14%), anorectal disease (4% to 10%), upper GI bleeding (1% to 11%), and small bowel bleeding (2% to 9%).[4]

Diverticular Bleeding

Diverticular bleeding is typically due to arterial bleeding, presents as painless hematochezia, and increases in prevalence with age. Most diverticula are in the left colon, but the majority of bleeding diverticula are in the right colon.[5] Although diverticular bleeding stops spontaneously in 80% of cases, the cumulative rebleeding rate is approximately 25% after 4 years.[6]

Angiodysplasia

Angiodysplasias (or vascular ectasias/angioectasias) appear as red, mucosal lesions on colonoscopy and account for up to 30% of LGIB. They commonly occur in the right colon and increase in frequency with age. Most angiodysplasias do not bleed; bleeding is precipitated by platelet dysfunction and coagulopathy and is more frequent in patients with renal failure.[5] Radiation proctopathy can result in telangiectasias, which can lead to rectal bleeding that is typically low volume and chronic. In a minority of patients, telangiectasias are due to hereditary hemorrhagic telangiectasia.[5]

Ischemic Colitis

Ischemic colitis classically presents with mild abdominal pain associated with self-limited hematochezia. The etiology of ischemic colitis is frequently a decrease in mesenteric blood flow in a watershed distribution due to low blood pressure or vasospasm.[5] Ischemic colitis risk factors include underlying cardiovascular disease, atherosclerosis, and advanced age.[5] Endoscopically, the colonic mucosa appears edematous and can show areas of submucosal hemorrhage or necrosis.

Mucosal Inflammation

Mucosal inflammation can be caused by IBD or an infectious colitis. In 50% of patients with inflammation-associated bleeding, bleeding will stop spontaneously; however, 35% will rebleed.[7] Nonsteroidal anti-inflammatory drug (NSAID) use has been noted to greatly increase the risk of bleeding in these conditions.[5]

Neoplasia and Postpolypectomy Bleeding

Two to nine percent of hematochezia is due to colon cancer and presents most commonly as occult or low-volume bleeding. Bleeding may occur up to 14 days after colonoscopic polypectomy, usually because of arterial bleeding from the stalk of the polyp.[5] Postpolypectomy bleeding accounts for 2% to 8% of acute LGIB.[3]

Anorectal Diseases

Hemorrhoids account for 2% to 9% of hemodynamically significant LGIB[4]. Solitary rectal ulcers resulting from internal rectal prolapse can also produce rectal bleeding. Rectal varices (enlarged blood vessels) can also cause hematochezia and significant GI bleeding.

Dieulafoy Lesion

A Dieulafoy lesion is an artery that is exposed through a colonic mucosal defect and can bleed profusely.[5] They are classically observed in the proximal stomach but can occur anywhere in the GI tract including the colon and rectum. These lesions can be difficult to locate endoscopically.

Initial Evaluation and Risk Stratification

A complete patient history and physical exam are essential during the initial emergency department (ED) evaluation. The reported color of the stool—maroon, bright red, or black and tarry (melena)—and confirmatory rectal exam are key to determining if the bleeding stems from an upper or lower gastrointestinal (UGI or LGI) source. The rectal exam also helps to assess rate of bleeding and the presence of anorectal pathology. Patient history should note duration and frequency of bleeding, associated symptoms (light-headedness, dizziness, palpitations, syncope, abdominal pain, and fevers), sick contacts, travel history, and prior episodes of GI bleeding.[8] The use of NSAIDs, family or personal history of colon cancer, prior radiation exposure, IBD history, liver disease, coagulopathy, and weight loss are important details to obtain.[5] In the setting of brisk hematochezia, clinicians must always maintain a high index of suspicion for the presence of a brisk upper GI bleed (UGIB), as 11% to 15% of patients with hematochezia are bleeding due to massive UGIB.[9]

Patients with brisk bleeding or showing signs of hemodynamic instability including orthostatic hypotension, chest pain, dyspnea, and tachypnea should be monitored in the intensive care unit (ICU). ICU placement should also be considered for LGIB patients with significant comorbidities or those requiring two or more units of packed red blood cells (PRBCs). Initial laboratory studies should include a complete blood count, serum chemistry including BUN and creatinine, and an international normalized ratio (INR).[5] In addition to volume resuscitation, patients with active bleeding and an INR > 1.5 or a platelet count <50,000/μL will require transfusion of fresh frozen plasma or platelets, respectively.[5] A recent randomized clinical trial (RCT) in patients with acute UGIB suggests that a restrictive strategy of transfusion for hemoglobin <7 g/dL may be optimal.[10] This study provides new guidelines for blood transfusion in the setting of GI bleeding and represents a departure from previous recommendations for transfusion in critically ill patients established by the Transfusion Requirements in Critical Care (TRICC) Investigators study.[11] Patients with underlying cardiac disease should still be transfused when the hemoglobin drops below 9 g/dL.[2]

To help identify patients with severe LGIB, the following validated risk factors should be assessed: heart rate > 100, systolic blood pressure < 115 mm Hg, syncope, nontender abdominal exam, bleeding within the first 4 hours of evaluation, aspirin use, and greater than two comorbid conditions (Charlson Comorbidity Index).[12,13] In a patient with a LGIB and hemodynamic instability, placement of a nasogastric tube (NGT) and evaluation of the aspirate for bile or blood help identify whether brisk UGIB is the cause of the patient's rectal bleeding. If NGT aspirate is clear, and an esophagogastroduodenoscopy (EGD) is not deemed necessary, colonoscopy should be planned within 12 to 48 hours of arrival to the ED. All patients should have a clear liquid diet until 4 hours before the procedure. Four liters of GoLytely or an equivalent polyethylene glycol solution should be administered at a rate of a liter per hour until 4 hours before the procedure.

Management Guidelines

Colonoscopy

Colonoscopy is the preferred modality for identifying the source of an LGIB and achieving hemostasis with the fewest complications.[5] The risk of serious complications from a colonoscopy is approximately 1 in 1,000 procedures.[5] In patients with severe LGIB due to diverticular bleeding, colonoscopic treatment may prevent recurrent bleeding and decrease the need for surgery.[9]

Timing of Colonoscopy The timing of colonoscopy has been the subject of several RCTs.[8,14] The most recent considered 85 patients with hematochezia with the following attributes: heart rate > 100 bpm, systolic blood pressure < 100 mm Hg, orthostatic change in heart rate or blood pressure > 20 mm Hg, hemoglobin drop > 1.5 g/dL, or requiring blood transfusion. These patients all underwent EGD within 6 hours to exclude brisk UGI bleeding; 13 (15%) were found to have an UGI source. Of the remainder, 36 patients were randomized to an urgent colonoscopy group (<12 hours) and 36 were randomized to an elective colonoscopy group (36 to 60 hours). There were no differences in clinical outcomes, including recurrent bleeding, units of blood transfused, hospital days, need for subsequent interventions, treatment of bleeding, hospital charges, or length of stay.[8] The study concluded that the timing of colonoscopy between 12 and 60 hours from initial ED evaluation made no difference in clinical or economic outcomes.[8]

In patients with brisk LGIBs unable to undergo colonoscopy due to hemodynamic instability or with bleeding that is too brisk to permit successful colon preparation, immediate angiography, radionucleotide scintigraphy (tagged red blood cell [RBC] scan), computed tomography (CT), or surgery may be necessary.[12,15]

Angiography

A minimum colonic bleeding rate of 0.5 to 1 mL/min is required to be detected by angiography; the higher the bleeding rate, the more likely the study will be able to localize its source.[12] A spontaneous bacterial peritonitis (SBP) < 90 and the need for more than 5 units of PRBCs in 24 hours are also predictors that angiography will locate the source of bleeding.[16] Therapeutically, angiography works by embolization of the arterial branches that feed the bleeding site. Embolization has been demonstrated to be more effective than vasoconstrictor infusion and carries a lower risk of bowel infarction.[12,15] Complications of angiography include contrast allergies, nephrotoxicity, hematomas, thrombosis, and vascular dissections.[15,12]

Radionucleotide Scintigraphy

Radionucleotide scintigraphy, or tagged RBC scanning, detects LGIB at rates as low as 0.05 to 0.1 mL/min[12]; source detection is improved when the scans are positive within 2 hours.[12] No randomized trials have compared tagged RBC scanning to angiography, and studies regarding the diagnostic advantage of performing tagged RBC scans prior to angiography are equivocal.[12,15] One RCT compared colonoscopy with tagged RBC scan following angiography and demonstrated colonoscopy to be the superior diagnostic test.[14] A tagged RBC scan has the advantage of being noninvasive and not requiring special patient preparation; its disadvantage, however, is that it provides no therapeutic option for controlling a bleeding site once identified. In the setting of a brisk LGI bleed, tagged RBC scans remain valuable when time-consuming colonoscopy preparation prevents urgent localization of the bleeding source. RBC scans are also useful at the time of colonoscopy if the bleeding site cannot be identified or hemostasis cannot be achieved endoscopically. In this setting, the tagged RBC scan would be used to localize the site of bleeding, followed by angiography for hemostasis.

Computed Tomography

Multidetector CTs have improved imaging time and the ability to detect arterial bleeds; in animal models, they have detected bleeding rates as low as 0.3 to 0.5 mL/min.[12] The main disadvantage of CT, as with the tagged RBC scan, is the inability to provide therapeutic options. Other disadvantages include radiation exposure, false-positive rates, contrast allergies, and potential contrast-induced nephrotoxicity.[12] CT appears to be highly effective in detecting vascular ectasias.[17]

Surgery

Surgery is performed when LGIB is recurrent and other measures, such as colonoscopy or angiography, have proven unsuccessful. Preoperative angiography can localize the bleeding source and appears to be associated with decreased rebleeding rates.[15]

NONVARICEAL UPPER GASTROINTESTINAL BLEEDING

Background

Nonvariceal upper gastrointestinal bleeding (NVUGIB) has a mortality rate of 10% to 14%[18] and imposes a significant clinical and economical burden on the U.S. health care system. Cases range from 48 to 160 per 100,000 adults per year,[19] with an associated mean length of hospital stay of 2.7 to 4.4 days.[20]

Initial Evaluation and Risk Stratification

Initial evaluation—as with any critically ill patient—begins with an assessment of airway, breathing, and circulation (ABC). Once the ABCs are attended to, patients may be stratified as either high- or low-risk for re-bleeding and mortality using clinical assessment, laboratory data, and endoscopic criteria for risk of rebleeding. This type of risk stratification can help the emergency physician and gastroenterologist determine the appropriate timing of endoscopy. Clinical predictors of increased risk include age over 65, multiple comorbidities, hemodynamic instability, melena, poor overall functional status, hematochezia, hematemesis, and bloody nasogastric aspirate. Concerning laboratory data include a low initial hemoglobin, and/or elevated BUN, creatinine, or serum aminotransferase.[19] Endoscopic predictors of increased risk for rebleeding include arterial bleeding, nonbleeding visible vessel or adherent clot, ulcer size greater than 2 cm, ulcer location in the posterior lesser gastric curvature or posterior duodenal wall, and varices or cancer.[19]

Management Guidelines

PPI Therapy

Initiation of intravenous proton pump inhibitor (PPI) therapy with an 80-mg bolus followed by an 8 mg/hour infusion rate is recommended for all NVUGIB. High-dose PPI therapy decreases the proportion of patients that will present with endoscopic findings that place them at risk of significant hemorrhage and/or in need of therapeutic intervention (e.g., active bleeding, nonbleeding visible vessel, or adherent clot). High-dose PPI therapy in NVUGIB does not reduce mortality, rebleeding rate, the need for blood transfusions, or the need for surgery.[21,22]

Blood Transfusion

The TRICC trial is a landmark study that has historically guided ICU blood transfusion strategies. This study stratified ICU-admitted patients who had been given blood transfusions into a restrictive (transfused when hemoglobin dropped below 7 g/dL) versus liberal (when hemoglobin dropped below 10 g/dL) transfusion strategy. The trial found that less critically ill patients (Acute Physiology and Chronic Health Evaluation II score < 20) and patients under the age of 55 had significantly decreased mortality rates when transfused with the restrictive transfusion strategy. Patients with significant underlying cardiac disease had improved mortality rates with the liberal transfusion strategy.[11]

A 2013 landmark RCT has provided strong new evidence, and established a new standard, for blood transfusion in patients with active GI bleeding.[10] Unlike the TRICC trial, which surveyed ICU-admitted patients requiring blood transfusions for all causes, this trial was performed exclusively in patients with acute UGI bleeding. Furthermore, the 2013 trial studied a lower hemoglobin cutoff for the liberal transfusion strategy. Of the 921 patients enrolled in the trial, 421 patients were randomized to a restrictive transfusion strategy when the hemoglobin dropped below 7 g/dL; and 460 patients were randomized to a liberal transfusion strategy when the hemoglobin dropped below 9 g/dL. Patients in the restrictive group had higher probability of survival at 6 weeks, lower recurrence of further bleeding, and lower risks of adverse events.[10] Patients with cardiovascular disease, hypotension (systolic blood pressure < 90 mm Hg), or thought to be hemoconcentrated due to low systemic volume should still be considered for more liberal transfusion strategies.[2]

Prokinetic Therapy

Infusion of erythromycin 250 mg 30 minutes before endoscopy stimulates gastric emptying and has been known to increase endoscopic visualization, increase diagnostic yield, and decrease the need for repeat endoscopy in randomized trials.[23] Only two small studies have evaluated the benefit of metoclopramide, with no significant benefits noted.[23]

Correction of Coagulopathy

Correction of coagulopathy is recommended but should not delay early endoscopy.[19] Data on the correction of coagulopathy for patients with NVUGIB are sparse and often contradictory. For patients on anticoagulation therapy, the threshold for correcting the INR varies widely in different studies.[19] The International Consensus on Nonvariceal Upper Gastrointestinal Bleeding, which stresses the importance of early endoscopic intervention in NVUGIB, provides a general recommendation to correct supratherapeutic INRs prior to endoscopy.[19]

Endoscopy

Endoscopic findings are useful in predicting an individual patients' risk of rebleeding. Initial endoscopic findings that place a patient at highest risk for rebleed and warrant intervention include ulcers with active bleeding, nonbleeding visible vessels, and adherent clot with an underlying vessel visualized after clot removal. Current guidelines recommend the use of clips or thermal coagulation alone and in combination with epinephrine; monotherapy with epinephrine alone is no longer recommended.[25] Patients with flat pigmented spots and clean-based ulcers are at low risk and generally do not benefit from endoscopic treatment.

Timing of Endoscopy In patients who are hemodynamically stable with no significant comorbidities, endoscopy should be performed within 24 hours, following which patients can often be discharged home if demonstrated to have low-risk endoscopic findings (clean-based ulcers or ulcers with flat pigmented spots).[2] In patients with a more concerning clinical profile (tachycardia, hypotension, bloody emesis on NG lavage), endoscopy within 12 hours is recommended, as this may improve clinical outcomes.[2] In low-risk hemodynamically stable patients, expedited endoscopy resulted in earlier hospital discharge and lowered costs. No clinical outcome data exist, however, to support emergent endoscopy in the low-risk group.

Discharge of Low-Risk Patients from the ED

Multiple assessment scoring systems exist to risk-stratify patients and to predict mortality and the need for clinical intervention such as blood transfusions, endoscopic treatment, or surgery. Some of these systems, such as the Rockall system, require endoscopic criteria to risk-stratify patients, making them less helpful in the ED; others, such as Glasgow-Blatchford Bleeding Score (GBS), require only clinical and laboratory data.[24] A prospective study performed in the United Kingdom compared the GBS to the Rockall system for predicting mortality and need for clinical intervention (blood transfusions, endoscopic treatment, or surgery). Of the 676 patients presenting with acute GI bleeding, 105 received a GBS score of 0, indicating a low risk of need for intervention and an ability to be safely discharged from the ED without endoscopy if they meet the following additional criteria: urea nitrogen < 18.2 mg/dL, hemoglobin > 13.0 g/dL for men and 12.0 g/dL for women, systolic blood pressure > 100 mm Hg, pulse < 100 bpm, and absence of melena, syncope, cardiac failure, and liver disease. The study used receiver operator characteristic (ROC) scores to compare each score's ability to predict mortality and the need for clinical intervention. The GBS outperformed the Rockall system in predicting both measures.[24] A follow-up study tested the GBS in clinical practice; of 123 patients with UGI bleeding, 84 (68%) were characterized as low risk (GBS score of 0) and were successfully managed in the outpatient setting. No clinical interventions were required and no deaths occurred.[24]

VARICEAL UPPER GASTROINTESTINAL BLEEDING

Background

Patients with suspected acute gastroesophageal variceal bleeding should be admitted to an ICU for management and resuscitation.[26] Gastric and esophageal varices are formed as an end result of cirrhosis. Cirrhosis results from advanced liver disease and is characterized by hepatic tissue fibrosis, which leads to a structural resistance to hepatic blood flow and intrahepatic vasoconstriction due to an associated decrease in nitric oxide production. These changes result in portal venous system hypertension and the formation of a collateral (gastric and esophageal) circulation. Elevated portal pressures persist, however, because of resistance to portal flow within the collateral circulation and increased portal venous blood flow from concurrent splanchnic vasodilation.[26] Fifty percent of patients with cirrhosis will have gastroesophageal varices, and variceal wall tension is the primary determinant of variceal rupture. Variceal hemorrhage typically occurs when the hepatovenous portal gradient is over 12 mm Hg.[26]

Management Guidelines

Blood Transfusions

Based on the findings of the 2013 trial discussed above, blood transfusions should now target a hemoglobin of 7 to 8 g/dL[10,26]; excessive transfusion and vigorous saline infusion should be avoided because of resulting increases in portal pressures and increased risk of variceal rebleed.[10,26] Data from the 2013 study recommended a similar restrictive transfusion strategy for cirrhotics with variceal bleeding as for patients with NVUGIB. Survival improved in all patients assigned to the lower transfusion threshold (<7 g/dL compared to 9 g/dL); this benefit was magnified in the subgroup of patients with cirrhosis and a Child-Pugh class A or B disease.[10,27] Compared to the restrictive strategy group, cirrhotics in the liberal transfusion strategy had significantly higher portal pressure gradients.[10]

Octreotide

Octreotide causes splanchnic vasoconstriction and is thought to decrease vasodilatory peptides such as glucagon, thereby helping to counteract the increased portal venous blood flow from splanchnic vasodilation seen in cirrhotics.[26] Current guidelines recommend octreotide be given as an initial 50-μg bolus followed by a 50 μg/h infusion for 3 to 5 days following initial presentation of variceal bleeding.[26]

Antibiotic Prophylaxis

Patients with cirrhosis with gastroesophageal variceal bleeding are at high risk of bacterial infections including SBP and bacterial peritonitis, which cause increased risk of variceal rebleed and increased overall mortality.[26] Current guidelines recommend that patients receive antibiotics pre-endoscopy to cover gram-negative bacteria and for a total of 7 days after initial GI bleed. Recommended antimicrobials include norfloxacin 400 mg PO BID or ciprofloxacin 500 mg IV BID for patients unable to tolerate oral intake. In areas of high fluoroquinolone resistance, ceftriaxone 1 g/day is preferred.[26]

Endoscopy

There are two endoscopic methods for treating esophageal varices. The first, endoscopic variceal band ligation (EVL), deploys bands across varices with stigmata of recent hemorrhage with subsequent necrosis and sloughing of the varix. The second, sclerotherapy, injects a sclerosing agent such as cyanoacrylate into a bleeding varix to obtain hemostasis. A meta-analysis of 10 RCTs demonstrated EVL to be superior in overall outcomes when compared to sclerotherapy (pooled relative risk of 0.53).[28] When EVL is not available or technically infeasible, sclerotherapy should be used.[26]

Data on endoscopic management of bleeding gastric varices are minimal. In contrast to esophageal varices, sclerotherapy is recommended over EVL. TIPS should be considered when bleeding continues despite endoscopic attempts for hemostasis.

Transjugular Intrahepatic Portosystemic Shunt

Transjugular intrahepatic portosystemic shunt (TIPS) is a procedure performed by interventional radiology. It utilizes an expandable metal stent that creates a connection between the hepatic vein and the intrahepatic portal vein to help decrease portal pressure in the setting of acute variceal GI bleeding. TIPS may be considered in patients who are Child-Pugh class A or B with variceal bleeding and have failed endoscopic and medical therapy.[26,27]

CONCLUSION

The management of gastroesophageal bleeding requires a focused patient history and physical exam, close hemodynamic monitoring, rapid resuscitation using a restrictive transfusion strategy, and prompt endoscopic evaluation. In variceal bleeding, an octreotide infusion to promote splanchnic vasoconstriction and prophylactic antibiotics to prevent bacterial translocation are also recommended. EVL, sclerotherapy, and TIPS are three validated management options for refractory variceal bleeding.

LITERATURE TABLE

TRIAL	DESIGN	RESULT
Lower GI Bleeding		
Laine et al., *Am J Gastroenterol.* 2010[8]	RCT of 72 patients with LGIB who received either urgent <12 h or elective (36–60 h) colonoscopy	No difference between urgent colonoscopy (<12 h) and routine colonoscopy (36–60 h) in further bleeding, transfusion requirement, or hospital stay.
Green et al., *Am J Gastroenterol.* 2005[14]	RCT of 100 patients comparing urgent colonoscopy to standard care (red cell scan followed by angiography for positive scan and colonoscopy within 4 days for negative scan)	Urgent colonoscopy identified a definite source of bleeding more often than the standard care group (OR = 2.6, 95% CI [1.1–6.2]), but there was no difference in mortality (2% vs. 4%), hospital stay (5.8 vs. 6.6 days), ICU stay (1.8 vs. 2.4 days), transfusion requirement (4.2 vs. 5 units), early rebleeding (22% vs. 30%), or need for surgery (14% vs. 12%)
Non-Variceal Upper GI Bleeding		
Villanueva et al., *N Engl J Med.* 2013[10]	RCT of 921 patients comparing a restrictive transfusion strategy (hemoglobin < 7) to a liberal transfusion strategy (hemoglobin < 9)	Patients in the restrictive group had higher probability of survival at 6 weeks (95% vs. 91%, hazard ratio of death in the restrictive strategy 0.55, 95% CI [0.33–0.92]), less recurrent bleeding (10% vs. 16%, $p = 0.01$), fewer adverse events (40% vs. 48%, $p = 0.02$)
Leontiadis et al., *Mayo Clin Proc.* 2007[21]	Meta-analysis of 24 RCTs evaluating the efficacy of PPIs in the treatment of peptic ulcer disease	Treatment with PPI did not affect mortality (OR = 1.01, 95% CI [0.74–1.40]) but did decrease the need for surgery (OR = 0.61, 95% CI [0.48–0.78] NNT 34), rebleeding rate (OR = 0.49, 95% CI [0.37–0.65] NNT 13), and need for repeat endoscopic treatment (OR = 0.32, 95% CI [0.20–0.51] NNT 10)
Lau et al., *N Engl J Med.* 2007[22]	RCT 638 patients comparing IV omeprazole (80-mg bolus followed by 8 mg/h) to placebo prior to endoscopy	Fewer patients in the omeprazole group required endoscopic treatment (19% in the omeprazole group vs. 28.4% in the placebo group, $p = 0.007$). No difference in transfusion requirements, recurrent bleeding, or need for surgery
Barkun et al., *Gastrointest Endosc.* 2010[23]	Meta-analysis of five RCTs, three studies using erythromycin and two studies using metoclopramide	Erythromycin 250 mg or 3 mg/kg given prior to endoscopy decreased the need for repeat endoscopy (OR = 0.55, 95% CI [0.32–0.94]), but there was no difference in the number of blood transfusions given, length of hospital stay, or need for surgery. No benefits of using metoclopramide were noted
Stanley et al., *Lancet.* 2009[24]	Prospective multicenter observational study comparing the use of the GBS to the Rockall system to determine which model better predicted mortality and/or the need for clinical intervention (blood transfusion, endoscopic treatment, or surgery)	The ROC score was used to compare ability to predict mortality and the need for clinical intervention. The GBS was superior to the Rockall system to predict both outcome measures (ROC = 0.9, 95% CI [0.88–0.93]) compared to the admission Rockall score (ROC = 0.70, 95% CI [0.65–0.75])[24]

CI, confidence interval; NNT, number needed to treat; OR, odds ratio.

REFERENCES

1. Zuccaro G, Jr. Management of the adult patient with acute lower gastrointestinal bleeding. American College of Gastroenterology. Practice Parameters Committee. *Am J Gastroenterol.* 1998;93:1202–1208.
2. Laine L, Jensen DM. Management of patients with ulcer bleeding. *Am J Gastroenterol.* 2012;107:345–360; quiz 361.
3. Farrell JJ, Friedman LS. Review article: the management of lower gastrointestinal bleeding. *Aliment Pharmacol Ther.* 2005;21:1281–1298.
4. Zuckerman GR, Prakash C. Acute lower intestinal bleeding. Part II: etiology, therapy, and outcomes. *Gastrointest Endosc.* 1999;49:228–238.
5. Barnert J, Messmann H. Diagnosis and management of lower gastrointestinal bleeding. *Nat Rev Gastroenterol Hepatol.* 2009;6:637–646.

6. Longstreth GF. Epidemiology and outcome of patients hospitalized with acute lower gastrointestinal hemorrhage: a population-based study. *Am J Gastroenterol.* 1997;92:419–424.
7. Robert JR, Sachar DB, Greenstein AJ. Severe gastrointestinal hemorrhage in Crohn's disease. *Ann Surg.* 1991;213:207–211.
8. Laine L, Shah A. Randomized trial of urgent vs. elective colonoscopy in patients hospitalized with lower GI bleeding. *Am J Gastroenterol.* 2010;105:2636–2641; quiz 2642.
9. Jensen DM, Machicado GA. Diagnosis and treatment of severe hematochezia. The role of urgent colonoscopy after purge. *Gastroenterology.* 1988;95:1569–1574.
10. Villanueva C, Colomo A, Bosch A, et al. Transfusion strategies for acute upper gastrointestinal bleeding. *N Engl J Med.* 2013;368:11–21.
11. Hebert PC, Wells G, Tweeddale M, et al. Does transfusion practice affect mortality in critically ill patients? Transfusion Requirements in Critical Care (TRICC) Investigators and the Canadian Critical Care Trials Group. *Am J Respir Crit Care Med.* 1997;155:1618–1623.
12. Strate LL, Naumann CR. The role of colonoscopy and radiological procedures in the management of acute lower intestinal bleeding. *Clin Gastroenterol Hepatol.* 2010;8:333–343; quiz e44.
13. Strate LL, Orav EJ, Syngal S. Early predictors of severity in acute lower intestinal tract bleeding. *Arch Intern Med.* 2003;163:838–843.
14. Green BT, Rockey DC, Portwood G, et al. Urgent colonoscopy for evaluation and management of acute lower gastrointestinal hemorrhage: a randomized controlled trial. *Am J Gastroenterol.* 2005;100:2395–2402.
15. Rockey DC. Lower gastrointestinal bleeding. *Gastroenterology.* 2006;130:165–171.
16. Abbas SM, Bissett IP, Holden A, et al. Clinical variables associated with positive angiographic localization of lower gastrointestinal bleeding. *ANZ J Surg.* 2005;75:953–957.
17. Junquera F, Quiroga S, Saperas E, et al. Accuracy of helical computed tomographic angiography for the diagnosis of colonic angiodysplasia. *Gastroenterology.* 2000;119:293–299.
18. van Leerdam ME, Vreeburg EM, Rauws EA, et al. Acute upper GI bleeding: did anything change? Time trend analysis of incidence and outcome of acute upper GI bleeding between 1993/1994 and 2000. *Am J Gastroenterol.* 2003;98:1494–1499.
19. Barkun A, Bardou M, Marshall JK. Consensus recommendations for managing patients with nonvariceal upper gastrointestinal bleeding. *Ann Intern Med.* 2003;139:843–857.
20. Viviane A, Alan BN. Estimates of costs of hospital stay for variceal and nonvariceal upper gastrointestinal bleeding in the United States. *Value Health.* 2008;11:1–3.
21. Leontiadis GI, Sharma VK, Howden CW. Proton pump inhibitor therapy for peptic ulcer bleeding: cochrane collaboration meta-analysis of randomized controlled trials. *Mayo Clin Proc.* 2007;82:286–296.
22. Lau JY, Leung WK, Wu JC, et al. Omeprazole before endoscopy in patients with gastrointestinal bleeding. *N Engl J Med.* 2007;356:1631–1640.
23. Barkun AN, Bardou M, Martel M, et al. Prokinetics in acute upper GI bleeding: a meta-analysis. *Gastrointest Endosc.* 2010;72:1138–1145.
24. Stanley AJ, Ashley D, Dalton HR, et al. Outpatient management of patients with low-risk upper-gastrointestinal haemorrhage: multicentre validation and prospective evaluation. *Lancet.* 2009;373:42–47.
25. Greenspoon J, Barkun A, Bardou M, et al. Management of patients with nonvariceal upper gastrointestinal bleeding. *Clin Gastroenterol Hepatol.* 2012;10:234–239.
26. Garcia-Tsao G, Sanyal AJ, Grace ND, et al. Prevention and management of gastroesophageal varices and variceal hemorrhage in cirrhosis. *Am J Gastroenterol.* 2007;102:2086–2102.
27. Child CG, Turcotte JG. Surgery and portal hypertension. *Major Probl Clin Surg.* 1964;1:1–85.
28. Garcia-Pagan JC, Bosch J. Endoscopic band ligation in the treatment of portal hypertension. *Nat Clin Pract Gastroenterol Hepatol.* 2005;2:526–535.

25

Acute Liver Failure and Hepatic Encephalopathy

Robert J. Wong and Glen A. Lutchman

BACKGROUND

Acute liver failure (ALF) is a rare condition characterized by a rapid decline in hepatic synthetic function, marked hepatocellular inflammation, and a high mortality rate. The incidence of ALF is approximately 2,000 cases per year in the United States; it accounts for 6% of all liver-related deaths and 6% of liver transplantations.[1–3] Differentiating acute from acute-on-chronic liver failure can be difficult, but is important when assessing patient prognosis and need for transfer to a liver transplant center. Early recognition of ALF allows for targeted supportive therapy, early evaluation for liver transplantation, and timely involvement of multidisciplinary specialties, including hepatologists, intensivists, and transplant surgeons.

DEFINITIONS

ALF is a general term used to define the development of jaundice, hepatic encephalopathy, and coagulopathy (international normalized ratio [INR] ≥ 1.5) in an individual without underlying liver disease with a disease course of <26 weeks. More accurate subclassifications are differentiated by elapsed time from development of jaundice to development of hepatic encephalopathy[1,3]:

- *Hyperacute liver failure*: development of hepatic encephalopathy 0 to 7 days after the onset of jaundice
- *Acute liver failure*: development of hepatic encephalopathy 8 to 21 days after the onset of jaundice
- *Subacute liver failure*: development of hepatic encephalopathy >21 days to <26 weeks after the onset of jaundice

While popular, these terms are not particularly useful since they do not have prognostic significance. For example, "hyperacute" disease generally carries a better prognosis because of a high prevalence in this cohort of acetaminophen-related disease, which tends to have better outcomes.[1,3–5] For the remainder of this chapter, we will use the more general definition of ALF.

DIAGNOSTIC EVALUATION

The initial approach to ALF (Fig. 25.1) involves determining the underlying etiology of disease and the implementing etiology-specific targeted therapy (Tables 25.1 and 25.2). A thorough patient history, including interviews with family and friends, can provide clues to specific ingestions, drugs, or toxins that may be implicated in the patient's disease and enables a review of the patient's prescribed medications for

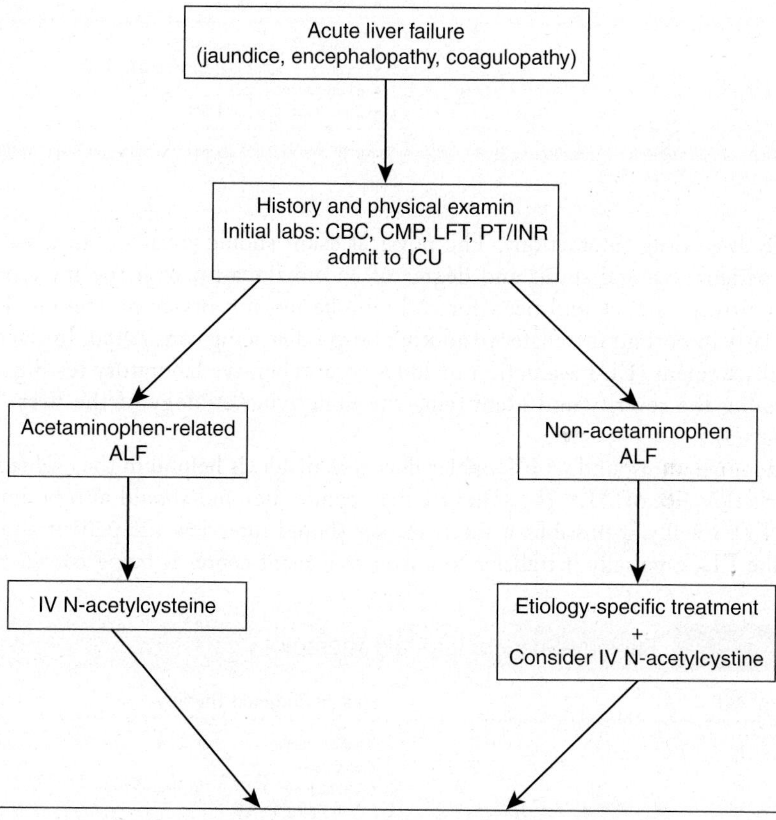

FIGURE 25.1 Initial evaluation of ALF.

TABLE 25.1 Common Etiologies of Acute Liver Failure

Drug-induced liver injury	• Acetaminophen (46%) • Other drug-induced liver injury (12%)
Acute viral hepatitis	• Hepatitis A infection (2.6%) • Hepatitis B infection (7.7%)
Vascular	• Acute ischemic hepatitis (4.6%) • Budd-Chiari syndrome (0.9%)
Metabolic	• Wilson disease (1.4%)
Other	• Autoimmune hepatitis (5.9%) • Pregnancy-related liver failure (0.8%) • Indeterminate (14%) • Other toxins (e.g., *Amanita*)

Data from the Acute Liver Failure Study Group Registry, 1998–2008. From Stravitz RT, Kramer DJ. Management of acute liver failure. *Nat Rev Gastroenterol Hepatol.* 2009;6:542–553.

possible drug–drug interactions. The physical exam should focus on an assessment of the patient's mental status and degree of encephalopathy, with specific attention paid to airway patency and need for early intubation for airway protection. This is particularly important if transfer to another hospital is being considered. Initial emergency department (ED) evaluation includes comprehensive laboratory testing aimed at assessing the severity and identifying the underlying etiology of the liver failure (Table 25.3).

Abdominal ultrasound with Doppler flow, if available, is helpful in the evaluation of vascular etiologies of ALF (i.e., Budd-Chiari syndrome) and should also be initiated in the ED. Finally, if possible, a social worker should interview the patient and family in the ED, especially if transfer to a liver transplant center is being considered, as

TABLE 25.2 Etiology-Specific Targeted Therapy

Etiology of ALF	Specific Targeted Therapy
Acetaminophen	*N*-acetylcysteine: Intravenous: • Loading dose of 150 mg/kg over 15 min • 12.5 mg/kg/h × 4 h • 6.25 mg/kg/h Enteral: • Loading dose of 140 mg/kg • 70 mg/kg every 4 h × 17 doses
Mushroom poisoning (e.g., *Amanita*)	• Silibinin 30–40 gm/kg/d IV (not available in the United States) • Penicillin G 300,000—1 million units/kg/d
Acute hepatitis B	Tenofovir 300 mg/d or entecavir 0.5 mg/d
Herpes simplex virus Varicella zoster virus	IV acyclovir 5–10 mg/kg/8 h
Autoimmune hepatitis	Prednisone 40–60 mg/d
Acute fatty liver of pregnancy HELLP syndrome	Delivery of the fetus

TABLE 25.3 Laboratory Evaluation in Patients with Acute Liver Failure

- Complete blood count, comprehensive metabolic panel, liver function tests, PT/INR
- Arterial blood gas for pH
- Acetaminophen level
- Viral hepatitis screening:
  - Hepatitis A (HAV): IgM
  - Hepatitis B (HBV): core IgM, surface antigen (Ag), surface antibody (Ab), DNA viral load
  - Hepatitis C (HCV): HCV Ab, RNA viral load
  - Hepatitis E (HEV): IgM
- Autoimmune hepatitis screening:
  - Antineutrophil antibody (ANA)
  - Anti–smooth muscle antibody (ASMA)
  - Serum total IgG
- Ceruloplasmin for Wilson Disease
- Other viral hepatitis:
  - Herpes simplex 1 and 2 (HSV): anti-HSV-1 IgM, anti-HSV-2 IgM, HSV DNA
  - Varicella-zoster (VSV): anti-VZV IgM, VZV DNA
  - Cytomegalovirus (CMV): CMV DNA
  - Epstein-Barr (EBV): EBV DNA
  - HIV Ab

information gained in these interviews can have significant bearing on liver transplant candidacy (e.g., recent alcohol or drug use, social support mechanisms, financial/insurance information).

SYSTEM-SPECIFIC CLINICAL COMPLICATIONS

Respiratory Complications

A common presenting symptom of ALF is hepatic encephalopathy (see Hepatic Encephalopathy). With more severe forms of encephalopathy, maintenance of airway protection may be compromised, necessitating endotracheal intubation. As a result, all patients presenting with ALF should be assessed for the need for ventilatory support. In addition to providing airway protection in patients with severe hepatic encephalopathy, mechanical ventilation also allows for targeted hyperventilation (i.e., hypocapnia) for treatment of cerebral edema and intracranial hypertension (see Neurologic Complications).[6,7] There are currently insufficient data to recommend a standard mode of mechanical ventilation in ALF patients. However, tidal volume and plateau pressure should be limited to prevent development of acute lung injury. As a result, respiratory rate should be adjusted to ensure adequate minute ventilation to prevent increasing PCO_2, which can further exacerbate intracranial hypertension.[8,9]

Neurologic Complications

One of the most feared complications of ALF, and a leading cause of mortality among these patients, is neurologic impairment—specifically, cerebral edema and intracranial hypertension. Both of these conditions are more common among patients with hyperacute liver failure and can result in hypoxic brain injury, permanent neurologic deficits, and death.[1,8,9] Failure to clinically recognize cerebral edema can lead to treatment delays and progression of neurologic complications, including uncal herniation. While the exact etiology of cerebral edema is unclear, it is hypothesized that ALF-induced systemic inflammation and hormonal dysregulation lead to osmotic disturbances in the brain and to heightened cerebral blood flow from autoregulation.[10] The risk of cerebral edema and subsequent herniation has been shown to correlate with both the severity of a patient's hepatic encephalopathy and the degree of serum ammonia elevation (see Hepatic Encephalopathy).[10–12]

Patients with ALF and evidence of neurologic impairments (e.g., cerebral edema) should be monitored in the intensive care unit (ICU). Management of cerebral edema and intracranial hypertension consists of endotracheal intubation when indicated for mental status compromise, close monitoring of intracranial pressure (ICP), and medical therapy to minimize further elevation in ICP. ICP should be maintained at <20 mm Hg and cerebral perfusion pressure (CPP) at >60 mm Hg. CPP is determined by the difference between mean arterial pressure (MAP) and ICP. The role of invasive ICP monitoring in ALF is under study and is only to be undertaken in collaboration with an intensivist and transplant hepatologist.[1,13–15] Alternative methods of ICP monitoring, such as transcranial Doppler, are under evaluation.[16]

In patients with ALF suspected of developing intracranial hypertension, several steps can be taken to treat the elevated pressures and prevent further deterioration. Minimizing patient stimuli, elevating the head of bed to 30°, and avoiding placement of central access in the neck region are initial precautions that can be taken.[1,8,9] Medical intervention includes osmotic therapy with either mannitol or hypertonic saline; this increases blood osmolality and induces fluid shift from the brain intracellular space to the intravascular space, thereby decreasing brain edema and pressure. An early randomized control trial of 34 patients with ALF evaluated the effect of intravenous mannitol (given as a rapid infusion of 1 g/kg body weight) in the treatment of patients with intracranial hypertension (ICP ≥30 mm Hg for >5 minutes). Compared to the 17 patients who did not receive mannitol therapy, those who underwent mannitol infusions had significantly higher overall survival (47.1% vs. 5.9%).[17] In a randomized controlled trial of 30% hypertonic saline in the management of 45 patients with ALF (using a target serum sodium level of between 145 and 150 mmol/L), a significantly lower incidence of intracranial hypertension was seen among the treatment group.[18]

For patients requiring mechanical ventilation, hyperventilation to a goal $PaCO_2$ of 25 to 30 mm Hg results in vasoconstriction and decreased ICP and cerebral edema. While mechanical hyperventilation has not been proven effective in the prevention of cerebral edema, it is commonly used for treatment of acute rises in ICP/cerebral edema.[6,7]

The role of hypothermia in the management of ALF patients is complex; it likely affects multiple factors responsible for the development of encephalopathy and intracranial hypertension.[19–21] An early clinical study evaluated the role of hypothermia in seven patients with uncontrolled intracranial hypertension despite the aforementioned therapies. Patients who were cooled to 32°C demonstrated a significant decline in ICP, from 45 to 16 mm Hg, with subsequent improvements in CPP.[21] Other studies have reported that hypothermia used as adjunct to standard therapy may be helpful in patients with persistent uncontrolled intracranial hypertension, especially as a bridge toward liver transplantation[19–21]; however, well-designed randomized clinical trials for this application are lacking.

Pharmacologic coma and sedation, another adjunctive therapy, reduce ICP by suppressing cerebral metabolic activity and decreasing CPP. Phenobarbital has been traditionally used for this purpose, but propofol has become the preferred sedative agent in many centers.[22,23]

Hepatic Encephalopathy

Hepatic encephalopathy is a neurologic complication of ALF that requires early identification and aggressive treatment. Accurate assessment (see grading system, below) of degree of encephalopathy helps inform the decision to initiate definitive ventilatory support and protect the patient's airway; prompt treatment helps prevent worsening cerebral edema. Serum ammonia will be elevated in ALF and is hypothesized play a role in the pathogenesis of worsening cerebral edema and intracranial hypertension. Lowering ammonia levels with lactulose and early dialysis may help treat or prevent the development of cerebral edema.[1,11,24,25] The U.S. Acute Liver Failure Study Group retrospectively evaluated the role of lactulose in the management of encephalopathy among ALF patients.[25] While the severity of encephalopathy did not differ between patients in the treated and untreated groups, overall survival was slightly higher for patients receiving lactulose therapy.[25] Care should be taken, however, to avoid lactulose therapy–associated dehydration and electrolyte disturbances. The role of nonabsorbable antibiotics (e.g., rifaximin) in the management of encephalopathy in patients with ALF is not well studied[26]; as a result, rifaximin is not considered standard of care, but may be considered on a case-by-case scenario in consultation with the hepatology service.

Hepatic Encephalopathy Grading System

- *Grade 1*—changes in behavior, minimal change in consciousness
- *Grade 2*—gross disorientation, drowsiness, asterixis, slowness of mentation
- *Grade 3*—marked confusions, incoherent speech, sleeping, arousable to vocal stimuli
- *Grade 4*—comatose, unresponsive to pain, decorticate or decerebrate positioning

Cardiovascular Complications

The systemic inflammation and hormonal dysregulation that result from ALF can lead to systemic vasodilation, contributing to decreased MAP and CPP. Adequate maintenance of cardiovascular perfusion directly affects the CPP and overall neurologic complications. Initial management with intravascular volume repletion is aimed at maintaining MAP > 80 mm Hg and CPP > 60 mm Hg. Patients should be resuscitated with normal saline first and switched to half-normal saline with 75 mEq/L of sodium bicarbonate if acidosis is present. Adjunctive therapy with vasopressor therapy may be needed to maintain/reach MAP and CPP targets. Norepinephrine is the vasopressor of choice, with the addition of vasopressin to permit titration of the norepinephrine infusion.[1,4]

Hematologic Complications

Coagulopathy is another common feature of ALF and correlates with a patient's degree of hepatic synthetic dysfunction. Aggressive correction of thrombocytopenia and elevated INR is not necessary if there is no evidence of bleeding.[27] Prior to invasive diagnostic or therapeutic interventions, however, coagulopathy may be corrected with fresh frozen plasma and platelets; goals for correction, however, are not well established.

In the setting of active gastrointestinal bleeding, more aggressive transfusion of cryoprecipitate may also be instituted. Recombinant factor VIIa is an option for life-threatening bleeding but carries risk of thrombosis.[28] Given the increased risk of gastrointestinal tract bleeding in the setting of coagulopathy and the risk of developing stress-induced ulcers, routine prophylactic acid suppression therapy is indicated. In a multicenter, randomized placebo-controlled trial of 1,200 mechanically ventilated patients, acid suppression therapy was associated with significantly reduced risk of gastrointestinal bleeding (relative risk 0.44).[29] While the study cohort was not limited to patients with ALF, the findings of this study have been used to support the routine use of acid suppression in ALF.

Renal Complications

Acute renal failure is a common complication in ALF. Hemodynamic alterations affecting adequate renal perfusion coupled with the direct nephrotoxicity of drugs and toxins such as acetaminophen and amanita poisoning contribute to worsening renal function. ALF-induced acidosis, electrolyte abnormalities, and uremia can further contribute to renal impairment. The renal failure, in turn, can exacerbate the systemic inflammatory response triggered by the ALF.

Fluid resuscitation to achieve optimal intravascular volume, coupled with vasopressor therapy to achieve MAP goals, can improve hypoperfusion-induced renal failure. Early recognition of renal failure and, when indicated, initiation of renal replacement therapy with continuous venovenous hemodialysis (CVVH) can also assist significantly in the overall management of ALF.[30,31] Early initiation of dialysis allows for more aggressive management of encephalopathy and elevated ICP by forced hypernatremia and lowering of blood ammonia levels. Furthermore, CVVH has been demonstrated to improve cardiovascular stability in patients with ALF.[30,31] In one study, 32 critically ill patients with ALF and acute renal failure were randomized to receive either intermittent or continuous modes of renal replacement therapy.[31] Patients treated with CVVH had improved overall cardiovascular parameters, as measured by cardiac output and tissue oxygen delivery.

Infectious Complications

Ninety percent of ALF patients develop some degree of infection, a result of the confluence of invasive monitoring and immune system dysfunction. Severe bacterial or fungal infections can preclude liver transplantation and/or complicate the posttransplantation recovery.[1,32–35] Pneumonia is the most common infection experienced by ALF patients, followed by urinary tract infections and catheter-related infections. Gram-positive organisms are the most common infectious culprits, followed by gram-negative organisms and fungi.[34,35]

Surveillance cultures of blood, urine, and sputum and chest radiography should be routinely evaluated in patients with ALF. In the absence of suspected infection, empiric prophylactic antibiotic or antifungal therapy has not been shown to provide a survival benefit.[32,33] In one study, ALF patients without evidence of acute infection were randomized to receive or not to receive prophylactic parenteral and enteral antimicrobial therapy.[33] While the treated group showed a significant reduction in the development of infections, overall survival was not significantly different between the treated and untreated groups. Gut decontamination with poorly absorbable antibiotics has also not been shown to improve survival outcomes among ALF patients.[36] Antibiotic or antifungal therapy should, however, be initiated if there is a clinical suspicion of infection or deteriorating clinical status (e.g., worsening hepatic encephalopathy or systemic inflammatory response syndrome).

Metabolic Complications

Severe metabolic and electrolyte abnormalities are common in patients with ALF, a result of multiorgan dysfunction. Early recognition and correction of these derangements can prevent further deterioration.[1] Some of the common metabolic complications that result from ALF include the following:

- *Acidemia and alkalemia*: Both are important predictors of mortality and need for liver transplantation. Acid–base status is also an important component of the King's College criteria (Table 25.4),[37] which is used to guide prognostication in patients with ALF.
- *Hypoglycemia*: Patients with ALF experience hypoglycemia because of impaired glucose metabolism. When hypoglycemia is identified, a continuous glucose infusion (e.g., 5% dextrose, half-normal saline) should be administered.
- *Hypophosphatemia, hypokalemia, and hypomagnesemia*: These electrolyte disturbances are commonly encountered in the ALF. Frequent monitoring of electrolytes with prompt repletion is needed to avoid associated complications.
- *Inadequate nutrition*: As with other ICU patients, early initiation of enteral nutrition is preferred over parenteral nutrition in patients with ALF.[40]

MANAGEMENT GUIDELINES

Acetaminophen

Acetaminophen toxicity is by far the most common cause of ALF in the United States, accounting for over 50% of all cases in the United States.[1,3,5] A detailed patient history is essential to diagnosing a deliberate or accidental overdose, especially given the multitude of both prescription and nonprescription medications that include acetaminophen. Acetaminophen-related hepatotoxicity is a dose-related adverse event; while ingestion of >10 to 15 g over a period of 24 hours is typically needed to induce ALF, concurrent disease or individual variations in hepatic metabolism may allow significant damage from ingestion of only 3 to 4 g.[41–43]

In toxic acetaminophen ingestions, aminotransferase levels are characteristically elevated several hundred-fold above normal values, with a peak in the rise of aminotransferases typically occurring 48 to 72 hours following ingestion. Use of the Rumack-Matthew acetaminophen nomogram can assist in prognosticating the risk of ALF in patients with less severe aminotransferase abnormalities.[3,43] The nomogram plots the serum concentration of acetaminophen against last known ingestion time in

TABLE 25.4 King's College Criteria for Assessment of Liver Failure Prognosis

Acetaminophen-Related ALF	Non-Acetaminophen-Related ALF
• pH < 7.30, or All three of the following: • INR > 6.5 (PT > 100 s), creatinine > 3.4 mg/dL, and grade 3–4 hepatic encephalopathy	• INR > 6.5 (PT >100 s), or Any three of the following: • Age < 10 or age > 40 • Non-A, non-B hepatitis, drug-induced, or indeterminate etiology • >7 d of jaundice prior to encephalopathy • INR > 3.5 (PT > 50 s) • Bilirubin > 17.6 mg/dL

From O'Grady JG, Alexander GJM, Hayllar KM, et al. Early indicators of prognosis in fulminant hepatic failure. *Gastroenterology*. 1989;97:439–455. Patients meeting the criteria are identified has having a poor prognosis.

an attempt to prognosticate hepatotoxicity and guide administration of therapy with *N*-acetylcysteine (NAC). Recently, acetaminophen–protein adducts, which have a longer half-life than acetaminophen, have been proposed as a means of identifying the cause of ALF in patients presenting without an identifiable etiology or undetectable acetaminophen levels.[43,44] A recent study evaluated sera from 110 subjects with indeterminate ALF enrolled in the Acute Liver Failure Study Group.[43] The sera of these patients, along with 199 positive controls of sera from patients with known acetaminophen-related ALF, were evaluated for acetaminophen–cysteine adducts. Over 94.5% of controls demonstrated levels of adducts that confirmed acetaminophen toxicity; 18% of the indeterminate cases tested positive, which confirmed previous reports citing the high prevalence of unrecognized acetaminophen toxicity among patients with indeterminate liver failure.[43]

If ingestion occurs within 3 to 4 hours, administration of activated charcoal at a dose of 1 g/kg orally may be of some benefit,[45] however, NAC therapy remains the most beneficial intervention.[46,47] One of the original studies evaluating the benefit of NAC in the treatment of acetaminophen-related ALF described the outcomes of 2,540 acetaminophen-toxic patients treated with oral NAC.[47] Patients treated with oral NAC had significantly lower rates of hepatotoxicity and significantly reduced mortality; patients treated within 8 hours of last ingestion had better outcomes that those who were treated at later intervals. NAC can be administered orally or intravenously; however, the intravenous route is preferred given the lower risk of aspiration. The dosing regimen for both oral and intravenous NAC is presented in Table 25.2.

Nonacetaminophen Drug/Toxins

Given the multitude of potentially hepatotoxic prescription and nonprescription drugs, a thorough patient history is essential. Common culprits of mixed-etiology ALF include antibiotics, antifungals, antituberculosis medications, sulfa-containing drugs, and psychiatric and neurologic medications including antiepileptics. In addition to pharmaceutical agents, nutritional and herbal supplements need to be carefully evaluated for potential hepatotoxicity. Early identification and removal of the offending agent, along with supportive care, are the mainstay of therapy in these cases.[48,49]

While NAC therapy has demonstrated greatest utility in patients with acetaminophen toxicity, it may also benefit patients with non–acetaminophen-related ALF.[50] In a prospective, double-blinded trial of 173 ALF patients without evidence of acetaminophen toxicity, a 72-hour infusion of NAC was compared to placebo (dextrose) in affecting survival outcomes. While there was no statistically significant difference in overall 3-week survival seen between the NAC group and the placebo group (70% vs. 66%), patients treated with NAC had significantly better 3-week transplant-free survival (40% vs. 27%).[50] The survival advantage was, however, limited to patients with less severe hepatic encephalopathy (grade 1 to 2).

Mushroom poisoning with *Amanita* toxin is a potentially lethal cause of ALF. As there is no serologic test to confirm exposure, a careful patient/observer history is essential, both to identify the fungus and to estimate the timing of exposure. Patients presenting with recent ingestion may benefit from nasogastric lavage to attempt removal of remaining toxic material. Silibinin and penicillin are accepted antidotes to mushroom poisoning. While greater evidence supports the efficacy of silibinin, this treatment is not available as a licensed drug in the United States.[51,52] However, when *Amanita* poisoning is suspected, an application to the Food and Drug Administration for emergency use of this agent is possible. Silibinin is administered orally or intravenously at a dose of 30 to 40 mg/kg/d for 3 to 4 days. Penicillin is an acceptable alternative in conjunction with NAC treatment. *Amanita* toxin is excreted in the bile, and the use of nasobiliary drainage or aspiration of the second portion of the duodenum (ideally performed in an ICU) may decrease enterohepatic circulation of the toxin.[53]

Viral Hepatitis

Acute viral hepatitis accounts for approximately 12% of all cases of ALF in the United States.[54,55] Several viruses have the potential to induce liver failure, each with its own unique risk factors, routes of transmission, diagnostic workup, and targeted treatment regimen. Acute hepatitis A infection (HAV) is a common ailment spread primarily through fecal–oral transmission. The diagnosis can be confirmed with positive anti-HAV IgM. Most HAV infections resolve with supportive therapy that includes fluid resuscitation and correction of electrolyte disturbances. However, any signs of hepatic dysfunction, including encephalopathy or coagulopathy, or signs of multiorgan dysfunction (e.g., renal failure or respiratory failure) require hospital admission and monitoring for development of ALF.

Acute hepatitis B infection (HBV) most often occurs as a result of intravenous drug use or sexual transmission. Acute HBV is confirmed by the presence of anti-HBV core Ab IgM. HBV antigen and HBV viral DNA may also be present. As in acute HAV, patient evaluation in acute HBV centers on assessment of organ function and identification of early symptoms of ALF that would require hospital admission. Following an initial diagnostic workup and appropriate resuscitation in the ED, inpatient treatment is generally guided by the hepatology service. First-line treatment for HBV consists of tenofovir 300 mg/d or entecavir 0.5 mg/d.[56] A randomized, placebo-controlled trial of patients with ALF secondary to HBV demonstrated that treatment with tenofovir was associated with significantly lower HBV viral DNA levels and improved liver disease severity, as measured by the model for end-stage liver disease (MELD) score and Child-Pugh score.[56] In addition, patients who were treated with tenofovir had significantly higher 3-month survival compared to patients who received placebo (57% vs. 15%).[56]

Acute hepatitis C infection (HCV) in the United States is associated primarily with intravenous drug use in the United States; the diagnosis can be confirmed with anti-HCV Ab and HCV viral RNA. ALF secondary to acute HCV is rare. The timing of antiviral therapy for acute HCV is unclear; current studies lack definitive data, and recently developed anti-HCV therapies have not undergone well-designed clinical trials. In patients with uncomplicated acute HCV, monitoring for spontaneous clearance of HCV RNA over a 12- to 16-week period is reasonable. The evidence for antiviral therapy in the setting of HCV-induced ALF is less clear, and general supportive measures should be instituted instead.[57]

Acute hepatitis D infection (HDV) is rare and occurs either as a coinfection with HBV or as superimposed acute HDV in a patient with chronic HBV. Diagnosis is conferred with the anti-HDV Ab and HDV antigen; supportive care occurs concurrently with treatment of the HBV infection. Acute hepatitis E infection (HEV) is transmitted via fecal–oral route, and diagnosis is confirmed with anti-HEV IgM and IgG. Treatment is supportive. With all the acute viral hepatitis infections, the initial evaluation and management in the ED focus on supportive care, including fluid and electrolyte resuscitation. The appropriate laboratory workup as previously described should be initiated; treatment is usually guided by the diagnosis and initiated by the inpatient team.

Autoimmune Hepatitis

Autoimmune hepatitis can present with a wide spectrum of clinical disease severity. While it is often diagnosed in the workup of mild elevations in aminotransferase levels and vague systemic complaints, autoimmune hepatitis can also present in a fulminant course with ALF.[58,59] A suspicion for autoimmune hepatitis is gleaned from a complete patient history of potential comorbid autoimmune disease states. Initial evaluation in the ED should include antinuclear antibodies (ANA), anti–smooth muscle antibodies (ASMA), and total serum IgG.

A thorough workup to exclude viral hepatitis and alcoholic liver disease further supports the diagnosis of autoimmune hepatitis. In patients with negative serologic markers in whom the suspicion for this etiology remains, liver biopsy may help to confirm diagnosis. Once ALF secondary to autoimmune hepatitis is confirmed, timely initiation of immunosuppressive therapy is critical and may reduce the progression of disease and need for liver transplantation.[59] The initial evaluation in the ED should focus on ensuring that the diagnostic workup is sufficient to evaluate for this process.

Wilson Disease

Wilson disease is a rare cause of liver disease; it is caused by a defect in copper metabolism and characterized by Kayser-Fleischer rings (secondary to copper deposition at the corneoscleral junction of the eye) and neuropsychiatric disease (secondary to copper deposition in the brain). Coombs-negative hemolytic anemia is a common associated presentation. A characteristic biochemical finding is an extremely low alkaline phosphatase (ALK) in the setting of marked elevation of aminotransferases. Early identification is important for prompt initiation of liver transplant evaluation. Initial diagnostic tests that can be sent from the ED include serum ceruloplasmin and routine liver function tests. Further diagnostic testing with urinary copper levels and liver biopsy with quantitative copper concentration in patients with high suspicion of Wilson disease can help confirm the diagnosis. The hepatology service should be consulted to evaluate the need for liver biopsy. In the setting of ALF, treatment in the ED should be supportive while the patient is rapidly evaluated for liver transplantation.[1]

Vascular Disease

"Shock liver" is a relatively common syndrome of ischemic hepatitis, characterized by acute elevation of aminotransferase levels. Precipitated by severe hypotension or hypovolemia resulting in hepatic ischemia, this syndrome is common in patients with underlying cardiac disease or severe congestive heart failure. Post–cardiac arrest patients who experience a period of hepatic hypoperfusion will often present with some degree of ischemic hepatitis. Correction of the underlying etiology and prompt initiation of cardiovascular support generally lead to recovery of hepatic function and usually prevent the need for liver transplant.[1,60] Overall prognosis, however, depends on the etiologies that precipitate the ischemic event.

Budd-Chiari syndrome is a rare disease precipitated by hepatic venous outflow obstruction resulting in hepatic decompensation and ALF.[60,61] Hepatic vein obstruction is generally secondary to thrombosis, and an underlying hypercoagulable state should be evaluated for. Acute abdominal pain, new-onset ascites, and marked hepatomegaly are often found on clinical presentation. The diagnostic approach relies on radiographic evidence of obstructive disease, preferably obtained through abdominal ultrasonography with Doppler flow. Contrast-enhanced computed tomography and magnetic resonance venography are alternative diagnostic tools, but should be used with caution, as many patients presenting with ALF have impaired renal function.

A diagnosis of Budd-Chiari requires a comprehensive workup to determine the underlying prothrombotic disorder. Potential culprits include hematologic disorders and hematologic malignancy (which, if diagnosed, may preclude the option of transplantation). Anticoagulation therapy and venous decompression (i.e., transjugular intrahepatic portosystemic shunting) have a role in the management of Budd-Chiari syndrome, but patients presenting with ALF as a result of this disease have a poorer prognosis, and liver transplantation may be the preferred therapeutic option.[60,61] In the ED, initial workup involves early resuscitation and the initiation of appropriate laboratory and radiographic diagnostic evaluation.

Pregnancy-Related Disease

Pregnancy-related liver disease is relatively rare, and the development of ALF in pregnant patients is even more rare.[62] Both acute fatty liver of pregnancy and HELLP syndrome (hemolysis, elevated liver enzymes, and low platelets) generally occur during the third trimester of pregnancy and can result in progressive hepatic injury leading to liver failure. In addition to abnormal aminotransferase levels and thrombocytopenia, jaundice, coagulopathy, preeclampsia, and hypoglycemia are often seen in the setting of pregnancy-related ALF. Treatment is supportive, and prompt delivery of the fetus in consultation with a high-risk obstetrics team generally results in rapid recovery of hepatic function.[62] While rare, liver transplantation may need to be considered in postpartum patients with persistent or progressively worsening hepatic dysfunction.

CONCLUSION

ALF is a significant cause of morbidity and mortality in the United States. Prompt recognition of ALF is important to initiate the appropriate diagnostic workup and to triage the patient toward an appropriate critical care setting. While the diagnostic evaluation and subsequent management of ALF are complicated, the emergency physician plays a key role in assessing the severity of disease and initiating the appropriate diagnostic testing required to confirm the underlying etiology. Severely ill ALF patients should always be admitted to an ICU or transferred to a liver transplantation center as needed.

LITERATURE TABLE

TRIAL	DESIGN	RESULT
Ostapowicz et al., *Ann Intern Med.* 2002[3]	Prospective cohort study of 17 tertiary care centers in the United States evaluating 308 consecutive patients with ALF	Acetaminophen-related toxicity (39%) and nonacetaminophen drug toxicity (13%) were the two leading causes of liver failure. Etiology of liver failure and hepatic encephalopathy coma grade at presentation correlated with survival outcome
Vaquero et al., *Liver Transpl.* 2005[13]	Retrospective cohort study of 332 patients with ALF and severe hepatic encephalopathy evaluating how outcomes are affected by use of ICP monitoring	Risk of intracranial hemorrhage decreased with ICP monitoring. Patients listed for liver transplantation with ICP monitoring appeared to be treated more aggressively to optimize ICP compared to patients without ICP monitoring
Cook et al., *N Engl J Med.* 1998[29]	Multicenter, randomized, placebo-controlled trial comparing sucralfate with H_2-receptor antagonist (ranitidine) for the prevention of upper gastrointestinal bleeding in 1,200 patients who required mechanical ventilation	Significantly lower risk of upper gastrointestinal bleeding was observed in the ranitidine-treated group compared to patients treated with sucralfate (RR, 0.44; 95% CI, 0.21–0.92, $p = 0.02$)
Rolando et al., *Hepatology.* 1993[32]	Prospective, randomized clinical trial comparing prophylactic antimicrobial therapy vs. supportive care in ALF patients without signs of infection	Patients treated with empiric antimicrobial therapy had lower rates of infection, but no significant difference in overall survival compared to patients who received standard supportive care
O'Grady et al., *Gastroenterology.* 1989[37]	Retrospective cohort study evaluating the prognostic predictors of mortality in 588 patients with ALF	Established King's College criteria for assessment of ALF prognosis (Table 25.2)
Keays et al., *BMJ.* 1991[46]	Prospective open-label, placebo-controlled trial evaluating the efficacy of IV *N*-acetylcysteine in patients with acetaminophen-related ALF	Higher overall survival among patients treated with *N*-acetylcysteine (48% vs. 20%, $p = 0.037$). Lower rates of cerebral edema and hypotension requiring inotropic among patients treated with *N*-acetylcysteine
Lee et al., *Gastroenterology.* 2009[50]	Prospective double-blinded, placebo-controlled trial evaluating the efficacy of IV *N*-acetylcysteine in patients with non–acetaminophen-related ALF	Higher transplant-free survival among patients treated with IV *N*-acetylcysteine (40% vs. 27%, $p = 0.04$). Benefits of therapy limited to patients with milder encephalopathy (grades 1–2)
Garg et al., *Hepatology.* 2011[56]	Prospective double-blinded, placebo-controlled trial evaluating the efficacy of tenofovir in patients with acute-on-chronic liver failure secondary to spontaneous reactivation of hepatitis B	Higher 3-mo survival among patients treated with tenofovir (57% vs. 15%, $p = 0.03$). More significant improvements in Child score, MELD score, and greater reduction in HBV DNA levels

CI, confidence interval; RR, relative risk.

REFERENCES

1. Lee WM, Stravitz RT, Larson AM. Introduction to the revised American Association for the Study of Liver Diseases Position Paper on acute liver failure 2011. *Hepatology*. 2012;55(3):965–967.
2. Lee WM, Squires RH Jr., Nyberg SL, et al. Acute liver failure: summary of a workshop. *Hepatology.* 2008;47:1401–1415.
3. Ostapowicz GA, Fontana RJ, Schiodt FV, et al. Results of a prospective study of acute liver failure at 17 tertiary care centers in the United States. *Ann Intern Med.* 2002;137:947–954.
4. Stravitz RT, Kramer DJ. Management of acute liver failure. *Nat Rev Gastroenterol Hepatol.* 2009;6:542–553.
5. Larson AM, Polson J, Fontana RJ, et al.; for the Acute Liver Failure Study Group. Acetaminophen-induced acute liver failure: results of a United States multicenter, prospective study. *Hepatology.* 2005;42:1364–1372.

6. Strauss G, Hansen BA, Knudsen GM, et al. Hyperventilation restores cerebral blood flow autoregulation in patients with acute liver failure. *J Hepatol.* 1998;28:199–203.
7. Ede RJ, Gimson AE, Bihari D, et al. Controlled hyperventilation in the prevention of cerebral oedema in fulminant hepatic failure. *J Hepatol.* 1986;2:43–51.
8. Stravitz RT, Kramer AH, Davern T, et al.; for the Acute Liver Failure Study Group. Intensive care of patients with acute liver failure: recommendations of the U.S. Acute Liver Failure Study Group. *Crit Care Med.* 2007;35:2498–2508.
9. Frontera JA, Kalb T. Neurological management of fulminant hepatic failure. *Neurocrit Care.* 2011;14:318–327.
10. Vaquero J, Chung C, Cahill ME, et al. Pathogenesis of hepatic encephalopathy in acute liver failure. *Semin Liver Dis.* 2003;23:259–269.
11. Bernal W, Hall C, Karvellas CJ, et al. Arterial ammonia and clinical risk factors for encephalopathy and intracranial hypertension in acute liver failure. *Hepatology.* 2007;46:1844–1852.
12. Munoz SJ. Difficult management problems in fulminant hepatic failure. *Semin Liver Dis.* 1993;13:395–413.
13. Vaquero J, Fontana RJ, Larson AM, et al. Complications and use of intracranial pressure monitoring in patients with acute liver failure and severe encephalopathy. *Liver Transpl.* 2005;11:1581–1589.
14. Munoz SJ, Robinson M, Northrup B, et al. Elevated intracranial pressure and computed tomography of the brain in fulminant hepatocellular failure. *Hepatology.* 1991;13:209–212.
15. Lidofsky SD, Bass NM, Prager MC, et al. Intracranial pressure monitoring and liver transplantation for fulminant hepatic failure. *Hepatology.* 1992;16:1–7.
16. Larsen FS, Hansen BA, Ejlersen E, et al. Cerebral blood flow, oxygen metabolism and transcranial Doppler sonography during high-volume plasmapheresis in fulminant hepatic failure. *Eur J Gastroenterol Hepatol.* 1996;8:261–265.
17. Canalese J, Gimson AES, Davis C, et al. Controlled trial of dexamethasone and mannitol for the cerebral oedema of fulminant hepatic failure. *Gut.* 1982;23:625–629.
18. Murphy N, Auzinger G, Bernal W, et al. The effect of hypertonic sodium chloride on intracranial pressure in patients with acute liver failure. *Hepatology.* 2002;39:464–470.
19. Stravitz RT, Larsen FS. Therapeutic hypothermia for acute liver failure. *Crit Care Med.* 2009;37:S258–S264.
20. Jalan R, Damink SWMO, Deutz NE, et al. Moderate hypothermia prevents cerebral hyperemia and increase in intracranial pressure in patients undergoing liver transplantation for acute liver failure. *Transplantation.* 2003;75:2034–2039.
21. Jalan R, Olde Damink SW, Deutz NE, et al. Moderate hypothermia in patients with acute liver failure and uncontrolled intracranial hypertension. *Gastroenterology.* 2004;127:1338–1346.
22. Forbes A, Alexander GJ, O'Grady JG, et al. Thiopental infusion in the treatment of intracranial hypertension complicating fulminant hepatic failure. *Hepatology.* 1989;10:306–310.
23. Wijdicks EF, Nyberg SL. Propofol to control intracranial pressure in fulminant hepatic failure. *Transplant Proc.* 2002;34:1220–1222.
24. Clemmesen JO, Larsen FS, Kondrup J, et al. Cerebral herniation in patients with acute liver failure is correlated with arterial ammonia concentration. *Hepatology.* 1999;29:648–653.
25. Alba L, Hay JE, Angulo P, et al. Lactulose therapy in acute liver failure. *J Hepatol.* 2002;36:33A.
26. Bass NM, Mullen KD, Sanyal A, et al. Rifaximin treatment in hepatic encephalopathy. *N Engl J Med.* 2010;362:1071.
27. Stravitz RT, Lisman T, Luketic VA, et al. Minimal effects of acute liver injury/acute liver failure on hemostasis as assessed by thromboelastography. *J Hepatol.* 2012;56:129–136.
28. Shami VM, Caldwell SH, Hespenheide EE, et al. Recombinant activated factor VII for coagulopathy in fulminant hepatic failure compared with conventional therapy. *Liver Transpl.* 2003;9:138–143.
29. Cook D, Guyatt G, Marshall J, et al. A comparison of sucralfate and ranitidine for the prevention of upper gastrointestinal bleeding in patients requiring mechanical ventilation: Canadian Critical Care Trials Group. *N Engl J Med.* 1998;338:791–797.
30. Ring-Larsen H, Palazzo U. Renal failure in fulminant hepatic failure and terminal cirrhosis: a comparison between incidence, types, and prognosis. *Gut.* 1981;22:585–591.
31. Davenport A, Will EJ, Davidson AM. Improved cardiovascular stability during continuous modes of renal replacement therapy in critically ill patients with acute hepatic and renal failure. *Crit Care Med.* 1993;21:328–338.
32. Rolando N, Harvey F, Brahm J, et al. Prospective study of bacterial infection in acute liver failure: an analysis of fifty patients. *Hepatology.* 1990;11:49–53.
33. Rolando N, Gimson A, Wade J, et al. Prospective controlled trial of selective parenteral and enteral antimicrobial regimen in fulminant liver failure. *Hepatology.* 1993;17:196–201.

34. Vaquero J, Polson J, Chung C, et al. Infection and the progression of encephalopathy in acute liver failure. *Gastroenterology.* 2003;125:755–764.
35. Rolando N, Harvey F, Brahm J, et al. Fungal infection: a common, unrecognized complication of acute liver failure. *J Hepatol.* 1991;12:1–9.
36. Rolando N, Wade J, Davalos M, et al. The systemic inflammatory response syndrome in acute liver failure. *Hepatology.* 2000;32:734–739.
37. O'Grady JG, Alexander GJM, Hayllar KM, et al. Early indicators of prognosis in fulminant hepatic failure. *Gastroenterology.* 1989;97:439–455.
38. Shakil AO, Kramer D, Mazariegos GV, et al. Acute liver failure: clinical features, outcome analysis, and applicability of prognostic criteria. *Liver Transpl.* 2000;6(2):163–169.
39. Anand AC, Nightingale P, Neuberger JM. Early indicators of prognosis in fulminant hepatic failure: an assessment of the King's criteria. *J Hepatol.* 1997;26(1):62–68.
40. Casaer MP, Mesotten D, Hermans G, et al. Early versus late parenteral nutrition in critically ill adults. *N Engl J Med.* 2011;365(6):506–517.
41. Schiodt FV, Rochling FJ, Casey DL, et al. Acetaminophen toxicity in an urban county hospital. *N Engl J Med.* 1997;337:1112–1117.
42. Zimmerman JH, Maddrey WC. Acetaminophen (paracetamol) hepatotoxicity with regular intake of alcohol: analysis of instances of therapeutic misadventure. *Hepatology.* 1995;22:767–773.
43. Khandelwal N, James LP, Sanders C, et al.; Acute Liver Failure Study Group. Unrecognized acetaminophen toxicity as a cause of indeterminate acute liver failure. *Hepatology.* 2011;53:567–576.
44. Heard KJ, Green JL, James LP, et al. Acetaminophen-cysteine adducts during therapeutic dosing and following overdose. *BMC Gastroenterol.* 2011;11:20–29.
45. Sato RL, Wong JJ, Sumida SM, et al. Efficacy of superactivated charcoal administration late (3 hours) after acetaminophen overdose. *Am J Emerg Med.* 2003;21:189–191.
46. Keays R, Harrison PM, Wendon JA, et al. A prospective controlled trial of intravenous N-acetylcysteine in paracetamol-induced fulminant hepatic failure. *BMJ.* 1991;303:1024–1029.
47. Smilkstein MJ, Knapp GL, Kulig KW, et al. Efficacy of oral N-acetylcysteine in the treatment of acetaminophen overdose. *N Engl J Med.* 1988;319:1557–1562.
48. Lee WM. Drug-induced hepatotoxicity. *N Engl J Med.* 2003;349:474–485.
49. Reuben A, Koch DG, Lee WM; and the Acute Liver Failure Study Group. Drug-induced acute liver failure: results of a U.S. multicenter, prospective study. *Hepatology.* 2010;52:2065–2076.
50. Lee WM, Hynan LS, Rossaro L, et al. Intravenous N-acetylcysteine improves transplant-free survival in early stage non-acetaminophen acute liver failure. *Gastroenterology.* 2009;137:856–864.
51. Hruby K, Csomos G, Fuhrmann M, et al. Chemotherapy of *Amanita phalloides* poisoning with intravenous silibinin. *Hum Toxicol.* 1983;2:183–195.
52. Schneider SM, Michelson EA, Vanscoy G. Failure of N-acetylcysteine to reduce alpha amanitin toxicity. *J Appl Toxicol.* 1992;12:141–142.
53. Klein AS, Hart J, Brems JJ, et al. Amanita poisoning: treatment and the role of liver transplantation. *Am J Med.* 1989;86:187–193.
54. Schiodt FV, Davern TA, Shakil O, et al. Viral hepatitis-related acute liver failure. *Am J Gastroenterol.* 2003;98:448–453.
55. Lok AS, McMahon BJ. Chronic hepatitis B: update 2009. *Hepatology.* 2009;50:661–662.
56. Garg H, Sarin SK, Kumar M, et al. Tenofovir improves the outcome in patients with spontaneous reactivation of hepatitis B presenting as acute-on-chronic liver failure. *Hepatology.* 2011;53:774–780.
57. Ghany MG, Strader DB, Thomas DL, et al.; American Association for the Study of Liver Diseases. Diagnosis, management, and treatment of hepatitis C: an update. *Hepatology.* 2009;49:1335–1374.
58. Czaja AJ, Freese DK; American Association for the Study of Liver Disease. Diagnosis and treatment of autoimmune hepatitis. *Hepatology.* 2002;36:479–497.
59. Stravitz RT, Lefkowitch JH, Fontana RJ, et al. Autoimmune acute liver failure: proposed clinical and histological criteria. *Hepatology.* 2011;53:517–526.
60. DeLeve LD, Valle D-C, Garcia-Tsao G. AASLD practice guidelines: vascular disorders of the liver. *Hepatology.* 2009;49:1729–1764.
61. Ringe B, Lang H, Oldhafer K-J, et al. Which is the best surgery for Budd-Chiari syndrome: venous decompression or liver transplantation? A single center experience with 50 patients. *Hepatology.* 1995;21:1337–1344.
62. Hay JE. Liver disease in pregnancy: a review. *Hepatology.* 2008;47:1067–1076.

26

Pancreatitis

Susan Y. Quan and Walter G. Park

BACKGROUND

The pancreas is approximately 6 to 10 inches long, is located directly behind the stomach, and has distinct endocrine and exocrine functions. The endocrine portion of the pancreas is composed of islets of Langerhans cells that constitute about 2% of the organ. These cells produce and secrete hormones including insulin, glucagon, and somatostatin. The exocrine portion of the pancreas is composed of acinar cells (80% of the organ) and ductal cells (18% of the organ). Acinar cells produce digestive enzymes that are sequestered until physiologic impulses stimulate their release into the pancreatic ductal system where they are transported to the small intestine. The digestive enzymes are enzymatically inert until activated in the small intestine by various peptides. Disruption of this physiologic process, by any of a variety of etiologies, is the basis for our current understanding of acute and chronic pancreatitis. This chapter primarily focuses on acute pancreatitis, which is more commonly seen in emergency care. Pertinent aspects of chronic pancreatitis are also addressed.

ACUTE PANCREATITIS

The incidence of acute pancreatitis is estimated to be as high as 38 per 100,000 patients and accounts for more than 220,000 hospital admissions in the United States annually.[1] Most cases are clinically mild and self-limited; a minority of cases are severe and are associated with critical illness, prolonged hospitalization, infection, organ failure, and death.

Acute pancreatitis occurs from premature activation of digestive enzymes within the pancreatic parenchyma leading to an autodigestive and inflammatory process. Evolution into a life-threatening systemic process begins when acinar cell injury leads to expression of endothelial adhesion molecules that further potentiates the inflammatory response. Local microcirculatory failure and ischemia–reperfusion injury ensue, with some patients developing systemic complications such as systemic inflammatory response syndrome (SIRS), acute respiratory distress syndrome, and multiorgan failure.

The most common causes of acute pancreatitis are gallstones and excess alcohol ingestion. These account for about 45% and 35% of cases, respectively.[2,3] Hypertriglyceridemia accounts for up to 5% of cases. Other causes include hypercalcemia, autoimmune diseases, infections, medications, trauma, and complications after endoscopic retrograde cholangiopancreatography (ERCP) (Table 26.1). Controversial etiologies include

TABLE 26.1 Causes of Acute Pancreatitis

Obstructive	Gallstones, tumors, altered ductal anatomy
Toxins/drugs	Alcohol, insecticides, drugs
Metabolic	Hypertriglyceridemia, hypercalcemia
Infections	Mumps, Coxsackie, HBV, cytomegalovirus, zoster
Vascular	Vasculitis, emboli
Trauma	Spine dissection of pancreas
Iatrogenesis	ERCP, surgery
Hereditary	PRSS1, CFTR, SPINK1 mutations
Idiopathic	

pancreatic divisum and sphincter of Oddi dysfunction. Idiopathic pancreatitis occurs in up to 20% of patients, and by definition, the cause is not established by history, physical exam, routine laboratory tests, or imaging.

History and Physical Exam

The typical presentation includes a constant (as opposed to waxing and waning) upper abdominal pain located primarily in the epigastric area with radiation to the back. The onset of pain is rapid and typically reaches maximum intensity within 10 to 20 minutes. Pain that lasts only a few hours is unlikely to be pancreatitis. About 90% of patients will also complain of nausea and vomiting.

Mild pancreatitis may involve minimal abdominal tenderness without guarding. In severe disease, abdominal tenderness can be elicited with superficial palpation. Abdominal distention and reduced bowel sounds can occur secondary to ileus. Extravasation of hemorrhagic pancreatic exudate can lead to ecchymosis in one or both flanks (Turner sign) or the periumbilical regions (Cullen sign). Severe disease should be suspected with abnormal vital signs that can include fever, tachycardia, tachypnea, and hypotension. These signs represent a transition from localized retroperitoneal inflammation to one of systemic inflammation. Pleural effusions and mental status changes are also hallmarks of severe disease. The presence of jaundice may suggest an underlying alcoholism or choledocholithiasis.

Diagnostic Evaluation

Acute pancreatitis is diagnosed when two of the following three criteria are met: (1) characteristic abdominal pain, (2) serum amylase or lipase greater than three times the upper limit of normal, and, if needed, (3) radiologic imaging consistent with the diagnosis.[4] Amylase and lipase are the most frequently used serum-based tests for pancreatitis. The most common source of amylase is not the pancreas, but salivary glands. In contrast, 90% of lipase is made from the pancreas, making it a more specific marker. Amylase rises within 6 to 24 hours of acute pancreatitis and peaks in 48 hours, normalizing in 3 to 7 days. Lipase has a longer half-life than amylase, with levels increasing within 4 to 8 hours, peaking at 24 hours, and falling over 8 to 14 days.[5] The degree of elevation is not a marker of disease severity, and mild elevation of these serum markers—less than three times the upper limit of normal—is not specific for pancreatitis.

The use of computed tomography (CT) or magnetic resonance imaging (MRI) should only be considered when the first two diagnostic criteria are not met and (1) the pretest probability for pancreatitis remains high or (2) there is a high pretest probability for another abdominal process. Otherwise, CT and MRI have no role and may exacerbate renal injury from use of intravenous contrast.[6] Such imaging can be considered 7 days later should the diagnosis remain uncertain or to assess disease severity and identify complications related to severe pancreatitis. Following clinical and laboratory parameters allows adequate initial assessment of disease severity. For patients with an established history of chronic pancreatitis or recent acute pancreatitis, imaging may be considered as part of the initial emergency department assessment for specific treatable complications of pancreatitis including, but not limited to, enlarging pseudocysts, arterial pseudoaneurysms, and/or new common bile stones.

Differential Diagnosis

The differential diagnosis includes biliary colic, acute cholecystitis, acute cholangitis, biliary dyskinesia, peptic ulcer disease, dyspepsia, acute mesenteric ischemic, and bowel obstruction. Nongastrointestinal disorders, including acute myocardial infarction, aortic dissection, pulmonary embolism, acute spinal disorders, and renal calculi, should also be considered.

Complications

The majority of cases (80% to 90%) of pancreatitis are mild and self-limiting; 10% of cases, however, develop severe disease, defined as the presence of significant fluid collections, infectious complications including abscess formation, infected necrosis, and/or extrapancreatic organ failure. These patients typically exhibit SIRS or sepsis physiology.

Fluid collections around the pancreas affect over half of patients. Most will resolve, but for those that persist, a fibrogenic anti-inflammatory response will lead to containment of these fluid collections, resulting in the formation of a pseudocyst. A pancreatic pseudocyst is a fluid collection that persists beyond 4 weeks. Other complications include infections (arising from pancreatic necrosis or within pseudocysts), thrombosis (splenic, superior mesenteric, and/or portal vein), arterial pseudoaneurysms, and gastrointestinal bleeding. The mortality rate for patients with severe pancreatitis is approximately 30%. Death within the first 2 weeks of illness is usually due to multiorgan failure. Death after 2 weeks typically stems from infection.

Management Guidelines

Once a diagnosis of acute pancreatitis is made, a risk stratification calculation should be performed. Clinical risk scoring systems, such as Ranson's and APACHE II, have traditionally been used. However, both are cumbersome and require 48 hours before a meaningful interpretation can be made. The Bedside Index for Severity in Acute Pancreatitis (BISAP) score is a newer validated scoring system that requires five data points of collection in the emergency room.[7,8] This includes a blood urea nitrogen (BUN) >25 mg/dL,

TABLE 26.2 Risk Stratification Scoring System for Severity of Acute Pancreatitis

Bedside **I**ndex for **S**everity of **A**cute **P**ancreatitis (BISAP)
- **B**UN >25 mg/dL - **I**mpaired mental status - **S**IRS - **A**ge >60 - **P**leural effusion
Estimated in-hospital mortality by number of positive criteria met: 0 = 0.1%, 1 = 0.5%, 2 = 2.0%, 3 = 5.3%, 4 = 12.7%, 5 = 22.5%.[7] ICU consultation should be considered for anyone with three or more met criteria.

impaired mental status, SIRS, age >60, and the presence of a pleural effusion (Table 26.2). The presence of three or more features at admission is associated with a 7- to 12-fold increase in organ failure. Such patients should be managed in the intensive care unit.

Initial treatment is primarily supportive and includes adequate fluid resuscitation, pain control, and bowel rest.[6] Fluid resuscitation is necessary to replace intravascular volume depletion that occurs from third-space losses. The amount of fluid should be calibrated to a urine output of 0.5 mL/kg/h. Initial resuscitation may begin with 1 to 2 L of normal saline within the first several hours of presentation. Early resuscitation appears to be clinically important in reducing downstream complications. In a large retrospective analysis of 434 patients with acute pancreatitis, early compared to late resuscitation was associated with less organ failure at 72 hours (5% vs. 10%), a lower rate of admission to the intensive care unit (6% vs. 17%), and a reduced length of hospital stay (8 vs. 11 days).[9] After early initial bolus treatment of intravenous fluids, maintenance fluids should be titrated (up or down) to urine output. In severe disease, aggressive fluid resuscitation is important to maintain adequate vascular volume in the setting of SIRS or sepsis physiology.[9] Pain can be controlled with intravenous short-acting narcotic pain medications. Nausea and vomiting can be controlled with antiemetic medications as needed.

Acute pancreatitis is a hypercatabolic state, and initiating nutrition at 48 hours from onset is important. In mild disease, patients can be started on an oral diet. For those with severe disease, enteral nutrition by nasojejunal feeding should be started. The current rationale for nasojejunal feeding is that bypassing the duodenum minimizes pancreatic stimulation. Enteral nutrition is superior to parenteral nutrition because it carries a lower risk for infectious complications and mortality.[10]

Documented infections associated with pancreatitis require prompt treatment with carbapenem-based antibiotics to ensure optimal penetration. Antibiotic prophylaxis, however, is not indicated.[11,12] Endoscopy is indicated for removing common bile duct stones and secondary cholangitis, and cholecystectomy should be planned during hospitalization for those with gallstone-related pancreatitis identified by right upper quadrant ultrasound.

For some patients who have no clinical or laboratory evidence to suggest severe disease (i.e., a BISAP score of 0, no other laboratory abnormalities), discharge from the emergency room can be considered. These patients should also have mild enough pain to be managed with PO pain medications, have the ability to consume liquids without vomiting, and be considered adequately competent and compliant to follow instructions to return to the emergency room for worsening signs and/or symptoms.

CHRONIC PANCREATITIS

Chronic pancreatitis is characterized by chronic inflammation and fibrosis with destruction of exocrine and endocrine cells. The incidence is estimated to be 6 cases per 100,000 people, and it affects about 0.04% of the US population.[13] Although relatively uncommon, chronic pancreatitis is associated with a high level of morbidity and use of health care resources.[14] In the United States, the most common cause is chronic alcohol use, accounting for nearly 70% of cases. It should be noted that only approximately 10% of heavy drinkers ever develop pancreatitis, suggesting an underlying genetic predisposition. In up to 20% of patients, the etiology is idiopathic. The remaining 10% are due to obstructive causes, metabolic derangements, autoimmune diseases, and hereditary disorders.[15]

History and Physical Exam

The most common complaint is chronic abdominal pain that is often associated with nausea and vomiting. In advanced disease, maldigestion develops from pancreatic exocrine insufficiency and presents as chronic diarrhea with unintentional weight loss. The stool is particularly odorous as most is maldigested fat (also known as steatorrhea). Other late findings include symptoms and signs of diabetes.

Mild abdominal tenderness with palpation may be elicited. An abdominal mass may represent a pseudocyst or splenomegaly. Splenomegaly occurs in the setting of splenic vein thrombosis—the result of chronic (or recurrent acute) pancreatic inflammation in proximity to the splenic vein—and can compromise venous return from the spleen with subsequent splenic engorgement and splenomegaly. As alcohol is the most common precipitating cause of pancreatitis, findings of liver disease including hepatomegaly, jaundice, ascites, and hepatic encephalopathy may also be observed. Because of chronic maldigestion of fat, these patients can be fat-soluble vitamin deficient (vitamins A, D, E, and K), and this can lead to related examination findings including peripheral neuropathy, fatigue, and signs of easy bruising and bleeding.

Diagnostic Evaluation

Diagnosis begins with an assessment of clinical symptoms, signs, and risk factors for chronic pancreatitis. CT can be used for diagnosing structural features associated with advanced disease including calcifications, atrophy, pancreatic duct dilation, and/or strictures. CT may also show common complications including pseudocysts, splenic vein thromboses, and inflammatory masses. Magnetic resonance cholangiopancreatography may be used to evaluate the pancreatic and biliary ducts without requiring ERCP. Endoscopic ultrasound currently offers the most sensitive imaging for diagnosis of chronic pancreatitis. Functional diagnostic tests for chronic pancreatitis include stool elastase, 72-hour fecal fat, and secretin stimulation test.

Differential Diagnosis

The differential diagnosis for chronic pancreatitis includes gastritis, dyspepsia, small bowel bacterial overgrowth, intestinal obstruction, neoplasms, mesenteric ischemia, biliary obstruction, celiac disease, inflammatory bowel disease, Zollinger-Ellison syndrome, and functional gut disorders such as irritable bowel syndrome.

Complications

Chronic pancreatitis is associated with a nearly fourfold increase in standardized mortality rate, which stems mostly from continued alcohol and tobacco abuse.[16] Common complications include pseudocysts, gastrointestinal bleeding, bile duct obstruction, duodenal obstruction, and pancreatic fistula formation.

Management Guidelines

Management of suspected chronic pancreatitis with increased abdominal pain should include prompt and adequate analgesia (often requiring narcotic pain medications) and assessment of hydration and nutrition status.[17] Evaluation of acute complications of chronic pancreatitis and nonpancreatic abdominal emergencies should also occur though with judicious use of imaging. When imaging suggests a main duct stricture, pancreatic ductal stones, and/or pseudocysts, an endoscopic intervention may be appropriate. During evaluation, patients should be counseled on smoking and alcohol cessation when applicable. Management of chronic pain and nutritional deficiencies from long-standing pancreatitis is primarily an outpatient issue, and a referral to gastroenterology is indicated.

CONCLUSION

Pancreatitis is a common presenting illness in the emergency department. Initial management centers on early aggressive fluid resuscitation, pain control, and bowel rest. All patients should be risk-stratified using a validated scoring system such as the BISAP to help direct appropriate disposition, including intensive care services. Advanced imaging, although generally not required, should be used when there is diagnostic uncertainty or when there is concern for the presence of associated complications including pseudocysts, arterial pseudoaneurysms, or common bile stones.

LITERATURE TABLE

TRIAL	DESIGN	RESULT
Prognosis		
Wu et al., *Gut.* 2008[7]	Data collected from between 17,992 and 18,256 cases of acute pancreatitis for the purpose of developing and validating a new clinical scoring system for prediction of in-hospital mortality	BISAP was derived from five variables identified for prediction of in-hospital mortality: BUN >25 mg/dL, impaired mental status, SIRS, age >60, and presence of pleural effusion. BISAP was validated against APACHE II with BISAP AUC 0.82 (95% CI 0.79–0.84) vs. APACHE II AUC of 0.83 (95% CI 0.80–0.85)
Papachristou et al., *Am J Gastroenterol.* 2010[8]	Comparison of BISAP, Ranson's, APACHE II, and CTSI scores in 185 patients with acute pancreatitis	The prognostic accuracy of BISAP is similar to those of the other scoring systems. Predictive accuracy rates as measured by AUCs for BISAP, Ranson's, APACHE II, and CTSI in predicting SAP were 0.81 (CI 0.74–0.87), 0.94 (CI 0.89–0.97), 0.78 (CI 0.71–0.84), and 0.84 (CI 0.76–0.89), respectively

LITERATURE TABLE (*Continued*)

TRIAL	DESIGN	RESULT
Supportive Care		
Warndorf et al., *Clin Gastroenterol Hepatol. 2011*[9]	Retrospective study of 434 patients with acute pancreatitis stratified by early vs. late resuscitation, which were defined as ≥ one third vs. ≤one third of total 72-h fluid volume within 24 h of presentation	Early as compared to late resuscitation was associated with decreased SIRS at 24 h (15% vs. 32%, $p = 0.001$), 48 h (14% vs. 33%, $p = 0.001$), and 72 h (10% vs. 23%, $p = 0.01$), as well as reduced organ failure at 72 h (5% vs. 10%, $p < 0.05$), a lower rate of admission to the intensive care unit (6% vs. 17%, $p < 0.001$), and a reduced length of hospital stay (8 vs. 11 d, $p = 0.01$)
Nutrition		
Petrov et al., *Arch Surg. 2008*[10]	Meta-analysis of five randomized controlled trial (RCTs) comparing enteral and parenteral nutrition in patients with predicted severe acute pancreatitis	Enteral feeding reduced the risk of infectious complications (RR 0.47; 95% CI 0.28–0.77; $p < 0.001$), pancreatic infections (RR 0.48; 95% CI 0.26–0.91; $p = 0.02$), and mortality (RR 0.32; 95% CI 0.11–0.98; $p = 0.03$). The risk reduction for organ failure was not statistically significant (RR 0.67; 95% CI 0.30–1.52; $p = 0.34$)
Use of Antibiotics		
Bai et al., *Am J Gastroenterol. 2008*[11]	Meta-analysis of seven RCTs involving 467 patients with acute necrotizing pancreatitis comparing prophylactic intravenous antibiotics with placebo or no treatment	Prophylactic antibiotics did not significantly reduce rates of infected pancreatic necrosis (antibiotics 17.8%, controls 22.9%; RR 0.81; 95% CI 0.54–1.22) and mortality (antibiotics 9.3%, controls 15.2%; RR 0.70; 95% CI 0.42–1.17) in patients with acute necrotizing pancreatitis
Jafri et al., *Am J Surg. 2009*[12]	Meta-analysis of eight RCTs pooling 502 patients with severe acute pancreatitis randomized to prophylactic antibiotics or placebo	No protective effect of antibiotic treatment with respect to mortality (RR 0.76; 95% CI 0.49–1.16), infected necrosis (RR 0.79; 95% CI 0.56–1.11), or surgical intervention (RR 0.88; 95% CI 0.65–1.20)

REFERENCES

1. DeFrances CJ, Hall MJ. 2005 National hospital discharge survey. *Adv Data.* 2007;385:1–19.
2. Sanders G, Kingsnorth AN. Gallstones. *BMJ.* 2007;335:295–299.
3. Steinberg W, Tenner S. Acute pancreatitis. *N Engl J Med.* 1994;330:1198–1210.
4. Banks PA, Freeman ML, Practice Parameters Committee of the American College of Gastroenterology. Practice Guidelines in Acute Pancreatitis. *Am J Gastroenterol.* 2006;101:2379–2400.
5. Yadav D, Agarwal N, Pitchumoni CS. A critical evaluation of laboratory tests in acute pancreatitis. *Am J Gastroenterol.* 2002;97:1309–1318.
6. Forsmark CE, Baillie J. AGA institute technical review on acute pancreatitis. *Gastroenterology.* 2007:132;2022–2044.
7. Wu BU, Johannes RS, Sun X, et al. The early prediction of mortality in acute pancreatitis: a large population-based study. *Gut.* 2008;57:1698–1703.
8. Papachristou GI, Muddana V, Yadav D, et al. Comparison of BISAP, Ranson's, APACHE-II, and CTSI scores in predicting organ failure, complications, and mortality in acute pancreatitis. *Am J Gastroenterol.* 2010;105:435–441.
9. Warndorf MD, Kurtzman JT, Bartel MJ, et al. Early fluid resuscitation reduces morbidity among patients with acute pancreatic. *Clin Gastroenterol Hepatol.* 2011;9:705–709.
10. Petrov MS, van Santvoort HC, Besselink MG, et al. Enteral nutrition and the risk of mortality and infectious complications in patients with severe acute pancreatitis: a meta-analysis of randomized trials. *Arch Surg.* 2008;143:1111–1117.
11. Bai Y, Gao J, Zou DW, et al. Prophylactic antibiotics cannot reduce infected pancreatic necrosis and mortality in acute necrotizing pancreatitis: evidence from a meta-analysis of randomized controlled trials. *Am J Gastroenterol.* 2008;103:104–110.
12. Jafri NS, Mahid SS, Idstein SR, et al. Antibiotic prophylaxis is not protective in severe acute pancreatitis: a systematic review and meta-analysis. *Am J Surg.* 2009;197:806–813.

13. Jupp J, Fine D, Johnson CD. The epidemiology and socioeconomic impact of chronic pancreatitis. *Best Pract Res Clin Gastroenterol.* 2010;24:219–231.
14. Gardner TB, Kennedy AT, Gelrud A. Chronic pancreatitis and its effect on employment and health care experience: results of a prospective America multicenter study. *Pancreas.* 2010;39:498–501.
15. Braganza JM, Lee SH, McCloy RF, et al. Chronic pancreatitis. *Lancet* 2011;377:1184–1197.
16. Lowenfels AB, Maisonneuve P, Cavallini G. Prognosis of chronic pancreatitis: an international multicenter study. International Pancreatitis Study Group. *Am J Gastroenterol.* 1994;89:1467–1471.
17. Warshaw AL, Banks PA, Fernández-Del Castillo C. AGA technical review: treatment of pain in chronic pancreatitis. *Gastroenterology.* 1998;115:765–776.

27

Acute Leukemia

Martina Trinkaus

ACUTE LEUKEMIA

Acute leukemia is a neoplasm of the stem cell that results in rapid accumulation of immature myeloid or lymphoid precursors (functionally inert blasts) in the bone marrow. This accumulation—termed clonal proliferation—takes up space necessary for normal hematopoiesis and causes secondary cytopenias. Leukemia affects different cell lineages in hematopoietic tissues, including erythrocytes, lymphocytes, granulocytes, and megakaryocytes. Individual leukemic cells do not divide more rapidly than do normal cells; however, at any given moment, a larger proportion of leukemic cells are dividing. Chemotherapy exploits this increase in mitotic activity.[1] When acute leukemia is left untreated, the accumulation of 10^{12} cells is fatal.[1]

The World Health Organization of Tumors of Hematopoietic and Lymphoid Tissues[2] defines leukemia as the presence of >20% blasts in the bone marrow or peripheral blood. Leukemia is subdivided by lineage into myeloid and lymphoid disease. Acute myeloid leukemia (AML) is further subdivided into seven subgroups based on cytology, cytogenetics, and molecular analysis. In some instances, a diagnosis of AML is made regardless of the percentage of bone marrow blasts—specifically, in patients with translocations between chromosome 8 and 21 or 15 and 17, inversions in chromosome 16, or myeloid sarcomas. Acute lymphoblastic leukemia (ALL) is divided into three major subgroups based on differences in treatment and prognosis: (1) precursor B- or T-cell ALL, with further subdivision made based on recurring molecular–cytogenetic abnormalities; (2) Burkitt leukemia/lymphoma; and (3) biphenotypic acute leukemia. Approximately 90% of leukemia is of myeloid origin, with 10% of lymphoid origin.[2]

The annual incidence of AML is 3.5 per 100,000; an estimated 13,780 patients were diagnosed in the United States in 2012.[3] AML incidence increases with age, with a median age at diagnosis of 67 according to the National Cancer Institute's Surveillance, Epidemiology, and End Results data.[4] If untreated, AML is fatal and confers an average overall survival of <20 weeks from time of diagnosis.[5] Six thousand and fifty total adult and pediatric cases of ALL were reported in the United States in 2012.[3] ALL is five times more likely to occur in the pediatric population than in the adult population; it represents 30% of all childhood neoplasms, with the average age at diagnosis of 13 years.[6] With improved treatment strategies, the 5-year overall cure rate for ALL in the pediatric population is over 80%; the lower adult cure rate of 30% to 40% is largely due to age-related adverse molecular features and resistance to therapy.[7]

RISK FACTORS

Most cases of acute leukemia are idiopathic. Known risks include exposure to cytotoxic chemotherapy (particularly topoisomerase II inhibitors and alkylating agents[8]), pesticides, benzene, or radiation.[9] Genetic disorders, including trisomy 21 and inherited bone marrow failure syndromes, have also been associated with AML.[2]

In AML, specific prognostic features guide patient survival prediction. These include, but are not limited to, advanced age[10]; previous exposure to chemotherapy[11]; cytogenetic features that stratify disease prognosis into favorable, intermediate, and poor[12]; and evolution of a patient's AML from a previous myelodysplasia or myeloproliferative neoplasms.[13] Molecular screening investigations can further delineate prognosis, with poor outcomes conferred by the presence of the FMS-like tyrosine kinase 3 (FLT-3)[14] and c-kit mutation,[15] and favorable outcomes conferred by nucleophosmin-1 and CEBPA[16] mutations. In ALL, as well, several prognostic factors—including age, leukocyte count, and molecular genotypes such as BCR-ABL1 positivity—guide selection of treatment.[17]

PATIENT HISTORY

Patient symptoms vary according to clinical stage of acute leukemia. Symptoms on initial presentation are due to increased tumor cell mass, factors released by leukemic cells, pancytopenia, and immunologic reactions. Later symptoms are usually secondary to either the sequelae of pancytopenia or complications of chemotherapy. Table 27.1 reviews pertinent clinical history and physical exam findings of patients on their initial presentation.

DIAGNOSTIC EVALUATION

The following studies are recommended for any patient in whom acute leukemia is suspected:

- CBC with peripheral blood film, ideally read by an experienced hematologist or pathologist. In cases of elevated blast counts, a manual platelet count should be made, as automated cell counters may erroneously count fragments of blast cells as platelets.
- Coagulation studies: PT, PTT, fibrinogen, D-dimer. Consider fibrinogen assays for the bleeding patient.
- Complete biochemical profile to assess for tumor lysis syndrome (TLS) (electrolytes, creatinine, calcium, magnesium, phosphate, uric acid, LDH).
- Liver enzymes and liver function tests.
- Viral serologies: HSV, VZV, CMV, hepatitis B and C.
- Screening for syphilis.
- In the case of fever: blood cultures, urine cultures, imaging guided by physical exam, and a complete evaluation of oral hygiene, as the mouth is a common site of bacterial seeding.
- In the case of significant CNS signs or symptoms: CT head or MRI imaging to rule out intracerebral hemorrhage, leptomeningeal disease, or extramedullary disease.

TABLE 27.1 Pertinent Findings on Patient History and Physical Exam with First Presentation

Etiology	Clinical Presentation
Tumor Mass	Hyperviscosity syndrome (retinopathy, CNS symptoms, hypoxia, priapism) Gingival hypertrophy (prominent in monocytic AML) Hepatosplenomegaly Arthralgias (chief complaint in 14% of pediatric leukemias) Tender sternum or long bones Leukemia cutis (prominent in monocytic AML) Chloroma Hypermetabolism leading to fevers, sweats, weight loss Tumor lysis syndrome Neurologic complaints (CNS involvement is rare; <3% of cases) Factitious laboratory results from increased metabolism of leukemic cells with: low PaO_2, increased K^+, and hypoglycemia Testicular recurrence of ALL
Factors released by leukemic cells	APL granules induce DIC Muramidase causes increased creatinine and hypokalemia
Pancytopenia	
Anemia	Pallor, fatigue With hemoglobin <5 g/dL, orbital bruits and retinal hemorrhage
Neutropenia	Patients with ANC < 500/μL are predisposed to infections • Line infections • Typhlitis • Oral mucositis, candidiasis, herpes
Thrombocytopenia	Bleeding with platelets <10,000/μL—worse if febrile or on antiplatelet drugs Petechiae, mucocutaneous bleeding (epistaxis, gingival bleeding, menorrhagia) Periosteal bleeding is a presenting cause in the pediatric population
Immunologic	TRALI (transfusion-related associated lung injury) TA-GvHD (transfusion-associated graft versus host disease)

From Miller KB, Daoust PR. Clinical manifestations of acute myeloid leukemia. In: Hoffman R, ed. *Hematology Basic Principles and Practice.* 4th ed. Philadelphia, PA: Elsevier Inc.; 2005:1071–1095; Zuckerman T, Ganzel C, Tallman M, et al. How I treat hematologic emergencies in adults with acute leukemia. *Blood.* 2012;120(10):1993–2002.[18]

Hematology should be consulted and will typically coordinate the following studies:

- CT chest to rule out occult fungal infection
- Bone marrow aspirate and biopsy
- Cardiac function test: if anthracyclines are to be administered, MUGA nuclear imaging is preferred over echocardiography because of cardiotoxicity risk
- Lumbar puncture: provided the patient is not coagulopathic and neuroimaging is normal
- HLA typing of the patient and siblings if considering a transplant

Acute leukemia is diagnosed when the peripheral blood or bone marrow contains >20% blasts. Typically, a bone marrow aspirate and biopsy are performed to distinguish AML from ALL and high-grade myelodysplasia. Alternative diagnoses to consider in the setting of severe pancytopenia include aplastic anemia, severe B_{12} deficiency, or drug-induced aplasia. In patients with blasts on peripheral blood film, myeloproliferative neoplasms, including myelofibrosis and chronic myelogenous leukemia, should also be considered.

EMERGENCIES IN ACUTE LEUKEMIA

Hyperleukocytosis

Hyperleukocytosis is a medical emergency that typically occurs when the blast count exceeds >100,000/μL. It is seen in 5% to 18% of acute leukemia, predominantly in disease of monocytic origin.[19] Increased blood viscosity in hyperleukocytosis is due to the rigidity of the myeloblast membrane and an up-regulation of blast adhesion molecules; this results in blasts occluding circulatory flow, with subsequent tissue hypoxia, tissue infiltration, and secondary hemorrhage. Hyperviscosity does not occur with similar elevations of neutrophils (as seen in severe infections) or lymphocytes (as seen in chronic lymphocytic leukemia). Presenting symptoms of hyperleukocytosis are variable and include respiratory distress and hypoxia, as well as seizure, confusion, abdominal pain, angina, priapism, and visual complaints. Funduscopy should be performed to rule out papilledema, dilated vessels, or hemorrhage. In circumstances of respiratory decline, it is important to consider alternative explanations, including pneumonia, volume overload, or transfusion complications, including transfusion-related acute lung injury (TRALI).[18] Pulse oximetry provides a more reliable measure of oxygen saturation for the hypoxic patient than does PaO_2, which can be misleadingly low because of blast consumption of oxygen in the collection medium.[20] If untreated, hyperleukocytosis confers a mortality of 20%; its most serious complications are pulmonary failure and intracerebral hemorrhage.[21]

Treatment of symptomatic hyperleukocytosis (aka leukostasis) varies by institution; a standard approach includes the prompt initiation of hydroxyurea for cytoreduction, with 2 to 5 g/day administered in divided doses.[22] The role of leukapheresis is controversial; most studies that support its impact on survival are retrospective in design.[23–25] Finally, caution should be used in transfusing patients with hyperleukocytosis because of the risk of worsening blood viscosity and aggravating symptoms.

Anemia and Transfusions

No clinical trials have evaluated a specific transfusion trigger in patients with acute leukemia. In critically ill patients without cardiac disease, the TRICC trial demonstrated that a restrictive transfusion strategy in the ICU (maintaining hemoglobin values between 7 and 9 g/dL) resulted in a reduced mortality rate at 30 days.[26] For the leukemic patient, this approach has unclear benefit; thus, the threshold for transfusion is often practice dependent, with most providers transfusing for hemoglobin levels below 8 g/dL or as warranted given clinical symptoms.[27] Caution must be exercised when transfusing patients with high blast counts in order to avoid inciting hyperviscosity. There is no role for erythropoietin-stimulating agents.

All transfused blood products should be irradiated and leukocyte depleted to minimize risk of transfusion-associated graft versus host disease (TA-GvHD). If a patient's cytomegalovirus (CMV) status is unknown, exclusively CMV-negative blood products should be used. TA-GvHD is seen in immunocompromised hosts, particularly those undergoing AML therapy, post–allogeneic stem cell transplantation, or post–purine analogue therapy. One to four weeks post-transfusion patients with TA-GvHD can present with severe cytopenias and with associated fever, hepatitis, rash, and/or diarrhea. A bone marrow biopsy will reveal complete bone marrow aplasia. No treatment is effective, and the mortality rate of TA-GvHD exceeds 95%; it is therefore imperative to provide these patients with blood products that are leukoreduced and irradiated.[18]

Coagulopathy and Thrombocytopenia

All patients with leukemia should be transfused to maintain a platelet count of >10,000/μL in cases of nonactive bleeding or >50,000/μL in cases of active bleeding.[28–31] All coagulopathic derangements should be promptly reversed with frozen plasma or cryoprecipitate. Note that patients with APL, acute monocytic, or myelomonocytic leukemias are at highest risk of disseminated intravascular coagulation (DIC); in these populations, coagulation screening should be performed at least twice daily to ensure proper replacement of platelets, coagulation factors, and fibrinogen.[32] As with red blood cell support, all products should be irradiated and CMV negative if a patient's CMV status is unknown.

Acute Promyelocytic Leukemia

APL is a subset of AML defined by the translocation of the retinoic acid receptor t(15;17); "PML;RAR-alpha" in 95% of patients. APL constitutes 10% of AML cases in the United States with most patients being diagnosed between ages 30 and 40. APL has an overall cure rate of 80% to 90%.[33] Unlike other leukemias, APL poses an increased risk of fatal hemorrhage from DIC or primary hyperfibrinolysis and has a pretreatment mortality rate reported to be as high as 10% to 17%.[34] Because of this, any patient suspected of having leukemia (i.e., blasts reported on their CBC differential) and a concurrent unexplained coagulopathy should be evaluated promptly for APL. A pathologist or hematologist should assess blast morphology; if APL is confirmed, treatment with all-trans retinoic acid (ATRA), which allows for differentiation of APL promyelocytes and restoration of coagulation, should begin immediately.[35] Doses in children may be modified because of the potential risk of pseudotumor cerebri.[36] Concurrent anthracycline chemotherapy is typically reserved for the patient with high-risk disease (i.e., WBC > 10,000/μL) to minimize the risk of leukocytosis, differentiation syndrome (previously ATRA syndrome), and provocation of coagulopathy—all potential risks when ATRA is administered alone.[37] Because of the risk of fatal coagulopathy and hyperfibrinolysis, the platelet count, PT, PTT, and fibrinogen should be closely monitored. There are scant data on the optimal trigger for platelet and plasma product infusion, but consensus opinion targets a platelet count of 30,000 to 50,000/μL and a fibrinogen level of >150 mg/dL.[32] Coagulopathy of APL can last for up to 20 days despite ATRA therapy.[38] Placement of a central venous catheter, or invasive procedures such as lumbar punctures, should be avoided until the coagulopathy has been corrected. The hypogranular variant, a subset of APL, is conversely associated with thrombosis in up to 5% of patients[39] and is typically managed with intravenous heparin and replacement of factor product as needed.

Tumor Lysis Syndrome

TLS occurs secondary to rapid cell death, as cellular products are excreted into the circulation. This can be observed at the time of leukemia diagnosis or after initiation of chemotherapy. TLS manifests biochemically either as increased uric acid that may result in concomitant renal failure or as marked hyperphosphatemia that leads to hypocalcemia and its attendant complications. Patients at highest risk of TLS include those with a high tumor burden, preexisting renal failure, chemotherapy-sensitive tumors with rapid lysis, and inadequate TLS prophylaxis (i.e., allopurinol).[40] Uncontrolled TLS places patients at risk of renal failure, cardiac dysrhythmias, seizure, and death.[41]

TLS-Associated Uric Acid Nephropathy

Treatment of TLS focuses on intravenous hydration to attain a urine output of 80 to 100 mL/m.[2,18] Patients often require more than 4 L of daily intravenous fluid support to achieve this goal.[40] Alkalinization of the urine is no longer a routine treatment, as it has the potential to cause calcium phosphate or xanthine precipitation in renal tubules.[42] Reduction in uric acid is typically achieved with renal-dosed allopurinol, a xanthine oxidase inhibitor, which generally lowers uric acid within 1 to 3 days. Rasburicase, a recombinant version of urate oxidase, has proven effective in cases of renal failure or allopurinol intolerance.[43] Allopurinol affects only further production of uric acid; rasburicase, by contrast, can convert existing uric acid to allantoin, which is 5 to 10 times more soluble than is uric acid. The standard rasburicase dose is 0.2 mg/kg IV infusion over 30 minutes. The use of rasburicase is contraindicated in patients with G6PD deficiency because of the increased risk of oxidative hemolysis and methemoglobinemia.[44]

TLS-Associated Metabolic Derangements

Hyperphosphatemia results in a secondary hypocalcemia. Because calcium phosphate crystals can precipitate in the renal parenchyma and lead to renal failure, calcium correction should occur only in the context of clinically severe hypocalcemia (e.g., tetany, seizures) or after correction of hyperphosphatemia.[37] If hypercalcemia is seen in the context of acute leukemia, the diagnoses of plasma cell leukemia or adult T-cell leukemia/lymphoma should be considered as alternate explanations.

Hyperkalemia should be monitored closely in the first 24 to 48 hours after initiation of chemotherapy (including hydroxyurea), when the risk of TLS is greatest. Potassium levels, however, should be interpreted with caution. Monocytic leukemias may present with significant hypokalemia due to renal tubular damage from high levels of muramidase (the lysozyme released by monoblasts), with subsequent renal potassium wasting.[1] In addition, measurement of potassium in samples can be factitious: when blast counts are significantly high, metabolically active blasts up-take residual potassium from the serum if a blood specimen is left standing too long, resulting in pseudohypokalemia. Conversely, pseudohyperkalemia may be caused by in vitro blast lysis in the sample. Treatment of hyperkalemia should, therefore, be pursued only after obtaining a heparinized—and more truly diagnostic—plasma potassium level.[45]

Infection

Because chemotherapy destroys dividing cells, it disproportionately affects those cells with increased mitotic potential—in the bone marrow, oral cavity, GI endothelium, nails, and hair. Chemotherapy patients thus carry a high risk of oral mucositis and ulcers, as well as enteric ulcers, resulting in multiple potential portals of entry for gram-negative bacteria.

In patients with febrile neutropenia, treatment should include broad-spectrum antibiotics including coverage for *Pseudomonas aeruginosa*. Antifungal therapy is recommended in the event of persistent fevers despite 4 to 7 days of antibiotic coverage or in the event of persistent neutropenia. Treatment should continue throughout the duration of neutropenia until the ANC exceeds 500 cells/mm^3.[46] The use of granulocyte colony–stimulating factor varies by institution; most literature specific to AML shows no impact or mixed results on duration of neutropenia, infection, antibiotic usage, hospitalization, or survival.[47,48]

The selection of antiviral, antifungal, and antibiotic prophylaxis is dependent on local levels of invasive fungal infections and is often institution specific. The Infectious Disease Society of America recommends acyclovir prophylaxis for HSV seropositive patients.[46] Posaconazole has been shown to significantly reduce fungal infections when compared to fluconazole and is increasingly being used in the leukemia population.[49]

Neutropenic Colitis/Typhylitis

Neutropenic colitis—termed typhlitis when only the ileocecal region is involved—typically occurs 10 to 14 days after initiation of chemotherapy and presents with neutropenia, right lower quadrant pain, and fever.[50] Patients may also have nausea, vomiting, and watery or bloody diarrhea. The pathogenesis of neutropenic colitis is likely related to chemotherapy-induced mucosal injury with bowel wall edema, ulceration, and secondary intestinal microbial infiltration. The cecum is particularly vulnerable because of its low blood supply. Patients will typically demonstrate gram-negative bacteremia; up to 15% of patients will have fungus isolated in blood or bowel specimens.[51] Along with testing and empirical treatment for *Clostridium difficile*, patients must undergo immediate CT imaging. Bowel wall thickening of >4 mm on imaging is consistent with the diagnosis.[52] Despite aggressive treatment with broad-spectrum antibiotics, bowel rest, volume resuscitation, and surgical consultation, the mortality rate of typhlitis is as high as 30% to 50%.[53]

Differentiation Syndrome of APL

Differentiation syndrome occurs in 15% to 25% of patients receiving ATRA or arsenic trioxide (ATO) and can occur between 2 and 47 days after exposure to ATRA or ATO.[54,55] Patients will present with cough, fever, or dyspnea and often with a white blood cell count of >10,000/μL. This cardiopulmonary syndrome is often mistaken for pulmonary edema or pneumonia. Patients must be monitored closely for hypoxia, pulmonary infiltrates, and pleural or pericardial effusions. In cases of APL with a WBC > 10,000/μL, or suspicion for differentiation syndrome, patients should receive dexamethasone 10 mg bid for 3 to 5 days with a taper over 2 weeks.[35] Treatment should commence immediately, rather than after abnormalities appear on chest radiograph. If differentiation syndrome is suspected, ATRA and/or ATO should be discontinued and not resumed until resolution of all signs and symptoms; steroid therapy should be given concurrently.[37]

Cytoreductive Therapy in AML and ALL

AML treatment is divided into two stages: induction chemotherapy to induce a remission and subsequent consolidation (postremission) therapy. The goal of therapy is to achieve a complete response (CR)—defined as having <5% of blasts in a repeat bone marrow aspirate with a count of 200 nucleated cells. To date, the cure rates for AML excluding APL are low; only 40% of young adults and 10% of elderly patients will be cured.[37] Treatment varies by institution; in patients who are transplant eligible (age <60 with good performance status), every effort should be made to enroll the patient into a clinical trial.

Induction chemotherapy has not changed considerably for over 30 years: it consists of anthracyclines such as daunorubicin (60 to 90 mg/m^2 × 3 days) and cytarabine (100 to 200 mg/m^2 continuous infusion × 7 days),[56] known as the "3+7" strategy. Studies have shown that varying the doses of chemotherapy can improve CR rates but can also precipitate considerable toxicity. Patients who achieve remission proceed to consolidation (postremission therapy), typically with high-dose cytarabine. Treatment regimens, including subsequent hematopoietic stem cell transplant, are dependent on prognostic factors and type of leukemia.

Treatment of ALL includes multiagent chemotherapies divided into induction, consolidation, and maintenance phases of treatment, with all patients receiving CNS prophylaxis. Treatment will always include anthracyclines, vincristine, L-asparaginase, cyclophosphamide, methotrexate, cytrarabine, mercaptopurine, and corticosteroids, all of which can result in significant toxicity. Imatinib is added in those patients who are Philadelphia chromosome positive. Due to their significant exposure to steroids, patients must also receive prophylaxis for *Pneumocystis jiroveci* and are often placed on viral and fungal prophylaxis as well. Impressively, with this regimen, most children with ALL included in clinical trials have 5-year survival rates that approach 85%; in adults, only a 30% 5-year survival rate is achieved.[57] Table 27.2 highlights the major toxicities associated with the standard chemotherapies used for AML, APL, and ALL.

TABLE 27.2 Selected Chemotherapy Drug Complications

Chemotherapy	Complication	Onset
Daunorubicin/idarubicin	Myelosuppression (risk of mucositis, colitis)	Onset: 7 d; nadir: 10–14 d; recovery: 21–28 d
	Cardiotoxicity	Delayed (dose related); weeks to years
	Alopecia	2–3 wk
High-dose cytarabine	Myelosuppression (risk of mucositis, colitis)	Onset: 7 d; nadir 10–14 d; recovery: 21–28 d
	Iritis (must ensure steroid eye drops provided to each eye q4h until 24 h after last dose)	Immediate
	Cytarabine Syndrome (flu, rash, myalgia, bone pain)	6–12 h post iv infusion (symptom resolution in 24 h)
	Cerebellar toxicity (nystagmus, dysmetria, gait disturbance); neuroimaging will be normal	Days 3 to 8 posttherapy (symptoms may take up to 10 d to resolve)
ATRA (all-trans retinoic acid)	Differentiation syndrome Hyperleukocytosis	2–49 d onset Immediate
ATO	Differentiation syndrome	2–49 d onset
Vincristine	Jaw pain Constipation/paralytic ileus, neuropathy	Days to weeks Days to weeks
L-Asparaginase	Hypersensitivity reactions Pancreatitis Thrombosis	Immediate days to weeks days to weeks
Allopurinol	Maculopapular rash to vasculitis	Immediate/early

From Cancer Drug Manual. British Columbia Cancer Agency. Available at: www.bccancer.bc.ca. Accessed January 29, 2013.[58]

CONCLUSION

Acute leukemia is a medical emergency. It should be suspected in any patient who presents with blasts on white cell differential or peripheral blood film or with undiagnosed pancytopenia. Patients should be referred promptly to the hematology service and screened for life-threatening complications (see Table 27.1). In patients with high blast counts (>100,000 μL) or symptoms of hyperleukostasis, a monitored setting should be considered, as these cases require aggressive cytoreduction with chemotherapy. Electrolytes must be also monitored with any leukemic diagnosis to rule out TLS and secondary renal failure. Coagulopathies should be aggressively reversed to avoid secondary hemorrhage, and platelet counts >10,000/μL should be maintained. Transfused blood products should be irradiated and, if possible, CMV negative. It should be emphasized that patients with acute leukemia are immunocompromised, and a full pan-culture with initiation of broad-spectrum antibiotics must be started in the event of fever or infection.

LITERATURE TABLE

TRIAL	DESIGN	RESULT
Selected Trials in the Acute Management of Acute Leukemia		
Cortes et al., *JCO.* 2010[43]	Phase III open-label trial with three treatment arms: (1) single-agent rasburicase (0.20 mg/kg/d IV infusion over 30 min) for 5 d, (2) sequential treatment with rasburicase (0.20 mg/kg/d IV infusion over 30 min) from days 1 through 3 followed by oral allopurinol (300 mg/d orally) from days 3 through 5 (overlap on day 3), and (3) single-agent oral allopurinol (300 mg/d orally) for 5 d	Primary end point was control of plasma uric acid levels (≤7.5 mg/dL) during days 3 to 7 post-AML treatment. Control achieved in 87%, 78%, and 66% for arms (1), (2), and (3), respectively ($p = 0.001$)
Wheatley et al., *BJH.* 2009[48]	RCT comparing GCSF support to placebo in AML patients postinduction chemotherapy	GCSF offered no benefit on overall survival, number, severity of duration of infection
Cornely et al., *NEJM.* 2007[49]	Blinded RCT in AML- or MDS-treated patients randomized to posaconazole (arm A) or fluconazole or itraconazole (arm B) for fungal prophylaxis	Posaconazole prevented invasive fungal infections more effectively than did either fluconazole or itraconazole (absolute reduction in the posaconazole group, −6%; 95% confidence interval, −9.7 to −2.5%; $p < 0.001$) and improved overall survival ($p = 0.04$)

REFERENCES

1. Miller KB, Daoust PR. Clinical manifestations of acute myeloid leukemia. In: Hoffman R, ed. *Hematology Basic Principles and Practice.* 4th ed. Philadelphia, PA: Elsevier Inc; 2005:1071–1095.
2. Swerdlow SH, Campo E, Harris NL, et al. (eds). *World Health Organization Classification of Tumours of Haematopoietic and Lymphoid Tissues.* Lyon, France: IARC Press; 2008.
3. Siegel R, Naishadham D, Jemal A. Cancer statistics, 2012. *CA Cancer J Clin.* 2012;62:10–29.
4. National Cancer Institute. *SEER Stat Fact Sheets: Acute Myeloid Leukemia.* Bethesda, MD: National Cancer Institute; 2011.
5. Deschler B, Lübbert M. Acute myeloid leukemia: epidemiology and etiology. *Cancer.* 2006;107(9): 2099–2107.
6. Jabbour EJ, Faderl S, Kantarjian HM. Adult acute lymphoblastic leukemia. *Mayo Clin Proc.* 2005;80: 1517–1527.
7. Annino L, Vegna ML, Camera A, et al. Treatment of adult acute lymphoblastic leukemia (ALL): long-term follow-up of the GIMEMA ALL 0288 randomized study. *Blood.* 2002;99:863–871.

8. Leone G, Pagano L, Ben-Yehuda D, et al. Therapy-related leukemia and myelodysplasia: susceptibility and incidence. *Haematologica.* 2007;92:1389–1398.
9. Smith M, Barnett M, Bassan R, et al. Adult acute myeloid leukemia. *Crit Rev Oncol Hematol.* 2004;50: 197–222.
10. Appelbaum FR, Gundacker H, Head DR, et al. Age and acute myeloid leukemia. *Blood.* 2006;107(5): 3481–3485.
11. Kayser S, Dohner K, Krauter J, et al. The impact of therapy-related acute myeloid leukemia (AML) on outcome in 2858 adult patients with newly diagnosed AML. *Blood.* 2011;117:2137–2145.
12. Byrd JC, Mrózek K, Dodge RK, et al. Pretreatment cytogenetic abnormalities are predictive of induction success, cumulative incidence of relapse, and overall survival in adult patients with de novo acute myeloid leukemia: results from Cancer and Leukemia Group B (CALGB 8461). *Blood.* 2002;100(13):4325–4336.
13. Kantarjian H, O Brien S, Cortes J, et al. Results of intensive chemotherapy in 998 patients age 65 years or older with acute myeloid leukemia or high-risk myelodysplastic syndrome: predictive prognostic models for outcome. *Cancer.* 2006;106(5):1090–1098.
14. Abu-Duhier FM, Goodeve AC, Wilson GA, et al. FLT3 internal tandem duplication mutations in adult acute myeloid leukemia defines a high-risk group. *Br J Haematol.* 2000;111(1):190–195.
15. Paschka P, Marcucci G, Ruppert AS, et al. Adverse prognostic significance of KIT mutations is adult acute myeloid leukemia with inv (16) and t (8:21): a Cancer and Leukemia Group B Study. *J Clin Oncol.* 2006;24(24):3904–3911.
16. Thiede C, Koch S, Creutzig E, et al. Prevalence and prognostic impact of NPM1 mutations in 1485 patients with AML. *Blood.* 2006;107(10):4011–4020.
17. Gokbuget N, Hoelzer D. Treatment of adult acute lymphoblastic leukemia. *Semin Hematol.* 2009;46: 64–75.
18. Zuckerman T, Ganzel C, Tallman M, et al. How I treat hematologic emergencies in adults with acute leukemia. *Blood.* 2012;120(10):1993–2002.
19. Porcu P, Cripe LD, Ng EW, et al. Hyperleukocytic leukemias and leukostasis: a review of pathophysiology, clinical presentation and management. *Leuk Lymphoma.* 2000;39:1–18.
20. Hess CE, Nichols AB, Hunt EB, et al. Peudohypoxemia secondary to leukemia and thrombocytosis. *N Engl J Med.* 1979;301(7):361–363.
21. Dutcher JP, Schiffer CA, Wiernik PH. Hyperleukocytosis in adult acute nonlymphocytic leukemia: impact on remission rate and duration, and survival. *J Clin Oncol.* 1987;5:1364–1372.
22. Grund FM, Armitage JO, Burns P. Hydroxyurea in the prevention of the effects of leukostasis in acute leukemia. *Arch Intern Med.* 1977;137(9):1246.
23. Bug G, Anargyrou K, Tonn T, et al. Impact of leukapheresis on early death rate in adult acute myeloid leukemia presenting with hyperleukocytosis. *Transfusion.* 2007;47(10):1843.
24. Giles FJ, Shen Y, Kantarjian HM, et al. Leukapheresis reduces early mortality in patients with acute myeloid leukemia with high white cell counts but does not improve long-term survival. *Leuk Lymphoma.* 2001;42(1–2):67.
25. De Santis CG, Oliverira de Oliveria LC, et al. Therapeutic leukapheresis in patients with leukostasis secondary to acute myelogenous leukemia. *J Clin Apher.* 2011;26:181–185.
26. Hebert PC, Wells G, Blajchman MA, et al. A multicenter, randomized, controlled clinical trial of transfusion requirements in critical care. Transfusion requirements in critical care investigators, Canadian Critical Care Trials Group. *N Engl J Med.* 1999;340(6):409–417.
27. Carson JL, Grossman BJ, Kleinman S, et al. Clinical Transfusion Medicine Committee of the AABB. Red blood cell transfusion: a clinical practice guideline from the AABB. *Ann Intern Med.* 2012;157(1):49.
28. Rebulla P, Finazzi G, Marangoni F, et al. The threshold for prophylactic platelet transfusions in adults with acute myeloid leukemia. Gruppo Italiano Malattie Ematologiche Maligne dell'Adulto. *N Engl J Med.* 1997;337(26):1870–1875.
29. Wandt H, Schaefer-Echart K, Wendelin K, et al. Therapeutic platelet transfusion versus routine prophylactic transfusion in patients with hematologic malignancies: an open-label, multicentre, randomised study. *Lancet.* 2012;380(9850):1309–1316.
30. Schiffer CA, Anderson KC, Bennett CL, et al. Platelet transfusion for patient with cancer: clinical practice guidelines of the American Society of Clinical Oncology. *J Clin Oncol.* 2001;19(5):1519.
31. Slichter SS, Kaufmann RM, McCullough J, et al. Dose of prophylactic platelet transfusions and prevention of hemorrhage. *N Engl J Med.* 2010;362;600–613.
32. Tallman MS, Brenner B, Serna Jde L, et al. Meeting report: acute promyelocytic leukemia associated coagulopathy, 21 January 2004, London, United Kingdom. *Leuk Res.* 2005;29(3):347–351.

33. Tallman MS, Nabhan C, Feusner JH, et al. Acute promyelocytic leukemia: evolving therapeutic strategies. *Blood.* 2002;99(3):759–767.
34. Jacomo RH, Melo RA, Souto FR, et al. Clinical features and outcomes of 134 Brazilians with acute promyelocytic leukemia who received ATRA and anthracyclines. *Haematologica.* 2007;92(10):1431–1432.
35. Sanz MA, Martin G, Gonzalez M, et al. Risk adapted treatment of acute promyelocytic leukemia with all-trans-retinoic acid and anthracycline monochemotherapy: a multicenter study by the PETHEMA group. *Blood.* 2004;103(4):1237–1243.
36. Testi AM, Biondi A, Lo Coco F, et al. GIMEMAAIEOPAIDA protocol for the treatment of newly diagnosed acute promyelocytic leukemia (APL) in children. *Blood.* 2005;106(2):447–453.
37. Tallman MS, Altman JK. How I treat acute promyelocytic leukemia. *Blood.* 2009;114(25):5126–5135.
38. Yanada M, Matsushita T, Asou N, et al. Severe hemorrhagic complications during remission induction therapy for acute promyelocytic leukemia: incidence, risk factors, and influence on outcome. *Eur J Haematol.* 2007;78(3):213–219.
39. Breccis M, Avvisati G, Latagliata R, et al. Occurrence of thrombotic events in acute promyelocytic leukemia correlates with consistent immunophenotypic and molecular features. *Leukemia.* 2007;21(1):79–83.
40. Abu-Alfa AK, Younes A. Tumor lysis syndrome and acute kidney injury: evaluation, prevention, and management. *Am J Kidney Dis.* 2010;55(5 suppl 3):S1–S13.
41. Cairo MD, Coiffier B, Reiter A, et al. Recommendations for the evaluation of risk and prophylaxis of tumor lysis syndrome in adults and children with malignant diseases: an expert TLS panel consensus. *Br J Haematol.* 2010;149(4):578–586.
42. Howard DC, Jones DP, Pui CH. The tumor lysis syndrome. *N Engl J Med.* 2011;364(19):1844–1854.
43. Cortes J, Moore JO, Maziarz ET, et al. Control of plasma uric acid in adults at risk of tumor lysis syndrome: efficacy and safety of rasburicase alone and rasburicase followed by allopurinol compared with allopurinol along: results of a multicenter phase III study. *J Clin Oncol.* 2010;28(27):4207–4213.
44. Yim BT, Sims-McCallum RP, Chong PH. Rasburicase for the treatment and prevention of hyperuricemia. *Ann Pharmacother.* 2003;37(7):1047–1054.
45. Adams PC, Woodhouse KW, Adela M, et al. Exaggerated hypokalaemia in acute myeloid leukaemia. *Br Med J (Clin Res Ed).* 1981;282(6269):1034.
46. Freifeld AG, Bow EJ, Sepkowitz KA, et al. Infectious Diseases Society of America. Clinical practice guideline for the use of antimicrobial agents in neutropenic patients with cancer: 2010 update by the infectious diseases society of america. *Clin Infect Dis.* 2011;52(4):e56.
47. Smith TJ, Khatcheressian J, Lyman GH, et al. 2005 update of recommendations for the use of white blood cell growth factors: an evidence-based clinical practice guideline. *J Clin Oncol.* 2006;24(19):3187–3205.
48. Wheatley K, Goldstone AH, Littlewood T, et al. Randomized placebo-controlled trial of granulocyte colony stimulating factor (G-CSF) as supportive care after induction chemotherapy in adult patients with acute myeloid leukemia: a study of the United Kingdom MRC Adult Leukaemia Working Party. *Br J Haematol.* 2009;146(1):54–63.
49. Cornely OA, Maetens J, Winston DJ, et al. Posoconazole vs. fluconazole or itraconazole prophylaxis in patients with neutropenia. *N Engl J Med.* 2007;356:348–359.
50. Wade DS, Nava HR, Douglass HO Jr. Neutropenic enterocolitis in adults: clinical diagnosis and treatment. *Cancer.* 1992;69(1):17–23.
51. Davila ML. Neutropenic enterocolitis: current issues in diagnosis and management. *Curr Infect Dis Rep.* 2007;9(2):116–120.
52. Gorschluter M, Mey U, Strehl J, et al. Neutropenic enterocolitis in adults: systematic analysis of evidence quality. *Eur J Haematol.* 2005;75(1):1–13.
53. Williams N, Scott AD. Neutropenic colitis: a continuing surgical challenge. *Br J Surg.* 1997;84(9): 1200–1205.
54. Tallman MD, Andersen JW, Schiffer CA, et al. Clinical description of 44 patients with acute promyelocytic leukemia who developed retinoic acid syndrome. *Blood.* 2000;95:90–95.
55. Sanz MA, Grimwade D, Tallman MS, et al. Management of acute promyelocytic leukemia: recommendations from an expert panel on behalf of the European Leukemia Net. *Blood.* 2009;113(9): 1875–1891.
56. Löwenberg B, Ossenkoppele GJ, van Putten W, et al. High-dose daunorubicin in older patients with acute myeloid leukemia. *N Engl J Med.* 2009;361:1235–1248.
57. Pui CH, Robison LL, Look AT. Acute lymphoblastic leukemia. *Lancet.* 2008;371:1030–1043.
58. Cancer Drug Manual. British Columbia Cancer Agency. Available at: www.bccancer.bc.ca. Accessed January 29, 2013.

28

Sickle Cell Disease

Richard Ward

BACKGROUND

Sickle cell disease (SCD) is one of the most common genetic disorders in North America, affecting an estimated 70,000 individuals. It results from a point mutation (valine for glutamate) at codon 6 of the beta-globin gene on chromosome 11. The most common genotype, HbSS (SCD-SS, sickle cell anemia), is due to mutation of both genes leading to the production of sickle hemoglobin (HbS) and no normal adult hemoglobin (HbA). HbSC and HbS/beta-thalassemia are two other commonly encountered genotypes of SCD.

Under physiologic stress, the HbS undergoes conformational change, creates polymers in the red blood cell (RBC), and deforms the cell to a sickle shape. This change has two consequences. First, it results in hemolysis of the RBC, which causes anemia and the release of free Hb into the circulation; this, in turn, produces a vasculopathy by triggering an abnormal increase in nitric oxide consumption and, by modulating arginine pathways, nitric oxide underproduction. Second, it results in vasoocclusion of microcirculatory organ beds and an ischemic–reperfusion pattern of injury.[1] It is this second consequence that produces bony pain, the most common clinical presentation of SCD.[2]

SCD is a lifelong, multisystem disorder with variable and intermittent severity. Many adult patients with SCD are not registered in a comprehensive care center and are therefore at risk of developing significant end-organ dysfunction over time. This inadequate access to care is made worse by the fact that hydroxyurea, the only U.S. FDA-approved disease-modifying treatment, is underutilized.[3]

DIAGNOSTIC EVALUATION

An acute sickle cell vasoocclusive episode or "crisis" (VOC) is a frequent complication of SCD and the most common reason these patients present to the emergency department (ED).[4] Patients typically present with limb, back, or chest pain caused by vasoocclusion in the bone marrow and resultant severe generalized bony pain.

Prompt clinical assessment and provision of rapid, adequate, and sustained analgesia are key to successful treatment. Clinical assessment should focus on the location of pain, severity of pain (using an objective pain scale such as the visual analogue scale), and duration of pain; precipitating factors (extremes of temperature, dehydration, infection, psychological distress, menstruation in females, excessive exercise); and home analgesic use. A systems-based patient history and physical exam should work to identify additional complications—related to SCD or to other general medical/surgical conditions—that may require specific treatment. Complications commonly associated with VOCs include infection (particularly respiratory tract), stroke, cholecystitis, sequestration syndrome (presenting with organomegaly), and, in males, priapism.

A detailed medical history can help identify SCD patients with severe sickle cell phenotype and should include the use of hydroxyurea, a history of multiple transfusions, previous exchange transfusion, prior acute chest syndrome (ACS), or intensive care unit admission. A thorough transfusion history will also assist the blood bank in sourcing safe units of blood, when required.

Laboratory and imaging testing rarely provide much assistance in the management algorithm of an uncomplicated VOC, with the exception of a complete blood count and reticulocyte count. The reticulocyte count is helpful in determining whether an unexpectedly severe anemia is due to marrow aplasia (usually viral in etiology) or simply brisk hemolysis. There is no indication for chest radiograph (CXR) in the absence of hypoxia or respiratory symptoms and signs. Routine biochemistry will usually confirm the hemolytic process and normal renal function. All SCD patients presenting with a fever, even if they otherwise appear well, should undergo a full septic screen, as they are predisposed to infection as a result of functional asplenia. In patients with new and unexplained hypoxia and an unremarkable CXR, a diagnosis of pulmonary embolism should be considered.[5]

MANAGEMENT OF AN UNCOMPLICATED PAIN EPISODE

The mainstay of the management of an acute, uncomplicated VOC is supportive care, including analgesia, hydration, and oxygenation.[6,7]

Analgesia

Rapid administration of adequate analgesia optimizes chances for patient discharge. Analgesia should be initiated within 30 minutes of presentation, with adequate pain control achieved ideally within 60 minutes.[8] Pain should be reassessed, and vital signs checked, on a frequent basis until pain is controlled. Patients with SCD usually have had previous exposure to opiate analgesia and often require higher doses of opiates to achieve analgesia when compared to opiate-naive patients. Despite a paucity of supporting clinical trials, multimodal analgesia is recommended, including combination of a nonsteroidal anti-inflammatory drug (NSAID) and acetaminophen with an opiate.[1,2,9] Consultation with a pain service may be helpful for patients with difficult-to-control pain (i.e., pain that cannot be controlled without inducing significant side effects or excessive sedation).

The route and formulation of analgesia depend on local institutional policies; there is little high-quality clinical trial evidence to guide specific recommendations. Analgesics are often administered intravenously, but this can be challenging in patients with poor venous access, and subcutaneous or oral administration can be equally effective.[10] Intramuscular administration is not recommended due to pain at the injection site and unpredictable absorption. Both morphine sulfate[11] and hydromorphone are available for intravenous and subcutaneous administration, as well as in both immediate-acting and slow-release oral liquid and tablet formulations. Using these agents in a combination of intravenous and oral administration allows for background analgesia with breakthrough dosing, permits patients to be discharged on a weaning dose of opiates, and removes the need to switch class of agent. If switching from one opiate to another is unavoidable, care should be taken to ensure bioequivalent dosing.

Certain analgesics have specific risks. Morphine sulfate has been weakly associated with an increased risk of developing ACS,[12] and oxycodone has been associated with an increased risk of opiate dependency. Meperidine is contraindicated due to cerebral agitation and risk of seizure. Adjunct laxatives and an antihistamine should be prescribed as required. Acute painful episodes in pregnancy should be managed as at other times but with close monitoring of fetal movements and avoidance of NSAIDs, especially in the first trimester and after 32 weeks' gestation.[13]

Fluid Replacement

Reduced renal tubular concentrating ability is common in patients with SCD and predisposes to dehydration. Continued fluid loss without adequate replacement causes a reduction in plasma volume with an increased blood viscosity and aggravation of the sickling process. However, the concurrent use of opiates for pain control can increase vascular leak and predisposes SCD patients to pulmonary edema. The goal of hydration should, therefore, be to replace estimated deficits and provide adequate maintenance while avoiding excessive hydration. Oral hydration, if tolerated, is preferred.

Other Measures

Patients often feel symptomatic benefit from supplemental oxygen, even when pulse oximetry is normal. Since SCD is a prothrombotic disorder, once a patient is admitted to the hospital, or in cases of extended ED stay, pharmacologic venous thromboembolism prophylaxis should be instituted.[14] In the absence of infection, current hydroxyurea treatment should not be withheld during a pain episode. Its efficacy in the treatment of VOC is thought to be due to its ability to increase fetal hemoglobin and reduce neutrophil and platelet activation.[15]

Limited data have shown dexamethasone therapy to be associated with reduced hospital length of stay and trends toward improvement in oxygen and opiate use; however, because of a potential to cause rebound pain, its use is currently not recommended. Various investigational and novel therapies—such tinzaparin, arginine, and inhaled nitric oxide—have been trialed in the setting of VOC, but there are insufficient supporting data at this time to formally recommend their use or their place in a treatment algorithm (see literature summary table for details of recent trials). These therapies remain an area of active research in SCD.

Common infectious organisms in SCD include *Streptococcus pneumoniae*, *Haemophilus influenzae*, and *Salmonella* spp., while atypical organisms such as *Mycoplasma*, *Chlamydia*, and *Legionella* spp. are common in patients with ACS. If there are signs of a lower respiratory tract infection, a macrolide antibiotic should be added to a broad-spectrum, third-generation cephalosporin. In suspected sepsis, hydroxyurea and iron chelation therapy should be avoided due to the risk of cytopenia and promoting growth of siderophore organisms, respectively. Transfusion therapy carries specific risks in patients with SCD, and in the great majority of cases, there is no role for transfusion therapy in management of uncomplicated acute pain.

Patients may be discharged from the ED if their pain can be adequately controlled with oral analgesia.[16] Due to the complex interrelationship between pain and psychosocial stressors in patients with SCD, a social work consultation can be very useful in coordinating patient disposition.

DIFFERENTIAL DIAGNOSIS OF AN UNCOMPLICATED PAIN EPISODE

Patients presenting with features other than simple bone pain should be referred to internal medicine and/or hematology.

Acute Chest Syndrome

ACS is an acute illness characterized by fever (>38.50°C), respiratory symptoms, and new pulmonary infiltrates on CXR. Precipitants are commonly infection, postoperative atelectasis, and pulmonary fat emboli (a known complication of marrow infarction in patients with SCD). ACS is the second most common cause of hospitalization in SCD and carries a mortality of approximately 5%.[17] Previous pulmonary events, including prior ACS, are risk factors. The pain of ACS is characterized by a "T-shirt" distribution; its severity will usually cause splinting of the diaphragm, further impairing oxygenation and resulting in progressive hypoxia. Signs of lung consolidation may varyingly accompany tachycardia and tachypnea; cough is a late symptom.

If ACS is suspected, the following laboratory tests should be ordered in addition to routine investigations and chest radiography: RBC transfusion crossmatch, hemoglobin electrophoresis, arterial blood gas, pan-culture, and an atypical organism infectious disease serology screen. Specific management of ACS should incorporate inspired O_2 to maintain oxygen saturations >96%, bronchodilators if there is history of obstructive/reversible airways disease or in the presence of bronchospasm or wheeze, antimicrobials, incentive spirometry, and blood transfusion.[18–20] Early transfusion is appropriate and can prevent the need for ventilator support. The purpose of transfusion is to enhance oxygen-carrying capacity, improve tissue oxygen delivery, and reduce HbS concentration and RBC sickling, all of which can together help prevent progression to acute respiratory failure. Transfusion commonly results in impressive improvement within hours. Patients presenting with mild or moderate ACS, or severe anemia, can be managed with a simple transfusion, aiming for a maximum Hb level of no more than 10 g/dL.[21]

For severe ACS, or in the presence of rapid or significant clinical deterioration, worsening chest radiography, a $pO_2 < 70$ mm Hg, or baseline Hb > 9 g/dL that preludes use of simple transfusion due to risk of hyperviscosity, consensus opinion is that an exchange transfusion is indicated. Under these circumstances, critical care support is advised. A randomized control trial on the use of exchange transfusion in this setting is still needed to provide more definitive evidence-based guidelines. To ensure that the most appropriate units of blood are selected (given the prevalence of alloimmunization in patients with SCD who have received multiple transfusions), it is imperative that the patient's diagnosis of SCD be communicated to the blood bank with any transfusion request.

Additional information may be available if the patient is carrying an antibody warning card documenting clinically significant antibodies whose titers have fallen below currently detectable levels.

Acute Stroke

Ischemic or hemorrhagic stroke is a common complication of SCD, and the diagnosis should be confirmed with a CT or MRI of the brain. The management of acute stroke in patients with SCD should include most aspects of care provided for non-SCD patients, including aggressive control of blood pressure, administration of antiplatelet therapy, and deep venous thrombosis (DVT) prophylaxis. Thrombolysis, however, is generally not used due to the increased risk of intracerebral hemorrhage. SCD patients with stroke should also undergo immediate exchange transfusion.[22] The goal of exchange transfusion support is to increase the HbA to 70% while keeping total Hb < 11 g/dL.

Gallbladder Disease

Chronic hemolysis with accelerated bilirubin turnover leads to a high incidence of pigment gallstones. Certain antimicrobials, such as ceftriaxone, are also known to promote biliary sludge formation and should be used with caution in patients with SCD. Management of acute cholecystitis in SCD patients is the same as for the general population.

Acute Sequestration

Hepatic sequestration presents as a rapidly enlarging liver with a significant drop in hemoglobin, accompanied by reticulocytosis. Exchange transfusion may be required, and simple transfusion should be performed judiciously as it carries a risk of hyperviscosity due to desequestering of the RBCs when the episode resolves. Splenic sequestration is less common in adults.

Priapism

Priapism—a sustained, painful, and unwanted erection of the penis—may go unrecognized by patients as a complication of SCD; they may be reluctant to discuss it and/or may present late to ED. Priapism is caused by vasoocclusion obstructing venous drainage of the penis and typically affects the corpora cavernosa. Penile ischemia and acidosis begin to occur approximately 6 hours into a sustained priapic episode, and recurrent episodes can result in fibrosis and impotence. Treatment centers on management of the underlying sickling process should include urologic consultation for penile aspiration and epinephrine irrigation if the condition persists beyond 6 hours.[23] There is little evidence to support transfusion for priapism, and there has been a reported association between priapism, exchange transfusion, and adverse neurologic events.[24]

CONCLUSION

SCD is a multisystem, inherited blood disorder characterized by ischemia–reperfusion injury and vasculopathy. The most common ED presentation is simple VOC causing generalized bone pain. Assessment of the patient is targeted to detection of complications that may warrant blood transfusion. Management of a VOC should be focused on rapid, adequate, and sustained multimodal analgesia.

LITERATURE TABLE		
TRIAL	**DESIGN**	**RESULT**
Acute pain episode		
Qari et al., *Thromb Haemost.* 2007[14]	RCT of 253 patients treated with adjuvant tinzaparin 175 IU/kg or placebo with acute pain	Tinzaparin-treated patients had significantly fewer total hospital days, overall days of pain, and pain declined or resolved more rapidly during the first 4 d of treatment in the tinzaparin group ($p = 0.05$ for each comparison)
Gladwin et al., *JAMA.* 2011[15]	RCT of inhaled nitric oxide for up to 72 h vs. nitrogen placebo for acute pain in SCD	Inhaled nitric oxide had no effect on the time to VOC resolution (primary outcome) or on length of hospitalization, change in VAS pain score, and total opioid use
Bellet et al., *N Engl J Med.* 1995[18]	RCT of 29 patients with acute chest or thoracic back pain	Incentive spirometer with 10 maximal inspirations every 2 h from 8 AM to 10 PM and when the patients were awake at night significantly decreased the incidence of pulmonary complications ($p = 0.019$)
Dampier et al., *Am J Hematol.* 2001[25]	RCT comparing 2 different opioid PCA therapies for acute pain in 38 subjects	Low demand, high basal infusion demonstrated faster, larger improvements in various measures of pain than did the high demand, low basal infusion strategy
Morris et al., *Haematologica.* 2013[26]	RCT of 38 children hospitalized with 56 pain episodes treated with arginine or placebo for acute pain	54% reduction in total opiate requirement during admission in intervention arm ($p = 0.02$)
Acute chest syndrome		
Quinn et al., *BJH.* 2011[19]	RCT of oral dexamethasone in 12 patients with ACS	Dexamethasone significantly reduced duration of hospitalization ($p = 0.024$) and trends toward reduced use of supplemental oxygen, hypoxemia, and total opioid usage
Knight-Madden and Hambleton, *Cochrane.* 2003[20]	Cochrane systematic review of inhaled bronchodilators for ACS	Lack of trials, but bronchodilators are likely to be helpful in those with ACS who have a history of asthma or wheezing during the episode
Blood transfusion		
Turner et al., *Transfusion.* 2009[21]	Retrospective cohort study of consecutive patients admitted with ACS who received simple transfusion or exchange transfusion	No meaningful benefit from exchange, relative to simple transfusion, including primary outcome of length of stay

RCT, randomized controlled trial.

REFERENCES

1. Ballas SK, Gupta K, Adams-Graves P. Sickle cell pain: a critical reappraisal. *Blood.* 2012;120(18):3647–3656.
2. Ballas SK. Current issues in sickle cell pain and its management. *Hematology.* 2007;2007(1):97–105.
3. Charache S, Terrin ML, Moore RD, et al. Effect of hydroxyurea on the frequency of painful crises in sickle cell anemia. Investigators of the Multicenter Study of Hydroxyurea in Sickle Cell Anemia. *N Engl J Med.* 1995;332(20):1317–1322.
4. Brousseau DC, Owens PL, Mosso AL, et al. Acute care utilization and rehospitalizations for sickle cell disease. *JAMA.* 2010;303(13):1288–1294.
5. Stein PD, Beemath A, Meyers FA, et al. Deep venous thrombosis and pulmonary embolism in hospitalized patients with sickle cell disease. *Am J Med.* 2006;119(10):897 e7–e11.

6. Mousa SA, Al Momen A, Al Sayegh F, et al. Management of painful vaso-occlusive crisis of sickle-cell anemia: consensus opinion. *Clin Appl Thromb Hemost.* 2010;16(4):365–376.
7. *NIH, The Management of Sickle Cell Disease.* US Department of Health and Human Services, Editor; 2002.
8. Rees DC, Olujohungbe AD, Parker NE, et al. Guidelines for the management of the acute painful crisis in sickle cell disease. *Br J Haematol.* 2003;120(5):744–752.
9. Bartolucci P, et al. A randomized, controlled clinical trial of ketoprofen for sickle-cell disease vaso-occlusive crises in adults. *Blood.* 2009;114(18):3742–3747.
10. Dunlop RJ, Bennett KC. Pain management for sickle cell disease. *Cochrane Database Syst Rev.* 2006(2):CD003350.
11. Darbari DS, Neely M, et al. Morphine pharmacokinetics in sickle cell disease: implications for pain management. *ASH Annual Meeting Abstracts.* 2009;114(22):2574.
12. Kopecky EA, Jacobson S, Joshi P, et al. Systemic exposure to morphine and the risk of acute chest syndrome in sickle cell disease. *Clin Pharmacol Ther.* 2004;75(3):140–146.
13. Marti-Carvajal AJ, Peña-Martí GE, Comunián-Carrasco G, et al. Interventions for treating painful sickle cell crisis during pregnancy. *Cochrane Database Syst Rev.* 2009(1):CD006786.
14. Qari MH, Aljaouni SK, Alardawi MS, et al. Reduction of painful vaso-occlusive crisis of sickle cell anaemia by tinzaparin in a double-blind randomized trial. *Thromb Haemost.* 2007;98(2):392–396.
15. Gladwin MT, Kato GJ, Weiner D, et al. Nitric oxide for inhalation in the acute treatment of sickle cell pain crisis: a randomized controlled trial. *JAMA.* 2011;305(9):893–902.
16. Tanabe P, Artz N, Mark Courtney D, et al. Adult emergency department patients with sickle cell pain crisis: a learning collaborative model to improve analgesic management. *Acad Emerg Med.* 2010;17(4):399–407.
17. Vichinsky EP, Neumayr LD, Earles AN, et al. Causes and outcomes of the acute chest syndrome in sickle cell disease. National Acute Chest Syndrome Study Group. *N Engl J Med.* 2000;342(25):1855–1865.
18. Bellet PS, Kalinyak KA, Shukla R, et al. Incentive spirometry to prevent acute pulmonary complications in sickle cell diseases. *N Engl J Med.* 1995;333(11):699–703.
19. Quinn CT, Stuart MJ, Kesler K, et al. Tapered oral dexamethasone for the acute chest syndrome of sickle cell disease. *Br J Haematol.* 2011;155(2):263–267.
20. Knight-Madden JM, Hambleton IR. Inhaled bronchodilators for acute chest syndrome in people with sickle cell disease. *Cochrane Database Syst Rev.* 2003; doi: 10.1002/14651858.CD003733
21. Turner JM, Kaplan JB, Cohen HW, et al. Exchange versus simple transfusion for acute chest syndrome in sickle cell anemia adults. *Transfusion.* 2009;49(5):863–868.
22. Adams RJ. Big strokes in small persons. *Arch Neurol.* 2007;64(11):1567–1574.
23. Mantadakis E, Ewalt DH, Cavender JD, et al. Outpatient penile aspiration and epinephrine irrigation for young patients with sickle cell anemia and prolonged priapism. *Blood.* 2000;95(1):78–82.
24. Merritt AL, Haiman C, Henderson SO. Myth: blood transfusion is effective for sickle cell anemia-associated priapism. *CJEM.* 2006;8(2):119–122.
25. Dampier CD, Smith WR, Kim HY, et al. Opioid patient controlled analgesia use during the initial experience with the IMPROVE PCA trial: a phase III analgesic trial for hospitalized sickle cell patients with painful episodes. *Am J Hematol.* 2011;86(12):E70–E73.
26. Morris CR, Kuypers FA, Lavrisha L, et al. A randomized, placebo-controlled trial of arginine therapy for the treatment of children with sickle cell disease hospitalized with vaso-occlusive pain episodes. *Haematologica.* 2013;98(9):1375–1382.

29

Platelet Disorders and Hemostatic Emergencies

Shawn K. Kaku and Catherine T. Jamin

BACKGROUND

Hemostasis is the process by which a blood clot is formed at a site of vessel injury. For simplicity, this process may be thought of as occurring in two steps. The first step, primary hemostasis, is the formation of a platelet aggregate at the site of injury. The second step, termed secondary hemostasis, is the activation of the coagulation cascade, which results in the formation of crossed-linked fibrin that strengthens the platelet aggregate. The fibrinolysis system limits the coagulation cascade, thus preventing excess clot formation. A properly functioning hemostatic system requires a functioning liver to synthesize coagulation factors, a sufficient number of platelets and cofactors, and appropriate coordination between the coagulation and fibrinolysis systems. This chapter provides an overview of the etiology and management of hemostatic dysfunction.

HISTORY AND PHYSICAL EXAM

A thorough history and physical will help to identify the etiology of the hemostatic or platelet disorder. In addition to a standard patient history, the provider should review the details of any bleeding events, including triggers, location, frequency, duration, and severity.[1] The physical exam should assess for bruising and petechiae, liver size and stigmata of cirrhosis, joint hemarthrosis, signs of anemia, and evidence of an infection.

Details of the history and physical can indicate a primary or secondary hemostatic disorder. Petechiae, bruising, mucosal bleeding, epistaxis, menorrhagia, and persistent bleeding are suggestive of disorders of platelets or primary hemostasis. Bleeding into soft tissues, muscles, and joints, or delayed bleeding, implies the presence of a coagulation factor deficiency or a disorder of secondary hemostasis.[2]

PLATELET DISORDERS

Idiopathic Thrombocytopenic Purpura

Idiopathic thrombocytopenic purpura (ITP) is an autoimmune disorder that results in the destruction of platelets through an IgG-mediated antibody. Platelets coated with the antibody are rapidly cleared by macrophages in the liver and spleen.[3] ITP is characterized by an isolated thrombocytopenia, defined as a platelet count $<100 \times 10^9/L$, in the absence of an obvious initiating or underlying cause.[4,5] As there is no gold standard for the diagnosis of ITP, it is considered a diagnosis of exclusion.[4,6] Therefore, a myriad of potential causes of thrombocytopenia must be evaluated prior to diagnosis, including systemic diseases, thrombotic thrombocytopenic purpura (TTP), drug reactions, primary hematologic disorders, liver dysfunction, infections, and recent transfusions.[6] A secondary form of ITP may also occur in association with underlying conditions such as human immunodeficiency virus, systemic lupus erythematosus, lymphoproliferative disorder, and antiphospholipid syndrome.[3]

In contrast to the self-limited presentation of ITP that is typical in children, ITP in adults is generally chronic, with a gradual onset.[3] Mucocutaneous bleeding, purpura, petechiae, epistaxis, and gum bleeding are the most common initial manifestations.[4]

No definitive evidence exists to guide an exact threshold at which to initiate medical therapy, such as glucocorticoids, in adults with ITP. Most patients will not require therapy; however, it is generally accepted that a platelet count $<30 \times 10^9$/L should be treated, regardless of the presence of bleeding.[5] Therapy must be individually tailored, and the decision to treat should weigh the patient's risk of bleeding—that is, previous bleeding episodes, age, presence of other comorbidities, level of activity, etc.[6]

In the critically ill patient with ITP and hemorrhage, initial therapy consists of high-dose intravenous steroids, such as methylprednisolone (30 mg/kg/d × 3 days for children and 1 g/day × 3 days for adults). Intravenous immunoglobulin (IVIG) 1 g/kg and transfusions may also be used.[5,6] Although the exact mechanism of IVIG in treating ITP remains to be elucidated, it is thought to play a role in preventing the uptake of antibody-coated platelets through the blockage of the Fc receptor on macrophages.[7] Platelet transfusion is not typically advised in the treatment of ITP, since any transfused platelets will eventually also be destroyed by circulating autoantibodies. However, platelet transfusions have been shown to help sustain the treatment response and may temporarily aid hemostasis in the bleeding patient.[7,8] The use of anti-Rho(D) immune globulin (anti-D) has been shown to be effective, though only in Rh-positive patients who have not had a splenectomy.[9] The anti-D binds Rh-positive erythrocytes, occupying the receptor in the splenic macrophages that would otherwise be used for removal of platelets. Emergency splenectomy may also be considered. As a nonemergent second-line therapy, splenectomy is associated with an 80% response rate.[6] Its use in an emergency situation must be individualized, as the bleeding thrombocytopenic patient makes a challenging ideal surgical candidate.

Heparin-Induced Thrombocytopenia

Heparin-induced thrombocytopenia (HIT) is a life-threatening disorder caused by antibodies against complexes of heparin bound to platelet factor IV. It should be suspected when a patient has a low platelet count, or at least a 50% drop in the platelet count, approximately 5 to 10 days after heparin exposure.[10,11] The frequency of HIT is 1% to 5% when unfractionated heparin is used and <1% with low molecular weight heparin (LMWH).[10] Although HIT causes thrombocytopenia, thrombosis—not bleeding—is the major clinical concern.[10] This is due to platelet activation and the generation of platelet microparticles that leads to thrombin generation and thrombosis.[11,12] Thrombotic complications develop in approximately 20% to 50% of patients and can persist for days to weeks after heparin therapy is stopped.[11] Complications include arterial and venous thrombosis, limb ischemia, and cerebral venous sinuses thrombosis.[11]

The laboratory testing for HIT includes a heparin–platelet factor 4 (H-PF4) ELISA antibody test and functional assay tests. The H-PF4 test is widely available and often the first diagnostic test sent. The functional assay tests, while becoming more common, are not always available and are often send-out tests that require up to a week to result. The H-PF4 test has a high sensitivity (>97%) but a poor specificity (74% to 86%), as only a subset of these detected antibodies can cause HIT.[11] This is especially true in surgical patients; up to 20% to 50% of postoperative cardiac patients and 81% of surgical ICU patients can have a false positive H-PF4.[10,12] Given the high negative predictive value of the H-PF4 test, patients deemed to have a high to intermediate risk of HIT with a negative H-PF4 should be evaluated for alternative diagnoses of their thrombocytopenia.[11]

The heparin-induced platelet aggregation test is a functional assay test, with a sensitivity of >90% and a specificity ranging from 77% to 100%.[11] The c-serotonin functional assay test measures serotonin release from activated platelets and is considered the "gold standard" for the diagnosis of HIT, with a sensitivity and specificity of >95%.[11,13–15] Unfortunately, this test is often not available in the emergency department (ED).

Waiting for the send-out test to confirm a diagnosis of HIT can be problematic, given both the dangers of treatment delay and the potentially serious side effects of the treatment itself. The "4Ts" clinical scoring system shown in Table 29.1 provides a real-time evaluation of HIT.[16] A recent meta-analysis confirmed its utility in a wide range of patient population, demonstrating a negative predictive value of 99.8% for those with a low score.[17]

Treatment of HIT—to suppress thrombotic events—consists of stopping all sources of heparin, including LMWH, and initiating an alternate form of systemic anticoagulation. There are currently three FDA-approved medications for the treatment of HIT:

TABLE 29.1 4T's Pretest Scoring System for HIT

4T's	2 Points	1 Point	0 Points
Thrombocytopenia	Platelet count fall >50% and nadir $\geq 20 \times 10^9$/L	Platelet count fall 30%–50% or platelet nadir 10–19 $\times 10^9$/L	Platelet count fall <30% or platelet nadir <10 $\times 10^9$/L
Timing of platelet count fall	Platelet count fall between days 5 and 10 after heparin exposure or Platelet count fall ≤1 d and prior heparin exposure within 30 d	Consistent with fall 5–10 d after heparin exposure, but not clear (e.g., missing platelet counts) or Platelet count fall > day 10 or Platelet count fall ≤1 d and prior heparin exposure within 30–100 d	Platelet count fall ≤4 d without recent heparin exposure
Thrombosis or other sequelae	New thrombosis (confirmed); skin necrosis; acute systemic reaction postintravenous unfractionated heparin bolus	Progressive or recurrent thrombosis; nonnecrotizing (erythematous) skin lesions; suspected thrombosis (not proven)	None
Other causes of thrombocytopenia	None apparent	Possible	Definite

Source: Lo GK, Juhl D, Warkentin TE, et al. Evaluation of pretest clinical score (4T's) for the diagnosis of heparin-induced thrombocytopenia in two clinical settings. *J Thromb Haemost.* 2006;4(4):759–765.

Test interpretation: 0 to 3, low probability; 4 to 5, intermediate probability; 6 to 8, high probability.

argatroban, bivalirudin, and lepirudin; however, the manufacture of lepirudin has recently been discontinued. While there are no prospective randomized studies examining their efficacy, argatroban has shown superior efficacy in two prospective trials compared to historical controls in reducing thrombotic events and death from thrombosis without an increase in bleeding rates.[18,19] Argatroban should be dose adjusted in patients with hepatic dysfunction. Bivalirudin is approved only for patients with HIT undergoing percutaneous coronary intervention. The American College of Chest Physician (ACCP) guidelines notes that fondaparinux may have a theoretical role in treating HIT; at this time, however, it is not approved for this use.[20]

Patients with HIT are in a prothrombotic state and should remain on anticoagulation for 4 to 12 weeks after diagnosis; this may be accomplished via transition to warfarin therapy.[20] The initiation of warfarin must be done cautiously, as warfarin rapidly decreases protein C levels, which can exacerbate the prothrombotic state and lead to skin necrosis and limb gangrene.[20] The 2012 ACCP guidelines recommend starting warfarin only after the patient shows platelet recovery of at least 150×10^9/L and stable anticoagulation on thrombin inhibitors; if warfarin has already been started when a patient is diagnosed with HIT, then vitamin K should be administered until the above criteria are met.[20] Finally, since spontaneous bleeding is uncommon with HIT, platelets should be transfused only in patients who are bleeding or during the performance of an invasive procedure with a high risk of bleeding.[20]

HELLP Syndrome

HELLP syndrome is a serious complication of pregnancy, characterized by hemolysis (H), elevated liver enzymes (EL), and low platelets (LP). Controversy exists as to whether HELLP is a severe manifestation of preeclampsia or a separate disease process. Although it can occur earlier, HELLP syndrome usually presents after 28 weeks' gestation.[10] Classic symptoms include epigastric or right upper quadrant abdominal pain, nausea, and vomiting.[21,22] Patients also may have nonspecific symptoms, such as malaise or headache, which can be mistaken for a viral syndrome.[21,22] Although there is no consensus on laboratory values for the diagnosis of HELLP syndrome, patients ideally should demonstrate all components of its acronym, namely, microangiopathic hemolytic anemia (MAHA), EL, and decreased platelets.[10,21,22]

HELLP syndrome increases the chance of maternal death and is associated with disseminated intravascular coagulopathy, abruptio placentae, severe postpartum bleeding, pulmonary and cerebral edema, liver infarct and rupture, and cerebral infarcts and hemorrhages.[21,22] While delivery of the fetus is the cornerstone of treatment, the exact timing of delivery is unclear and is dependent on the gestational age as well as the stability and condition of the mother and fetus.[21,22] Laboratory abnormalities may reverse in a subgroup of patients who are managed expectantly; however, this approach needs to be more rigorously investigated.[23,24] All patients with HELLP syndrome should be admitted to the hospital and treated for severe preeclampsia, with intravenous magnesium as prophylaxis against convulsions and antihypertensive medications to keep systolic blood pressure below 160 mm Hg, diastolic blood pressure below 105 mmHg, or both.[22] Corticosteroid administration to aid fetal lung maturation is often recommended if the fetus is between 24 and 34 weeks' gestational age.[22] Platelets should be transfused for significant bleeding or platelet counts <20 × 10^9/L.[22] The use of corticosteroids to improve maternal outcome remains controversial and experimental, as the benefits seen by early small randomized and observational studies could not be reproduced in two larger, randomized, double-blind, placebo-controlled trials.[25,26]

Thrombotic Thrombocytopenic Purpura and Hemolytic Uremic Syndrome

TTP and hemolytic uremic syndrome (HUS) describe two diseases of a broader category called thrombotic microangiopathies. The thrombotic microangiopathies are microvascular occlusive disorders characterized by aggregation of platelets, thrombocytopenia, and mechanical injury to erythrocytes.[27] While sharing similar characteristics, the adult form of TTP and the childhood form of diarrheal HUS are two separate disorders.

TTP is thought to be due to a deficiency of the ADAMTS13 enzyme, with an inhibitory antibody being the cause in the majority of the classic cases.[10] The ADAMTS13 enzyme is responsible for cleaving the newly synthesized von Willebrand factor (vWF) multimer. When not cleaved, these unusually large vWF multimers lead to spontaneous platelet aggregation and the clinical syndrome of TTP.[10] TTP can be both congenital and acquired, with the congenital form being extremely rare. While the majority of acquired causes are idiopathic, examples of secondary causes of TTP include medications, infections, pregnancy, lupus, malignancy, and transplantation.[28]

The classic pentad of TTP is thrombocytopenia, MAHA, fluctuating neurologic signs, renal impairment, and fever[27] MAHA is caused by erythrocytes passing through areas of the microcirculation that are partially occluded by aggregated platelets.[27] This causes fragmented erythrocytes, termed schistocytes or helmet cells, as well as elevated lactate dehydrogenate and indirect bilirubin.[27,28] Some patients, however, may not present with neurologic symptoms, renal failure, or fever. Therefore, the diagnosis of TTP may be made in the presence of an MAHA and thrombocytopenia in the absence of any other identifiable cause.[28]

Treatment for TTP should be initiated even if diagnostic uncertainty exists, as the untreated mortality rate can be as high as 95% to 100%.[29–31] Plasma exchange, or the removal of a patient's plasma and replacement with another fluid (donor plasma, colloid, etc.), is the mainstay of treatment, as it removes the inhibitory antibody and supplies new ADAMTS13. Plasma exchange has decreased the TTP mortality rate to <20%.[10,27–31] While not as effective as plasma exchange, plasma infusion alone has been shown to decrease the mortality rate to 37%.[28,32] Therefore, plasma infusion (30 mL/kg/d) may be indicated as the initial treatment if there is to be an unavoidable delay in plasma exchange.[28] Although steroids have been widely used for TTP as an adjunctive immunosuppressive treatment, there is minimal evidence for their efficacy and no consensus on dosing or route.[28] Since patients may benefit from their use, steroids can be given as adjuvant therapy. A reasonable approach is methylprednisolone 2 mg/kg/d, although pulse doses of 1 g/day × 3 days may also be used.[28] Rituximab, an anti-CD20 antibody, should be considered for patients refractory to plasma exchange.[33,34] Platelet transfusions are contraindicated as they can worsen the platelet aggregation and effects of TTP. They should be reserved for life-threatening hemorrhage or for invasive procedure preparation.[28]

HUS is characterized by MAHA, thrombocytopenia, and acute renal failure. HUS is commonly associated with a prodrome of bloody diarrhea caused by the Shiga toxin–producing *Escherichia coli* 0157:H7.[27,28] The toxin damages endothelial cells, causing platelet aggregation and intravascular thrombogenesis. Much of the treatment for HUS is supportive in nature. The optimal care requires careful management of fluid and electrolyte balance and blood pressure. The use of hemodialysis may be required if renal failure is severe.[28] Antibiotics and antimotility agents should be avoided as they can worsen the outcome.[27,28] Two prospective studies on plasma infusion in HUS failed to show any outcome benefit.[35,36] There are no randomized controlled prospective studies evaluating the use of therapeutic plasma exchange for HUS caused by Shiga toxin–producing *Escherichia coli*, and it is currently reserved only for severe cases, often those involving the nervous system. As in the case of TTP, blood transfusion for HUS should be given based on clinical evaluation and need, rather than on a strict hemoglobin threshold; platelet transfusions should be avoided if possible.

DISORDERS OF COAGULATION

Disseminated Intravascular Coagulation

Disseminated intravascular coagulation (DIC) is characterized by the widespread activation of the coagulation cascade, which results in fibrin formation, thrombotic occlusion of small and midsize vessels, and subsequent organ failure. Simultaneously, the consumption of platelets and coagulation proteins can induce severe bleeding.[37] DIC is not a disease in itself but is instead a complication of an underlying disorder. These disorders include sepsis, trauma, organ dysfunction (pancreatitis), obstetric emergencies, malignancy, and toxic and transfusion reactions.[38]

No single laboratory test can diagnose or rule out DIC. Instead, in a patient at risk for DIC, a combination of test results can be used to diagnose the disorder with reasonable certainty.[37] Common laboratory abnormalities include thrombocytopenia, elevated fibrin degradation products, prolongation of clotting times including the prothrombin time (PT) and the activated partial thromboplastin time (PTT), and a low fibrinogen.[37,39] Schistocytes may also be present on the blood smear.[37] Caution must be exercised when interpreting fibrinogen levels, as it is an acute-phase reactant that can remain within the normal range or elevated for a long period of time.[37,39]

The cornerstone of treatment of DIC is treatment of the precipitating condition.[37–39] Transfusion of platelets or plasma should be reserved for patients with active or high risk of bleeding. Platelet transfusion is indicated in bleeding patients with platelet counts $<50 \times 10^9$/L and in nonbleeding patients with platelet counts <10 to 20×10^9/L.[39] Fresh frozen plasma (FFP) and/or cryoprecipitate are recommended for patients who are bleeding with an INR > 2 or a fibrinogen level <100 mg/dL.[40] In cases of DIC where a thrombotic picture predominates (e.g., arterial or venous thromboembolism, severe purpura fulminans, or vascular skin infarctions), therapeutic doses of heparin should be considered.[39] In critically ill, nonbleeding patients with DIC, prophylaxis for venous thromboembolism with heparin or LMWH is recommended.[39] The use of antithrombin (formerly antithrombin III) has not improved outcomes in DIC, and further investigation is warranted in the use of recombinant human factor VIIa.[41,42] For patients with inherited or acquired protein C deficiencies, protein C concentrate has demonstrated some benefit.[43]

HEMOPHILIA

Hemophilia is an X-linked heritable coagulopathy, most often referring to a deficiency of factor VIII (hemophilia A) or factor IX (hemophilia B, Christmas disease). While these deficiencies are difficult to distinguish clinically, factor VIII deficiency comprises approximately 80% of cases and factor IX deficiency the remaining 20%.[44,45] The severity of hemophilia is defined by the level of serum clotting factors as compared to the general population: <1% of normal is defined as severe, 1% to 5% of normal as moderate, and >5% of normal as mild.[44,46] Patients with hemophilia are at risk for hemarthrosis (especially knee, ankle, and elbow joints), soft tissue hematomas, bruising, retroperitoneal bleed, intracranial hemorrhage, and postsurgical bleeding.[44,47]

Due to the heritability of the disease, a family history of hemophilia or abnormal bleeding is extremely helpful in making the diagnosis. Approximately 30% of cases, however, have no known family history and are caused by spontaneous mutations. Laboratory values for patients with hemophilia A and B will demonstrate normal platelets and PT, with a prolonged PTT. Specific assays for each factor can be used to identify the type of hemophilia.

Administration of the deficient factor is needed to limit or stop an episode of bleeding. The amount of factor replaced is dependent on the location of the bleeding. According to the guideline from the World Federation of Hemophilia, a factor level of 40% to 60% is recommended for deep lacerations, joint, and most muscle bleeding, and a factor level of 80% to 100% is recommended for CNS, throat and neck, GI, and iliopsoas muscle bleeding.[48] The formulas for estimating the dose of factor required to be administered are shown in Table 29.2. If unknown, the baseline factor should be presumed to be 0%. The patient's replaced factor level should be measured approximately 15 minutes after infusion to verify calculated doses.[48] The half-life of factors VIII and IX is 8 to 12 hours and 18 to 24 hours, respectively. Redosing will be needed at that time.[48]

When specific factor replacement is unavailable, other options do exist. FFP contains all coagulation factors, in a concentration of 1 unit of factor in 1 mL, and can be used for both hemophilia A and B.[48] Concerns with use of FFP include the large volume required and the inherent risks of transfusion (e.g., transfusion reaction, volume overload, and TRALI). Cryoprecipitate contains about 70 to 80 units of factor VIII and can be used as an alternative for treatment of hemophilia A.[48] However, similar safety concerns make it second-line therapy. Other treatment options include prothrombin

TABLE 29.2 Formulas for Calculating Dosage of Required Factor

Type of Replacement Factor	Dosing
Factor VIII	Weight (kg) × desired % increase × 0.5
Factor IX	Weight (kg) × desired % increase
Recombinant factor IX—adult dose	Weight (kg) × desired % increase × 1.25
Recombinant factor IX—child dose	Weight (kg) × desired % increase × 1.43

Source: Srivastava A, Brewer AK, Mauser-Bunschoten EP, et al. Treatment Guidelines Working Group on behalf of The World Federation of Hemophilia. Guidelines for the management of hemophilia. *Haemophilia.* 2013;19(1):e1–e47.

complex concentrates, recombinant factor VII, and antifibrinolytic agents. These treatments should be used in consultation with a hematologist.

LIVER DISEASE

The liver's essential contribution to maintenance of normal hemostasis is severely disrupted in advanced liver disease, which can lead to coagulopathy and severe bleeding. The loss of hepatic parenchymal cells leads to decreased production of the hemostatic factors II, V, VII, IX, X, XI, XII, and fibrinogen (both the liver and endothelium synthesize factor VIII, allowing for a normal to elevated level in liver disease).[49] Impaired bile production decreases the absorption of vitamin K, an essential cofactor for factors II, VII, IX, and X. Although its clinical significance is unclear, vitamin K deficiency may also contribute to the coagulopathy.[49,50] Finally, decreased clearance of tissue plasminogen activator and diminished production of fibrinolytic inhibitors are thought to be responsible for the low-grade fibrinolysis found in 30% to 46% of patients with end-stage liver disease.[49,51]

Platelet number and function are also affected in advanced liver disease. Thrombocytopenia (in the setting of liver disease) is thought to be multifactorial, with factors including excessive trapping and clearing of platelets from portal hypertension–induced hypersplenism; impaired platelet production from decreased synthesis of thrombopoietin; and immune and nonimmune platelet destruction.[49–51] Immune-mediated platelet destruction is often seen with chronic liver disease, and particularly in hepatitis C, a disease state associated with antiplatelet antibodies, including the glycoprotein autoantibody associated with ITP.[49,50]

In addition to decreasing the quantity of platelets, advanced liver disease impairs platelet function through a variety of mechanisms. Increased circulating platelet inhibitors, excess nitric oxide synthesis, a deficiency of platelet receptors, defective signal transduction, and impaired thromboxane A2 synthesis all contribute to impaired platelet aggregation, defective platelet–vessel wall interaction, and enhanced platelet inhibition associated with liver disease.[49,51]

While liver disease is most often associated with bleeding disorders, hypercoagulability can also be present. Liver disease results in the decreased production of anticoagulation factors such as antithrombin and proteins C and S; in turn, this may either balance the disruption of the pro- and anticoagulation systems or may result in a hypercoagulable state.[50–52] In fact, the notion that elevated PT/INR levels in patients with liver disease reflect "autoanticoagulation" may be unfounded.[51,53,54] An elevated PT does not necessarily reflect a uniform decrease in vitamin K clotting factors, as in warfarin therapy; it can also reflect an unbalanced decrease of the short-lived factor VII without the concomitant protection from thrombosis.[51] Moreover, INR and PT results vary widely in patients with liver disease based on the reagent and device used.[50] Thus, clinical context—such as sepsis, recent surgery, or bleeding—is more important than any single laboratory value in assessing coagulation balance in these patients.

In the acutely bleeding patient with liver disease, aggressive treatment of hemostatic deficits is essential. Therapy should be aimed not at complete correction of abnormal laboratory values but at achieving hemostatic competence.[51] To guide therapy, laboratory testing should include PT/INR, PTT, platelet count, and fibrinogen level. FFP should be administered to correct an elevated PT/INR and PTT levels as it contains all coagulation factors; however, this correction can be difficult to achieve and may have only transient effect.[50,51] Also, note again that an elevated PT/INR may not reflect an increased bleeding risk; and transfusion of FFP may lead to volume overload and other transfusion-related complications. Cryoprecipitate should be used to keep the fibrinogen level >100 mg/dL, and platelets transfused to keep a level $>50 \times 10^9$/L.[51] A trial of desmopressin may be used to aid platelet function in cases of refractory bleeding.[51] The mechanism of action of desmopressin is unclear, but it is thought to improve platelet adhesiveness through its release of vWF.[51] As previously noted, vitamin K deficiency may also contribute to coagulopathy, and a 3-day trial of vitamin K (5 to 10 mg/day) may be given.[51] The efficacy and safety of recombinant factor VIIa is currently under study, and it should be reserved as a rescue therapy.[50,51]

CONCLUSION

Emergency departments and intensive care units frequently admit patient with platelet disorders and hemostatic emergencies. While many of these conditions share common laboratory values, they vary widely in pathology and appropriate course of treatment. Proper identification of, and tailored therapy for, the platelet disorders ITP, HIT, HELLP, HUS, and TTP, as well as the coagulopathies of hemophilia, DIC, and liver disease, is an essential skill for the emergency physician.

LITERATURE TABLE

TRIAL	DESIGN	RESULT
Heparin-Induced Thrombocytopenia		
Lo et al., *J Thromb Haemost.* 2006[16]	Prospective study evaluating the 4Ts clinical scoring system on 336 patients	A low pretest clinical score seems to be suitable for ruling out HIT in most situations
Cuker et al., *Blood.* 2012[17]	Systematic review and meta-analysis of the predictive value of the 4Ts scoring system. Included 13 studies and 3,068 patients	Low probability score on the 4Ts clinical scoring system had a 99.8% negative predictive value (95% CI, 0.970–1.000) for HIT across a broad patient population
Lewis et al., *Arch Intern Med.* 2003[18]	Multicenter, nonrandomized prospective study of 418 patients with HIT treated with argatroban	Compared to historical controls, argatroban reduced composite of all-cause death, all-cause amputation, or new thrombosis (OR 0.61, $p = 0.04$). No difference in bleeding rates
Lewis et al., *Circulation.* 2001[19]	Prospective, multicenter, nonrandomized, open-label, historical-controlled study of 304 patients with HIT treated with argatroban	Argatroban therapy, relative to control subjects, significantly reduced the composite of all-cause death, all-cause amputation, or new thrombosis (25.6% vs. 38.8%, $p = 0.014$). No difference in bleeding rates
HELLP Syndrome		
Fonseca et al., *Am J Obstet Gynecol.* 2005[25]	Prospective, double-blind, placebo-controlled randomized study of 132 patients with HELLP treated with dexamethasone vs. placebo	No significant differences in duration of hospitalization, time to recovery of platelet counts confidence interval, lactate dehydrogenase, aspartate aminotransferase, or to the development of complications

(*Continued*)

LITERATURE TABLE (*Continued*)

TRIAL	DESIGN	RESULT
Katz et al., *Am J Obstet Gynecol.* 2008[26]	Prospective, randomized, double-blind, placebo-controlled study of 105 patients with HELLP treated with dexamethasone vs. placebo	No difference in mortality, duration of hospital stay, platelet recovery, aspartate aminotransferase, lactate dehydrogenase, hemoglobin, or diuresis
Thrombotic Thrombocytopenic Purpura		
Rock et al., *N Engl J Med.* 1991[32]	Randomized prospective study of 102 patients with TTP treated with plasma exchange vs. infusion	6-mo mortality for plasma exchange was 22% vs. 37% ($p = 0.036$) for plasma infusion. 6-mo response rate for plasma exchange was 78% vs. 49% for plasma infusion ($p = 0.002$). Historical control mortality of 95%
Liver Disease		
Dabbagh, *Chest.* 2010[53]	Retrospective cohort study. Evaluated incidence of VTE in 190 patients admitted with a primary diagnosis of chronic liver disease over a 7-y period	An elevated INR in the setting of chronic liver disease does not appear to protect against the development of hospital-acquired VTE
Northup, *Am J Gastroenterol.* 2006[54]	Retrospective case–control study. 113 hospitalized patients with cirrhosis with a documented new venous thromboembolism were compared to controls	Approximately 0.5% of admissions involving cirrhosis patients resulted in a new thromboembolic event, with INR and platelet counts not predictive of events

CI, confidence interval; OR, odds ratio.

REFERENCES

1. Rydz N, James PD. Why is my patient bleeding or bruising? *Hematol Oncol Clin North Am.* 2012;26(2):321–344.
2. van Ommen CH, Peters M. The bleeding child. Part I: primary hemostatic disorders. *Eur J Pediatr.* 2012;171(1):1–10.
3. Cines DB, Blanchette VS. Immune thrombocytopenic purpura. *N Engl J Med.* 2002;346(13):995–1008.
4. Liebman HA, Pullarkat V. Diagnosis and management of immune thrombocytopenia in the era of thrombopoietin mimetics. *Hematology Am Soc Hematol Educ Program.* 2011;2011:384–390.
5. Bussel JB, Cines DB, Kelton JG, et al. Idiopathic thrombocytopenic purpura: a practice guideline developed by explicit methods for the American Society of Hematology. *Blood.* 1996;88(1):3–40.
6. Provan D, Stasi R, Newland AC, et al. International consensus report on the investigation and management of primary immune thrombocytopenia. *Blood.* 2010;115(2):168–186.
7. Baumann MA, Menitove JE, Aster RH, et al. Urgent treatment of idiopathic thrombocytopenic purpura with single-dose gammaglobulin infusion followed by platelet transfusion. *Ann Intern Med.* 1986;104:808.
8. Carr JM, Kruskall MS, Kaye JA, et al. Efficacy of platelet transfusion in immune thrombocytopenia. *Am J Med.* 1986;80:1051.
9. Ramadan KM, El-Agnaf M. Efficacy and response to intravenous anti-D immunoglobulin in chronic idiopathic thrombocytopenic purpura. *Clin Lab Haematol.* 2005;27:267.
10. DeLoughery TG. Critical care clotting catastrophies. *Crit Care Clin.* 2005;21(3):531–562.
11. Arepally GM, Ortel TL. Clinical practice. Heparin-induced thrombocytopenia. *N Engl J Med.* 2006;355(8):809–817.
12. Berry C, Tcherniantchouk O, Ley EJ, et al. Overdiagnosis of heparin-induced thrombocytopenia in surgical ICU patients. *J Am Coll Surg.* 2011;213(1):10–17.
13. Sheridan D, Carter C, Kelton JG. A diagnostic test for heparin-induced thrombocytopenia. *Blood.* 1986;67(1):27–30.
14. Napolitano LM, Warkentin TE, Almahameed A, et al. Heparin-induced thrombocytopenia in the critical care setting: diagnosis and management. *Crit Care Med.* 2006;34(12):2898–2911.
15. Warkentin TE. Platelet count monitoring and laboratory testing for heparin-induced thrombocytopenia. *Arch Pathol Lab Med.* 2002;126(11):1415–1423.

16. Lo GK, Juhl D, Warkentin TE, et al. Evaluation of pretest clinical score (4 T's) for the diagnosis of heparin-induced thrombocytopenia in two clinical settings. *J Thromb Haemost.* 2006;4(4):759–765.
17. Cuker A, Gimotty PA, Crowther MA, et al. Predictive value of the 4Ts scoring system for heparin-induced thrombocytopenia: a systematic review and meta-analysis. *Blood.* 2012;120(20):4160–4167.
18. Lewis BE, Wallis DE, Leya F, et al. Argatroban-915 Investigators. Argatroban anticoagulation in patients with heparin-induced thrombocytopenia. *Arch Intern Med.* 2003;163(15):1849–1856.
19. Lewis BE, Wallis DE, Berkowitz SD, et al. ARG-911 Study Investigators. Argatroban anticoagulant therapy in patients with heparin-induced thrombocytopenia. *Circulation.* 2001;103(14):1838–1843.
20. Linkins LA, Dans AL, Moores LK, et al. Treatment and prevention of heparin-induced thrombocytopenia: Antithrombotic Therapy and Prevention of Thrombosis, 9th ed.: American College of Chest Physicians Evidence-Based Clinical Practice Guidelines. *Chest.* 2012;141(2 Suppl):e495S–530S.
21. Haram K, Svendsen E, Abildgaard U. The HELLP syndrome: clinical issues and management. A Review. *BMC Pregnancy Childbirth.* 2009;9:8.
22. Sibai BM. Diagnosis, controversies, and management of the syndrome of hemolysis, elevated liver enzymes, and low platelet count. *Obstet Gynecol.* 2004;103(5 Pt 1):981–991.
23. Visser W, Wallenburg HC. Temporising management of severe pre-eclampsia with and without the HELLP syndrome. *Br J Obstet Gynaecol.* 1995;102(2):111–117.
24. van Pampus MG, Wolf H, Westenberg SM, et al. Maternal and perinatal outcome after expectant management of the HELLP syndrome compared with pre-eclampsia without HELLP syndrome. *Eur J Obstet Gynecol Reprod Biol.* 1998;76(1):31–36.
25. Fonseca JE, Méndez F, Cataño C, et al. Dexamethasone treatment does not improve the outcome of women with HELLP syndrome: a double-blind, placebo-controlled, randomized clinical trial. *Am J Obstet Gynecol.* 2005;193(5):1591–1598.
26. Katz L, de Amorim MM, Figueiroa JN, et al. Postpartum dexamethasone for women with hemolysis, elevated liver enzymes, and low platelets (HELLP) syndrome: a double-blind, placebo-controlled, randomized clinical trial. *Am J Obstet Gynecol.* 2008;198(3):283.e1–e8.
27. Moake JL. Thrombotic microangiopathies. *N Engl J Med.* 2002;347(8):589–600.
28. Allford SL, Hunt BJ, Rose P, et al. Haemostasis and Thrombosis Task Force, British Committee for Standards in Haematology. Guidelines on the diagnosis and management of the thrombotic microangiopathic haemolytic anaemias. *Br J Haematol.* 2003;120(4):556–573.
29. von Baeyer H. Plasmapheresis in thrombotic microangiopathy-associated syndromes: review of outcome data derived from clinical trials and open studies. *Ther Apher.* 2002;6(4):320–328.
30. Lara PN Jr, Coe TL, Zhou H, et al. Improved survival with plasma exchange in patients with thrombotic thrombocytopenic purpura-hemolytic uremic syndrome. *Am J Med.* 1999;107(6):573–579.
31. Bell WR, Braine HG, Ness PM, et al. Improved survival in thrombotic thrombocytopenic purpura-hemolytic uremic syndrome–clinical experience in 108 patients. *N Engl J Med.* 1991;325:398–403.
32. Rock GA, Shumak KH, Buskard NA, et al. Comparison of plasma exchange with plasma infusion in the treatment of thrombotic thrombocytopenic purpura. Canadian Apheresis Study Group. *N Engl J Med.* 1991;325(6):393–397.
33. Fakhouri F, Vernant JP, Veyradier A, et al. Efficiency of curative and prophylactic treatment with rituximab in ADAMTS13-deficient thrombotic thrombocytopenic purpura: a study of 11 cases. *Blood.* 2005;106(6):1932.
34. Scully M, Cohen H, Cavenagh J, et al. Remission in acute refractory and relapsing thrombotic thrombocytopenic purpura following rituximab is associated with a reduction in IgG antibodies to ADAMTS-13. *Br J Haematol.* 2007;136(3):451.
35. Rizzoni G, Claris-Appiani A, Edefonti A, et al. Plasma infusion for hemolytic uremic syndrome in children: results of a multicenter controlled trial. *J Pediatr.* 1988;12:284–290.
36. Loirat C, Sonsino E, Hinglais N, et al. Treatment of childhood haemolytic uraemic syndrome with plasma. A multicentre randomised controlled trial. *Pediatr Nephrol.* 1988;2:279–285.
37. Levi M, Ten Cate H. Disseminated intravascular coagulation. *N Engl J Med.* 1999;341(8):586–592.
38. Levi M, de Jonge E, van der Poll T. New treatment strategies for disseminated intravascular coagulation based on current understanding of the pathophysiology. *Ann Med.* 2004;36(1):41–49.
39. Levi M, Toh CH, Thachil J, et al. Guidelines for the diagnosis and management of disseminated intravascular coagulation. British Committee for Standards in Haematology. *Br J Haematol.* 2009;145(1):24–33.
40. Wada H, Asakura H, Okamoto K, et al. Japanese Society of Thrombosis Hemostasis/DIC subcommittee. Expert consensus for the treatment of disseminated intravascular coagulation in Japan. *Thromb Res.* 2010;125(1):6–11.

41. Warren BL, Eid A, Singer P, et al. Caring for the critically ill patient. High-dose antithrombin III in severe sepsis: a randomized controlled trial. *JAMA.* 2001;286(15):1869.
42. Franchini M, Manzato F, Salvagno GL, et al. Potential role of recombinant activated factor VII for the treatment of severe bleeding associated with disseminated intravascular coagulation: a systematic review. *Blood Coagul Fibrinolysis.* 2007;18(7):589.
43. Smith OP, White B, Vaughan D, et al. Use of protein-C concentrate, heparin, and haemodiafiltration in meningococcus-induced purpura fulminans. *Lancet.* 1997;350(9091):1590.
44. Knobe K, Berntorp E. Haemophilia and joint disease: pathophysiology, evaluation, and management. *J Comorbidity.* 2011;1:51–59.
45. Coppola A, Di Capua M, Di Minno MN, et al. Treatment of hemophilia: a review of current advances and ongoing issues. *J Blood Med.* 2010;1:183–195.
46. White GC II, Rosendaal F, Aledort LM, et al. Factor VIII and Factor IX Subcommittee. Definitions in hemophilia. Recommendation of the scientific subcommittee on factor VIII and factor IX of the scientific and standardization committee of the International Society on Thrombosis and Haemostasis. *Thromb Haemost.* 2001;85(3):560.
47. Ljung R, Petrini P, Nilsson IM. Diagnostic symptoms of severe and moderate haemophilia A and B. A survey of 140 cases. *Acta Paediatr Scand.* 1990;79(2):196–200.
48. Srivastava A, Brewer AK, Mauser-Bunschoten EP, et al. Treatment Guidelines Working Group on behalf of The World Federation of Hemophilia. Guidelines for the management of hemophilia. *Haemophilia.* 2013;19(1):e1–e47.
49. Senzolo M, Burra P, Cholongitas E, et al. New insights into the coagulopathy of liver disease and liver transplantation. *World J Gastroenterol.* 2006;12(48):7725–7736.
50. Trotter JF. Coagulation abnormalities in patients who have liver disease. *Clin Liver Dis.* 2006;10(3):665–678.
51. Kujovich JL. Hemostatic defects in end stage liver disease. *Crit Care Clin.* 2005;21(3):563–587.
52. Tripodi A, Mannucci PM. The coagulopathy of chronic liver disease. *N Engl J Med.* 2011;365(2):147–156.
53. Dabbagh O, Oza A, Prakash S, et al. Coagulopathy does not protect against venous thromboembolism in hospitalized patients with chronic liver disease. *Chest.* 2010;137(5):1145–1149.
54. Northup PG, McMahon MM, Ruhl AP, et al. Coagulopathy does not fully protect hospitalized cirrhosis patients from peripheral venous thromboembolism. *Am J Gastroenterol.* 2006;101(7):1524–1528.

30

Transfusion Therapy

Michael P. Jones and John E. Arbo

BACKGROUND

The use of blood product transfusion in the critically ill is commonplace, with more than 40% of all ICU admissions receiving some form of transfusion therapy.[1] Patients with acute hemorrhage from trauma or gastrointestinal bleed, with severe coagulopathy, sepsis, and toxicologic syndromes may all require blood product administration. While blood products may confer benefit to the critically ill patient, the emergency physician and intensivist must also consider the potential risks of transfusion—which are numerous—when choosing to employ this therapy. This chapter reviews the indications and associated complications of the most commonly transfused blood products, namely packed red blood cells (PRBCs) and whole-blood derivatives such as fresh frozen plasma (FFP), cryoprecipitate, and platelets. Use of the synthetic antifibrinolytic tranexamic acid is also discussed.

INDICATIONS FOR BLOOD PRODUCT TRANSFUSION

Packed Red Blood Cells

The use of red blood cells in the critically ill patient has evolved in recent years. Prior to the Transfusion Requirements in Critical Care (TRICC) trial, PRBCs transfusion was used aggressively in patients with a hemoglobin (Hgb) concentration below 10 g/dL; this cutoff was based largely on physiologic and clinical assumptions and lacked significant evidentiary support.[2] The results of the TRICC trial and subsequent follow-up studies suggested a more restrictive threshold of 7 g/dL for PRBC transfusion. The TRICC trial was a multicenter randomized controlled trial (RCT) of 838 patients admitted to the ICU (without evidence of active bleeding) and randomized to a restrictive (Hgb goal 7–9) or liberal (Hgb goal 10–12) transfusion strategy. Enrolled patients were euvolemic and had Hgb levels of <9 within 72 hours. The primary outcome, 30-day mortality, was similar in the two groups; however, the restrictive group's 30-day mortality was significantly lower among a subset of less acutely ill patients (APACHE II scores = <20, 8.7% vs. 16.1%) as well as among patients older than 55 years. There was also a significant reduction in in-hospital mortality for the restrictive group (22.2% vs. 28.1%).

Exceptions to the restrictive transfusion strategy recommendation include patients with acute hemorrhage and hemodynamic instability; and septic patients with evidence of inadequate tissue oxygen delivery (guided by trauma and sepsis literature respectively).

The optimal transfusion threshold for patients with acute myocardial ischemia or unstable angina is unknown, as these patients have typically been excluded from these trials.[3] In a subgroup analysis of the TRICC trial, however, patients with active ischemic cardiac disease had better outcomes when a transfusion threshold of <10 g/dL was used.

Plasma Products: Fresh Frozen Plasma and Cryoprecipitate

Plasma products, including FFP and cryoprecipitate, represent the liquid portion of human blood that remains after cellular components such as red and white blood cells have been removed. Guidelines for plasma use in critically ill patients are poorly established due to a paucity of data. Based on clinical experience and biologic rationale, plasma transfusion is generally recommended in patients with inadequate hemostasis, particularly in those with known or suspected coagulation abnormalities. The current accepted indication for plasma is: any abnormality on coagulation tests (prothrombin time, international normalized ratio (INR), or partial thromboplastin time) in patients slated for invasive procedures carrying a high risk of bleeding complications; and severe coagulation abnormality in patents slated for invasive procedures carrying a low risk of bleeding complications.[4] Additionally, any patient with abnormal coagulation tests and life-threatening bleeding should receive FFP.

Fresh frozen plasma (FFP) is a plasma product that contains all coagulation factors in normal concentrations. In the average patient, 1 unit of FFP will raise coagulation factors by 5% to 8% and fibrinogen by 13 mg/dL. FFP is used to reverse severe coagulopathy or excessive anticoagulation resulting from warfarin use in patients with active bleeding or in need of immediate invasive procedures.[5] FFP is not effective at reversing minor elevations in the INR (1.3 to 1.8).[6]

Cryoprecipitate, also derived from plasma, contains fibrinogen, von Willebrand factor, factor VIII, and factor XIII. It is packaged in six concentrated units, each unit taken from a separate donor. Cryoprecipitate is indicated for patients with severe hypofibrinogenemia (<100 mg/dL) immediately prior to any invasive procedure. Its chief advantage is that it provides these factors in substantially less volume than an equivalent transfusion of FFP. Cryoprecipitate is not commonly used in patients with von Willebrand disease or hemophilia A (factor VIII deficiency), as other therapies, such as desmopressin (DDAVP) and concentrated factor VII, are more specifically targeted to these conditions.

Platelets

Platelet transfusion in the critically ill may be used to help stop or prevent bleeding in patients with thrombocytopenia. Current guidelines recommend platelet transfusions in patients with platelet counts <10,000/μL for the prevention of spontaneous bleeding; in patients with counts <50,000/μL with active bleeding or requiring invasive procedures; and in those with counts <100,000/μL with central nervous system (CNS) injury, major trauma, or requiring neurosurgical intervention.[7,8]

Tranexamic Acid

Tranexamic acid is a synthetic derivative of the amino acid lysine and an antifibrinolytic that inhibits the activation of plasminogen to plasmin. It is commonly used in surgeries with high risk of blood loss. Several recent studies have advocated its use in acute care

TABLE 30.1	Summary of Indications for Blood Product Transfusion
Packed red cells	• Hemoglobin concentration below 7 g/dL. (Some data suggest patients with active ischemic cardiac disease should have a threshold of below 10 g/dL)
Fresh frozen plasma and cryoprecipitate	• Any patient with any abnormality on coagulation tests (prothrombin time, international normalized ratio, or partial thromboplastin time) prior to invasive procedures carrying a high risk of bleeding complications or with current life-threatening bleeding • For those with severe coagulation abnormality prior to invasive procedures carrying a low risk of bleeding complications • Cryoprecipitate is indicated for patients with severe hypofibrinogenemia (<100 mg/dL) immediately prior to any invasive procedure
Platelets	• Platelet counts <10,000/μL for the prevention of spontaneous bleeding • Platelet counts below 50,000/μL with active bleeding or requiring invasive procedures • Platelet counts below 100,000/μL with CNS injury, major trauma, or requiring neurosurgical intervention

settings; data suggest that when given to trauma patients within 3 hours of acute injury, tranexamic acid confers a mortality benefit.[9–11] In the CRASH-2 study—an RCT of 20,211 adult trauma patients with, or at risk of, significant bleeding—patients received either tranexamic acid (loading dose 1 g over 10 minutes and then infusion of 1 g over 8 hours) or matching placebo. Tranexamic acid was associated with a 1.5% absolute reduction in mortality (14.5% vs. 16%) compared to placebo. A separately published but prespecified subgroup analysis demonstrated that early administration of tranexamic acid (within 1 hour of injury) was associated with greater reductions in death due to bleeding, while delayed administration (>3 hours from injury) was associated with increased bleeding deaths. All-cause mortality was reduced in the <1 hour and 1–3 hour strata, but not in the >3 hour stratum. Further studies are needed to clarify these results, as this trial did not specifically measure innate fibrinolytic activity of participants and lacked complete data in the subgroup of all-cause mortality.

Transfusion in Massive Hemorrhage

Several recent and ongoing studies advocate for a more balanced approach to the ratio of blood product transfusion in the acutely hemorrhaging patient, specifically in cases of hemorrhage due to trauma. Hemorrhaging patients lose red cells, platelets, and coagulation factors, so replacement with PRBCs alone can lead to a dilution of platelets and coagulation factors, blunting the effects of the clotting cascade. A more appropriate strategy in these patients is to replace red blood cells, platelets, and plasma simultaneously. The exact ratio of these products is the subject of ongoing clinical trials, but data suggest a ratio of 1:1:1 confers a survival benefit at 24 hours and 30 days (Table 30.1).[12–14]

COMPLICATIONS

Blood product transfusion is not without risk; however, adverse reactions with significant morbidity and mortality have steadily declined, due in large part to advances in screening techniques for infectious disease.[15] Transmission of serious infectious disease, once the most common cause of blood transfusion mortality, has been supplanted in frequency by transfusion-related acute lung injury (TRALI), transfusion-related circulatory overload (TACO), and transfusion-associated immunologic complications.

Transfusion-Transmitted Infection

Transfusion-transmitted infections have a variety of bacterial and viral etiologies. Platelet transfusions carry the highest risk of bacterial contamination because they are stored at room temperature. If bacteremia—which may present with typical findings of fever, rigors, tachycardia, and hypotension—is suspected, the transfusion should be stopped, and the patient and blood products broadly cultured and evaluated for an immunologic-related transfusion reaction (discussed below). HIV infection from blood transfusions has steadily declined, mostly because of donor behavior screening and sophisticated testing of blood products for HIV antibody and nucleic acid. However, HIV contamination may occur if the donor is tested during the window period of infection or is infected with a variant strain that eludes current assays. The risk of HIV transmission from transfusion is estimated to be 1 in 1.4 million units.[16]

Transmission of the hepatitis C virus via blood transfusion once accounted for 0.5% to 10% of HCV infections; now, with increasingly sensitive blood donor screening assays (including nucleic acid testing) and with behavioral screening, the transmission rate from transfusion is estimated to be 1 per 2 million units.[17]

Transfusion-Related Acute Lung Injury

Transfusion Related Acute Lung Injury (TRALI) is a rare but serious complication of blood transfusion. The diagnosis of TRALI is made in patients receiving transfusions who develop hypoxemia, fever, and bilateral infiltrate on chest radiograph within 2 to 6 hours of blood product transfusion. The condition must be determined not to be the result of circulatory overload or preexisting acute lung injury. TRALI is considered a form of acute respiratory distress syndrome (ARDS), caused when HLA antibodies in the donor serum trigger activation of the complement system and result in lung injury. Aggressive respiratory support is warranted in these patients and may include noninvasive positive pressure ventilation; most patients eventually require intubation and mechanical ventilation.[18,19] With appropriate supportive care, complete recovery is usually made within 24 to 48 hours.

Transfusion-Associated Circulatory Overload

Transfusion-Associated Circulatory Overload (TACO) occurs following large-volume blood transfusion and is more common in the elderly, children, and those with preexisting cardiac dysfunction. Clinical presentation is similar to TRALI and includes acute dyspnea and hypoxemia, but TACO is uniquely accompanied by hypertension, which can help distinguish the two entities. Additionally, B-type natriuretic peptide levels are likely to be elevated in TACO. Prevention is paramount and includes slow transfusion rates and smaller volumes of transfusion. TACO should be treated similarly to cardiogenic pulmonary edema, with noninvasive ventilatory support and diuresis.[20]

Immunologic Complications

Immunologic complications of blood transfusion include acute and delayed hemolytic reactions, febrile nonhemolytic transfusion reactions (FNHTR), transfusion-associated graft versus host disease (TA-GvHD) and allergic reactions.

Hemolytic reactions are rare, and occur in <0.01% of transfusions. These reactions, caused most often by ABO-incompatible blood, may be immediate or delayed. Immediate reaction is characterized by fevers, hypotension, pain, and oliguria; delayed reactions by fever, Coombs-positive hemolytic anemia, jaundice, and lack of expected rise in Hgb levels. Treatment includes immediate cessation of transfusion, aggressive hydration, supportive care, and blood bank notification.

FNHTRs, caused by the presence of leukocyte debris and cytokines in the donated blood, are more common and occur in up to 7% of red blood cell transfusions.[21] Patients will present with a spectrum of symptoms including fevers, pain at the infusion site, hypotension, mental status changes, and bleeding diathesis. Laboratory tests used to differentiate hemolytic reaction from nonhemolytic reaction include a peripheral blood smear, haptoglobin, and Coombs' testing. Mainstays of therapy include acetaminophen and diphenhydramine. In patients who have had FNHTRs, future transfusions require use of leukoreduced blood specimens.

TA-GvHD is a rare and commonly fatal complication of blood transfusion.[22] TA-GvHD results when donor lymphocytes mount an immune response to the blood recipient's antigen presenting tissues. TA-GvHD is typically limited to immunosuppressed patients (e.g., Hodgkin disease and leukemia, but notably not with HIV), and presents with dysfunction of the liver, skin, and bone marrow 4 to 30 days following blood transfusion. Since no effective therapy exists, prevention in susceptible patients—achieved by use of leukoreduced or irradiated blood products—is essential.[17]

Allergic reactions are also common in blood product transfusion and do not require previous sensitization to blood products. Like all allergic reactions, they range from urticaria to bronchospasm to anaphylaxis, and should be treated with the immediate cessation of transfusion and antihistamines, steroids, volume replacement, and, when necessary, epinephrine.

Citrate Toxicity

Citrate toxicity may occur following large-volume blood transfusion. Citrate is an anticoagulant added to preserved PRBCs in order to chelate calcium and prevent clotting. Large-volume infusions can cause a metabolic alkalosis from citrate metabolism, as well as a reduction in ionized calcium resulting from calcium complex formation. Symptoms of severe hypocalcemia include tetany, cardiac dysrhythmias, and hypotension, and require treatment with calcium gluconate or calcium chloride. Importantly, if required, calcium therapy should be administered in a separate vein from the transfusion line to prevent clotting.

CONCLUSION

Transfusion therapy, while commonplace in the critically ill population, is not without its accompanying risks. Adherence to established guidelines for transfusion enables appropriate patient care and minimization of adverse outcome.

LITERATURE TABLE

TRIAL	DESIGN	RESULT
Hébert et al., *N Engl J Med.* 1999[2]; TRICC	RCT of 838 patients admitted to ICU without evidence of active bleeding, randomized to a restrictive transfusion strategy (transfusion to maintain hemoglobin >7 g/dL) vs. a liberal strategy (transfusion to maintain hemoglobin ≥10 g/dL)	The restrictive transfusion strategy was associated with decreased rates of in-hospital mortality. This benefit was highest among the less critically ill patients (APACHE II score ≤20) and <55 y old. In the restrictive group, there was a trend toward improved outcomes in patients with active cardiac ischemia
Shakur et al., *Lancet.* 2010[9];	RCT of 20,211 adult trauma patients with, or at risk of, significant bleeding received either tranexamic acid (loading dose 1 g over 10 min then infusion of 1 g over 8 h) or matching placebo	Tranexamic acid was associated with a 1.5% absolute reduction in mortality (14.5% vs. 16%) compared to placebo. A separately published but prespecified subgroup analysis demonstrated that early administration of tranexamic acid (within 1 h of injury) was associated with greater reductions in death due to bleeding, while delayed administration (>3 h from injury) was associated with increased bleeding deaths. All-cause mortality was reduced in the <1 h and 1–3 h strata, but not in the >3 h stratum

REFERENCES

1. Corwin HL, Gettinger A, Pearl RG, et al. The CRIT Study: anemia and blood transfusion in the critically ill—current clinical practice in the United States. *Crit Care Med.* 2004;32:39.
2. Hébert PC, Wells G, Blajchman MA, et al. A multicenter, randomized, controlled clinical trial of transfusion requirements in critical care. Transfusion Requirements in Critical Care Investigators, Canadian Critical Care Trials Group. *N Engl J Med.* 1999;340:409.
3. Napolitano LM, Kurek S, Luchette FA, et al. Clinical practice guideline: red blood cell transfusion in adult trauma and critical care. *Crit Care Med.* 2009;37:3124.
4. Yang L, Stanworth S, Hopewell S, et al. Is fresh-frozen plasma clinically effective? An update of a systematic review of randomized controlled trials. *Transfusion.* 2012;52:1673.
5. Gajic O, Dzik WH, Toy P. Fresh frozen plasma and platelet transfusion for nonbleeding patients in the intensive care unit: benefit or harm? *Crit Care Med.* 2006;34:S170.
6. Abdel-Wahab OI, Healy B, Dzik WH. Effect of fresh-frozen plasma transfusion on prothrombin time and bleeding in patients with mild coagulation abnormalities. *Transfusion.* 2006;46:1279–1285.
7. Fresh-Frozen Plasma, Cryoprecipitate, and Platelets Administration Practice Guidelines Development Task Force of the College of American Pathologists. Practice parameter for the use of fresh-frozen plasma, cryoprecipitate, and platelets. *JAMA.* 1994;271:777.
8. Slichter SJ. Evidence-based platelet transfusion guidelines. *Hematology Am Soc Hematol Educ Program.* 2007:172–178.
9. Shakur H, et al. Effects of tranexamic acid on death, vascular occlusive events, and blood transfusion in trauma patients with significant haemorrhage. *Lancet.* 2010;376(9734):23–32.
10. Roberts I, et al. The importance of early treatment with tranexamic acid in bleeding trauma patients: an exploratory analysis of the CRASH-2 randomised controlled trial. *Lancet.* 2011;377(9771):1096–1010.
11. Morrison JJ, et al. Military Application of Tranexamic Acid in Trauma Emergency Resuscitation (MATTERs) Study. *Arch Surg.* 2012;147(2):113–119.
12. Borgman MA, Spinella PC, Perkins JG, et al. The ratio of blood products transfused affects mortality in patients receiving massive transfusions at a combat support hospital. *J Trauma.* 2007;63:805.
13. Holcomb JB, Wade CE, Michalek JE, et al. Increased plasma and platelet to red blood cell ratios improves outcome in 466 massively transfused civilian trauma patients. *Ann Surg.* 2008;248:447.
14. Shaz BH, Dente CJ, Nicholas J, et al. Increased number of coagulation products in relationship to red blood cell products transfused improves mortality in trauma patients. *Transfusion.* 2010;50:493.
15. Vamvakas EC, Blajchman MA. Transfusion-related mortality: the ongoing risks of allogeneic blood transfusion and the available strategies for their prevention. *Blood.* 2009;113:3406.

16. Zou S, Dorsey KA, Notari EP, et al. Prevalence, incidence, and residual risk of human immunodeficiency virus and hepatitis C virus infections among United States blood donors since the introduction of nucleic acid testing. *Transfusion.* 2010;50:1495.
17. www.cdc.gov/hepatitis/HCV/index.htm. Accessed September 16, 2013.
18. Kleinman S, Caulfield T, Chan P, et al. Toward an understanding of transfusion-related acute lung injury: statement of a consensus panel. *Transfusion.* 2004;44:1774.
19. Toy P, Popovsky MA, Abraham E, et al. Transfusion-related acute lung injury: definition and review. *Crit Care Med.* 2005;33:721.
20. Li G, Rachmale S, Kojicic M, et al. Incidence and transfusion risk factors for transfusion-associated circulatory overload among medical intensive care unit patients. *Transfusion.* 2011;51:338.
21. Raghavan M, Marik PE. Anemia, allogenic blood transfusion, and immunomodulation in the critically ill. *Chest.* 2005;127:295.
22. Fast LD. Developments in the prevention of transfusion-associated graft-versus-host disease. *Br J Haematol.* 2012;158(5):583–588.

SECTION 8

Sepsis and Septic Shock

31

Sepsis

Michael C. Scott and Michael E. Winters

BACKGROUND

Approximately 650,000 cases of sepsis are diagnosed each year in the United States, making it one of the most common causes of critical illness encountered by the emergency physician.[1] Despite significant advances in management, more than 200,000 patients die annually from this devastating disease.[2] It is therefore imperative that the emergency physician be expert in the recognition and treatment of patients with sepsis, severe sepsis, and septic shock.

DEFINITIONS

The most widely used definition of sepsis is the presence of infection (presumed or confirmed) combined with signs of a systemic inflammatory response.[3] Traditionally, an inflammatory response is diagnosed by the presence of at least two of the four criteria for the systemic inflammatory response syndrome (SIRS). Recently, updated international guidelines for the management of severe sepsis and septic shock expand upon the traditional SIRS criteria (Table 31.1). The clinical spectrum of sepsis includes patients with severe sepsis and septic shock. Severe sepsis is defined as sepsis with evidence of organ dysfunction or tissue hypoperfusion (Table 31.2).[3] The simplest and most objective marker of the onset of severe sepsis is an elevated lactate level. Lactate levels >4 mmol/L suggest significant tissue hypoperfusion and warrant aggressive resuscitation. Although an elevated lactate level is not specific to sepsis, it has been used as an inclusion criterion for severe sepsis in the majority of studies of patients with severe sepsis or septic shock. Septic shock is defined as the presence of arterial hypotension despite adequate fluid resuscitation, commonly defined as at least 20 to 30 mL/kg of a crystalloid solution.[3]

TABLE 31.1 Criteria for Sepsis

Presumed or documented infection plus *some* of the following:

General
- Temperature >38.3°C or <36°C
- Heart rate >90 beats/min (or more than two standard deviations above normal rate for age)
- Tachypnea
- Altered mental status
- Hyperglycemia (>140 mg/dL) in the absence of diabetes

Inflammatory Variables
- WBC count >12,000 cells/μL or <4,000 cells/μL
- Normal WBC count with >10% immature forms
- C-reactive protein more than two standard deviations above the normal value
- Procalcitonin more than two standard deviations above the normal value

WBC, white blood cell.
Modified from Dellinger RP, Levy MM, Rhodes A, et al. Surviving Sepsis Campaign: International Guidelines for Management of Severe Sepsis and Septic Shock: 2012. *Crit Care Med.* 2013;41:580–637.

HISTORY AND PHYSICAL EXAM

The clinical presentation of patients with sepsis depends on the source of infection. For patients with suspected sepsis, the history and physical exam should be directed toward the most common sources of infection (Table 31.3). Patients with sepsis do not always present with overt signs of arterial hypotension and shock. Many, notably the elderly, will present with more subtle signs of illness, including altered mental status, fatigue, and lethargy. A complete physical exam, including assessment of mental status, a thorough skin examination, and complete neurologic examination, should be performed in any patient with suspected infection. Septic shock is a form of distributive shock. Patients in the early stages of this illness may have warm, seemingly well-perfused extremities rather than the cool, dusky appearance of patients with other forms of circulatory shock.

TABLE 31.2 Markers of Severe Sepsis (Sepsis-Induced Organ Dysfunction and Tissue Hypoperfusion)

Hemodynamic Variable
- Arterial hypotension (SBP < 90 mm Hg, MAP < 70 mm Hg, or SBP decrease >40 mm Hg from the patient's baseline)

Organ Dysfunction Variables
- Acute lung injury
  - PaO_2/FiO_2 < 250 in the absence of pneumonia
  - PaO_2/FiO2 < 200 in the presence of pneumonia
- Acute oliguria (urine output <0.5 mL/kg/h for at least 2 h despite IVFs)
- Acute kidney injury (creatinine > 2.0 mg/dL)
- Thrombocytopenia (platelets < 100,000 cells/μL)
- Hyperbilirubinemia (total bilirubin > 2 mg/dL)
- Coagulopathy (INR > 1.5)

Tissue Hypoperfusion Variable
- Elevated lactate (above upper limits of laboratory normal)

SBP, systolic blood pressure; MAP, mean arterial pressure; IVFs, intravenous fluids; INR, international normalized ratio.
Modified from Dellinger RP, Levy MM, Rhodes A, et al. Surviving sepsis campaign: international guidelines for management of severe sepsis and septic shock: 2012. *Crit Care Med.* 2013;41:580–637.

TABLE 31.3 Most Common Sources of Infection in Sepsis (*in Descending Order*)

1. Pulmonary system (pneumonia, lung abscess)
2. Genitourinary system (urinary tract infection, pyelonephritis)
3. Gastrointestinal system (cholecystitis, appendicitis, abscess, colitis, diverticulitis)
4. Skin and soft tissue (cellulitis, necrotizing fasciitis, abscess)
5. Indwelling intravascular devices (peripherally inserted central venous catheters)

DIAGNOSTIC EVALUATION

Initial laboratory and radiographic testing should be directed toward the most likely source of infection (Table 31.3). Current guidelines recommend obtaining at least two sets of blood cultures before initiating antimicrobial therapy, provided that the time needed to draw these cultures does not delay the initiation of therapy more than 45 minutes.[3] For patients with indwelling catheters, at least one blood culture should be obtained from the vascular device.[3] Obtaining timely blood cultures is essential for identifying the pathogenic organism and narrowing the spectrum of antimicrobial therapy. Additional blood samples should be sent for a complete blood count, a comprehensive metabolic panel, a coagulation profile, serum lactate measurement, venous blood gas analysis to determine pH, and central venous oxygen saturation if an internal jugular or subclavian central line has been placed. In addition to blood work, urinalysis and urine culture should also be obtained in any patient with suspected sepsis.

Radiographic studies should be obtained to determine if source control of an infection is required. Because the pulmonary system is the most common source of infection in patients with sepsis, unless there is another clear location of infection, a chest radiograph is essential. Additional testing, such as computed tomography or ultrasound, may be obtained based on the suspected location of infection. In critically ill patients without an obvious source of infection, an intra-abdominal infection is likely, and diagnostic testing with computed tomography or ultrasound should be considered.

MANAGEMENT GUIDELINES

Management of the critically ill ED patient with sepsis includes early administration of antimicrobial therapy; quantitative, protocol-guided hemodynamic resuscitation; and critical adjunctive therapy, including the use of corticosteroids, blood product transfusion, glucose control, and mechanical ventilation. The recently updated international guidelines for the management of patients with severe sepsis and septic shock are summarized in the following sections.[3]

Antimicrobial Therapy and Source Control

Early administration of appropriate antibiotics is paramount to improving survival in patients with severe sepsis or septic shock. In 2006, a landmark study demonstrated a 7.6% decrease in mortality for every hour delay in administering effective antimicrobial therapy for patients with septic shock.[4] As a result of this study and several others demonstrating similar findings, current guidelines recommend that effective antimicrobial therapy be administered within 1 hour after the recognition of septic shock and severe sepsis.[3] Initial antimicrobial therapy should be broad spectrum and effective against the most likely causative organism. When selecting empiric antimicrobial medications, the emergency physician must take into account the site of infection, local hospital and community susceptibility patterns, the presence of comorbid illnesses, recent antibiotic exposure (within the previous 3 months), and the patient's medical history.[3] Despite the fact that many patients with severe sepsis or septic shock have evidence of acute kidney injury (AKI), all patients should receive an initial full loading dose of antimicrobial medications.[3] For neutropenic patients or those with multidrug-resistant organisms, combination antimicrobial therapy (i.e., a beta-lactam antibiotic and either an aminoglycoside or fluoroquinolone) is recommended.[3] Combination therapy is also recommended for patients with septic shock and respiratory failure.[3]

A confirmed nidus of infection (e.g., intra-abdominal abscess, empyema, infected device, or necrotizing soft tissue infection) may be resistant to antimicrobial agents. In these cases, source control is essential and should be undertaken within 12 hours of diagnosis, provided the patient can safely undergo the required procedure.[3]

Protocol-Guided Hemodynamic Resuscitation

In 2001, a landmark study demonstrated significantly reduced mortality with use of a protocol-guided resuscitation with quantitative endpoints, delivered to patients with sepsis-induced hypotension within 6 hours of their presentation to an emergency department.[5] The hemodynamic targets of their study were central venous pressure (CVP), mean arterial pressure (MAP), urine output, and central venous oxygen saturation ($ScvO_2$). While the findings of the study are still being debated, current guidelines have remained consistent in their recommended hemodynamic targets (Table 31.4) within the first 6 hours of therapy for patients with sepsis-induced hypotension.[3]

Though current guidelines recommend protocol-guided therapy for patients with severe sepsis and septic shock, a recently published multi-center trial has questioned the utility of this approach. The ProCESS trial[6] was a randomized, controlled, multi-center study designed to evaluate three treatment groups in patients with severe sepsis and septic shock: 1) protocol-based early goal-directed therapy (identical to the original EGDT protocol), 2) protocol-based standard therapy (derived from current literature and expert consensus), and 3) standard therapy (no predetermined resuscitation protocol). In the standard therapy group, care was left to the discretion of the treating physician. Importantly, investigators found no difference in 60-day, 90-day, and 1-year mortality

TABLE 31.4 Initial Resuscitation Targets

- Central venous pressure 8–12 mm Hg
- Mean arterial pressure ≥65 mm Hg
- Urine output ≥0.5 mL/kg/h
- Central venous oxygen saturation ≥70%

Modified from Dellinger RP, Levy MM, Rhodes A, et al. Surviving sepsis campaign: international guidelines for management of severe sepsis and septic shock: 2012. *Crit Care Med.* 2013;41:580–637.

between the three groups. While many clinicians have cited this trial to debate the utility of early goal-directed therapy, it is important to note that ProCESS was carried out in large, academic centers throughout the United States. These centers were required to adhere to the non-resuscitative aspects of care recommended by the Surviving Sepsis Campaign (e.g., prompt administration of antibiotics). Furthermore, baseline mortality was significant different between these two trials. Given these limitations, it is unclear whether "standard therapy" can be expected to be the same at centers outside of those involved in the ProCESS trial. Pending the publication of two additional trials (ARISE and PROMISE), protocol-based resuscitation should focus on early identification of patients with sepsis, early antibiotics, adequate fluid administration, and an appropriate assessment of the adequacy of circulation.

The continuous assessment of tissue perfusion is another essential component of the initial resuscitation of septic patients. In recent years, significant emphasis has been placed on global markers of tissue perfusion, namely, serum lactate and $ScvO_2$. Current guidelines continue to recommend continuous or intermittent monitoring of $ScvO_2$ as a marker of tissue perfusion[3] using either a subclavian or internal jugular central venous catheter. Depending on the patient and resources available to the emergency physician, central venous access may not be feasible. In these patients, guidelines recommend monitoring serial serum lactate values.[3] In patients with elevated values (i.e., lactate >4 mmol/L), resuscitation should target the normalization of serum lactate. Currently, there is no consensus on the optimal interval to measure serial lactate values. It is the authors' opinion that serum lactate (venous or arterial) should be measured every 2 to 3 hours in the septic patient.

Intravenous Fluids

The administration of intravenous fluids to restore intravascular volume is central to the hemodynamic resuscitation of the septic patient. Currently, isotonic crystalloid solutions are the fluid of choice for patients with severe sepsis or septic shock.[3] For patients with sepsis-induced hypoperfusion, a minimum of 30 mL/kg of crystalloids should be administered.[3] While there is no evidence that clearly demonstrates the superiority of a particular crystalloid fluid, there is mounting evidence of the harm of normal saline. The supra-physiologic concentration of chloride in normal saline has been associated with increased kidney injury and need for renal replacement therapy (RRT).[7] Recent literature has focused on the use of "balanced" fluids (e.g., lactated Ringer's, Plasma-Lyte) for resuscitation in sepsis, particularly in patients with significant acidosis.[8] When large amounts of crystalloid solution are required, guidelines allow for the consideration of albumin. The addition of albumin to crystalloid fluid resuscitation is based on the results of the 2004 SAFE trial, in which the use of albumin in a subgroup of patients with severe sepsis demonstrated a trend toward an improved mortality rate.[9] Hydroxyethyl starch solutions are not recommended as a result of several studies demonstrating their harmful effects.[3,10–12]

Current guidelines recommend titration of intravenous fluids to achieve a CVP of 8 to 12 mm Hg—with a higher goal of 12 to 15 mm Hg for those receiving mechanical ventilation—as a physiologic target for resuscitation in patients with severe sepsis or septic shock.[3] CVP, however, is a poor marker of fluid status and responsiveness in the critically ill patient. Recent studies have focused on the use of dynamic markers of fluid responsiveness, such as pulse pressure variation, stroke volume variation, passive leg raise, and respirophasic changes in the diameter of the inferior vena cava as measured by bedside ultrasound. While no one dynamic technique has been proven superior, most provide better assessment of fluid responsiveness than the CVP. For this reason, current guidelines do allow for the use of dynamic indices to guide intravenous fluid therapy.[3]

Vasopressors

When intravenous fluid therapy fails to maintain adequate arterial perfusion pressure (MAP ≥ 65 mm Hg), a vasopressor medication should be administered. Historically, norepinephrine and dopamine have been the most common first-line agents. However, recent publications suggest that dopamine is associated with a higher rate of tachyarrhythmias and may result in increased mortality when given to patients in cardiogenic shock.[13] A subsequent related meta-analysis demonstrated that for patients in septic shock, dopamine is associated with increased mortality when compared with norepinephrine.[14] As a result of these reports, norepinephrine is recommended as the initial vasopressor agent of choice for patients with fluid-refractory septic shock.[3] When an additional vasopressor agent is required to maintain sufficient perfusion pressure, either epinephrine or vasopressin is recommended.[3] Vasopressin should not be used as a single agent. Rather, it should be used in combination with norepinephrine and maintained at a stable dose of 0.03 to 0.04 units/min. Because of its higher incidence of tachyarrhythmias and association with an increased mortality rate, dopamine should be avoided, except in patients with absolute or relative bradycardia.[3] Phenylephrine is another popular vasopressor used to maintain adequate perfusion pressure in patients with a number of critical illnesses, especially given its presumed decreased risk of adverse events compared to other vasopressor medications when given peripherally. However, its use in patients with septic shock is not recommended, except as salvage therapy or in those with documented high cardiac output and low MAP.[3]

Inotropes

Inotropic therapy should be considered in the presence of myocardial dysfunction (i.e., elevated cardiac filling pressures with a low cardiac output) or when evidence suggests persistent tissue hypoperfusion (i.e., rising or unchanged serum lactate, low $ScvO_2$) despite augmentation of intravascular volume and optimization of MAP. With studies suggesting the rate of sepsis-induced myocardial dysfunction to be as high as 44%,[15] the availability of rapid assessment with bedside ultrasound allows the early institution of appropriate inotropic therapy. Dobutamine is the initial inotropic agent of choice, up to a maximum dose of 20 μg/kg/min. Titration to a predefined, supranormal level of cardiac output is not recommended.[3]

Glucocorticoids

Research findings differ as to the effect of glucocorticoids on mortality rates in patients with sepsis. Current guidelines recommend low-dose glucocorticoids (hydrocortisone 200 mg/d) in patients with persistent hypotension despite optimal fluid and vasopressor therapy.[3] This recommendation is based on the drug's benefit in earlier reversal of shock. Continuous (rather than intermittent) administration of hydrocortisone is recommended to decrease the incidence of hypernatremia and hyperglycemia, both of which are associated with increased morbidity and mortality. A patient's response to an adrenocorticotropic hormone stimulation test has not been found to be predictive of his/her response to glucocorticoids; therefore, this test is not recommended.

Blood Transfusion

In the early goal-directed therapy (EGDT) protocol, administration of blood transfusion to a goal hemoglobin of 10 g/dL was an important step in the management of patients with persistent tissue hypoperfusion (low $ScvO_2$) despite achieving the goals for CVP and MAP.[5] The use of this transfusion threshold has become one of the most controversial components of the protocol. Currently, there are several ongoing trials evaluating individual components of the EGDT protocol including blood transfusion. The results of these studies are not available at the time of this publication. While the optimal hemoglobin during early resuscitation of the patient with severe sepsis or septic shock has not been clearly defined, it is clear that blood transfusions in the critically ill patient can be harmful. As a result, guidelines recommend maintaining a hemoglobin concentration between 7 and 9 g/dL in patients who have been resuscitated and no longer have evidence of tissue hypoperfusion.[3] It may be reasonable to target a higher hemoglobin level for those with active myocardial ischemia or hemorrhage.

Mechanical Ventilation

Patients with severe sepsis and septic shock are at significant risk for developing acute respiratory distress syndrome (ARDS). Guidelines strongly recommend the use of low tidal volume ventilation in patients who have sepsis-induced ARDS and who require mechanical ventilation. Specifically, an initial tidal volume of 6 mL/kg of predicted body weight should be used, and plateau pressures should be kept under 30 cm H_2O.[3]

NEW DIRECTIONS

Historically, the pathophysiology of severe sepsis and septic shock was thought to result primarily from inflammatory mediators that, on a macrovascular level, cause a maldistribution of blood flow, resulting in impaired tissue oxygen delivery. Recent research, focusing on microcirculatory and mitochondrial dysfunction, suggests that it is, rather, the ability to increase oxygen consumption in response to increased oxygen delivery that best predicts which patients with septic shock will survive and which will not.[16]

Microcirculatory dysfunction in sepsis is thought to result from two distinct mechanisms. First, sepsis produces significant heterogeneity in blood flow even within a particular tissue, organ, or vascular bed. This maldistribution at the microcirculatory level can result in significant cellular hypoxia, despite a seemingly normal systemic perfusion pressure. Second, sepsis is associated with endothelial damage. Whether due to the direct effect of select microorganisms or to inflammatory mediators, endothelial dysfunction inhibits the ability of oxygen to move from the vessel lumen to the tissues. The result is a relative hypoxia despite adequate blood flow. Endothelial dysfunction has been the target of recent sepsis research, though no promising therapies have yet proved beneficial.

Markers of microcirculatory dysfunction, such as elevated lactate levels, have been shown to correlate with poor outcomes in patients with sepsis.[17,18] It also appears that microvascular resuscitation (i.e., increased capillary recruitment) correlates with improved global perfusion (e.g., decreased lactate levels) despite little to no improvement in macrovascular assessments (e.g., improved MAP). These results have led to investigations of a variety of microcirculatory monitoring and resuscitative techniques.[19,20]

Evidence indicates that sepsis also results in mitochondrial dysfunction,[21] leading to impaired oxidative phosphorylation. This results in "cytopathic hypoxia," the inability to use delivered oxygen and produce adenosine triphosphate. Sepsis-induced mitochondrial dysfunction is another emerging area of study.[22]

CONCLUSION

The past decade has seen great leaps forward in the management of sepsis, although this disease continues to impose a tremendous burden in terms of mortality rates. Many of these advances apply directly to the emergency physician's management of these patients. It is vital that emergency physicians continue to embrace their role as the frontline managers of this deadly disease.

LITERATURE TABLE

TRIAL	DESIGN	RESULT
Dellinger et al., *Crit Care Med.* 2013[3] Surviving Sepsis Campaign Guidelines	Consensus committee of 68 international experts representing 30 international organizations, providing an update of existing guidelines for the management of severe sepsis and septic shock	Developed key recommendations and suggestions based on existing evidence for the management of patients with severe sepsis and septic shock
Kumar et al., *Crit Care Med.* 2006[4]	Multicenter retrospective cohort study of 2,154 patients with septic shock, who received antimicrobial therapy after the onset of shock; evaluated the relationship between timing of appropriate antimicrobial administration and survival	Each hour delay to initiation of appropriate antimicrobials in the first 6 h after shock increased the mortality rate by a mean of 7.6%. Adjusted OR for death of 1.119/h of delay to appropriate therapy (95% CI, 1.103–1.136, $p < 0.001$). Delay to appropriate antimicrobial therapy was more strongly associated with outcome than APACHE II score at admission or amount of fluids received in the first hour of hypotension
Rivers et al., *N Engl J Med.* 2001[5]	Single-center, prospective, randomized controlled trial of 263 patients with severe sepsis or septic shock; compared standard care with early goal-directed therapy for the first 6 h prior to admission to an intensive care unit	The early goal-directed therapy group had a 16% absolute reduction in in-hospital mortality compared with the control group (30.5% vs. 46.5%, $p = 0.009$)
Yealy et al., *N Engl J Med.* 2014[6] ProCESS	Multi-center, randomized controlled trial comparing protocol-based Early Goal Directed Therapy, protocol-based standard therapy, and usual care in treatment of severe sepsis and septic shock	No difference in 60-day in-hospital mortality between the three groups (21.0% in the EGDT group vs. 18.2% in the protocol-based standard therapy vs. 18.9% in the usual care group, $p = 0.83$ for the two protocol-based groups compared to usual care)
Yunos et al., *JAMA.* 2012[7]	Prospective, sequential period single-center pilot study; during study period, patients received chloride rich fluids (0.9% saline, 4% succinylated gelatin solution, or 4% albumin solution) only given with attending-specialist approval)	During study period (limitation of chloride-rich fluids), lower incidence of AKI (8.4% vs. 14%, $p < 0.001$) and use of RRT (6.3% vs. 10%, $p = 0.005$) compared with control

(*Continued*)

LITERATURE TABLE (*Continued*)

TRIAL	DESIGN	RESULT
Raghunathan et al., *Crit Care Med.* 2014[8]	Retrospective cohort study comparing ICU patients with sepsis treated with "balanced" crystalloid solutions (e.g., lactated Ringer's) and "no-balanced" fluids (e.g., normal saline)	Group treated with balanced solutions had significantly lower in-hospital mortality (19.6% vs. 22.8%, relative risk, 0.86; 95% CI, 0.78–0.94)
Finfer et al., *N Engl J Med.* 2004[9] SAFE	Multicenter, prospective, randomized, double-blind trial of 6,997 patients; compared the use of saline with albumin for fluid resuscitation of ICU patients	No significant differences in primary (28-day mortality, RR 0.99, 95% CI, 0.91–1.09, $p = 0.87$) or secondary outcomes between the two groups. However, predefined subgroup analysis of patients with severe sepsis suggested a trend toward improved survival with albumin (absolute mortality reduction of 4.6%, $p = 0.09$)
Myburgh et al., *N Engl J Med.* 2012[10] CHEST	Multicenter, randomized controlled trial comparing use of 6% hydroxyethyl starch (molecular weight 130 kD) in 0.9 % normal saline to 0.9% normal saline alone for fluid resuscitation in 7,000 ICU patients	No significant difference in mortality between hydroxyethyl starch and normal saline group (18% vs. 17%, $p = 0.26$), but higher rate of need for renal replacement therapy in starch group (7% vs. 5.8%, $p = 0.04$)
Perner et al., *N Engl J Med.* 2012[11]	Multicenter, randomized controlled trial comparing the use of Ringer acetate to hydroxyethyl starch 130/0.42 for fluid resuscitation in 804 ICU patients with severe sepsis	Ringer acetate group had lower 90-d mortality (43% vs. 51%, $p = 0.03$) and lower rates of renal replacement therapy (16% vs. 22%, $p = 0.04$) compared to hydroxyethyl starch group
DeBacker et al., *Crit Care Med.* 2012[14]	Meta-analysis of trials comparing outcomes after the use of dopamine vs. norepinephrine in patients with septic shock	In pooled randomized trials and in observational trials lacking heterogeneity, dopamine use was associated with increased risk of death (RR 1.23, 95% CI, 1.05–1.43, $p < 0.01$ in observational trials, RR 1.12, CI 1.01–1.2, $p = 0.035$ in randomized trials). In the two trials reporting rate of arrhythmias, dopamine was associated with an increased rate of arrhythmias (RR 2.34, 95% CI, 1.46–3.77, $p = 0.001$)
Sprung et al., *N Engl J Med.* 2008[23] CORTICUS	Multicenter, prospective, randomized, double-blind study of 499 patients; compared the use of hydrocortisone (50 mg IV every 6 h) with placebo	No difference in mortality rate between the two groups (39.2% vs. 36.1%, $p = 0.69$). The hydrocortisone group had faster resolution of shock compared with placebo but higher rates of superinfection. Response or lack of response to corticotropin stimulation had no significant effect on response to hydrocortisone
Russell et al., *N Engl J Med.* 2008[24] VASST	Multicenter, prospective, randomized, double-blind study of 778 patients with septic shock requiring at least 5 μg/min of norepinephrine; compared the addition of low-dose vasopressin with the addition of norepinephrine	No difference in mortality rates between the two groups (35.4% vs. 39.3%, $p = 0.26$ for 28-day mortality). The vasopressin group saw a rapid decrease in the total norepinephrine dose while maintaining the same MAP. The norepinephrine group showed a trend toward higher rate of cardiac arrest; the vasopressin group showed a trend toward higher rate of digital ischemia
Jones et al., *JAMA.* 2010[25]	Multicenter, randomized, noninferiority trial of 300 patients; compared central venous oxygen saturation to lactate clearance as the third resuscitation goal in patients with severe sepsis and evidence of hypoperfusion or septic shock	Use of lactate clearance as a treatment goal was found to be noninferior to $ScvO_2$ (mortality rates of 17% and 23%, respectively)

CI, confidence interval; RR, relative risk.

REFERENCES

1. Jawad I, Lukšić I, Rafnsson SB. Assessing available information on the burden of sepsis: global estimates of incidence, prevalence and mortality. *J Glob Health.* 2012;2:10404.
2. Angus DC, Linde-Zwirble WT, Lidicker J, et al. Epidemiology of severe sepsis in the United States: analysis of incidence, outcome, and associated costs of care. *Crit Care Med.* 2001;29:1303–1310.
3. Dellinger RP, Levy MM, Rhodes A, et al. Surviving Sepsis Campaign: International Guidelines for Management of Severe Sepsis and Septic Shock: 2012. *Crit Care Med.* 2013;41:580–637.
4. Kumar A, Roberts D, Wood KE, et al. Duration of hypotension before initiation of effective antimicrobial therapy is the critical determinant of survival in human septic shock. *Crit Care Med.* 2006;34:1589–1596.
5. Rivers E, Nguyen B, Havstad S, et al. Early goal-directed therapy in the treatment of severe sepsis and septic shock. *N Engl J Med.* 2001;345:1368–1377.
6. ProCESS Investigators, Yealy DM, Kellum JA, Huang DT, et al. A randomized trial of protocol-based care for early septic shock. *N Engl J Med.* 2014;370(18):1683–1693.
7. Yunos NM, Bellomo R, Hegarty C, et al. Association between a chloride-liberal vs chloride-restrictive intravenous fluid administration strategy and kidney injury in critically ill adults. *JAMA.* 2012;308(15):1566–1572.
8. Raghunathan K, Shaw A, Nathanson B, et al. Association between the choice of IV crystalloid and in-hospital mortality among critically ill adults with sepsis. *Crit Care Med* 2014; Mar 26, epub ahead of print.
9. Finfer S, Bellomo R, Boyce N, et al. A comparison of albumin and saline for fluid resuscitation in the intensive care unit. *N Engl J Med.* 2004;350:2247–2256.
10. Myburgh JA, Finfer S, Bellomo R, et al. Hydroxyethyl starch or saline for fluid resuscitation in intensive care. *N Engl J Med.* 2012;367:1901–1911.
11. Perner A, Haase N, Guttormsen AB, et al. Hydroxyethyl starch 130/0.42 versus Ringer's acetate in severe sepsis. *N Engl J Med.* 2012;12;367:124–134.
12. Guidet B, Martinet O, Boulain T, et al. Assessment of hemodynamic efficacy and safety of 6% hydroxyethylstarch 130/0.4 vs. 0.9% NaCl fluid replacement in patients with severe sepsis: the CRYSTMAS study. *Crit Care* 2012;16:R94.
13. De Backer D, Biston P, Devriendt J, et al. Comparison of dopamine and norepinephrine in the treatment of shock. *N Engl J Med.* 2010;362:779–789.
14. De Backer D, Aldecoa C, Njimi H, et al. Dopamine versus norepinephrine in the treatment of septic shock: a meta-analysis. *Crit Care Med.* 2012;40:725–730.
15. Charpentier J, Luyt CE, Vinsonneau C, et al. Brain natriuretic peptide: a marker of myocardial dysfunction and prognosis during severe sepsis. *Crit Care Med.* 2004;32:660–665.
16. Hayes MA, Timmins AS, Yau EH, et al. Oxygen transport patterns in patient with sepsis syndrome or septic shock: influence of treatment and relationship to outcome. *Crit Care Med.* 1997;25:926–936.
17. Sakr Y, Dubois MJ, De Backer D, et al. Persistent microcirculatory alterations are associated with organ failure and death in patients with septic shock. *Crit Care Med.* 2004;32:1825–1831.
18. Trzeciak S, Dellinger RP, Parrillo JE, et al. Early microcirculatory perfusion derangements in patients with severe sepsis and septic shock: relationship to hemodynamics, oxygen transport, and survival. *Ann Emerg Med.* 2007;49:88–98.
19. De Backer D, Ospina-Tascon G, Salgado D, et al. Monitoring the microcirculation in the critically ill patient: current methods and future approaches. *Intensive Care Med.* 2010;36:1813–1825.
20. De Backer D, Donadello K, Taccone FS, et al. Microcirculatory alterations: potential mechanisms and implications for therapy. *Ann Intensive Care.* 2011;1(1):27.
21. Crouser ED. Mitochondrial dysfunction in septic shock and multiple organ dysfunction syndrome. *Mitochondrion.* 2004;4:729–741.
22. Dare AJ, Phillips AR, Hickey AJ, et al. A systematic review of experimental treatments for mitochondrial dysfunction in sepsis and multiple organ dysfunction syndrome. *Free Radic Biol Med.* 2009;47:1517–1525.
23. Sprung CL, Annane D, Keh D, et al. CORTICUS Study Group. Hydrocortisone therapy for patients with septic shock. *N Engl J Med.* 2008;358(2):111–124.
24. Russell JA, Walley KR, Singer J, et al. VASST Investigators. Vasopressin versus norepinephrine infusion in patients with septic shock. *N Engl J Med.* 2008;358(9):877–887.
25. Jones AE, Shapiro NI, Trzeciak S, et al. Emergency Medicine Shock Research Network (EMShockNet) Investigators. Lactate clearance vs. central venous oxygen saturation as goals of early sepsis therapy: a randomized clinical trial. *JAMA.* 2010;303(8):739–746.

32

Vasopressors and Inotropes

Matthew C. Strehlow

BACKGROUND

Vasopressors and inotropes are vasoactive agents used to improve cardiac output and distribution of blood flow in patients suffering from shock. Vasopressors act by inducing vasoconstriction, while inotropes increase cardiac contractility; many vasoactive agents exhibit properties of both. Vasopressors and inotropes have been in widespread use since the 1940s, when Dr. Raymond Ahlquist differentiated alpha- and beta-adrenergic receptors, but to date, there is surprisingly little high-quality evidence demonstrating that vasoactive agents improve outcomes. Vasopressors and inotropes nevertheless continue to be fundamental to shock management, and an understanding of their individual pharmacodynamics is crucial for appropriate drug selection in critically ill patients.

Historically, vasopressors and inotropes have been used to improve global markers of hypoperfusion. Recent advances in tissue perfusion monitoring and use of biomarkers have expanded both the targeted goals of resuscitation and, consequently, the range of clinical scenarios in which vasoactive agents are employed. As our understanding of the physiologic response to shock states improves, tailoring resuscitative therapy to specific clinical scenarios and individual patients will become feasible.

PHYSIOLOGY

The categories of receptors targeted by vasopressors and inotropes include alpha-1, beta-1, and beta-2 adrenergic receptors and dopamine receptors (see Table 32.1). Alpha-1 receptor activation in vascular smooth muscle causes a rise in intracellular calcium and, correspondingly, smooth muscle contraction; the latter is manifested by vasoconstriction, mydriasis, and contraction of GI and urinary bladder sphincters. Beta-1 receptors are located primarily in the heart; activation of beta-1 receptors increases intracellular cyclic adenosine monophosphate (cAMP), which augments cardiac chronotropy, dromotropy, and inotropy. Beta-2 receptor activation in vascular smooth muscle leads to an elevation in cAMP and relaxation of vascular smooth muscle, producing peripheral vasodilation. Dopamine receptors exist in many body tissues; stimulation of these receptors causes vasodilation and increased blood flow to cerebral, coronary, renal, and mesenteric tissues, among others.

TABLE 32.1 Sympathomimetic Agents Effect Upon Adrenergic Receptors

	Receptor			
	α_1	β_1	β_2	DA
Dobutamine	+	+++++	+++	0
Dopamine	+++	++++	++	+++++
Epinephrine	+++++	++++	+++	0
Isoproterenol	0	+++++	+++++	0
Norepinephrine	+++++	+++	++	0
Phenylephrine	+++++	0	0	0

SPECIFIC VASOPRESSORS

Norepinephrine

Norepinephrine is recommended as the first-line vasopressor for septic shock once volume resuscitation has been achieved and for severe cardiogenic shock. It causes potent vasoconstriction with a corresponding increase in systolic, diastolic, and pulse pressure and has minimal net impact on cardiac output and heart rate. Coronary perfusion is augmented by elevated diastolic blood pressure and indirect release of local vasodilators.[1] Prolonged use of exogenous norepinephrine can have direct toxic effects on cardiac myocytes (see Table 32.2).[2]

Epinephrine

Epinephrine is recommended as the first-line vasopressor for cardiac arrest and anaphylaxis and as a second-line agent for septic shock. At low doses, epinephrine stimulates beta-1 receptors, subsequently increasing cardiac output by augmenting cardiac contractility and heart rate. Peripherally, epinephrine's alpha-1 and beta-2 stimulation offset. Epinephrine enhances coronary blood flow by dilating coronary vessels and increasing diastolic blood pressure.[3] At higher doses, epinephrine produces potent alpha-adrenergic stimulation, in addition to the increase in cardiac output, leading to peripheral vasoconstriction and an increase in systemic vascular resistance. Prolonged use of epinephrine can cause cardiac dysrhythmias and direct cardiac toxicity. Epinephrine also produces splanchnic vasoconstriction—to a greater degree than equipotent doses of norepinephrine and dopamine—although the clinical importance of this feature is unknown.

Dopamine

Dopamine is recommended for symptomatic bradycardia unresponsive to atropine and as a second-line agent for septic shock in patients who are at a low risk for dysrhythmias. Additionally, dopamine is an alternative to norepinephrine in patients with acute decompensated heart failure who have persistent hypotension and corresponding end-organ dysfunction. All patients receiving dopamine should be monitored for cardiac dysrhythmias; therapy should be discontinued if dysrhythmia is present.

TABLE 32.2 Commonly Used Vasopressors and Inotropes

Drug	Clinical Indication	Dose	Clinical Effect	Major Side Effects
Catecholamines				
Dobutamine	Low cardiac output (decompensated heart failure, cardiogenic shock, septic shock with ongoing hypoperfusion despite fluid and vasopressor therapy)	Infusion: 2–20 μg/kg/min (max 40 μg/kg/min)	Increases cardiac output by increasing contractility and a less dramatic increase in heart rate	Tachycardia Ventricular arrhythmias Cardiac ischemia Hypotension
Dopamine	Symptomatic bradycardia Shock (septic, cardiogenic, neurogenic)	Infusion: 2–20 μg/kg/min	Moderate doses increase cardiac output and systemic vascular resistance and higher doses provide an additional increase in systemic vascular resistance	Ventricular arrhythmias Cardiac ischemia
Epinephrine	Shock (anaphylactic, septic, cardiogenic, neurogenic) Cardiac arrest Bronchospasm Symptomatic bradycardia	Infusion: 0.01–0.1 μg/kg/min Bolus: 1 mg IV every 3–5 min (max 0.2 mg/kg) IM: (1:1,000): 0.1–0.5 mg (max 1 mg)	Lower doses increase cardiac output and higher doses add an increase in systemic vascular resistance	Ventricular arrhythmias Cardiac ischemia Sudden cardiac death
Isoproterenol	Symptomatic bradycardia Polymorphic ventricular tachycardia (torsades de pointes) Brugada syndrome	Infusion: 0.01–0.05 μg/kg/min	Increases heart rate and contractility and decreases systemic vascular resistance	Ventricular arrhythmias Cardiac ischemia Hypotension
Norepinephrine	Shock (septic, cardiogenic, neurogenic, undifferentiated)	Infusion: 0.01–3 μg/kg/min	Increase in systemic vascular resistance with a net neutral effect on cardiac output and heart rate	Arrhythmias Bradycardia Peripheral ischemia
Phenylephrine	Severe hypotension (vagally mediated or medication induced) Shock (septic or spinal) with a low systemic vascular resistance	Infusion: 0.4–9.1 μg/kg/min Bolus: 0.1–0.5 mg IV every 10–15 min	Increase in systemic vascular resistance with a neutral to small increase in cardiac output if preserved cardiac function (decrease if preexisting cardiac dysfunction)	Reflex bradycardia Severe peripheral and visceral vasoconstriction
PDIs				
Milrinone	Low cardiac output (decompensated heart failure, cardiogenic shock)	Bolus: 50 μg/kg over 10–30 min Infusion: 0.375–0.75 μg/kg/min (adjust dose for renal impairment)	Increase in cardiac output with a reduction in preload, afterload, and systemic vascular resistance	Ventricular arrhythmias (including torsades des pointes) Cardiac ischemia Hypotension

(*Continued*)

TABLE 32.2 Commonly Used Vasopressors and Inotropes (*Continued*)

Drug	Clinical Indication	Dose	Clinical Effect	Major Side Effects
PDIs (Continued)				
Inamrinone	Low cardiac output (decompensated heart failure, cardiogenic shock)	Bolus: 0.75 mg/kg over 2–3 min Infusion: 5–10 μg/kg/min	Increase in cardiac output with a reduction in preload, afterload, and systemic vascular resistance	Arrhythmias Enhanced AV conduction (increased ventricular response rate in atrial fibrillation) Hypotension Thrombocytopenia Hepatotoxicity
Other Agents				
Vasopressin	Shock (septic, anaphylactic) Cardiac arrest	Infusion: 0.01–0.1 units/min Infusion low dose to augment norepinephrine in septic shock: 0.03 units/min Bolus: 40 units IV	Increase systemic vascular resistance with a neutral effect on cardiac output and decrease in heart rate	Arrhythmias Decreased cardiac output (at doses >0.4 units/min) Cardiac, skin, and mesenteric ischemia

When administered therapeutically, dopamine acts on dopaminergic and adrenergic receptors to elicit a multitude of distinct clinical effects, depending on the dose given. At lower doses (0.5 to 3 mcg/kg/min), dopamine causes selective vasodilation of the renal, mesenteric, cerebral, and coronary vascular beds through its action on dopamine receptors. Note that when dopamine is used at these low doses, hypotension can occur.[4] The clinical benefit of this "renal dose" dopamine has not been demonstrated, and use for renal protection is not recommended.[5] At moderate doses (3 to 10 mcg/kg/min), dopamine predominantly stimulates beta-1 adrenergic receptors, augmenting cardiac output by increasing stroke volume and, somewhat variably, heart rate. Systemic vascular resistance is minimally elevated, and the overall effect is an increase in mean arterial pressure (MAP). At higher doses (>10 mcg/kg/min), stimulation of alpha-adrenergic receptors dominates, leading to vasoconstriction and increased systemic vascular resistance. Note that higher doses of dopamine can result in rapid development of tachyphylaxis.

Vasopressin

Vasopressin and its analog, terlipressin, are used primarily as second-line agents for refractory vasodilatory shock that is poorly responsive to epinephrine. In addition, sepsis management guidelines indicate that low-dose vasopressin can be added to norepinephrine, either to increase MAP or to decrease the required dose of norepinephrine. Vasopressin use as a single agent for septic shock, however, is not recommended.[5] Vasopressin is a nonadrenergic peripheral vasoconstrictor that acts on V1 and V2 receptors, located in vascular smooth muscle and the renal collecting system, respectively. Administration of vasopressin causes marked vasoconstriction and increased systemic vascular resistance, with a neutral effect on cardiac output and a decrease in heart rate.[6] Potential advantages of vasopressin include less direct cerebral vasoconstriction than with the use of catecholamines and relatively preserved vasopressor effects during hypoxemic and acidemic conditions. A fixed dose of vasopressin at 0.03 units/min is recommended; higher doses, while potentially more effective at restoring blood pressure, have been associated with coronary and mesenteric ischemia and skin necrosis.[5,7,8] Since rapid withdrawal from vasopressin can result in rebound hypotension, a slow taper of 0.01 units/min every 30 minutes should be employed.

Phenylephrine

Phenylephrine is used in patients suffering severe hypotension with a low systemic vascular resistance (SVR <700 dynes × sec/cm^5), as seen in hyperdynamic sepsis and traumatic neurogenic shock. International sepsis guidelines, however, do not recommend phenylephrine unless other combinations of vasopressors are ineffective or cannot be used due to serious dysrhythmias.[9] Phenylephrine is also recommended in patients with severe aortic stenosis and significant hypotension or to decrease the outflow tract gradient in patients with obstructive hypertrophic cardiomyopathy. In the setting of anesthetic or other iatrogenic-induced hypotension, bolus administration is often used for rapid blood pressure correction.

Phenylephrine causes potent vasoconstriction and a rise in systemic vascular resistance through alpha-adrenergic receptor activation. It produces almost no stimulation of beta-adrenergic receptors, and as a result, cardiac stroke volume may be decreased.[10] Severe peripheral and visceral vasoconstriction can occur, and phenylephrine is contraindicated in patients with an elevated systemic vascular resistance (>1,200 dyne × sec/cm^5).

SPECIFIC INOTROPES

Dobutamine

Dobutamine is primarily used for three indications: (a) acute decompensated heart failure due to systolic dysfunction with signs of hypoperfusion and mild to moderate hypotension; (b) low-output cardiogenic shock, most often secondary to an acute myocardial infarction; and (c) septic shock patients who have ongoing signs of hypoperfusion despite appropriate fluid resuscitation and vasopressors. Surviving Sepsis Campaign Guidelines specifically recommend a trial of dobutamine for patients with myocardial dysfunction (demonstrated by an elevated cardiac filling pressure and persistently low cardiac output) or for patients with ongoing signs of hypoperfusion (e.g., low $ScVO_2$ or high lactate) despite adequate intravascular volume and MAP.[5]

Dobutamine primarily stimulates beta-1 adrenergic receptors, which leads to increased inotropy and moderately increased chronotropy. The result is a rise in cardiac output. At low doses, ≤5 mcg/kg/min, dobutamine also produces beta-2 and mild alpha-1 receptor stimulation, which leads to a mild net peripheral vasodilation. Higher doses of 5 to 15 mcg/kg/min have a minimal net effect on systemic vascular resistance, and at doses >15 mcg/kg/min, alpha-medicated vasoconstriction predominates peripherally—in addition to the primary effect of beta-1 stimulation. Even at low doses, dobutamine markedly increases myocardial oxygen consumption, and myocardial ischemia may result. Furthermore, dobutamine can lead to critical dysrhythmias. Likely as a result of these adverse side effects, dobutamine has never been demonstrated to decrease mortality in heart failure patients.[11] It does, however, remain first-line therapy in low-output cardiogenic shock patients when inotropy is required.[12]

Phosphodiesterase Inhibitors

Milrinone and inamrinone are used comparably to dobutamine in patients with acute decompensated heart failure due to systolic dysfunction with signs of hypoperfusion and mild to moderate hypotension and in patients with low-output cardiogenic shock. These agents, termed phosphodiesterase inhibitors (PDIs), act by blocking an enzyme that degrades cAMP in the cell, augmenting myocardial contractility, systemic vasodilation, and diastolic relaxation. The net clinical effect is a rise in cardiac output with a reduction in preload, afterload, and systemic vascular resistance. Milrinone is the most commonly used parenteral PDI, due in part to inamrinone's significant side effects, including dose-related thrombocytopenia. To date, PDIs have not been shown to improve mortality in acute decompensated heart failure or cardiogenic shock.[13] PDIs are second-line inotropic agents in most emergency settings, but may be considered in cases where dobutamine is not effective due to downregulation or desensitization of adrenergic receptors, as seen in (1) chronic heart failure patients, (2) chronic beta-agonist administration, or (3) outpatient beta-antagonist therapy.

Isoproterenol

Isoproterenol is infrequently administered; its use is primarily limited to second-line therapy for symptomatic bradycardia. It can be considered, however, for patients with polymorphic ventricular tachycardia, specifically for torsades de pointes associated with bradycardia and drug-induced QT prolongation, or Brugada syndrome. Isoproterenol should be avoided in polymorphic ventricular tachycardia associated with familial long QT syndrome.[14] Through its isolated beta-adrenergic stimulation, isoproterenol causes increased heart rate and contractility and decreased systemic vascular resistance.

Calcium-Sensitizing Agents

Calcium sensitizers (e.g., levosimendan) are not approved for use in the United States, but are used in multiple other countries for acute decompensated heart failure. They act by increasing the responsiveness of contractile proteins to calcium without increasing intracellular calcium levels and by opening adenosine triphosphate–dependent potassium channels. Clinically, this leads to increased myocardial contractility, arteriolar and venous dilation, and preserved diastolic relaxation. The result is increased cardiac output and decreased preload, afterload, and systemic vascular resistance.[15] Studies of levosimendan have not demonstrated a consistent mortality or other major outcome benefit when compared to dobutamine or placebo.[16,17]

THERAPEUTIC APPROACH IN SHOCK

The majority of patients suffering shock in the emergency department are undifferentiated (e.g., septic shock vs. cardiogenic shock) at the time of their arrival. Caring for these patients requires immediate intervention to restore perfusion to critical organs and rapid identification of the underlying etiology of the patient's illness. In patients who do not present with obvious signs of pulmonary edema, initial resuscitation focuses on rapid fluid administration to restore intravascular volume. If patients continue to display signs of shock following adequate fluid resuscitation, vasoactive agents should be initiated. Generally, vasopressors are indicated if the MAP is <60 mm Hg or the systolic blood pressure is >30 mm Hg below baseline in patients with signs of end-organ dysfunction due to hypoperfusion. In patients with severe hypotension and impending cardiopulmonary arrest, it is appropriate to begin vasopressors concurrently with fluid administration.

For patients presenting with undifferentiated or septic shock, norepinephrine is recommended as first-line therapy. Meta-analysis of six studies comparing norepinephrine to dopamine in septic shock patients demonstrated a modest improvement in survival in the norepinephrine group and an increase in cardiac dysrhythmias in the dopamine cohort.[18–23] In contrast, multiple studies comparing benefits of other vasopressors in shock states have demonstrated equivalence in terms of mortality and length of stay.[9,24–34]

An estimate of cardiac output can help to guide therapy in patients that remain hypotensive despite norepinephrine administration. If cardiac output is persistently low (i.e., "cold shock"), dobutamine should be added as a second agent or therapy switched to epinephrine to improve cardiac performance.[35] If cardiac output is normal or high (i.e., "warm shock"), vasopressin or phenylephrine can be added to norepinephrine therapy. Phenylephrine is also appropriate for patients who have significant tachycardia or dysrhythmias that preclude the use of norepinephrine or other agents with beta-adrenergic activity. Patients unresponsive to two vasopressors rarely benefit from the addition of a third. Instead, switching to alternative vasopressors is recommended.

If other forms of shock are suspected, the choice of vasoactive agent should be tailored appropriately. In cardiogenic shock patients, norepinephrine is the preferred initial agent if patients are significantly hypotensive (systolic blood pressure <80 mm Hg). In patients who respond to norepinephrine or whose systolic blood pressure is low but >80 mm Hg, a trial of dobutamine is indicated. Anaphylactic shock should be treated with epinephrine, while patients with neurogenic shock due to spinal cord injury should be treated with an agent that has both alpha-1 and beta-1 adrenergic activities (e.g., norepinephrine, epinephrine, dopamine).[36]

CONCLUSION

Vasopressors and inotropes are used to improve tissue perfusion during shock when volume resuscitation alone proves insufficient. Norepinephrine is the initial vasopressor of choice in most forms of shock, including patients lacking a clear etiology. When a low cardiac output exists and inotropy is desired, dobutamine is the recommended first-line therapy. Vasoactive agents should be titrated based on bedside and laboratory markers of tissue perfusion.

LITERATURE TABLE

TRIAL	DESIGN	RESULT
Vasopressors		
De Backer et al., *NEJM.* 2010[19]	Multicenter RCT of 1,679 patients with vasopressor-dependent shock for <4 h assigned to receive norepinephrine or dopamine	No significant difference in mortality between groups at 28 days (dopamine OR 1.17; 95% CI 0.97–1.42). Arrhythmias were more common in the dopamine group (24.7% vs. 12.4%, $p = 0.001$)
Patel et al., *Shock.* 2010[21]	Single-center quasi-randomized controlled trial (250 patients) evaluating protocolized use of dopamine and norepinephrine in vasopressor-dependent septic shock	No significant difference in 28-day mortality in patients receiving dopamine (RR 1.16; 95% CI 0.886–1.51). Arrhythmias were more common in the dopamine group (38% vs. 11.8%, RR 3.21; 95% CI 1.88–5.49)

(*Continued*)

LITERATURE TABLE (*Continued*)

TRIAL	DESIGN	RESULT
De Backer et al., *Crit Care Med.* 2012[24]	Meta-analysis of six RCT (1,408 patients) comparing norepinephrine to dopamine in patients with septic shock	Mortality was higher in patients receiving dopamine (RR 1.12; 95% CI 1.01–1.20)
Annane et al., *Lancet.* 2007[25]	Multicenter RCT of 230 patients with vasopressor-dependent septic shock for <24 h assigned to norepinephrine plus dobutamine or epinephrine	No significant difference in mortality between groups at 28 d (norepinephrine plus dobutamine RR 0.86; 95% CI 0.65–1.14). Serious adverse events were similar between groups
Polito et al., *Intensive Care Med.* 2012[30]	Meta-analysis of six randomized trials (973 patients) evaluating use of vasopressin/terlipressin in adults with vasopressor-dependent shock	No significant difference in short-term mortality in patients receiving vasopressin/terlipressin (RR 0.91; 95% CI 0.79–1.05) or either agent individually. Use of vasopressin/terlipressin resulted in lower doses of norepinephrine
Russel et al., *NEJM.* 2008[31]	Multicenter RCT of 778 patients with vasopressor-dependent septic shock receiving norepinephrine assigned to receive norepinephrine or vasopressin in addition to open-label vasopressors	No significant difference in 28-day mortality in patients receiving vasopressin (RR 0.90; 95% CI 0.75–1.08). Serious adverse events were similar between groups
Inotropes		
Cuffe et al., *JAMA.* 2002[13]	Multicenter RCT of 951 patients with acute decompensated heart failure comparing milrinone to placebo (patients requiring inotropic support were excluded)	No significant difference in primary outcome of days in hospital due to cardiovascular cause with milrinone (6 vs. 7 d, $p = 0.71$). Secondary outcomes were similar including in-hospital mortality (milrinone 3.8% vs. placebo 2.3%, $p = 0.19$)
Mebazaa et al., *JAMA.* 2007[16] SURVIVE	Multicenter RCT of 1,327 hospitalized patients with acute decompensated heart failure that required inotropic support comparing levosimendan to dobutamine	No significant difference in 180-day mortality in patients receiving levosimendan (RR 0.91; 95% CI 0.74–1.13). Secondary outcomes such as 28-day mortality did not show significant differences either
Rivers et al., *NEJM.* 2001[35]	Single-center RCT of 263 patients with early severe sepsis/septic shock comparing protocolized care, which included dobutamine to standard care	In-hospital mortality was lower in the protocolized care group (RR 0.58, 95% CI 0.38–0.87). During the 6-hour study period, patients in the protocolized care arm received dobutamine more frequently (13.7% vs. 0.8%, $p < 0.001$)

CI, confidence interval; OR, odds ratio; RR, relative risk.

REFERENCES

1. Tune JD, Richmond KN, Gorman MW, et al. Control of coronary blood flow during exercise. *Exp Biol Med (Maywood).* 2002;227(4):238–250.
2. Communal C, Singh K, Pimentel DR, et al. Norepinephrine stimulates apoptosis in adult rat ventricular myocytes by activation of the beta-adrenergic pathway. *Circulation.* 1998;98(13):1329–1334.
3. Jones CJ, DeFily DV, Patterson JL, et al. Endothelium-dependent relaxation competes with alpha 1- and alpha 2-adrenergic constriction in the canine epicardial coronary microcirculation. *Circulation.* 1993;87(4):1264–1274.
4. Duke GJ, Briedis JH, Weaver RA. Renal support in critically ill patients: low-dose dopamine or low-dose dobutamine? *Crit Care Med.* 1994;22(12):1919–1925.
5. Dellinger RP, Levy MM, Rhodes A, et al. Surviving sepsis campaign: international guidelines for management of severe sepsis and septic shock: 2012. *Crit Care Med.* 2013;41(2):580–637.
6. Gordon AC, Wang N, Walley KR, et al. The cardiopulmonary effects of vasopressin compared with norepinephrine in septic shock. *Chest.* 2012;142(3):593–605.
7. Dünser MW, Mayr AJ, Tür A, et al. Ischemic skin lesions as a complication of continuous vasopressin infusion in catecholamine-resistant vasodilatory shock: incidence and risk factors. *Crit Care Med.* 2003;31(5):1394–1398.
8. Malay M-B, Ashton JL, Dahl K, et al. Heterogeneity of the vasoconstrictor effect of vasopressin in septic shock. *Crit Care Med.* 2004;32(6):1327–1331.

9. Morelli A, Ertmer C, Rehberg S, et al. Phenylephrine versus norepinephrine for initial hemodynamic support of patients with septic shock: a randomized, controlled trial. *Crit Care.* 2008;12(6):R143.
10. Williamson AP, Seifen E, Lindemann JP, et al. WB4101- and CEC-sensitive positive inotropic actions of phenylephrine in rat cardiac muscle. *Am J Physiol.* 1994;266(6 Pt 2):H2462–H2467.
11. Tacon CL, McCaffrey J, Delaney A. Dobutamine for patients with severe heart failure: a systematic review and meta-analysis of randomised controlled trials. *Intensive Care Med.* 2011;38(3):359–367.
12. Hunt SA, Abraham WT, Chin MH, et al. 2009 Focused update incorporated into the ACC/AHA 2005 Guidelines for the Diagnosis and Management of Heart Failure in Adults. *J Am Coll Cardiol.* 2009;53(15):e1–e90.
13. Cuffe, MS, Califf RM, Adams KF, et al. Short-term intravenous milrinone for acute exacerbation of chronic heart failure. *JAMA* 2002;287(12):1541–1547.
14. Neumar RW, Otto CW, Link MS, et al. Part 8: adult advanced cardiovascular life support: 2010 American Heart Association Guidelines for Cardiopulmonary Resuscitation and Emergency Cardiovascular Care. *Circulation.* 2010;122(18 suppl 3):S729–S767.
15. Slawsky MT, Colucci WS, Gottlieb SS, et al. Acute hemodynamic and clinical effects of levosimendan in patients with severe heart failure. Study Investigators. *Circulation.* 2000;102(18):2222–2227.
16. Mebazaa A, Nieminen MS, Packer M, et al. Levosimendan vs dobutamine for patients with acute decompensated heart failure: the SURVIVE Randomized Trial. *JAMA.* 2007;297(17):1883–1891.
17. Packer M, Colucci W, Fisher L, et al. Effect of levosimendan on the short-term clinical course of patients with acutely decompensated heart failure. *JACC: Heart Fail.* 2013;1(2):103–111.
18. Martin C, Papazian L, Perrin G, et al. Norepinephrine or dopamine for the treatment of hyperdynamic septic shock? *Chest.* 1993;103(6):1826–1831.
19. De Backer D, Biston P, Devriendt J, et al. Comparison of dopamine and norepinephrine in the treatment of shock. *N Engl J Med.* 2010;362(9):779–789.
20. Marik PE, Mohedin M. The contrasting effects of dopamine and norepinephrine on systemic and splanchnic oxygen utilization in hyperdynamic sepsis. *JAMA.* 1994;272(17):1354–1357.
21. Patel GP, Grahe JS, Sperry M, et al. Efficacy and safety of dopamine versus norepinephrine in the management of septic shock. *Shock.* 2010;33(4):375–380.
22. Ruokonen E, Takala J, Kari A, et al. Regional blood flow and oxygen transport in septic shock. *Crit Care Med.* 1993;21(9):1296–1303.
23. De Backer D, Aldecoa C, Njimi H, Vincent J. Dopamine versus norepinephrine in the treatment of septic shock: a meta-analysis. *Crit Care Med.* 2012;40(3):725–730.
24. Mathur S, Dhunna R, Chakraborty A. Comparison of dopamine and norepinephrine in the management of septic shock using impedance cardiography. *Indian J Crit Care Med.* 2007;11:186.
25. Annane, D, Vignon P, Renault A, et al. Norepinephrine plus dobutamine versus epinephrine alone for management of septic shock: a randomized trial. *Lancet* 2007;370:676–684.
26. Myburgh JA, Higgins A, Jovanovska A, et al. A comparison of epinephrine and norepinephrine in critically ill patients. *Intensive Care Med.* 2008;34(12):2226–2234.
27. Russell JA, Walley KR, Gordon AC, et al. Interaction of vasopressin infusion, corticosteroid treatment, and mortality of septic shock. *Crit Care Med.* 2009;37(3):811–818.
28. Luckner G, Dünser MW, Stadlbauer K-H, et al. Cutaneous vascular reactivity and flow motion response to vasopressin in advanced vasodilatory shock and severe postoperative multiple organ dysfunction syndrome. *Crit Care.* 2006;10(2):R40.
29. Lauzier F, Lévy B, Lamarre P, et al. Vasopressin or norepinephrine in early hyperdynamic septic shock: a randomized clinical trial. *Intensive Care Med.* 2006;32(11):1782–1789.
30. Polito A, Parisini E, Ricci Z, et al. Vasopressin for treatment of vasodilatory shock: an ESICM systematic review and meta-analysis. *Intensive Care Med.* 2012;38:9–19.
31. Russell JA, Walley KR, Singer J, et al. Vasopressin versus norepinephrine infusion in patients with septic shock. *NEJM* 2008;358(9):877–887.
32. Boccara G, Ouattara A, Godet G, et al. Terlipressin versus norepinephrine to correct refractory arterial hypotension after general anesthesia in patients chronically treated with renin-angiotensin system inhibitors. *Anesthesiology.* 2003;98(6):1338–1344.
33. Albanèse J, Leone M, Delmas A, et al. Terlipressin or norepinephrine in hyperdynamic septic shock: a prospective, randomized study. *Crit Care Med.* 2005;33(9):1897–1902.
34. Morelli A, Ertmer C, Rehberg S, et al. Continuous terlipressin versus vasopressin infusion in septic shock (TERLIVAP): a randomized, controlled pilot study. *Crit Care.* 2009;13(4):R130.
35. Rivers E, Nguyen B, Havstad S, et al. Early goal-directed therapy in the treatment of severe sepsis and septic shock. *NEJM* 2001;345(19):1368–1377.
36. Wing P, Dalsey W, Alvarez E, et al. Early acute management in adults with spinal cord injury: a clinical practice guideline for health-care providers. *J Spinal Cord Med.* 2008;31(4):403–479.

33

Principles of Antimicrobial Therapy

Chanu Rhee and Michael Klompas

BACKGROUND

In the past several decades, advances in the development of antimicrobial agents have supplied the physician with dozens of drugs effective against bacterial, fungal, and viral pathogens. Unfortunately, these advances have been paralleled by increasing antibiotic resistance and the emergence of new pathogens. More than half of *Staphylococcus aureus* bloodstream infections in the United States now derive from methicillin-resistant strains, and hospitalizations due to vancomycin-resistant *Enterococcus* (VRE) infections doubled between 2003 and 2006.[1,2] In recent years, infections due to extended-spectrum beta-lactamase (ESBL)-producing gram-negative organisms and *Clostridium difficile* have increased in frequency, while carbapenemase-producing pathogens have emerged and spread worldwide.[3–5] The incidence of sepsis also appears to be increasing,[6–9] driven by an aging population and an intensified use of immunosuppressive medications. Overall, the prevalence and complexity of infectious diseases are greater than ever. The appropriate, rational use of antibiotics in the emergency department and intensive care unit requires a thorough understanding of principles of therapy and our current arsenal of antibiotics.

CHOOSING AN INITIAL EMPIRIC REGIMEN

Clinical Factors to Consider

Presumptive Diagnosis

Because microbiologic data generally take 24 to 72 hours to return, clinicians are usually forced to choose an empiric antibiotic regimen when encountering a patient with a likely infection. Making a presumptive infectious disease diagnosis is a critical step in deciding on an antimicrobial regimen, as many diagnoses tend to be associated with a predictable set of pathogens. The clinician should take into account the patient's signs and symptoms, physical exam, and basic workup including labs, urinalysis, chest x-ray, and other imaging studies as appropriate. Suggested empiric regimens for common serious infectious syndromes are described in Table 33.1.

Comorbidities

The choice of antibiotics depends in large part on the presence of comorbidities, especially the degree of immunosuppression. A history of HIV, corticosteroid or immunomodulator therapy, chemotherapy, organ transplant, malignancy, or congenital immunodeficiency

TABLE 33.1 Recommendations for Initial Empiric Therapy for Common Serious Infections

Condition	Likely Pathogens	Recommended Antibiotic Regimens and Dose (For Normal Renal/ Hepatic Function)	Typical Duration
Pulmonary			
Community-acquired pneumonia	*Streptococcus pneumoniae, Haemophilus influenzae,* intracellular atypical organisms (*Mycoplasma pneumoniae, Chlamydophila pneumoniae, Legionella*), respiratory viruses **S. aureus* if IV drug user, recent influenza **Pseudomonas* if structural lung disease (e.g., bronchiectasis, chronic obstructive lung disease [COPD] with frequent steroid use)	1. Ceftriaxone 1–2 g IV q24h + azithromycin 500 mg, then 250 mg PO/IV q24h, or 2. Moxifloxacin 400 mg PO/IV or Levofloxacin 750 mg PO/IV q24h (switch to PO as soon as can tolerate) *For severely ill patients, consider adding vancomycin or linezolid for MRSA coverage *Consider antipseudomonal coverage if risk factors present *Consider adding oseltamivir if flu-like syndrome	7–10 d Azithromycin can be given for 5 d, but longer if confirmed *Legionella*
Hospital, health care–associated, or ventilator-associated pneumonia	*S. aureus* (including MRSA) and aerobic GNRs, including *Pseudomonas, E. coli, K. pneumoniae,* and *Enterobacter.* Multidrug-resistant gram-negatives are common in ICU patents *Role of anaerobes, even in nosocomial aspiration pneumonia, is unclear (but reasonable to add anaerobic coverage in that scenario)	1. Anti-MRSA agent: Vancomycin 15–20 mg/kg IV q12h or linezolid 600 mg PO/IV q12h + 2. Antipseudomonal beta-lactam: Ceftazidime 2 g IV q8h, cefepime 2 g IV q8h, piperacillin/tazobactam 4.5 g IV q6h, imipenem 500 mg IV q6h, or meropenem 1–2 g IV q8h; aztreonam 1–2 g IV q8h if severe penicillin allergy *For severely ill patients, or if high risk of resistant gram-negative infection, also consider addition of "double coverage" with antipseudomonal fluoroquinolone (ciprofloxacin or levofloxacin), or aminoglycoside	7–8 d, but potentially longer for MRSA or *Pseudomonas* or immunocompromised 15-d course for *Pseudomonas* associated with decreased recurrence of disease (vs. 8 d)
Aspiration pneumonia	Oral anaerobes, enteric GNRs, *S. aureus, Streptococcus* species	1. Levofloxacin 750 mg PO/IV q24h + metronidazole 500 mg PO/IV q8h, or 2. Clindamycin 600 mg PO/IV q8h (add levofloxacin if concern for community-acquired pneumonia), or 3. Ampicillin/Sulbactam 3 g IV q6h *If nosocomial—treat as hospital-acquired pneumonia, with preference for piperacillin/tazobactam, imipenem, or meropenem for anaerobic coverage, or add clindamycin or metronidazole	7–10 d

Gastrointestinal			
Appendicitis, diverticulitis, intra-abdominal abscess, secondary peritonitis	Polymicrobial GI flora including GNRs (especially *E. coli*) and anaerobes (especially *Bacteroides*) For bowel perforation, microbiology depends on site. Upper GI tract (e.g., perforated duodenal ulcer) mainly *Streptococcus* species. Lower GI tract mainly GNRs and anaerobes *Enterococcus* and *Candida* species usually less important, except in health care–associated cases	1. Ceftriaxone 1–2 g IV q24h + metronidazole 500 mg IV q8h, or 2. Ciprofloxacin 400 mg IV q12h or levofloxacin 500 mg IV 24h + Metronidazole (caution with Cipro due to poor *Streptococcus* coverage), or 3. Piperacillin/tazobactam 3.375 g IV q6h, or 4. Imipenem 500 mg IV q6h or meropenem 1 g IV q8h (if high risk for resistant infections) *For severely ill or health care–/hospital-acquired disease, consider addition of Enterococcal and *Candida* coverage (especially if not responding to therapy) *Caution with ampicillin/sulbactam alone due to high rates of *E. coli* resistance at some institutions	4–7 d for appendicitis or diverticulitis Duration for abscesses depends on adequate drainage, but typically minimum 4–7 d after drainage
Spontaneous bacterial peritonitis (SBP) in patients with ascites	GNRs including *E. coli, Klebsiella, Enterobacter*. Also, enteric *Streptococcus* species and *Enterococcus*	Cefotaxime 2 g IV q8h or ceftriaxone 1–2 g IV q24h + Albumin 1.5 g/kg on day 1 and 1 g/kg on day 3 (shown to reduce renal failure and mortality)	5–7 d
Cholangitis	Polymicrobial GI flora. Anaerobes if biliary–enteric anastomosis *Enterococcus* coverage usually not required	Ceftriaxone 1–2 g IV q24h, ciprofloxacin 400 mg IV q12h, or levofloxacin 500 mg IV q24h + Metronidazole 500 mg IV q8h if biliary–enteric anastomosis If severe or health care–associated infection, consider piperacillin/tazobactam or imipenem or meropenem	4–7 d assuming adequate source control
Urinary			
Acute pyelonephritis	*E. coli* is most common, followed by other gram-negatives (*Proteus, Klebsiella, Serratia, Enterobacter*) and *Staphylococcus saprophyticus*	1. Ceftriaxone 1–2 g IV q24h, or 2. Ciprofloxacin 400 mg IV q12h or levofloxacin 500 mg IV q24h (caution due to rising *E. coli* resistance), or 3. Cefepime 1–2 g IV q12h (especially if prior resistant organisms or *Pseudomonas*)	7–10 d
Complicated UTI (defined by presence of anatomic or functional abnormality in the genitourinary tract, or urinary catheter)	More likely to be due to resistant gram-negatives, including ESBLs and *Pseudomonas*. *S. aureus* is possible if chronic urinary catheters or stents. Also: *Enterococcus, Candida*	1. If mildly ill—ceftriaxone 1–2 g IV q24h or ciprofloxacin 400 mg IV q12h or levofloxacin 500 mg IV q24h 2. If severely ill—cefepime 1–2 g IV q12h, or ceftazidime 1 g IV q8h, or carbapenem if high risk for ESBL, or history of prior infections. Consider adding vancomycin especially if history of prior MRSA infection, chronic urinary catheters, or stents	10–14 d (longer if suspect prostatitis)

(*Continued*)

TABLE 33.1 Recommendations for Initial Empiric Therapy for Common Serious Infections (*Continued*)

Condition	Likely Pathogens	Recommended Antibiotic Regimens and Dose (For Normal Renal/Hepatic Function)	Typical Duration
Skin and Soft Tissue			
Cellulitis	*Streptococcus* species (most commonly Group A), *S. aureus* including MRSA More unusual pathogens are possible depending on risk factors (i.e., water exposures, animal bites, neutropenia)	1. IV options for *Streptococcus*, low suspicion for MRSA: cefazolin 2 g IV q8h, clindamycin 600 mg IV q8h 2. IV options with MRSA coverage: vancomycin 15–20 mg/kg IV q12h, linezolid 600 mg PO/IV q12h, daptomycin 4–6 mg/kg IV q24h, clindamycin 600 mg IV/PO q8h (but MRSA often resistant)	7–14 d
Infected diabetic foot ulcer	*Streptococcus* species, *S. aureus* including MRSA, GNRs (*E. coli, Klebsiella, Proteus, Pseudomonas*), anaerobes	1. Moderate disease—ceftriaxone 2 g IV q24h, levofloxacin 750 mg PO/IV q24h, or cefepime 1–2 g IV q8h, all with metronidazole 500 mg po/IV q8h 2. Severe disease: vancomycin 15–20 mg/kg IV q12h with antipseudomonal beta-lactam (ceftazidime 2 g IV q8h, cefepime 2 g IV q12h), or aztreonam 2 g IV q8h with metronidazole 500 mg q8h, or piperacillin/tazobactam 4.5 g IV q6h, imipenem 500 mg IV q6h, or meropenem 1 g IV q8h)	7–21 d if no evidence of osteomyelitis
Necrotizing fasciitis	Type I is polymicrobial (gram-positives, gram-negatives and anaerobes) Type II is due to beta-hemolytic streptococci (usually group A Streptococcus), less commonly community-acquired MRSA	In addition to emergent surgical debridement: 1. Anti-MRSA agent: Vancomycin 15–20 mg/kg IV q12h, consider loading dose of 25–30 mg/kg, or linezolid 600 mg IV q12h, or daptomycin 6 mg/kg IV q24h + 2. Broad-spectrum beta-lactam: Piperacillin/tazobactam 4.5 g IV q6h, imipenem 500 mg IV q6h, meropenem 1 g IV q8h alone, or Cefepime 2 g IV q8–12 h + metronidazole 500 mg IV q8h * Consider addition of clindamycin 600–900 mg IV q8h for antitoxin effect versus streptococci and staphylococci. Intravenous immunoglobulin (IVIG) may be beneficial in cases due to group A *Streptococcus*	Depends on clinical course but should continue at least until no more surgical debridement necessary and minimum of 10–14 d

Musculoskeletal			
Septic arthritis	*S. aureus* including MRSA, *Streptococcus* species (especially group B *Streptococcus* in diabetics), *N. gonorrhoeae* (triad of pustular skin lesions, tenosynovitis, and arthritis), GNRs (*Pseudomonas* if IVDU)	In addition to surgical drainage, empiric antibiotics based on Gram stain: 1. Gram-positive cocci in clusters (likely *S. aureus*): Vancomycin 15–20 mg IV q12h 2. Gram-negative cocci (likely *Neisseria*): Ceftriaxone 1–2 g IV q24h 3. GNRs: Cefepime 2 g IV q8–12h or ceftazidime 2 g IV q8h 4. Negative Gram stain: Vancomycin + ceftriaxone, or vancomycin + cefepime or ceftazidime if risk factors for *Pseudomonas*	2–4 wk
Central Nervous System			
Bacterial meningitis, community acquired	*S. pneumoniae, Neisseria meningitidis, H. influenza* species *Listeria* if risk factors: Immunocompromised or age > 50 *Pseudomonas* if immunocompromised	Ceftriaxone 2 g IV q12h + vancomycin 15–20 mg/kg IV q8h (target trough ~20 mcg/mL) *Add ampicillin 2 g IV q4h if at risk for *Listeria* *Substitute Ceftriaxone with cefepime 2 g IV q8h or meropenem 2 g IV q8h if immunocompromised *If severe beta-lactam allergies: Vancomycin + moxifloxacin or chloramphenicol (+ bactrim if risk for *Listeria*) *Consider dexamethasone 0.15 mg/kg IV q6h, 15–20 min prior to antibiotics, in adults with suspected pneumococcal meningitis	Duration depends on pathogen (range 7–21 d) Steroids should be stopped after 4 d, or if the patient found to have another organism
Nosocomial meningitis	*S. aureus*, coagulase-negative staphylococci, GNRs including *P. aeruginosa* and *Acinetobacter* sp	Vancomycin 15–20 mg/kg IV q8h + Cefepime 2 g IV q8h or Ceftazidime 2 g IV q8h or Meropenem 2 g IV q8h (Meropenem preferred over Imipenem due to less risk of seizures)	Duration depends on pathogen
Bloodstream			
Catheter-associated bloodstream infection	*S. aureus*, coagulase-negative staphylococci, Enterococci, GNRs (more likely with femoral lines or ICU patient), *Candida* (especially if receiving total parenteral nutrition)	Vancomycin 15–20 mg/kg IV q12h *Consider adding cefepime 1–2 g IV q8–12h, piperacillin–tazobactam 4.5 g IV q6h, imipenem 500 mg IV q6h, or meropenem 1 g IV q8h if severely ill, if suspected source is a femoral line, or otherwise at risk for resistant gram negatives *Consider echinocandin (Caspofungin, Micafungin, or Anidulafungin) if severely ill and high risk of *Candida* (e.g., TPN, immunocompromised, prolonged exposure to antibiotics)	Depends on pathogen and clinical course (usually 7 d for Coag-neg Staph, 14 d for most other pathogens). 14 d is a minimum for *S. aureus* infections

(*Continued*)

TABLE 33.1 Recommendations for Initial Empiric Therapy for Common Serious Infections (*Continued*)

Condition	Likely Pathogens	Recommended Antibiotic Regimens and Dose (For Normal Renal/ Hepatic Function)	Typical Duration
Other Syndromes			
Neutropenic fever	Oral and enteric streptococci, gram-negative rods including *Pseudomonas, Candida. S. aureus,* or coagulase-negative staphylococci in patients with indwelling lines	1. Cefepime 2 g IV q8h 2. Alternatives: Piperacillin/tazobactam 4.5 g IV q6h, imipenem 500 mg IV q6h, or meropenem 1 g IV q8h *If severe beta-lactam allergy: Levofloxacin + aztreonam *Add Vancomycin if hypotensive or severely ill, pneumonia, suspected catheter-related infection, known colonization with MRSA or penicillin-resistant streptococci, recent prophylaxis with fluoroquinolones. Discontinue vancomycin if no evidence of MRSA after 48h *Add antifungal (Echinocandin, Voriconazole, or Amphotericin B) if persistently febrile after 4–7 d despite antibacterial therapy	Depends on duration of neutropenia and resolution of fever
Severe sepsis of unknown source	Target both gram-positive and gram-negative organisms	Anti-MRSA agent: Vancomycin 15–20 mg IV q12h with loading dose of 25–30 mg/kg IV, or linezolid 600 mg PO/IV if contraindication to vancomycin. Alternative is daptomycin 6 mg/kg IV q24h if pulmonary source unlikely + Antipseudomonal beta-lactam (cefepime 2 g IV q8h, ceftazidime 2 g IV q8h, piperacillin/tazobactam 4.5 g IV q6h, imipenem 500 mg IV q6h, or meropenem 1 g IV q8h) +/− Antipseudomonal fluoroquinolone (ciprofloxacin 400 mg IV q12h or levofloxacin 750 mg IV q24h), or aminoglycoside, or aztreonam 1–2 g IV q8h	Depends on clinical course and identification of source

Organism Abbreviations: MSSA, methicillin-sensitive *Staphylococcus aureus*; MRSA, methicillin-resistant *Staphylococcus aureus*; CA-MRSA, community-acquired MRSA; ESBL, extended-spectrum beta-lactamase producer; VRE, vancomycin-resistant *Enterococcus*.

drastically increases the range of pathogens that could be causing disease. Infections in immunocompromised hosts are discussed in detail in a separate chapter.

Clinical Setting and Local Resistance Patterns

It is important to determine whether the patient is likely to have a community-acquired or hospital-/health care–associated infection, as the latter is associated with more resistant organisms. For example, methicillin-resistant *S. aureus* (MRSA) and *Pseudomonas* are leading causes of hospital-acquired pneumonia, while they are rare in community-acquired cases.[10] For patients with a health care–associated infection, knowledge of local resistance patterns can be very helpful in choosing an appropriate regimen.

Recent Antibiotic Exposure

A history of the patient's recent antibiotic exposure should be elicited. A recent study of critically ill patients with gram-negative sepsis showed that patients who received antibiotics within the past 90 days were more likely to have resistant organisms, receive inappropriate initial therapy, and die.[11] In particular, recent broad-spectrum antibiotic exposure is a risk factor for MRSA and multidrug-resistant *Pseudomonas*, *Acinetobacter*, and *Enterobacteriaceae*.

Known History of Resistant Organism

A history of colonization (or prior infection) with resistant pathogens should also be noted. Patients colonized with MRSA are at higher risk for developing MRSA-invasive infection. In one study of patients in whom nares cultures were obtained on hospital admission, 19% of those colonized with MRSA developed MRSA infection in the following year, compared to 2% whose were not colonized.[12] Similar results have been noted in patients colonized with VRE.[13]

Level of Illness

The acuity of the presentation dictates the breadth of coverage of the initial regimen, as well as the timing of therapy (discussed later in this chapter). Inappropriate initial antibiotic therapy (i.e., when the pathogen is later shown to be resistant in vitro) in patients with severe sepsis is associated with a fivefold increase in mortality risk.[14] Therefore, when patients are severely ill, it is preferable to start with a broad-spectrum regimen; de-escalation can and should occur later as guided by microbiologic data. Conversely, a patient with a very mild presentation of an infection may not warrant broad-spectrum antibiotics at the onset.

Antibiotic Allergies

Taking an accurate allergy history prior to administration of antibiotics is necessary to avoid serious iatrogenic events. When assessing allergies, be sure to determine the severity of reaction and how long ago it occurred. For example, a history of anaphylaxis usually precludes reexposure under any circumstance, but patients with a remote history of mild rash or other vague symptoms can often be safely rechallenged. Penicillin allergies are common examples of this phenomenon, as fewer than 10% of patients who report penicillin allergies have a positive skin test.[15] Avoid inappropriately labeling mild toxicities (e.g., gastrointestinal [GI] upset) as drug "allergies," as this may prevent future providers from administering drugs that may be vitally important. Skin testing and desensitization are not typically practical in the acute setting, and so with a history of a potential allergy, the clinician must weigh the risks and benefits of administering that antibiotic. In most scenarios, however, a reasonable alternate choice is available.

Pharmacologic Factors to Consider

Bactericidal Versus Bacteriostatic Therapy

A common distinction is made based on the mechanism of action of antimicrobial agents. Agents that act on the cell wall tend to be bactericidal and cause cell death; beta-lactams are the classic example. Other bactericidal drugs include daptomycin (which causes cell membrane depolarization) and fluoroquinolones (which disrupt bacterial DNA). Drugs that act on protein synthesis, such as tetracyclines, macrolides, and clindamycin, tend to be bacteriostatic and inhibit growth of the organism without killing it. However, these distinctions are not absolute, and clinical outcomes do not necessarily parallel the mechanism of action. Furthermore, the relative bactericidal or static nature of an antibiotic depends on the organism and the minimum inhibitory concentration (MIC), defined as the lowest concentration of an antibiotic that inhibits growth of the organism. For example, vancomycin is considered to be a slowly bactericidal agent but is generally considered bacteriostatic against *Enterococcus*. As a general rule, bactericidal agents are preferred for serious infections such as endocarditis and meningitis.[16]

Mechanism of Killing

The two major types of "killing" exhibited by antibiotics are time-dependent killing, where efficacy depends on maximizing the time the antibiotic concentration is above the MIC, and concentration-dependent killing, where efficacy depends on achieving peak concentrations far above the MIC. Drugs that act via time-dependent killing include beta-lactams and vancomycin; those that act via concentration-dependent killing include aminoglycosides, fluoroquinolones, metronidazole, and daptomycin. The mechanism of killing has implications for dosing strategies. For time-dependent beta-lactams, there is increasing evidence that continuous or prolonged infusion strategies (to maximize time above the MIC) may lead to better microbiologic and possibly clinical outcomes in critically ill patients with resistant organisms.[17–19] For concentration-dependent aminoglycosides, once-daily dosing strategies are in many circumstances as efficacious and less toxic than traditional q8h dosing.[20]

Sites of Penetration

Choosing an initial appropriate regimen requires knowledge of the distribution and penetration of antibiotics into different tissue compartments, as well as determination of the patient's most likely site of infection. A particular antibiotic may match a pathogen under most circumstances, but if it does not act at the site of the infection, it will be clinically ineffective. Important examples of deficiencies in site penetration include the following:

- **Central nervous system**: First- and second-generation cephalosporins, macrolides, clindamycin, daptomycin, and aminoglycosides tend to have poor penetration and are suboptimal for treatment of meningitis.[21] Third-generation cephalosporins and carbapenems are better choices.

- **Lungs**: Daptomycin is inactivated by surfactant, making it ineffective for pneumonia.[22] Beta-lactams and fluoroquinolones are better choices.
- **Urine**: Moxifloxacin does not achieve adequate levels in the urine, making it ineffective for urinary tract infections (UTIs). Levofloxacin and ciprofloxacin are better choices among the fluoroquinolones.

Antibiotic Metabolism

The kidneys or the liver metabolize most antibiotics, and dysfunction in those organs may affect the dose or force the clinician to choose another drug class entirely. Dose adjustment for renal dysfunction in particular is frequently necessary; in these cases, creatinine should be routinely checked prior to antibiotic administration. Antibiotics whose dosing is dependent on renal function include vancomycin, aminoglycosides, and some beta-lactams; failure to account for this can lead to serious toxicities.

Combination Therapy

In critically ill patients, it is common to use two or more antibiotics in an empiric regimen to cover a broad range of pathogens (e.g., combining vancomycin and cefepime to cover gram-positive and gram-negative infections). Other than this, the reasons to consider combination therapy are as follows:

- **To increase the likelihood of empiric therapy being active against the pathogen**: In severely ill patients in whom microbiologic data are still pending and who are at risk for resistant organisms, administration of two antibiotics with similar spectrum of activity (typically gram-negative activity) increases the chance that at least one antibiotic will be active against the suspected organism. This is the rationale for the use of two gram-negative agents in nosocomial pneumonia and is often considered in patients in whom *Pseudomonas* is suspected (see "Empiric *Pseudomonas* Therapy" below).
- **To achieve synergistic activity against an organism:** Combinations of antibiotics can be synergistic in vitro, where the combined effect of the agents is greater than each alone. This scenario, however, is relatively uncommon in clinical practice and is mainly limited to endocarditis due to aminoglycoside-susceptible strains of *Enterococcus* and some streptococci (the synergistic agents in those cases are beta-lactams and aminoglycosides).[23] Use of aminoglycosides for synergy in *S. aureus* infections and endocarditis was more common in the past, but is used less commonly now due to weak evidence of benefit and strong evidence of nephrotoxicity.[24]
- **To prevent emergence of resistance:** Certain organisms are prone to develop resistance when exposed to antimicrobial agents, and the simultaneous administration of several antimicrobials can decrease this risk. Examples include HIV and tuberculosis. This practice tends to be the exception rather than the norm in cases of routine bacterial pathogens, although it is often considered for *Pseudomonas*.

When combination therapy is used, antibiotics should be chosen from different classes (e.g., a beta-lactam plus a fluoroquinolone) in order to minimize overlapping toxicities as well as possible pharmacologic antagonism. In particular, double beta-lactams should be avoided whenever possible.

Empiric *Pseudomonas* Therapy

An important consideration in choosing an empiric antimicrobial regimen is the need to cover *Pseudomonas*, a nonfermenting gram-negative bacillus notorious for both its inherent resistance to most antibiotics as well as its propensity to develop resistance. *Pseudomonas* is responsible for many nosocomial infections, including pneumonia, catheter-related infections, UTIs, and postsurgical infections. It also commonly affects immunocompromised patients (commonly causing neutropenic fever), those with cystic fibrosis, and burn patients. For immunocompetent patients, invasive *Pseudomonas* bacteremia at the time of hospital admission is rare. Based on a review of 4,114 episodes of gram-negative rod (GNR) bacteremia on admission, empiric antipseudomonal treatment in patients without immunodeficiency is warranted for patients with two or more of the following predictors: age >90 years, antimicrobial therapy within the preceding 30 days, presence of a central venous catheter, or presence of a urinary device.[26] In this study, the percentage of episodes of GNR bacteremia that were due to *Pseudomonas* was 2% with no risk factors, 8% with one risk factor, and 28% with two risk factors.

For serious infections due to suspected *Pseudomonas*, it is generally recommended to "double cover" empirically with two antibiotics from different classes until susceptibilities are available, and then narrow to one drug. The rationale (as discussed in the "Combination Therapy" section above) is to increase the chance that one of the agents will be active against the isolate; this approach has been associated with improved mortality in patients with severe sepsis and gram-negative bacteremia.[27]

The benefit of continuing double coverage after antibiotic susceptibilities are identified for *Pseudomonas* remains a long-standing point of controversy. Two meta-analyses published in 2004 reached conflicting results for the combination of beta-lactams and aminoglycosides in gram-negative and pseudomonal infections. One study showed no clinical benefit and increased nephrotoxicity; the other showed a mortality benefit in the subset of GNR bacteremia due to *Pseudomonas*.[28,29] Despite this uncertainty, several experts do recommend continuing combination therapy for serious infections due to *Pseudomonas*, including bacteremia in neutropenic patients, endocarditis, meningitis, and possibly pneumonia. If double coverage is utilized, as either empiric or definitive therapy, the regimen should include a beta-lactam plus either a fluoroquinolone or an aminoglycoside. The antibiotics with activity against *Pseudomonas* are described in further detail later in this chapter.

Empiric MRSA Therapy

Choice of an appropriate empiric regimen is often driven by the need to cover MRSA, which is feared for both its virulence and its resistance to many antibiotics. Failure to initially include an agent with activity against MRSA, in those who turn out to have a MRSA infection, is associated with increased mortality.[25] MRSA is typically categorized as community acquired or health-care associated; the two strains have different genetics and epidemiology, although the difference between them has begun to blur. Risk factors for MRSA include known colonization or prior disease with MRSA, indwelling lines or hardware, prior antibiotic use, residence in a long-term care facility, immunosuppression, injection drug use, hemodialysis, and prolonged hospital stay. Therapy directed at MRSA should be considered in patients with risk factors, as well as in patients presenting with severe illness. Specific drugs with MRSA activity are detailed later in this chapter.

Timing of Antimicrobial Therapy

In critically ill patients, timely administration of antibiotics is essential. A retrospective study of 2,731 patients with septic shock found that time to appropriate antibiotic therapy was the factor most strongly associated with survival; each hour of delay after the onset of hypotension until administration of effective antibiotic therapy increased mortality by 7.6%.[30] Similar results were reported in a recent single-center prospective cohort study of patients with severe sepsis or septic shock, where a delay in starting antibiotics more than 1 hour from hospital triage, or from the moment the patient qualified for early goal-directed therapy, increased in-hospital mortality risk by more than 50%.[31] Administration of appropriate antibiotic therapy is also a medical emergency in bacterial meningitis and neutropenic fever. Practitioners should make every effort to obtain diagnostic blood (+/− cerebrospinal fluid, sputum, and urine) cultures prior to initiating antibiotics, but not at the cost of significant delay in starting antibiotics for critically ill individuals. In contrast, for stable patients, especially those for whom prolonged antimicrobial therapy is likely, it is crucial to obtain adequate specimen cultures prior to antibiotics. This sometimes requires invasive diagnostic tests and biopsies. Classic examples include subacute bacterial endocarditis and osteomyelitis, where symptoms have usually been present for weeks to months. In these situations, starting antibiotics before obtaining specimens for culture ultimately proves harmful, as the lack of a microbiologic diagnosis may lead to long treatment courses of excessively broad-spectrum antibiotics.

CONTINUING ANTIMICROBIAL THERAPY

Definitive Therapy and De-escalation

Once the organism causing an infection has been identified, the antibiotic regimen should be narrowed in order to reduce costs, toxicities, and emergence of resistance. Failure to de-escalate antibiotics is unfortunately common in clinical practice, and in certain scenarios, such as hospital-acquired pneumonia, it may be associated with worse outcomes.[32] The decision to de-escalate for a specific infection may be complicated by other concurrent infections; in the absence of multiple infections, every effort should be made to narrow to the simplest regimen possible.

An important principle of therapy is the appropriate discontinuation of anti-MRSA therapy after 48 to 72 hours of negative cultures, assuming that adequate cultures were drawn prior to antibiotics. MRSA is a pathogen that grows easily on culture medium, so failure to recover MRSA strongly suggests an alternate organism. A similar rationale should be used to discontinue or narrow broad-spectrum gram-negative agents, such as the carbapenems, in the absence of positive cultures.

Interpretation of Antibiotic Susceptibility Results

After a pathogenic organism is identified on culture, it is usually subjected to antimicrobial susceptibility testing, whereby the ability of the organism to grow in the presence of various antibiotics in vitro is measured and interpreted using guidelines established by the Clinical and Laboratory Standards Institute. A report of "susceptible" indicates likely inhibition of the organism when the antimicrobial agent is used at the recommended dosage; a report of "resistant" indicates the opposite. A report of "intermediate" indicates that the MIC of the drug falls within attainable blood and tissue levels, but the response rates may be reduced compared to susceptible organisms (and may even be ineffective in sequestered body sites). MICs of different agents for an organism are not directly comparable; an antibiotic with an MIC of 1 is not necessarily superior to a different antibiotic with a reported MIC of 2. The susceptibility data are very useful but are subject to important limitations:

- **Not all antibiotics to which an organism is susceptible are equally effective:** Although an organism may be susceptible to multiple antibiotics, clinical evidence often points to a superior match. For example, methicillin-susceptible *S. aureus* (MSSA) is susceptible to both vancomycin and nafcillin; however, nafcillin (and cefazolin) has a much higher clinical success rate than vancomycin for serious infections.[33,34] Only in the case of a severe beta-lactam allergy should vancomycin be used over nafcillin or cefazolin. Similarly, *C. difficile* is uniformly susceptible to intravenous or oral metronidazole and oral vancomycin; however, oral vancomycin is associated with superior cure rates, especially in severe infections.[35]
- **Some organisms carry enzymes that mediate resistance in vivo to antibiotics that are active in vitro**: For example, ESBLs, which are enzymes that confer resistance to almost all beta-lactams except carbapenems, may not be apparent on routine testing. One prospective study of patients with bacteremia from ESBL *Klebsiella pneumoniae* showed that use of carbapenems was associated with significantly lower short-term mortality than was use of other antibiotics that were active in vitro.[36]
- **Inducible chromosomal resistance may not be detected on initial susceptibility testing:** Some Enterobacteriaceae produce an inducible chromosomal beta-lactamase that can be expressed during antimicrobial therapy. Although initial tests may report susceptibility, clinical failure and development of resistance to beta-lactams occasionally occur with agents other than fourth-generation cephalosporins and carbapenems.[37] This is a risk with the so-called "SPICE A" group of organisms: *Serratia, Pseudomonas,* Indole-positive *Proteus*, *Citrobacter*, *Enterobacter*, and *Acinetobacter*.

Duration of Therapy

The optimal duration of therapy for many types of infections *is* based on expert opinion rather than well-designed studies. There are, however several important publications that have defined optimal courses of therapy, usually with an emphasis on shorter courses. One frequently cited study compared 8 versus 15 days of therapy for ventilator-associated pneumonia (VAP) diagnosed by bronchoalveolar lavage and found similar outcomes between the courses.[38] Another meta-analysis of studies examining antibiotic courses for community-acquired pneumonia reported successful treatment of mild to moderate cases within 7 days or fewer.[39] The appropriate duration of therapy will ultimately be determined by the clinical response to therapy, pathogen-specific factors, and host factors. For example, the study that examined the 8-day course of antibiotics for VAP excluded immunocompromised patients, and the optimal duration of therapy for this population remains unknown. Furthermore, patients in that study with *Pseudomonas* as the pathogen causing VAP had increased recurrence rates with the shorter course; this has led to recommendations that longer courses of therapy be used in this scenario.[40] Although many studies have emphasized short durations of therapy, certain deep-seated infections (such as endocarditis and osteomyelitis) clearly require prolonged courses of therapy to minimize relapse and treatment failure.

Clinical improvement is usually monitored by resolution of symptoms and normalization of laboratory values. Radiologic improvement can sometimes be misleading and lag behind clinical improvement. The importance of microbiologic cure depends on the type of infection; it is a crucial factor in bacteremia where failure to clear blood cultures generally indicates inadequate antimicrobial therapy and/or source control.

Route of Administration

For critically ill patients, an initial intravenous route of administration is generally preferable. However, several antibiotic classes have excellent bioavailability, making transition to oral therapy easy. These include fluoroquinolones, trimethoprim–sulfamethoxazole, metronidazole, clindamycin, azithromycin, and linezolid. Beta-lactams tend to have poor bioavailability, making the oral route for this class inappropriate for most serious or deep-seated infections. Even for those drugs with good bioavailability, an oral route is generally considered to be less effective than intravenous therapy for certain serious infections such as endocarditis, meningitis, and *S. aureus* bacteremia.

OVERVIEW OF MAJOR ANTIBIOTIC CLASSES

An overview of the mechanism, spectrum, common indications, and side effects of the major antibiotic classes is presented in Tables 33.2 to 33.5.

CONCLUSION

Today, our armamentarium of antibiotics is greater than ever, but so is the diversity of pathogens and their resistance to many common antibiotics. Choosing an empiric initial regimen and subsequently deciding on appropriate therapy can be complicated, but both are vital in determining patient outcome. After making a presumptive diagnosis, the physician must consider factors such as the patient's setting (community vs. nosocomial), degree of immunosuppression, level of illness, prior history of infections or colonization with resistant organisms, and recent antibiotic exposure. Knowledge of the pharmacologic characteristics of available antimicrobial agents may mean the difference between life and death, particularly in critically ill patients with sepsis. Although infectious disease problems are rarely straightforward, there are few things in medicine more satisfying than seeing a sick patient rapidly brought back to health by wise and informed decisions on the use of antimicrobial therapy.

TABLE 33.2 Major Antibiotic Classes: Beta-Lactams

- Mechanism: bind penicillin-binding proteins in the cell membrane and inhibit cell wall cross-linking (bactericidal). Beta-lactams exhibit time-dependent killing
- Highly variable spectrum depending on antibiotic, but in general none have activity against MRSA (except Ceftaroline), and none have activity against atypical intracellular organisms (e.g., *Legionella, Mycoplasma, Chlamydia*)
- Most oral beta-lactams have poor bioavailability and achieve low serum concentrations. Intravenous therapy should be given for serious or deep-seated infections
- Among patients with reported penicillin allergy, >85% will actually tolerate it (either because they were never truly allergic, or due to resolution of a remote prior allergy)
- Clinical cross-reactivity with penicillin and cephalosporins/carbapenems is very low: of those with a positive penicillin skin test, ~2% will have a cephalosporin reaction, and <1% will have a carbapenem reaction
- There is no cross-reactivity between penicillin and aztreonam; however, cross-reactivity between aztreonam and ceftazidime has been reported (due to an identical side chain)

Antibiotic	Spectrum	Common Indications	Authors' Notes
Penicillins			
Penicillin (IV or PO)	Gram-positives (many strains of streptococci, minority of staphylococci, some *Enterococcus*), most oral anaerobes, syphilis. Limited gram-negative coverage	Strep throat and other infections due to group A *Streptococcus*, Syphilis, bacteremia/endocarditis due to sensitive *Streptococcus*, *Enterococcus*, or *S. aureus* (<10% of *S. aureus* strains are penicillin sensitive)	For most situations, generally start with broader antibiotics until pathogen and susceptibilities identified
***Aminopenicillins*:** **Amoxicillin** (PO) **Ampicillin** (IV)	Some gram-positives (*Streptococcus, Enterococcus, Listeria*) but *not S. aureus*, and limited gram-negative coverage	Upper respiratory infections, sinusitis, otitis media, cellulitis, *Listeria* infections, UTIs, early Lyme disease (alternative to Doxycycline), and more. Drug of choice for most enterococcal infections	Often combined with aminoglycosides for synergy in serious enterococcal infections and endocarditis
***Antistaphylococcal Penicillins*:** **Nafcillin, Oxacillin** (IV) **Dicloxacillin** (PO)	Gram positives (MSSA and streptococci). Drug of choice for MSSA infections. No MRSA coverage and coagulase-negative staphylococci are usually resistant. No gram-negative or anaerobic coverage	Cellulitis, other infections from MSSA (osteomyelitis, endocarditis, bacteremia, etc.)	For all serious MSSA infections, the entire course of therapy should be given intravenously
Penicillin/Beta-Lactamase Inhibitors			
Note: Beta-lactamase inhibitor confers broader spectrum against common beta-lactamase–producing organisms (such as MSSA, some gram negatives including *H. influenza, Moraxellae*, and virtually all anaerobes)			
Amoxicillin/ **Clavulanate** (PO)	Gram positives (MSSA, streptococci, enterococci), some gram negatives, and anaerobes. Notable lack of activity against *Pseudomonas* and *Acinetobacter*	Sinusitis, respiratory infections, otitis media, some skin/soft tissue infections (including bite wounds), and more	Fairly broad-spectrum oral agent with good bioavailability

Ampicillin/Sulbactam (IV)	Similar spectrum to amoxicillin/clavulanate, except has activity against most *Acinetobacter* (sulbactam component has activity)	Similar situations as for amoxicillin/clavulanate but where IV form is desirable; also, some intra-abdominal and GYN infections, aspiration pneumonia and lung abscesses, and more	Caution for polymicrobial intra-abdominal infections due to high rate of resistance of *E. coli*
Piperacillin/Tazobactam (IV)	Similar spectrum to ampicillin/sulbactam (gram-positive, gram-negative, anaerobic coverage), but better overall gram-negative coverage, including *Pseudomonas*	Hospital-acquired/health care–associated pneumonia, severe skin/soft tissue infections, including diabetic foot ulcers, intra-abdominal infections, and severe UTIs, due to suspected resistant organisms	Note higher dosing for *Pseudomonas* coverage: 4.5 g q6h (vs. 3.375 g q6h for other indications)
Cephalosporins			
Note: No cephalosporin covers *Enterococcus* (except Ceftaroline). Only ceftazidime and cefepime cover *Pseudomonas*. Only cefoxitin and cefotetan have good anaerobic coverage			
First Generation **Cefazolin** (IV) **Cephalexin** (PO)	Good gram-positive coverage (MSSA and streptococci). Limited gram negative (*Proteus, E. coli, Klebsiella*). No anaerobic activity	Mild–moderate nonpurulent cellulitis (if MRSA not suspected). Cefazolin often used for prophylaxis prior to surgery. Can be used for UTIs (especially during pregnancy)	Cefazolin is first-line option for severe MSSA infections in patients allergic to nafcillin (for non-severe allergies)
Second Generation **Cefuroxime** (PO or IV)	Gram positives and more gram-negatives than first generation (gains activity against *H. influenzae, Enterobacter, Neisseria*). No anaerobic activity	Respiratory infections (upper and lower tract), gonorrhea, UTIs, Lyme disease (alternative to doxycycline)	Useful oral option for community-acquired pneumonia caused by penicillin-susceptible *S. pneumoniae*
Cephamycins: **Cefoxitin** (IV) **Cefotetan** (IV)	Gram negatives and anaerobes, but no *Pseudomonas* and poor gram-positive coverage	UTIs, nonsevere intra-abdominal infections, pelvic/gynecologic infections	*Bacteroides fragilis* has high rates of resistance, so avoid for serious intra-abdominal infections
Third Generation **Ceftriaxone** (IV) **Cefotaxime** (IV) **Cefpodoxime** (PO)	Gram-positives (MSSA, streptococci) and good gram-negative coverage (but not *Pseudomonas*). Limited anaerobic activity	Ceftriaxone used for community-acquired pneumonia (with azithromycin), community-acquired meningitis, spontaneous bacterial peritonitis, some skin/soft tissue infections, bacteremia/endocarditis from susceptible streptococci, UTIs and pyelonephritis, bone and joint infections, late Lyme disease, gonorrhea, pelvic infections, and more	Small but important rate of resistance in *S. pneumoniae* Ceftriaxone usually once-daily dosing (1–2 g) except for meningitis (2 g IV q12h)
Third/fourth Generation **Ceftazidime** (IV)	Covers *Pseudomonas* and other gram negatives. Virtually no gram-positive or anaerobic coverage	Used for many situations where *Pseudomonas* infection is suspected	Option for empiric neutropenic fever treatment, but lack of streptococcal and staphylococcal coverage makes cefepime a better choice

(*Continued*)

TABLE 33.2 Major Antibiotic Classes: Beta-Lactams (*Continued*)

Fourth Generation **Cefepime** (IV)	Broad spectrum: Gram positives (MSSA, streptococci) and gram-negatives (including *Pseudomonas*), but lacks anaerobic coverage	Empiric neutropenic fever, hospital-acquired pneumonia, complicated UTIs, nosocomial meningitis, and more	Beware central nervous system (CNS) toxicity: encephalopathy, altered mental status, and seizures in the elderly and those with renal failure
Fifth Generation **Ceftaroline** (IV)	Broad gram-positive coverage, including MRSA, vancomycin-intermediate and vancomycin-resistant *S. aureus*, streptococci, and *Enterococcus faecalis* including vancomycin-resistant strains (less activity against *E. faecium*). Similar gram-negative coverage as ceftriaxone (no *Pseudomonas*). Limited anaerobic activity	FDA approved only for complicated skin/soft tissue infections and community-acquired pneumonia (but increasingly being used for other indications—bone/joint infections, refractory MRSA bacteremia, etc.)	Newest cephalosporin (approved in 2010) and only beta-lactam with activity against MRSA. Only cephalosporin with activity versus *Enterococcus* (but rarely used for this purpose)
Carbapenems			
Imipenem/Cilastin **Meropenem** **Doripenem** **Ertapenem** (all IV)	Broadest-spectrum antibiotics that cover gram positives (MSSA, streptococci, some enterococci), gram-negatives including *Pseudomonas* (except Ertapenem) and ESBLs, and anaerobes	Many serious infections due to resistant gram negatives including hospital and health care–associated pneumonia, meningitis, intra-abdominal infections, complicated skin and soft tissue infections. The most reliable class of antibiotics against ESBL organisms	Ertapenem has no activity against *Pseudomonas* but has the advantage of once-daily dosing Imipenem has highest risk of seizures
Monobactam			
Aztreonam (IV)	Active against aerobic gram negatives including *Pseudomonas* (but high rates of resistance). No activity against gram positives or anaerobes	Hospital-acquired/health care–associated pneumonia, UTIs, intra-abdominal infections, sepsis, skin and soft tissue infections. Often used in combination with other agents with gram-positive activity	No cross-reactivity with penicillin allergy and minimal toxicity Consider second agent for empiric double coverage for *Pseudomonas*

Side effects for all beta-lactams: Hypersensitivity reactions including anaphylaxis and rash, bone marrow suppression, interstitial nephritis, GI effects (nausea, diarrhea, and *C. difficile*), and seizures (mainly with high doses in renal failure)

Organism Abbreviations: MSSA, methicillin-sensitive *Staphylococcus aureus*; MRSA, methicillin-resistant *Staphylococcus aureus*; CA-MRSA, community-acquired MRSA; ESBL, extended-spectrum beta-lactamase producer; VRE, vancomycin-resistant *Enterococcus*.

TABLE 33.3 Major Antibiotic Classes: Non–Beta Lactam Antibiotics

Antibiotic	Spectrum	Common Indications	Authors' Notes
Macrolides—Mechanism: Reversibly bind to the 50S ribosomal subunit (static)			
Azithromycin **Erythromycin** **Clarithromycin** (PO or IV)	Excellent for atypical intracellular organisms (*Chlamydia, Mycoplasma, Legionella*). Limited activity against gram-positives (staphylococci, streptococci), some gram-negatives, and syphilis. Also have activity against some nontuberculous mycobacteria	Azithromycin most commonly used: bronchitis, COPD exacerbations, community-acquired pneumonia (combined with ceftriaxone for patients ill enough to require hospitalization), sinusitis, strep throat in penicillin-allergic patients, and more	Azithromycin is the drug of choice for atypical organisms Erythromycin now used mostly as GI motility agent
Side effects: QT prolongation, GI side effects, and rash			
Tetracyclines and Glycylcycline—Mechanism: Reversibly bind to 30S ribosomal subunit (static)			
Doxycycline **Tetracycline** **Minocycline** (PO or IV)	Gram positives (MSSA and community-acquired MRSA), some gram-negative coverage, and atypical organisms. Active against many unusual pathogens (*Rickettsia*, Lyme disease, Tularemia, *Vibrio, Brucella*, Q fever, Anthrax)	Skin and soft tissue infections when suspect community-acquired MRSA, respiratory tract infections, early Lyme disease, and other unusual infections. Often part of empiric therapy in toxic-appearing patients with fever and rash	Poor streptococcal coverage, combine with beta-lactam when using for cellulitis Doxycycline is generally the preferred tetracycline due to bid dosing, and no food interactions
Tigecycline (IV)	Member of glycylcycline class that is structurally similar to tetracyclines Broad coverage—gram positives (including streptococci, MRSA and vancomycin-resistant enterococci [VRE]), gram-negatives, anaerobes, and atypicals. Lacks activity against *Pseudomonas, Proteus*, and *Providencia*	Complicated intra-abdominal infections, skin/soft tissue infections, and pneumonia Can occasionally be used against multidrug-resistant gram-negative pathogens, including some ESBL and carbapenemase-producing strains (check sensitivities)	Caution: Overall increased risk of death when used for severe infections, and high rate of failure for hospital-acquired and VAP Low serum concentration (distributes widely into tissues)—poor choice for bacteremia
Side effects: Photosensitivity, GI discomfort, teeth discoloration, inhibition of bone growth in children, teratogenicity, hepatosteatosis, and hepatotoxicity			
Lincosamide—Mechanism: Reversibly binds to the 50S ribosomal subunit (static)			
Clindamycin (PO or IV)	Excellent activity against anaerobes (but resistance common in *Bacteroides*) and gram-positive cocci (streptococci and staphylococci), including some community-acquired MRSA, but *not* enterococci. No gram-negative activity	Skin/soft tissue infections, pelvic infections, lung abscess, sinusitis. Also used often for its antitoxin effect in toxic shock syndrome or necrotizing fasciitis due to group A *Streptococcus* (less evidence for MRSA)	High rate of resistance among *Bacteroides* so avoid for intra-abdominal infections Check D-test for *S. aureus* infections to rule out inducible resistance. No CNS penetration, so avoid for brain abscesses
Side effects: GI intolerance and high rate of *C. difficile*			

(*Continued*)

TABLE 33.3 Major Antibiotic Classes: Non-Beta Lactam Antibiotics (*Continued*)

Antibiotic	Spectrum	Common Indications	Authors' Notes
Aminoglycosides—Mechanism: Irreversibly bind to the 30S ribosomal subunit (cidal)			
Gentamicin **Tobramycin** **Amikacin** (All IV)	Aerobic gram negatives including *Pseudomonas*. No activity against gram positives (except when used for synergy) or anaerobes	Usually used in combination with other agents for serious gram-negative infections, especially when *Pseudomonas* is suspected (pneumonia, bacteremia, UTIs). Used with beta-lactams against gram-positive organisms for synergistic effect (mainly endocarditis) Multiple dosing strategies exist (once/daily, traditional multiple times/daily, synergy dosing)	Avoid as monotherapy for *Pseudomonas* bacteremia due to associated high mortality Evidence for synergy is best for enterococcal and streptococcal infections (depending on the MIC). Weak clinical evidence for synergy against *S. aureus*
Side effects: Nephrotoxicity (manifests after 3–5 d, usually reversible), vestibular and ototoxicity (irreversible). If using long-term, check baseline audiology test and ~q2 wk			
Fluoroquinolones—Mechanism: DNA gyrase and topoisomerase inhibitors (bactericidal) • The fluoroquinolones described in this section have good atypical activity (moxifloxacin and levofloxacin > ciprofloxacin) • All have excellent bioavailability, so use oral form if possible • All have activity versus tuberculosis (moxifloxacin > levofloxacin > ciprofloxacin), so avoid in patients presenting with pneumonia if TB is a possibility (to avoid development of resistance on monotherapy) • Levofloxacin and moxifloxacin have good streptococcal and some staphylococcal coverage, but avoid for *S. aureus* infections as resistance develops quickly			
Ciprofloxacin (PO or IV)	Best gram-negative coverage of quinolones (including *Pseudomonas*), but virtually no gram-positive coverage. Lacks anaerobic coverage. Good atypical coverage	UTIs and pyelonephritis, double coverage of *Pseudomonas* including for hospital-acquired pneumonia, bone and joint infections, prostatitis, GI/intra-abdominal coverage (often with Flagyl), traveler's diarrhea. Also effective against anthrax	Not used for community-acquired pneumonia due to lack of *S. pneumoniae* coverage Due to availability of alternate agents (fosfomycin, nitrofurantoin), should be second line for uncomplicated UTIs (also due to rising *E. coli* resistance)
Levofloxacin (PO or IV)	Gram-positive coverage: mainly streptococci (especially *S. pneumoniae*), limited staphylococcal coverage. Good gram-negative coverage including *Pseudomonas*. Excellent for atypicals	Used for community-acquired pneumonia (can use as monotherapy), sinusitis/bronchitis, UTIs, pyelonephritis, and double coverage of *Pseudomonas* including hospital-acquired pneumonia	Gram-negative coverage is comparable to ciprofloxacin Dose at 750 mg PO/IV for pneumonia to increase *S. pneumoniae* coverage
Moxifloxacin (PO or IV)	Similar to levofloxacin but no *Pseudomonas* activity Best gram-positive, atypical, and anaerobic coverage out of the quinolones	Community-acquired pneumonia as monotherapy, sinusitis/bronchitis Cannot use for UTIs due to poor urine penetration	Although approved for intra-abdominal infections, rising resistance in *Bacteroides*. Therefore, do not use as monotherapy for intra-abdominal infections
Side effects: QT prolongation, tendon rupture (especially if on steroids), GI intolerance, cartilage damage, rare dysglycemias, dizziness/HAs, rashes, teratogenicity, transaminitis. Fluoroquinolones also recently associated with increased risk of retinal detachment. High rate of *C. difficile*			

Sulfonamides—Mechanism: Inhibit sequential steps in folate synthesis. Individually, components are static, but combination often cidal			
Trimethoprim/ Sulfamethoxazole (PO or IV)	Gram positives (*S. aureus* including most CA-MRSA, some *S. pneumoniae*), and some gram-negatives, but not *Pseudomonas*. No anaerobic activity. Notable differences from other agents are its activity against *Pneumocystis jiroveci* (PCP), *Nocardia, Toxoplasma, Listeria, Isospora*, and *Stenotrophomonas*	Many purposes including PCP pneumonia (drug of choice, both for treatment and prophylaxis), CA-MRSA skin/soft tissue infections, UTIs, nocardiosis, *Listeria* infections in penicillin-allergic patients, *Salmonella* infections, traveler's diarrhea, acute bronchitis, and otitis media	Best oral agent for CA-MRSA (except for Linezolid), but for empiric cellulitis, consider combining with a beta-lactam due to poor streptococcal coverage. Excellent bioavailability, so use oral form whenever possible. Dosing is highly variable depending on indication and patient weight
Side effects: Common—hypersensitivity (sulfas) and rashes, GI side effects, dose-dependent bone marrow suppression, increased creatinine (both from pseudocreatinine elevation due to blocked creatinine secretion into tubules, and true kidney injury from interstitial nephritis and acute tubular necrosis), hyperkalemia (dose dependent, especially in chronic kidney disease). Uncommon—aseptic meningitis, methemoglobinemia and hemolysis in glucose-6-phosphate deficiency, transaminitis and cholestasis, and pancreatitis			
Nitroimidazole—Mechanism: selectively taken up by anaerobic bacteria and reduced by proteins in the electron transport chain, leading to DNA disruption (cidal)			
Metronidazole (PO or IV)	Anaerobes (including *C. difficile*), and protozoans: *Giardia, Trichomonas, Entameba histolytica*, also *Helicobacter pylori* (part of triple therapy). No activity against aerobic gram-positive or gram-negative organisms	Anaerobic infections, usually in conjunction with other agents (since anaerobes generally part of a polymicrobial infection). Also used for mild–moderate *C. difficile*, and for the listed protozoal infections	Excellent anaerobic drug, but with notable lack of activity against *Propionibacterium acnes*. Excellent oral bioavailability. Not well tolerated long term due to side effects
Side effects: Nausea, diarrhea, metallic taste, dose-dependent and possibly cumulative peripheral neuropathy, and also disulfiram effect with ethanol			

Organism Abbreviations: MSSA, methicillin-sensitive *Staphylococcus aureus*; MRSA, methicillin-resistant *Staphylococcus aureus*; CA-MRSA, community-acquired MRSA; ESBL, extended-spectrum beta-lactamase producer; VRE, vancomycin-resistant *Enterococcus*.

TABLE 33.4 Major Antibiotic Classes: Anti-MRSA Antibiotics

- Other intravenous antibiotics with activity against MRSA, but not listed in the table, include ceftaroline, tigecycline, quinupristin–dalfopristin, and telavancin
- In general, community-acquired MRSA has broader susceptibility to antibiotics, including trimethoprim–sulfamethoxazole, doxycycline, and clindamycin
- The antibiotics listed below also have reliable activity against coagulase-negative staphylococci. Daptomycin, linezolid, tigecycline, and quinupristin–dalfopristin also have activity against most vancomycin-resistant enterococci (VRE)

Antibiotic	Spectrum	Common Indications	Authors' Notes
Glycopeptide—Mechanism: Inhibits cell wall synthesis in gram positives by binding to a protein that is distinct from the penicillin-binding proteins (cidal)			
Vancomycin (IV)	Purely gram-positive agent with activity against staphylococci (including MRSA), streptococci, and non-VRE *Enterococcus*. Considered the gold standard for MRSA infections. Oral form is not absorbed and is used for severe *C. difficile*. No activity against gram negatives or anaerobes	Many situations with suspected or proven gram-positive infections including bacteremia, meningitis, pneumonia, skin/soft tissue, and more. Drug of choice for gram-positive infections in patients with severe beta-lactam allergy	Slowly bactericidal drug that is inferior to nafcillin and cefazolin for MSSA infection. Avoid for MRSA if MIC ≥2 (increased treatment failure). Typical dosing = 15–20 mg/kg q12h (actual body weight), higher in critically ill patients. Adjust for renal function. Goal trough for serious infection 15–20 mg/L
Side effects: Red man syndrome due to histamine release, nephrotoxicity (acute tubular necrosis), ototoxicity (reversible), and bone marrow suppression (leukopenia > thrombocytopenia)			
Oxazolidinone—Mechanism: Ribosomal inhibitor—different site than other protein synthesis inhibitors (static)			
Linezolid (PO or IV)	Virtually all gram positives including streptococci, MRSA, and VRE Also has good activity against tuberculosis No gram-negative coverage. Limited anaerobic activity	Skin/soft tissue infections, hospital-acquired pneumonia with proven or suspected MRSA, and various VRE infections Sometimes used as part of a second-line regimen for tuberculosis	Oral form is virtually 100% bioavailable Cost of drug (and long-term toxicity) is often prohibitive for outpatient use
Side effects: Bone marrow suppression, especially thrombocytopenia. Linezolid is a monoamine oxidase (MAO) inhibitor—risk of serotonin syndrome with selective serotonin reuptake inhibitors (SSRIs), so avoid coadministration. Long-term usage can lead to mitochondrial toxicity (lactic acidosis, peripheral neuropathy, optic neuritis, and blindness).			
Lipopeptide—Mechanism: Forms transmembrane channels and depolarizes cells (cidal).			
Daptomycin (IV)	Purely gram-positive activity including MRSA, streptococci, and *Enterococcus* including VRE No activity against gram negatives or anaerobes	Complicated skin/soft tissue infections, also being used more for MRSA bacteremia/endocarditis, and various infections due to VRE	Cannot use for pneumonia (lacks activity in lung parenchyma due to inactivation by surfactant)
Side effects: Muscle toxicity (myalgias, rhabdomyolysis) so need to check baseline and weekly creatine kinase level, and discontinue statins. Also, peripheral neuropathy, GI side effects, and pain at injection site			

Organism Abbreviations: MSSA, methicillin-sensitive *Staphylococcus aureus*; MRSA, methicillin-resistant *Staphylococcus aureus*; CA-MRSA, community-acquired MRSA; ESBL, extended-spectrum beta-lactamase producer; VRE, vancomycin-resistant *Enterococcus*.

TABLE 33.5 Major Antibiotic Classes: Antipseudomonal Antibiotics

- Resistance rates vary by institution and are important to consider when choosing an agent
- Double coverage should be strongly considered for empiric therapy, but the benefit of continuing two active agents once susceptibilities are known is controversial
- Double coverage should consist of a beta-lactam plus either a fluoroquinolone or an aminoglycoside. Aztreonam should be used in the case of severe beta-lactam allergy

Antipseudomonal Beta-Lactams	Non–Beta Lactam Antipseudomonal Drugs
Piperacillin/Tazobactam and Ticarcillin/Clavulanate Note higher rates of resistance to ticarcillin than piperacillin	**Fluoroquinolones—Ciprofloxacin and Levofloxacin** Moxifloxacin does not have activity against *Pseudomonas*. Ciprofloxacin and levofloxacin are usually used as second agents, not as monotherapy for empiric *Pseudomonas* treatment due to relatively high rates of resistance
Carbapenems (Meropenem, Imipenem, Doripenem) Note: Ertapenem has no pseudomonal activity. Doripenem has greater in vitro potency against *Pseudomonas*, but clear clinical benefit has yet to be demonstrated	**Aminoglycosides** On average, amikacin > tobramycin > gentamicin for antipseudomonal activity. Should not be used as monotherapy for serious *Pseudomonas* infections due to worse outcomes
Ceftazidime, Cefepime Both have reliable activity against *Pseudomonas*	**Polymyxins—Colistin (Polymyxin E) and Polymyxin B** Generally last-line agents when the pathogen has become resistant to all other options (historically high rates of renal and neurologic toxicities)
Aztreonam High rates of resistance at most institutions, so use only if penicillin allergic, and empirically double-cover with a second agent (fluoroquinolone or aminoglycoside)	

LITERATURE TABLE

TRIAL	DESIGN	RESULT
Importance of Timing and Appropriateness of Empiric Antibiotic Therapy in Severe Sepsis/Septic Shock		
Kumar et al., *Chest.* 2009[14]	Multicenter retrospective cohort study of 5,715 patients with septic shock	Survival in the group that received initial appropriate antimicrobial therapy was five times as high as in the initial inappropriate antimicrobial therapy group; inappropriateness of initial antimicrobial therapy was the factor most highly associated with death
Kumar et al., *Crit Care Med.* 2006[30]	Retrospective cohort study of 2,731 adult patients with septic shock in 14 ICUs	Effective antimicrobial administration within the first hour of documented hypotension was associated with increased survival, with each hour of delay over the ensuing 6 h associated with an increase in mortality of 7.6% per hour. Time to initiation of effective antimicrobial therapy was the single strongest predictor of outcome
Gaieski et al., *Crit Care Med.* 2010[31]	Single-center prospective cohort study of 261 patients with severe sepsis or septic shock undergoing early goal-directed therapy	A delay of 1 h or more from triage or time from qualification for early goal-directed therapy to appropriate antibiotics was associated with an increase in mortality risk by >50%

(*Continued*)

LITERATURE TABLE (*Continued*)		
TRIAL	**DESIGN**	**RESULT**
Gram-Negative Infections: Combination Therapy, Resistance, and Risk Factors for *Pseudomonas*		
Johnson et al., *Crit Care Med.* 2011[11]	Retrospective single-center cohort study of 754 consecutive patients with gram-negative bacteremia complicated by severe sepsis or septic shock	Patients with recent antibiotic exposure (within 90 days) had significantly higher rates of resistance to broad-spectrum gram-negative agents, with greater rates of inappropriate initial antimicrobial therapy (45% vs. 21%, $p < 0.001$) and hospital mortality (51% vs. 34%, $p < 0.001$)
Schechner et al., *Clin Infec Dis.* 2009[26]	Multicenter retrospective study of 4,114 episodes of GNR bacteremia upon hospital admission	Predictors of *Pseudomonas aeruginosa* bacteremia in patients without severe immunodeficiency presenting with GNR bacteremia were age >90 years, receipt of antimicrobial therapy within the past 30 d, central venous catheter, or urinary device. With zero risk factors, the risk was 2%; one risk factor—8%; two risk factors—28%
Micek et al., *Antimicrob Agents Chemother.* 2010[27]	Retrospective single-center cohort study of 760 patients with severe sepsis or septic shock associated with gram-negative bacteremia	Patients treated with an empiric combination antibiotic regimen were less likely to receive inappropriate initial antimicrobial therapy compared to monotherapy (22% vs. 36%, $p < 0.001$), which was an independent predictor of hospital mortality
Optimal Therapy for Specific Infections		
MSSA bacteremia: Schweizer et al., *BMC Infect Dis.* 2011[34]	Retrospective cohort study of 267 patients with MSSA bacteremia, examining outcomes with vancomycin, nafcillin, and cefazolin	Patients receiving nafcillin or cefazolin had 79% lower mortality compared to those who received vancomycin alone (adjusted hazard ratio 0.21, 95% CI 0.09, 0.47). Those who initially received vancomycin empirically but were switched to nafcillin or cefazolin still had 69% lower mortality than those who remained on vancomycin (adjusted HR 0.31, 95% CI 0.10, 0.95)
***Clostridium difficile*:** Zar et al., *Clin Infect Dis.* 2007[35]	Single-center randomized trial of 172 patients with *C. difficile*–associated diarrhea comparing oral metronidazole versus oral vancomycin for 10 days. Patients were stratified by disease severity	No significant difference in those with mild-moderate disease, but in the predefined subgroup of patients with severe disease, oral vancomycin was associated with superior clinical cure rates compared to metronidazole (97% vs. 76%, $p = 0.02$)
ESBL-Producing Organisms: Paterson et al., *Clin Infect Dis.* 2004[36]	Multicenter prospective study of 455 consecutive episodes of *Klebsiella pneumoniae* bacteremia (85 due to ESBL-producing organisms)	Use of a carbapenem was associated with significantly lower 14-d mortality than use of other antibiotics active in vitro (4.8% vs. 27.6%, $p = 0.012$)
MRSA pneumonia: Wunderink et al., *Clin Infect Dis.* 2012[41]	Prospective, double-blind, controlled, multicenter trial involving hospitalized adult patients with hospital-acquired or health care–associated MRSA pneumonia, randomized to intravenous linezolid or vancomycin (adjusted on the basis of trough levels)	Linezolid was associated with a higher rate of clinical and microbiologic cure with lower rate of nephrotoxicity on per protocol analysis. However, no difference in clinical cure, microbiologic cure, or 60-d mortality on intention-to-treat analysis
Duration of Therapy in VAP		
Chastre et al., *JAMA.* 2003[38] PneumA Trial Group	Prospective, randomized, double-blind trial in 51 French ICUs of 401 patients with VAP as diagnosed by quantitative culture results of bronchoscopic specimens, comparing 8 vs. 15 d of therapy	No difference in mortality or 28-d recurrence in the 8-d group, with increased antibiotic-free days. The exception was in those with *P. aeruginosa*) who had a higher recurrence rate in the 8 day group (40.6% vs. 25.4%; difference of 15.2%, 90% CI 3.9–26.6%) although still no difference in mortality. Multiresistant pathogens emerged less frequently in those who received 8 days of antibiotics

CI, confidence interval; HR, hazard ratio.

REFERENCES

1. Wisplinghoff H, Bischoff T, Tallent SM, et al. Nosocomial bloodstream infections in US hospitals: analysis of 24,179 cases from a prospective nationwide surveillance study. *Clin Infect Dis.* 2004;39(3):309.
2. Ramsey AM, Zilberberg MD. Secular trends of hospitalization with vancomycin-resistant enterococcus infection in the United States, 2000–2006. *Infect Control Hosp Epidemiol.* 2009;30(2):184.
3. Won SY, Munoz-Price LS, Lolans K, et al.; Centers for Disease Control and Prevention Epicenter Program. Emergence and rapid regional spread of Klebsiella pneumonia carbapenemase-producing Enterobacteriaceae. *Clin Infect Dis.* 2011;53(6):532.
4. Gupta N, Limbago BM, Patel JB, et al. Carbapenem-resistant Enterobacteriaceae: epidemiology and prevention. *Clin Infect Dis.* 2011;53(1):60–67.
5. Bartlett JG. Narrative review: the new epidemic of Clostridium difficile-associated enteric disease. *Ann Intern Med.* 2006;145(10):758.
6. Martin GS, Mannino DM, Eaton S, et al. The epidemiology of sepsis in the United States from 1979 through 2000. *N Engl J Med.* 2003;348(16):1546–1554.
7. Dombrovskiy VY, Martin AA, Sunderram J, et al. Rapid increase in hospitalization and mortality rates for severe sepsis in the United States: a trend analysis from 1993 to 2003. *Crit Care Med.* 2007;35(5):1244–1250.
8. Kumar G, Kumar N, Taneja A, et al.; Milwaukee Initiative in Critical Care Outcomes Research Group of Investigators. Nationwide trends of severe sepsis in the 21st century (2000–2007). *Chest.* 2011;140(5):1223–1231.
9. Hall MJ, Williams SN, DeFrances CJ, et al. Inpatient care for septicemia or sepsis: a challenge for patients and hospitals. *NCHS Data Brief.* 2011;(62):1–8.
10. Jones RN. Microbial etiologies of hospital-acquired bacterial pneumonia and ventilator-associated bacterial pneumonia. *Clin Infect Dis.* 2012;51(suppl 1):S81–S87.
11. Johnson MT, Reichley R, Hoppe-Bauer J, et al. Impact of previous antibiotic therapy on outcome of Gram-negative severe sepsis. *Crit Care Med.* 2011;39(8):1859.
12. Davis KA, Stewart JJ, Crouch HK, et al. Methicillin-resistant *Staphylococcus aureus* (MRSA) nares colonization at hospital admission and its effect on subsequent MRSA infection. *Clin Infect Dis.* 2004;39(6):776.
13. Calfee DP, Giannetta ET, Durbin LJ, et al. Control of endemic vancomycin-resistant Enterococcus among inpatients at a university hospital. *Clin Infect Dis.* 2003;37(3):326.
14. Kumar A, Ellis P, Arabi Y, et al.; Cooperative Antimicrobial Therapy of Septic Shock Database Research Group. Initiation of inappropriate antimicrobial therapy results in a fivefold reduction of survival in human septic shock. *Chest.* 2009;136(5):1237–1248.
15. Gadde J, Spence M, Wheeler B, et al. Clinical experience with penicillin skin testing in a large inner-city STD clinic. *JAMA.* 1993;270(20):2456.
16. Leekha S, Terrell CL, Edson RS. General principles of antimicrobial therapy. *Mayo Clin Proc.* 2011;86(2):156–167.
17. Dulhunty JM, Roberts JA, Davis JS, et al. Continuous infusion of beta-lactam antibiotics in severe sepsis: a multicenter double-blind, randomized controlled trial. *Clin Infect Dis.* 2013;56(2):236–244.
18. Chytra I, Stepan M, Benes J, et al. Clinical and microbiological efficacy of continuous versus intermittent application of meropenem in critically ill patients: a randomized open-label controlled trial. *Crit Care.* 2012;16(3):R113.
19. Roberts JA, Boots R, Rickard CM, et al. Is continuous infusion ceftriaxone better than once-a-day dosing in intensive care? A randomized controlled pilot study. *J Antimicrob Chemother.* 2007;59(2):285–291.
20. Barza M, Ionnidis JP, Cappelleri JC, et al. Single or multiple daily doses of aminoglycosides: a meta-analysis. *BMJ.* 1996;312(7027):338.
21. Nau R, Sorgel F, Eiffert H. Penetration of drugs through the blood-cerebrospinal fluid/blood–brain barrier for treatment of central nervous system infections. *Clin Microbiol Rev.* 2010;23(4):858–883.
22. Silverman JA, Mortin LI, Vanpraagh AD, et al. Inhibition of daptomycin by pulmonary surfactant: in vitro modeling and clinical impact. *J Infect Dis.* 2005;191(12):2149–2152.
23. Baddour LM, Wilson WR, Bayer AS, et al. Infective endocarditis: diagnosis, antimicrobial therapy, and management of complications: a statement for healthcare professions from the Committee on Rheumatic Fever, Endocarditis, and Kawasaki Disease, Council on Cardiovascular Disease in the Young, and the Councils on Clinical Cardiology, Stroke, and Cardiovascular Surgery and Anesthesia, American Heart Association: endorsed by the Infectious Diseases Society of America. *Circulation.* 2005;111(23):e394–e434.
24. Cosgrove SE, Vigliani GA, Fowler VG Jr, et al. Initial low-dose gentamicin for *Staphylococcus aureus* bacteremia and endocarditis is nephrotoxic. *Clin Infect Dis.* 2009;48(6):713–721.

25. Gomez J, Garcia-Vazquez E, Banos R, et al. Predictors of mortality in patients with methicillin-resistant *Staphylococcus aureus* (MRSA) bacteraemia: the role of empiric antibiotic therapy. *Eur J Clin Microbiol Infect Dis.* 2007;26(4):239–245.
26. Schechner V, Nobre V, Kaye KS, et al. Gram-negative bacteremia upon hospital admission: when should *Pseudomonas aeruginosa* be suspected? *Clin Infect Dis.* 2009;48(5):580.
27. Micek ST, Welch EC, Khan J, et al. Empiric combination antibiotic therapy is associated with improved outcome against sepsis due to Gram-negative bacteria: a retrospective analysis. *Antimicrob Agents Chemother.* 2010;54(5):1742–1748.
28. Paul M, Benuri-Silbiger I, Soares-Weiser K, et al. Beta lactam monotherapy versus beta lactam-aminoglycoside combination therapy for sepsis in immunocompetent patients: systematic review and meta-analysis of randomized trials. *BMJ.* 2004;328(7441):668.
29. Safdar N, Handelsman J, Maki DG. Does combination antimicrobial therapy reduce mortality in Gram-negative bacteraemia? A meta-analysis *Lancet Infect Dis.* 2004;4(8):519.
30. Kumar A, Roberts D, Woods KE, et al. Duration of hypotension before initiation of effective antimicrobial therapy is the critical determinant of survival in human septic shock. *Crit Care Med.* 2006;34(6):1589.
31. Gaieski DF, Mikkelsen ME, Band RA, et al. Impact of time to antibiotics on survival in patients with severe sepsis or septic shock in whom early goal-directed therapy was initiated in the emergency department. *Crit Care Med.* 2010;38(4):1045.
32. Ewig G. Nosocomial pneumonia: de-escalation is what matters. *Lancet Infect Dis.* 2011;11(3):155.
33. Chang FY, Peacock JE Jr, Musher DM, et al. Staphylococcus aureus bacteremia: recurrence and the impact of antibiotic treatment in a prospective multicenter study. *Medicine (Baltimore).* 2003;82(5):333.
34. Schweizer ML, Furuno JP, Harris AD, et al. Comparative effectiveness of nafcillin or cefazolin versus vancomycin in methicillin-susceptible *Staphylococcus aureus* bacteremia. *BMC Infect Dis.* 2011;11:279.
35. Zar FA, Bakkangagari SR, Moorthi KM, et al. A comparison of vancomycin and metronidazole for the treatment of Clostridium difficile-associated diarrhea, stratified by disease severity. *Clin Infect Dis.* 2007;45(3):302.
36. Paterson DL, Ko WC, Von Gottberg A, et al. Antibiotic therapy for Klebsiella pneumonia bacteremia: implications of production of extended-spectrum beta-lactamases. *Clin Infect Dis.* 2004;39(1):31.
37. Jacobson KL, Cohen SH, Inciardi JF, et al. The relationship between antecedent antibiotic use and resistance to extended-spectrum cephalosporins in group I beta-lactamase-producing organisms. *Clin Infect Dis.* 1995;21(5):1107.
38. Chastre J, Wolff M, Fagon JY, et al.; PneumA Trial Group. Comparison of 8 vs 15 days of antibiotic therapy for ventilator-associated pneumonia in adults: a randomized trial. *JAMA.* 2003;290(19):2588.
39. Li JZ, Winston LG, Moore DH, et al. Efficacy of short-course antibiotic regimens for community-acquired pneumonia: a meta-analysis. *Am J Med.* 2007;120(9):783.
40. American Thoracic Society; Infectious Diseases Society of America. Guidelines for the management of adults with hospital-acquired, ventilator-associated, and healthcare-associated pneumonia. *Am J Respir Crit Care Med.* 2005;171(4):388.
41. Wunderink RG, Rello J, Cammarata SK, et al. Linezolid vs vancomycin: analysis of two double-blind studies of patients with methicillin-resistant *Staphylococcus aureus* nosocomial pneumonia. *Chest.* 2003;124(5):1789.

34

Infections in the Immunocompromised Host

M. Cristina Vazquez-Guillamet, Joshua J. Mooney, and Joe L. Hsu

BACKGROUND

Recent decades have challenged the emergency physician to manage an evolving spectrum of infections in immune-compromised patients. This comes as a result of an increased use of immune suppression and infectious disease prophylaxis, as well as the improved survival of patients with human immunodeficiency virus (HIV), cancer, and following solid organ transplant (SOT) and hematopoietic stem cell transplantation (HSCT). Early diagnosis and treatment of these individuals with appropriate antimicrobial agents are essential for successful clinical outcomes.

DIAGNOSTIC EVALUATION

The frequent absence of early signs and symptoms traditionally used to define infection presents a major challenge in the care of immune-compromised patients. Cultures—the gold standard for guiding choice of antimicrobial agents—are positive in <50% of patients with invasive fungal diseases (IFDs) or febrile neutropenia and take several days for detection.[1,2] This diagnostic uncertainty is particularly concerning since delay in starting appropriate antimicrobial therapy is well established as a cause of increased mortality.[3]

When performing a targeted evaluation of an immune-compromised patient, the emergency physician should begin with an assessment of the "net state of immune suppression," including an evaluation of the type of immune suppression, current immune suppressive therapy, level of immune suppression (myeloablative vs. nonmyeloablative regimen prior to HSCT, ongoing immune suppressive therapy), duration (transplant date, last chemotherapy, time from diagnosis of underlying malignancy), and anti-infective prophylaxis. Immune-suppressed patients will typically have unique pathogen susceptibilities based on their underlying immune defect (e.g., defects in T and/or B cells, neutropenia). A thorough patient history should document recent infections, including multidrug-resistant infections (MDRIs), latent and opportunistic infections, and recent surgical procedures including indwelling central venous catheters (CVC). In the patients with HIV, knowledge of a recent CD4 cell count and the use or lack of use of antiretroviral therapy (ART) and anti-infective prophylaxis is essential. The immune-compromised patient may have multiple potential infectious sources including donor acquired, nosocomial, reactivation, and environmental, and community acquired, all of which should be investigated.

In addition to standard infectious laboratory testing, non–culture-based methods including polymerase chain reaction (PCR) assays, antigen and antibody capture assays (*Aspergillus* galactomannan [GM], (1–3)-β-D-glucan, direct fluorescent antibody [DFA] stains), and microscopy with special stains, if available, should be ordered in consultation with infectious disease. Early use of computed tomography (CT) to identify an infectious source is also indicated since plain radiographs are known to lack sensitivity in the detection of infections in immune-suppressed patients.[4–8]

INFECTIONS IN PATIENTS WITH HUMAN IMMUNODEFICIENCY VIRUS

The mortality of critically ill HIV-infected patients has decreased to the point that survival rates now approach those seen in non-HIV patients.[9,10] Although survival in critically ill patients is independent of ART at the time of admission, the use of ART is associated with higher CD4 counts, increased virologic suppression, and lower rates of opportunistic infections (such as *Pneumocystis jirovecii* pneumonia [PJP] and others) that independently correlate with survival.[11] These changes have shifted the epidemiology of critically ill HIV-infected patients beyond opportunistic infections to include nosocomial and community-acquired infections, comorbid chronic diseases, and medication-related toxicities, including the immune reconstitution inflammatory syndrome (IRIS).[12] In general, ART should be continued in critically ill HIV-infected patients with known prior virologic suppression; at the same time, these patients should be monitored for drug side effects (although rare, nucleoside analog reverse transcriptase inhibitors can cause lactic acidosis), proper dosing, and pharmacologic interactions.[13]

Sepsis in HIV-Positive Patients

The incidence of sepsis in ICU admissions of HIV-infected patients increased from 12% in 1995 to 20% in 2000, but mortality continues to improve.[11,14] More than half of these septic episodes were due to respiratory infections, followed by bacteremia, catheter-related blood stream infections (CRBSIs), and urinary tract infections (UTIs). Nosocomial pathogens, including *Staphylococcus aureus* and *Pseudomonas aeruginosa*, were the organisms implicated in up to 60% of all infections, followed by opportunistic and community-acquired pathogens.[15] Sepsis-associated mortality among HIV-infected patients is correlated to illness severity, rather than degree of immune deficiency; however, an increased risk of nosocomial and opportunistic pathogen infection is observed with CD4 cell counts <200 cells/mm^3 and with the absence of ART.[15]

Treatment of Infection in the HIV-Positive Patient

Treatment of infection in any immune-compromised patient includes goal-directed therapy and broad-spectrum antimicrobials, including empiric coverage for nosocomial organisms in patients at risk for severe sepsis. In HIV-infected patients with suspected sepsis and recent initiation of ART, the possibility of IRIS should be considered. IRIS presents as either a localized or systemic inflammatory reaction that develops after initiation of ART (typically 90 d later) and is due to recovery of the patient's immune response. The syndrome results from either the inflammatory reaction to a recognized preexisting infection (e.g., *Pneumocystis jirovecii*) or the unmasking of an unrecognized preexisting infection (e.g., *Mycobacterium avium complex [MAC], Mycobacterium tuberculosis* [MTB], endemic fungal infections) with clinical features related to the prior infection. The diagnosis is one of exclusion. Active infection and drug reaction (e.g., abacavir hypersensitivity) must first be excluded. Management of IRIS is supportive, with continued treatment of the underlying infection and ART. In moderate to severe cases of IRIS, the use of prednisone (1 mg/kg/d) has been employed, although no controlled trials definitively support its benefit.

Respiratory Infections in HIV-Positive Patients

Respiratory infections are the most common reason HIV-infected patients are admitted to the ICU. The clinical presentation, radiographic appearance, and CD4 count help narrow the differential diagnosis (Table 34.1). *Streptococcus pneumoniae* is the most common etiologic agent.[35] Risk factors for MDRIs include CD4 cell counts <200 cells/mm^3, underlying lung disease, neutropenia, and recent health care exposures.[15]

The incidence of PJP has declined with the use of prophylactic antibiotics and ART, but it remains the most common opportunistic respiratory infection and should be considered in those with a CD4 cell count <200 cells/mm^3. The sputum immunofluorescent antibody (IFA) test, the presence of ground-glass opacities on high-resolution chest CT scan, and/or elevated serum (1,3)-β-D-glucan[36] are reliable noninvasive tests for diagnosing PJP.[19,20,22] All patients should undergo arterial blood gas (ABG) sampling on ambient air to determine if adjunct corticosteroids (typically prednisone 40 mg q12h) and low tidal volume ventilation (employed in mechanically ventilated patients to minimize the risk for pneumothorax) are indicated. A $PaO_2 < 70$ mm Hg on ABG or an alveolar–arterial difference (A-a gradient) of >35 mm Hg is the standard cutoff used for corticosteroid initiation.[37]

HIV-infected patients are also at an increased risk of primary and reactivation of MTB infection. Those with a clinical syndrome suggestive of MTB should be placed in respiratory isolation, and three serial acid-fast bacillus (AFB) sputum samples should be collected. Common radiographic patterns of MTB include upper lung cavitation at higher CD4 cell counts and middle-to-lower lobe infiltrates at lower CD4 cell counts, but any radiographic pattern may be encountered. Severely immune-compromised HIV-infected patients (CD4 cell count <50 to 100 cells/mm^3) are also at risk for pulmonary infections from endemic (e.g., *Histoplasma capsulatum, Coccidioides immitis*) and geographic (e.g., *Cryptococcus neoformans*) fungi and *M. avium complex*.

Altered Mental Status in HIV-Positive Patients

Altered mental status is a common presenting symptom in critically ill HIV-infected patients and results from both infectious and noninfectious etiologies. The following factors can help narrow the differential diagnosis: level of CD4 cell count, status of virologic suppression, toxoplasma serology, and ART regimen and timeline (Table 34.1).

While any infection may result in an altered sensorium, dangerous infections of the central nervous system (CNS) include meningitis (bacterial, cryptococcal, tuberculous, syphilitic), viral encephalitis (Cytomegalovirus [CMV], herpes simplex virus

TABLE 34.1 Common Infectious Conditions for Patients Infected with Human Immunodeficiency Virus

Condition	CD4 Cell Count (Cells/mm³)	Clinical Presentation	Diagnostic Tests (Sensitivity/Specificity)	Recommended Antibiotic Regimens[a,16]
Pulmonary Infections				
Pneumonia	Any CD4 count Risk of nosocomial infection increased if <200	Acute onset Cough Purulent sputum Fever, chills Dyspnea	• Blood, sputum culture • Endotracheal aspirate culture • *Legionella* urine antigen (70%–80%/>99%)[17,18] • Imaging: CXR—unilateral focal, segmental, or lobar consolidation ± pleural effusion	1. Ceftriaxone 1 g IV q24h + azithromycin 500 mg PO/IV q24h or levofloxacin 750 mg PO/IV q24h 2. If nosocomial risk factors, CD4 count <200, or critically ill: Vancomycin 15–20 mg/kg IV q12h or linezolid 600 mg IV q12h + piperacillin–tazobactam 4.5 g IV q6h or cefepime 1 g IV q8h + levofloxacin 750 mg IV q24h

Pneumocystis pneumonia	<200	Subacute onset
		Nonproductive cough
		Dyspnea
		Fever
			• (1,3)-β-D-glucan (92%/65%)[19,20]
			• ABG
			• Induced sputum (>55%/>90%)[21]
			• IFA sputum (91%–100%/95%–100%)[19]
			• IFA BAL (>90%/99%)[21]
			• Imaging:
			  ○ CXR—normal or diffuse interstitial pattern
			  ○ High-resolution CT—bilateral ground-glass opacities (100%/89%)[22]
				1. TMP–SMX 15–20 mg/kg/d IV divided q6–8 h
				2. TMP–SMX DS 2 tablets PO q8h, or clindamycin 450 mg q6h + primaquine 15 mg PO q24h[23]
				3. If PaO_2 < 70 mm Hg or A-a gradient >35 mm Hg: Prednisone 40 mg PO q12h

M. tuberculosis Pneumonia	Any CD4 count	Subacute onset
		Cough
		Fever
		Night sweats
			• Sputum AFB smear and culture
			• Imaging: *CXR*—alveolar infiltrates and adenopathy, nodules, or pleural effusion
			  ○ Lower CD4: lower lobe opacity
			  ○ Higher CD4: upper lobe, cavitary opacity
				Isoniazid, rifabutin or rifampin, pyrazinamide, and ethambutol at weight-based dosing[b]

Pneumonia due to severe immune suppression
• *Mycobacterium avium complex (MAC)*
• CMV
• Endemic fungi
• *Cryptococcus*
	<50–100	Cough
		Fever
		Dyspnea
		Night sweats
		Weight loss
			• MAC
			  ○ AFB smear/culture/ nucleic acids hybridization tests—sputum and blood
			• CMV
			  ○ CMV quantitative PCR
			• Endemic fungi
			• Histoplasma *Blastomyces* antibodies
			  ○ *Blastomycosis*
			    □ Sputum culture (75%–86%)[24]
			    □ Urine antigen (89%–93%/79%)[25]
			  ○ *Coccidioidomycosis* antibodies
			  ○ *Histoplasma* urine antigen (75%–97%)[19]
			• *Cryptococcus*
			  ○ Serum *Cryptococcus* antigen (56%–96%/93%–100%)[26,27]
			  ○ Fungal culture
				1. MAC: Clarithromycin 500 mg PO q12h, ethambutol (weight-based dosing)[b] and rifabutin 450 mg q24h[28]
				2. CMV: Ganciclovir 5 mg/kg IV q12h
				3. Endemic fungi
				  i. Mild to moderate: fluconazole 400 mg PO/IV q24h (blastomycosis, coccidioidomycosis) or itraconazole 200 mg PO q8h (blastomycosis, coccidioidomycosis, histoplasmosis)
				  ii. Severe: Liposomal amphotericin IV 3–5 mg/kg q24h
				4. *Cryptococcus*
				  i. Mild to moderate: fluconazole 400 mg PO/IV q24h
				  ii. Severe: See below treatment for CNS disease

CNS Infections				
Bacterial meningitis	Any CD4 count	Acute onset Headache Fever Meningismus	• Blood cultures • LP: Neutrophilic pleocytosis, elevated protein, low glucose, positive Gram stain or culture • Imaging: Head CT/MRI—Should be performed in HIV-infected patients prior to LP	1. Ceftriaxone 2 g IV q12h + Vancomycin 15–20 mg/kg IV q8–12 h + Ampicillin 2 g IV q4h Prior to antibiotics: Dexamethasone 0.15 mg/kg IV q6h × 4 d if suspected or proven pneumococcal infection
Cryptococcal meningitis	<100	Subacute onset Headache Fever Malaise Confusion Coma	• Serum *Cryptococcal* antigen (83%–97%/93%–100%)[29] • LP: CSF studies may be normal. CSF *Cryptococcal* antigen (93%–100%/93%–98%), check opening pressure, India ink stain[29] • Imaging: Head CT/MRI—normal, hydrocephalus or edema	1. Liposomal amphotericin 5 mg/kg IV q24h + flucytosine 25 mg/kg/dose PO q6h 2. If CSF pressure >25 cm reduce opening pressure by 50% or to normal pressure of <20 cm
Toxoplasmosis	<100	Subacute onset Seizure Focal neurologic deficit Headache Confusion, stupor Coma	• Serum toxoplasma IgG positive • LP: CSF toxoplasmosis PCR (>33%/100%)[30] • Imaging: Head CT and/or MRI: Ring-enhancing lesions with surrounding edema	1. Pyrimethamine 200 mg PO once, then 75 mg PO q24h + sulfadiazine 1 g (<60 kg) or 1.5 g (>60 kg) PO q6h + leucovorin 10–25 mg PO q24h
Syphilitic meningitis	Any CD4 count	Subacute to chronic onset Headache Confusion Impaired visual acuity Seizure Focal cerebral symptoms	• Serum RPR, VDRL, FTA-ABS • LP: Lymphocytic pleocytosis (>20 cell/mL), elevated protein, CSF VDRL (53%–70%/>99%)[31,32] • Imaging: Head CT/MRI—Normal, basilar, or temporal enhancement	1. Penicillin G 3–4 million units IV q4h, or penicillin 24 million units as a continuous infusion
Tuberculous meningitis	Any CD4 count <200, poor prognosis	Subacute Headache Fever Confusion Cranial nerve involvement	• LP: Bland or mild neutrophilic pleocytosis (early) lymphocytic pleocytosis (later), elevated protein, low glucose • Serial LPs: AFB and culture • MTB PCR CSF (56%/98%)[33] • Imaging: Head CT/MRI—Hydrocephalus, basilar enhancement, cerebral infarct, tuberculoma	1. Isoniazid, rifampin or rifabutin, pyrazinamide, and ethambutol at weight-based dosing[c] 2. Dexamethasone 12 mg/d or Prednisone 60 mg/d

[a]Dosing based on normal renal and hepatic function.

[b]Initiate in conjunction with an ID specialist or pharmacist due to drug interactions.

BAL, bronchoalveolar lavage; CSF, cerebral spinal fluid; FTA-ABS, fluorescent treponemal antibody absorption; IFA, immunofluorescence assay; LP, lumbar puncture; MRI, magnetic resonance imaging; PCR, polymerase chain reaction; RPR, rapid plasma regain; TMP–SMX, trimethoprim–sulfamethoxazole; VDRL, venereal disease research laboratory.

From *The Sanford guide to antimicrobial therapy*. Sperryville, VA: Antimicrobial Therapy; 2012. Ref.[34]

[HSV]), or parenchymal lesions including parasitic infection (toxoplasmosis) and brain abscess (bacterial, fungal). All patients with CD4 cell counts <200 cells/mm^3 and focal findings should undergo a CT head with intravenous contrast to evaluate for presence of cerebral toxoplasmosis (characterized by ring-enhancing lesions on CT imaging), CNS lymphoma (usually single lesion), and progressive multifocal leukoencephalopathy (plaques in the white matter). Following head imaging, lumbar puncture should be performed to evaluate for bacterial and fungal meningitis or more indolent CNS processes such as syphilitic and tuberculous meningitis.

Noninfectious etiologies in HIV-infected patients with mental status changes include primary CNS lymphoma, HIV-associated dementia, toxins or medication-side effects (e.g., efavirenz), IRIS, and metabolic encephalopathy.

INFECTIONS IN PATIENTS WITH HEMATOLOGIC MALIGNANCIES AND FOLLOWING HEMATOPOIETIC STEM CELL TRANSPLANTATION

For patients with hematologic malignancies, the primary malignancy dictates the immune defect and pathogen susceptibilities. For example, patients with acute lymphoblastic leukemia have more profound cellular defects than those with acute myeloid leukemia. Multiple myeloma is associated with a reduced humoral immunity. Chronic lymphocytic leukemia is characterized by a prolonged course of T-cell and antibody deficiency. Chemotherapy for hematologic malignancies is uniformly myelosuppressive, resulting in profound neutropenia, which increases susceptibility to bacterial and fungal pathogens. Among chemotherapeutic agents, daunorubicin and cytarabine can produce severe, prolonged neutropenia, while fludarabine and alemtuzumab decrease the T- (especially CD4 cells) and B-cell function.[38]

For HSCT patients, the preparative regimen for transplantation determines the level of immune suppression. Myeloablative regimens completely suppress the host bone marrow, resulting in profound immune compromise; nonmyeloablative regimens are less suppressive. Posttransplant hematopoietic immune recovery follows a predictable sequence: pre-engraftment (0–1 month), early postengraftment (1 to 3 months) with gradual return of the host's humoral response, and late postengraftment (>3 months) during which cellular immunity returns. In some patients, cellular immune defects may persist 1 to 2 years posttransplant. If graft versus host disease (GVHD) ensues, prolonged and aggressive immune suppression will be required, increasing the risk of infections.

Febrile Neutropenia

Neutropenia is defined as an absolute neutrophil count (ANC) < 1,500 cells/mm^3; severe neutropenia as an ANC < 500 cells/mm^3 (ANC = [% Neutrophils + % Bands] × [WBC]/100). Febrile neutropenia is defined as one episode of fever >38.3°C or fever >38°C for ≥1 hour with an absolute neutrophil count (ANC) <500 cells/mm^3 or with an expected ANC drop to <500 cells/mm^3 within 48 hours. The ANC nadir, duration of neutropenia, and rapidity of decline determine infection risk. Table 34.2 provides criteria for risk-stratifying patients with febrile neutropenia.[39,40]

TABLE 34.2 Classification Scheme for Risk in Patients with Neutropenic Fever

Risk Category	Duration of Neutropenia	Clinical Presentation	Comorbidities	Treatment
Low	<7 d	Fever, stable	None	Outpatient: Augmentin 875 mg PO BID + ciprofloxacin 750 mg PO BID
High	>7 d	Localizing signs,hypotension, respiratory failure	Present	Inpatient: IV antibiotics

Duthie R, Denning DW. Aspergillus fungemia: report of two cases and review. *Clin Infect Dis.* 1995;20:598–605.
Freifeld AG, Bow EJ, Sepkowitz KA, et al. Clinical practice guideline for the use of antimicrobial agents in neutropenic patients with cancer: 2010 Update by the Infectious Diseases Society of America. *Clin Infect Dis.* 2011;52:427–431; *The Sanford guide to antimicrobial therapy.* Sperryville, VA: Antimicrobial Therapy; 2012. Ref.[34].

Patients with febrile neutropenia are susceptible to CRBSI, as well as infections that originate in the gastrointestinal tract (most commonly due to bacterial translocation in the setting of mucositis or enterocolitis), lung, kidneys, or soft tissues. The epidemiology of these infections has shifted from gram-negative rods (GNRs) to gram-positive cocci (GPCs, 60% to 75% of positive blood cultures) due to widespread use of antimicrobial prophylaxis that targets GNRs.[41] Common pathogens include coagulase-negative *Staphylococcus, S. aureus, Streptococcus* spp, *Enterococcus, Corynebacterium jeikeium, P. aeruginosa*, and Enterobacteriaceae. For patients with enterocolitis, potential pathogens include anaerobes (*Clostridium septicum, Clostridium tertium*, and *Bacillus cereus*). Neutropenic patients are also at risk for breakthrough infections, resulting from a gap in the pathogen coverage of prophylactic antibiotics (typically fluoroquinolones) leading to infections with *Streptococcus* spp and anaerobic spp. Breakthrough infection, for example, from *Streptococcus viridans*, can rapidly lead to severe sepsis and acute respiratory distress syndrome (ARDS).

Diagnostic Evaluation for Febrile Neutropenia

Laboratory Studies Although only 30% to 40% of neutropenic fever episodes will prove to have a documented infection,[42] the clinician must assume an infectious etiology, even when the patient presents with no signs of inflammation (e.g., no meningeal signs, nonproductive cough, no leukocytosis). Table 34.3 highlights diagnostic tests to consider based on the clinical presentation. In a neutropenic host with sepsis, a procalcitonin level may be useful in considering a bacterial etiology (serum cutoff level >0.5 μg/L); it should not be used in localized bacterial or fungal infections, or those due to viral pathogens.[55,56] The serum concentration of procalcitonin peaks at 24 hours after development of fever.

Imaging CT imaging should be obtained for patients with focal CNS findings and respiratory or abdominal complaints. For patients with lower quadrant abdominal symptoms, typhlitis, also known as neutropenic enterocolitis, should be suspected. Typhlitis is a chemotherapy-related colonic inflammation that leads to bacterial translocation, resulting in diffuse wall edema and perforation. Abdominal CT imaging determines the extent of typhlitis and the presence of local complications.

TABLE 34.3 Common Infectious Conditions for Patients with Hematologic Malignancies and after Hematopoietic Stem Cell Transplantation

Timing	Condition	Pathogens	Diagnostic Tests (Sensitivity/ Specificity)	Recommended Antibiotic Regimens[a,43]	Noninfectious Mimics
Febrile Neutropenia					
7 d after chemotherapy, 2 wk after HSCT	GI: neutropenic enterocolitis CRBSI Skin Mucositis Pneumoniac UTI	• GNRs • GPCs • Anaerobes • *Candida spp*	• Blood, sputum, urine, CSF cultures, as appropriate • Non–culture-based tests, as appropriate • Procalcitonin (cutoff >0.5 μg/L) • Imaging: CT—imaging method of choice, plain radiograph insensitive	1. Meropenem 1 g IV q8h or Piperacillin–tazobactam 4.5 g IV q6h ± Vancomycin 15 mg/kg IV q12h or Linezolid 600 mg IV q12h ± echinocandin 2. Vancomycin for CRBSI, pneumonia, severe sepsis, mucositis, known colonization with MRSA 3. Echinocandin (e.g., Micafungin 100 mg IV q24 or Caspofungin 75 mg IV × 1 then 50 mg IV q24h) for prolonged use of CVC, TPN, or prior antibiotic use	Engraftment syndrome
Pulmonary Infections					
Early postengraftment (1–3 mo)	Bacterial pneumonia	• Community acquired • Nosocomial ○ MRSA ○ *P. aeruginosa* • *Legionella* • *M. tuberculosis*	• Blood, Sputum culture • *Legionella* urine antigen for serotype I (85% in severe pneumonia/99%)[44] • AFB smear and culture • Imaging: CXR—Focal, segmental, or lobar consolidation ± pleural effusion	1. Vancomycin 15–20 mg/kg IV q 8–12h + Piperacillin–tazobactam 4.5 g IV q6h / Meropenem 1 g IV q8h + Azithromycin 500 mg IV q24h ○ Consider double coverage with ciprofloxacin/ gentamicin until susceptibilities are known 2. *M. tuberculosis*: Isoniazid, Rifampin or Rifabutin, Pyrazinamide, and Ethambutol at weight based dosing	Diffuse Alveolar Hemorrhage Drug toxicity Radiation pneumonitis Idiopathic pneumonia syndrome
	Fungal pneumonia	• *Aspergillus* • Non-*Aspergillus* molds	• *Aspergillus* GM serum (70%–82%/86%–92%) BAL (88%/87%)[19,45] • Imaging: CT—nodules (>1 cm) with "halo," crescent sign	1. Voriconazole 6 mg/kg IV q12 × 2 doses then 4 mg/kg IV q12h 2. Liposomal Amphotericin 5 mg/kg IV q24h	
		• *P. jirovecii*	See Tables 1 and 4, section on *Pneumocystis* pneumonia		
	Viral pneumonia	• CMV	• Serum CMV quantitative PCR • BAL CMV immunohistochemical stain and culture • Imaging: CT—reticular infiltrates, ground glass opacities, small nodules	1. Ganciclovir 5 mg/kg IV q12h	

		Respiratory viruses: • RSV • Influenza • Parainfluenza • Human metapneumovirus	• Nasopharyngeal viral swab: ○ DFA RSV (15%/97%)[49] ○ DFA Influenza (54%/98%)[50] • Specific Viral PCR • Imaging: CT—diffuse ground glass opacities	1. Influenza: Oseltamivir 75 or 150 mg PO q12h depending on severity 2. RSV, human metapneumovirus, ± parainfluenza: inhaled Ribavirin 2 g nebulized over 2 h q8h	
Late postengraftment (>3 mo)	Bacterial Pneumonia	• Community acquired	As above (Early postengraftment section on bacterial pneumonia)		BOS (bronchiolitis obliterans syndrome)
		• *Nocardia* • MRSA • *P. aeruginosa*	• Macroscopic examination of granules • Gram stain and modified AFB stain of sputum, biopsy specimens, wounds, cultures (invasive specimens: 85%–90% positive[51]) and PCR or 16S rRNA-based PCR (90%–100%)[52] • Imaging: CT—nodular lesions with cavitation	1. *Nocardia*: Double coverage: TMP–SMX 5 mg/kg IV q8h + imipenem 500 mg IV q6h 2. MRSA: Vancomycin 15–20 mg/kg IV q12h or linezolid 600 mg IV q12h 3. P. aeruginosa: Piperacillin–tazobactam 4.5 g IV q6h or meropenem 1 g IV q8h/cefepime 1 g IV q8h ○ Consider double coverage with ciprofloxacin/ gentamicin until susceptibilities are known	Radiation fibrosis
	Disseminated Varicella Infection[b]	• VZV	• VZV PCR—serum and/or noncrusted lesions • VZV culture: BAL • Imaging: CT—ground-glass opacities, reticular, small nodules	1. Acyclovir 10 mg/kg IV q8h	
	Fungal Pneumonia	• *Aspergillus* • Non-*Aspergillus* molds	As above (early postengraftment section on fungal pneumonia)		
Gastrointestinal Infections					
Early postengraftment (1–3 mo)	Diarrhea, Abdominal pain	• CMV • *C. difficile* • Enteric viruses	• CMV quantitative PCR • *C difficile* toxin: EIA for toxins A and B (75%–100%/ 83%–100%),[53] PCR (87%/96%)[54] • Stool culture • Colonoscopy with biopsy • Imaging: CT—evaluate extent of colitis	1. CMV: Ganciclovir 5 mg/kg IV q12h 2. *C. difficile:* ○ Mild: Metronidazole 500 mg q8h IV/PO ○ Severe: Vancomycin 125 mg PO q6h ○ Septic shock: Vancomycin 500 mg PO q6h + metronidazole 500 mg IV/PO q8	Venoocclusive disease (VOD) Mucositis GVHD MMF side effect
Late postengraftment (>3 mo)	Diarrhea, Abdominal pain	Same as above Decreased incidence	Same as above		GVHD, MMF side effects

(*Continued*)

TABLE 34.3 Common Infectious Conditions for Patients with Hematologic Malignancies and after Hematopoietic Stem Cell Transplantation (*Continued*)

Timing	Condition	Pathogens	Diagnostic Tests (Sensitivity/ Specificity)	Recommended Antibiotic Regimens[a,43]	Noninfectious Mimics
Early postengraftment (1–3 mo)	⇑LFTs	• CMV, HSV, VZV, adenovirus • Hepatosplenic Candida • Bacterial sepsis • Rare: EBV, *Ehrlichia* in summer • HCV	• CMV, HSV, VZV PCR: serum • Adenovirus: serum PCR, stool antigen • Blood cultures • *Ehrlichia* PCR • Imaging: CT—nodular lesions in the liver and spleen in hepatosplenic candidiasis	1. CMV: Ganciclovir 5 mg/kg IV q12h 2. HSV, VZV: Acyclovir 10 mg/kg IV q8h 3. *Candida*: Echinocandin (e.g., micafungin 100 mg IV q24 or caspofungin 75 mg IV × 1 then 50 mg IV q24h) 4. Antibiotics as appropriate in bacterial sepsis: Meropenem 1 g IV q8h or piperacillin–tazobactam 4.5 g IV q6h ± vancomycin 15 mg/kg IV q12h or linezolid 600 mg IV q12h	GHVD Medication side effect Malignancy recurrence VOD—early
Late postengraftment	⇑LFTs	• Accelerated cirrhosis with HCV • Same as above	• Imaging: Ultrasound Doppler—liver nodularity, evaluate for hepatocellular cancer	1. Multiple drug–drug interactions, ID consultation	Same as above except for VOD
Genitourinary Infections					
Early postengraftment (1–3 mo)	Hematuria Dysuria Fever Abdominal pain	BK virus Gram Negative Rods Adenovirus CMV HSV	• BK PCR in urine and serum • Decoy cells in urine sediment • Urinalysis, microscopy, and urine culture • CMV, HSV PCR serum	1. Bladder irrigation 2. Meropenem 1 g IV q8h	Cyclophosphamide toxicity (usually in the first 2 wk posttransplant)
Late postengraftment (>3 mo)	Hematuria	Same as above	Same as above		

CNS Infections					
Early postengraftment (1–3 mo)	Altered mental status Focal deficits ± Meningeal signs	• HSV • Fungal • Listeria • Community-acquired bacteria • HHV6[c] • CMV • VZV	• LP with opening pressure, WBC, gram stain, bacterial and AFB cultures, HSV PCR, cryptococcal CSF antigen, HHV6 PCR • Imaging: CT—encephalitis (especially temporal lobe involvement in HSV), nodular parenchymal lesions with fungal etiologies	1. Vancomycin 15 mg/kg IV q12h + ceftriaxone 2 g IV q12h + acyclovir 10 mg/kg IV q8h + ampicillin 2 g IV q4h 2. Cryptococcal meningitis: Liposomal amphotericin 5 mg/kg IV q24h + Flucytosine 25 mg/kg/dose PO q6h	Posterior reversible encephalopathy syndrome (drug toxicity—calcineurin inhibitors) Malignancy recurrence
Late postengraftment (>3 mo)	Altered mental status Focal deficits Seizures ± Meningeal signs	• *S. pneumoniae* • *H. influenzae* • HSV • *Nocardia* • Toxoplasmosis • Brain Abscess • Cryptococcus spp	• LP with opening pressure, cells, Gram stain, bacterial and AFB cultures, HSV PCR, cryptococcal CSF antigen • Toxoplasma PCR CSF, toxoplasma serology • Imaging: CT, MRI—encephalitis, focal lesions (± enhancement) with *Nocardia*, brain abscess, toxoplasmosis, and fungal etiologies	Same as above 1. *Nocardia*: TMP–SMX 5 mg/kg IV q8h + imipenem 500 mg IV q6h 2. Toxoplasmosis: Pyrimethamine 200 mg PO once then 75 mg PO q24h + sulfadiazine 1 g (<60 kg) or 1.5 g (>60 kg) PO q6h + leucovorin 10–5 mg PO q24h	

[a]Dosing based on normal renal and hepatic function.

[b]VZV infection may disseminate, causing hepatitis, pneumonitis, encephalitis, disseminated intravascular coagulation, and thrombocytopenia without necessarily causing a rash.

[c]HHV6 causes PALE (posttransplant acute limbic encephalitis) characterized by antegrade amnesia, clinical or subclinical seizures, and syndrome of inappropriate antidiuretic hormone secretion.

BAL, bronchoalveolar lavage; CMV, cytomegalovirus virus; CRBSI, catheter-related blood stream infection; CSF, cerebrospinal fluid; DFA, direct fluorescent antibody; EBV, Epstein-Barr virus; EIA, enzyme immunoassay; GNRs, gram-negative rods; GPCs, gram-positive cocci; GVHD, graft versus host disease; HCV, hepatitis C virus; HHV6, human herpes virus 6; HSV, herpes simplex virus; MRSA, methicillin-resistant *S. aureus*; PCR, polymerase chain reaction; RSV, respiratory syncytial virus; TMP–SMX: trimethoprim–sulfamethoxazole; VOD, venoocclusive disease; VZV, varicella-zoster virus.

From *The Sanford guide to antimicrobial therapy*. Sperryville, VA: Antimicrobial Therapy; 2012. Ref.[34].

Treatment of Infection in Patients with HSCT

Antibacterial Therapy

Initial workup and antibiotic administration should occur as soon as possible after presentation to the emergency department. The Infectious Diseases Society of America (IDSA) guidelines recommend an antipseudomonal β-lactam as the initial regimen.[39] Cefepime should be avoided, as it is associated with (a) higher all-cause mortality compared with other β-lactams[57]; (b) inferior efficacy compared with piperacillin–tazobactam or carbapenems[58]; and (c) a failure to cover relevant anaerobic pathogens (*Bacteroides* spp).[59] If there is a low index of suspicion for multidrug-resistant GNRs (e.g., extended-spectrum beta-lactamase (ESBL) producing organisms), piperacillin–tazobactam is favored over carbapenems, as carbapenems are associated with higher rates of antibiotic- and *C. difficile*-associated diarrhea.[58] Among the carbapenems, ertapenem should be avoided as it fails to cover *P. aeruginosa*. The addition of an aminoglycoside, typically gentamicin, to any of the initial β-lactam regimens may be considered for the neutropenic patient in septic shock until culture results are available that will allow more selective antibiotic choice. Vancomycin should be initiated in HSCT critically ill patients or in those with risk factors for resistant GPC infections (oral mucositis, an indwelling catheter, or colonization with methicillin-resistant *S. aureus* [MRSA]).

Antifungal Therapy

Antifungals are added for HSCT patients at high risk for candidemia; risk factors include prolonged neutropenia, frequent hospitalizations, a protracted antibiotic course, and the presence of CVC, particularly for the administration of total parenteral nutrition. Antifungals are also indicated if fever persists after 5 days of adequate antimicrobial treatment and negative cultures. To date, there are no compelling studies favoring a specific antifungal agent. The initial use of an echinocandin, however, is now recommended given the rising incidence of azole-resistant *Candida* spp (*Candida glabrata, Candida krusei*) and the safer side effect profile of echinocandins compared to liposomal amphotericin.[60] A suitable alternative would be voriconazole. Both drugs also cover *Aspergillus*.[61]

Generally, CVCs should be replaced upon presentation in severe sepsis or septic shock, given the paucity of symptoms in CRBSI. In the presence of barriers to immediate line exchange, emergency physicians may consider sending blood cultures before antibiotic administration to assess "time-to-positivity" cultures (see CRBSIs in Patients with Solid Tumors).[47]

Adjunctive Therapies

If treatment with colony-stimulating factors has already been initiated, it should be continued. However, a recent meta-analysis did not demonstrate a benefit of colony-stimulating factors in established febrile neutropenia.[62] Current guidelines suggest their use in high-risk patients: age >65 years, prolonged and severe neutropenia, and septic shock.[63] Surgical consultation should be obtained promptly in enterocolitis, biliary sepsis, necrotizing fasciitis, and gynecologic sepsis.

Timing of Infections Following HSCT

Knowledge of the time since transplantation, use of ongoing immune suppression, and previous antimicrobial prophylaxis can help the emergency physician differentiate

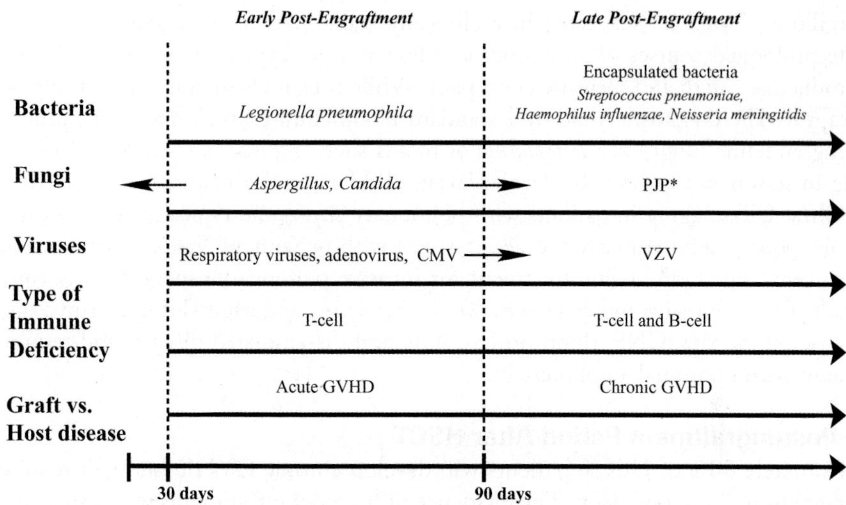

FIGURE 34.1 Timeline of infections after hematopoietic stem cell transplantation.

between noninfectious and infectious etiologies, as well as identify likely pathogens (Fig. 34.1).

Early Postengraftment Period After HSCT

Since the preengraftment period occurs while admitted to the hospital, we will only review the following stages in HSCT that are more relevant to the emergency physician. In the immediate postengraftment period, if no GVHD is encountered, immune suppression is gradually tapered. During this period, respiratory infections predominate. In addition to community-acquired pathogens, HSCT patients are at increased risk from respiratory viruses, including respiratory syncytial virus (RSV), influenza, parainfluenza, and human metapneumovirus.[64] Prompt diagnosis is essential in initiating respiratory isolation and appropriate antiviral therapy (e.g., ribavirin or oseltamivir). For RSV and influenza, rapid viral antigen tests are recommended, in conjunction with PCR-based detection (Table 34.3). Prophylaxis for CMV with ganciclovir delays the presentation of CMV syndromes. In addition to fever, interstitial pneumonia, and enteritis, CMV reactivation may manifest indirectly (e.g., concurrent infection such as PJP).[65] If CMV is suspected, PCR testing for quantitative CMV viral load is recommended. Adenovirus infection is also encountered in the early postengraftment period and may result in fulminant hepatitis, pneumonitis, and encephalitis.

Fungal Infections in the Early Postengraftment Period

Hepatosplenic candidiasis (chronic disseminated candidiasis) can develop in patients not receiving antifungal prophylaxis and should be considered in a patient recovering from neutropenia who presents with abdominal pain, fever, and increased alkaline phosphatase.

Aspergillosis should be suspected in a clinically stable patient with persistent fevers despite prolonged courses of antibiotics and fluconazole. Typical symptoms include a nonproductive cough and pleuritic chest pain. While fungal blood cultures typically do not improve the diagnostic yield over standard blood cultures, they may be helpful in isolating endemic fungi like *Histoplasma* or molds such as *Fusarium*.[19] *Aspergillus* GM testing in serum and/or bronchoalveolar lavage (BAL) can also help make the diagnosis.[66] Chest CT imaging in patients with pulmonary *Aspergillus* typically demonstrates multiple, poorly defined macronodules (>1 cm) with or without "halo," cavitation, or "air-crescent" sign.[67] First-line treatment for invasive pulmonary aspergillosis is voriconazole. Other invasive molds (*Fusarium, Scedosporium,* and agents of mucormycosis) can cause pulmonary, CNS, rhino-orbital, skin, and disseminated disease, and require treatment with liposomal amphotericin.

Late Postengraftment Period After HSCT

Approximately 50% of HSCT patients will develop chronic GVHD and will require prolonged immune suppression. The incidence of bacterial infection decreases substantially in the late posttransplant period, with the exception of infection by encapsulated organisms (e.g., *S. pneumoniae*) (Fig. 34.1, Table 34.3). Varicella zoster virus (VZV) and PJP also commonly occur in patients receiving corticosteroids for GVHD. Without trimethoprim–sulfamethoxazole (TMP–SMX) prophylaxis, patients are at risk for *Nocardia* and *Toxoplasma* infection. Failure of TMP–SMX prophylaxis also can occur (Table 34.3).

INFECTIONS IN PATIENTS WITH SOLID TUMORS

Immune Defect in Patients with Solid Tumors

While at a lower overall risk for infection than those with hematologic malignancies, patients with solid tumors are at risk from infections due to tumor-related immune dysfunction (e.g., mucocutaneous barrier disruption, cellular or humoral deficiencies) or treatment-related immune deficiency resulting from chemotherapy, radiation, or other immune-modulating therapy. Advanced age, malnutrition, comorbid conditions (e.g., chronic obstructive pulmonary disease [COPD]), and frequent health care exposures also increase infection risk.

Catheter-Related Blood Stream Infections in Patients with Solid Tumors

CVCs are essential for the administration of chemotherapeutic agents, but may result in CRBSIs. Local inflammatory changes (e.g., warmth, erythema, or purulent exudate) are unreliable (sensitivity <3%); confirmation with a "time-to-positivity" microbiologic culture, simultaneously drawn from a peripheral site and the CVC, is recommended.[68] The "time-to-positivity" diagnosis is established either quantitatively by a greater than threefold bacterial colony-forming unit (CFU) yield from the catheter versus the peripheral culture or temporally by catheter culture positivity ≤120 minutes before peripheral culture.[47,48] Typical infecting organisms include coagulase-negative *Staphylococcus* (31%), *S. aureus* (20%) with increasing rates of methicillin resistance, *Candida* (9%), and enterococci (9%) with increasing rates of vancomycin resistance.[46,69]

Treatment of CRBSIs

Antibiotic Therapy Antibiotic therapy should include vancomycin or daptomycin, and, in the presence of neutropenic fever and/or severe illness, an antipseudomonal β-lactam, such as a carbapenem (recommended if the patient has a history of ESBL infection).[70] Based on risk factors for candidemia, empiric treatment may also include an echinocandin.

Catheter Management Per the IDSA guidelines, long-term CVCs should be removed in the setting of infection with *S. aureus, P. aeruginosa,* or *Candida.* However, in the presence of alternative organisms (coagulase-negative *S. aureus, Enterococcus*) and in the absence of severe sepsis or complicating tunnel or exit-site infection, a trial of antibiotic lock therapy (ALT) and systemic antibiotics may allow for catheter salvage.[70,71]

Neutropenic Fever in Patients with Solid Tumors

In patients with solid tumors, repeated chemotherapy cycles lead to milder and briefer periods of neutropenia, compared to those with hematologic malignancies. Patients with solid tumors have a lower incidence of fungal infections, including *Candida* and *Aspergillus,* compared to patients with hematologic malignancies.

Corticosteroid Use and Risk of Opportunistic Infections in Patients with Solid Tumors

Prolonged corticosteroid use is common among solid tumor patients, particularly those with CNS lesions, increasing the risk for opportunistic infections including oropharyngeal candidiasis, *Nocardia, Legionella,* MTB, *Aspergillus,* endemic fungi, and *P. jirovecii. Pneumocystis* pneumonia occurs in <2% of non-HIV, solid tumor patients and is associated with daily prednisone doses (or corticosteroid equivalent) >15 mg for 4 weeks' duration.[72,73]

Diagnosis of PJP in HIV-Negative Patients with Solid Tumors

Due to a decreased *P. jiroveci* burden in HIV-Negative patients, the diagnostic yield of induced sputum, even with indirect fluorescent antibody (IFA) staining, is low. Recommended initial screening tests include (1–3)-β-D-glucan, PCR-based assays, and high-resolution chest CT imaging evaluating for ground-glass opacities.[74–76] BAL is the gold standard for obtaining diagnostic samples and should be performed in patients with a high clinical suspicion for PJP.[77]

PJP Treatment in HIV-Negative Patients with Solid Tumors

TMP–SMX is the treatment of choice for non–HIV-infected PJP patients. Despite limited evidence in HIV-negative patients, adjunctive corticosteroids (prednisone 40 mg q12h) are recommended in patients with moderate to severe PJP characterized by $PaO_2 \leq 70$ mm Hg on ambient air.

Sepsis in Patients with Solid Tumors

Sepsis is a common cause for ICU admission in patients with solid tumors, particularly in the presence of neutropenia caused by respiratory, blood stream, abdominal, and urinary infections. Although these patients do benefit from ICU admission, it is important to note that common prognostic models, including APACHE II or III and the Simplified Acute Physiology Score (SAPS) II, generally underestimate hospital mortality in cancer patients.[78] In patients with advanced cancer, preferences regarding the extent of therapeutic intervention(s) should be elicited early in their ICU course.

GENERAL CONSIDERATIONS BY TYPE OF SOLID TUMOR

Infections in nonneutropenic cancer patients include community-acquired and nosocomial infections with specific predilections by the type of malignancy (Table 34.4).

Lung Cancer

Pneumonia occurs in up to 24% of patients with lung cancer; 27% of these are postobstructive.[79] Postobstructive pneumonias are generally polymicrobial; however, there is an increasing incidence of *S. aureus* and enteric GNR infections due to nosocomial exposures. Antimicrobial treatment should include staphylococcal, anaerobic, and GNR coverage (e.g., vancomycin + piperacillin–tazobactam) to minimize progression to lung abscess or empyema.[80]

Breast Cancer

Patients with breast cancer are at risk for postoperative skin and soft tissue infections (incidence of 4% to 12%). Lymphedema can also cause delayed episodes of streptococcal cellulitis.[81,82] Antimicrobial treatment should include vancomycin, with consideration of antipseudomonal coverage for those with recent chemotherapy or neutropenia. Ultrasound evaluation for an underlying fluid collection should be considered if there is no clinical improvement within 72 hours of antibiotic treatment.

Gastrointestinal Cancer

Persons with gastrointestinal cancers are at risk for bowel obstruction and postsurgical complications, including anastomotic leaks, intra-abdominal abscesses, and peritonitis. Anaerobes (*Bacteroides*, *Clostridium*) are common copathogens. Antimicrobial treatment should include broad-spectrum GNR and anaerobic coverage (e.g., piperacillin–tazobactam or a carbapenem). Empiric coverage of *Candida* with an echinocandin is also recommended. When infectious collections are recognized, percutaneous or surgical drainage (source control) should be initiated within 12 hours.

Genitourinary Cancer

Genitourinary cancer patients have lower rates of infection (<5%); infections in this group are often related to urinary obstruction and/or diversion. Antimicrobial treatment should include coverage of GNRs, including ESBL organisms and vancomycin-resistant enterococci in those with risk factors (urinary procedures, uncontrolled diabetes, colonization with VRE). Urine cultures obtained from ileal conduit are rarely useful. These patients also may experience postsurgical wound infections, ranging from localized cellulitis to extensive infections resulting in pyometra and tuboovarian, intra-abdominal, or pelvic abscesses.

Head and Neck Cancer

For patients with head and neck cancers, wound infections secondary to loss of the protective oral mucosa barrier and subsequent oral anaerobic flora contamination

TABLE 34.4 Common Infectious Conditions for Patients with Solid Tumors

Condition	Pathogens	Diagnostic Tests (Sensitivity/Specificity)	Recommended Antibiotic Regimens[a,43]	Non-infectious Mimics
Catheter-Related Blood Stream Infections				
Bacteremia	• Coagulase-negative *Staphylococcus* (31%) • *S. aureus* (20%) including MRSA • Enterococci (9%) including VRE[41,46]	• "Time-to-positivity" blood/CVC culture, positive defined by ○ Threefold CFU: CVC versus peripheral (75%–93%/97%–100%)[47,48] ○ CVC culture "+" <120 min prior to + peripheral culture (81%–93%/75%–92%)[30,44]	1. Vancomycin 15 mg/kg IV q12h or daptomycin 4–6 mg/kg q24h (if vancomycin MIC ≥ 2 mcg/mL) 2. Consider piperacillin-tazobactam 4.5 g IV q6h or meropenem 1 g IV q8h (based on risk factors for MDRI)	None
Fungemia	• *Candida* (9%)	• Workup for endocarditis based on surveillance cultures or organism	1. Echinocandin (e.g., caspofungin 75 mg IV once then 50 mg IV q24h)	
Neutropenic Fever (see Table 34.3)				
Infections Associated with Corticosteroid Use				
Pneumonia	• *P. jirovecii*	• β-D-glucan >31.1 pg/mL (92%/86%)[19] • ABG • Induced sputum IFA (50%–67%)[19] • BAL IFA performance less than in HIV patients • Imaging: ○ CXR—Normal or diffuse interstitial pattern ○ High-resolution CT—bilateral ground-glass opacities < HIV-positive, focal consolidations	See Table 34.1 *Pulmonary infections* section on *Pneumocystis* pneumonia	Radiation Pneumonitis Lymphangitic tumor spread Drug toxicity
	• *Aspergillus*/non-*Aspergillus* molds	See Table 34.3 *Pulmonary infections,* Early postengraftment section on Fungal pneumonia		
	Endemic fungal infections • *H. capsulatum* • *Coccidioides immitis* • *Blastomyces dermatitis*	• Endemic fungi ○ *Histoplasma* urine antigen (75%–97%)[19] ○ *Coccidioidomycosis* antibodies ○ *Blastomycosis* □ Sputum culture (75%–86%)[24] □ Urine antigen (89%–93%/79%)[25]	1. Mild to moderate: Fluconazole 400 mg PO/IV q24h or itraconazole 200 mg PO q8h for 3 d followed by q12h 2. Severe: Liposomal amphotericin 3–5 mg/kg IV q24h	
	• *Nocardia*	See Table 34.3 Pulmonary infections, Late postengraftment section on Bacterial pneumonia, *Nocardia*		
	• *M. tuberculosis*	See Table 34.1 Pulmonary infections section on *M. tuberculosis* pneumonia		

(*Continued*)

TABLE 34.4 Common Infectious Conditions for Patients with Solid Tumors (*Continued*)

Condition	Pathogens	Diagnostic Tests (Sensitivity/Specificity)	Recommended Antibiotic Regimens[a,43]	Non-infectious Mimics
Lung Cancer–Related Infections				
Pneumonia	• Polymicrobial • *S. aureus* • *S. pneumoniae* • Enteric GNRs	• Blood culture • Sputum culture • Imaging: ○ CXR—Recurrent lobar consolidation ○ CT—lobar Consolidation ± bronchial "cutoff sign"	Health care–associated pneumonia: Vancomycin 15 mg/kg IV q12h + piperacillin–tazobactam 4.5 g IV q6h. Consider double coverage with ciprofloxacin/gentamicin until susceptibilities are known 1. Community-acquired: Ceftriaxone 1 g IV q24h + azithromycin 500 mg IV q24h or levofloxacin 750 mg PO/IV q24h	Radiation Pneumonitis Lymphangitic Tumor Spread Drug Toxicity
Breast Cancer–Related Infections				
Cellulitis	• *S. aureus* • *Streptococcus* • Nosocomial ○ *MRSA* ○ *P. aeruginosa*	• Blood culture • Imaging: Ultrasound—if evidence of fluid collection or persistence despite 72 h of antibiotics	1. Vancomycin 15 mg/kg IV q12h 2. Add piperacillin–tazobactam 4.5 g IV q6h if *P. aeruginosa* risk factors, specifically neutropenia 3. Surgical consultation for incision and drainage (as needed)	Radiation Skin Damage Lymphedema Inflammatory Breast Cancer
Gastrointestinal Cancer–Related Infections				
Secondary peritonitis **Intra-abdominal abscess**	• Polymicrobial • Enteric GNRs • Anaerobic (*Bacteroides, Clostridium*) • *S. bovis* • *Candida,* in neutropenic or health care–associated cases	• Blood cultures • Abdominal fluid culture (ascites, abscess) • Imaging: CT abdominal/pelvic	1. Ceftriaxone 1–2 g IV q24h + metronidazole 500 mg IV q8h, or 2. Piperacillin–tazobactam 4.5 g IV q6h, or meropenem 1 g IV q8h 3. Percutaneous catheter or surgical drainage	Bowel Obstruction/ Ileus Anastomotic Stricture(s)

Genitourinary Cancer–Related Infections				
Cystitis **Pyelonephritis** **Prostatitis**	• Gram negatives ○ *E. Coli* ○ *Proteus* ○ *Klebsiella* ○ Enterobacter ○ ESBL ○ *P. aeruginosa* ○ Enterococcus ○ *Candida*	• Urine culture • Blood culture	Complicated UTI or pyelonephritis: 1. Mild—ceftriaxone 1–2 g IV q24h or ciprofloxacin 400 mg IV q12h or levofloxacin 500 mg IV q24 h 2. Severe—cefepime 1 g IV q8h, or ceftazidime 1 g IV q8h, or carbapenem (imipenem 500 mg IV q6h or meropenem 1 g IV q8h) if high risk for ESBL, or history of prior ESBL infections 3. Consider adding vancomycin (15 mg/kg IV q12h) if history of prior susceptible enterococcus infection, chronic urinary catheters, or stents	Percutaneous renal radiofrequency (RF) post-ablation syndrome Medication-induced cystitis
Head and Neck Cancer–Related Infections				
Wound infection **Odontogenic infection**	• Polymicrobial • Anaerobic • *Streptococcus* spp	• Blood culture • Wound culture	1. Immune competent—ampicillin–sulbactam 3 g IV q6h 2. Immune compromised—vancomycin 15 mg/kg IV q12h and + piperacillin–tazobactam 4.5 g IV q6h 3. Surgical debridement and/or drainage	Airway obstruction Osteoradionecrosis or Soft Tissue Necrosis Vascular Injury and/or Invasion

ESBL, extended-spectrum beta-lactamase; MRSA, methicillin-resistant *S. aureus;* UTI, urinary tract infection.
From *The Sanford guide to antimicrobial therapy.* Sperryville, VA: Antimicrobial Therapy; 2012. Ref.[34]

commonly occur (6% to 20% incidence).[83] Management includes antimicrobials against oral flora and, where indicated, surgical drainage, which provides diagnostic culture and source control. Pneumonia, from oropharyngeal aspiration, remains a leading cause of death and should be tested for with routine chest radiography.[84]

INFECTIONS IN PATIENTS AFTER SOLID ORGAN TRANSPLANTATION

Immune Defect in Patients After SOT

For SOT recipients, intensified immune suppression has improved survival by reducing rejection, but it also increased the risk for infectious complications. Immune suppression may be divided into discrete phases: *induction* (high-dose corticosteroids ± antilymphocyte antibodies/IL-2 receptor antibodies), *maintenance* (corticosteroids, antimetabolites, calcineurin inhibitors), and *treatment for episodes of rejection* (high-dose corticosteroids, plasmapheresis, antilymphocyte antibodies). During the maintenance phase, immune suppression is gradually tapered; however, continued high levels may be required for transplanted organs with increased environmental exposure, such as the small bowel and lung. Despite continued high level of immune suppression, small bowel and lung recipients still experience the highest rates of acute rejection during the first year (70% and 30%, respectively).[85,86] Treatment for acute rejection greatly increases the risk for infection. Plasmapheresis, for example, removes antibodies, increasing the risk for encapsulated bacterial infections. Lymphocyte-depleting therapies result in prolonged B- and T-cell defects, increasing the risk for viral and fungal infections. In general, SOT patients are rarely neutropenic, unless they are receiving chemotherapy for posttransplant lymphoproliferative disease.

Timeline of Infections in SOT

As is the case with patients post-HSCT, knowledge of the timing since transplantation, intensity of immune suppression, and prophylaxis will allow clinicians to differentiate among likely infectious pathogens for solid organ recipients (Fig. 34.2).[87] Typical prophylaxis includes TMP–SMX against *P. jirovecii*, *Nocardia*, *Listeria*, and *Toxoplasma* and valganciclovir against CMV and HSV. Lung transplant patients often receive antimold prophylaxis with itraconazole or voriconazole.

Early to Intermediate Posttransplantation Period

The early posttransplant period (1 month) is dominated by donor-derived infections, nosocomial pathogens (MRSA, *P. aeruginosa*, *Candida*, *C. difficile*), and surgical complications. Postoperative infectious complications may persist into the intermediate posttransplantation period, requiring prolonged antimicrobial treatment. During the intermediate posttransplant period (1 to 6 months), patients are the most vulnerable to opportunistic pathogens, as they are recovering from major surgery and are increasingly immune suppressed as induction therapy is taking effect.

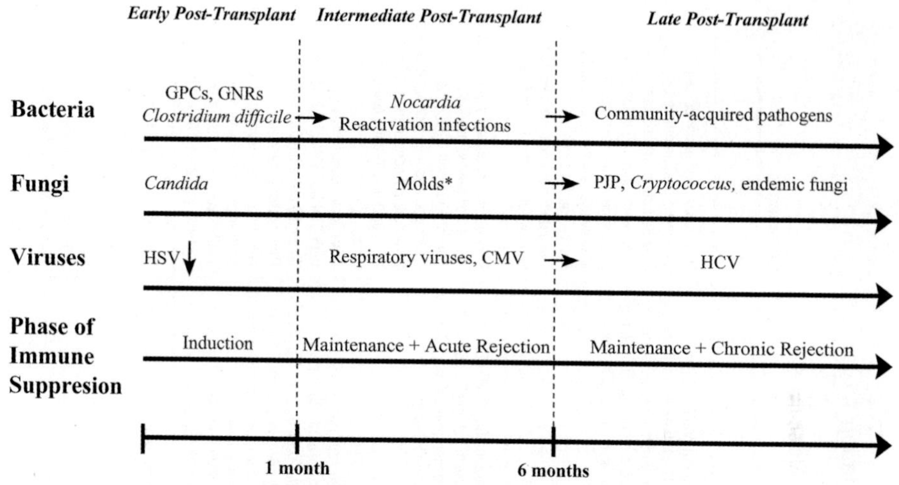

FIGURE 34.2 Timeline of infections after solid organ transplantation.

Fungal Infections in the Early to Intermediate Posttransplant Period

For SOT recipients, the incidence of IFD varies by the organ transplanted. Incidence is highest in lung, small bowel, and liver transplant patients and is lowest in renal transplant patients.[88] In liver transplants, the incidence of *Candida* infections ranges from 62% to 91% with risk factors including multiple surgical interventions, use of broad-spectrum antibiotics, and the use of TPN.[89] In small bowel transplants, the incidence of *Candida* infections is 85%.[90] In lung transplants, *Aspergillus* is the most common fungal infection, affecting up to 44% of patients and portending a high mortality (65% to 80%).[89–91] Among heart transplant patients, the rate of IFD is 3%.[90] During the intermediate post-transplant period, the clinician also must consider geographic and endemic mycoses. For example, disseminated cryptococcus with brain and lung manifestations; disseminated histoplasmosis to the lung, bone marrow, liver, and spleen; and disseminated coccidioidomycosis to the skin, skeletal system, and brain. The incidence of *P. jiroveci* has decreased with TMP–SMX prophylaxis but can present atypically with negative BAL, requiring biopsy for diagnosis in patients taking non–TMP-SMX–based prophylaxis.[92] Infections caused by *Aspergillus* spp tend to be localized to the lung compared to non-*Aspergillus* molds that will disseminate in 50% of the cases.[93]

Diagnosis of Invasive Fungal Diseases

The diagnosis of IFD is particularly difficult in lung transplant patients, who are frequently colonized with *Aspergillus*. Antifungal treatment is initiated based on clinical presentation, radiographic findings, and results of culture and non–culture-based assays (Table 34.5). *Aspergillus* (GM) from serum, with an index cutoff of 0.5 in SOT recipients, is not a reliable test to rule out infection.[45] *Aspergillus* GM from BAL has a higher

TABLE 34.5 Common Infectious Conditions for Patients After Solid Organ Transplantation

Condition	Pathogen	Clinical Presentation	Diagnostic Tests (Sensitivity/ Specificity)	Recommended Antibiotic Regimens[a,43]	Comments
Bacterial Infections in SOT Recipients					
Postoperative complications **Nosocomial infections**	• MRSA • *P. aeruginosa* • GNRs • *Candida*	Fever, cough, AMS Abdominal pain Surgical wound infection, dehiscence	• Blood, sputum or wound culture • Check donor cultures • Imaging—CXR or CT scan chest and/ or abdomen	1. Vancomycin 15 mg/kg IV q 8–12h or linezolid 600 mg IV q12h + Piperacillin–tazobactam 4.5 g IV q6h or meropenem 1 g IV q8h ± echinocandin (micafungin 100 mg IV daily or caspofungin 70 mg IV X1 then 50 mg IV q24h)	Nosocomial and donor-derived pathogens predominate early to intermediate posttransplant. Community-acquired pathogens predominate late posttransplant. May evolve rapidly to respiratory failure and septic shock. Evaluate for surgical complications: airway dehiscence, biliary leak
GI infection —fulminant colitis (13%) **Ileus**	• *C. difficile*	Diarrhea ± ileus Abdominal pain *Severe*—high fever, marked leukocytosis, poor nutritional state, and acute kidney injury	• *C. difficile* toxin detection PCR or EIA • Imaging: CT—colitis, colonic distension	1. Mild—metronidazole 500 mg PO q8h 2. Severe—vancomycin 125 mg PO q6h 3. Septic shock—vancomycin 500 mg PO every 6 h + metronidazole PO or IV	May not be preceded by antibiotics as also associated with MMF. May present with abdominal distension and pain without diarrhea. Early surgical consultation: 13% of SOT recipients require colectomy
Pneumonia	• Hospital-acquired pathogens (MRSA, *P. aeruginosa*, *K. pneumoniae*) • *Nocardia*	Cough ± sputum Late posttransplant Course: Subacute (weeks)	• Blood cultures • Sputum stain and culture: modified AFB for *Nocardia* • *Nocardia* PCR • Imaging: CT—macronodules ± cavitary	1. Hospital-acquired: Vancomycin 15 mg/ kg IV q 8–12h or linezolid 600 mg IV q 12h + piperacillin–tazobactam 4.5 g IV q6h or meropenem 1 g IV q8h. Consider double coverage with ciprofloxacin/gentamicin until susceptibilities are known 2. *Nocardia*: TMP–SMX 5 mg/kg IV q8h + imipenem 500 mg IV q6h	Always evaluate for CNS involvement with CT/MRI (50% of pulmonary *Nocardia* disseminates to the brain). Other sites: Cutaneous. Nocardiosis can develop despite bactrim prophylaxis: Increase. TMP–SMX dose to 5 mg/kg IV q8h and add imipenem 500 mg IV q6h
Pneumonia **Disseminated infection**	• *M. tuberculosis*	Fever, night sweats, weight loss, cough 6–12 mo posttransplant Course: Subacute	• AFB × 3 smear and culture • *M. tuberculosis* PCR • Tissue biopsy (e.g., pleura) for pathology, smear and cultures • Imaging: CT—miliary pattern, consolidation, rarely cavities, pleural effusion	Rifampin, isoniazid, pyrazinamide, ethambutol at weight-based dosing	Suspect in immigrants from *M. tuberculosis* endemic area or previous *M. tuberculosis* exposure. Skin test not useful. Frequent disseminated disease: lymph nodes, skin, CNS, bone marrow, etc

Fungal Infections in SOT Recipients					
Fungal pneumonia Disseminated infection	Invasive mold infections: • *Aspergillus spp* • Non-*Aspergillus* molds	Dry cough, fever, pleuritic chest pain No complaints Course: Subacute	• *Aspergillus* GM: serum >0.5[a] (22%/84%)[45] • *Aspergillus* GM: BAL (88%/87%)[19] • Fungal cultures • Imaging: CT—Nodules ± halo • consolidation, cavitation	1. *Aspergillus spp*: Voriconazole 6 mg/kg IV q12 × 2 doses then 4 mg/kg IV q12h[b] 2. Non-*Aspergillus* molds: Liposomal amphotericin 5 mg/kg IV q24h	Tracheobronchial aspergillosis may cause anastomotic site dehiscence in lung transplant patients. Other sites: CNS, skin, sinuses, orbits
Disseminated infection	• *Candida spp*		• Blood cultures; do not need fungal isolator • Ophthalmology evaluation for fungal endophthalmitis	1. Echinocandin (e.g., caspofungin 70 mg IV × 1 then 50 mg IV q24h)	Incidence: Highest in liver and small bowel transplants
Fungal pneumonia **Disseminated infection**	Endemic fungal infections	See Table 34.4 *Infections associated with corticosteroid use,* Pneumonia, section on Endemic fungal infections			Disseminated histoplasmosis—lung, bone marrow, liver, and spleen. Disseminated coccidioidomycosis—skin, skeletal system, and brain. Disseminated blastomycosis—lung, bone, skin, CNS, GU (prostatitis)
Pneumonia Disseminated infection (CNS—see below)	Geographic fungal infections: • *C. neoformans* • *C. gattii*	Pulmonary disease: Asymptomatic to ARDS CNS disease: AMS, fever, headache, focal deficits, meningeal signs may be absent	• *Cryptococcus* ○ Serum and CSF *Cryptococcus* antigen (>90% especially in disseminated disease)[94] ○ Fungal CSF culture	1. Liposomal amphotericin 5 mg/kg IV q24h + flucytosine 25 mg/kg/dose PO q6h. 2. If CSF pressure >25 cm, reduce opening pressure by 50% or to normal pressure of <20 cm	Increased incidence of *C. gattii* infections in the Pacific Northwest causing cryptococcomas. Asymptomatic lung infection can be portal for meningeal dissemination. Serum cryptococcal antigen becomes positive earlier than CSF antigen. IRIS can present similarly to a worsening infection. Higher incidence with T-cell depleting immune suppression and higher antigenemia at diagnosis[94]
***Pneumocystis* pneumonia**	• *P. jiroveci*	See Table 34.4 *Infections associated with corticosteroid use* section on Pneumonia, *Pneumocystis jiroveci*			Occurs when TMP–SMX prophylaxis stopped
Viral Infections in SOT Recipients					
Pneumonia	• CMV	Dry cough, low-grade fever, shortness of breath Course: Days	• CMV PCR—serum, BAL—standardization across laboratories in progress • Bronchoscopy (shell vial culture) ± biopsy • Imaging: CT—reticular infiltrates, ground-glass opacities, small nodules	Mild to moderate: Valganciclovir 900 mg PO q12h Severe disease: Ganciclovir 5 mg/kg IV q12h ± CMV Ig	CMV triggers rejection and reactivates with rejection. CMV may promote opportunistic infections. CMV: Donor positive/recipient negative have the highest risk

(*Continued*)

TABLE 34.5 Common Infectious Conditions for Patients after Solid Organ Transplantation (*Continued*)

Condition	Pathogen	Clinical Presentation	Diagnostic Tests (Sensitivity/Specificity)	Recommended Antibiotic Regimens[a,43]	Comments
Pneumonia	• Influenza • Parainfluenza • RSV • Human metapneumovirus	URI symptoms Mild to severe shortness of breath Seasonality except for parainfluenza Late posttransplant Course: Acute	For diagnosis and treatment see Table 34.3 Viral pneumonia section on Respiratory viruses		Influenza vaccine decreased efficacy in lung transplant recipients. 25% of the patients will have bacterial superinfection. Inhaled ribavirin can cause bronchospasm. See www.cdc.gov for updated yearly influenza susceptibilities. Initiate droplet isolation
CNS Infections in SOT Recipients					
Meningitis	• *S. pneumoniae* • *P. aeruginosa* • *Listeria* • *Cryptococcus* • *H. influenzae* • *M. tuberculosis*	Headache Fever Meningeal signs may be absent *M. tuberculosis:* Basilar meningitis with cranial nerve deficits	• LP: Opening pressure, glucose, protein, WBC, gram stain, cultures, cryptococcal antigen, • HSV and VZV PCR-CSF • AFB smear and cultures • Blood cultures	1. Empiric therapy: Cefepime 2 g IV q8h or meropenem 2 g IV q8h + vancomycin 15 mg/kg IV q12h + acyclovir 10 mg/kg IV q8h + ampicillin 2 g IV q4h 2. Dexamethasone 0.15 mg/kg IV q6h × 4 d if suspected or proven pneumococcal infection 3. See Table 34.1 for treatment of *Cryptococcus* or *M. tuberculosis* meningitis	Consider GNRs (e.g., *P. aeruginosa*). Cryptococcal antigen has 2–3 h turnaround time. Consider tacrolimus side effects as alternative cause
Encephalitis	• HSV • VZV	AMS Fever Headache Focal deficits	• LP: Opening pressure, glucose, protein, cell count • HSV and VZV PCR: CSF • CT, MRI: Temporal lobe involvement	1. Acyclovir 10 mg/kg IV q8h	
Parenchymal lesions	• *Aspergillus* spp[a] • Non-*Aspergillus* molds • *Nocardia* • Toxoplasmosis	Headache Focal deficits Seizures Altered mental status	• Brain biopsy if feasible • *Aspergillus* GM: CSF[95] • *Toxoplasma* serologies • Imaging: CT head, sinuses and chest; MRI head	1. *Aspergillus* spp: Voriconazole 6 mg/kg IV q12h × 2 doses then 4 mg/kg IV q12h[b] ± echinocandin (e.g., caspofungin 75 mg IV × 1, then 50 mg IV q24h) 2. Non-*Aspergillus* molds: Liposomal amphotericin 5 mg/kg IV q24h 3. *Nocardia*: TMP–SMX 5 mg/kg IV q8h + imipenem 500 mg IV q6h 4. Toxoplasmosis: Pyrimethamine 200 mg PO once then 75 mg PO q24h + sulfadiazine 1 g (<60 kg) or 1.5 g (>60 kg) PO q6h + leucovorin 10–25 mg PO q24h	CNS involvement in aspergillosis has a high mortality. Voriconazole is superior to liposomal amphotericin[95,96] Toxoplasma reactivation can occur after stopping TMP–SMX prophylaxis Toxoplasmosis presents usually without focal neurologic findings

Infections Specific for Liver Transplant Recipients					
1. Intra-abdominal abscesses 2. Bacteremia especially in patients on HD 3. Viral hepatitis 4. HCV recurrence	1 & 2: GI flora including *Candida*, VRE 1 & 2: Skin flora 3: CMV 3: HHV6 3 & 4: HCV	Abdominal pain Fever, chills Diarrhea Increased LFTs	• Blood cultures • Cultures from aspirates, drains • CMV PCR • HHV6 PCR • HCV PCR • Imaging: CT abdomen	1. Daptomycin 8–10 mg/kg IV q24h + meropenem 1 g q8h ± echinocandin (e.g., caspofungin 70 mg IV once then 50 mg IV q24h or micafungin 100 mg IV q24h)	Always consider VRE and *Candida*. CMV, HHV6 can accelerate HCV recurrence. HCV recurs in 90% of the patients during the first year
Infections Specific for Renal Transplant Recipients					
1. 50% have UTIs 2. Bacteremia from urinary source 3. CMV colitis 4. Hepatitis	1 & 2: GNRs 1 & 2: *Enterococcus* 1: *Candida* 1: BK virus 1: *C. urealyticum* 3: CMV	Asymptomatic to pyelonephritis Increased creatinine Abdominal pain, diarrhea, increased LFTs	• UA, microscopy (decoy cells with BK), urine culture • BK PCR: urine and blood • Imaging: Ultrasound: evaluate for anatomic defects: obstruction, leak • CMV PCR serum • Colonoscopy with biopsy	1. Cefepime 1 g IV q8h 2. VRE: Daptomycin 8 mg/kg IV q24h 3. Candiduria: Fluconazole 200–400 mg PO q24h or liposomal amphotericin 3 mg/kg IV q24h 1. Nonsevere: Valganciclovir 900 mg PO q12h 2. Severe: Ganciclovir 5 mg/kg IV q12h	High mortality with *Candida* pyelonephritis. Linezolid and echinocandin (e.g., micafungin, caspofungin) have poor urinary penetration. Avoid urinary catheters
Infections Specific for Pancreatic Transplant Recipients					
1. UTIs 2/2 alkaline urine 2. Pancreatic pseudocyst 3. Peritonitis 4. Anastomotic bowel leak	1, 2, & 3: GNRs 1, 2, & 3: GPCs 1, 2, & 3: *Candida*	Abdominal pain Pneumaturia Rise in amylase and creatinine	• UA, urine microscopy, urine culture • Paracentesis with WBC, amylase, gram stain, and cultures • Imaging: CT abdomen with IV contrast	1. Vancomycin 15 mg/kg IV q12h + piperacillin–tazobactam 4.5 g IV q6h + fluconazole 400 mg PO q24h	Pancreas exocrine secretions are drained in the bladder or small bowel. Aspirate pseudocyst if considered infected. Fluconazole has excellent penetration in the peritoneal cavity
Infections Specific for Small Bowel Transplant Recipients					
1. Enteritis 2. Bacteremia secondary to bacterial translocation 3. Peritonitis due to leak	1: CMV 1: Adenovirus 1: *C. difficile* 1: Cryptosporidium 1, 2, & 3: GNRs 1, 2, & 3: Anaerobes	Abdominal pain Fever, chills Increased ostomy output	• CMV serum PCR • *C. difficile* toxin PCR • Stool for ova and parasites • Blood cultures • Paracentesis • Endoscopy with biopsy • Imaging: CT abdomen with IV contrast	1. Piperacillin–tazobactam 4.5 g IV q6h or (cefepime 1 g IV q8h and metronidazole 500 mg IV q8h) + echinocandin (e.g., caspofungin 70 mg IV × 1 then 50 mg IV q24h or micafungin 100 mg IV q24h)	

(*Continued*)

TABLE 34.5 Common Infectious Conditions for Patients after Solid Organ Transplantation (*Continued*)

Condition	Pathogen	Clinical Presentation	Diagnostic Tests (Sensitivity/ Specificity)	Recommended Antibiotic Regimens[a,43]	Comments
Infections Specific for Heart Transplant Recipients					
1. Pneumonia 2. Pleural space infections 3. Anastomotic site infections 4. Wound site infections 5. *C. difficile* colitis	1. Bacteria: *S. aureus*, *Pseudomonas* spp., MDR GNRs, *Burkholderia cepacia*, *Streptococcus pneumoniae*, *M. hominis*, *C. pneumoniae* Viruses: CMV, respiratory viruses Fungi: Aspergillus and non-*Aspergillus* molds 2. Same bacteria + *Candida* spp. 3. *Aspergillus* spp. 4. MRSA, *Candida* spp., *Pseudomonas* spp.	Dyspnea Cough Chest pain Fever, chills Wound drainage/ dehiscence Diarrhea Abdominal pain	• Sputum cultures • Galactomannan antigen from serum and BAL • Viral naso-pharyngeal DFA • Thoracentesis with fluid analysis and cultures • Wound cultures • *C. difficile* PCR • Imaging: CT thorax	See bacterial, viral, and fungal pneumonia treatment See *C. difficile* treatment based on severity	Cystic fibrosis patients are colonized with *S. aureus* (especially MRSA), *Pseudomonas*, and *Burkholderia* spp. so empiric antibiotics should be based on prior susceptibility patterns. Double coverage for MDR GNR is often warranted Rejection can mimic pneumonia Consider CNS and sinuses imaging in fungal pneumonias
Infections Specific for Heart Transplant Recipients					
1. Pneumonia 2. Wound infections including mediastinitis	1 & 2: MRSA 1 & 2: *Pseudomonas* 1 & 2: *E. coli* 2: CMV 1 & 2: *Aspergillus spp.* 2: *P. jirovecii*	Cough Dyspnea Fever, chills Chest pain Wound drainage/dehiscence	• Sputum cultures • Serum CMV PCR • *P. jirovecii* DFA sputum • Imaging: CT thorax	See treatment of bacterial, viral and fungal pneumonias	Much lower infectious risk than in heart-lung transplant recipients

[a]Dosing based on normal renal and hepatic function.
[b]Initiate in conjunction with an ID specialist or pharmacist due to drug interactions: Voriconazole may interact with tacrolimus and antiepileptic medications.
AFB, acid-fast bacilli; AMS, altered mental status; BAL, bronchoalveolar lavage; CMV, cytomegalovirus; CNS, central nervous system; CSF, cerebrospinal fluid; ELISA, enzyme-linked immunoassay; GI, gastrointestinal; GM, galactomannan; GNRs, gram-negative rods (e.g., *K. pneumonia, E. Coli*); GPCs, gram-positive cocci; HCV, hepatitis C virus; HD, hemodialysis; HHV6, human herpes virus 6; HSV, herpes simplex virus; IS, immune suppression; LFT, liver function tests; LP, lumbar puncture; MMF, mycophenolate mofetil; MRI, magnetic resonance imaging; MRSA, methicillin-resistant *S. aureus*; Non-*Aspergillus* molds, mucormycosis, *Scedosporium, Fusarium*; PCR, polymerase chain reaction; RSV, respiratory syncytial virus; SOT, solid organ transplant; TMP–SMX, trimethoprim–sulfamethoxazole; UA, urinalysis; URI, upper respiratory infection; UTI, urinary tract infection; VRE, vancomycin-resistant enterococcus; VZV, varicella zoster virus.
From *The Sanford guide to antimicrobial therapy*. Sperryville, VA: Antimicrobial Therapy; 2012. Ref.[34].

diagnostic yield. For pulmonary aspergillosis, noncontrast CT scans of the thorax often demonstrates multiple pulmonary nodules with or without a "halo sign," cavitation, or consolidation. For endemic mycoses, such as *Cryptococcus* and *PJP*, non–culture-based techniques are available and generally have good test performance (Table 34.5).[19]

Treatment of Invasive Fungal Diseases

Candida prophylaxis is reserved for high-risk patients, including patients with a history of multiple abdominal surgeries and recipients of small bowel, pancreas, and liver transplants. Lung transplant centers differ in their use of antimold prophylaxis with triazoles, which are thought to promote infections with resistant molds (mucormycosis, *Scedosporium*).[93] Non-*Aspergillus* molds account for 27% of the mycelial infections in SOTs.[93] Rapid microbiologic diagnosis of invasive mold infections is key, given the high mortality rates, medication interactions, and variable susceptibility patterns. Voriconazole is the drug of choice in treating *Aspergillus* spp. Liposomal amphotericin should be used for almost all other non-*Aspergillus* molds. Transplant pharmacy consultation should be considered before initiating therapy with antifungal agents, macrolides, metronidazole, and norfloxacin, given significant drug interactions with the immunosuppressive medications.

Clostridium difficile Infections in the Early to Intermediate Posttransplant Period

C. difficile can persist into the intermediate posttransplant period, producing diarrhea and fulminant colitis in 13% of patients.[97] The incidence of *C. difficile* infections varies by type of SOT ranging from 6% in kidney transplants to as high as 15% in heart and lung recipients.[43,98,99] Since mycophenolate mofetil (MMF)—an immunosuppressant used extensively in transplant patients—has antibacterial properties and has been associated with *C. difficile* infections, prior antibiotic exposure is not mandatory. The clinical symptoms (diarrhea, abdominal pain ± fever, ± ileus) can occur while receiving antimicrobials or even weeks after stopping them. Diagnosis is based upon *C. difficile* toxin detection in the stool using an enzyme immunoassay (EIA) or PCR assay coupled with EIA for *C. difficile* glutamate dehydrogenase. In the atypical presentation of *C. difficile* with induced ileus, abdominal CT imaging can demonstrate colitis. In mild cases, metronidazole PO can be used while monitoring for signs of colonic distension. In severe disease characterized by high fever, marked leukocytosis, poor nutritional state, and acute kidney injury, vancomycin PO should be started. For patients with septic shock, treatment requires both high-dose vancomycin PO and metronidazole either PO or IV.[100] Surgical consultation should be obtained, as 13% of SOT recipients with *C. difficile* colitis will require colectomy.[101]

Viral Infections in the Early to Intermediate Posttransplant Period

Respiratory Viruses

Weeks after transplant, most patients have returned to the community and are exposed to respiratory viruses. Potential pathogens include parainfluenza (no seasonality), influenza, RSV, and human metapneumovirus, but virtually any respiratory virus can cause pneumonia. Incidence of community-acquired respiratory virus disease ranges from

2% to 16%.[102] Symptoms vary from a mild viral prodrome to respiratory failure. The protective antibody response to influenza vaccination is not as robust as in immune-competent hosts, and transplant patients can develop respiratory disease even after vaccination. For RSV, influenza, and parainfluenza, rapid viral antigen tests are recommended, in conjunction with PCR-based detection (Table 34.5). The yield is higher with samples obtained from lower in the respiratory tract, and a negative DFA from a nasopharyngeal swab does not rule out viral pneumonia (DFA nasal swab sensitivity is 15%). Respiratory viruses also may contribute to bacterial superinfection and rejection.[103] Appropriate antiviral therapy (oseltamivir for influenza and inhaled ribavirin for RSV and human metapneumovirus) should be started and respiratory isolation initiated. Ribavirin therapy in parainfluenza infections remains controversial; however, its use in lung and heart–lung transplant patients in conjunction with methylprednisolone and IVIG has been associated with improved maintenance of lung function.[104]

Cytomegalovirus Infections

Posttransplantation, most patients receive prophylaxis with valganciclovir to prevent CMV disease. For SOT patients, a donor with a history of CMV and a recipient without previous exposure to CMV (donor positive/recipient negative (D+/R–)) is the combination that carries the highest risk of reactivating CMV. In contrast among HSCT patients, D–/R+ has the highest risk because the recipient losses his or her previous immunity against CMV after bone marrow transplantation. CMV "infection" is viral replication detected in the serum. CMV "disease" is defined as end-organ dysfunction attributed to the virus. This may involve invasive disease (colitis, pneumonitis, hepatitis, retinitis) or CMV viral syndrome (fever, malaise, leucopenia, or thrombocytopenia).[105] Patients treated with both universal and preemptive prophylactic therapy can develop late-onset CMV disease. After stopping the prophylactic regimen (usually 3 to 6 months posttransplantation), 25% of the D+/R– SOT patients will develop active CMV infection. Because CMV may affect the allograft, it can cause nephropathy in kidney recipients and pneumonitis in lung recipients. Because of its immune modulatory effects, CMV increases the risk of bacterial and fungal infection, as well as graft rejection and loss.[106]

Diagnosis of CMV CMV infection (viremia without end-organ damage) is characterized by nonspecific symptoms of fatigue and low-grade fever. CMV pneumonitis often manifests with dry cough and shortness of breath. CMV colitis presents with abdominal pain and diarrhea. Quantitative PCR-CMV viral load should be obtained in patients at risk for infection (D+/R–, D+/R+, D–/R+). Some patients may require invasive testing and biopsy in cases of normal serum PCR (commonly seen in CMV colitis) or to identify invasive disease.

Treatment and Follow-up of CMV Disease Based on severity, patients may receive outpatient treatment with oral valganciclovir[107] or inpatient therapy with IV ganciclovir. In a patient with stable or worsening viremia after >2 weeks of adequate CMV treatment, infection with a ganciclovir-resistant virus should be suspected and CMV genotype sent.

Reactivation Infections in the Intermediate Posttransplantation Period

Given a patient's intense state of immune suppression during this period, latent infections may reactivate, including MTB, toxoplasmosis (if not on prophylaxis), and leishmaniasis. The risk of MTB varies widely depending on the country of origin, with an incidence (1.2% to 15%) approximately 50 times higher than in the immune-competent population.[108] Tuberculosis presents with dry cough, fevers, night sweats, and weight loss, with frequent dissemination to the skin, soft tissues, and lymph nodes. Given that the mortality rate of MTB is 30%, these symptoms demand high suspicion in certain epidemiologic scenarios. The efficacy of pretransplant skin testing and interferon (IFN)-γ release assays is under investigation in transplant patients. Diagnosis of MTB is made by AFB smear and culture. Four-drug therapy is recommended along with immediate respiratory isolation (Table 34.5).

Leishmaniasis is a very uncommon disease in SOT population (62 cases reported)[109] and usually arises from reactivation (but can also be transmitted by blood transfusion or organs).

Toxoplasmosis may be acquired via transplanted organs (especially the heart), reactivation, or from exposure to feline excrements. It develops in patients not on TMP–SMX prophylaxis. Infection can occur in the CNS (4% to 29% of the CNS lesions in transplant patients can be attributed to toxoplasmosis),[110] heart (myocarditis), lung (pneumonitis), and retina (choroiditis). Fever is present along with headache and altered mental status. Diagnosis relies on positive serologies, presence of the parasite in the histologic specimen, and/or PCR technology.

Late Posttransplantation Period

The late posttransplantation period begins >6 months postoperatively. During this time, most infections are community acquired, with typical pathogens including *S. pneumoniae* and respiratory viruses. Community-acquired pneumonia presents similarly in both immune-compromised and immune-competent hosts, but in transplant patients, it can evolve rapidly into respiratory failure. The initial antimicrobial regimen should cover nosocomial pathogens (MRSA, *P. aeruginosa, Klebsiella pneumoniae*) until finalized sputum cultures and blood cultures allow de-escalation or until the patient is clinically improving. This period is also characterized by late-onset infections with CMV, *Nocardia*, and/or PJP after the discontinuation of prophylaxis, but while the patient is still receiving active immune suppression. Cryptococcosis, with a prevalence of 0.2% to 5% and a mortality of 40%, is an important IFD in the transplant population.[89] It usually occurs at approximately 1.5 years posttransplantation.[90] Patients can present with localized pulmonary disease (cough and shortness of breath) or with disseminated disease affecting the CNS. Because of the lack of inflammation, meningeal signs may be absent; fever, headache, and altered mentation may be the only findings. Lumbar puncture studies should include a record of the opening pressure and cerebrospinal fluid (CSF) cryptococcal antigen. *Cryptococcal* meningitis is treated as disseminated disease with liposomal amphotericin and 5-flucytosine for the first 2 weeks. In endemic regions of the United States, emergency physicians should also evaluate for endemic mycoses: *histoplasmosis* in the Ohio and Mississippi river valleys, *coccidioidomycosis* in the Southwest, and *blastomycosis* in the Midwest, Southeast, and South Central states. Serologic studies and antigens along with histopathologic examination provide the diagnosis.

CONCLUSION

Immune-compromised persons are a highly specialized patient subset whose management is increasingly being returned to community-based physicians. This chapter serves as a guide to their initial management, but the emergency physician is encouraged to consult with infectious disease specialists, oncologists, and transplant physicians familiar with ongoing disease management. In addition, the early involvement of pulmonologists, gastroenterologists, and surgeons may facilitate early diagnosis and improve targeted therapy. Optimization of patient outcomes requires an understanding of pathogen susceptibilities, appropriate empiric anti-infective regimens, and a multidisciplinary approach to patient care.

LITERATURE TABLE

TRIAL	DESIGN	RESULT
Infections in Patients with Human Immune Deficiency Virus		
Gruden et al., *Am J Roentgenol.* 1997[22]	Single-center prospective study of 51 HIV-infected adults with high clinical probability for PJP who underwent high-resolution chest tomography (HRCT) imaging. Inter-interpreter variability assessed in PJP diagnosis compared to BAL or clinical follow-up	PJP was diagnosed in 12% of patients. HRCT sensitivity was 100% and specificity of 89% for PJP with the radiographic findings defined as presence of patchy or nodular ground-glass opacities
Hirschtick et al., *N Engl J Med.* 1995[35]	Multicenter, prospective, observational study of 1,130 HIV-infected adults and non–HIV-infected adults monitored for up to 64 mo for occurrence of pulmonary disease	Bacterial pneumonia occurred more frequently in HIV-infected patients (5.5 per 100 person y) versus matched non–HIV-infected controls (0.9 per 100 person years) ($p < 0.001$). There was an association with decreasing CD4 cell count and incidence of pneumonia
Bozzette et al., *N Engl J Med.* 1990[37]	Multicenter nonblinded trial of 353 HIV-infected adults with PJP receiving standard therapy randomly assigned to corticosteroids (40 mg twice daily, followed by taper) vs. no additional therapy	Treatment with corticosteroids resulted in a lower risk of respiratory failure (14% vs. 30%, $p = 0.004$) and death at 31 d (11% vs. 23%, $p = 0.009$) and 84 d (16% vs. 26%, $p = 0.026$). There was no clinical benefit in the subgroup of patients with mild disease defined as $PaO_2 < 74$ on ambient air
Infections in Patients with Hematologic Malignancies and After HSCT		
Paul et al., *Cochrane Database Syst Rev.* 2010[58]	Analysis of all RCTs (only two double-blinded) published up to 2010 that compared antipseudomonal beta-lactams (cefepime, ceftazidime, piperacillin–tazobactam, imipenem, meropenem). Primary outcome was all-cause mortality	There was a higher risk of mortality when using cefepime compared to other beta-lactams (RR, 1.39, 95% CI, 1.04–1.86). There was a higher rate of bacterial superinfections with cefepime. Piperacillin–tazobactam had a lower mortality compared to other antibiotics (RR, 0.56, 95% CI, 0.34–0.92). Carbapenems had a higher rate of *C difficile* diarrhea
Walsh et al., *N Engl J Med.* 2004[60]	Randomized, double-blinded multicenter trial evaluating caspofungin vs. amphotericin B in patients with persistent febrile neutropenia. Outcome was a composite clinical end point	In the caspofungin group, there was a statistically significant better response if baseline fungal infection present (51.9% vs. 25.9%, $p = 0.04$) and better survival at 7 d into treatment (92.6% vs. 89.2%, $p = 0.05$). They also had less treatment discontinuation (10.3% vs. 14.5%, $p = 0.03$) and experienced less nephrotoxicity (2.6% vs. 11.5%, $p < 0.001$)
Freifeld et al., *N Engl J Med.* 1999[111]	Singe-center, randomized controlled, double-blinded placebo trial in patients with low-risk febrile neutropenia randomized to PO antibiotics (ciprofloxacin + amoxicillin–clavulanate) or IV antibiotics (ceftazidime)	Adjusted data showed that treatment was successful in 71% of the episodes in the oral therapy group and 67% of the episodes in the intravenous therapy group. Failure resulted from addition of a second drug in the IV group (32% vs. 13%, $p < 0.0001$) and intolerance to the PO regimen (16% vs. 8%, $p = 0.07$). Extrapolated current guidelines recommend PO outpatient antibiotics in low-risk febrile neutropenia

LITERATURE TABLE *(Continued)*

TRIAL	DESIGN	RESULT
Infections in Patients with Solid Tumors		
Tasaka et al. *Chest.* 2007[36]	Single-center retrospective study of 295 patients who underwent BAL for diagnosis of PJP with 57 PJP-positive (77% non–HIV-infected) and 222 PJP-negative patients	(1,3)-β-D-glucan is the most reliable serum marker and, when using a cutoff of 31.1 pg/mL, has a sensitivity of 92.3% and a specificity of 86.1% for PJP
Raad et al., *Ann Intern Med.* 2004[47]	Single-center prospective study evaluating the differential time to positivity of 191 patients with identification of the same organism from blood cultures drawn from CVC and peripheral vein. Catheter-tip colonization or quantitative blood cultures were used as the gold standard to define CRBSIs	A differential time to positivity of 120 min or more between the CVC blood culture and the peripheral vein blood culture has an 81% sensitivity and 92% specificity for short-term CRBSI and 93% sensitivity and 75% specificity for long-term CRBSI
Fernandez-Hidalgo et al., *J Antimicrob Chemother.* 2006[71]	Single-center, mixed retrospective and prospective study of 98 patients with 115 episodes of CRBSI were studied to assess the effectiveness of ALT. Primary outcome was evidence of negative blood cultures at 1 mo	ALT combined with systemic antibiotics resulted in an 82% cure rate and was particularly effective in treating coagulase-negative staphylococci CRBSI (84% cure rate). ALT was less effective in treating *S. aureus* CRBSI with only a 55% cure rate
Infections in Patients After Solid Organ Transplantation		
Asberg et al., *Am J Transplant.* 2007[107]	Randomized, open-label, parallel-group, active drug-controlled, multicenter trial to assess the noninferiority of valganciclovir compared to ganciclovir in adult SOT recipients with CMV disease. Primary outcome was treatment success: eradication of viremia at day 21. After that, both groups were treated with valganciclovir	321 patients randomized to either ganciclovir 5 mg/kg IV or valganciclovir 900 mg PO q12h. More than 70% of the patients were kidney transplant recipients who had gastrointestinal CMV disease (28%–29%). In the intention-to-treat analysis, viral eradication was achieved in 45.1% of the valganciclovir-treated patients and in 48.4% of the ganciclovir group. Treatment success at day 49 was 85.4% vs. 84.1%. Side effects were also comparable

CI, confidence interval; RR, relative risk.

REFERENCES

1. Bodey GP. The emergence of fungi as major hospital pathogens. *J Hosp Infect.* 1988;11(suppl A):411–426.
2. Duthie R, Denning DW. Aspergillus fungemia: report of two cases and review. *Clin Infect Dis.* 1995;20:598–605.
3. Morrell M, Fraser VJ, Kollef MH. Delaying the empiric treatment of candida bloodstream infection until positive blood culture results are obtained: a potential risk factor for hospital mortality. *Antimicrob Agents Chemother.* 2005;49:3640–3645.
4. Blum U, Windfuhr M, Buitrago-Tellez C, et al. Invasive pulmonary aspergillosis. MRI, CT, and plain radiographic findings and their contribution for early diagnosis. *Chest.* 1994;106:1156–1161.
5. Caillot D, Casasnovas O, Bernard A, et al. Improved management of invasive pulmonary aspergillosis in neutropenic patients using early thoracic computed tomographic scan and surgery. *J Clin Oncol.* 1997;15:139–147.
6. Kuhlman JE, Fishman EK, Siegelman SS. Invasive pulmonary aspergillosis in acute leukemia: characteristic findings on CT, the CT halo sign, and the role of CT in early diagnosis. *Radiology.* 1985;157:611–614.
7. Mori M, Galvin JR, Barloon TJ, et al. Fungal pulmonary infections after bone marrow transplantation: evaluation with radiography and CT. *Radiology.* 1991;178:721–726.
8. Staples CA, Kang EY, Wright JL, et al. Invasive pulmonary aspergillosis in AIDS: radiographic, CT, and pathologic findings. *Radiology.* 1995;196:409–414.
9. Adlakha A, Pavlou M, Walker DA, et al. Survival of HIV-infected patients admitted to the intensive care unit in the era of highly active antiretroviral therapy. *Int J STD AIDS.* 2011;22:498–504.
10. Dickson SJ, Batson S, Copas AJ, et al. Survival of HIV-infected patients in the intensive care unit in the era of highly active antiretroviral therapy. *Thorax.* 2007;62:964–968.

11. Powell K, Davis JL, Morris AM, et al. Survival for patients With HIV admitted to the ICU continues to improve in the current era of combination antiretroviral therapy. *Chest.* 2009;135:11–17.
12. Akgun KM, Pisani M, Crothers K. The changing epidemiology of HIV-infected patients in the intensive care unit. *J Intensive Care Med.* 2011;26:151–164.
13. Huang L, Quartin A, Jones D, et al. Intensive care of patients with HIV infection. *N Engl J Med.* 2006;355:173–181.
14. Nickas G, Wachter RM. Outcomes of intensive care for patients with human immunodeficiency virus infection. *Arch Intern Med.* 2000;160:541–547.
15. Greenberg JA, Lennox JL, Martin GS. Outcomes for critically ill patients with HIV and severe sepsis in the era of highly active antiretroviral therapy. *J Crit Care.* 2012;27:51–57.
16. Kaplan JE, Benson C, Holmes KH, et al. Guidelines for prevention and treatment of opportunistic infections in HIV-infected adults and adolescents: recommendations from CDC, the National Institutes of Health, and the HIV Medicine Association of the Infectious Diseases Society of America. *MMWR Recomm Rep.* 2009;58:1–207; quiz CE201-204.
17. Den Boer JW, Yzerman EP. Diagnosis of Legionella infection in Legionnaires' disease. *Eur J Clin Microbiol Infect Dis.* 2004;23:871–878.
18. Helbig JH, Uldum SA, Bernander S, et al. Clinical utility of urinary antigen detection for diagnosis of community-acquired, travel-associated, and nosocomial legionnaires' disease. *J Clin Microbiol.* 2003;41:838–840.
19. Hsu JL, Ruoss SJ, Bower ND, et al. Diagnosing invasive fungal disease in critically ill patients. *Crit Rev Microbiol.* 2011;37:277–312.
20. Sax PE, Komarow L, Finkelman MA, et al. Blood (1- > 3)-beta-D-glucan as a diagnostic test for HIV-related Pneumocystis jirovecii pneumonia. *Clin Infect Dis.* 2011;53:197–202.
21. Cruciani M, Marcati P, Malena M, et al. Meta-analysis of diagnostic procedures for Pneumocystis carinii pneumonia in HIV-1-infected patients. *Eur Respir J.* 2002;20:982–989.
22. Gruden JF, Huang L, Turner J, et al. High-resolution CT in the evaluation of clinically suspected Pneumocystis carinii pneumonia in AIDS patients with normal, equivocal, or nonspecific radiographic findings. *AJR Am J Roentgenol.* 1997;169:967–975.
23. Smego RA, Jr., Nagar S, Maloba B, et al. A meta-analysis of salvage therapy for Pneumocystis carinii pneumonia. *Arch Intern Med.* 2001;161:1529–1533.
24. Martynowicz MA, Prakash UB. Pulmonary blastomycosis: an appraisal of diagnostic techniques. *Chest.* 2002;121:768–773.
25. Durkin M, Witt J, Lemonte A, et al. Antigen assay with the potential to aid in diagnosis of blastomycosis. *J Clin Microbiol.* 2004;42:4873–4875.
26. Meyohas MC, Roux P, Bollens D, et al. Pulmonary cryptococcosis: localized and disseminated infections in 27 patients with AIDS. *Clin Infect Dis.* 1995;21:628–633.
27. Pappas PG, Perfect JR, Cloud GA, et al. Cryptococcosis in human immunodeficiency virus-negative patients in the era of effective azole therapy. *Clin Infect Dis.* 2001;33:690–699.
28. Benson CA, Williams PL, Currier JS, et al. A prospective, randomized trial examining the efficacy and safety of clarithromycin in combination with ethambutol, rifabutin, or both for the treatment of disseminated Mycobacterium avium complex disease in persons with acquired immunodeficiency syndrome. *Clin Infect Dis.* 2003;37:1234–1243.
29. Tanner DC, Weinstein MP, Fedorciw B, et al. Comparison of commercial kits for detection of cryptococcal antigen. *J Clin Microbiol.* 1994;32:1680–1684.
30. Cingolani A, De Luca A, Ammassari A, et al. PCR detection of Toxoplasma gondii DNA in CSF for the differential diagnosis of AIDS-related focal brain lesions. *J Med Microbiol.* 1996;45:472–476.
31. Castro R, Prieto ES, da Luz Martins Pereira F. Nontreponemal tests in the diagnosis of neurosyphilis: an evaluation of the Venereal Disease Research Laboratory (VDRL) and the Rapid Plasma Reagin (RPR) tests. *J Clin Lab Anal.* 2008;22:257–261.
32. Hart G. Syphilis tests in diagnostic and therapeutic decision making. *Ann Intern Med.* 1986;104:368–376.
33. Pai M, Flores LL, Pai N, et al. Diagnostic accuracy of nucleic acid amplification tests for tuberculous meningitis: a systematic review and meta-analysis. *Lancet Infect Dis.* 2003;3:633–643.
34. *The Sanford guide to antimicrobial therapy.* Sperryville, VA: Antimicrobial Therapy; 2012.
35. Hirschtick RE, Glassroth J, Jordan MC, et al. Bacterial pneumonia in persons infected with the human immunodeficiency virus. *Pulmonary Complications of HIV Infection Study Group. N Engl J Med.* 1995;333(13):845–851.
36. Tasaka S, Hasegawa N, Kobayashi S, et al. Serum indicators for the diagnosis of pneumocystis pneumonia. *Chest.* 2007;131(4):1173–1180.

37. Bozzette SA, Sattler FR, Chiu J, et al. A controlled trial of early adjunctive treatment with corticosteroids for *Pneumocystis carinii* pneumonia in the acquired immunodeficiency syndrome. *N Engl J Med.* 1990;323(21):1451–1457.
38. Hillmen P, Skotnicki AB, Robak T, et al. Alemtuzumab compared with chlorambucil as first-line therapy for chronic lymphocytic leukemia. *J Clin Oncol.* 2007;25:5616–5623.
39. Freifeld AG, Bow EJ, Sepkowitz KA, et al. Clinical practice guideline for the use of antimicrobial agents in neutropenic patients with cancer: 2010 Update by the Infectious Diseases Society of America. *Clin Infect Dis.* 2011;52:427–431.
40. Klastersky J. Management of fever in neutropenic patients with different risks of complications. *Clin Infect Dis.* 2004;39(suppl 1):S32–S37.
41. Wisplinghoff H, Seifert H, Wenzel RP, et al. Current trends in the epidemiology of nosocomial bloodstream infections in patients with hematological malignancies and solid neoplasms in hospitals in the United States. *Clin Infect Dis.* 2003;36:1103–1110.
42. Pizzo PA. Evaluation of fever in the patient with cancer. *Eur J Cancer Clin Oncol.* 1989;25(2):S9–S16
43. Munoz P, Giannella M, Alcala L, et al. Clostridium difficile-associated diarrhea in heart transplant recipients: is hypogammaglobulinemia the answer? *J Heart Lung Transplant.* 2007;26:907–914.
44. Blazquez RM, Espinosa FJ, Martinez-Toldos CM, et al. Sensitivity of urinary antigen test in relation to clinical severity in a large outbreak of Legionella pneumonia in Spain. *Eur J Clin Microbiol Infect Dis.* 2005;24:488–491.
45. Pfeiffer CD, Fine JP, Safdar N. Diagnosis of invasive aspergillosis using a galactomannan assay: a meta-analysis. *Clin Infect Dis.* 2006;42:1417–1427.
46. Edwards JR, Peterson KD, Mu Y, et al. National Healthcare Safety Network (NHSN) report: data summary for 2006 through 2008, issued December 2009. *Am J Infect Control.* 2009;37:783–805.
47. Raad I, Hanna HA, Alakech B, et al. Differential time to positivity: a useful method for diagnosing catheter-related bloodstream infections. *Ann Intern Med.* 2004;140:18–25.
48. Flynn PM, Shenep JL, Barrett FF. Differential quantitation with a commercial blood culture tube for diagnosis of catheter-related infection. *J Clin Microbiol.* 1988;26:1045–1046.
49. Englund JA, Piedra PA, Jewell A, et al. Rapid diagnosis of respiratory syncytial virus infections in immunocompromised adults. *J Clin Microbiol.* 1996;34:1649–1653.
50. Chartrand C, Leeflang MM, Minion J, et al. Accuracy of rapid influenza diagnostic tests: a meta-analysis. *Ann Intern Med.* 2012;156:500–511.
51. Couble A, Rodriguez-Nava V, de Montclos MP, et al. Direct detection of Nocardia spp. in clinical samples by a rapid molecular method. *J Clin Microbiol.* 2005;43:1921–1924.
52. Palmer DL, Harvey RL, Wheeler JK. Diagnostic and therapeutic considerations in Nocardia asteroides infection. *Medicine (Baltimore).* 1974;53:391–401.
53. Planche T, Aghaizu A, Holliman R, et al. Diagnosis of Clostridium difficile infection by toxin detection kits: a systematic review. *Lancet Infect Dis.* 2008;8:777–784.
54. van den Berg RJ, Bruijnesteijn van Coppenraet LS, Gerritsen HJ, et al. Prospective multicenter evaluation of a new immunoassay and real-time PCR for rapid diagnosis of Clostridium difficile-associated diarrhea in hospitalized patients. *J Clin Microbiol.* 2005;43:5338–5340.
55. Kim DY, Lee YS, Ahn S, et al. The usefulness of procalcitonin and C-reactive protein as early diagnostic markers of bacteremia in cancer patients with febrile neutropenia. *Cancer Res Treat.* 2011;43:176–180.
56. Schuttrumpf S, Binder L, Hagemann T, et al. Utility of procalcitonin concentration in the evaluation of patients with malignant diseases and elevated C-reactive protein plasma concentrations. *Clin Infect Dis.* 2006;43:468–473.
57. Sanz MA, Lopez J, Lahuerta JJ, et al. Cefepime plus amikacin versus piperacillin-tazobactam plus amikacin for initial antibiotic therapy in haematology patients with febrile neutropenia: results of an open, randomized, multicentre trial. *J Antimicrobial Chemotherapy.* 2002;50:79–88.
58. Paul M, Yahav D, Bivas A, et al. Anti-pseudomonal beta-lactams for the initial, empirical, treatment of febrile neutropenia: comparison of beta-lactams. *Cochrane Database Syst Rev.* 2010:CD005197.
59. King A, Boothman C, Phillips I. Comparative in vitro activity of cefpirome and cefepime, two new cephalosporins. *Eur J Clin Microbiol Infect Dis.* 1990;9:677–685.
60. Walsh TJ, Teppler H, Donowitz GR, et al. Caspofungin versus liposomal amphotericin B for empirical antifungal therapy in patients with persistent fever and neutropenia. *N Engl J Med.* 2004;351: 1391–1402.
61. Walsh TJ, Pappas P, Winston DJ, et al. Voriconazole compared with liposomal amphotericin B for empirical antifungal therapy in patients with neutropenia and persistent fever. *N Engl J Med.* 2002;346: 225–234.

62. Berghmans T, Paesmans M, Lafitte JJ, et al. Therapeutic use of granulocyte and granulocyte-macrophage colony-stimulating factors in febrile neutropenic cancer patients. A systematic review of the literature with meta-analysis. *Support Care Cancer.* 2002;10:181–188.
63. Smith TJ, Khatcheressian J, Lyman GH, et al. 2006 update of recommendations for the use of white blood cell growth factors: an evidence-based clinical practice guideline. *J Clin Oncol.* 2006;24:3187–3205.
64. Chemaly RF, Ghosh S, Bodey GP, et al. Respiratory viral infections in adults with hematologic malignancies and human stem cell transplantation recipients: a retrospective study at a major cancer center. *Medicine.* 2006;85:278–287.
65. Freeman RB, Jr. The 'indirect' effects of cytomegalovirus infection. *Am J Transplant.* 2009;9:2453–2458.
66. Walsh TJ, et al. Treatment of aspergillosis: clinical practice guidelines of the Infectious Diseases Society of America. *Clin Infect Dis.* 2008;46(3):327–360.
67. Greene RE, Schlamm HT, Oestmann JW, et al. Imaging findings in acute invasive pulmonary aspergillosis: clinical significance of the halo sign. *Clin Infect Dis.* 2007;44:373–379.
68. Safdar N, Maki DG. Inflammation at the insertion site is not predictive of catheter-related bloodstream infection with short-term, noncuffed central venous catheters. *Crit Care Med.* 2002;30:2632–2635.
69. Wisplinghoff H, Bischoff T, Tallent SM, et al. Nosocomial bloodstream infections in US hospitals: analysis of 24,179 cases from a prospective nationwide surveillance study. *Clin Infect Dis.* 2004;39:309–317.
70. Mermel LA, Allon M, Bouza E, et al. Clinical practice guidelines for the diagnosis and management of intravascular catheter-related infection: 2009 Update by the Infectious Diseases Society of America. *Clin Infect Dis.* 2009;49:1–45.
71. Fernandez-Hidalgo N, Almirante B, Calleja R, et al. Antibiotic-lock therapy for long-term intravascular catheter-related bacteraemia: results of an open, non-comparative study. *J Antimicrob Chemother.* 2006;57(6):1172–1180.
72. Sepkowitz KA. Opportunistic infections in patients with and patients without Acquired Immunodeficiency Syndrome. *Clin Infect Dis.* 2002;34:1098–1107.
73. Yale SH, Limper AH. Pneumocystis carinii pneumonia in patients without acquired immunodeficiency syndrome: associated illness and prior corticosteroid therapy. *Mayo Clin Proc.* 1996;71:5–13.
74. Azoulay E, Bergeron A, Chevret S, et al. Polymerase chain reaction for diagnosing pneumocystis pneumonia in non-HIV immunocompromised patients with pulmonary infiltrates. *Chest.* 2009;135:655–661.
75. Hardak E, Brook O, Yigla M. Radiological features of Pneumocystis jirovecii Pneumonia in immunocompromised patients with and without AIDS. *Lung.* 2010;188:159–163.
76. Tasaka S, Tokuda H, Sakai F, et al. Comparison of clinical and radiological features of pneumocystis pneumonia between malignancy cases and acquired immunodeficiency syndrome cases: a multicenter study. *Intern Med.* 2010;49:273–281.
77. LaRocque RC, Katz JT, Perruzzi P, et al. The utility of sputum induction for diagnosis of Pneumocystis pneumonia in immunocompromised patients without human immunodeficiency virus. *Clin Infect Dis.* 2003;37:1380–1383.
78. den Boer S, de Keizer NF, de Jonge E. Performance of prognostic models in critically ill cancer patients—a review. *Crit Care.* 2005;9:R458–R463.
79. Kohno S, Koga H, Oka M, et al. The pattern of respiratory infection in patients with lung cancer. *Tohoku J Exp Med.* 1994;173:405–411.
80. Perlman LV, Lerner E, D'Esopo N. Clinical classification and analysis of 97 cases of lung abscess. *Am Rev Respir Dis.* 1969;99:390–398.
81. Keidan RD, Hoffman JP, Weese JL, et al. Delayed breast abscesses after lumpectomy and radiation therapy. *Am Surg.* 1990;56:440–444.
82. Olsen MA, Chu-Ongsakul S, Brandt KE, et al. Hospital-associated costs due to surgical site infection after breast surgery. *Arch Surg.* 2008;143:53–60; discussion 61.
83. Papac RJ. Medical aspects of head and neck cancer. *Cancer Invest.* 1985;3:435–444.
84. Weber RS, Hankins P, Rosenbaum B, et al. Nonwound infections following head and neck oncologic surgery. *Laryngoscope.* 1993;103:22–27.
85. Abu-Elmagd K, Reyes J, Bond G, et al. Clinical intestinal transplantation: a decade of experience at a single center. *Ann Surg.* 2001;234:404–416; discussion 416–407.
86. Christie JD, Edwards LB, Kucheryavaya AY, et al. The Registry of the International Society for Heart and Lung Transplantation: 29th adult lung and heart-lung transplant report-2012. *J Heart Lung Transplant.* 2012;31:1073–1086.
87. Fishman JA. Infection in solid-organ transplant recipients. *N Engl J Med.* 2007;357:2601–2614.
88. Singh N. Fungal infections in the recipients of solid organ transplantation. *Infect Dis Clin North Am.* 2003;17:113–134, viii

89. Silveira FP, Husain S. Fungal infections in solid organ transplantation. *Med Mycol.* 2007;45:305–320.
90. Pappas PG, Alexander BD, Andes DR, et al. Invasive fungal infections among organ transplant recipients: results of the Transplant-Associated Infection Surveillance Network (TRANSNET). *Clin Infect Dis.* 2010;50:1101–1111.
91. Singh N, Paterson DL. Aspergillus infections in transplant recipients. *Clin Microbiol Rev.* 2005;18:44–69.
92. Fishman JA. Prevention of infection caused by Pneumocystis carinii in transplant recipients. *Clin Infect Dis.* 2001;33:1397–1405.
93. Husain S, Alexander BD, Munoz P, et al. Opportunistic mycelial fungal infections in organ transplant recipients: emerging importance of non-Aspergillus mycelial fungi. *Clin Infect Dis.* 2003;37:221–229.
94. Singh N, Forrest G. Cryptococcosis in solid organ transplant recipients. *Am J Transplant.* 2009;9(suppl 4):S192–S198.
95. Herbrecht R, Denning DW, Patterson TF, et al. Voriconazole versus amphotericin B for primary therapy of invasive aspergillosis. *N Engl J Med.* 2002;347:408–415.
96. Schwartz S, Ruhnke M, Ribaud P, et al. Improved outcome in central nervous system aspergillosis, using voriconazole treatment. *Blood.* 2005;106:2641–2645.
97. Riddle DJ, Dubberke ER. Clostridium difficile infection in solid organ transplant recipients. *Curr Opin Organ Transplant.* 2008;13:592–600.
98. Gunderson CC, Gupta MR, Lopez F, et al. Clostridium difficile colitis in lung transplantation. *Transplant Infect Dis.* 2008;10:245–251.
99. Keven K, Basu A, Re L, et al. Clostridium difficile colitis in patients after kidney and pancreas-kidney transplantation. *Transplant Infect Dis.* 2004;6:10–14.
100. Cohen SH, Gerding DN, Johnson S, et al. Clinical practice guidelines for Clostridium difficile infection in adults: 2010 update by the society for healthcare epidemiology of America (SHEA) and the infectious diseases society of America (IDSA). *Infect Control Hosp Epidemiol.* 2010;31:431–455.
101. Dallal RM, Harbrecht BG, Boujoukas AJ, et al. Fulminant Clostridium difficile: an underappreciated and increasing cause of death and complications. *Ann Surg.* 2002;235:363–372.
102. Kim YJ, Boeckh M, Englund JA. Community respiratory virus infections in immunocompromised patients: hematopoietic stem cell and solid organ transplant recipients, and individuals with human immunodeficiency virus infection. *Semin Respir Crit Care Med.* 2007;28:222–242.
103. Ison MG. Respiratory viral infections in transplant recipients. *Antivir Ther.* 2007;12:627–638.
104. Liu V, Dhillon GS, Weill D. A multi-drug regimen for respiratory syncytial virus and parainfluenza virus infections in adult lung and heart-lung transplant recipients. *Transplant Infect Dis.* 2010;12:38–44.
105. Humar A, Michaels M. American Society of Transplantation recommendations for screening, monitoring and reporting of infectious complications in immunosuppression trials in recipients of organ transplantation. *Am J Transplant.* 2006;6:262–274.
106. Rubin RH. The pathogenesis and clinical management of cytomegalovirus infection in the organ transplant recipient: the end of the 'silo hypothesis'. *Curr Opin Infect Dis.* 2007;20:399–407.
107. Asberg A, Humar A, Rollag H, et al. Oral valganciclovir is noninferior to intravenous ganciclovir for the treatment of cytomegalovirus disease in solid organ transplant recipients. *Am J Transplant.* 2007;7(9):2106–2113.
108. Munoz P, Rodriguez C, Bouza E. Mycobacterium tuberculosis infection in recipients of solid organ transplants. *Clin Infect Dis.* 2005;40:581–587.
109. Basset D, et al. Visceral leishmaniasis in organ transplant recipients: 11 new cases and a review of the literature. *Microbes Infect.* 2005;7(13):1370–1375
110. Singh N, et al. Infections of the central nervous system in transplant recipients. *Transpl Infect Dis.* 2000;2(3):101–111
111. Freifeld A, Marchigiani D, Walsh T, et al. A double-blind comparison of empirical oral and intravenous antibiotic therapy for low-risk febrile patients with neutropenia during cancer chemotherapy. *N Engl J Med.* 1999;341(5):305–311.

35

Burns and Soft Tissue Infections

Carla M. Carvalho and Paul Maggio

BURNS

Background

Each year in the United States, 450,000 people require medical treatment for burns, with 40,000 requiring hospitalization and 30,000 requiring specialty care in a Burn Center. 2012 data estimated the number of deaths from thermal injuries at 3,400 per year.[1] The three most common causes of residential fire deaths are believed to be careless smoking, arson, and defective or improperly used heating devices.[2,3] Factors affecting mortality include patient age >60 years, total body surface area (TBSA%) burned >40%, and the presence of inhalation injury (IHI).[4]

Diagnostic Evaluation

The size and depth of a thermal injury are often challenging to accurately determine, but these parameters are important in guiding in the resuscitation and triage of the injured patient. The depth of injury is typically heterogeneous, and the extent of tissue injury may not be visually apparent, particularly in the acute setting. In addition, the extent of a burn injury may deepen over time in a process known as burn wound progression.

Traditionally, burns were classified as first, second, third, and fourth degree. While this nomenclature still exists, a clinically more meaningful classification consists of superficial (or epidermal), superficial partial thickness, deep partial thickness, and full thickness (Table 35.1). Both classifications are based on the depth of skin penetration of the burn. Superficial, or first-degree burns, involve only the epidermis. Second-degree burns include superficial partial thickness and deep partial-thickness burns, which extend, respectively, into the superficial and deep layers of the hypodermis. Full-thickness, or third-degree, burns involve the epidermis, hypodermis, and the subcutaneous fat beneath the skin.

Calculating the TBSA involved in a burn injury helps to identify patients who require a higher level of care. This can be done using the "rule of nines" for adults and the Lund-Browder chart for children and infants.[5] For smaller or patchy burns, the patient's palmar surface can be used. The patient's palmar surface, including fingers, represents approximately 1% TBSA. Table 35.2 outlines the American Burn Association criteria for burn center referral.[6]

IHI—which has a reported incidence of 1.5% to 19.6% among all burn patients—is an independent predictor of mortality and a leading cause of death in burn patients.[7–9]

TABLE 35.1 Burn Depth

Depth	Cause	Appearance	Sensation	Healing Time
Superficial	Ultraviolet exposure Short flash	Skin intact, pink or red Blanches with pressure	Painful	3–6 d
Superficial partial thickness	Scald (spill or splash) Contact	Blisters (intact or ruptured) Moist, weeping Blanches with pressure	Painful to temperature and air	7–14 d
Deep partial thickness	Scald (spill) Flame Contact Oil/Grease Chemical Electrical	Blisters (easily unroofed) Weeping or dry Variable color (patchy to cheesy white to red) No color change with pressure	Mostly perceptive of pressure only; may have pain	>14 d
Full thickness	Water immersion Flame Contact Oil/Grease Chemical Electrical	Waxy white to leathery gray to charred and black Dry and inelastic Does not blanch with pressure	Deep pressure only	Never (if >2% TBSA)

Modified from Mertens DM, Jenkins ME, Warden GD. Outpatient burn management. *Nurs Clin North Am.* 1997;32:343–364; and Peate WF. Outpatient management of burns. *Am Fam Physician.* 1992;45:1321–1330.

IHI should be suspected in burn patients presenting with persistent cough, stridor, facial burns, or singed nasal hair, particularly if the patient was injured in an enclosed space. Injury to the upper airway from direct thermal exposure or chemical irritation results in upper airway edema and may lead to early airway obstruction. This differs from the parenchymal lung injury seen in patients with IHI, which is the result of chemical by-products of combustion transported to the lower airways on particles of soot. Airway injury varies from mild desquamation to complete disruption of the epithelial lining, cast formation, and airway obstruction. Fiberoptic laryngoscopy and bronchoscopy are the standard for diagnosing injury to the upper airway, and findings include soot, erythema, edema, and inflammation.

Management Guidelines

The management of burns is complex and involves integrated and prolonged care from teams, including physicians, nurses, therapists, and nutritionists. In the acute setting,

TABLE 35.2 American Burn Association Criteria for Referral to a Burn Center

1. Partial-thickness burns >10% TBSA
2. Burns that involve the face, hands, feet, genitalia, perineum, or major joints
3. Third-degree burns in any age group
4. Electrical burns, including lightning injury
5. Chemical burns
6. Inhalation injury
7. Burn injury in patients with preexisting medical disorders that could complicate management, prolong recovery, or affect mortality
8. Any patient with burns and trauma injury in whom the burns present the most life-threatening injury. In patients where the trauma is most life threatening, the patient is first stabilized
9. Burned children in hospitals without qualified personnel or equipment for the care of children
10. Burn injury in patients who will require special social, emotional, or rehabilitative intervention

Burn Center Referral Criteria. American Burn Association.

treatment strategies must incorporate a high suspicion for an IHI, maintenance of normal hemodynamics, and appropriate volume resuscitation.

IHI may result in the rapid compromise of a patient's airway. Early endotracheal intubation is indicated in the following situations: if upper airway patency is threatened; if gas exchange or compliance is impaired; if there are significant signs of worsening airway edema (e.g., new hoarseness); if there is clinical expectation of worsening edema (e.g., circumferential neck burns); or if the patient's mental status precludes airway protection. There is no indication in inhalational injury for prophylactic steroids or antibiotics.

Patients who suffer IHI are at higher risk of pneumonia, which is a major cause of morbidity and mortality in the ICU. Correctly diagnosing pneumonia in a patient with IHI can be challenging; chest radiographs can be hard to interpret, and carbonaceous sputum can mask purulent secretions, so careful consideration of white blood cell count (WBC), patient temperature, chest radiograph findings, and sputum culture results is required. Antibiotics are likely overprescribed in IHI. In one study, a 20% false-positive rate for pneumonia was observed in IHI patients whose pneumonia diagnosis was established using the Clinical Pulmonary Infection Score.[10] Patients with IHI who develop ventilator-associated pneumonia are at higher risk of acquiring multidrug-resistant (MDR) pathogens. Routine surveillance cultures from endotracheal aspirates have been shown to predict MDR etiology in IHI-associated ventilator-associated pneumonia (VAP) with a sensitivity and specificity of 83% and 96.2%, respectively.[11]

In patients suffering significant thermal injury, total body water typically remains constant, although fluid shifts result in greater intracellular and interstitial volumes and decreased circulating plasma volume. Initial volume resuscitation of burn patients with >20% TBSA should be guided by one of several well-known formulas that address the need to replace sequestered fluid. The commonly used Parkland formula calls for 4 mL of crystalloid per kilogram per percent TBSA burned, with half of the required 24-hour volume given in the first 8 hours, and the remaining half is given in the second 16 hours.[12]

Although formulas help to establish initial goals for resuscitation in the acute setting, administered fluids should ultimately be titrated based on organ perfusion. Military guidelines for burn resuscitation that incorporate hourly fluid input and output significantly improve the combined outcome of mortality and abdominal compartment syndrome.[13] Use of the electronic medical record to guide resuscitation has been shown to decrease total IV crystalloid volumes infused and better maintain targeted urine output.[14]

Recent studies have looked at the role of B-type natriuretic peptide (BNP) in guiding volume resuscitation. A recent prospective study studied 38 burn patients prospectively and followed BNP levels.[15] Those patients with higher BNP levels at day 3 received less fluid resuscitation and had significantly lower Sequential Organ Failure Assessment (SOFA) scores. The study suggested this finding could be explained by lower capillary leakage in these patients, resulting in greater intravascular fluid retention and consequently higher levels of BNP. These findings suggest a potential role for markers such as BNP to help adjust volume infused during resuscitation.

Burn patients epitomize the physiologic stress response because burn injury is often of longer duration and of greater severity than other critical illness. Alterations in immunologic and endocrinologic function characterize the intense stress response in burn injury, and glucose control has emerged as an important early management strategy in this setting.[15–18] Recently, preliminary results from a prospective study of 40 burn patients (24 diabetic and 16 nondiabetic) showed delayed closure of index burn wounds, despite grafting, in diabetic patients.[19] The NICE-SUGAR study, which showed an increase in 90-day mortality for those patients receiving insulin therapy to maintain a target blood glucose level of 81 to 108 mg/dL compared to those with a goal blood glucose level of <180 mg/dL, provides a useful guide for glucose management in burn patients.[20]

A patient with chemical burns presents unique challenges for the treating physician. In addition to skin damage or loss, there is potential for systemic toxicity. For most acids, copious fluid irrigation, often hours in duration, is indicated. Evaluation of skin pH at onset and periodically during irrigation treatment may or may not be useful. In the case of hydrofluoric acid, fluoride ions may be absorbed systemically and bind with positive ions such as calcium, causing potentially lethal effects. Treatment depends on clinical scenario; for patients with signs of locally isolated symptoms, a calcium gluconate slurry applied topically may suffice. In patients with signs of systemic toxicity, intra-arterial injection of calcium gluconate is necessary (see Chapter 49).

SKIN AND SOFT TISSUE INJURY

Background

Skin and soft tissue infections (SSTIs) account for more than 14 million outpatient visits and 869,000 hospital admissions in the United States each year. The number of hospital admissions related to SSTIs increased by 29% between 2000 and 2004, a fact likely explained by the emergence of community-acquired methicillin-resistant *Staphylococcus aureus* (MRSA).[21] Surveillance of MRSA is carried out by the U.S. Centers for Disease Control and Prevention, and this information is accessible online.[22]

SSTIs include a spectrum of diseases, ranging from superficial cellulitis to life-threatening necrotizing soft tissue infection (NSTI). A classification scheme developed in 1998 by the U.S. Food and Drug Administration (FDA) divided SSTIs into two broad categories: uncomplicated skin and soft tissue infections and complicated skin and soft tissue infections.[23] In general, uncomplicated infections could be treated with antibiotics or surgical drainage alone. Complicated infections were those that penetrated tissues more deeply and required more extensive surgery. Although the terms uncomplicated and complicated continue to be used, the FDA revised its classification in 2010. These infections are now known as, respectively, milder skin infections and acute bacterial skin and skin structure infections (ABSSSI). Milder skin infections include superficial cutaneous abscesses and impetigo; ABSSSIs include cellulitis, major cutaneous abscesses, wound infections, and burn infections and are defined by a minimum of 75 cm^2 of redness, induration, or erythema.

Another important classification for SSTIs differentiates non-NSTIs from NSTIs. NSTIs include necrotizing fasciitis, synergistic necrotizing cellulitis, clostridial myonecrosis, and Fournier gangrene. A diagnosis of NSTI need not be preceded by a diagnosis of SSTI, as patients sometimes present to emergency departments with infections that have progressed beyond the superficial tissue. NSTIs progress rapidly and can lead to severe sepsis, multiorgan failure, and death, and carry mortality rates of 20% to 60%.[24,25] Although the factors that lead to higher mortality rates remain incompletely defined, WBC > 30 and patient transfer from an outside institution (e.g., skilled nursing facility) prior to delivery of definitive therapy have been shown to be independent predictors of mortality by multivariable analysis.[26]

Diagnostic Evaluation

ABSSSIs and milder skin infections are often identified in emergency departments. Cellulitis is a common mild skin infection characterized by spreading erythema localized to the skin or superficial soft tissues. It is typically the result of a break in the skin or superficial wound, and patients are usually afebrile. Common pathogens include beta-hemolytic streptococci and, less commonly, *Staphylococcus aureus*. Treatment consists of antibiotics alone. Cutaneous or deep abscesses are pockets of pus within the dermis or soft tissues, which may or may not have associated cellulitis or erythema. Abscesses may develop spontaneously, particularly in the immunocompromised patient, or they may represent the progression of a superficial bite wound, skin injury, or surgical incision. Abscesses are typically polymicrobial, with *S. aureus* occurring as a single pathogen in only 25% of cases. Treatment consists of incision and drainage and antibiotics. Inadequate drainage places the patient at risk of developing NSTI.

The diagnosis of NSTIs can be difficult, and clinical suspicion should be high in a patient with risk factors such as IV drug use, obesity, diabetes, immunosuppression, malignancy, and cirrhosis.[27] Clinical findings may be subtle and nonspecific, and the classic symptoms of crepitus, epidermolysis, and erythema may not occur in the first 24 to 48 hours of the disease. In subacute forms of NSTIs, symptoms may be mild and limited to drainage from the wound's edge. Pain, edema, fever, and an elevated WBC often manifest as the disease progresses and are the findings commonly reported in large series. Pain may be out of proportion to examination, or it may be blunted in patients with diabetic or other associated neuropathies.

NSTIs require immediate and aggressive surgical intervention, making rapid diagnosis essential to optimize outcomes. Because "hard signs" of NSTI (bullae, crepitus, skin necrosis, gas on radiograph) may be absent in over 50% of patients, several laboratory adjuncts are useful in establishing the diagnosis. One study comparing patients with non-NSTIs and NSTIs found a WBC > 15,400 and a serum sodium <135 mmol/L to be associated with NSTIs.[26] In this study, these values were highly sensitive, with a negative predictive value (NPV) of 99%, but poorly specific, with a positive predictive value (PPV) of only 26%. In 2004, the Laboratory Risk Indicator for Necrotizing Fasciitis (LRINEC) score was developed as an adjunct to clinical evaluation for establishing a diagnosis of NSTI.[27] The LRINEC score is based on independent laboratory variables associated with NSTI: C-reactive protein, WBC, hemoglobin, sodium, glucose, and serum creatinine. A LRINEC score of ≥6 had a PPV of 92% and a NPV of 96% for NTSI. These results have been subsequently validated in other studies, including a multicenter study of 209 patients that showed a higher rate of mortality and amputation in patients with LRINEC scores of ≥6.[28,29]

Imaging may be helpful in diagnosing NSTI and in delineating the extent of infection, particularly in the stable patient with subtle findings. Plain radiographs uncommonly show subcutaneous gas, and these studies must be interpreted with caution. Computed tomography may also be helpful, but magnetic resonance imaging remains the most sensitive imaging modality.[30] Importantly, since a diagnosis of NSTI can often be made by clinical exam and laboratory data, imaging should not delay operative intervention.

Management Guidelines

The successful treatment of patients with SSTIs relies on four management principles: (a) prompt diagnosis with differentiation between nonnecrotizing and necrotizing SSTI; (b) early initiation of empiric broad-spectrum antibiotics, with coverage for specific pathogens based on risk and coverage for MRSA for all patients; (c) early debridement of NSTIs and surgical drainage for abscesses; and (d) definition of pathogen (by culture) and subsequent de-escalation of antimicrobial therapy.[31]

MRSA has emerged as the most common identifiable cause of severe SSTIs.[32] A multi-institutional study across the United States recently reported MRSA in 320 out of 422 enrolled patients who arrived in emergency departments with skin infections. Community-acquired MRSA (CA-MRSA) is now commonly responsible for SSTIs and NSTIs seen in emergency departments. In one study, SSTIs accounted for 74% of all CA-MRSA infections.[33] Timely treatment with empiric anti-MRSA antimicrobials such as vancomycin, linezolid, or daptomycin is warranted in all cases of severe SSTIs and improves outcomes.[34] Several other SSTI and NSTI pathogens have been associated with rapid clinical deterioration. These include *Streptococcus pyogenes, Clostridium* spp., and *Vibrio* spp.[35] SSTIs and NSTIs can also be polymicrobial. Specific antibiotic regimens for non-MRSA organisms have not been studied rigorously, but treatment should cover gram-positive, gram-negative, and anaerobic organisms. Typical antibiotics for these cases (combined with an anti-MRSA agent) include imipenem, meropenem, and piperacillin–tazobactam. Finally, streptococcal and staphylococcal infections are associated with toxin production, and the addition of antitoxin antimicrobials such as linezolid or clindamycin should be incorporated in all patients with severe SSTIs or NSTIs.

The mainstay of treatment for NSTIs has been surgical debridement. Multiple studies support early aggressive debridement as predictive of better outcome.[36,37] A recent retrospective study showed a median 8.6-hour time to operation when NSTI patients were treated by the emergency general surgery service, and an overall mortality of 9.6% in 52 patients.[38] Both the time to operation and mortality rate were lower than in other studies, which may suggest that early identification and surgical intervention of NSTI could reduce mortality. Surgical debridement includes excision of all nonviable tissue to achieve adequate source control; however, no prospective data exist to guide specific surgical therapy as pertains to number or size of incisions. The fundamental principles that guide surgical therapy include (a) the extent of the resection, which is usually determined intraoperatively upon gross inspection of the tissues; (b) full-thickness soft tissue or fascial excision for necrotizing fasciitis; (c) serial wound inspections and debridements; and (d) fecal diversion (e.g., colostomy) if there is involvement of the perineum and scrotum. Several authors advocate for return to the operating room within 24 hours for further debridement, if necessary, of devitalized tissue.[39] In patients with NSTIs, serial operations are not uncommon.

For patients with NSTIs, critical care management is an important component in treatment. Patients often present with accompanying severe sepsis or septic shock. In addition to antibiotic and surgical therapy, early goal-directed therapy, including aggressive resuscitation, appropriate hemodynamic monitoring, and glucose control, is recommended.[40,41]

CONCLUSION

Thermal injuries and soft tissue infections present unique challenges for the treating physician. The true extent of the burn injury may be difficult to ascertain at initial presentation and its treatment remains complex. Targeted resuscitation, early excision of burn wounds, topical antimicrobials, advances in ICU care, and a multidisciplinary integrated treatment approach have all contributed to a steady improvement in the survival rate of burn patients over the last half century.

Early diagnosis of soft tissue infections, and the differentiation of non-NSTIs from NSTIs, is essential in guiding management. Whereas the treatment of non-NSTIs requires an understanding of the microbiology to guide antibiotic therapy, treatment of NSTIs requires immediate and aggressive surgical intervention.

LITERATURE TABLE

TRIAL	DESIGN	RESULT
Burns		
Ryan et al., *N Engl J Med.* 1998[4]	Retrospective review of 1,665 patients with acute burn injuries (1990–1994) Derived mortality formula subsequently applied prospectively to 530 patients from 1995 to 1996	Overall, 96% lived to discharge. Three risk factors associated with death were age >60, more than 40% TBSA involved, and IHI. Predicted mortality is 0.3%, 3%, 33%, and ~90% based on whether zero, one, two, or three risk factors are present
Brusselaers et al., *Burns.* 2012[11]	Retrospective review of 53 burn patients with IHI requiring mechanical ventilation in a single burn unit (2002–2010)	Seventy episodes of VAP in 46 patients (86.8%). Median duration of mechanical ventilation prior to VAP was 7 d. In 23 episodes (32.9%), at least one MDR pathogen was involved Sensitivity and specificity of surveillance cultures (three times a wk) to predict MDR in subsequent VAP were 83% and 96.2%, respectively
Salinas et al., *Crit Care Med.* 2011[14]	Prospective study of the resuscitation of 39 patients with TBSA burns >20% was used to develop a fluid-response model. This model was subsequently incorporated into a computer decision support system (CDSS) and used in resuscitation of 32 subsequent patients with severe burns	Total crystalloid volume post–ICU admission over the initial 24 h reduced from 14,973 ± 10,681 mL in the control group to 9,679 ± 4,776 mL in the CDSS group ($p < 0.05$). Total crystalloid volume after ICU admission over the entire resuscitation reduced from 21,316 ± 12,974 mL in the control group to 13,088 ± 5,644 mL in the CDSS group ($p < 0.05$). The number of patients meeting their urine output goals was higher in the CDSS group
SSTIs		
Wong et al., *Crit Care Med.* 2004[27]	Retrospective observational study divided into developmental ($N = 314$) and validation ($N = 140$) cohorts of patients with SSTIs and NSTIs	Univariate and multivariate logistic regression identified significant predictors: WBC, hemoglobin, sodium, glucose, serum creatinine, and C-reactive protein. A LRINEC score >6 produced a PPV of 92% and NPV of 96% in predicting NSTI. Area under the receiver-operating curve 0.976 in the validation cohort

(*Continued*)

LITERATURE TABLE (*Continued*)

TRIAL	DESIGN	RESULT
Moet et al., *Diag Microbiol Infect Dis.* 2007[32]	Report from the SENTRY Antimicrobial Surveillance Program (1998–2004). Pathogens from SSTIs of hospitalized patients from three continents (Europe, Latin America, and North America) collected and analyzed prospectively	Predominant pathogens identified were *S. aureus* (most common pathogen in all regions), *Pseudomonas aeruginosa*, *Escherichia coli*, and *Enterococcus* spp. Considerable variation in MRSA rate between continents, with the highest rate of MRSA noted in North America (35.9%), followed by Latin America (29.4%) and Europe (22.8%)
Moran et al., *N Engl J Med.* 2006[42]	Prospective, multicenter trial of 422 patients presenting to emergency departments with SSTIs	MRSA was the most common pathogen identified in emergency room patients with SSTIs. *S. aureus* was isolated from 320 of 422 patients (76%) with SSTI. 249 of the *S. aureus* isolates (78%) were MRSA. Overall, MRSA was isolated from 59% of patients

REFERENCES

1. Burn Incidence and Treatment in the United States: 2012 Fact Sheet. American Burn Association; 2012.
2. Fast Facts About Smoke Alarms and Fires, National Fire Protection Association. National Fire Protection Association.
3. Fire in the United States 2003–2007. In: FEMA, ed. 15th ed. 2009.
4. Ryan CM, Schoenfeld DA, Thorpe WP, et al. Objective estimates of the probability of death from burn injuries. *N Engl J Med.* 1998;338:362–366.
5. Lund CC, Browder NC. The estimation of areas of burns. *Surg Gynecol Obstet.* 1944;79:352–358.
6. Burn Center Referral Criteria. American Burn Association.
7. Haik J, Liran A, Tessone A, et al. Burns in Israel: demographic, etiologic and clinical trends, 1997–2003. *Isr Med Assoc J.* 2007;9:659–662.
8. Shirani KZ, Pruitt BA Jr, Mason AD, Jr. The influence of inhalation injury and pneumonia on burn mortality. *Ann Surg.* 1987;205:82–87.
9. Smith DL, Cairns BA, Ramadan F, et al. Effect of inhalation injury, burn size, and age on mortality: a study of 1447 consecutive burn patients. *J Trauma.* 1994;37:655–659.
10. Pham TN, Neff MJ, Simmons JM, et al. The clinical pulmonary infection score poorly predicts pneumonia in patients with burns. *J Burn Care Res.* 2007;28:76–79.
11. Brusselaers N, Logie D, Vogelaers D, et al. Burns, inhalation injury and ventilator-associated pneumonia: value of routine surveillance cultures. *Burns.* 2012;38:364–370.
12. Baxter CR, Shires T. Physiological response to crystalloid resuscitation of severe burns. *Ann N Y Acad Sci.* 1968;150:874–894.
13. Ennis JL, Chung KK, Renz EM, et al. Joint theater trauma system implementation of burn resuscitation guidelines improves outcomes in severely burned military casualties. *J Trauma.* 2008;64:S146–S151; discussion S51–S52.
14. Salinas J, Chung KK, Mann EA, et al. Computerized decision support system improves fluid resuscitation following severe burns: an original study. *Crit Care Med.* 2011;39:2031–2038.
15. de Leeuw K, Nieuwenhuis MK, Niemeijer AS, et al. Increased B-type natriuretic peptide and decreased proteinuria might reflect decreased capillary leakage and is associated with a better outcome in patients with severe burns. *Crit Care.* 2011;15:R161.
16. Atiyeh BS, Gunn SW, Dibo SA. Metabolic implications of severe burn injuries and their management: a systematic review of the literature. *World J Surg.* 2008;32:1857–1869.
17. Jeschke MG, Chinkes DL, Finnerty CC, et al. Pathophysiologic response to severe burn injury. *Ann Surg.* 2008;248:387–401.
18. Wolfe RR, Durkot MJ, Allsop JR, et al. Glucose metabolism in severely burned patients. *Metabolism.* 1979;28:1031–1039.
19. Schwartz SB, Rothrock M, Barron-Vaya Y, et al. Impact of diabetes on burn injury: preliminary results from prospective study. *J Burn Care Res.* 2011;32:435–441.
20. Finfer S, Chittock DR, Su SY, et al. Intensive versus conventional glucose control in critically ill patients. *N Engl J Med.* 2009;360:1283–1297.

21. Edelsberg J, Taneja C, Zervos M, et al. Trends in US hospital admissions for skin and soft tissue infections. *Emerg Infect Dis.* 2009;15:1516–1518.
22. MRSA Surveillance. Centers for Disease Control and Prevention. http://www.cdc.gov/mrsa
23. Guidance for industry acute bacterial skin and skin structure infections: developing drugs for treatment. In: Administration USFaD, ed. 2010.
24. Cuschieri J. Necrotizing soft tissue infection. *Surg Infect (Larchmt).* 2008;9:559–562.
25. Salcido RS. Necrotizing fasciitis: reviewing the causes and treatment strategies. *Adv Skin Wound Care.* 2007;20:288–293; quiz 94–95.
26. Wall DB, de Virgilio C, Black S, et al. Objective criteria may assist in distinguishing necrotizing fasciitis from nonnecrotizing soft tissue infection. *Am J Surg.* 2000;179:17–21.
27. Wong CH, Khin LW, Heng KS, et al. The LRINEC (Laboratory Risk Indicator for Necrotizing Fasciitis) score: a tool for distinguishing necrotizing fasciitis from other soft tissue infections. *Crit Care Med.* 2004;32:1535–1541.
28. Chao WN, Tsai SJ, Tsai CF, et al. The Laboratory Risk Indicator for Necrotizing Fasciitis score for discernment of necrotizing fasciitis originated from *Vibrio vulnificus* infections. *J Trauma Acute Care Surg.* 2012;73:1576–1582.
29. Su YC, Chen HW, Hong YC, et al. Laboratory risk indicator for necrotizing fasciitis score and the outcomes. *ANZ J Surg.* 2008;78:968–972.
30. Brothers TE, Tagge DU, Stutley JE, et al. Magnetic resonance imaging differentiates between necrotizing and non-necrotizing fasciitis of the lower extremity. *J Am Coll Surg.* 1998;187:416–421.
31. Napolitano LM. Severe soft tissue infections. *Infect Dis Clin North Am.* 2009;23:571–591.
32. Moet GJ, Jones RN, Biedenbach DJ, et al. Contemporary causes of skin and soft tissue infections in North America, Latin America, and Europe: report from the SENTRY Antimicrobial Surveillance Program (1998–2004). *Diagn Microbiol Infect Dis.* 2007;57:7–13.
33. Naimi TS, LeDell KH, Como-Sabetti K, et al. Comparison of community- and health care-associated methicillin-resistant *Staphylococcus aureus* infection. *JAMA.* 2003;290:2976–2984.
34. Ruhe JJ, Smith N, Bradsher RW, et al. Community-onset methicillin-resistant *Staphylococcus aureus* skin and soft-tissue infections: impact of antimicrobial therapy on outcome. *Clin Infect Dis.* 2007;44:777–784.
35. May AK. Skin and soft tissue infections: the new surgical infection society guidelines. *Surg Infect (Larchmt).* 2011;12:179–184.
36. Freischlag JA, Ajalat G, Busuttil RW. Treatment of necrotizing soft tissue infections. The need for a new approach. *Am J Surg.* 1985;149:751–755.
37. Sudarsky LA, Laschinger JC, Coppa GF, et al. Improved results from a standardized approach in treating patients with necrotizing fasciitis. *Ann Surg.* 1987;206:661–665.
38. Gunter OL, Guillamondegui OD, May AK, et al. Outcome of necrotizing skin and soft tissue infections. *Surg Infect (Larchmt).* 2008;9:443–450.
39. McHenry CR, Piotrowski JJ, Petrinic D, et al. Determinants of mortality for necrotizing soft-tissue infections. *Ann Surg.* 1995;221:558–563; discussion 63–65.
40. Dellinger RP, Levy MM, Rhodes A, et al. Surviving sepsis campaign: international guidelines for management of severe sepsis and septic shock: 2012. *Crit Care Med.* 2013;41:580–637.
41. Rivers E, Nguyen B, Havstad S, et al. Early goal-directed therapy in the treatment of severe sepsis and septic shock. *N Engl J Med.* 2001;345:1368–1377.
42. Moran GJ, Krishnadasan A, Gorwitz RJ, et al. Methicillin-resistant *S. aureus* infections among patients in the emergency department. *N Engl J Med.* 2006;355:666–674.

36

Biomarkers in Sepsis

David M. Maslove

BACKGROUND

According to the Biomarkers Definition Working Group, a biomarker is any "...characteristic that is objectively measured and evaluated as an indicator of normal biological processes, pathogenic processes, or pharmacologic responses to a therapeutic intervention."[1] While this definition admits such basic signs as fever and leukocytosis, it most commonly refers to a blood test or histologic finding that can be used to suggest a particular diagnosis, estimate disease severity, or inform the decision to prescribe specific treatments. In cardiology, for instance, an elevated serum troponin level indicates myocardial injury, while in cancer care, a breast tumor biopsy that is positive for the HER2 receptor indicates disease that is more likely to respond to treatment with trastuzumab.

The role of biomarkers in sepsis is not as well established as in cardiology and oncology, but has garnered increasing attention in recent years. In 2001, the revised consensus conference definition of sepsis was expanded to acknowledge the utility of certain biomarkers, including C-reactive protein (CRP) and procalcitonin (PCT).[2] More recently, biomarkers have been used to stratify septic patients according to disease severity and to direct the timing and duration of fluid administration, antibiotic therapy, and other treatments. There are now more than 170 proposed biomarkers for sepsis, although only a few have been studied adequately in prospective clinical trials.[3]

Biomarkers may prove to play an important role in the diagnosis of sepsis, a syndrome that is traditionally defined by a set of highly sensitive but nonspecific clinical parameters.[4] Current clinical criteria have shown a limited capacity to unambiguously identify patients with sepsis or to provide risk stratification. Ultimately, the goal of using biomarkers in sepsis is to bring quantification and exactitude to a diagnostic task that remains in many ways subjective. Toward this end, more than 2 dozen clinical trials investigating the role of biomarkers in sepsis are currently under way, with more still examining their use in guiding therapy.[5]

SPECIFIC BIOMARKERS IN SEPSIS

Lactate

Lactate is widely used as a biomarker to identify septic patients in need of fluid resuscitation.[6] The mechanism by which serum lactate levels increase in sepsis is multifaceted; it includes stimulation of glycolysis, increases in cytokine and catecholamine activity, and up-regulation of lactate production by bacterial endotoxin.[7–9]

In septic shock, inadequate tissue oxygen delivery results in anaerobic cellular metabolism, in which glycolysis terminates in the conversion of pyruvate to lactic acid, rather than its entry into the tricarboxylic acid cycle. Hyperlactatemia can also be seen in sepsis despite adequate tissue oxygenation because of thiamine deficiency, the presence of bacterial endotoxin, and diminished lactate clearance secondary to liver failure.[8–10] On its own, hyperlactatemia is a nonspecific finding, as it can occur in other shock states, including hemorrhagic and cardiogenic shock.

Arterial blood lactate levels reflect the weighted sum of lactate production from all tissue sources. Venous lactate samples are easier to collect and have been shown to correlate well with arterial samples drawn simultaneously, being on average higher by about 0.18 mmol/L.[11] In patients with infection, there is a linear relationship between serum lactate level and mortality.[12] The current Surviving Sepsis guidelines recommend fluid resuscitation in patients with blood lactate levels ≥4 mmol/L, a value beyond which mortality risk has been shown to increase precipitously.[12,13] More recent studies have suggested that lactate levels are prognostic for 28-day mortality even within the range considered normal.[14]

A recent systematic review of the role of lactate in predicting outcome examined 28 studies, concluding that although elevated lactate levels were associated with sequential organ failure and 28-day mortality, the overlap in lactate values between survivors and nonsurvivors meant that a specific cutoff with adequate performance characteristics could not be defined.[15] Of greater prognostic value in the emergency management of sepsis is the rate of lactate clearance, usually defined as

$$\left(\text{Lactate}_{\text{admission}} - \text{Lactate}_{\text{follow-up}}\right) / \text{Lactate}_{\text{admission}}$$

In one retrospective study of prospectively collected data, mortality was 19% among patients with lactate clearance of at least 10% after 6 hours, compared to 60% in those whose lactate remained elevated.[16] A prospective study of lactate clearance found that a decrease of ≥10% following 6 hours of resuscitation significantly predicted survival, with every 10% reduction corresponding to an 11% reduction in mortality.[17] As such, serial lactate levels are often used as part of a "quantitative" resuscitation strategy, in which intravenous fluid boluses are given serially until lactate levels normalize. One study has shown this strategy to be noninferior to a resuscitation strategy that targets normalization of central venous oxygen saturation ($ScvO_2$).[18] Patients in the lactate clearance arm of this trial still had central venous lines placed and received most elements of early goal-directed therapy, including a target central venous pressure of ≥8 mm Hg.[19] Lactate clearance may correlate better with survival in septic shock than with survival in other shock states.[20]

Cortisol

As a physiologically stressful state, sepsis is associated with activation of the hypothalamic–pituitary–adrenal axis, leading to an increase in cortisol levels.[21] In a prospective study designed specifically to assess the predictive value of cortisol levels in sepsis, three prognostic groups were defined based on baseline cortisol levels and on patient response to a short adrenocorticotropic hormone (ACTH) stimulation test (250 μg).[22] Patients with a favorable prognosis (26% mortality) had low baseline cortisol levels, which responded appropriately (increase of >9 μg/dL) to ACTH stimulation, while those with the worst prognosis (82% mortality) had high baseline cortisol levels that did not respond to ACTH. Patients in the intermediate group (67% mortality) had either low baseline levels without adequate ACTH response or high baseline levels with adequate ACTH response.

A subsequent study demonstrated that in patients with septic shock, ACTH nonresponders benefited from treatment with hydrocortisone and fludrocortisone (mortality rate 63% vs. 53%, $p = 0.02$)[23]; however, the subsequent CORTICUS trial, which included patients who were less sick overall, failed to reproduce this result.[24] Current Surviving Sepsis guidelines recommend against the routine use of ACTH stimulation to identify patients likely to respond to glucocorticoids, but do recommend administering steroids to patients who remain hypotensive despite adequate fluid resuscitation and vasopressor support.[13]

C-Reactive Protein

C-reactive protein is a pentameric protein secreted mostly by the liver, that activates the complement cascade and stimulates cell-mediated immunity.[25] As an acute-phase reactant, CRP is nonspecifically increased in the setting of acute or chronic inflammation. Thus in addition to sepsis, other causes of elevated CRP levels include trauma, burns, surgery, chronic immune-mediated inflammatory diseases, and cancer.[25]

In diagnosing sepsis, a number of small, older studies have shown CRP levels to be sensitive (71% to 100%) but to lack specificity (40% to 85%).[25] CRP levels begin to rise within 4 to 6 hours of an inflammatory stimulus and, in the case of sepsis, track the effectiveness of antimicrobial therapy.[25,26] Early, adequate antibiotics produce a sharp decrease in CRP levels, which predicts a positive outcome; an increase, or even a slow decrease, should prompt consideration of broader spectrum coverage and a search for an uncontrolled source of infection.[26–28]

CRP levels have been shown to correlate with severity of sepsis, differing significantly in the settings of systemic inflammatory response syndrome (SIRS), sepsis, severe sepsis, and septic shock.[25,29] In a prospective study of patients admitted to the ICU, increasing CRP levels correlated directly with length of stay, number of failing organ systems, incidence of infection, and mortality. Compared to patients with a CRP level <1 mg/dL on admission, those with levels >10 mg/dL had higher incidences of respiratory failure (65% vs. 28.8%), renal failure (16.6% vs. 3.6%), coagulopathy (6.4% vs. 0.9%), and death (36% vs. 21%).[30] CRP levels have greater diagnostic performance than traditional signs of infection, such as fever and leukocytosis, and may be of particular value in elderly patients.[27,28,31]

Procalcitonin

Calcitonin, a hormone central to skeletal homeostasis that is expressed in the thyroid gland, is not known to play a significant role in infection and inflammation.[32] By contrast, its larger precursor PCT has been shown to be ubiquitously expressed throughout the body in response to bacterial infection.[33,34] Under such conditions, production of this "hormokine" can increase up to several thousandfold, a finding that has led to extensive investigation of its potential use as a sepsis biomarker.[32]

In experimental models, PCT levels rise within 3 hours of exposure to endotoxin, peak at around 24 hours, and persist in the circulation for up to 1 week.[35] Importantly, PCT levels stabilize and then decrease in response to adequate antimicrobial therapy, while a failure to normalize reflects inadequate coverage and portends a worse outcome.[36,37]

In the setting of renal failure, PCT levels may be elevated in the absence of sepsis, but decrease with initiation of hemodialysis.[38] Unlike other nonspecific markers of inflammation, such as white blood cells, CRP, and erythrocyte sedimentation rate, PCT levels are not typically affected in the settings of chronic inflammation or glucocorticoid use,[34] but may be elevated in shock states, whether or not these are related to infection.[39] Certain drugs can interfere with the measurement of PCT levels, most notably poly- and monoclonal antibody preparations.[34] PCT levels typically are measured from serum samples, by means of an automated immunohistochemistry method.[40] Healthy individuals typically have undetectable plasma PCT values (<0.05 μg/L). Infection is suggested by a level >0.25 μg/L to >0.5 μg/L, depending on the patient population and assay used. In severe sepsis and septic shock, levels in excess of 10 μg/L can be seen.

Some of the first clinical studies on PCT focused on its use in differentiating sepsis from noninfectious SIRS. A meta-analysis of these early works[41] pooled 18 studies and showed that in critically ill adult patients, PCT had poor diagnostic performance. The value of both sensitivity and specificity was 71%, with an area under the summary receiver operating characteristic curve of 0.78. Likelihood ratios (LR + = 3.03, LR − = 0.43) were insufficient to confidently rule in or out a diagnosis of sepsis, based on a moderate pretest probability.

Despite these early findings, newer studies have correlated PCT levels with severity of illness in sepsis.[34] One prospective study of 255 patients admitted to the ICU found that PCT levels were significantly correlated with the clinical subtypes of sepsis (median PCT = 1.5 μg/L), severe sepsis (median PCT = 4.5 μg/L), and septic shock (median PCT = 13.1 μg/L).[42] A multicenter study of 1,156 immunocompetent hospital inpatients with sepsis, including patients admitted to the emergency department (ED), showed that PCT levels correlated with mortality both outside the ICU (8% vs. 20% for PCT < vs. > 0.12 μg /L) and in the ICU (26% vs. 45% for PCT < vs. > 0.85 μg /L).[43] PCT has also been shown to be useful in identifying sepsis among immunocompromised ICU patients (sensitivity 100% and specificity 63% for PCT >0.5 μg/L).[44]

The finding that PCT directly reflects the effectiveness of antimicrobial therapy has led to an exploration of its role within a broader movement toward antibiotic stewardship in the ICU.[45–47] Large studies, such as the PRORATA trial,[48] provided evidence that basing the timing and duration of antibiotic administration on daily PCT levels could reduce the overall duration of therapy. In this study, 630 medical and surgical ICU patients with suspected bacterial infections were randomized to have antibiotics started and stopped either according to PCT levels (see Fig. 36.1) or at the discretion of the supervising clinician using local and international guidelines. Noninferiority analysis revealed no difference in 28-day and 60-day mortality between groups. Patients receiving PCT-guided antibiotic therapy received antibiotics for a total of 10.3 days (SD 7.7) and those in the control group for 13.3 days (SD 7.6) (23% relative reduction in days of antibiotic exposure). Analysis of secondary endpoints showed no difference between groups in terms of relapse, superinfection, or emergence of multidrug-resistant bacteria. A systematic review of 14 randomized clinical trials (RCTs) examining PCT algorithms for prescribing antibiotics came to similar conclusions, showing no significant differences in mortality between PCT-guided therapy and standard therapy, but a significant decrease in antibiotic exposure.

The current Surviving Sepsis Campaign guidelines have been revised to reflect newer evidence regarding the use of PCT in diagnosing and managing sepsis. These guidelines

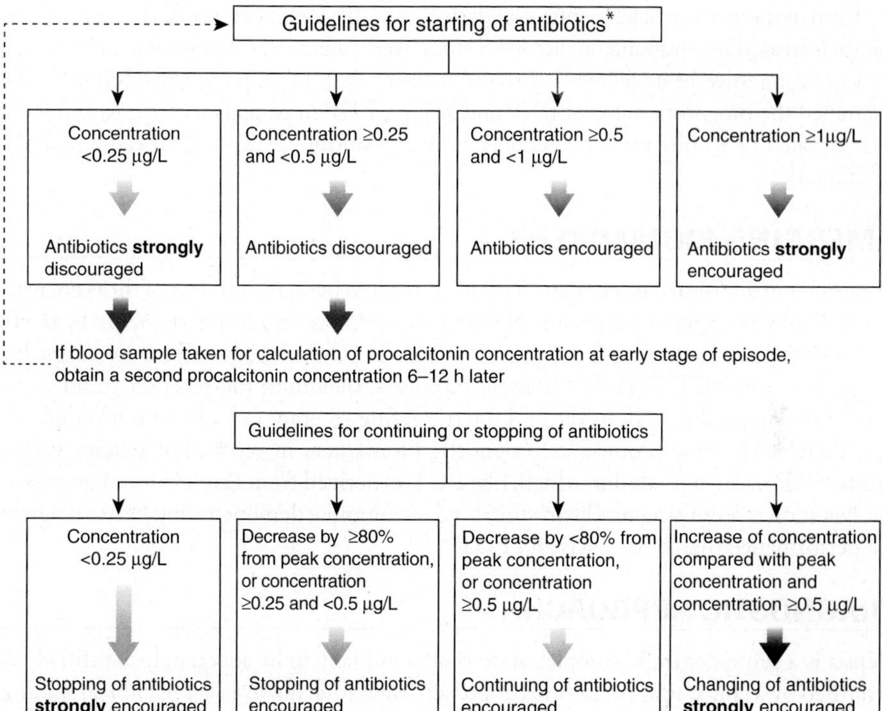

FIGURE 36.1 From: Bouadma L, Luyt CE, Tubach F, et al. Use of procalcitonin to reduce patients' exposure to antibiotics in intensive care units (PRORATA trial): a multicentre randomised controlled trial. *Lancet.* 2010;375:463–474.

include a weak recommendation for using low PCT levels in deciding to discontinue empiric antibiotics in patients without evidence of infection. The authors do not, however, endorse the use of PCT in distinguishing sepsis from noninfectious SIRS, citing an inadequate evidence base for its use in this regard.

CARDIAC MARKERS

Some degree of reversible myocardial dysfunction is known to affect up to half of all patients with sepsis and septic shock, even in the absence of preexisting cardiac disease.[49–51] Cardiac biomarkers including troponon I (TnI), which is known to correlate with myocardial injury, and the brain natriuretic peptides (BNP and NT-proBNP), which are known to correlate with ventricular stretch, have therefore been studied as biomarkers in sepsis.[52]

In a subgroup of 598 patients with severe sepsis from the PROWESS study, 75% had positive TnI levels at the time of enrollment into the trial.[53] The multivariate logistic regression model derived showed that a positive TnI at baseline was an independent predictor of 28-day mortality (32.2% vs. 13.6%). Another prospective study found that in patients with septic shock, a positive TnI correlated with reduced left ventricular ejection fraction (46% vs. 62%), greater need for inotropic or vasopressor support (94% vs. 53%), and increased mortality (56% vs. 24%).[54]

Even in the absence of left ventricular dysfunction, BNP and NT-proBNP can be significantly increased in sepsis and, in one small study, were found to be comparable to levels seen in acute congestive heart failure.[55] A recent meta-analysis of 12 prospective cohort studies examined the prognostic value of BNP and NT-proBNP in patients with sepsis and found that elevated levels of natriuretic peptides were a powerful predictor of all-cause mortality (OR 8.65).[56]

EMERGING BIOMARKERS

A number of additional biomarkers have been studied in sepsis, but few of these are readily available as commercial assays. Numerous cytokines, including IL-6, IL-8, IL-10, and MCP-1, have been found to predict survival in sepsis, but offer little diagnostic advantage over PCT levels.[57,58] Soluble receptors, including the receptor of advanced glycation end products (sRAGE) and the triggering receptor expressed on myeloid cells 1 (sTREM-1), show promise as prognostic biomarkers in sepsis, but require further study.[57,59] Proadrenomedullin, which, like PCT, is derived from the calcitonin gene family, has shown promising results in studies of pneumonia, demonstrating better diagnostic performance than both CRP and PCT.[6,60,61]

DIAGNOSTIC APPROACH

Sepsis is a physiologically complex state that is unlikely to be adequately identified and stratified by a single test. A reasoned approach, therefore, involves using clinical findings to develop a pretest probability of sepsis and then deploying the biomarker tests best suited to answer the question at hand.

In the ED, traditional markers such as hyper- or hypothermia and leukocytosis or leukopenia remain useful in distinguishing infectious from noninfectious processes, but may lack specificity in older or immunocompromised patients. In these cases, PCT levels >0.5 μg/L are suggestive of bacterial infection, with higher values being more specific and suggesting more severe disease. Since timely initiation of appropriate antibiotics is crucial, treatment decisions may have to be made in the absence of complete biomarker data. Much like the results of microbial culture samples, baseline values of PCT or CRP may play a key role in decision making over the first few days of hospital admission, and serial levels may prove useful in reassessing ED patients within the first 24 hours.

Serial lactate measurements are useful in guiding the initial resuscitation of the septic patient and in identifying those with persistently elevated lactate levels that are at risk of worse outcomes and may benefit from ICU admission. While studies on lactate clearance have used a 10% cutoff to define patients with improved survival, most survivors had clearance of approximately 40% or greater, with mortality lowest among those whose levels normalized.

In the ICU, the emergence of sepsis may be less obvious, as SIRS criteria are very frequently met. In septic patients who fail to improve or deteriorate anew, markers such as CRP and PCT may be useful in prompting either a change in antimicrobial coverage or a search for persistent or new sources of infection. The specificity of PCT in this setting, however, may be lower. ICU patients with sepsis from nosocomial infections have significantly lower PCT values than those with community-acquired infections (2.9 μg/L vs. 6.6 μg/L, respectively).[37]

In addition to the tests described above, newer technologies are being explored for their potential in diagnosing sepsis. Examples include the computational analysis of heart rate variability,[62] PCR amplification of bacterial DNA,[63] and high-throughput genomic technologies.[64–66] Ultimately, the most valuable use of biomarkers in sepsis will come not from their ability to predict severity of illness or mortality, but from matching individual patients with the specific therapies to which they are most likely to respond.

LITERATURE TABLE

TRIAL	DESIGN	RESULT
Lactate		
Nguyen et al., *Crit Care Med.* 2004[17]	Prospective observational study of 111 patients presenting to the ED with severe sepsis and septic shock	6-h lactate clearance of survivors significantly greater than nonsurvivors (38% vs. 12%, $p = 0.005$). 11% decrease in risk of death for every 10% decrease in lactate
Jones et al., *JAMA.* 2010[18] EMShockNet	Multicenter RCT of 300 patients presenting to the ED with severe sepsis and septic shock	No difference in mortality between resuscitation guided by lactate clearance vs. $ScvO_2$ targets
Cortisol		
Annane et al., *JAMA.* 2000[22]	Prospective cohort study to evaluate prognostic value of cortisol levels in sepsis, both before and after ACTH stimulation	Mortality highest for high baseline cortisol (>34 μg/dL) with minimal post-ACTH increment (<9 μg/dL) and lowest for low baseline cortisol (≤34 μg/dL) with increment >9 μg/dL
Sprung et al., *N Eng J Med.* 2008[24] CORTICUS	Multicenter RCT of hydrocortisone in 499 patients with septic shock	No difference in mortality between hydrocortisone and placebo (34.3% vs. 31.5%, $p = 0.51$). Response to ACTH did not correlate with response to hydrocortisone
CRP		
Lobo et al., *Chest.* 2003[30]	Prospective cohort study of 313 patients admitted to mixed ICU	Mortality higher for patients with CRP levels >10 mg/dL compared to those with CRP <1 mg/dL (36% vs. 21%, $p < 0.05$). A decrease in CRP after 48 h predicted increased survival rate
PCT		
Tang et al., *Lancet.* 2007[41]	Meta-analysis of 18 studies, mostly in ICU, examining role of PCT in differentiating sepsis from noninfectious SIRS	Diagnostic accuracy of PCT for sepsis vs. noninfectious SIRS: sensitivity 71%, specificity 71%, area under summary ROC 0.78
Giamarellos-Bourboulis et al., *J Hosp Infection.* 2011[43]	Multicenter prospective observational study of 1,156 patients in hospital, including ED, with sepsis	PCT levels correlated with mortality both outside the ICU (8% vs. 20% for PCT ≤ vs. > 0.12 μg /L) and in the ICU (26% vs. 45% for PCT ≤ vs. >0.85 μg /L). PCT levels were higher in the ICU, necessitating a higher cutoff value
Boudama et al., *Lancet.* 2010[48] PRORATA	PCT-guided vs. clinician-guided prescribing of antibiotics in 630 ICU patients with suspected bacterial infection	No difference in 28-d mortality (21% vs. 20%). More days without antibiotics in PCT group (14.3 vs. 11.6, $p < 0.0001$)

LITERATURE TABLE (*Continued*)

TRIAL	DESIGN	RESULT
Cardiac Biomarkers		
John et al., *J Crit Care.* 2010[53] PROWESS subgroup	Retrospective analysis of patients from the PROWESS trial, a large RCT of rhAPC (recombinant human activated protein C) vs. placebo for severe sepsis	598 patients (75% of total study population) had positive TnI ($\geq$0.06 ng/mL), which was an independent predictor of 28-d mortality (OR 2.0, 95% CI 1.15–3.54, $p < 0.0001$)
Wang et al., *Crit Care.* 2012[56]	Meta-analysis of 12 prospective cohort studies ($n = 1{,}865$) of patients with sepsis in the ED and ICU	Elevated BNP/NT-proBNP associated with increased mortality (OR 8.65, 95% CI 4.94–15.13, $p < 0.00001$). Pooled sensitivity 79%, specificity 60%

OR, odds ratio; CI, confidence interval.

REFERENCES

1. Biomarkers and surrogate endpoints: preferred definitions and conceptual framework. *Clin Pharmacol Ther.* 2001;69:89–95.
2. Levy MM, Fink MP, Marshall JC, et al. 2001 SCCM/ESICM/ACCP/ATS/SIS International Sepsis Definitions Conference. *Crit Care Med.* 2003;31:1250–1256.
3. Pierrakos C, Vincent JL. Sepsis biomarkers: a review. *Crit Care.* 2010;14:R15.
4. Zhao H, Heard SO, Mullen MT, et al. An evaluation of the diagnostic accuracy of the 1991 American College of Chest Physicians/Society of Critical Care Medicine and the 2001 Society of Critical Care Medicine/European Society of Intensive Care Medicine/American College of Chest Physicians/American Thoracic Society/Surgical Infection Society sepsis definition. *Crit Care Med.* 2012;40:1700–1706.
5. ClinicalTrials.gov. ClinicalTrials.gov. http://clinicaltrials.gov (Accessed 5 Oct 2012).
6. Schuetz P, Haubitz S, Mueller B. Do sepsis biomarkers in the emergency room allow transition from bundled sepsis care to personalized patient care? *Curr Opin Crit Care.* 2012;18:341–349.
7. Gibot S. On the origins of lactate during sepsis. *Crit Care.* 2012;16:151.
8. Kjelland CB, Djogovic D. The role of serum lactate in the acute care setting. *J Intensive Care Med.* 2010;25:286–300.
9. Michaeli B, Martinez A, Revelly JP, et al. Effects of endotoxin on lactate metabolism in humans. *Crit Care.* 2012;16:R139.
10. Leverve XM. Energy metabolism in critically ill patients: lactate is a major oxidizable substrate. *Curr Opin Clin Nutr Metab Care.* 1999;2:165–169.
11. Younger JG, Falk JL, Rothrock SG. Relationship between arterial and peripheral venous lactate levels. *Acad Emerg Med.* 1996;3:730–734.
12. Trzeciak S, Dellinger RP, Chansky ME, et al. Serum lactate as a predictor of mortality in patients with infection. *Intensive Care Med.* 2007;33:970–977.
13. Dellinger RP, Levy MM, Rhodes A, et al. Surviving Sepsis Campaign: international guidelines for management of severe sepsis and septic shock: 2012. *Crit Care Med.* 2013;41:580–637.
14. Wacharasint P, Nakada T, Boyd JH, et al. Normal-range blood lactate concentration in septic shock is prognostic and predictive. *Shock.* 2012;38:4–10.
15. Borthwick H-A, Brunt LK, Mitchem KL, et al. Does lactate measurement performed on admission predict clinical outcome on the intensive care unit? A concise systematic review. *Ann Clin Biochem.* 2012;49:391–394.
16. Arnold RC, Shapiro NI, Jones AE, et al. Multicenter study of early lactate clearance as a determinant of survival in patients with presumed sepsis. *Shock.* 2009;32:35–39.
17. Nguyen HB, Rivers EP, Knoblich BP, et al. Early lactate clearance is associated with improved outcome in severe sepsis and septic shock. *Crit Care Med.* 2004;32:1637–1642.
18. Jones AE, Shapiro NI, Trzeciak S, et al. Lactate clearance vs central venous oxygen saturation as goals of early sepsis therapy: a randomized clinical trial. *JAMA.* 2010;303:739–746.
19. Rivers E, Nguyen B, Havstad S, et al. Early goal-directed therapy in the treatment of severe sepsis and septic shock. *N Engl J Med.* 2001;345:1368–1377.
20. Jansen TC, van Bommel J, Mulder PG, et al. Prognostic value of blood lactate levels: does the clinical diagnosis at admission matter? *J Trauma.* 2009;66:377–385.

21. Bendel S, Karlsson S, Pettilä V, et al. Free cortisol in sepsis and septic shock. *Anesth Analg.* 2008;106:1813–1819.
22. Annane D, Sébille V, Troché G, et al. A 3-level prognostic classification in septic shock based on cortisol levels and cortisol response to corticotropin. *JAMA.* 2000;283:1038–1045.
23. Annane D, Sébille V, Charpentier C, et al. Effect of treatment with low doses of hydrocortisone and fludrocoritsone on mortality in patients with septic shock. *JAMA.* 2002;288:862–871.
24. Sprung CL, Annane D, Keh D, et al. Hydrocortisone therapy for patients with septic shock. *N Engl J Med.* 2008;358:111–124.
25. Póvoa P. C-reactive protein: a valuable marker of sepsis. *Intensive Care Med.* 2002;28:235–243.
26. Schmit X, Vincent JL. The time course of blood C-reactive protein concentrations in relation to the response to initial antimicrobial therapy in patients with sepsis. *Infection.* 2008;36:213–219.
27. Cox ML, Rudd AG, Gallimore R, et al. Real-time measurement of serum C-reactive protein in the management of infection in the elderly. *Age Ageing.* 1986;15:257–266.
28. Lobo SM. Sequential C-reactive protein measurements in patients with serious infections: does it help? *Crit Care.* 2012;16:130.
29. Luzzani A, Polati E, Dorizzi R, et al. Comparison of procalcitonin and C-reactive protein as markers of sepsis. *Crit Care Med.* 2003;31:1737–1741.
30. Lobo SMA, Lobo FRM, Bota DP, et al. C-reactive protein levels correlate with mortality and organ failure in critically ill patients. *Chest.* 2003;123:2043–2049.
31. Póvoa P, Coelho L, Almeida E, et al. C-reactive protein as a marker of infection in critically ill patients. *Clin Microbiol Infect.* 2005;11:101–108.
32. Müller B, Becker KL. Procalcitonin: how a hormone became a marker and mediator of sepsis. *Swiss Med Wkly.* 2001;131:595–602.
33. Müller B, White JC, Nylén ES, et al. Ubiquitous expression of the calcitonin-i gene in multiple tissues in response to sepsis. *J Clin Endocrinol Metab.* 2001;86:396–404.
34. Foushee JA, Hope NH, Grace EE. Applying biomarkers to clinical practice: a guide for utilizing procalcitonin assays. *J Antimicrobial Chemotherapy.* Published Online First: 24 July 2012.
35. Becker KL, Nylén ES, White JC, et al. Procalcitonin and the calcitonin gene family of peptides in inflammation, infection, and sepsis: a journey from calcitonin back to its precursors. *J Clin Endocrinol Metab.* 2004;89:1512–1525.
36. Charles PE, Tinel C, Barbar S, et al. Procalcitonin kinetics within the first days of sepsis: relationship with the appropriateness of antibiotic therapy and the outcome. *Crit Care.* 2009;13:R38.
37. Karlsson S, Heikkinen M, Pettilä V, et al. Predictive value of procalcitonin decrease in patients with severe sepsis: a prospective observational study. *Crit Care.* 2010;14:R205.
38. Dahaba AA, Rehak PH, List WF. Procalcitonin and C-reactive protein plasma concentrations in nonseptic uremic patients undergoing hemodialysis. *Intensive Care Med.* 2003;29:579–583.
39. Reynolds SC, Shorr AF, Muscedere J, et al. Longitudinal changes in procalcitonin in a heterogeneous group of critically ill patients*. *Crit Care Med.* 2012;40:2781–2787.
40. de Wolf HK, Gunnewiek JK, Berk Y, et al. Comparison of a new procalcitonin assay from roche with the established method on the Brahms Kryptor. *Clin Chem.* 2009;55:1043–1044.
41. Tang BMP, Eslick GD, Craig JC, et al. Accuracy of procalcitonin for sepsis diagnosis in critically ill patients: systematic review and meta-analysis. *Lancet Infect Dis.* 2007;7:210–217.
42. Castelli GP, Pognani C, Cita M, et al. Procalcitonin, C-reactive protein, white blood cells and SOFA score in ICU: diagnosis and monitoring of sepsis. *Minerva Anestesiol.* 2006;72:69–80.
43. Giamarellos-Bourboulis EJ, Tsangaris I, Kanni T, et al. Procalcitonin as an early indicator of outcome in sepsis: a prospective observational study. *J Hosp Infect.* 2011;77:58–63.
44. Bele N, Darmon M, Coquet I, et al. Diagnostic accuracy of procalcitonin in critically ill immunocompromised patients. *BMC Infect Dis.* 2011;11:224.
45. Riedel S. Procalcitonin and antibiotic therapy: can we improve antimicrobial stewardship in the intensive care setting? *Crit Care Med.* 2012;40:2499–2500.
46. Schuetz P, Chiappa V, Briel M, et al. Procalcitonin algorithms for antibiotic therapy decisions: a systematic review of randomized controlled trials and recommendations for clinical algorithms. *Arch Intern Med.* 2011;171:1322–1331.
47. Schuetz P, Müller B, Christ-Crain M, et al. Procalcitonin to initiate or discontinue antibiotics in acute respiratory tract infections. *Cochrane Database Syst Rev.* 2012;9:CD007498.
48. Bouadma L, Luyt CE, Tubach F, et al. Use of procalcitonin to reduce patients' exposure to antibiotics in intensive care units (PRORATA trial): a multicentre randomised controlled trial. *Lancet.* 2010;375:463–474.

49. Vieillard-Baron A, Caille V, Charron C, et al. Actual incidence of global left ventricular hypokinesia in adult septic shock. *Crit Care Med.* 2008;36:1701–1706.
50. Smeding L, Plötz FB, Groeneveld ABJ, et al. Structural changes of the heart during severe sepsis or septic shock. *Shock.* 2012;37:449–456.
51. Court O, Kumar A, Parrillo JE, et al. Clinical review: Myocardial depression in sepsis and septic shock. *Crit Care.* 2002;6:500–508.
52. Noveanu M, Mebazaa A, Mueller C. Cardiovascular biomarkers in the ICU. *Curr Opin Crit Care.* 2009;15:377–383.
53. John J, Woodward DB, Wang Y, et al. Troponin-I as a prognosticator of mortality in severe sepsis patients. *J Crit Care.* 2010;25:270–275.
54. Mehta NJ, Khan IA, Gupta V, et al. Cardiac troponin I predicts myocardial dysfunction and adverse outcome in septic shock. *Int J Cardiol.* 2004;95:13–17.
55. Maeder M, Ammann P, Kiowski W, et al. B-type natriuretic peptide in patients with sepsis and preserved left ventricular ejection fraction. *Eur J Heart Fail.* 2005;7:1164–1167.
56. Wang F, Wu Y, Tang L, et al. Brain natriuretic peptide for prediction of mortality in patients with sepsis: a systematic review and meta-analysis. *Crit Care.* 2012;16:R74.
57. Lichtenstern C, Brenner T, Bardenheuer HJ, et al. Predictors of survival in sepsis: what is the best inflammatory marker to measure? *Curr Opin Infect Dis.* 2012;25:328–336.
58. Harbarth S, Holeckova K, Froidevaux C, et al. Diagnostic value of procalcitonin, interleukin-6, and interleukin-8 in critically ill patients admitted with suspected sepsis. *Am J Respir Crit Care Med.* 2001;164:396–402.
59. Su L, Han B, Liu C, et al. Value of soluble TREM-1, procalcitonin, and C-reactive protein serum levels as biomarkers for detecting bacteremia among sepsis patients with new fever in intensive care units: a prospective cohort study. *BMC Infect Dis.* 2012;12:157.
60. Courtais C, Kuster N, Dupuy AM, et al. Proadrenomedullin, a useful tool for risk stratification in high Pneumonia Severity Index score community acquired pneumonia. *Am J Emerg Med.* 2013;31(1):215–221.
61. Christ-Crain M, Morgenthaler NG, Stolz D, et al. Pro-adrenomedullin to predict severity and outcome in community-acquired pneumonia. *Crit Care.* 2006;10:R96.
62. Bravi A, Green G, Longtin A, et al. Monitoring and Identification of Sepsis Development through a Composite Measure of Heart Rate Variability. *PLoS ONE.* 2012;7:e45666.
63. Dierkes C, Ehrenstein B, Siebig S, et al. Clinical impact of a commercially available multiplex PCR system for rapid detection of pathogens in patients with presumed sepsis. *BMC Infect Dis.* 2009;9:126.
64. Srinivasan L, Harris MC. New technologies for the rapid diagnosis of neonatal sepsis. *Curr Opin Pediatr.* 2012;24:165–171.
65. Wong HR, Cvijanovich NZ, Allen GL, et al. Validation of a gene expression-based subclassification strategy for pediatric septic shock. *Crit Care Med.* 2011;39:2511–2517.
66. Wong HR, Salibury S, Xiao Q, et al. The pediatric sepsis biomarker risk model. *Crit Care.* 2012;16:R174.

SECTION 9

Disorders of Acid-Base, Electrolytes, and Fluid Balance

37

Acid–Base Disorders

Tara Scherer and Corey Slovis

BACKGROUND

Acid–base homeostasis influences protein function, which in turn affects tissue and organ performance. Disturbances of the acid–base system are common in the critically ill patient and must be promptly identified and corrected to prevent harm. Optimal cellular function occurs with a pH of 7.35 to 7.45, and the body employs several compensatory mechanisms to tightly regulate its pH. It is helpful to use accurate terminology when describing acid–base disturbances. Acidemia refers to a pH $\leq$ 7.35, while alkalemia refers to a pH $\geq$ 7.45. Acidosis denotes a process that increases hydrogen ion concentration, while alkalosis denotes a process that decreases hydrogen ion concentration. Patients with an acid–base disorder will either be acidemic or alkalemic or have a normal pH.[1,2]

Acid–base disturbances are classified as either primarily respiratory or metabolic in origin. Respiratory disturbances are caused by changes in the partial pressure of carbon dioxide (pCO_2). The pCO_2 is elevated in a respiratory acidosis and decreased in a respiratory alkalosis. Metabolic disturbances are caused by primary changes in the bicarbonate concentration (HCO_3^-). The HCO_3^- is elevated in a metabolic alkalosis and decreased in a metabolic acidosis. Each primary disturbance has a compensatory mechanism that leads to a change in pH opposite of the primary problem. For example, a metabolic acidosis is compensated for by hyperventilation, leading to a decrease in pCO_2 and a compensatory respiratory alkalosis, resulting in a corrective increase in pH. The approaches described in this chapter allow rapid detection of acid–base disturbances and identification of their underlying etiology.

AN APPROACH TO ACID–BASE PROBLEMS

Blood Gas Analysis

Analyzing blood gas results is a rapid way to determine a patient's acid–base status. Blood gas values include pH, pCO_2, and partial pressure of oxygen (pO_2).

Traditionally, blood gases have been obtained via arterial puncture. Normal arterial blood gas (ABG) values are a pH of 7.36 to 7.44, HCO_3^- of 21 to 27 mEq/L, pCO_2 of 35 to 45 mm Hg, and pO_2 of 80 to 100 mm Hg. In an ABG, the pH, pCO_2, and pO_2 are measured directly, while the HCO_3^- is calculated using the Henderson-Hasselbalch equation. Recently, venous blood gas (VBG) measurements have been suggested as a less invasive alternative to arterial blood sampling. Studies have shown that both venous pH and bicarbonate levels can serve as substitutes for arterial pH in normotensive patients.[3–8] Values from arterial and venous samples are not identical, but their differences are thought to be minimal. In a large prospective study of 246 emergency department (ED) patients, simultaneous arterial and venous samples demonstrated high correlation between pH and bicarbonate ($r = 0.97$ and $r = 0.95$, respectively).[7] In another study, arterial and central venous samples were obtained from 26 patients with normal cardiac output, 36 patients with moderate cardiac output, 5 patients with severe circulatory failure, and 38 patients in cardiac arrest. In patients with normal cardiac output, the venous pH was 0.03 less than the arterial pH, and venous pCO_2 was higher than arterial values by 5.7 mm Hg. In severe circulatory failure and cardiac arrest, there were substantial differences between pH and pCO_2.[5] Observed differences were thought to be due to the divergence of the arterial and venous systems that occur as a patient becomes more hypotensive. Specifically, hypotension leads to hypoperfusion at the tissue level, which causes an increased proportion of CO_2 to enter the blood at the capillary level. In a separate study that compared arterial and venous blood gas results in 16 patients in cardiac arrest, venous pH was shown to be 0.3 less than a simultaneously drawn arterial sample.[9] As a rule of thumb, arterial samples should be obtained in any patient with shock, respiratory distress leading to cardiovascular collapse, or cardiac arrest, while venous measurements can be used in all other patients, including those with diabetic or alcoholic ketoacidosis (AKA).

The pO_2 has not been shown to correlate accurately between arterial and venous samples. A prospective study of 95 pathologically diverse ED patients demonstrated venous pH, pCO_2, and HCO_3^- to be reliable substitutes for ABG analysis (pH lower by 0.02 to 0.04, pCO_2 higher by 3 to 8 mm Hg, and HCO_3^- higher by 1 to 2 mEq/L) but reported poor agreement in pO_2.[6]

The following is a simple, three-step approach to the interpretation of blood gas values.[10]

1. **Does the patient have an acidosis or alkalosis?**
   A pH of 7.35 or less indicates the presence of an acidosis. A pH > 7.45 indicates the presence of an alkalosis.
2. **Is the acidosis/alkalosis a respiratory or metabolic process?**
   If the pCO_2 and pH move in opposite directions, then there is a primary respiratory process. If the pCO_2 and pH move in the same direction, then there is a primary metabolic process.
3. **If a respiratory acidosis or alkalosis is present, is it a pure respiratory process or is there a concurrent metabolic component?**
   In a pure acute respiratory process, for every 10 mm Hg change in pCO_2, the pH should move in the opposite direction by 0.08 ± 0.02. For example, if the pCO_2 is

50 mm Hg (a 10 mm Hg increase), the pH should be 7.32 (a decrease of 0.08). If this rule is not followed, a simultaneous metabolic process is present: If the pH is higher than expected, there is a simultaneous metabolic alkalosis; if the pH is lower than expected, there is a simultaneous metabolic acidosis.

METABOLIC ACIDOSIS

The rapid identification and interpretation of acid–base disorders permits optimal patient management and disposition. Historically, physicians have been poor at acid–base analysis[11–13] despite multiple approaches to interpreting acid–base disorders being available.[14–16] Metabolic acidosis is the most common acid–base abnormality encountered in the ED. The following is a simplified five-step approach to interpretation and management of metabolic acidoses using the basic metabolic panel (BMP) and blood gas values as described below.

1. **Identify abnormal values on the BMP:** Prior to calculating the anion gap, be sure to identify other abnormalities (e.g., hyperkalemia) that commonly accompany acid–base disorders.
2. **Calculate the anion gap:** The anion gap is the difference in the measured serum cations and anions.[17–19] Using the values from the BMP, the anion gap is calculated using the following formula:

$$\text{Anion Gap} = Na^+ - \left(HCO_3^- + Cl^-\right)$$

   A normal anion gap ranges from 8 to 12 ± 2. Values above this indicate the presence of unmeasured anions. An elevated, or wide, anion gap indicates the presence of a metabolic acidosis regardless of the serum bicarbonate or pH value.
3. **If a wide or normal gap acidosis is present, apply the Rule of 15 to evaluate for a "hidden" respiratory process.**[20]

   When an acidosis is identified, further evaluation must be performed to determine if there is an appropriate respiratory compensatory process or a concurrent primary respiratory process. If an appropriate respiratory compensation for a metabolic acidosis is present, the respiratory rate will be increased in order to lower the pCO_2 and correct the low serum pH.

   The Rule of 15 is used to predict a patient's expected compensatory pCO_2 and pH based on the bicarbonate concentration. The rule states that HCO_3^- + 15 should equal the pCO_2 and the last two digits of the pH as described below:

$$HCO_3^- + 15 = pCO_2 \pm 2$$
$$HCO_3^- + 15 = \text{last 2 digits of the pH} \pm 0.02$$

   If the pCO_2 and pH equal to the predicted values, there is a pure metabolic acidosis with appropriate secondary respiratory alkalosis. If the Rule of 15 is not followed, a simultaneous primary respiratory process must be present. If the pCO_2 is lower than predicted, a primary respiratory alkalosis exists in addition to a metabolic acidosis. If the pCO_2 is higher than predicted, a primary respiratory acidosis exists in addition to the metabolic acidosis.

The following is an example in which the Rule of 15 is satisfied:

$$HCO_3^- = 20; \quad pCO_2 = 35; \quad pH = 7.35$$
$$HCO_3^- + 15 = pCO_2 \pm 2 \rightarrow 20 + 15 = 35$$

Because the actual pCO_2 is within ± 2 of predicted pCO_2 using the Rule of 15, this is a pure metabolic acidosis with appropriate respiratory compensation. The last two digits of the pH are also within 0.02 of the predicted pH.

The following is an example in which the Rule of 15 is not satisfied:

$$HCO_3^- = 10; \quad pCO_2 = 20; \quad pH = 7.32$$
$$HCO_3^- + 15 = pCO_2 \pm 2 \rightarrow 10 + 15 = 25$$

The expected pCO_2 is 25 (± 2), but the actual pCO_2 is 20. Therefore, the Rule of 15 is not followed, and a simultaneous respiratory process is also present. Because the actual pCO_2 is lower than the expected pCO_2, there is a concurrent primary respiratory alkalosis in addition to the metabolic acidosis.

A corollary to the Rule of 15 is that as HCO_3^- falls below 10 and approaches 5, then the pCO_2 should equal 15. Recall that on an ABG, the HCO_3^- is estimated using the Henderson-Hasselbalch equation, while on a BMP, it is the directly measured total serum CO_2 that is used in lieu of HCO_3^- (total serum CO_2 represents both serum bicarbonate and other forms of CO_2 such as dissolved CO_2 and carbonic acid (H_2CO_3)). A bicarbonate buffering system exits to maintain the balance between CO_2 and HCO_3, as described by the following equation:

$$CO_2 + H_2O \leftrightarrow H_2CO_3 \leftrightarrow H^+ + HCO_3^-$$

In a patient with metabolic acidosis (i.e., increased H^+), this equation is driven to the left as compensatory hyperventilation increases the loss of CO_2. In a patient with a respiratory acidosis (i.e., increased CO_2), this process is driven to the right with a concomitant increase in bicarbonate. Winter's formula (below) is used to evaluate respiratory compensation—the change in pCO_2 for a given HCO_3^-—in the setting of a metabolic acidosis[20]:

$$pCO_2 = 1.5 \times HCO_3^- + 8 \pm 2$$

The Rule of 15 is extrapolated from this formula. The maximal fall in pCO_2 in adults, however, is approximately 15; thus, once HCO_3^- drops below 10, the Rule of 15 can no longer be applied, and Winter's formula should be used instead. For example, in a patient with a HCO_3^- of 8, the pCO_2 should be 20.

4. **If an acidosis is present, check the delta gap to evaluate for a "hidden" metabolic process.**

The next step is to evaluate for the presence of an additional primary metabolic process by calculating the delta gap. In an uncomplicated anion gap acidosis, for every 1 mmol/L rise in the anion gap, there should be a concomitant fall of 1 mmol/L in the HCO_3^- ± 4.[21–23] The delta gap (Δ gap) is defined as the difference between the rise in the anion gap and the fall in the bicarbonate concentration[24]:

$$\Delta \text{gap} = \Delta \text{AG} - \Delta \text{HCO}_3^-$$
$$\Delta \text{AG} = \text{observed anion gap} - \text{upper normal anion gap}$$
$$\Delta \text{HCO}_3^- = \text{lower normal HCO}_3^- - \text{observed HCO}_3^-$$

For this approach, the upper normal anion gap is defined as 15 mmol/L, and the lower normal bicarbonate concentration is 25 mmol/L. If the Δ HCO_3^- equals the Δ AG and the delta gap is zero, then there is no hidden metabolic process. If the bicarbonate is higher than expected, leading to a positive delta gap, then there is an additional metabolic alkalosis. If the bicarbonate is lower than expected, leading to a negative delta gap, then there is a concomitant primary non–anion gap metabolic acidosis.

5. **For an unexplained wide gap metabolic acidosis, check the osmolar gap.**
   In an unexplained anion gap metabolic acidosis, or in a patient with a history of toxic alcohol ingestion, the osmol gap should be calculated to determine the presence of substances with osmotic activity omitted from the calculated osmolarity, such as ethylene glycol or methanol:

$$\text{Osmolar gap} = \text{Measured osmolarity} - \text{calculated osmolarity}$$
$$\text{Calculated osmolarity} = (\text{Na} \times 2) + (\text{Glucose}/18) + (\text{BUN}/2.8) + (\text{EtOH}/4.6)$$

   Traditional teaching is that a normal osmolar gap is 10 or less and that in the setting of an elevated anion gap metabolic acidosis, an osmol gap of >10 indicates the presence of a toxic alcohol. While this is a good general guide, a more accurate calculation of a normal osmol gap is approximately -2 ± 6, the range that accounts for 95% of the population, which has a baseline osmol gap of −10 to +14. As such, a normal gap measurement can be misleading. For example, in a patient with a baseline osmol gap of −5 and a calculated osmol gap of 12, the true osmol gap would be 17.[25] Since a patient's baseline osmol gap is not known, it can be difficult to be certain whether the calculated gap is in fact elevated.

Management Guidelines

Metabolic acidosis is frequently seen in the ED and results from either a loss of bicarbonate or an accumulation of a nonvolatile acid. Severe acidemia can be devastating to the cardiovascular system (producing arrhythmias, decreased cardiac contractility, and arteriolar vasodilation) and the neurologic system (producing coma and seizures). Severe acidemia is often accompanied by profound hypotension and shock, which only further exacerbate acid production.

Anion Gap Metabolic Acidosis

Anion gap acidosis results from the presence of unaccounted-for anions such as sulfate, phosphate, and organic anions or weak acid proteins not measured on a basic metabolic profile.[26] Common etiologies of an elevated anion gap acidosis can be recalled using the mnemonics **KULT** (**k**etones, **u**remia, **l**actate, and **t**oxins) or the more comprehensive **MUDPILES** (**m**ethanol, **u**remia, **D**KA (and AKA along with starvation ketoacidosis), **p**henformin (and metformin), **p**aracetamol (acetaminophen), **I**soniazid (INH) and **i**ron, **l**actic acidosis, **e**thylene glycol, **s**alicylates, and **s**olvents.

Causes of Anion Gap Acidosis

1. **Lactic acidosis:**
   a. **Type A lactic acidosis**: Impaired systemic perfusion due to shock, severe hypoxemia, or severe anemia
   b. **Type B lactic acidosis:**
      i. **Type B1 (underlying disease)**: Impaired clearance of lactate due to liver or renal dysfunction or increased production of lactate due to seizures, hypothermic shivering, strenuous exercise, and ischemic colitis
      ii. **Type B2 (medication/intoxication)**: Metformin, linezolid, isoniazid (INH), HIV medications
      iii. **Type B3 (inborn errors of metabolism)**
2. **Ketoacidosis**: Diabetic ketoacidosis (DKA), AKA, starvation ketoacidosis
3. **Renal failure**: Decreased excretion of organic anions (urea, phosphates, sulfates)
4. **Toxic ingestions**: Methanol, ethylene glycol, toluene, salicylates

Lactic Acidosis Lactic acidosis is the most common cause of an anion gap metabolic acidosis and is defined as a pH of <7.35 with a lactate concentration of >5 mmol/L.[27] Lactate is most commonly a product of anaerobic metabolism (i.e., a type A lactic acidosis), and elevated levels can be observed in a variety of conditions, including severe hypoxia, seizures, sepsis, shock, and cyanide poisoning. Patients with severe lactic acidosis have mortality rates as high as 80% at 10 days.[28] The mainstay of lactic acidosis treatment is correction of the underlying or precipitating illness and aggressive patient resuscitation. The role of supplemental therapeutic buffers, such as sodium bicarbonate ($NaHCO_3$), is controversial. In a prospective randomized study, 14 hemodynamically unstable patients with lactic acidosis were given $NaHCO_3$- and sodium chloride–containing infusions. While the $NaHCO_3$ infusions helped correct the patient's acidemia, the hemodynamic response, including response to catecholamines, was the same to both solutions.[29] A second similarly designed study in 10 patients yielded comparable results.[30] As a consequence of these and other studies, current guidelines recommend avoiding $NaHCO_3$ treatment in patients with lactic acidosis unless the pH falls below 7.15 or when bicarbonate levels fall below 5 mEq/L, at point at which small changes in bicarbonate concentration can lead to profound and potentially fatal decreases in serum pH.[26]

Diabetic Ketoacidosis and Alcoholic Ketoacidosis In DKA and AKA, an anion gap metabolic acidosis occurs as the result of decreased availability of cellular glucose, leading to fatty acid metabolism and associated ketoacid production. DKA occurs because of a relative insulin deficiency; AKA is the result of a starvation state. In DKA, treatment centers on the provision of fluid resuscitation and insulin. The role of $NaHCO_3$ in DKA management is controversial. In a prospective study, 21 patients with severe DKA (defined as pH of 6.9 to 7.14) were randomized to either receive or not receive supplemental $NaHCO_3$.[31] The group receiving $NaHCO_3$ showed no benefit in terms of clinical recovery.[31] No randomized prospective studies have examined the effect of $NaHCO_3$ on DKA patients with a pH of <6.9. In these cases, careful, judicious $NaHCO_3$ administration is recommended to prevent possible cardiovascular collapse.[32]

In AKA, treatment centers on volume resuscitation; repletion of glucose, potassium, and magnesium; and provision of intravenous vitamins, most importantly thiamine. It should be noted that a similar starvation ketoacidosis can be seen early in pregnancy in women with hyperemesis gravidarum.

Uremia As kidneys fail, they lose their ability to excrete ammonium and hydrogen ions, leading to a non–anion gap metabolic acidosis. Ammonia is converted to urea in the liver, and the urea is subsequently excreted in the urine. As the renal dysfunction progresses, the kidneys lose the ability to effectively excrete urea, phosphates, sulfates, and other organic acids, which results in an anion gap metabolic acidosis.[33] Treatment is hemodialysis, which corrects the acidosis by removing nitrogenous waste products.

Toxic Alcohols Ingestion of toxic alcohols such as methanol or ethylene glycol can result in the accumulation of toxic metabolites and an associated anion gap metabolic acidosis. The metabolism of methanol, a substance found in products such as windshield wiper fluid and "moonshine," leads to the formation of formate, an organic acid that can cause acidosis, blindness, and pancreatic injury. The formation of formate is catalyzed by the enzyme alcohol dehydrogenase. The acidosis in methanol toxicity leads to the protonation of formate to formic acid, an uncharged molecule that is more likely to penetrate tissues. Treatment begins with administration of $NaHCO_3$ to reverse the acidosis, which decreases formic acid production and results in less tissue penetration and damage. Another treatment modality is 4-methylpyrazole (trade name Fomepizole). Fomepizole is a competitive inhibitor of alcohol dehydrogenase, and thus serves to block the formation of formate. Hemodialysis to remove the toxic metabolite is indicated in severe cases.[34]

Ethylene glycol, the primary ingredient of antifreeze, is another important toxic alcohol capable of producing an anion gap metabolic acidosis. Following ingestion, alcohol dehydrogenase metabolizes ethylene glycol to glycolic and oxalic acids, which result in metabolic acidosis and renal injury, respectively. The treatment for ethylene glycol ingestion is the same as for methanol (bicarbonate, 4-methylpyrazole, and hemodialysis). A recent study evaluated available treatment algorithms for toxic alcohol ingestion by combining therapeutic interventions with a physiologically based pharmacokinetic model. The study found that if administered early enough, fomepizole was more effective than hemodialysis. However, if renal injury had already occurred or toxic metabolites had already formed, then hemodialysis was the appropriate treatment.[35]

Other Toxins INH, a drug used to treat tuberculosis, inhibits GABA synthesis and lowers the seizure threshold. Frequently, patients with INH overdoses will present with refractory seizures. The anion gap metabolic acidosis is a result of both the seizure activity and INH's interference with nicotine adenine dinucleotide, an essential cofactor in the conversion of lactate to pyruvate. INH also binds to pyridoxine, making it inactive. Pyridoxine is a necessary cofactor for the production of GABA, and in the setting of an INH overdose, GABA stores are depleted, which leads to seizure activity. Treatment of INH overdoses requires pyridoxine therapy to replete the GABA stores.[36]

Acute iron poisoning can also lead to an anion gap metabolic acidosis. This is due in part to the hydration of ferric ions, a process that results in the release of three protons. Iron also causes mitochondrial dysfunction, which leads to anaerobic metabolism and subsequent lactic acid formation. Treatment of iron overdose is chelation with deferoxamine.[37]

An anion gap metabolic acidosis may also be seen with salicylate overdose. Salicylates uncouple oxidative phosphorylation, which results in an increase in anaerobic metabolism and an associated lactic acidosis and ketoacidosis. Treatment focuses on administration of $NaHCO_3$ to alkalinize the urine and on hemodialysis when indicated. Urine alkalinization enhances the renal elimination of salicylates; in alkaline urine, salicylates will ionize and become "ion trapped," limiting reabsorption.[38]

Finally, inhalation of solvents such as toluene can lead to an anion gap metabolic acidosis when they are metabolized to hippuric acid. Treatment is supportive.[39]

Non–Anion Gap Metabolic Acidosis

Non–anion gap metabolic acidoses are rarely life threatening and typically resolve with correction of the underlying etiology. The most common causes of a non–anion gap acidosis are loss of base from either the kidneys or the gastrointestinal system. Etiologies of an elevated anion gap acidosis may be recalled using the mnemonic **HARDUP**: **h**yperalimentation or **h**yperventilation, **a**cetazolamide, **r**enal tubular acidosis (RTA), **d**iarrhea, **u**reteral diversions, and **p**ancreatic fistula.

Gastrointestinal Etiologies Gastrointestinal loss of bicarbonate-rich fluid occurs in diarrhea, ureteral diversions, and pancreatic fistulas. In severe diarrhea, excessive loss of this fluid can result in a non–anion gap metabolic acidosis. Therapy consists of fluid replacement and prevention of further loss. Ureteral diversions (e.g., ileal conduits) lead to a non–anion gap metabolic acidosis when chloride from the urine enters the colon. The colonic mucosa has an anion exchanger to reabsorb chloride in exchange for bicarbonate. This leads to increased gastrointestinal loss of bicarbonate.[40] Pancreatic fluids are also high in bicarbonate, and when a pancreatic fistula is present, this fluid is lost. Treatment consists of repairing the fistula.[41]

Renal Etiologies An RTA results when the kidneys are unable to adequately manage the body's acid. A distal, or type 1 RTA, occurs in the setting of impaired H^+ secretion. There are many causes of a distal RTA. The most common etiologies in adults are autoimmune disorders such as lupus. In children, distal RTAs are frequently hereditary. A proximal, or type 2 RTA, occurs when there is a defect in bicarbonate reabsorption leading to excessive bicarbonate loss. Type 2 RTAs can be caused by multiple myeloma, familial disorders, amyloidosis, heavy metal toxicity, and renal transplantation. Medications, notably carbonic anhydrase inhibitors such as acetazolamide, can mimic a proximal RTA by inhibiting the renal absorption of bicarbonate.[42] A type 4 RTA occurs in the setting of hypoaldosteronism and decreased ammonium secretion and is associated with electrolyte disturbances including hyperkalemia (type 3 RTA is now excluded from modern classifications). Renal losses of bicarbonate can also occur in the setting of prolonged hyperventilation—for example, in patients with severe asthma or COPD—leading to a compensatory metabolic acidosis. If the respiratory condition is corrected quickly (e.g., with sedation and mechanical ventilation), the underlying metabolic acidosis will be unmasked.[43]

Iatrogenic Etiologies Rapid administration of chloride-rich and bicarbonate-poor solutions, such as normal saline, can also produce a non–anion gap metabolic acidosis. Normal saline has a chloride concentration of 154 to 155 mmol/L and a pH of 5.5. Normal plasma has a chloride concentration of 100 mmol/L and a pH of 7.4. Administration of a large amount of normal saline during volume resuscitation can result in a hyperchloremic non–anion gap metabolic acidosis. No anion gap is seen because chloride is accounted for in the anion gap formula. Resolution occurs after stopping administration of high–chloride content fluids and/or switching to a more pH neutral alternative such as lactated Ringer's.[44,45] Iatrogenic addition of acids, such as hydrochloric acid and ammonium chloride, can also lead to a non–anion gap metabolic acidosis.

METABOLIC ALKALOSIS

Metabolic alkalosis is defined by a primary elevation in the serum bicarbonate concentration. While not as common as metabolic acidosis, severe alkalemia can be equally dangerous. Neurologic complications include altered mental status, coma, and seizures. Cardiovascular complications include increased risk of arrhythmias and arteriolar vasoconstriction, which can cause decreased coronary blood flow. Alkalemia is also associated with hypokalemia, hypocalcemia, and hypophosphatemia.

Metabolic alkalosis occurs in the setting of acid loss by gastrointestinal or renal routes or exogenous base administration. Metabolic alkalosis may be categorized as either chloride responsive or chloride unresponsive:

1. **Chloride responsive**
   - **a.** GI losses: vomiting, gastric drainage
   - **b.** Contraction alkalosis
   - **c.** Diuretics
2. **Chloride unresponsive**
   - **a.** Hyperaldosteronism
   - **b.** Hypokalemia
   - **c.** Exogenous alkali load

Chloride-/Saline-Responsive Conditions

Gastric fluid contains a high concentration of hydrochloric acid. Loss of this fluid through vomiting and nasogastric suctioning can lead to a metabolic alkalosis. Therapy is directed at fluid replacement and preventing future loss of gastric fluid. Potassium repletion may also be required. A rare congenital chloride-losing diarrhea results from a defect in the chloride/bicarbonate transporter; in this case, large amounts of chloride are lost in the stool, leading to a metabolic alkalosis that is refractory to antidiarrheal agents.

Contraction alkalosis can occur with the setting of thiazides or loop diuretics use. These diuretics result in enhanced sodium and chloride excretion without a proportional loss of bicarbonate. Treatment involves administration of IV fluids.

Saline-/Chloride-Unresponsive Conditions

Hyperaldosteronism results in renal acid loss. Aldosterone directly enhances sodium and chloride resorption in the cortical collecting tubule. This creates a more electronegative environment promoting hydrogen and potassium secretion. It also stimulates the apical H-ATPase in the collecting tubule. Primary hyperaldosteronism is seen with adrenal hyperplasia and adrenal adenomas. Secondary hyperaldosteronism occurs in the setting of congestive heart failure, chronic renal insufficiency, and hepatic failure. Aldosterone excess is also seen in Bartter syndrome. In patients with concurrent hypokalemia, potassium repletion will improve alkalosis due to transcellular hydrogen/potassium ion exchange.[46]

Acetazolamide decreases the proximal tubule's reabsorption of bicarbonate and is commonly used to correct a metabolic alkalosis in critically ill patients.[47] Case reports exist of large bicarbonate ingestions causing severe metabolic alkalosis. If a patient has a severe alkalosis with a pH > 7.7 or experiences arrhythmias, dilute hydrochloric acid is indicated. When administering hydrochloric acid, it should be given through a central line at 100 mL/h with hourly pH checks.[48]

RESPIRATORY ACIDOSIS

Respiratory acidosis is defined as a primary increase in pCO_2. Etiologies stem from disturbances in the airway, pulmonary system, central nervous system, and neuromuscular system. Airway causes include obstruction and spasm. Pulmonary etiologies include COPD, asthma, pulmonary edema, pneumothorax, mass, and infection. Narcotics, sedative hypnotics, and brain tumors can suppress the central respiratory center. Neuromuscular disorders, including myopathies and neuropathies, can also lead to respiratory acidosis. Treatment aims to remove or correct the underlying cause while ensuring adequate oxygenation and ventilation using either noninvasive positive pressure ventilation or orotracheal intubation.[1]

RESPIRATORY ALKALOSIS

Respiratory alkalosis occurs when the primary disturbance is a decrease in pCO_2. The differential diagnosis is broad and includes a variety of benign and pathologic causes. Normal pregnancy, high-altitude residence, anxiety, pain, and withdrawal can all lead to a respiratory alkalosis. Pathologic causes of respiratory alkalosis include sepsis, pulmonary embolus, hypoxia, and salicylate overdose. The respiratory alkalosis from salicylate toxicity occurs due to the stimulation of the respiratory center. Management of respiratory alkalosis is directed toward correction of its underlying cause.[2]

MIXED ACID–BASE DISORDERS

There are myriad potential mixed acid–base disturbances. The most important are (1) an anion gap metabolic acidosis and primary respiratory alkalosis, (2) an anion gap metabolic acidosis and respiratory acidosis, and (3) an anion gap metabolic acidosis and metabolic alkalosis.

An anion gap metabolic acidosis accompanied by a primary respiratory alkalosis is most commonly seen in patients with hypotension from traumatic blood loss and hyperventilation due to pain. This mixed disorder can also be seen in patients with AKA and withdrawal leading to hyperventilation. Aspirin toxicity (salicylic acid) and sepsis (lactic acidosis) should also be considered with this acid–base abnormality.

An anion gap metabolic acidosis accompanied by a primary respiratory acidosis is seen in patients unable to appropriately compensate for their acidosis. This may be seen in patients with severe acidosis or cerebral edema and/or elevated intracranial pressure or in the presence of CNS depressants (e.g., opiates). Treatment focuses on correction of the underlying disease process with accompanying supportive care and, frequently, ventilatory assistance.

Finally, an anion gap metabolic acidosis accompanied by a primary metabolic alkalosis is seen in patients with renal failure (RTA) or DKA and emesis (contraction alkalosis) or in similarly acidemic patients receiving intravenous $NaHCO_3$ therapy.

CONCLUSION

Acid–base disturbances are common in critically ill patients. The systematic approach outlined in this chapter is designed to enable prompt recognition and response to these disorders in order to optimize cellular function and improve patient outcomes.

LITERATURE TABLE

TRIAL	DESIGN	RESULT
ABG vs. VBG		
Gennis et al., *Ann Emerg Med.* 1985[3]	Prospective study of 171 ED patients to determine the usefulness of peripheral venous blood gas sampling	Mean venous pH was 0.056 less than the mean arterial pH demonstrating a linear relationship between ABG and VBG
Kelly et al., *Emerg Med J.* 2001[4]	Prospective study of 246 ED patients to determine correlation of arterial and venous pH	Arterial and venous pH highly correlated ($r = 0.92$); venous pH is an acceptable substitute for arterial pH
Adrogue et al., *N Engl J Med.* 1989[5]	Prospective study of 26 patients with normal cardiac output, 41 patients with moderate to severe circulatory failure, and 38 patients with cardiac arrest to assess arteriovenous difference	Patients with normal cardiac output had venous pH lower by 0.03 ($p < 0.05$) and PCO_2 higher by 0.8 ($p < 0.05$); patients with severe circulatory failure and cardiac arrest demonstrated large differences between arterial and venous pH and PCO_2
Malatesha et al., *Emerg Med J.* 2007[6]	Prospective study of 95 ED patients to determine the agreement between arterial and venous samples	Venous values of pH, bicarbonate, and PCO_2 are reliable substitute for ABG analysis. Agreement in PO_2 was poor (95% limits of agreement 145.3 to −32.9)
Brandenburg et al., *Ann Emerg Med.* 1998[7]	Prospective study of 38 patients with DKA to determine if VBG can replace ABG	Arterial and venous pH and bicarbonate results were highly correlated ($r = 0.9689$ and $r = 0.9543$, respectively) with a high measure of agreement
McCanny et al., *Am J Emerg Med.* 2012[8]	Prospective study of 89 patients with acute COPD exacerbations to investigate the correlation between ABG and VBG values	Moderate agreement between arterial and venous PCO_2 with average difference of 8.6 mm Hg (−7.84 to 25.05); analysis of pH showed near equivalence; insufficient agreement to determine degree of hypercarbia using VBG
Weil et al., *N Engl J Med.* 1986[9]	Prospective study of 16 patients with cardiac arrest to assess the difference in arterial and venous blood gas	Arterial pH was 7.41, while venous pH was 7.15 ($p < 0.001$); arterial blood gas is not an appropriate guide for acid–base status in patients with cardiac arrest

(*Continued*)

LITERATURE TABLE (*Continued*)

TRIAL	DESIGN	RESULT
Role of $NaHCO_3$ Therapy in Lactic Acidosis		
Cooper et al., *Ann Intern Med.* 1990[29]	Prospective, randomized, blinded, crossover study of 14 patients with lactic acidosis to determine if $NaHCO_3$ improves hemodynamics	$NaHCO_3$ does not improve hemodynamics in patients with lactic acidosis. The mean arterial pressure was unchanged
Mathieu et al., *Crit Care Med.* 1991[30]	Prospective, randomized, blinded, crossover study of 10 patients with lactic acidosis to determine if $NaHCO_3$ improves hemodynamics and tissue oxygenation	$NaHCO_3$ does not improve hemodynamics or tissue oxygenation in patients with lactic acidosis
Role of $NaHCO_3$ Therapy in DKA		
Morris et al., *Ann Intern Med.* 1986[31]	Prospective, randomized study of 21 patients with severe diabetic ketoacidosis to determine if $NaHCO_3$ affects recovery outcome variables	$NaHCO_3$ does not increase the rate of glucose or ketone decline and does not shorten the time to resolution of DKA

REFERENCES

1. Adrogue HJ, Madias NE. Management of life-threatening acid–base disorders. First of two parts. *N Engl J Med.* 1998;338:26–34.
2. Adrogue HJ, Madias NE. Management of life-threatening acid–base disorders. Second of two parts. *N Engl J Med.* 1998;338:107–111.
3. Gennis PR, Skovron ML, Aronson ST, et al. The usefulness of peripheral venous blood in estimating acid–base status in acutely ill patients. *Ann Emerg Med.* 1985;14:845–849.
4. Kelly AM, McAlpine R, Kyle E. Venous pH can safely replace arterial pH in the initial evaluation of patients in the emergency department. *Emerg Med J.* 2001;18:340–342.
5. Adrogue H, et al. Assessing acid–base status in circulatory failure: differences between arterial and central venous blood. *N Engl J Med.* 1989;320:1312–1316.
6. Malatesha G, et al. Comparison of arterial and venous pH, bicarbonate, PCO_2 and PO_2 in initial emergency department assessment. *Emerg Med J.* 2007;24(8):569–571.
7. Brandenburg MA, Dire DJ. Comparison of arterial and venous blood gas values in the initial emergency department evaluation of patients with diabetic ketoacidosis. *Ann Emerg Med.* 1998;31:459–465.
8. McCanny P, Bennett K, et al. Venous vs arterial blood gases in the assessment of patients presenting with an exacerbation of chronic obstructive pulmonary disease. *Am J Emerg Med.* 2012;30:896–900.
9. Weil M, Rachow E, et al. Difference in acid–base state between venous and arterial blood during cardiopulmonary resuscitation. *N Engl J Med.* 1986;315:153–156.
10. Isenhour JL, Slovis CM. Arterial blood gas analysis: a simple, 3-step approach: When should you suspect a mixed acid–base disturbance? *J Respir Dis.* 2008;29:74–82.
11. O'Sullivan I, Jeavons R. Survey of blood gas interpretation. *Emerg Med J.* 2005;22:391–392.
12. Schreck D, et al. Diagnosis of complex acid–base disorders: physician performance versus the microcomputer. *Ann Emerg Med.* 1986;15:164–170.
13. Austin K, Jones P. Accuracy of interpretation of arterial blood gases by emergency medicine doctors. *Emerg Med Australas.* 2010;22:159–165.
14. Haber R. A practical approach to acid–base disorders. *West J Med.* 1991;155(2):146–151.
15. Palmer B. Approach to fluid and electrolyte disorders and acid–base problems. *Prim Care.* 2008;35(2):195–213.
16. Carmody JB, Norwood VF. A clinical approach to paediatric acid–base disorders. *Postgrad Med J.* 2012:88:143–151.
17. Emmett M, Narins R. Clinical use of the anion gap. *Medicine.* 1977;56:38–54.
18. Gabow P, et al. Diagnostic importance of an increased serum anion gap. *N Engl J Med.* 1980;303:854–858.
19. Oh M, Carroll H. The anion gap. *N Engl J Med.* 1977;297:814–817.
20. Albert MS, Dell RB, Winters RW. Quantitative displacement of acid base equilibrium in metabolic acidosis. *Ann Intern Med.* 1967;66:312–322.

21. Narins R, Emmett M. Simple and mixed acid–base disorders: a practical approach. *Medicine.* 1980;59:161–187.
22. Dubose T. Clinical approach to patients with acid–base disorders. *Med Clin North Am.* 1983;67:799–813.
23. Goodkin D, et al. The role of the anion gap in detecting and managing mixed metabolic acid–base disorders. *Clin Endocrinol Metab.* 1984;13:333–349.
24. Wrenn K. The delta gap: an approach to mixed acid–base disorders. *Ann Emerg Med.* 1990;19:1310–1313.
25. Hoffman RS, Smilkstein MJ, Howland MA, et al. Osmol gaps revisited: normal values and limitations. *J toxicol Clin toxicol.* 1993;31(1):81–93.
26. Gauthier P, Szerlip H. Metabolic acidosis in the intensive care unit. *Crit Care Clin.* 2002;18:289–308.
27. Mizock B, Falk J. Lactic acidosis in critical illness. *Crit Care Med.* 1992;20:80–93.
28. Stacpoole P, Wright E, et al. Natural history and course of acquired lactic acidosis in humans: the DCA-lactic acidosis study group. *Am J Med.* 1994;97:47–54.
29. Cooper DJ, et al. Bicarbonate does not improve hemodynamics in critically ill patients who have lactic acidosis. *Ann Intern Med.* 1990;112:492–498.
30. Mathieu D, et al. Effects of bicarbonate therapy on hemodynamics and tissue oxygenation in patients with lactic acidosis: a prospective, controlled clinical study. *Crit Care Med.* 1991;19(11):1352–1356.
31. Morris LR, et al. Bicarbonate therapy in severe diabetic ketoacidosis. *Ann Intern Med.* 1986;105:836–840.
32. Kitabchi A, et al. Hyperglycemic crises in adult patients with diabetes: a consensus statement from the American Diabetes Association. *Diabetes Care.* 2006;29(12):2739–2748.
33. Walls J. Metabolic acidosis and uremia. *Perit Dial Int.* 1995;15(5):S36–S38.
34. Burns M, et al. Treatment of methanol poisoning with intravenous 4-methylpyrazole. *Ann Emerg Med.* 1997;30(6):829–832.
35. Corley R, McMartin K. Incorporation of therapeutic interventions in physiologically based pharmacokinetic modeling of human clinical case reports of accidental or intentional overdosing with ethylene glycol. *Toxicol Sci.* 2005;85(1):491–501.
36. Morrow L, et al. Acute isoniazid toxicity and the need for adequate pyridoxine supplies. *Pharmacotherapy.* 2006;26(10):1529–1532.
37. Britton R, et al. Iron toxicity and chelation therapy. *Int J Hematol.* 2002;76(3):219–228.
38. O'Malley G. Emergency department management of the salicylate-poisoned patient. *Emerg Med Clin North Am.* 2007;25(2):333–346.
39. Dickson R, Luks A. Toluene toxicity as a cause of elevated anion gap metabolic acidosis. *Respir Care.* 2009;54(8):1115–1117.
40. Davidsson T, et al. Long-term metabolic and nutritional effects of urinary diversion. *Urology.* 1995;46:804–809.
41. Callery M, et al. Prevention and management of pancreatic fistula. *J Gastrointest Surg.* 2009;13(1):163–173.
42. Heller I, et al. Significant metabolic acidosis induced by acetazolamide. Not a rare complication. *Arch Intern Med.* 1985;145(10):1815–1817.
43. Morris C, Low J. Metabolic acidosis in the critically ill: Part 2. Causes and treatment. *Anaesthesia.* 2008;63:396–411.
44. Kellum J. Saline induced hyperchloremic metabolic acidosis. *Crit Care Med.* 2002;30:259–261.
45. Prough D, Bidani A. Hyperchloremic metabolic acidosis is a predictable consequence of intraoperative infusion of 0.9% saline. *Anesthesiology.* 1999;90:1247–1249.
46. Khanna A, Kurtzman N. Metabolic alkalosis. *J Nephrol.* 2006;19(suppl 9):S86–S96.
47. Mazur J, et al. Single versus multiple doses of acetazolamide for metabolic alkalosis in critically ill medical patients: a randomized, double-blind trial. *Crit Care Med.* 1999;27:1257–1261.
48. Mennen M, Slovis C. Severe metabolic alkalosis in the emergency department. *Ann Emerg Med.* 1988;17(4):354–357.

38

Electrolyte Disorders

Katy M. Deljoui and Michael T. McCurdy

BACKGROUND

Electrolyte disorders are frequently observed in critically ill patients and are associated with increased morbidity and mortality. This chapter reviews the most common electrolyte disturbances and provides a systematic approach to their management.

DISORDERS OF SODIUM

Hyponatremia

Epidemiology

Hyponatremia is a common electrolyte abnormality and may be seen in isolation or as a complication of other medical problems. Its prevalence varies according to the patient population, clinical setting, and serum sodium level used to define it. A normal serum sodium range is generally considered to be 135 to 145 mEq/L; hyponatremia is typically defined as a serum sodium level of <135 mEq/L.

Sodium is the dominant extracellular cation and does not move freely across cell membranes. Therefore, in order for hyponatremia to occur, water intake must exceed water excretion. In healthy individuals, water intake rarely overwhelms the kidneys' ability to excrete sodium, and hyponatremia most commonly results from either impaired renal function or inappropriate antidiuretic hormone (ADH) or vasopressin release.[1]

History and Physical Exam

Manifestations of hyponatremia include headache, seizures, coma, and, if brain edema results from associated fluid shift, even death. Symptom severity correlates with the rapidity of onset and the magnitude of drop in serum sodium.[2]

Diagnostic Evaluation

True hyponatremia is always hypoosmolar, but hyperosmolar and iso-osmolar hyponatremia may also occur. Hyperosmolar hyponatremia (>295 mOsm/kg) is due to the presence of another effective osmole, typically excess serum glucose or an osmotic diuretic (e.g., mannitol). Treatment includes stopping the offending infusion, and/or targeting a decrease in glucose concentration of 75 to 100 mg/dL/h. Iso-osmolar hyponatremia (280 to 295 mOsm/kg), also termed pseudohyponatremia, represents artifact due to hyperlipidemia or hyperproteinemia. It is usually asymptomatic and does not require specific treatment. The remainder of this review will focus on hypoosmolar hyponatremia (<280 mOsm/kg).

Hypoosmolar hyponatremia can exist in the setting of elevated (hypervolemic), normal (isovolemic), or low (hypovolemic) plasma volumes. Hypovolemic hyponatremia results from either renal or extrarenal losses of water and salt. Extrarenal hypovolemic hyponatremia typically results from vomiting and diarrhea. Other notable etiologies include burns, trauma, and pancreatitis. In cases of extrarenal losses, the body attempts to retain sodium while simultaneously releasing ADH. Ultimately, however, more water than salt is retained, resulting in low serum sodium levels as well as hypertonic urine (urine sodium <10 mEq/L). Renal causes of sodium and water loss include mineralocorticoid insufficiency, excessive use of diuretics, osmotic diuresis, and cerebral salt wasting syndrome.[3] In cases of renal loss, inappropriate elevations in both urine sodium (>20 mEq/L, usually >40 mEq/L) and urine osmolality (>100 mOsm/kg, and frequently >300 mOsm/kg) exist.

Isovolemic hyponatremia results from retention of water without salt. Although a diagnosis of exclusion, the classic example of isovolemic hyponatremia is the syndrome of inappropriate antidiuretic hormone (SIADH) secretion. SIADH is defined as hypotonic hyponatremia that occurs in the face of clinical euvolemia and in the absence of diuretic use, hypothyroidism, or adrenal insufficiency. In SIADH, both urine sodium concentration (>20 mEq/L) and urine osmolality (>100 mOsm/kg and generally >300 mOsm/kg) are elevated.[4] SIADH has multiple etiologies, including meningitis, malignancy (e.g., cervical cancer, lymphoma, leukemia, bronchogenic cancers), medications (e.g., cyclophosphamide, vincristine, vinblastine, selective serotonin reuptake inhibitors), and pulmonary or granulomatous diseases.[5] Other less common causes of isovolemic hyponatremia include psychogenic polydipsia, hypothyroidism, and adrenal or glucocorticoid insufficiency.

Hypervolemic hyponatremia occurs when the quantity of water retained is greater than that of sodium; it most commonly occurs with congestive heart failure, cirrhosis, and nephrotic syndrome.[6] In these disorders, the body attempts to retain sodium, resulting in a low urine sodium level (<20 mEq/L) and a high urine osmolality (>500 mOsm/kg). Of note, acute or chronic renal failure can also lead to hypervolemic hyponatremia, but in these cases the urine sodium level is generally elevated (>20 mEq/L) and the urine isotonic.[7]

Management Guidelines

Correction of hypovolemic hyponatremia requires both salt and water supplementation. Factors to consider in management include the severity and duration of symptoms. Chronic hyponatremia (or asymptomatic hyponatremia of unknown duration) should be treated with water restriction and avoidance of extra sodium, with a goal to correct the serum sodium at a rate of ≤0.5 mEq/L/h and avoid neurologic complications associated with overly rapid correction rates. In mild and acute hyponatremia, the sodium correction should not exceed 1 mEq/L/h[8] or approximately 8 mEq/L/24 h.[9] In acute symptomatic cases (e.g., seizures, altered mental status), hypertonic saline should be used to raise the serum sodium by 2 mEq/L/h, preserving a target increase of ≤12 mEq/L/24 h.[10] The most feared consequence of overly rapid correction of chronic hyponatremia is central pontine myelinolysis (CPM), which develops when water abruptly leaves the intracellular space of brain cells to equalize intra- and extracellular osmolalities.[11,12]

CPM will typically present as paraparesis or quadriparesis with dysarthria and dysphagia. On autopsy, patients with CPM will often demonstrate diffuse demyelinating lesions.

Once the severity and duration of symptoms are clarified, the next steps are to calculate the sodium deficit, total body water (TBW), and the target rate of rise of sodium.

- Sodium deficit = TBW × (desired serum sodium - measured serum sodium)
- TBW = body weight (kg) × factor Y

  (Y = 0.6 L/kg in children/adult males, 0.5 L/kg in adult females/elderly males, 0.4 L/kg in elderly females)

For example, in a symptomatic 50-kg female with a serum sodium of 112 mEq/L, raise the serum sodium by approximately 10 mEq in the first 24 hours (target serum sodium of 122 mEq/L). The sodium deficit is calculated as follows: (50 kg × 0.5 L/kg) × (122 mEq/L – 112 mEq/L) = 250 mEq. Because the patient is symptomatic, 3% hypertonic saline, containing 500 mEq of sodium per liter, can be used. Therefore, 500 mL (i.e., 250 mEq × [1,000 mL/500 mEq]) of 3% hypertonic saline would be given in the first 24 hours, resulting in an infusion rate of approximately 20 mL/h.

As a general guideline, the increase in serum sodium in mEq/L produced by giving 1 L of any fluid can be estimated as follows:

- Increase in sodium with 1 L of fluid = (infused sodium - measured sodium)/(TBW + 1)

If the above patient's symptoms are not severe and normal saline (154 mEq/L) was used instead, the expected rise in serum sodium would be (154 – 112)/(25 + 1) = 1.6 mEq/L.

Correction of isovolemic hyponatremia is usually achieved with water restriction and correction of the underlying cause of the imbalance (e.g., SIADH, hypothyroidism, adrenal insufficiency). The use of salt tablets may be considered, and loop diuretics may be needed in cases where urine output is low. In refractory cases, vasopressin antagonists, referred to as vaptans, may be used. ADH has multiple receptors, including V_{1a}, V_{1b}, and V_2. The V_{1a} and V_{1b} receptors are largely responsible for vasoconstriction, while the V_2 receptors mediate the antidiuretic response.[13,14] Vaptans work by selectively causing water diuresis without affecting sodium. The loss of free water corrects the hyponatremia, although the resulting increase in thirst may lead patients to drink more free water, thereby limiting the anticipated rise in sodium. Only two vaptans are currently available in the United States: tolvaptan and conivaptan. Tolvaptan, an oral formulation selective for the V_2 receptors, has been shown to increase serum sodium levels significantly when compared to placebo. However, a potential significant adverse effect of tolvaptan is overly rapid correction of hyponatremia.[15] In contrast, conivaptan, available either intravenously (IV) or orally (PO), blocks both the V_2 and V_{1a} receptors. Trials with the IV[16] and oral[17] forms have shown statistically significant increases in serum sodium when compared to placebo. Concerns, however, exist about conivaptan's ability to lower blood pressure and potential to increase the risk of variceal bleed in cirrhotic patients via its V_{1a} effect. More research is needed before the regular use of vaptans can be recommended. Additional treatment options include demeclocycline (600 to 1,200 mg/d), a tetracycline antibiotic that renders the collecting ducts unresponsive to ADH, effectively inducing a state of nephrogenic diabetes insipidus (DI), or diphenylhydantoin (40 mg/kg every 6 hours), which prevents the release of ADH and mimics central DI.[18,19]

Correction of hypervolemic hyponatremia centers on fluid restriction (600 to 1,000 mL/d), treatment of the underlying disorder (e.g., cardiac failure, renal failure, cirrhosis, nephrotic syndrome), and avoidance of extra sodium. Vaptans may also be considered along with loop diuretics.[20]

Hypernatremia

Epidemiology

Hypernatremia occurs when sodium exceeds water in the body. As previously noted, hyponatremia can be associated with hypo-, iso-, or even hyperosmolality. Hypernatremia, on the other hand, always results in hyperosmolality.[21,22] Because hyperosmolality stimulates thirst and water ingestion, hypernatremia only occurs when either a defect in the thirst mechanism or restricted water access exists. Therefore, the elderly or otherwise disabled patients, as well as critically ill hospitalized patients, are at greatest risk. Between 2% and 6% of newly admitted ICU patients are hypernatremic,[23] and between 6% and 26% of patients in medical intensive care units (ICUs) and 4% to 10% of patients in surgical ICUs will become hypernatremic during the hospitalization, usually in the first week after admission. This is important because the development of hypernatremia in hospitalized patients has been shown to be an independent risk factor for mortality.[24–29]

History and Physical Exam

Manifestations of hypernatremia occur as a result of neuronal dehydration as intracellular water shifts to the more hypertonic extracellular space. Lethargy, altered level of consciousness, irritability, hyperreflexia, and spasticity are common. Hypernatremia may be associated with impaired glucose metabolism leading to hyperglycemia,[30,31] and, in severe cases, can cause rhabdomyolysis with consequent acute renal failure.[32,33] Finally, hypernatremia has been associated with a decrease in cardiac function.[34]

Diagnostic Evaluation

Like hyponatremia, hypernatremia can coexist with decreased, normal, or elevated plasma volumes. Hypovolemic hypernatremia occurs when the body loses hypotonic fluids (water deficit exceeds sodium deficit). This is commonly seen with gastrointestinal losses (e.g., vomiting, diarrhea) and renal losses (e.g., intrinsic renal disease, use of diuretics). Physical exam abnormalities usually are not evident until dehydration reaches ≥10% to 15% (expressed as percentage of body weight) because fluid shifts from the intracellular to the extracellular space to preserve plasma volume.

Isovolemic hypernatremia typically occurs when a patient is unable to sense thirst, usually the result of a congenital or acquired disorder of the hypothalamus (e.g., craniopharyngiomas, primary or metastatic hypothalamic tumors [usually breast or lung], vascular lesions, trauma).[35] Other causes of isovolemic hypernatremia include central and nephrogenic DI. Central DI results from either impaired production or release of ADH, and it often follows head trauma or pituitary surgery. Nephrogenic DI results from a defect in the kidneys' response to ADH. In either case, urine output can be as high as 3 mL/kg/h, and the specific gravity will usually be between 1.000 and 1.003.

Hypervolemic hypernatremia is usually iatrogenic in nature and secondary to large infusions of hypertonic fluids, such as 3% saline or sodium bicarbonate

($NaHCO_3$), as well as replacing hypotonic insensible losses (e.g., febrile illness, respiratory distress, gastrointestinal loss) with 0.9% (normal) saline. It can also be seen in accidental salt ingestions and, rarely, with mineralocorticoid excess (e.g., Cushing syndrome).

Management Guidelines

The first step in the management of hypernatremia is determination of volume status, as hypovolemic hypernatremia is treated differently from isovolemic or hypervolemic hypernatremia. Clinical signs of low volume status include increased thirst, sunken eyes, dry mucous membranes, resting or orthostatic tachycardia, and hypotension, as well as oliguria. Hemodynamic monitoring may reveal a very low central venous pressure, arterial pressure variation in ventilated patients, or increase in arterial pressure with passive leg raise in spontaneously breathing patients. Biochemistries may show rising hematocrit, high serum uric acid, high urine osmolarity, and low urine sodium (extrarenal cases).

Management of hypovolemic hypernatremia begins with fluid resuscitation with a balanced crystalloid solution to correct volume deficit. Fluid resuscitation should be guided by symptom resolution, including improvement in orthostasis, tachycardia, and urine output. Once the volume deficit is corrected, the next step is to calculate the free water deficit, obtained with the following formula:

- Free Water Deficit (L) = TBW × [(measured serum Na/140)−1]

The free water deficit can then be corrected with 5% dextrose in water (D5W) or a low-sodium crystalloid solution (e.g., half-normal saline).[36] As with hyponatremia, a gradual rate of replacement is essential, as overly rapid correction can cause cerebral edema.[37,38] In chronic cases, or cases of unknown duration, the rate of correction should not exceed 0.5 mEq/L/h or 8 to 10 mEq/L/24 h. The diagnosis of acute hypernatremia should only be made if the rise in sodium has a documented onset within the last 48 hours prior to presentation. In these cases, rapid correction at a rate of 2 to 3 mEq/L/h or 12 mEq/L/24 h is appropriate.[39] For example, in a 50-kg 40-year-old female patient with a serum sodium of 160 mEq/L, the TBW would be 50 kg × 0.5 L/kg = 25 L. Total water deficit would be 25 L × [160/140) −1] = 3.6 L. Thus, a total positive water balance of 3.6 L must be achieved for the sodium to decrease from 160 to 140 mEq/L, or by 20 mEq. However, assuming that the case is not acute, the rate of correction should be ≤0.5 mEq/h, which would require replacement of the water deficit over 40 hours, or approximately 90 mL/h, to which insensible water losses should be added—generally about 30 mL/h—for a total of 120 mL/h.

In the particular case of hypernatremia caused by DI, water loss should be replaced at a rate of 0.5 to 0.75 mL for every 1 mL of urine made. In cases of central DI, vasopressin (5 to 10 units IM q6-12h) and desmopressin acetate or DDAVP (1 to 2 mcg SC/IV q12h) may be considered. These agents are ADH analogs that increase water reabsorption by the renal collecting ducts.

In cases of isovolemic and hypervolemic hyponatremia, treatment requires only replacement of the free water (e.g., D5W) with or without the use of loop diuretics. In renal failure, dialysis may be necessary.

Sodium treatment summary: Tables 38.1 and 38.2

TABLE 38.1 Treatment of Hyponatremia

	Treatment	Rate of Correction or Dosage
Hypovolemic hyponatremia • Mild acute • Severe acute • Chronic	• Isotonic saline • Hypertonic saline • Water restriction	• 1 mEq/L/h or 8–10 mEq/L/d • 2 mEq/L/h or 12 mEq/L/d • 0.5 mEq/L/h or 4–6 mEq/L/d
Isovolemic hyponatremia	• Treat underlying cause • Water restriction • Salt supplementation • Vaptans • Demeclocycline • Diphenylhydantoin	• Tolvaptan 15–60 mg/d PO • 300 mg q6–12h PO • 600–1,200 mg/d PO
Hypervolemic hyponatremia	• Treat underlying cause • Water restriction • Vaptans • Loop diuretics	• 50%–60% of daily fluid requirements

TABLE 38.2 Treatment of Hypernatremia

	Treatment	Rate of Correction or Dosage
Hypovolemic hypernatremia • Acute • Chronic	• Free water replacement • Free water replacement • Pitressin • Desmopressin	• 2 mEq/L/h or 12 mEq/L/d • 0.5 mEq/L/h or 4–6 mEq/L/d • 5–10 units q6–12h IM • 1–2 mcg q12h SC/IV
Isovolemic hypernatremia	• Water replacement • Loop diuretics	
Hypervolemic hypernatremia	• Water replacement • Loop diuretics • Dialysis	

POTASSIUM

Hypokalemia

Epidemiology

While sodium is the major extracellular cation, potassium is the dominant intracellular one. The concentration differences of these positively charged particles create a difference in electrical potential between the inside and outside of cells, known as the membrane potential. The membrane potential allows the cells to generate an action potential, an electrical discharge, which is critical for neurotransmission and muscle contraction. For this reason, the serum potassium level is maintained within a very narrow range. In the setting of hypokalemia, where serum levels are low, potassium shifts from the intracellular to the extracellular space. As a result, the cell membranes become hyperpolarized and thus more resistant to depolarization, which makes them less likely to generate an action potential.

History and Physical Exam

Hypokalemia can manifest as generalized muscle weakness, paralytic ileus, and abnormalities in cardiac conduction. Electrocardiogram (ECG) changes that accompany hypokalemia include ST depressions, small amplitude of T waves, and increased height of U waves.[40] In severe cases, prolonged PR intervals and wide QRS complexes may also be seen.

Diagnostic Evaluation

Three broad mechanisms lead to hypokalemia: increased intracellular shifts, decreased potassium intake, and increased potassium loss. Insulin, epinephrine, β_2 agonists, and α agonists all shift potassium intracellularly[41,42]; starvation and malnutrition can lead to inadequate potassium intake; and diuretics and gastrointestinal disorders increase potassium loss. Diuretic therapy is the most common cause of potassium wasting. By blocking sodium reabsorption, thiazide and loop diuretic increase sodium delivery to the collecting tubules, creating a favorable electrochemical gradient for potassium secretion in exchange for sodium reabsorption.[43] Contrary to popular belief, hypokalemia complicating vomiting or nasogastric suctioning actually results from renal potassium loss, not gastric fluid loss. Intravascular volume depletion from gastric fluid loss stimulates the renin–angiotensin pathway and aldosterone release. Aldosterone, in turn, increases renal sodium absorption at the expense of potassium excretion, similar to other primary or secondary aldosteronism–induced hypokalemia.

Management Guidelines

Management of asymptomatic hypokalemia is safely achieved with slow enteral correction over several days. For patients with severe hypokalemia, parenteral replacement is preferred with a maximum recommended rate of correction of 10 to 20 mEq/h. Potassium chloride is commonly used, but potassium phosphate is also acceptable. In life-threatening cases, up to 40 mEq/h of potassium chloride can be given through a central line, preferably in an ICU setting.[44] Because severe transient hyperkalemia can easily occur during correction of hypokalemia, care must be taken to closely monitor telemetry data as treatment proceeds.[45] Low phosphate and magnesium levels often accompany hypokalemia and must also be treated in order for potassium levels to be successfully corrected.[46]

Hyperkalemia

Epidemiology

Hyperkalemia is a potentially lethal electrolyte disturbance. Expeditious recognition and prompt treatment are paramount. Like hypokalemia, hyperkalemia can be caused by increased intake, intracellular-to-extracellular potassium shifts, or defects in renal excretion. Increased intake in hospitalized patients is typically iatrogenic in nature and the result of accidental overdose of IV potassium. Shifts between the intracellular and extracellular fluids occur in the setting of acidosis or cell destruction. Decreased excretion is often the result of renal failure or adrenal insufficiency.

History and Physical Exam

Severe hyperkalemia can present with paresthesias, muscle weakness leading to flaccid paralysis but typically with sparing of the diaphragm, and depressed deep tendon reflexes. Cranial nerves are rarely affected.[47] Electrocardiographic changes include peaked and narrow T waves, widened QRS complexes, sine waves, and shortened

QT intervals, which, when left untreated, can progress to ventricular fibrillation and asystole.[48]

Diagnostic Evaluation

Although commonly relied upon for diagnosis, the sensitivity of the ECG to reveal changes related to hyperkalemia has been estimated at around 80%, according to one retrospective review of 90 hyperkalemic patients.[49] ECG sensitivity for hyperkalemia increases with the severity of electrolyte derangement, but normal ECGs have been reported even with profound hyperkalemia.[50] ECG changes should, therefore, not be considered sine qua non to initiate treatment of severe hyperkalemia.

Management Guidelines

Immediate treatment of hyperkalemia is needed if ECG changes are noted, irrespective of serum potassium level, or if the serum potassium level is >6.5 to 7 mEq/L.[51] The goals of therapy are threefold: (1) antagonize the effect of potassium on excitable cell membranes; (2) shift potassium from the extracellular milieu into cells; and (3) enhance elimination of potassium from the body.

Calcium gluconate or calcium chloride should be given first to antagonize the myocardial effects of hyperkalemia and prevent dysrhythmias. Classic teaching recommends an ampule of calcium gluconate, which represents 1 g or 4.6 mEq in 10 mL of a 10% solution, infused over 2 to 5 minutes with expected effect in 2 to 3 minutes.[52,53] Calcium gluconate is preferred over calcium chloride—although calcium chloride is more concentrated (13.6 mEq in 10 mL of a 10% solution)—because it is less likely to cause tissue necrosis in the event of extravasation from the peripheral IV.[54] A second ampule may be repeated after 5 minutes if there is no improvement in the ECG or if the ECG deteriorates after an initial improvement. The duration of action of 1 ampule is 30 to 60 minutes.[55] Of note, reports exist of sudden death in patients taking digitalis glycosides who were given given IV calcium.[56,57] Although these cases were anecdotal, prudence warrants either avoidance of IV calcium entirely in this subset of patients or at least very close monitoring during calcium administration.

Insulin lowers potassium levels by shifting potassium into cells. The effect is dose dependent[58] and is mediated by the sodium/potassium ATPase pump in the plasma membrane of cells.[59] An IV 10-unit dose of regular insulin is standard, and will shift potassium from the extracellular fluid to the intracellular fluid within 15 to 30 minutes, with the effect lasting 4 to 6 hours.[60] Studies have shown that this dose will reduce serum potassium level by approximately 0.6 mEq/L. A bolus of 25 g of IV dextrose (50% solution) is generally given with the insulin to prevent hypoglycemia. However, because the effect of insulin on serum potassium levels peaks at 60 minutes, a single bolus of dextrose may be inadequate to prevent later hypoglycemia. For this reason, some advocate starting a dextrose infusion after the initial bolus.[61] Insulin should be used without dextrose in hyperglycemic patients (baseline glucose level >250 mg/dL), as the hyperglycemia itself may the cause of hyperkalemia in these patients.[62]

$NaHCO_3$ use in the emergent treatment of hyperkalemia remains controversial. $NaHCO_3$ is typically formulated as an 8.4% solution (1 mEq/mL) and given in ampules of 50 mL (50 mEq per ampule) infused over 5 minutes. Like insulin, $NaHCO_3$ has been postulated to shift potassium from the extracellular to the intracellular space. In theory, the administration of $NaHCO_3$ should prompt hydrogen ions to move out of the cells via the Na^+/H^+ exchanger. This, in turn, leads to more sodium entering the cells to maintain electroneutrality. In the setting of hyperkalemia, this increase in intracellular sodium would subsequently activate the Na^+/K^+ ATPase pump, driving potassium from the extracellular to the intracellular space. Of critical importance, the Na^+/H^+ exchanger appears to be inactive in a steady state but active in the setting of acidosis.[63] Arguments for the benefit of $NaHCO_3$ in hyperkalemia originated with a few small clinical studies conducted in the 1950s and 1970s.[64,65] Subsequent research has suggested that short-term infusions or boluses of $NaHCO_3$ are ineffective in the acute setting,[66–69] whereas a prolonged (4 to 6 hours) infusion of $NaHCO_3$ decreased potassium levels by about 0.6 mEq/L.[70] Given its limited efficacy acutely, while not contraindicated in hyperkalemic patients with acidemia, no significant or rapid change in potassium levels should be expected with $NaHCO_3$ therapy.

The effect of β_2-adrenergic stimulation effectively lowers serum potassium.[71–78] β_2 agonists (e.g., albuterol), like insulin, stimulate the Na^+/K^+ ATPase pump to shift potassium from the extracellular to the intracellular space. The recommended dose is 10 to 20 mg in 4 to 8 mL of saline, nebulized over 10 to 20 minutes. IV and metered-dose inhaler doses are also sometimes used. The onset of action is typically within 30 minutes, and the effect is maintained for up to 2 hours. Serum potassium will usually decrease by 0.5 to 1.2 mEq/L per 10- to 20-mg dose of albuterol.

Sodium polystyrene sulfonate (Kayexalate) is a cation-exchange resin that removes potassium from the body by exchanging sodium for secreted potassium in the gastrointestinal tract. Kayexalate is generally given as an oral dose of 1 to 2 g/kg or as a retention enema with sorbitol to prevent constipation. Each gram of sodium polystyrene removes approximately 0.65 mEq/L of potassium, although the effect can be variable.[79,80] Two important concerns exist with the use of Kayexalate. The first is its slow onset; when given orally, the onset of action is >2 hours and the maximum effect may not occur for 6 hours. As a retention enema, the effect is more rapid, but the magnitude of effect is less because of a shorter transit time through the gut lumen.[81] The second potential problem is the possibility of toxicity. Numerous reports of Kayexalate-induced intestinal necrosis exist, both with the enema[82–85] and oral forms.[86–90] Although the true incidence of necrosis is unknown, estimates are 0.1% to 0.3% in the general population given the medication, and it occurs almost exclusively in "at-risk" patients (i.e., post–abdominal surgery, bowel injury, other gastrointestinal dysfunction).[91] The Food and Drug Administration (FDA) first approved Kayexalate in 1958 after a small case series published in 1953 showed potassium binding in the stool and a hypokalemic effect in four patients with renal failure and a normal volunteer.[92] The reported effectiveness of the drug, however, is largely based on the 1961 study, in which Kayexalate suspended in water was used orally or rectally in patients with acute and chronic kidney disease. In 22 of 32 cases, the plasma potassium fell by a mean of 1 mEq/L with the oral formulation versus 0.8 mEq/L with the rectal.[93] Soon after, however, it was recognized that Kayexalate could cause life-threatening intestinal impactions, which then led to the practice of concomitantly administering 70% sorbitol, an osmotic laxative. A follow-up study showed a decrease in intestinal impactions with this combination[94]; however, reports of gastrointestinal necrosis continued to accumulate.

TABLE 38.3 Treatment of Hypokalemia

	Treatment	Rate of Correction or Dosage
Hypokalemia		
• Asymptomatic	• PO potassium chloride	• 20–80 mEq/d
• Symptomatic	• IV potassium chloride	• 10–20 mEq/h
• Life-threatening	• IV potassium chloride	• 40 mEq/h via central line

Treat concomitant low magnesium and phosphate.

With the precise mechanism of injury unclear, it was postulated that the 70% sorbitol rather than Kayexalate itself could be the culprit.[95] Since 2007, the FDA has asked all manufacturers of premixed resin to reformulate their products to contain 33%, rather than 70%, sorbitol.

Studies have now called into questions the safety of even the 33% formulation.[96] For all these reasons, consensus recommendations are to exhaust alternatives (e.g., diuretics, dialysis) before considering Kayexalate use.[97,98] Importantly, Kayexalate continues to play a key role in the treatment of acute hyperkalemia under austere conditions, for example, after a natural or manmade disaster. In situations like these, where dialysis is not available, Kayexalate may be the only option for potassium removal, especially in chronic renal patients in whom diuretics are expected to have no effect. In the recent past, it was used in military facilities in Iraq, in the aftermath of Hurricane Katrina, and after the Haitian earthquake.[99–102]

If the potassium levels remain elevated despite the aforementioned therapies, a trial of loop diuretics in patients with preserved renal function may be attempted. In patients with end-stage renal disease and refractory cases, dialysis should be considered. Hemodialysis against a potassium-free dialysate can decrease the serum potassium level by as much as 1.5 mEq/h.[66] However, a rebound in serum levels will always occur following dialysis, with 35% of the decrease in potassium negated after just 1 hour and nearly 70% after 6 hours as intracellular levels equilibrate with those of the serum. The magnitude of the rebound is thought to be proportional to the predialysis potassium level.[103] Due to the risk of ventricular dysrhythmias during dialysis for severe hyperkalemia, which may result from the substantial intravascular volume shifts in the presence of a dysrhythmogenic potassium level, such patients are recommended to undergo continuous ECG monitoring[104] during the session.

Potassium treatment summary: Tables 38.3 and 38.4

TABLE 38.4 Treatment of Hyperkalemia

	Treatment	Rate of Correction or Dosage
Hyperkalemia	• Calcium gluconate • Insulin and dextrose • Sodium bicarbonate • Albuterol • Kayexalate • Loop diuretics • Dialysis	• 1 amp IV over 2–5 min • 10 units of regular insulin and 25 g of D50 IV • 1 amp IV over 3–5 min • 10 mg in 4 mL NS INH • 1–2 g/kg orally or enema • Furosemide 40 mg IV

CALCIUM

Hypocalcemia

Epidemiology

Calcium is the most abundant electrolyte in the body and exists in three forms: (1) a chelated form; (2) an ionized form; and (3) a protein-bound form. The ionized form is the most physiologically active form and is therefore the one needing measurement. Two hormones—parathyroid hormone (PTH) and calcitonin—are responsible for regulating the body's calcium balance. PTH is released in response to hypocalcemia and increases calcium levels by stimulating osteoclasts, enhancing intestinal absorption, and decreasing renal excretion. Calcitonin, conversely, inhibits osteoclast activity and promotes renal excretion of calcium.

History and Physical Exam

Because calcium plays a major role in muscle contraction–excitation, nerve conduction, myocardial function, and coagulation, the effects of hypocalcemia can be varied. Paresthesias in the hands and feet, circumoral numbness, muscle spasms, seizures, anxiety, irritability, psychosis, hypotension, low cardiac output, and QT interval prolongation may all be observed. QT interval prolongation can progress to bradycardia, heart block, or ventricular fibrillation.[105]

Diagnostic Evaluation

Hypocalcemia is diagnosed by measurement of serum levels. Because serum protein levels affect total serum calcium levels, the ionized calcium level provides a more accurate assessment of the physiologic active calcium available. Ionized calcium of <1.1 mmol/L confirms hypocalcemia (physiologic range is 1.1 to 1.4 mmol/L, or 4.5 to 5.6 mg/dL; 1 mmol/L is roughly equivalent to 4 mg/dL). Common causes of hypocalcemia include hypoparathyroidism; hyperphosphatemia, in which excess phosphate chelates circulating calcium (e.g., rhabdomyolysis, kidney disease); and massive transfusion, in which the preservative citrate binds calcium.[106]

Management Guidelines

In severe symptomatic cases, hypocalcemia is treated with 200 mg of elemental calcium given slowly over 10 to 20 minutes. Calcium gluconate can be given through a peripheral IV, but calcium chloride infused through a central line provides three times as many ionized calcium molecules (10 mL of calcium gluconate 10% contains 94 mg of elemental calcium; 10 mL of calcium chloride 10% contains 272 mg of elemental calcium). In less emergent cases, infusions containing 0.5 to 1.5 mg elemental calcium/kg/h may also be used, diluted in dextrose or saline, and given over 4 to 6 hours.[107]

A magnesium level must be concurrently checked and repleted because hypomagnesemia can impair PTH secretion and induce end-organ resistance to PTH, thus rendering hypocalcemia correction difficult.[108] Finally, ionized calcium and H^+ ions compete to bind to negatively charged sites on protein molecules, such as albumin. This binding is pH dependent, such that a sudden increase in pH—in the setting of, for example, alkali therapy—would cause proteins to release H^+ and then bind calcium instead, potentially precipitously decreasing ionized calcium levels.[109] For this reason, if a metabolic acidosis exists concomitantly with hypocalcemia, calcium replacement must take place before attempting to correct the acidosis.

Hypercalcemia

Epidemiology

Hypercalcemia is usually encountered in the setting of malignancy or primary hyperparathyroidism. Hyperparathyroidism is the culprit in 90% of ambulatory patients, while cancer causes 65% of hypercalcemia in hospitalized patients.[110,111] Other causes of hypercalcemia include hyperthyroidism, Addison disease, and use of thiazide diuretics.

History and Physical Exam

Manifestations of hypercalcemia are varied and frequently nonspecific. Patients will often report nausea, vomiting, and constipation. Weakness and fatigue are common, and altered mental status and coma may also be observed. Dysrhythmias can result from PR interval prolongation and QT interval shortening. Reports of heart block and cardiac arrest exist but are rare.[112]

Diagnostic Evaluation

As with hypocalcemia, hypercalcemia is generally diagnosed by measuring serum levels. Mild hypercalcemia is defined as total serum level of 12 mg/dL and is usually asymptomatic. Levels between 12 and 16 mg/dL can produce the nonspecific symptoms of weakness, nausea, vomiting, and abdominal pain. Cognitive dysfunction, personality changes, confusion, hallucinations, psychosis, stupor, and coma are expected with concentrations >16 mg/dL.

Management Guidelines

Because hypercalcemic patients are frequently volume-depleted from the associated polyuria (hypercalciuria) and poor oral intake, IV fluids are usually indicated initially. As with hypovolemic hypernatremia, the volume deficit must first be calculated and corrected using isotonic saline (generally 1 to 2 L IV over 1 hour). By increasing the glomerular filtration rate, renal calcium excretion also increases. Once the patient is determined to be euvolemic, a loop diuretic may be added to accelerate calcium excretion by the kidneys.[113] Furosemide, 20 to 40 mg IV every 2 hours after correction of dehydration, is commonly used.

Calcitonin may also be used if first-line treatments are ineffective. A standard dose of 4 IU/kg is given either subcutaneously or intramuscularly every 12 hours. Its mechanism of action is inhibition of bone resorption and enhancement of renal excretion of calcium. Its main advantage is its fast onset of action; a response is usually noted within 2 to 4 hours. Unfortunately, its impact is mild (expected lowering in serum calcium level is 1 to 3 mg/dL after 4 to 6 hours, with a nadir within 12 to 24 hours), and tachyphylaxis is known to occur after 2 to 3 days.[114,115] Bisphosphonates are good alternatives and inhibit osteoclast activity. The bisphosphonate pamidronate has been used for many years and is generally well tolerated, even in patients with renal disease. Pamidronate is a pyrophosphate analog that binds to hydroxyapatite and inhibits bone crystal dissolution as well as osteoclastic resorption.[116] Standard dosing is 60 to 90 mg in 500 mL of isotonic saline given as an infusion over 1 to 2 hours. Unfortunately, it can take up to 48 hours to take effect, and the duration of action is 2 to 4 weeks. For these reasons, it is more appropriate for long-term rather than acute management of hypercalcemia.[117]

Additional therapies include mithramycin, an antibiotic that works by inhibiting RNA synthesis in osteoclasts. Its calcium-lowering effect is seen after 24 to 48 hours, but its use is limited by its poor side effect profile, including hepatotoxicity, renal failure,

TABLE 38.5 Treatment of Hypocalcemia

	Treatment	Rate of Correction or Dosage
Hypocalcemia		
• Mild	• Calcium gluconate 10% sol (10 mL= 94 mg elemental calcium)	• Elemental calcium 0.5–1.5 mg/kg/h IV run over 4–6 h ~0.1 mL/kg/h
• Severe	• Calcium chloride 10% sol (10 mL= 272 mg elemental calcium)	• Elemental calcium 200 mg (~7.5 mL) through central line over 10–20 min

Correct simultaneous hypomagnesemia.

TABLE 38.6 Treatment of Hypercalcemia

	Treatment	Rate of Correction or Dosage
Hypercalcemia	• Normal saline	• 1–2-L bolus
	• Loop diuretic	• Furosemide 20–40 mg IV
	• Calcitonin	• 4 IU/kg q12h SC/IM
	• Pamidronate	• 60–90 mg in 500 mL NS over 1–2 h
	• Mithramycin	• 25–50 mcg/kg IV
	• Dialysis	

and bone marrow suppression.[118] In severe or refractory cases of hypercalcemia, dialysis may be considered.[119]

Calcium treatment summary: Tables 38.5 and 38.6

MAGNESIUM

Hypomagnesemia

Epidemiology

Hypomagnesemia is seen in as many as 12% of hospitalized patients, and 60% to 65% of critically ill patients in the ICU.[120] Common etiologies include nutritional deficiency, intestinal losses, renal losses, as well as endocrine and metabolic derangements. Like calcium, magnesium exists in three forms: (1) ionized (61%), (2) protein-bound (33%), and (3) complexed (6%). The kidney is primarily responsible for magnesium homeostasis and, because magnesium reabsorption is proportional to urine flow, volume expansion can lead to magnesium wasting. In addition, thiazides and loop diuretics are well known for inhibiting magnesium reabsorption in the kidneys. Finally, many drugs, most notably alcohol, cause renal magnesium loss.[121]

History and Physical Exam

Magnesium deficiency is often seen in conjunction with hypokalemia, hypocalcemia, and metabolic alkalosis. Thus, signs and symptoms are often varied and nonspecific. Cardiac manifestations include prolonged PR and QT intervals, as well as a widened QRS complex, which can lead to dysrhythmias, notably torsades de pointes.[122] Neuromuscular manifestations include generalized weakness, seizures, tetany, lethargy, and coma.

Diagnostic Evaluation

A normal serum magnesium concentration is 1.7–2.1 mg/dL (1.4–1.8 mEq/L) in most cases, a diagnosis of hypomagnesemia can be made from patient history, as magnesium depletion is usually the result of either gastrointestinal or renal losses. In obscure cases, however, calculating the fractional excretion of magnesium or measuring the magnesium excretion over a 24-hour period can help to distinguish between the two causes of wasting. A daily excretion of more than 10 to 30 mg, or a fractional excretion of more than 2%, suggests renal wasting.[123,124]

Management Guidelines

If the patient is asymptomatic, oral supplementation is generally sufficient with a daily maintenance requirement of 0.4 mEq/kg/d. Magnesium oxide (49.6 mEq/g) is commonly used for repletion. If the patient is symptomatic, IV magnesium sulfate (8.12 mEq/g) is preferred at a dose of 1 to 2 mEq/kg administered over 8 to 24 hours. In the event of life-threatening dysrhythmias, the patient should be loaded with 25 to 50 mg/kg of magnesium sulfate over 3 to 5 minutes, followed by an infusion of 25 to 50 mg/kg/h for 4 to 6 hours.[125]

Hypermagnesemia

Epidemiology

Hypermagnesemia is rare and typically iatrogenic in nature. It tends to occur because of overzealous correction of hypomagnesemia, or in the treatment of preeclampsia and preterm labor.[126] However, it may also be seen with parenteral hyperalimentation, use of laxatives and enemas, or use of antacids. Patients with kidney disease are particularly at risk.[127]

History and Physical Exam

Signs and symptoms of hypermagnesemia are flushing, respiratory depression, pulmonary edema, hypotension, weakness with loss of deep tendon reflexes, or paralysis. ECG manifestations associated with hypermagnesemia include prolonged PR and ST intervals, which may lead to bradycardia, complete heart block, and even cardiac arrest.

Diagnostic Evaluation

Except in severely symptomatic cases, the diagnosis of hypermagnesemia is made on laboratory evaluation. It is usually defined by a serum magnesium concentration >0.95 mmol/L, or 2.2 mg/dL.

Management Guidelines

Because most cases of hypermagnesemia are iatrogenic, the first-line treatment is to remove the exogenous source of magnesium. Diuretics can also promote renal excretion. In severe cases, calcium gluconate can temporarily antagonize the cardiac and neurologic symptoms. Dialysis may also be considered if initial therapies are unsuccessful.[128]

Magnesium treatment summary: Tables 38.7 and 38.8.

TABLE 38.7 Treatment of Hypomagnesemia

	Treatment	Correction Rate or Dosage
Hypomagnesemia		
• Mild	• Magnesium oxide (49.6 mEq/g)	• 0.4 mEq/kg/d PO ~8 mg/kg/d PO
• Moderate	• Magnesium sulfate (8.12 mEq/g)	• 1–2 mEq/kg IV ~125–250 mg/kg over 8–24 h
• Severe	• Magnesium sulfate (8.12 mEq/g)	• Load 25 to 50 mg/kg IV over 3–5 min; then 25–50 mg/kg/h for 4–6 h

TABLE 38.8 Treatment of Hypermagnesemia

	Treatment
Hypermagnesemia	• Remove exogenous source • Diuretics • Dialysis

LITERATURE TABLE

TRIAL	DESIGN	RESULT
Use of Vaptans		
Schrier et al., *N Engl J Med.* 2006[15] SALT-1 and SALT-2	Multicenter, prospective, randomized, double-blind, placebo-controlled trials of 448 euvolemic and hypervolemic patients; compared oral tolvaptan 15 mg, 30 mg or 60 mg daily × 30 d vs. placebo	Serum Na^+ concentrations were significantly higher in the oral tolvaptan group vs. placebo in the first 4 days ($p < 0.001$) and after the full 30 d ($p < 0.001$)
Zeltser et al., *Am J Nephrol.* 2007[16]	Multicenter, prospective, randomized, double-blind, placebo-controlled trial of 84 euvolemic and hypervolemic patients; compared 20 mg IV loading dose of conivaptan followed by 4-day infusion of either 40 mg/d or 80 mg/d vs. placebo	Serum Na^+ concentrations were significantly higher with both doses of the IV conivaptan groups vs. placebo ($p < 0.0001$)
Annane et al., *Am J Med Sci.* 2009[17]	Multicenter, prospective, randomized, double-blind, placebo-controlled trial of 83 euvolemic and hypervolemic patients; compared oral conivaptan 20 mg twice daily or 40 mg twice daily × 5 d vs. placebo	Increase in serum Na^+ concentrations were higher, achieved significantly faster, and maintained longer with either dose of the oral conivaptan groups vs. placebo ($p = 0.0001$)
Bicarbonate in hyperkalemia		
Schwarz CK et al., *Circulation.* 1959[64]	Case reports of 4 uremic patients with acidosis, hyperkalemia, and ECG changes; received infusion of 5% $NaHCO_3$	Serial determinations showed fall in potassium, rise in pH, and regression of ECG changes toward normal
Allon et al., *Am J Kid Dis.* 1996[68]	Single-center, prospective, crossover design, of 8 dialysis patients; compared potassium at 1 h after: (1) $NaHCO_3$ infusion, (2) saline infusion, (3) bicarbonate in D10 + insulin, (4) saline in D10 + insulin, (5) bicarbonate + nebulized albuterol, and (6) saline + nebulized albuterol	Neither bicarbonate nor saline decreased potassium significantly ($p = 0.6$). Insulin decreased potassium by same degree when given with bicarbonate or saline ($p = 0.65$). Nebulized albuterol decreased potassium levels by same degree with bicarbonate or saline ($p = 0.18$)
Blumberg A et al. *Kidney Int.* 1992[70]	Observational study of 12 hyperkalemic end-stage renal disease patients on hemodialysis; received infusion of 8.4% $NaHCO_3$ for 1 h, followed by infusion of 1.4% for 5 h; compared bicarbonate, pH, and potassium at 1 h, 4 h, and 6 h	Bicarbonate and pH rose. Decline in plasma potassium noted only at 4 h ($p < 0.05$) and 6 h ($p < 0.01$), half of which was attributed to volume expansion
Kayexalate in hyperkalemia		
Evans et al., *Lancet.* 1953[92]	Case reports of 4 renal failure patients and 1 normal volunteer, given a sulfonate resin charged with sodium orally (precursor of modern Kayexalate)	Showed potassium binding in the stool and hypokalemic effect

LITERATURE TABLE (*Continued*)

TRIAL	DESIGN	RESULT
Scherr et al., *N Engl J Med.* 1961[93]	Report of 32 hyperkalemic patients; 22 received a range dose 20–60 g/d of a sulfonate resin charged with sodium, orally in water, for a range period 1–6 d; 8 received a range dose 10–160 g/d rectally for a range period 1–4 d	Mean decline in potassium at 24 h of 1 mEq/L with the oral formulation vs. 0.8 mEq/L with the rectal. No serious toxic effects observed
Harel et al., *Am J Med.* 2013[98]	Systematic review of adverse effects associated with Kayexalate, 1948–2011, MEDLINE, EMBASE, CENTRAL, 30 reports identified	58 cases described: 41 preparations with sorbitol, 17 without. Colon, the most common site injured (76%), and transmural necrosis most common lesion (62%). Mortality 33% due to gastrointestinal injury

REFERENCES

1. Anderson RJ, Chung H-M, Kluge R, et al. Hyponatremia: a prospective analysis of its epidemiology and the pathogenetic role of vasopressin. *Ann Intern Med.* 1985;102:164–168.
2. Arieff AI, Llach F, Massry SG. Neurologic manifestations and morbidity of hyponatremia, correlation of brain water and electrolytes. *Medicine (Baltimore).* 1976;55:121–129.
3. Wijdicks EF, Ropper AH, Hunnicutt EJ, et al. Atrial natriuretic factor and salt wasting after aneurysmal subarachnoid hemorrhage. *Stroke.* 1991;22:1519–1524.
4. Fried LF, Palevsky PM. Hyponatremia and hypernatremia. *Med Clin North Am.* 1997;81:585–609.
5. Kapoor M, Chan GZ. Fluid and electrolyte abnormalities. *Crit Care Clin.* 2001;17:503–529.
6. Schrier RW. Pathogenesis of sodium and water retention in high output and low output cardiac failure, nephrotic syndrome, cirrhosis, and pregnancy. *N Engl J Med.* 1988;319:1127–1134.
7. Spalding HK, Goodwin SR. Fluids and electrolyte disorders in the critically ill. *Semin Anesth Perioper Med Pain.* 1999;18:15–26.
8. Cluitmans FH, Meinders AE. Management of severe hyponatremia: rapid or slow correction? *Am J Med.* 1990;88:161–166.
9. Adrogue HJ, Madias NE. Hyponatremia. *N Engl J Med.* 2000;342:1581–1589.
10. Rose BD. *Clinical Physiology of Acid–base and Electrolyte Disorders.* 4th ed. New York: McGraw-Hill; 1994:651–694.
11. Sterns RH, Thomas DJ, Herndon RH. Brain dehydration and neurologic deterioration after rapid correction of hyponatremia. *Kidney Int.* 1989;35:69–75.
12. Sterns RH, Riggs JE, Schochet SS Jr. Osmotic demyelination syndrome following correction of hyponatremia. *N Engl J Med.* 1986;314:1535–1542.
13. Verbalis JG, Goldsmith SR, Greenberg A, et al. Hyponatremia treatment guidelines 2007: expert panel recommendations. *Am J Med.* 2007;120:S1.
14. Greenberg A, Verbalis JG. Vasopressin receptor antagonists. *Kidney Int.* 2006;69:2124–2130.
15. Schrier RW, Gross P, Gheorghiade M, et al.; SALT Investigators. Tolvaptan, a selective oral vasopressin V2-receptor antagonist, for hyponatremia. *N Engl J Med.* 2006;355:2099–2112.
16. Zeltser D, Rosansky S, van Rensburg H, et al.; Conivaptan Study Group. Assessment of the efficacy and safety of intravenous conivaptan in euvolemic and hypervolemic hyponatremia. *Am J Nephrol.* 2007;27:447–457.
17. Annane D, Decaux G, Smith N. Efficacy and safety of oral conivaptan, a vasopressin-receptor antagonist, evaluated in a randomized, controlled trial in patients with euvolemic or hypervolemic hyponatremia. *Am J Med Sci.* 2009;337:28–36.
18. White MG, Fetner CD. Treatment of the syndrome of inappropriate secretion of antidiuretic hormone with lithium carbonate. *N Engl J Med.* 1975;292:390–392.
19. Forrest JN, Cox M, Hong C, et al. Superiority of demeclocycline over lithium in the treatment of chronic syndrome of inappropriate secretion of antidiuretic hormone. *N Engl J Med.* 1978;298:173–177.
20. Chawla R. Hyponatremia. In: Chawla R, Subhash T, eds. *ICU Protocols: A Stepwise Approach.* India: Springer; 2012:433–440.
21. Rose BD. *Clinical Physiology of Acid–Base and Electrolyte Disorders.* 5th ed. New York: McGraw-Hill; 2001.

22. Kumar S, Berl T. Sodium. *Lancet.* 1998;352:220–228.
23. Funk GC, Lindner G, Druml W, et al. Incidence and prognosis of dysnatremias present on ICU admission. *Intensive Care Med.* 2010;36:304–311.
24. Lindner G, Funk GC, Schwarz C, et al. Hypernatremia in the critically ill is an independent risk factor for mortality. *Am J Kidney Dis.* 2007;50:952–957.
25. Darmon M, Timsit JF, Francais A, et al. Association between hypernatremia acquired in the ICU and mortality: a cohort study. *Nephrol Dial Transplant.* 2010;25:2510–2515.
26. Lindner G, Funk GC, Lassnigg A, et al. Intensive care-acquired hypernatremia after major cardiothoracic surgery is associated with increased mortality. *Intensive Care Med.* 2010;36:1718–1723.
27. Stelfox HT, Ahmed SB, Khandwala F, et al. The epidemiology of intensive care unit-acquired hyponatremia and hypernatremia in medical-surgical intensive care units. *Crit Care.* 2008;12:R162.
28. Stelfox HT, Ahmed SB, Zygun D, et al. Characterization of intensive care unit acquired hyponatreamia and hypernatremia following cardiac surgery. *Can J Anaesth.* 2010;57:650–658.
29. O'Donoghue SD, Dulhunty JM, Bandeshe HK, et al. Acquired hypernatremia is an independent predictor of mortality in critically ill patients. *Anesthesia.* 2009;64:514–520.
30. Bratusch-Marrain PR, DeFronzo RA. Impairment of insulin-mediated glucose metabolism by hyperosmolality in man. *Diabetes.* 1983;32:1028–1034.
31. Hoorn EJ, de Vogel S, Zietse R. Insulin resistance in an 18-year-old patient with Down syndrome presenting with hyperglycemia coma, hypernatremia, and rhabdomyolysis. *J Intern Med.* 2005;528:285–288.
32. Alonso PC, Matute SS, Urena SF, et al. Rhabdomyolysis secondary to hypernatremia. *An Pediatr (Barc).* 2010;73:223–224.
33. Denman JP. Hypernatremia and rhabdomyolysis. *Med J Aust.* 2007;187:527–528.
34. Kozeny GA, Murdock DK, Euler DE, et al. In vivo effects of acute changes in osmolality and sodium concentration on myocardial contractility. *Am Heart J.* 1985;109:290–296.
35. Robertson GL, Aycinena P, Zerbe RL. Neurogenic disorders of osmoregulation. *Am J Med.* 1982;72: 339–353.
36. Chawla R. Hypernatremia. In: Chawla R, Subhash T, eds. *ICU Protocols: A Stepwise Approach.* India: Springer; 2012:441–446.
37. Haddow JE, Cohen DL. Understanding and managing hypernatremic dehydration. *Pediatr Clin North Am.* 1974;21:435–441.
38. Adrogue HJ, Madias NE. Hypernatremia. *N Engl J Med.* 2000;342:1493–1499.
39. Lindner G, Funk GC. Hypernatremia in critically ill patients. *J Crit Care.* 2013;28:216.e11–216.e20.
40. Gennari F. Hypokalemia. *N Engl J Med.* 1998;339:451–458.
41. Fulop M. Hyperkalemia in diabetic ketoacidosis. *Am J Med Sci.* 1990;299:164–169.
42. Williams ME, Gervino EV, Rosa RM, et al. Catecholamine modulation of rapid potassium shifts during exercise. *N Engl J Med.* 1985;312:823–827.
43. Tannen RL. Potassium disorders. In: Kokko JP, Tannen RL, eds. *Fluids and Electrolytes.* 3rd ed. Philadelphia, PA: WB Saunders; 1996:111–199.
44. Subhash T. Hypokalemia and Hyperkalemia. In: Chawala R, Subhash T, eds. *ICU Protocols: A Stepwise Approach.* India: Springer; 2012.
45. Kruse JA, Carlson RW. Rapid correction of hypokalemia using concentrated intravenous potassium chloride infusions. *Arch Intern Med.* 1990;150:613–617.
46. Dyckner T. Relation of cardiovascular disease to potassium and magnesium deficiencies. *Am J Cardiol.* 1990;65:44–46.
47. Weiner ID, Wingo CS. Hyperkalemia: a potential silent killer. *J Am Soc Nephrol.* 1998;9:1535–1543.
48. Fisch C. Relation of electrolyte disturbances to cardiac arrhythmias. *Circulation.* 1973;47:408–419.
49. Montague BT, Ouellette JR, Buller GK. Retrospective review of the frequency of ECG changes in hyperkalemia. *Clin J Am Soc Nephrol.* 2008;3:324–330.
50. Szerlip HM, Weiss J, Singer I. Profound hyperkalemia without electrocardiographic manifestations. *Am J Kidney Dis.* 1986;7:461–465.
51. Weisberg LS. Potassium Homeostasis. In: Carlson RW, Geheb MA, eds. *Principle and Practice of Medical Intensive Care.* Philadelphia, PA: Saunders; 1993.
52. Schwartz AB. Potassium-related cardiac arrhythmias and their treatment. *Angiology.* 1978;29:194–205.
53. Bisogno JL, Langley A, Von DMM. Effect of calcium to reverse the electrocardiographic effects of hyperkalemia in the isolated rat heart: a prospective, dose–response study. *Crit Care Med.* 1994;22:697–704.
54. Semple P, Booth C. Calcium chloride: a reminder. *Anesthesia.* 1996;51:93.
55. Weisberg LS. Management of severe hyperkalemia. *Crit Care Med.* 2008;36:3246–3251.

56. Bower JO, Mengle HAK. The additive effect of calcium and digitalis. A warning with a report of two deaths. *JAMA.* 1936;106:1151–1153.
57. Shrager MW. Digitalis intoxication: a review and report of forty cases, with emphasis on etiology. *AMA Arch Intern Med.* 1957;100:881–893.
58. DeFronzo RA, Felig P, Ferrannini E, et al. Effects of graded doses of insulin on splanchnic and peripheral potassium metabolism in man. *Am J Physiol.* 1980;238:E421–E427.
59. Clausen T, Everts ME. Regulation of the Na/K-pump in skeletal muscle. *Kidney Int.* 1989;35:1–13.
60. Allon M, Takeshian A, Shanklin N. Effect of insulin-plus-glucose infusion with or without epinephrine on fasting hyperkalemia. *Kidney Int.* 1993;43:212–217.
61. Allon M, Copkney C. Albuterol and insulin for treatment of hyperkalemia in hemodialysis patients. *Kidney Int.* 1990;38:869–872.
62. Goldfarb S, Cox M, Singer I, et al. Acute hyperkalemia induced by hyperglycemia: hormonal mechanisms. *Ann Intern Med.* 1976;84:426–432.
63. Kamel KS, Wei C. Controversial issues in the treatment of hyperkalemia. *Nephrol Dial Transplant.* 2003;18:2215–2218.
64. Schwarz KC, Cohen BD, Lubash GD, et al. Severe acidosis and hyperpotassemia treated with sodium bicarbonate infusion. *Circulation.* 1959;19:215–220.
65. Fraley DS, Adler S. Correction of hyperkalemia by bicarbonate despite constant blood pH. *Kidney Int.* 1977;12:354–360.
66. Blumberg A, Weidmann P, Shaw S, et al. Effect of various therapeutic approaches on plasma potassium and major regulating factors in terminal renal failure. *Am J Med.* 1988;85:507–512.
67. Gutierrez R, Schlessinger F, Oster JR, et al. Effect of hypertonic versus isotonic sodium-bicarbonate on plasma potassium concentration in patients with end-stage renal disease. *Miner Electrolyte Metab.* 1991;17:297–302.
68. Allon M, Shanklin N. Effect of bicarbonate administration on plasma potassium in dialysis patients: interactions with insulin and albuterol. *Am J Kidney Dis.* 1996;28:508–514.
69. Kim HJ. Combined effect of bicarbonate and insulin with glucose in acute therapy of hyperkalemia in end-stage renal disease patients. *Nephron.* 1996;72:476–482.
70. Blumberg A, Weidmann P, Ferrari P. Effect of prolonged bicarbonate administration on plasma potassium in terminal renal failure. *Kidney Int.* 1992;41:369–374.
71. Brown MJ, Brown DC, Murphy MB. Hypokalemia from beta2-receptor stimulation by circulating epinephrine. *N Engl J Med.* 1983;309:1414–1419.
72. Montoliu J, Lens XM, Revert L. Potassium-lowering effect of albuterol for hyperkalemia in renal failure. *Arch Intern Med.* 1987;147:713–717.
73. Allon M, Dunlay R, Copkney C. Nebulized albuterol for acute hyperkalemia in patients on hemodialysis. *Ann Intern Med.* 1989;110:426–429.
74. Montoliu J, Lens XM, Revert L. Treatment of hyperkalemia in renal failure with salbutamol inhalation. *J Intern Med.* 1990;228:35–37.
75. Liou HH, Chiang SS, Wu SC, et al. Hypokalemic effects of intravenous infusion or nebulization of salbutamol in patients with chronic renal failure. *Am J Kidney Dis.* 1994;23:266–270.
76. Kemper MJ, Harps E, Müller-Wieffel DE. Hyperkalemia: therapeutic options in acute and chronic renal failure. *Clin Nephrol.* 1996;46:67–69.
77. Halperin ML. Potassium. *Lancet.* 1998;352:135–142.
78. Mandelberg A, Krupnik Z, Houri S, et al. Salbutamol metered-dose inhaler with spacer for hyperkalemia: how fast? How safe? *Chest.* 1999;115:617–622.
79. Frohnert PP, Johnson WJ, Mueiier GJ, et al. Resin treatment of hyperkalemia I. Exchange properties of a cation exchange resin (calcium cycle). *J Lab Clin Med.* 1968;71:834–839.
80. Frohnert PP, Johnson WJ, Mueiier GJ, et al. Resin treatment of hyperkalemia II. Clinical experience with a cation exchange resin (calcium cycle). *J Lab Clin Med.* 1968;71:840–846.
81. Emmett M, Hootkins RE, Fine KD, et al. Effect of three laxatives and a cation exchange resin on fecal sodium and potassium excretion. *Gastroenterology.* 1995;108:752–760.
82. Rogers RB, Li SC. Acute colonic necrosis associated with sodium polystyrene sulfonate (Kayexalate) enemas in critically-ill patients: case report and review of the literature. *J Trauma.* 2001;51: 395–397.
83. Rashid A, Hamilton SR. Necrosis of the gastrointestinal tract in uremic patients as a result of sodium polystyrene sulfonate (Kayexalate) in sorbitol: an under-recognized condition. *Am J Surg Pathol.* 1997;21: 60–69.

84. Scott TR, Graham SM, Schweitzer EJ, et al. Colonic necrosis following sodium polystyrene sulfonate (Kayexalate)–sorbitol enema in a renal transplant patient. Report of a case and review of the literature. *Dis Colon Rectum.* 1993;36:607–609.
85. Wootton FT, Rhodes DF, Lee WM, et al. Colonic necrosis with kayexalate-sorbitol enemas after renal transplantation. *Ann Intern Med.* 1989;111:947–949.
86. Abraham SC, Bhagavan BS, Lee LA, et al. Upper gastrointestinal tract injury in patients receiving kayexalate (sodium polystyrene sulfonate) in sorbitol: clinical, endoscopic, and histopathologic findings. *Am J Surg Pathol.* 2001;25:637–644.
87. Cheng ES, Stringer KM, Pegg SP. Colonic necrosis and perforation following oral sodium polystyrene sulfonate (resonium A/kayexalate) in a burn patient. *Burns.* 2002;28:189–190.
88. Dardik A, Moesinger RC, Efron G, et al. Acute abdomen with colonic necrosis induced by kayexalate-sorbitol. *South Med J.* 2000;93:511–513.
89. Gardiner GW. Kayexalate (sodium polystyrene sulfonate) in sorbitol associated with intestinal necrosis in uremic patients. *Can J Gastroenterol.* 1997;11:573–577.
90. Roy-Chaudhury P, Meisels IS, Freedman S, et al. Combined gastric and ileocecal toxicity (serpiginous ulcers) after oral kayexalate in sorbitol therapy. *Am J Kidney Dis.* 1997;30:120–122.
91. Watson M, Abbott KC, Yuan CM. Damned if you do, damned if you don't: potassium binding resins in hyperkalemia. *Clin J Am Soc Nephrol.* 2010;5:1723–1726.
92. Evans BM, Evans BM. Ion-exchange resins in the treatment of anuria. *Lancet.* 1953;262:791–795.
93. Scherr L, Ogden DA, Mead AW, et al. Management of hyperkalemia with a cation-exchange resin. *N Engl J Med.* 1961;264:115–119.
94. Flinn RB, Merrill JP, Welzan WR. Treatment of the oliguric patient with a new sodium ion-exchange resin and sorbitol: a preliminary report. *N Engl J Med.* 1961;264:111–115.
95. Lillemoe KD, Romolo JL, Hamilton SR, et al. Intestinal necrosis due to sodium polystyrene (Kayexalate) in sorbitol enemas: clinical and experimental support for the hypothesis. *Surgery.* 1987;101:267–272.
96. McGowan CE, Saha S, Chu G, et al. Intestinal necrosis due to sodium polystyrene sulfonate (Kayexalate) in sorbitol. *South Med J.* 2009;102:493–497.
97. Sterns RH, Rojas M, Bernstein P, et al. Ion-exchange resins for the treatment of hyperkalemia: are they safe and effective? *J Am Soc Nephrol.* 2010;21:733–735.
98. Harel Z, Harel S, Shah PS, et al. Gastrointestinal adverse events with sodium polystyrene sulfonate (Kayexalate) use: a systematic review. *Am J Med.* 2013;126:264e.
99. Kopp JB, Ball LK, Cohen A. Kidney patient care in disasters: lessons from hurricanes and earthquakes of 2005. *Clin J Am Soc Nephrol.* 2007;2:814–824.
100. Centers for Medicare and Medicaid Services. *Preparing For Emergencies: A Guide for People on Dialysis.* CMS publication No. 10150. Baltimore, MD: Department of Health and Human Services, Centers for Medicare and Medicaid Services; 2007.
101. Miller AC, Arquilla B. Chronic diseases and natural hazards: impact of disasters on diabetic, renal and cardiac patients. *Prehosp Disaster Med.* 2008;23:185–194.
102. Amundson D, Dadekian G, Etienne M, et al. Practicing internal medicine onboard the USNS COMFORT in the aftermath of the Haitian earthquake. *Ann Intern Med.* 2010;152:733–737.
103. Zehnder C, Gutzwiller JP, Huber A, et al. Low-potassium and glucose-free dialysis maintains urea but enhances potassium removal. *Nephrol Dial Transplant.* 2001;16:78–84.
104. Ahmed J, Weisberg LS. Hyperkalemia in dialysis patients. *Semin Dial.* 2001;14:348–356.
105. Shane E, Irani D. Hypercalcemia: pathogenesis, differential diagnosis, and management. In: Favus MJ, ed. *Primer on the Metabolic Bone Diseases and Disorders of Mineral Metabolism.* Philadelphia, PA: Lippincott-Raven; 1996:217–219.
106. Wilson RF, Binkley LE, Sabo FM Jr, et al. Electrolyte and acid–base changes with massive blood transfusions. *Am Surg.* 1992;9:535–544.
107. Weiss-Guillet E-M, Takala J, Jakob SM. Diagnosis and management of electrolyte emergencies. *Best Pract Res Clin Endocrinol Metab.* 2003;17(4):623–651.
108. Cholst IN, Steinberg SF, Tropper PJ, et al. The influence of hypermagnesemia on serum calcium and parathyroid hormone levels in human subjects. *N Engl J Med.* 1984;310:1221–1225.
109. Suki WN, Massry MG, eds. *Therapy of Renal Diseases and Related Disorders.* 2nd ed. Norwell, MA: Kluwer Academic Publishers; 1991.
110. Fisken RA, Heath DA, Somers S, et al. Hypercalcemia in hospital patients: clinical and diagnostic aspects. *Lancet.* 1981;1:202–207.
111. Klee GG, Kao, PC, Heath, H III. Hypercalcemia. *Endocrinol Metab Clin North Am.* 1988;17:573–600.

112. Bajorunas DR. Clinical manifestations of cancer-related hypercalcemia. *Semin Oncol* 1990;17(2)(suppl 5): 16–25.
113. Suki WN, Yium JJ, Von Minden M, et al. Acute treatment of hypercalcemia with furosemide. *N Engl J Med.* 1970;283:836–840.
114. Kammerman S, Canfield RE. Effect of porcine calcitonin on hypercalcemia in man. *J Clin Endocrinol Metabol.* 1970;31:70–75.
115. Wisneski LA. Salmon calcitonin in the acute management of hypercalcemia. *Calcif Tissue Int.* 1990;46(suppl):S26–S30.
116. McCurdy MT, Shanholtz CB. Oncologic Emergencies. *Crit Care Med.* 2012;40:2212–2222.
117. Wimalawansa SJ. Optimal frequency of administration of pamidronate in patients with hypercalcemia of malignancy. *Clin Endocrinol (Oxf).* 1994;41:591–595.
118. Smith IE, Powles TJ. Mithramycin for hypercalcemia associated with myeloma and other malignancies. *BMJ.* 1975;1:268–269.
119. Bilezikian JP. Management of acute hypercalcemia. *N Engl J Med.* 1992;326:1196–1203.
120. Wong ET, Rude RK, Singer FR, et al. A high prevalence of hypomagnesemia and hypermagnesemia in hospitalized patients. *Am J Clin Pathol.* 1983;79:348–352.
121. Elisaf M, Merkouropoulos M, Tsianos EV, et al. Pathogenetic mechanisms of hypomagnesemia in alcoholic patients. *J Trace Elem Med Biol.* 1995;9:210–214.
122. Dyckner T. Serum magnesium in acute myocardial infarction. Relation to arrhythmias. *Acta Med Scand.* 1980;207:59–66.
123. Al Ghamdi SM, Cameron EC, Sutton RA. Magnesium deficiency: pathophysiologic and clinical overview. *Am J Kidney Dis.* 1994;24:737–752.
124. Elisaf M, Panteli K, Theodorou J, et al. Fractional excretion of magnesium in normal subjects and in patients with hypomagnesemia. *Magnes Res.* 1997;10:315–320.
125. Agus ZA, Wasserstein A, Gold Farb S. Disorders of calcium and magnesium homeostasis. *Am J Med.* 1982;72:473–488.
126. Morisaki H, Yamamoto S, Morita Y, et al. Hypermagnesemia-induced cardiopulmonary arrest before induction of anesthesia for emergency cesarean section. *J Clin Anesth.* 2000;12:224–226.
127. Schelling JR. Fatal hypermagnesemia. *Clin Nephrol.* 2000;53:61–65.
128. Mordes JP, Wacker WE. Excess magnesium. *Pharmacol Rev.* 1977;29:273–300.

39

Rhabdomyolysis

Audrey K. Wagner and Deborah M. Stein

BACKGROUND

Rhabdomyolysis is a syndrome characterized by the necrosis of striated muscle and the subsequent release of intracellular contents—including myoglobin, electrolytes, creatine kinase (CK), and other sarcoplasmic proteins—into the systemic circulation.[1] Rhabdomyolysis has multiple etiologies, including physical, metabolic, toxicologic, and genetic. Presentation ranges from an asymptomatic elevation in diagnostic markers to a life-threatening emergency characterized by hypovolemic shock, renal failure, severe electrolyte abnormalities, cardiac dysrhythmias, compartment syndrome, and disseminated intravascular coagulopathy (DIC).

EPIDEMIOLOGY

While the true incidence of rhabdomyolysis is unknown, it is reported to occur in up to 85% of patients with traumatic injuries.[2] It affects patients of all ages and does not demonstrate a gender bias.[3–5] Because of their greater muscle mass, men do tend to experience a more severe clinical course and a greater alteration in diagnostic markers; however, outcomes do not differ significantly between genders.[6] Interestingly, studies of nondisaster hospital admissions for rhabdomyolysis reveal a predominance of male patients,[7–12] which likely reflects the greater incidence of traumatic injury in males.

Approximately 15% to 50% of patients with rhabdomyolysis will develop acute kidney injury (AKI), the syndrome's most feared complication.[7,9,11,13] The incidence of rhabdomyolysis-associated AKI accounts for 7% to 10% of all cases of AKI in the United States.[14] Development of AKI in the setting of rhabdomyolysis portends a poor prognosis and is associated with a mortality of 40% to 59%.[7,8,10] Fortunately, most of those who survive will recover renal function and not require long-term dialysis.[1]

ETIOLOGY

Rhabdomyolysis is caused by a broad range of injuries, illnesses, toxins, and genetic influences. Table 39.1 lists the categories of common causes with representative examples of each.[2,13,14] The five most commonly reported causes are (1) trauma, (2) drugs/alcohol, (3) compression/immobilization, (4) ischemia, and (5) seizures.[7–11,13,15]

TABLE 39.1 Causes of Rhabdomyolysis

Excessive muscle activity
  Exercise/exertion
  Seizures
 	
Trauma
  Crush injury/syndrome
 	
Burns
 	
Compartment syndrome
 	
Ischemia
  Vascular occlusion
  Sickle cell disease
 	
Electrical injury
  Lightening
  Electrical shock
  Cardioversion
 	
Hypo/hyperthermia
  Malignant hyperthermia
  Neuroleptic malignant syndrome
	Metabolic disorders
	  Diabetic ketoacidosis
	  Hyperosmolar
	  Hyperglycemic state
	  Hypothyroidism
	  Hyper/hyponatremia
	  Hypokalemia
	  Hypophosphatemia
	
	Autoimmune disease
	  Polymyositis
	  Dermatomyositis
	
	Genetic disorders
	  McArdle disease
	  Carnitine deficiency
	  Phosphofructokinase deficiency
	  Muscular dystrophies
	
	Compression
	  Prolonged immobilization (including long surgeries)
	
	Idiopathic
		Drugs
		  Cocaine
		  Heroin
		  Amphetamine
		  Phencyclidine
		
		Medications
		  Statins
		  Antipsychotics
		  Sedatives
		  Salicylates
		
		Toxins
		  Alcohol
		  Toxic alcohols
		  Insect bites
		  Snake bites
		
		Infections/sepsis
		  Tetanus
		  Legionella
		  Streptococcus
		  Staphylococcus

HISTORY AND PHYSICAL EXAM

In patients with obvious trauma or crush injuries, the signs and symptoms concerning for the development of rhabdomyolysis are usually readily apparent. For patients with nontraumatic rhabdomyolysis, exam findings and reported symptoms may be subtler.

Classic rhabdomyolysis symptoms include muscle pain and swelling, weakness, and dark-colored urine.[2,13,14] Commonly involved muscle groups include the calves, thighs, and lower back.[2,16] Muscle pain may be generalized or localized to a specific muscle group. It may be mild, severe, or—importantly—absent, as it is in up to 50% of patients eventually diagnosed with rhabdomyolysis.[11,13] Systemic complaints can include fever, malaise, nausea, and vomiting.[2,16]

In patients without history of trauma, the physical exam is frequently nonspecific. Swelling, if present, may be apparent on presentation or may develop only after the patient has received fluid resuscitation.[13] Patients may be tachycardic due to pain, dehydration, or fluid shifts into injured muscles. Other suggestive findings include signs of limb ischemia, such as pain, pallor, paresthesias, and pulselessness, with or without associated compartmental swelling. Dermatologic findings, including skin bruising and signs of pressure necrosis, may indicate compression injury, a frequent cause of rhabdomyolysis. Given the wide variability in presentation, it is always reasonable to consider the diagnosis of rhabdomyolysis in a patient found immobile or unresponsive for an unknown or prolonged period of time.

A special note about compartment syndrome is warranted, as it can be both the cause and the result of rhabdomyolysis. In the patient being treated for rhabdomyolysis, continued monitoring of fixed compartments is necessary as exam findings consistent with compartment syndrome may be delayed in presentation until resuscitative fluids shift into the injured muscles. Any concern for compartment syndrome should trigger the measurement of pressures and a surgical consultation for possible fasciotomy.

DIAGNOSTIC EVALUATION

The diagnostic challenge of rhabdomyolysis is remembering to include it as part of one's differential. Once considered, the diagnostic workup is relatively straightforward.

Creatine Kinase

Serum CK—and specifically the muscle isoenzyme CK-MM—is the most sensitive marker of muscle injury and the universally accepted test for rhabdomyolysis.[17] Serum CK begins to rise within 2 to 12 hours of the onset of muscle injury, peaks in 1 to 3 days, and declines 3 to 5 days after muscle injury has stopped.[14] Rhabdomyolysis does not have a diagnostic CK cutoff value; however, a level five times the upper limit of normal is strongly suggestive.[17] CK levels that do not decline as expected raise the likelihood of continued injury and compartment syndrome.

Urinalysis

Myoglobinuria is found almost exclusively as a result of rhabdomyolysis and begins to occur when plasma levels of myoglobin reach 0.5 to 1.5 mg/dL.[1,13] When rhabdomyolysis is suspected in the emergency department (ED), the initial test of choice is a urine dipstick and microscopic analysis. A urine dipstick positive for blood, combined with an absence of red blood cells on microscopy, is suggestive of rhabdomyolysis. However, the utility of this diagnostic method is limited, as the reported sensitivities of dipsticks for blood range from 14% to 82%[13,18] and because the presence of red blood cells on microscopy does not exclude concomitant myoglobinuria, especially in the setting of trauma.

CK and Serum Myoglobin

Although CK is generally accepted as the most sensitive test for diagnosis and monitoring of rhabdomyolysis, some investigators argue that serum myoglobin, as the pathogenic entity, is the preferred marker to follow over time. Studies correlating CK and myoglobin levels with the incidence of renal failure have had widely disparate results.[8,9,19,20] Debate about their efficacy hinges on elimination kinetics; myoglobin has a half-life of 12 hours, versus 42 hours for CK.[21] Some authors argue that the rapid clearance of myoglobin makes it a less sensitive marker for muscle injury[22] and that longer and more consistent elevations of CK make it more reliable.[12] Others argue that myoglobin is more accurate precisely because of its faster elimination kinetics.[19] Test cost and availability are additional considerations; while assays exist for testing serum myoglobin directly, they are expensive and not readily available or expedient in most hospitals. For these reasons, CK remains the more commonly used diagnostic marker.

Additional Studies

Additional studies that assess for complications of rhabdomyolysis include an electrocardiogram (ECG), complete blood count, basic metabolic profile, calcium, phosphate, uric acid, albumin, coagulation studies, troponin, and an arterial blood gas.

Potassium

Hyperkalemia is a life-threatening complication of rhabdomyolysis. It is caused by the release of high levels of potassium from the intracellular space of the necrotic muscle cells.[14] AKI and metabolic acidosis sustained as part of rhabdomyolysis may exacerbate this complication.

Phosphate and Calcium

In the early phase of rhabdomyolysis, phosphorus released from the cells results in hyperphosphatemia, which, in turn, causes calcium deposition in damaged tissues and subsequent hypocalcemia.[16] Later in the course of the disease, calcium is released from the cells; this, together with secondary hyperparathyroidism from the initial hypocalcemia, may result in hypercalcemia. Consequently, calcium should not be given to treat the initial hypocalcemia—except in cases of tetany or hyperkalemia-induced ECG changes—as doing so may result in metastatic calcification.[14,16,23]

BUN/Creatinine

Renal function should be monitored in all patients with either suspected or established rhabdomyolysis, as AKI is a serious and common complication of the disease. As a rule, any rise in creatinine should be interpreted as a sign of worsening renal clearance and should raise concern for AKI. It has been suggested that elevated creatinine may relate to both renal injury and to the release of preformed creatinine from damaged muscles, although several studies have failed to support this hypothesis.[13,14]

Anion Gap/Coagulation

Other lab abnormalities may include an elevated anion gap and hypoalbuminemia. Anion gap elevations result from the release of lactate, uric acid, and other organic acids from muscle cells. A falling serum albumin, which portends a poor prognosis, occurs because of leakage of albumin from damaged capillaries into interstitial tissues.[16] Finally, DIC is a common complication of severe rhabdomyolysis; high-risk patients should be screened for DIC with a complete blood count and coagulation studies.[14]

MANAGEMENT GUIDELINES

The management of rhabdomyolysis consists of (1) identifying and treating the underlying cause and (2) minimizing subsequent complications. As a complete discussion of etiologies of rhabdomyolysis lies outside the scope of this chapter, the discussion here will focus on minimizing complications.

The pathogenesis of AKI in rhabdomyolysis is a prerenal state caused by (1) the sequestration of fluid in injured muscles and an associated intravascular volume depletion and (2) intrinsic disease, caused both by myoglobin's cytotoxic effects on the tubular epithelial cells and by the formation of obstructing casts in the distal nephrons. Patients with AKI require fluid administration not only to achieve and maintain hemodynamic stability but also to limit the myoglobinuric injury to the kidney by increasing renal perfusion, urine flow, and toxin clearance.

There is no strong evidence to guide the treatment of rhabdomyolysis as it relates to the prevention of AKI. Much of the available data come from retrospective analyses and case series. The strength of these studies is limited and the results difficult to compare because of population heterogeneity and the lack of control groups. Additionally, investigators employ differing definitions of rhabdomyolysis and renal failure (ranging from creatinine >1.5 mg/dL to the need for hemodialysis) and recommend significantly variable treatment approaches.

Timing and Volume of Fluids

Based on available data, it is recommended that fluid resuscitation be initiated as early as possible, ideally within 6 hours of evidence of injury and, when appropriate, in the prehospital setting.[1,2,17,24] Several case series support early and aggressive hydration to lower renal failure risk.[25–27] In a report of the sixteen crush victims from the 2003 earthquake in Turkey, those patients requiring hemodialysis had a significantly longer wait time between rescue and initiation of fluid resuscitation (average 9.2 hours) compared to those who did not require hemodialysis (average 3.7 hours). Victims who required hemodialysis also received significantly less fluid volume (11 ± 2.5 L vs. 21.8 ± 2.7 on day 1).[28] Case studies of other earthquake victims have reported similar outcomes.[5,29]

The optimal fluid volume for resuscitation is unknown. No controlled studies compare specific volumes or targeted urine goals, and there are no established formulas (such as the Parkland formula for burn victims) to help direct resuscitation. Guidelines for fluid administered generally advise an initial 2 to 3 L at 1 to 1.5 L per hour, followed by an ongoing infusion of 200 to 700 mL per hour until diuresis is established, at which point fluid administration should be titrated for a urine output of about 300 mL per hour.[17,24,30,31]

It is important to remember that elderly patients and those suffering from congestive heart failure may not tolerate aggressive volume resuscitation and should be closely monitored for signs of volume overload. Either invasive or noninvasive hemodynamic monitoring may be useful to help guide fluid administration. All critically ill patients should have a urinary catheter placed to facilitate careful monitoring of urine output.

Choice of Fluid

The only prospective randomized single-blind study addressing the question of crystalloid choice compared the use of normal saline (NS) to lactated Ringer's (LR) in 28 patients with rhabdomyolysis caused by doxylamine overdose (a first generation antihistamine).[32] Although the NS group used more bicarbonate and diuretics, there was no significant difference in median time to CK normalization between the groups (96 h in LR group, 120 h in NS group). The study's small size may, however, have left it underpowered to detect a difference. Of note, no problems with hyperkalemia were noted in the LR group, and lactate seemed to be protective against—and not causal of—metabolic acidosis.

Sodium Bicarbonate and Mannitol

The most controversial aspect of rhabdomyolysis management is the role, if any, for sodium bicarbonate and mannitol. Few studies address this question directly, in part because the majority of rhabdomyolysis studies report using both therapies and provide limited data on patients administered only crystalloid. Additionally, there are no controlled studies evaluating the efficacy of bicarbonate and mannitol individually, making it difficult to determine the relative importance of either in the prevention of AKI.[28,33]

Both sodium bicarbonate and mannitol have theoretical benefits in the treatment of rhabdomyolysis. Sodium bicarbonate alkalinizes the urine, which is thought to minimize tubular damage and cast formation by increasing myoglobin's solubility and limiting its precipitation with the Tamm-Horsfall protein, a principal urinary glycoprotein.[1,34] A nonreabsorbed solute, sodium bicarbonate, also promotes diuresis and may be beneficial in managing the hyperkalemia often seen in rhabdomyolysis.[34] In addition to these proposed benefits, sodium bicarbonate can ameliorate metabolic acidosis, which may be present in patients with severe rhabdomyolysis and which may be compounded by administration of large volumes of NS.[1,31]

Mannitol has been used in rhabdomyolysis management as an osmotic agent to extract fluid from injured muscles and expand plasma volume and increase urinary flow, theoretically increasing the excretion of myoglobin and limiting its blockage of renal tubules. Through its osmotic effects on muscles, mannitol may aid in the prevention and treatment of compartment syndrome.[26] Studies suggest that mannitol may also protect the kidney from oxidant injury by scavenging free radicals,[35] although in at least one animal model, this did not prove true.[36]

There are two English-language controlled studies that have evaluated the efficacy of bicarbonate/mannitol (BIC/MAN) versus crystalloid alone. The first was a retrospective review of all adult trauma ICU admissions over 5 years at a level 1 trauma center; of these, 382 patients had a peak CK > 5,000. At the surgeon's discretion, 154 (40%) of these patients were treated with bicarbonate and mannitol and 228 (60%) were not. There was no statistical difference in the incidence of acute renal failure (defined as creatinine >2.0 mg/dL), dialysis, or mortality between the two groups. It is notable, however, that there was a significant difference in the peak CK between the two groups, with the BIC/MAN group having an average peak CK of about 23.5 K and the no BIC/MAN group having an average peak CK of 9.8 K. A subsequent subgroup analysis of patients by peak CK level revealed no statistically significant difference in the incidence of AKI, need for dialysis, or mortality, but among patients with CK > 30 K, there was a strong trend toward improved outcomes for those treated with BIC/MAN. This finding suggests that patients with severe rhabdomyolysis may benefit from BIC/MAN; however, the authors concluded that overall, BIC/MAN does not prevent AKI, need for dialysis, or mortality in patients with CK > 5 K and recommend that its use in post-traumatic rhabdomyolysis patients be reevaluated.[12]

The strengths of this study include its size and the presence of a control group. It was not, however, a randomized trial, and data regarding the type, quantity, and timing of volume resuscitation were not made available, making it difficult to draw conclusions about the relative importance of BIC/MAN versus quality of fluid resuscitation.

A second smaller study evaluated the efficacy of saline versus saline/bicarbonate/mannitol (SBM) in preventing rhabdomyolysis. This retrospective review of ICU patients at risk for developing renal failure (not defined) from rhabdomyolysis (defined as CK > 500) included only 24 patients; 15 were treated with SBM, and 9 received saline only. Both groups had similar demographics and similar average initial creatinine values, but significantly different initial CK levels (SBM's average CK 3,351 IU/L, saline group 1,747 IU/L). Outcomes between the groups were not significantly different: No patients developed worsening AKI, and all had resolution of their mild azotemia.[37] The authors concluded that the progression to renal failure can be completely avoided with prophylactic treatment and that once appropriate saline expansion is provided, the addition of mannitol and bicarbonate is unnecessary.[37] However, this study reported on patients with a mild degree of rhabdomyolysis, which limits its applicability to more severe cases.

Summary of Fluid Administration Recommendations

The absence of a randomized controlled study addressing ideal fluid composition in the treatment of rhabdomyolysis makes it difficult to advocate for or against a specific resuscitative regimen. A 2013 systematic review of 27 studies evaluating therapies used to prevent AKI in rhabdomyolysis concluded that no high-level evidence exists to suggest fluid therapy combined with sodium bicarbonate and/or mannitol is superior to fluid therapy alone.[24] The review offers the following recommendations regarding the timing, volume, and type of fluid used in the prevention of AKI in rhabdomyolysis[24]:

1. Fluid administration should be initiated as soon as possible, preferably within the first 6 hours after muscle injury.
2. Fluids should be administered at a rate that maintains a urine output of 300 mL per hour or more for at least the first 24 hours, unless a medical condition precludes giving enough fluids to meet this goal.
3. Intravenous sodium bicarbonate should only be administered if necessary to correct systemic acidosis.
4. Mannitol should only be administered when fluid administration fails to maintain a urine output of 300 mL per hour and should be discontinued in patients in whom it does not augment urine output.

Given the theoretical benefit of mannitol and bicarbonate, and the trends in some studies that suggest possible benefit, many published reviews, recommendations, and guidelines still do advocate for their use, especially in severely affected patients.[1,24,31,38]

Dosing

There are no standardized regimens for the administration of sodium bicarbonate and mannitol. For sodium bicarbonate, a common approach is to add either 44 to 50 mEq to 1 L 0.45% saline or 88 to 132 mEq to 1 L of 0.5% dextrose in water. Recommended infusion rates vary from 100 mL per hour[17] to alternating 1 L of the above regimen with a liter of 0.9% saline but at a rate closer to 500 mL per hour.[1,38] For mannitol, a 20% solution is added at a dose of 0.04 to 0.1 g/kg/h to each liter of fluid administered up to 200 g per day, with a cumulative dose of up to 800 g.[1,17,38] Doses higher than this have been associated with AKI due to osmotic nephrosis.[1]

Risks

The use of bicarbonate and/or mannitol has attendant risks. The primary risk of alkalinization is worsening of hypocalcemia in the early stages of rhabdomyolysis.[34] To minimize this, it is recommended to keep serum pH below 7.5, by either administering acetazolamide or discontinuing the bicarbonate infusion. Calcium should not be administered except in cases of symptomatic hypocalcemia, as discussed above.

The use of mannitol risks the precipitation of a hyperosmolar state and requires monitoring of serum osmolality and osmolal gap. Treatment with mannitol is contraindicated in anuric patients as well as in persistently or progressively oliguric patients; mannitol should be stopped if the osmol gap rises above 55 mOsm/kg or if treatment does not effect an adequate diuresis.[1]

Renal Replacement Therapy

There are two indications for renal replacement therapy (RRT) in the setting of rhabdomyolysis. The first is the standard indication for initiating RRT in any patient: development of oliguric AKI, symptomatic volume overload, severe electrolyte disturbances (particularly hyperkalemia), or acidosis. The second is particular to rhabdomyolysis and involves the removal of myoglobin from the plasma, so as to reduce the injurious effects on the kidney.

Conventional hemodialysis (HD) effectively and efficiently corrects electrolyte abnormalities, metabolic acidosis, and volume overload. HD is unable, however, to effectively remove myoglobin because of its molecular weight (15.7 kDa) and its steric properties.[39] Continuous RRT modes have been shown to successfully remove myoglobin in several case report series[40–43]; this is attributable to their convective (vs. diffusive) method of filtration. The use of super high-flux or "high-cutoff" hemofilters has been shown to remove myoglobin even more effectively.[44–46]

Few of these case reports, however, provide any data on outcomes. In the absence of prospective studies, it is not known whether myoglobin removal through RRT affects the clinical course of rhabdomyolysis.[19] Complicating matters is that the metabolism of myoglobin is poorly understood; some studies suggest that renal function does not affect the rate of myoglobin clearance and point toward an extrarenal removal mechanism.[21,47] While removing pathogenic myoglobin from plasma is in theory beneficial, and perhaps has a role in the prophylaxis of AKI in rhabdomyolysis, it is not currently a recommended intervention.

CONCLUSION

The diagnostic challenge of rhabdomyolysis is remembering to look for it. Once suspected, diagnosis and treatment is relatively straightforward. Given the highly variable presentation of this disease, the emergency physician should consider its presence in any patient found immobilized for a prolonged or unknown period of time. A familiarity with the therapeutic concepts discussed in this chapter, most importantly early and aggressive fluid resuscitation, will help optimize patient outcomes.

LITERATURE TABLE

TRIAL	DESIGN	RESULT
Prevention of AKI		
Brown et al., *J Trauma.* 2004[12]	Retrospective cohort study of 2,083 trauma ICU patients of which 1,771 had abnormal CK (>520). Patients received either crystalloid alone or together with bicarbonate and mannitol (BIC/MAN), based on surgeon's discretion	Among patients with CK > 5,000, there was no significant difference in rates of renal failure (22% vs. 18% $p = 0.27$), dialysis (7% vs. 6%, $p = 0.57$), or mortality (15% vs. 18%, $p = 0.37$) between the group who received BIC/MAN and the group that did not. However, CK levels between the groups varied significantly (24.5 K vs. 9.8 K, respectively, $p < 0.0001$), and among those with CK > 30,000, there was a nonsignificant trend toward better outcomes with BIC/MAN (AKI 46% vs. 63%, $p = 0.41$; need for dialysis 13% vs. 38%, $p = 0.12$; mortality 29% vs. 63%, $p = 0.09$)
Scharman and Troutman, *Ann Pharmacother.* 2013[24]	Systematic analysis of 27 studies evaluating fluid administration approaches in prevention of acute renal injury/failure in patients with rhabdomyolysis	Early fluid administration (within 6 h) is important. No evidence supporting a preferred fluid type or use of bicarbonate (with or without mannitol) over crystalloid alone. No studies evaluating appropriate volume

(Continued)

LITERATURE TABLE (*Continued*)

TRIAL	DESIGN	RESULT
Cho et al., *Emerg Med J.* 2007[32]	Prospective, randomized, single-blind study comparing effectiveness of NS vs. LR in 28 patients with rhabdomyolysis induced by doxylamine intoxication	No significant time difference in normalization of urine creatinine (96 h in LR group vs. 120 h in NS group ($p = 0.058$). However, patients in LR group required significantly less bicarbonate and diuretic and had significantly more alkaline urine than did the NS group
Homsi et al., *Ren Fail.* 1997[37]	Retrospective cohort study of 24 ICU patients with rhabdomyolysis of whom 15 received saline with bicarbonate and mannitol (SMB) and 9 received only saline	Maximum CK was 3,351 ± 1,693 in the SMB group and 1,747 ± 2,345 in the saline group. Admission creatinine similar in both (1.6 vs. 1.5). Both groups had resolution of renal insufficiency without initial worsening of renal function. SMB did not appear to improve outcomes, but study limited due to small sample size and low CK ranges

REFERENCES

1. Bosch X, Poch E, Grau JM. Rhabdomyolysis and acute kidney injury. *N Engl J Med.* 2009;361(1):62–72.
2. Huerta-Alardín AL, Varon J, Marik PE. Bench-to-bedside review: rhabdomyolysis – an overview for clinicians. *Crit Care.* 2005;9(2):158–169.
3. Sever MS, Erek E, Vanholder R, et al. Lessons learned from the Marmara disaster: time period under the rubble. *Crit Care Med.* 2002;30(11):2443–2449.
4. Hatamizadeh P, Najafi I, Vanholder R, et al. Epidemiologic aspects of the Bam earthquake in Iran: the nephrologic perspective. *Am J Kidney Dis.* 2006;47(3):428–438.
5. Oda J, Tanaka H, Yoshioka T, et al. Analysis of 372 patients with Crush syndrome caused by the Hanshin-Awaji earthquake. *J Trauma.* 1997;42(3):470–475.
6. Sever MS, Erek E, Vanholder R, et al. Effect of gender on various parameters of crush syndrome victims of the Marmara earthquake. *J Nephrol.* 2004;17(3):399–404.
7. Ward MM. Factors predictive of acute renal failure in rhabdomyolysis. *Arch Intern Med.* 1988;148(7):1553–1557.
8. de Meijer AR, Fikkers BG, de Keijzer MH, et al. Serum creatine kinase as predictor of clinical course in rhabdomyolysis: a 5-year intensive care survey. *Intensive Care Med.* 2003;29(7):1121–1125. Epub May 24, 2003.
9. Melli G, Chaudhry V, Cornblath DR. Rhabdomyolysis: an evaluation of 475 hospitalized patients. *Medicine (Baltimore).* 2005;84(6):377–385.
10. Veenstra J, Smit WM, Krediet RT, et al. Relationship between elevated creatine phosphokinase and the clinical spectrum of rhabdomyolysis. *Nephrol Dial Transplant.* 1994;9(6):637–641.
11. Woodrow G, Brownjohn AM, Turney JH. The clinical and biochemical features of acute renal failure due to rhabdomyolysis. *Ren Fail.* 1995;17(4):467–474.
12. Brown CV, Rhee P, Chan L, et al. Preventing renal failure in patients with rhabdomyolysis: do bicarbonate and mannitol make a difference? *J Trauma.* 2004;56(6):1191–1196.
13. Gabow PA, Kaehny WD, Kelleher SP. The spectrum of rhabdomyolysis. *Medicine (Baltimore).* 1982;61(3):141–152.
14. Bagley WH, Yang H, Shah KH. Rhabdomyolysis. *Intern Emerg Med.* 2007;2(3):210–218.
15. Fernandez WG, Hung O, Bruno GR, et al. Factors predictive of acute renal failure and need for hemodialysis among ED patients with rhabdomyolysis. *Am J Emerg Med.* 2005;23(1):1–7.
16. Giannoglou GD, Chatzizisis YS, Misirli G. The syndrome of rhabdomyolysis: pathophysiology and diagnosis. *Eur J Intern Med.* 2007;18(2):90–100.
17. Khan FY. Rhabdomyolysis: a review of the literature. *Neth J Med.* 2009;67(9):272–283.
18. Young SE, Miller MA, Docherty M. Urine dipstick testing to rule out rhabdomyolysis in patients with suspected heat injury. *Am J Emerg Med.* 2009;27(7):875–877.
19. Mikkelsen TS, Toft P. Prognostic value, kinetics and effect of CVVHDF on serum of the myoglobin and creatine kinase in critically ill patients with rhabdomyolysis. *Acta Anaesthesiol Scand.* 2005;49(6):859–864.

20. Shigemoto T, Rinka H, Matsuo Y, et al. Blood purification for crush syndrome. *Ren Fail.* 1997;19(5):711–719.
21. Lappalainen H, Tiula E, Uotila L, et al. Elimination kinetics of myoglobin and creatine kinase in rhabdomyolysis: implications for follow-up. *Crit Care Med.* 2002;30(10):2212–2215.
22. Beetham R. Biochemical investigation of suspected rhabdomyolysis. *Ann Clin Biochem.* 2000;37(Pt 5): 581–587.
23. Knochel JP. Serum calcium derangements in rhabdomyolysis. *N Engl J Med.* 1981;305(3):161–163.
24. Scharman EJ, Troutman WG. Prevention of kidney injury following rhabdomyolysis: a systematic review. *Ann Pharmacother.* 2013;47(1):90–105.
25. Reis ND, Michaelson M. Crush injury to the lower limbs. Treatment of the local injury. *J Bone Joint Surg Am.* 1986;68(3):414–418.
26. Better OS, Stein JH. Early management of shock and prophylaxis of acute renal failure in traumatic rhabdomyolysis. *N Engl J Med.* 1990;322(12):825–829.
27. Ron D, Taitelman U, Michaelson M, et al. Prevention of acute renal failure in traumatic rhabdomyolysis. *Arch Intern Med.* 1984;144(2):277–280.
28. Gunal AI, Celiker H, Dogukan A, et al. Early and vigorous fluid resuscitation prevents acute renal failure in the crush victims of catastrophic earthquakes. *J Am Soc Nephrol.* 2004;15(7):1862–1867.
29. Shimazu T, Yoshioka T, Nakata Y, et al. Fluid resuscitation and systemic complications in crush syndrome: 14 Hanshin-Awaji earthquake patients. *J Trauma.* 1997;42(4):641–646.
30. Slater MS, Mullins RJ. Rhabdomyolysis and myoglobinuric renal failure in trauma and surgical patients: a review. *J Am Coll Surg.* 1998;186(6):693–716.
31. Malinoski DJ, Slater MS, Mullins RJ. Crush injury and rhabdomyolysis. *Crit Care Clin.* 2004;20(1): 171–192.
32. Cho YS, Lim H, Kim SH. Comparison of lactated Ringer's solution and 0.9% saline in the treatment of rhabdomyolysis induced by doxylamine intoxication. *Emerg Med J.* 2007;24(4):276–280.
33. Altintepe L, Guney I, Tonbul Z, et al. Early and intensive fluid replacement prevents acute renal failure in the crush cases associated with spontaneous collapse of an apartment in Konya. *Ren Fail.* 2007;29(6):737–741.
34. Zager RA. Rhabdomyolysis and myohemoglobinuric acute renal failure. *Kidney Int.* 1996;49(2):314–326.
35. Odeh M. The role of reperfusion-induced injury in the pathogenesis of the crush syndrome. *N Engl J Med.* 1991;324(20):1417–1422.
36. Zager RA. Combined mannitol and deferoxamine therapy for myohemoglobinuric renal injury and oxidant tubular stress. Mechanistic and therapeutic implications. *J Clin Invest.* 1992;90(3):711–719.
37. Homsi E, Barreiro MF, Orlando JM, et al. Prophylaxis of acute renal failure in patients with rhabdomyolysis. *Ren Fail.* 1997;19(2):283–288.
38. Vanholder R, Sever MS, Erek E, et al. Rhabdomyolysis. *J Am Soc Nephrol.* 2000;11(8):1553–1561.
39. Bellomo R, Daskalakis M, Parkin G, et al. Myoglobin clearance during acute continuous hemodiafiltration. *Intensive Care Med.* 1991;17(8):509.
40. Cruz DN, Bagshaw SM. Does continuous renal replacement therapy have a role in the treatment of rhabdomyolysis complicated by acute kidney injury? *Semin Dial.* 2011;24(4):417–420. doi: 10.1111/j.1525-139X.2011.00892.x. Epub Jul 29, 2011.
41. Bastani B, Frenchie D. Significant myoglobin removal during continuous veno-venous haemofiltration using F80 membrane. *Nephrol Dial Transplant.* 1997;12(9):2035–2036.
42. Amyot SL, Leblanc M, Thibeault Y, et al. Myoglobin clearance and removal during continuous venovenous hemofiltration. *Intensive Care Med.* 1999;25(10):1169–1172.
43. Zhang L, Kang Y, Fu P, et al. Myoglobin clearance by continuous venous-venous haemofiltration in rhabdomyolysis with acute kidney injury: a case series. *Injury.* 2012;43(5):619–623.
44. Naka T, Jones D, Baldwin I, et al. Myoglobin clearance by super high-flux hemofiltration in a case of severe rhabdomyolysis: a case report. *Crit Care.* 2005;9(2):R90–R95.
45. Heyne N, Guthoff M, Krieger J, et al. High cut-off renal replacement therapy for removal of myoglobin in severe rhabdomyolysis and acute kidney injury: a case series. *Nephron Clin Pract.* 2012;121(3–4): c159–c164.
46. Premru V, Kovač J, Buturović-Ponikvar J, et al. High cut-off membrane hemodiafiltration in myoglobinuric acute renal failure: a case series. *Ther Apher Dial.* 2011;15(3):287–291.
47. Wakabayashi Y, Kikuno T, Ohwada T, et al. Rapid fall in blood myoglobin in massive rhabdomyolysis and acute renal failure. *Intensive Care Med.* 1994;20(2):109–112.

40

Acute Kidney Injury and Renal Replacement Therapy

Emilee Willhem-Leen and Glenn Chertow

BACKGROUND

Acute kidney injury (AKI) is common in critical illness. A recent, large, multinational prospective study reported that 5.7% of critically ill patients will develop AKI during their illness.[1] AKI in the setting of critical illness also confers a poor prognosis. In-hospital or short-term (90-day) mortality rates for critically ill patients who develop AKI range from 45% to 60%.[1–3] Fortunately, the majority of critically ill patients who develop AKI during their hospitalization and who survive to discharge do not require long-term dialysis.[1] This chapter reviews common definitions and classifications of AKI, etiologies of the disease, and appropriate emergency department (ED) diagnostic and therapeutic interventions for patients with AKI.

DEFINITIONS

Critically ill patients may have AKI at presentation or may develop it during the course of their illness. While there is no consensus definition for AKI, the diagnosis is commonly made based on the following:

- Decreased urine output (<200 mL/12 hours) despite fluid resuscitation or diuresis
- Uremia (elevated serum urea nitrogen [BUN > 80 mg/dL]) or clinical signs of uremia (e.g., pericardial effusion, pericarditis, altered mental status)
- Serum creatinine (sCr) elevated above baseline. Of note, sCr may not rise for 12 to 24 hours following renal injury and may not be dramatically elevated at the time of presentation to the ED.

Classification of AKI

sCr concentration is not an optimal early marker of AKI because (1) it does not accurately reflect kidney function in patients whose glomerular filtration rate (GFR) is acutely changing and (2) it may be lowered by muscle wasting that accompanies critical illness. Given this limitation, several criteria have been proposed to classify the severity of AKI.

RIFLE Criteria

The RIFLE criteria (*R*isk, *I*njury, *F*ailure, *L*oss, *E*SRD [end-stage renal disease]) consist of three levels of injury that are useful in ED assessment of kidney injury (R, I, and F) and two levels (L and E) that are more typically applied during inpatient evaluation:

- *RISK*: 1.5 times increase in sCr, GFR decrease by 25%, or urine output <0.5 mL/kg/h for 6 hours
- *INJURY*: 2 times increase in sCr, GFR decrease by 50%, or urine output <0.5 mL/kg/h for 12 hours
- *FAILURE*: 3 times increase in sCr, GFR decrease by 75%, or urine output <0.3 mL/kg/h for 24 hours or anuria for 12 hours
- *LOSS*: Complete loss of kidney function for more than 4 weeks
- *ESRD*: Complete loss of kidney function for more than 3 months

Acute Kidney Injury Network Criteria

The Acute Kidney Injury Network (AKIN) criteria are based on the RIFLE criteria but simplify the system for ease of use and clarity:

- AKIN criteria definition of AKI:
  - *Stage 1*: 1.5 times increase in sCr from baseline, ≥0.3 mg/dL increase in sCr, or urine output of <0.5 mL/kg/h for 6 hours
  - *Stage 2*: 2 times increase in sCr or urine output of <0.5 mL/kg/h for 12 hours
  - *Stage 3*: 3 times increase in sCr, sCr of ≥4 mg/dL (with an acute rise of ≥0.5 mg/dL), or urine output of <0.3 mL/kg/h for 24 hours or anuria for 12 hours
- The AKIN and RIFLE criteria compare as follows:
  - *Stage 1* equivalent to RIFLE RISK
  - *Stage 2* equivalent to RIFLE INJURY
  - *Stage 3* equivalent to RIFLE FAILURE

The Kidney Disease Improving Global Outcome Criteria

The Kidney Disease Improving Global Outcome (KDIGO) criteria consist of three levels of renal injury based on either sCr or urine output:

- *Stage 1*: 1.5 to 1.9 times increase in sCr from baseline, ≥0.3 mg/dL increase in sCr, or urine output <0.5 mL/kg/h for 6 to 12 hours
- *Stage 2*: 2.0 to 2.9 times increase in sCr from baseline and urine output <0.5 mL/kg/h for >12 hours
- *Stage 3*: 3 times increase in sCr from baseline, increase in sCr to ≥4.0 mg/dL, or initiation of renal replacement and urine output <0.3 mL/kg/h for ≥24 hours or anuria for ≥12 hours

For simplicity, we recommend use of either the AKIN or KDIGO classification. Unfortunately, precise classification of AKI stage may not be possible in the ED setting; often, baseline sCr is not available, and observation of urine output takes 6 to 24 hours. However, providing critical care or nephrology colleagues with this information, as available, aids in rapid triage and prognosis. For example, if a patient with a known baseline sCr of 1.0 mg/dL presents to the ED with sepsis and an initial sCr of 2.5 mg/dL and makes <50 mL of urine during the first 2 hours of evaluation and management, he or she likely has sustained at least a stage 2 AKI (per AKIN and KDIGO criteria). No stage of AKI, alone, necessitates admission to the intensive care unit, but nephrology consultation in the ED should be considered for patients presenting with likely stage 2 or 3 AKI.

ETIOLOGY OF AKI

AKI is a heterogeneous disease that can be caused by many factors. Typically, these factors are grouped into prerenal, intrarenal, and postrenal etiologies.

Prerenal

Prerenal AKI is caused by a reduction in renal perfusion. Precipitating conditions include hypovolemic shock (usually from gastrointestinal losses or severe burns), cardiogenic shock (usually from left-sided or biventricular failure), cirrhosis (including hepatorenal syndrome), and sepsis/systemic inflammatory response syndrome. Diuretic therapy and other drugs like ACE inhibitors and NSAIDs can exacerbate a prerenal state, especially in patients with additional risk factors. Typically, the urine sodium is low (<20 mmol/L), with a fractional excretion of sodium (FENa) <1% indicating a sodium-avid state in which the body is attempting to retain or replace lost volume.

Intrarenal

Etiologies of intrarenal AKI include vascular, glomerular, and tubular/interstitial disease. Common vascular diseases associated with AKI include atheroemboli (typically associated with angiographic or surgical/endovascular procedures), vasculitis, thromboembolic disease including hemolytic uremic syndrome (HUS) and thrombotic thrombocytopenic purpura (TTP) malignant hypertension, and scleroderma renal crisis. Glomerular diseases that result in AKI include the nephritic (generally accompanied by active sediment on urinalysis [UA], i.e., red cells, white cells, and/or cellular casts) and nephrotic (generally accompanied by heavy proteinuria) syndromes (Table 40.1). Tubular and interstitial diseases are the most common causes of AKI in hospitalized patients; they include acute tubular necrosis (ATN), acute interstitial nephritis (AIN), and, less commonly, multiple myeloma cast nephropathy and tumor lysis syndrome.

ATN is the most common cause of AKI in hospitalized patients and accounts for nearly 45% of in-hospital AKI.[2] Renal ischemia, sepsis, and nephrotoxins, including radiocontrast media, heme pigment (e.g., in patients with rhabdomyolysis or hemolysis), selected cancer chemotherapeutic agents (e.g., platinum-based agents), and antibiotics (e.g., amphotericin B, aminoglycosides), are all common causes of ATN. Because ATN can occur after prolonged or severe prerenal physiology, it can at times be difficult to distinguish the two processes. In general, prerenal disease, unless it is due to hemodynamic derangements associated with heart failure, cirrhosis, or sepsis, will resolve with the correction of hypovolemia or hypotension. When the cause of injury is uncertain, urine studies can help distinguish the two etiologies; ATN will demonstrate an FENa >1% (as opposed to <1% seen in prerenal conditions) and the presence of muddy brown casts. In the future, ATN may be more rapidly identified by the detection of urinary neutrophil gelatinase-associated lipocalin (NGAL) and other renal tubular injury markers, discussed below.

TABLE 40.1 Clinical Significance of Findings on UA or Urine Microscopy

Finding on UA or Urine Microscopy	Clinical Significance
Dipstick heme	If the sample is negative for RBCs, it suggests the presence of either free hemoglobin or free myoglobin
Leukocyte esterase	Lysed neutrophils—suggestive of pyuria
Nitrite positivity	Signifies the presence of nitrate reductase, produced by many Enterobacteriaceae species
Red blood cells (RBCs)	Suggestive of glomerular injury especially if dysmorphic. Nondysmorphic RBCs are commonly the result of nephrolithiasis or malignancy
White blood cells	Neutrophils suggest bacterial infection or colonization or acute interstitial nephritis
	Eosinophils suggest allergic acute interstitial nephritis but are neither sensitive nor specific for this diagnosis
Cellular casts	
Hyaline casts	Nonspecific, but may suggest dehydration
Muddy brown	Suggestive of ATN
RBC casts	Diagnostic of glomerular hematuria. Suggestive of glomerulonephritis
White blood cell casts	Diagnostic of kidney inflammation. Suggestive of pyelonephritis or noninfectious interstitial nephritis

AIN is another cause of tubular/interstitial AKI, but it is significantly less common than ATN. AIN is typically the result of exposure to drugs; common offenders include NSAIDs and antibiotics, including penicillins and cephalosporins. Less commonly, AIN can result from infection or systemic illness (e.g., sarcoidosis, Sjogren's, systemic lupus erythematosus [SLE]). A diagnosis of AIN requires the presence of pyuria and white cell casts on UA or urine microscopy.

Postrenal

Postrenal AKI is caused by obstruction to the flow of urine, typically from ureteral compression and occasionally from other causes (e.g., stones, papillary necrosis). Pelvic malignancies (e.g., colorectal carcinoma, ovarian or cervical carcinoma, retroperitoneal lymphadenopathy) are relatively common culprits. Generally, unless the patient has preexisting chronic kidney disease (CKD), the obstruction must affect both kidneys in order for changes in sCr to be detected.

HISTORY AND PHYSICAL EXAM

Because renal disease can impact all organ systems, a comprehensive history and physical exam should be taken. Special priority should be given to the assessment of urgent or emergent indications for dialysis, such as volume overload (shortness of breath, edema) and clinical uremia (myoclonus or asterixis, pericardial rub) (Table 40.2).

DIAGNOSTIC EVALUATION

ED patients with AKI require the following diagnostic workup:

- Accurate measurement of urine output, including catheter placement if necessary
- Metabolic panel including sCr, potassium, chloride, bicarbonate, and urea nitrogen

TABLE 40.2 Targeted Medical History and Physical Exam

Medical History	Physical Exam
History: • CKD or ESRD • DM, especially long-standing, poorly controlled, known micro- or macrovascular complications (e.g., diabetic retinopathy) • HTN, especially long standing and/or poorly controlled • Autoimmune disease especially SLE or systemic sclerosis • Toxic ingestion (e.g., ethylene glycol) • Urinary obstruction or benign prostatic hypertrophy active abdominal malignancy or lymphoma *Symptoms*: • Active infection • Uncontrolled HTN: headache, blurry vision, chest pain, altered mentation • Volume overload: shortness of breath, orthopnea, edema • Uremia: weakness, anorexia, vomiting, twitching, altered mentation *Other*: • Changes in urination: hematuria, reduced urine volume, increase in urine froth or foam • Flank pain	• Abnormal vital signs: hypotension or HTN, hypoxia (suggestive of pulmonary edema) • Volume overload: elevated JVP, rales, edema, S3 gallop • Uremia: altered mentation, asterixis, pericardial friction rub, uremic fetor • Systemic illness: fever, arthralgias, pulmonary findings

- UA including microscopic evaluation and reflex urine culture, as appropriate
- Urine electrolytes including creatinine and sodium (or urine urea for patients treated with loop diuretics)
- Quantification of urinary protein with a spot urine protein to creatinine ratio
- Bedside evaluation of postvoid residual, if concern for urinary retention
- Renal ultrasound

EMERGING BIOMARKERS FOR AKI

Cystatin C

Cystatin C is an alternative filtration marker to sCr for the estimation of GFR that is being evaluated for its ability to improve the accuracy of prognosis and prediction of mortality in CKD.[4] Although a recent study did not demonstrate improved estimation of GFR using cystatin C alone when compared to sCr, the combined use of the two markers did provide a more accurate estimation of GFR.[5] Cystatin C is currently not available for clinical use in the United States.

Neutrophil Gelatinase-Associated Lipocalin

Urinary and serum NGAL is another promising potential biomarker for AKI. Produced by renal tubular epithelial cells, NGAL is released into the serum and urine in response to cellular injury; NGAL levels rise in the serum and in the urine in AKI. NGAL is currently not available for clinical use in the United States.

MANAGEMENT GUIDELINES

Hyperkalemia

In patients with severe AKI and hyperkalemia, a rapidly rising serum potassium, or a reasonable clinical expectation of impending hyperkalemia (e.g., patients with crush injury or an ischemic limb), medical therapy is an important, but temporizing, intervention that is followed in the majority of cases by hemodialysis (HD) or continuous renal replacement therapy (CRRT). Medical therapy includes antagonism of the effect of potassium on the cardiac myocyte (e.g., intravenous administration of calcium), extra- to intracellular flux of potassium (e.g., insulin and glucose, sodium bicarbonate, β2-agonism), and removal of potassium from the body via the kidneys and gut (e.g., loop diuresis and use of cation exchange resins). In some patients with hyperkalemia and AKI, these therapies may actually perform multiple functions; for example, the use of loop diuretics helps correct hyperkalemia, hyperchloremic metabolic acidosis, and volume overload.

Volume Overload in a Patient Responsive to Diuresis

Patients with AKI who are oliguric or anuric may present to the ED already volume overloaded. The degree of kidney injury and associated metabolic abnormalities determine which patients require immediate dialysis. If dialysis is not immediately indicated, the patient should be given a trial of intravenous loop diuretics; a nonresponse (urine output of <0.5 mL/kg/h or insufficient urine output to improve volume overload) usually indicates more severe renal injury and a greater diagnostic and therapeutic urgency. In patients with evolving renal injury, the sCr may not reflect the extent of impaired function, and the required dose of diuretics may be higher than expected.

Acidemia in a Nonanuric Patient

Metabolic acidosis is a common finding in patients with AKI. The metabolic acidosis observed in AKI can mimic that seen in genetic or chronic tubular dysfunction, with the location of the tubular dysfunction determined by the etiology of the AKI. For example, patients with obstructive nephropathy can develop distal (type 2) RTA. Fortunately, in the acute setting, the treatment of the patient with AKI and metabolic acidosis is nearly always the same.

While HD or CRRT can rapidly correct metabolic acidosis (of any etiology), patients with AKI who develop hyperchloremic metabolic acidosis as a result of impaired acid secretion or bicarbonate regeneration (common in the setting of low GFR) may be conservatively managed with intravenous sodium bicarbonate–containing solutions. For a mild to moderate bicarbonate deficit, one strategy is to administer an isotonic solution containing three amps of bicarbonate (150 mEq) per liter, at a rate of 1 to 2 mL/kg/h. For patients with more severe metabolic acidosis who are awaiting dialysis, bolus administration of sodium bicarbonate may be necessary. Administering sodium bicarbonate to patients with severe lactic acidosis is generally not advised; rather, attention should be focused on reversing the primary cause of lactic acidosis (e.g., septic shock).

INDICATIONS FOR DIALYSIS IN AKI

The decision to initiate dialysis from the ED is generally made in conjunction with a consulting nephrologist. The following are the commonly accepted indications for dialysis in a patient with AKI:

- Hyperkalemia or rapidly rising serum potassium
- Acidemia in an oliguric or anuric patient

- Alcohol and drug toxicities
- Volume overload refractory to diuresis
- Clinical uremia (e.g., pericarditis, mental status change)

Although there are no studies comparing outcomes for patients who have dialysis initiated in the ED to those who have dialysis initiated later in their hospital course, several high-quality observational and randomized controlled trials (RCTs) suggest that earlier initiation of dialysis or hemofiltration in critically ill patients may improve short-term outcomes such as length of ICU stay and overall survival. In one study of ICU patients from several academic ICUs, the odds ratio for survival to hospital discharge was 1.85 in the group that received dialysis at a lower BUN target (≤76 mg/dL) when compared to those whose BUN was allowed to climb to a higher target (>76 mg/dL).[6]

TYPES OF RENAL REPLACEMENT

Hemodialysis

HD is the most common form of renal replacement for hospitalized patients. Dialysis is an intermittent therapy; typically, it is performed three times per week, but it can be performed daily if necessitated by acute illness or other clinical indication. Electrolytes, solutes, and uremic toxins are removed via diffusion; the patient's blood is pumped in a countercurrent fashion along a semipermeable membrane, on the other side of which flows dialysate solution containing precise concentrations of various electrolytes. Dialysis requires venous access, typically in the form of a fistula or graft, but may also be performed by means of a temporary or permanent dialysis catheter. Dialysis rapidly addresses electrolyte, acid–base, and volume derangements; however, removal of intravascular volume in large amounts may be limited by the patient's blood pressure.

Continuous Renal Replacement Therapy

CRRT is a low-flow, continuous therapy used for critically ill patients when adequate volume removal cannot be achieved via a short intermittent session or for those patients who will not tolerate the large fluid shifts associated with dialysis. CRRT also may allow for adequate solute clearance in a patient who is highly catabolic, where intermittent dialysis may be insufficient. Clearance can be obtained via diffusion (dialysis), convection (hemofiltration), or a combination of the two. Access generally requires a catheter; CRRT cannot be performed via a patient's preexisting fistula or graft. CRRT is almost always performed in an intensive care setting.

Sustained Low-Efficiency Daily Dialysis

Sustained low-efficiency daily dialysis (SLEDD) is a hybrid therapy that combines the long treatment times and slower blood flow rates used in CRRT with the purely diffusive clearance of HD. It is used for patients who require a therapy that can provide a slower removal of volume, reduced hemodynamic perturbation, and significant solute clearance. SLEDD is used in place of CRRT in some hospitals; clinical outcomes are generally similar between the two therapies.

SPECIAL CONSIDERATIONS

Contrast-Associated Nephropathy

For many ED practitioners, the perceived risk of contrast-associated nephropathy will influence the decision to limit the use of certain imaging modalities, especially for patients with CKD or AKI. However, the true risk of contrast-associated nephropathy is likely overestimated in practice, and there is evidence that patients with kidney dysfunction are being inappropriately denied necessary and potentially lifesaving diagnostic and therapeutic procedures.[7] The decision to administer or forgo contrast in a patient with AKI should be made in conjunction with a nephrologist. If contrast is administered to patients at highest risk for contrast-associated nephropathy (e.g., patients with preexisting CKD or AKI or patients with diabetes mellitus [DM]), it is reasonable to consider prophylactic pretreatment. One strategy for pretreatment is to administer a bicarbonate-containing isotonic solution at a rate of 1 mL/kg for 6 to 12 hours prior to contrast administration, continuing for 12 hours after contrast administration. Given the lack of risk, it is also reasonable to administer acetylcysteine, either by mouth or intravenously, on the day prior to, and on the day of, contrast administration. It should be noted that the evidence for this strategy is mixed and comes with little expert consensus.[8]

LITERATURE TABLE

TRIAL	DESIGN	RESULT
Uchino et al., *JAMA.* 2006[1]	Prospective observational study of 1,738 ICU patients with AKI from 54 hospitals in 23 countries	Severe AKI occurred in 5.7% of ICU patients. Hospital mortality among critically ill patient with AKI was 60.3%. Among survivors, dialysis dependence at hospital discharge was 13.8%
Liu et al., *Clin J Am Soc Nephrol.* 2006[6] PICARD	Prospective observational study comparing low blood urea nitrogen (BUN ≤ 76 mg/dL) at initiation of renal replacement therapy to high BUN (>76 mg/dL) in 243 critically ill patients with AKI and no preexisting CKD	Relative risk for death in high BUN group was 1.85 (95% CI 1.16–2.96) after adjustment for age and severity of illness
Zhang et al., *Am J Kidney Dis.* 2011[9]	Meta-analysis of 13 studies of the use of serum and urinary cystatin C to predict AKI	Sensitivity of serum cystatin C to predict AKI was 86%; sensitivity was 82%. Urinary cystatin C was less useful as a predictor than serum cystatin C
Elahi et al., *Eur J Cardiothorac Surg.* 2004[10]	Retrospective cohort of 43 consecutive cardiac surgery patients who developed postoperative AKI requiring CRRT; for analysis, cases divided into "early" CRRT (indication was urine output <100 mL over 8 h despite furosemide administration) and "late" CRRT (indication was BUN > 30 mmol/L, creatinine >250 mmol/L, or potassium >6 mEq/L)	"Early" CRRT patients demonstrated shorter ICU stays, shorter hospital stays, and decreased mortality (22% vs. 43%, $p < 0.05$) when compared to "late" CRRT patients
Demirkilic et al., *J Cardiac Surg.* 2004[11]	Prospective nonrandomized clinical trial of 61 postcardiac surgery patients enrolled consecutively in either an early CRRT arm (1996–2001; defined as urine output <100 mL over a 8-h period despite furosemide administration) or a late CRRT arm (1992–1996; defined as sCr >5.5 mg/dL or sK ≥5.5, refractory to medical management)	Patients who received early CRRT had shorter ICU and total hospital stays, decreased ICU mortality, and decreased overall mortality, all statistically significant. Specifically, hospital mortality for early CRRT was 24% compared to 56% in late CRRT patients ($p = 0.016$)
Sugahara and Suzuki, *Hemodial Int.* 2004[12]	RCT comparing early vs. conventional initiation of CRRT in 28 post-CABG patients. Early start patients received CRRT when urine output fell below 30 mL/h for 3 consecutive hours; late-start patients received CRRT when urine output fell below 20 mL/h for 2 consecutive hours	Survival to 14 d in the early initiation group was 86%, compared with 14% in the conventional start group ($p < 0.01$)

CI, confidence interval.

CONCLUSION

AKI is common in critically ill patients and confers a poor prognosis. Identifying these patients early and determining who will require HD is a priority for the emergency physician. Application of the grading systems discussed in this chapter and—since acute AKI may not mount a significant elevation in sCr in the ED—close attention to urine output can greatly expedite achieving this goal.

REFERENCES

1. Uchino S, Kellum JA, Bellomo R, et al. Acute renal failure in critically ill patients: a multinational, multicenter study. *JAMA.* 2005;294(7):813–818.
2. Prescott GJ, Metcalfe W, Baharani J, et al. A prospective national study of acute renal failure treated with RRT: incidence, aetiology and outcomes. *Nephrol Dial Transplant.* 2007;22(9):2513–2519.
3. Liano F, Pascual J. Epidemiology of acute renal failure: a prospective, multicenter, community-based study. Madrid Acute Renal Failure Study Group. *Kidney Int.* 1996;50(3):811–818.
4. Shlipak MG, Sarnak MJ, Katz R, et al. Cystatin C and the risk of death and cardiovascular events among elderly persons. *N Engl J Med.* 2005;352(20):2049–2060.
5. Inker LA, Schmid CH, Tighiouart H, et al. Estimating glomerular filtration rate from serum creatinine and cystatin C. *N Engl J Med.* 2012;367(1):20–29.
6. Liu KD, Himmelfarb J, Paganini E, et al. Timing of initiation of dialysis in critically ill patients with acute kidney injury. *Clin J Am Soc Nephrol.* 2006;1(5):915–919.
7. Chertow GM, Normand SL, McNeil BJ. "Renalism": inappropriately low rates of coronary angiography in elderly individuals with renal insufficiency. *J Am Soc Nephrol.* 2004;15(9):2462–2468.
8. Kshirsagar AV, Poole C, Mottl A, et al. *N*-acetylcysteine for the prevention of radiocontrast induced nephropathy: a meta-analysis of prospective controlled trials. *J Am Soc Nephrol.* 2004;15(3):761–769.
9. Zhang Z, Lu B, Sheng X, et al. Cystatin C in prediction of acute kidney injury: a systemic review and meta-analysis. *Am J Kidney Dis.* 2011;58(3):356–365.
10. Elahi MM, Lim MY, Joseph RN, et al. Early hemofiltration improves survival in post-cardiotomy patients with acute renal failure. *Eur J Cardiothorac Surg.* 2004;26(5):1027–1031.
11. Demirkilic U, Kuralay E, Yenicesu M, et al. Timing of replacement therapy for acute renal failure after cardiac surgery. *J Card Surg.* 2004;19(1):17–20.
12. Sugahara S, Suzuki H. Early start on continuous hemodialysis therapy improves survival rate in patients with acute renal failure following coronary bypass surgery. *Hemodial Int.* 2004;8(4):320–325.

SECTION 10

Endocrine Critical Care

41

Glycemic Control in the Critically Ill

Daniel Runde and Jarone Lee

BACKGROUND

Glycemic control is one of the most controversial topics in critical care. A large body of evidence demonstrates a clear association between elevated blood glucose levels and increased morbidity and mortality.[1–4] Persistent hyperglycemia also correlates with poor outcomes in all subtypes of critically ill patients: postoperative, myocardial infarction, ischemic and hemorrhagic stroke, neurologic trauma, and sepsis.[5–10] Pathophysiologic changes caused by hyperglycemia affect a wide variety of biologic responses, from immune function to wound healing. Despite extensive research, however, it is yet to be determined whether hyperglycemia is a marker of disease severity; whether it directly causes poor outcomes; and whether interventions to control and regulate blood glucose levels result in improved outcomes in critically ill patients. The controversy surrounding glycemic control is driven in large part by the fact that, in contrast to hyperglycemia, even transient hypoglycemic episodes, which commonly occur in the setting of strict blood glucose control, can have potentially disastrous consequences for the critically ill patient.[11]

PATHOPHYSIOLOGY OF HYPERGLYCEMIC STATES

Stress hyperglycemia is common in the acutely ill and in both diabetic and nondiabetic patients. Hyperglycemia occurs as a response to a range of events that result in physiologic stress, including, but not limited to, trauma, hemorrhage, hypoxia, myocardial ischemia, and infection.[12–16] This stress response is mediated by a complex interaction of hormones and proinflammatory cytokines, including a dramatic increase in the production of cortisol, epinephrine, and norepinephrine, as well as tumor necrosis factor-alpha and interleukins 1 and 6. The hypothalamic–pituitary–adrenal axis plays a key role, as does the sympathoadrenal system.[17–19] Metabolically, these changes produce increases in gluconeogenesis, glycogenolysis, and insulin resistance.[2,20]

Short-term hyperglycemia may be an adaptive response to stress, resulting in improved glucose delivery to tissue that is poorly perfused at the microvascular level.[21] Macrophages, which play a key role in immune response, rely on glucose as a means of energy production, and adequate glucose delivery is necessary to ensure optimal function.[22,23] Furthermore, laboratory, animal, and human studies have demonstrated that hyperglycemia may initially limit ischemic myocardial injury.[24,25]

In contrast, chronic hyperglycemia appears to be associated with a variety of negative effects at the cellular level. In vitro models have found that hyperglycemia inhibits glucose-6-phosphate dehydrogenase activity, which in turn decreases oxygen radical production by neutrophils.[26,27] It has been theorized that this could result in impaired bactericidal activity and immune function.[28] Chronic hyperglycemia is also associated with increased myocardial cell death in the setting of cardiac ischemia.[29]

HYPERGLYCEMIA AND CLINICAL OUTCOMES

There is ample evidence that hyperglycemia is associated with poor clinical outcomes in a wide variety of patients who present to the emergency department. Among these are patients with acute coronary syndrome, neurologic injuries, and sepsis.

Acute Coronary Syndrome

In patients with acute myocardial infarction (AMI), several studies suggest that elevated serum glucose on admission is associated with increased risk of reinfarction, the development of congestive heart failure, the incidence of future cardiac events, and increased mortality.[30,31] A related study tracked long-term outcomes in patients with AMI (either known diabetics or those with elevated serum glucose at the time of their event) and demonstrated a significant decrease in mortality in the group with more strict blood sugar regulation.[32]

Neurologic Injury

In several studies of patients presenting with ischemic strokes, hyperglycemia on admission was independently associated with worse long-term neurologic outcomes and increased mortality.[7–10,33,34] Hyperglycemia is also associated with an increased rate of hemorrhagic transformation in patients receiving thrombolytic therapy.[35] Again, these findings were independent of the patient's diabetic status at the time of the event.

Similarly, patients with traumatic brain injury with elevated blood glucose on admission experience worse neurologic outcomes and increased mortality, both in the short and in the long term. In one study of severely brain-injured patients, the degree of hyperglycemia was inversely proportional to Glasgow Coma Scale score and to favorable outcome.[9]

Sepsis

In patients with sepsis, even moderate hyperglycemia is associated with increased rates of complication, length of stay, and unfavorable clinical outcomes.[3,16,19,36–38]

PATHOPHYSIOLOGY OF HYPOGLYCEMIC STATES

In contrast to hyperglycemia, whose negative effects occur over hours to days, even transient hypoglycemia can result in profound morbidity and potential mortality in the critically ill patient. The brain, in particular, is dependent on a near-continuous supply of glucose, and any interruption or decrease in glucose delivery can result in impaired judgment, confusion, seizures, coma, and even death. While there are no definitive cutoffs for the degree or duration of hypoglycemia required to produce permanent neurologic damage, the correlation between the two is clear.[39,40] The heart is similarly sensitive to hypoglycemia. One of the initial adaptive responses to hypoglycemia is an increase in heart rate, myocardial contractility, and stroke volume, with the end result being a dramatic increase in cardiac workload over a short period of time. This increase, while of little concern to a healthy patient, can produce demand ischemia in critically ill patients with coronary artery disease. In addition, hypoglycemia can result in cardiac conduction abnormalities, specifically a prolonged QT interval, and an increase in myocyte repolarization time. These changes are associated with an increased risk of arrhythmias, including atrial fibrillation and ventricular tachycardias.[41]

HYPOGLYCEMIA AND CLINICAL OUTCOMES

There is a convincing body of evidence, from both observational studies and randomized control trials, that even a moderate degree of hypoglycemia is associated with worse clinical outcomes and increased mortality. These findings are seen in both medical and surgical patients, and they appear to be independent of patients' underlying pathology or reason for admission.[42–45] In a recent retrospective, case–control study examining the effects of mild hypoglycemia on medical ICU patients, even a single episode of mild hypoglycemia independently predicted increased mortality (OR 2.98).[46]

CONTROVERSY REGARDING GLYCEMIC CONTROL IN THE CRITICALLY ILL

Given the observed relationship between hyperglycemia and poor clinical outcomes, the notion that strict control of a patient's glycemic state would result in improved outcomes has been actively investigated for more than 20 years. Early studies were often limited to patients with diabetes undergoing the same treatment or procedure (e.g., therapy for acute MI or cardiac surgery). The DIGAMI study included patients with hyperglycemia, regardless of diabetic status, who presented with acute MI.[32] This study demonstrated that patients who were randomized to receive intravenous insulin infusions during their inpatient stay and subsequently received 3 months of subcutaneous outpatient insulin therapy had dramatically improved survival at 1 year follow-up (7.5% ARR, NNT = 13 for survival). It should be noted, however, that there were no significant differences in mortality during the in-hospital period, or at 3-month follow-up, and it remains unclear the extent to which inpatient glycemic control affected outcomes. Though it did not involve glycemic targets, the CREATE-ECLA trial enrolled 20,000 subjects in a multicenter investigation of the effect of insulin and glucose infusion on patients with acute MI; it found no changes in mortality, cardiac arrest, recurrent MI, or cardiogenic shock.[47] A similar trial randomized nearly 2,500 patients undergoing cardiac surgery to receive either continuous insulin infusion or intermittent subcutaneous insulin injections for glycemic control. While the authors did not find any mortality benefit in the intervention group, they did note a small, but statistically significant decrease in deep sternal wound infections in the intervention group (0.8 vs. 2.0%).[48]

In 2001, the Lueven intensive insulin therapy trial enrolled 1,548 critically ill surgical ICU patients and reported a 42% relative reduction in mortality (3.4% ARR, NNT = 30 for survival) and a 46% reduction in septicemia (3.6% ARR, NNT = 28 for preventing bloodstream infection) for patients targeted to tight glycemic control (70 to 110 mg/dL).[49]

Following the study's publication, strict glycemic control was rapidly adopted as the standard of care in many ICUs worldwide. In 2006, the same research group enrolled 1,200 subjects and examined the effects of tight glycemic control in critically patients in the medical ICU setting.[50] Unlike their previous trial, this investigation did not find any overall difference in mortality between the intervention and control groups, nor did it find any difference in the rate of bloodstream infections. In a subgroup analysis, the authors noted that for patients with ICU stays <3 days, there was decreased mortality in the intervention group. Unfortunately, this benefit was offset by an increase in deaths among intervention patients with ICU stays longer than 3 days.

There have been multiple subsequent attempts to reproduce the results of the original 2001 Leuven trial. Ensuing investigations failed to demonstrate any mortality benefit for patients receiving tight glycemic control. The majority of these trials did, however, again demonstrate intensive insulin therapy to be associated with an increase in hypoglycemic events, with at least one trial stopped early because of an increase in mortality in the intervention group.[51–59] High-quality systematic reviews have likewise failed to demonstrate a benefit for tight glycemic control in more defined populations, such as perioperative patients with diabetes or in patients following ischemic stroke. These reviews also reinforced the finding of increased hypoglycemic events in intervention groups.[38,60–62] As a result of these studies, there has been a trend away from tight glycemic control in the treatment of the critically ill.[24,63,64]

Follow-up studies investigating the effect of tight glycemic control in critically ill patients culminated in the 2009 NICE-SUGAR study, a landmark multicenter trial that randomized over 6,000 medical and surgical ICU subjects expected to require ICU care for 3 or more days to either intensive (goal 80 to 110 mg/dL) or conventional (goal <180 mg/dL) glycemic control.[45] In stark contrast to the results of the Lueven trial and in agreement with the smaller studies discussed above, all-cause mortality at 90 days (the primary endpoint) was actually higher in the intensive glucose control group (27.5% vs. 24.9%, NNH = 38 for death). The rate of severe hypoglycemic episodes was also found to be dramatically increased in the intervention group (6.9% vs. 0.5%, NNH = 15).[65] Importantly, there was no difference in outcomes for medical or surgical patients and no difference in secondary outcomes (ICU/hospital days, days requiring mechanical ventilation, need for renal replacement therapy). As a result of this study, aggressive glucose control in the ICU to goal <110 mg/dL is definitively no longer recommended. Although an ideal target serum glucose remains unclear and prolonged hyperglycemia remains, in general, undesirable, the risks associated with hypoglycemia have led most centers to target 140 to 180 mg/dL for patients in the critically care setting.

CONCLUSION

The majority of data on glycemic control in the critically ill are derived from studies performed in an ICU setting. At this time, there are little data on glycemic control among critically ill patients in the ED.[66,67] Extrapolating current evidence from the ICU-based studies, targeting a blood glucose target of 140 to 180 mg/dL is recommended.

Many emergency departments, however, lack the staffing, protocols, and resources to safely ensure even this level of glycemic control. Data clearly suggest hypoglycemic events to be of greater danger to the patient than modest increases in blood glucose, and insulin continues to be a top five "high-risk" medications, with one in three fatal medical errors being linked to insulin therapy.[68] As such, in emergency departments in which resources are limited, targeting a more liberal blood glucose target of 160 to 220 mg/dL may be appropriate.

In summary, while an abundance of data demonstrates a clear association between hyperglycemia and worsened outcomes for critically ill patients of all types (sepsis, acute MI, ischemic and hemorrhagic stroke, postsurgical), it is unclear whether this association is causal. It remains a distinct possibility that hyperglycemia is in fact an independent marker of disease severity—similar to lactate in severe sepsis—rather than a cause of increased morbidity and mortality.[69] Causality notwithstanding, it appears that hyperglycemia is associated with worsened outcomes when present on the scale of hours to days. In contrast, even very brief episodes of hypoglycemia may be catastrophic for a critically ill patient. Despite the development of well-defined protocols, the introduction of continuous serum glucose monitoring devices, and highly trained and attentive ICU staff, modern medicine is still unable to adequately anticipate or avoid hypoglycemic events in patients targeted to tight—or even moderate—glycemic control. Acknowledging these limitations, as well as the near-zero tolerance for harm from iatrogenic hypoglycemia, helps justify the current trend away from tight glycemic control despite the known association between hyperglycemia and poor clinical outcomes.

LITERATURE TABLE

TRIAL	DESIGN	RESULT
Medical–surgical ICU patients		
NICE-SUGAR Investigators, *N Engl J Med.* 2009[45]	Multicenter RCT of 6,104 patients in the ICU evaluating intensive vs. conventional glucose control	3.4% increase in risk of death with intervention (OR = 1.14). A 6.3% increase in reported hypoglycemic events in intervention group. No difference in ICU LOS, hospital LOS, need for RRT
Preiser et al. *Intensive Care Med.* 2009[52] Glucontrol Study	Multicenter RCT of 1,101 patients in the ICU evaluating tight glycemic control (80–110 mg/dL) vs. loose control (140–200 mg/dL) from 2004 to 2006	Trial stopped early. A 6.0% increase in hypoglycemic events in the tight control group (8.7% vs. 2.7%). No difference in mortality, ICU LOS, hospital LOS, days on ventilator, need for RRT
De La Rosa et al. *Crit Care.* 2008[55]	Prospective, single-centered, RCT of 504 ICU patients evaluating intensive vs. conventional glucose control	6.8% increase in hypoglycemic events in the intervention group (8.5% vs. 1.7%). No difference in mortality, ICU LOS, hospital LOS, days on ventilator, need for RRT, or rates of infection
Treggiari et al. *Crit Care.* 2008[56]	Prospective, Observational Study of intensive insulin therapy in 10,456 ICU patients from 2001 to 2005	Fourfold increase in hypoglycemic events after adoption of intensive insulin therapy. A trend toward increased mortality
Arabi et al. *Crit Care.* 2008[57]	Prospective, single-centered, RCT of 523 ICU patients evaluating intensive vs. conventional glucose control	25.5% increase in hypoglycemic events in the tight glycemic control group (28.6% vs. 3.1%). No difference in mortality, ICU LOS, hospital LOS, days on ventilator, need for RRT, or rates of infection
Surgical ICU patients		
Van den Berghe et al. *N Engl J Med.* 2001[49]	Prospective, single-centered, RCT of 1,548 patients in the surgical ICU evaluating intensive vs. conventional glucose control	At 1 y, a 3.4% decrease in mortality among intervention patients. Overall in-hospital mortality decreased by 34%, blood stream infection by 46%, and critical illness polyneuropathy by 44% in the intervention group

(*Continued*)

LITERATURE TABLE *(Continued)*

TRIAL	DESIGN	RESULT
Medical ICU patients		
Park et al., *Crit Care.* 2012[46]	Retrospective, case–control study of 313 medical ICU patients and effect of mild hypoglycemia on mortality	Mild hypoglycemia independently associated with increased hospital mortality (OR = 3.43). One episode of mild hypoglycemia associated with increased mortality (OR = 2.98)
Brunkhorst et al., *N Engl J Med.* 2008[54]	Prospective, multicentered, RCT of 537 patients in the medical ICU evaluating intensive vs. conventional glucose control, as well as pentastarch vs. Ringer lactate for fluid resuscitation	Trial stopped early for harm. 12.9% increase in hypoglycemic events in the tight glycemic control group (17% vs. 4.1%). With a 3.2% increase in life-threatening hypoglycemic events and a 2.1% increase in hypoglycemic events resulting in a prolonged hospital stay
Van den Berghe et al., *N Engl J Med.* 2006[56]	Prospective, single-centered, RCT of 1,200 patients in the medical ICU evaluating intensive vs. conventional glucose control	No difference in mortality, reduced morbidity as defined by new kidney injury, improved weaning from ventilator, and decreased ICU and hospital LOS
Cardiothoracic ICU patients		
Furnary et al., *Ann Thorac Surg.* 1999[48]	Prospective, intervention study of 2,467 diabetic patients undergoing open heart surgery that compared insulin infusion vs. conventional therapy to maintain glucose <200 mg/dL	Decreased incidence of deep sternal infections (RR = 0.34) in the continuous infusion group
Agus et al., *N Engl J Med.* 2012[58]	Multicenter RCT of 980 children undergoing cardiopulmonary bypass surgery evaluating intensive vs. conventional glucose control	No difference in mortality, infection rate, LOS, organ failure scores

RR, relative risk; OR, odds ratio.

REFERENCES

1. Badawi O, Waite MD, Fuhrman SA, et al. Association between intensive care unit-acquired dysglycemia and in-hospital mortality. *Crit Care Med.* 2012;40:3180–3188.
2. Dungan K, Braithwaite SS, Preiser JC. Stress hyperglycemia. *Lancet.* 2009;373:1798–1807.
3. Falciglia M, Freyberg RW, Almenoff PL, et al. Hyperglycemia-related mortality in critically ill patients varies with admission diagnosis. *Crit Care Med.* 2009;37:3001–3009.
4. Bagshaw SM, Egi M, George C, et al. Australia New Zealand Intensive Care Society Database Management Committee: early blood glucose control and mortality in critically ill patients in Australia. *Crit Care Med.* 2009;37:463–470.
5. Yendamuri S, Fulda GJ, Tinkoff GH. Admission hyperglycemia as a prognostic indicator in trauma. *J Trauma.* 2003;55:33–38.
6. Bruno A, Levine SR, Frankel MR, et al. Admission glucose level and clinical outcomes in the NINDS rt-PA Stroke Trial. *Neurology.* 2002;59:669–674.
7. Capes SE, Hunt D, Malmberg K, et al. Stress hyperglycemia and prognosis of stroke in nondiabetic and diabetic patients: a systematic overview. *Stroke.* 2001;32:2426–2432.
8. Capes SE, Hunt D, Malmberg K, et al. Stress hyperglycaemia and increased risk of death after myocardial infarction in patients with and without diabetes: a systematic overview. *Lancet.* 2000;355:773–778.
9. Young B, Ott L, Dempsey R, et al. Relationship between admission hyperglycemia and neurologic outcome of severely brain-injured patients. *Ann Surg.* 1989;210:466–472.
10. Rovlias A, Kotsou S. The influence of hyperglycemia on neurological outcome in patients with severe head injury. *Neurosurgery.* 2000;46:335–342.
11. Fahy BG, Sheehy AM, Coursin DB. Glucose control in the intensive care unit. *Crit Care Med.* 2009;37(5):1769–1776.
12. Bochicchio GV, Bochicchio KM, Joshi M, et al. Acute glucose elevation is highly predictive of infection and outcome in critically injured trauma patients. *Ann Surg.* 2010;252:597–602.
13. Gale SC, Sicoutris C, Reilly PM, et al. Poor glycemic control is associated with increased mortality in critically ill trauma patients. *Am Surg.* 2007;73:454–460.

14. Melamed E. Reactive hyperglycaemia in patients with acute stroke. *J Neurol Sci.* 1976;29:267–275.
15. Kernan WN, Viscoli CM, Inzucchi SE, et al. Prevalence of abnormal glucose tolerance following a transient ischemic attack or ischemic stroke. *Arch Intern Med.* 2005;165:227–233.
16. Marik PE, Raghavan M. Stress-hyperglycemia, insulin and immunomodulation in sepsis. *Intensive Care Med.* 2004;30(5):748–756.
17. Marik PE. Critical illness related corticosteroid insufficiency. *Chest.* 2009;135:181–193.
18. Chernow B, Rainey TR, Lake CR. Endogenous and exogenous catecholamines in critical care medicine. *Crit Care Med.* 1982;10:409–416.
19. Oswald GA, Smith CC, Betteridge DJ, et al. Determinants and importance of stress hyperglycaemia in non-diabetic patients with myocardial infarction. *Br Med J (Clin Res Ed).* 1986;293:917–922.
20. Marik PE, Bellomo R. Stress hyperglycemia: an essential survival response! *Crit Care.* 2013;17(2):305.
21. Losser MR, Damoisel C, Payen D. Bench-to-bedside review: glucose and stress conditions in the intensive care unit. *Crit Care.* 2010;14:231.
22. Lang CH, Dobrescu C. Gram-negative infection increases noninsulin-mediated glucose disposal. *Endocrinology.* 1991;128:645–653.
23. Meszaros K, Lang CH, Bagby GJ, et al. In vivo glucose utilization by individual tissues during nonlethal hypermetabolic sepsis. *FASEB J.* 1988;2:3083–3086.
24. Malfitano C, Alba Loureiro TC, Rodrigues B, et al. Hyperglycaemia protects the heart after myocardial infarction: aspects of programmed cell survival and cell death. *Eur J Heart Fail.* 2010;12:659–667.
25. Frustaci A, Kajstura J, Chimenti C, et al. Myocardial cell death in human diabetes. *Circ Res.* 2000;87:1123–1132.
26. Lin Y, Rajala MW, Berger JP, et al. Hyperglycemia-induced production of acute phase reactants in adipose tissue. *J Biol Chem.* 2001;276:42077–42083.
27. Perner A, Nielsen SE, Rask-Madsen J. High glucose impairs superoxide production from isolated blood neutrophils. *Intensive Care Med.* 2003;29:642–645.
28. Rassias AJ, Marrin CA, Arruda J, et al. Insulin infusion improves neutrophil function in diabetic cardiac surgery patients. *Anesth Analg.* 1999;88:1011–1016.
29. Fiordaliso F, Leri A, Cesselli D, et al. Hyperglycemia activates p53 and p53-regulated genes leading to myocyte cell death. *Diabetes.* 2001;50:2363–2375.
30. Wahab NN, Cowden EA, Pearce NJ, et al. Is blood glucose an independent predictor of mortality in acute myocardial infarction in the thrombolytic era? *J Am Coll Cardiol.* 2002;40:1748–1754.
31. Norhammar AM, Ryden L, Malmberg K. Admission plasma glucose. Independent risk factor for long-term prognosis after myocardial infarction even in nondiabetic patients. *Diabetes Care.* 1999;22:1827–1831.
32. Malmberg K. Prospective randomised study of intensive insulin treatment on long term survival after acute myocardial infarction in patients with diabetes mellitus. DIGAMI (Diabetes Mellitus, Insulin Glucose Infusion in Acute Myocardial Infarction) Study Group. *BMJ.* 1997;314:1512–1515.
33. Yang S, Zhang S, Wang M. Clinical significance of admission hyperglycemia and factors related to it in patients with acute severe head injury. *Surg Neurol.* 1995;44:373–377.
34. Weir CJ, Murray GD, Dyker AG, et al. Is hyperglycaemia an independent predictor of poor outcome after acute stroke? Results of a long-term follow up study. *BMJ.* 1997;314:1303–1306.
35. Demchuk AM, Morgenstern LB, Krieger DW, et al. Serum glucose level and diabetes predict tissue plasminogen activator-related intracerebral hemorrhage in acute ischemic stroke. *Stroke.* 1999;30:34–39.
36. Whitcomb BW, Pradhan EK, Pittas AG, et al. Impact of admission hyperglycemia on hospital mortality in various intensive care unit populations. *Crit Care Med.* 2005;33(12):2772–2777.
37. Krinsley JS. Association between hyperglycemia and increased hospital mortality in a heterogeneous population of critically ill patients. *Mayo Clin Proc.* 2003;78(12):1471–1478.
38. Ling Y, Li X, Gao X. Intensive versus conventional glucose control in critically ill patients: a meta-analysis of randomized controlled trials. *Eur J Intern Med.* 2012;23(6):564–574.
39. Raichle ME. The pathophysiology of brain ischemia. *Ann Neurol.* 1983;13(1):2–10.
40. Fujioka M, Okuchi K, Hiramatsu KI, et al. Specific changes in human brain after hypoglycemic injury. *Stroke.* 1997;28(3):584–587.
41. Frier BM, Schernthaner G, Heller SR. Hypoglycemia and cardiovascular risks. *Diabetes Care.* 2011;34(suppl 2):S132–S137.
42. Duning T, van dH I, Dickmann A, et al. Hypoglycemia aggravates critical illness-induced neurocognitive dysfunction. *Diabetes Care.* 2010;33:639–644.
43. D'Ancona G, Bertuzzi F, Sacchi L, et al. Iatrogenic hypoglycemia secondary to tight glucose control is an independent determinant for mortality and cardiac morbidity. *Eur J Cardiothorac Surg.* 2011;40(2):360–366. doi: 10.1016/j.ejcts.2010.11.065

44. Vespa P, McArthur DL, Stein N, et al. Tight glycemic control increases metabolic distress in traumatic brain injury: a randomized controlled within-subjects trial. *Crit Care Med.* 2012;40:1923–1929.
45. NICE-SUGAR Study Investigators; Finfer S, Liu B, et al. Hypoglycemia and risk of death in critically ill patients. *N Engl J Med.* 2012;367(12):1108–1118.
46. Park S, Kim DG, Suh GY, et al. Mild hypoglycemia is independently associated with increased risk of mortality in patients with sepsis: a three year retrospective observational study. *Crit Care.* 2012;16:R189.
47. Mehta SR, Yusuf S, Diaz R, et al. Effect of glucose-insulin-potassium infusion on mortality in patients with acute ST-segment elevation myocardial infarction: the CREATE-ECLA randomized controlled trial. *JAMA.* 2005;293:437–446.
48. Furnary AP, Zerr KJ, Grunkemeier GL, et al. Continuous intravenous insulin infusion reduces the incidence of deep sternal wound infection in diabetic patients after cardiac surgical procedures. *Ann Thorac Surg.* 1999;67(2):352–360; discussion 360–362.
49. Van den Berghe G, Wouters P, Weekers F, et al. Intensive insulin therapy in critically ill patients. *N Engl J Med.* 2001;345(19):1359–1367.
50. Van den Berghe G, Wilmer A, Hermans G, et al. Intensive insulin therapy in the medical ICU. *N Engl J Med.* 2006;354(5):449–461.
51. Ingels C, Debaveye Y, Milants I, et al. Strict blood glucose control with insulin during intensive care after cardiac surgery: impact on 4-years survival, dependency on medical care, and quality-of-life. *Eur Heart J.* 2006;27:2716–2724.
52. Preiser JC, Devos P, Ruiz-Santana S, et al. A prospective randomized multicenter controlled trial on tight glucose control by intensive insulin therapy in adult intensive care units: the Glucontrol study. *Intensive Care Med.* 2009;35:1738–1748.
53. Brunkhorst F, Kuhnt E, Engel C, et al. Intensive insulin therapy in patient with severe sepsis and septic shock is associated with an increased rate of hypoglycemia—results from a randomized multicenter study (VISEP). *Infection.* 2005;33:19.
54. Brunkhorst FM, Engel C, Bloos F, et al. Intensive insulin therapy and pentastarch resuscitation in severe sepsis. *N Engl J Med.* 2008;358:125–139.
55. De La Rosa Gdel C, Donado JH, Restrepo AH, et al. Grupo de Investigacion en Cuidado intensivo: GICI-HPTU. Strict glycaemic control in patients hospitalised in a mixed medical and surgical intensive care unit: a randomised clinical trial. *Crit Care.* 2008;12(5):R120.
56. Treggiari MM, Karir V, Yanez ND, et al. Intensive insulin therapy and mortality in critically ill patients. *Crit Care.* 2008;12(1):R29.
57. Arabi YM, Dabbagh OC, Tamim HM, et al. Intensive versus conventional insulin therapy: a randomized controlled trial in medical and surgical critically ill patients. *Crit Care Med.* 2008;36(12):3190–3197.
58. Agus MS, Steil GM, Wypij D, et al. SPECS Study Investigators. Tight glycemic control versus standard care after pediatric cardiac surgery. *N Engl J Med.* 2012;367(13):1208–1219.
59. Buchleitner AM, Martínez-Alonso M, Hernández M, et al. Perioperative glycaemic control for diabetic patients undergoing surgery. *Cochrane Database Syst Rev.* 2012;9:CD007315.
60. Bellolio MF, Gilmore RM, Stead LG. Insulin for glycaemic control in acute ischaemic stroke. *Cochrane Database Syst Rev.* 2011;(9):CD005346.
61. Kansagara D, Fu R, Freeman M, et al. Intensive insulin therapy in hospitalized patients: a systematic review. *Ann Intern Med.* 2011;154(4):268–282.
62. Jacobi J, Bircher N, Krinsley J, et al. Guidelines for the use of an insulin infusion for the management of hyperglycemia in critically ill patients. *Crit Care Med.* 2012;40(12):3251–3276.
63. Samokhvalov A, Farah R, Makhoul N. Glycemic control in the intensive care unit: between safety and benefit. *Isr Med Assoc J.* 2012;14(4):260–266.
64. NICE-SUGAR Study Investigators; Finfer S, Chittock DR, Su SY. Intensive versus conventional glucose control in critically ill patients. *N Engl J Med.* 2009;360(13):1283–1297.
65. Cohen J, Goedecke E, Cyrkler JE, et al. Early glycemic control in critically ill emergency department patients: pilot-trial. *West J Emerg Med.* 2010;11(1):20–23.
66. Lee JH, Kim K, Jo YH, et al. Feasibility of continuous glucose monitoring in critically ill emergency department patients. *J Emerg Med.* 2012;43(2):251–257.
67. Hellman R. A systems approach to reducing errors in insulin therapy in the inpatient setting. *Endocr Pract.* 2004;10(suppl 2):100–108.
68. Henderson WR, Chittock DR, Dhingra VK, et al. Hyperglycemia in acutely ill emergency patients—cause or effect? *CJEM.* 2006;8(5):339–343.

42

Diabetic Ketoacidosis and Hyperosmolar Hyperglycemic State

Catherine T. Jamin and Jeffrey Manko

BACKGROUND

Diabetic ketoacidosis (DKA) and the hyperosmolar hyperglycemic state (HHS) are two potentially devastating complications of diabetes. Although the number of patients diagnosed with DKA or HHS has nearly doubled in recent decades, the age-adjusted mortality of these patients has declined by almost half within the same time period.[1,2] This improvement in outcomes is due in large part due to the early recognition and therapeutic interventions delivered in the emergency department.

DKA and HHS are characterized by an imbalance between the effective action of insulin and of counterregulatory hormones such as glucagon, cortisol, catecholamines, and growth hormone.[3] This imbalance results in increased gluconeogenesis, impaired peripheral glucose utilization, lipolysis, and increased ketoacid production. In DKA, this produces the triad of hyperglycemia, ketonemia, and metabolic acidosis. In HHS, it is thought that there is sufficient effective insulin to limit lipolysis and ketogenesis, but not enough to facilitate glucose uptake in the tissues (Fig. 42.1). In both conditions, patients undergo a significant osmotic diuresis—HHS with total body water (TBW) deficit of 8 to 10 L and DKA with a TBW deficit of 3 to 6 L—resulting in dehydration and electrolyte shifts.

HISTORY AND PHYSICAL EXAM

Classically reported findings in a patient with DKA or HHS include polyuria, polydipsia, weakness, and dehydration. The onset of HHS is usually insidious, occurring over days to weeks, while DKA tends to manifest over a period of hours. Patients with DKA may complain of abdominal pain, nausea, or vomiting, while HHS patients often report mental status changes or confusion. The physical exam in both conditions will reveal evidence of hypovolemia, including hypotension, tachycardia, decreased capillary refill, and poor skin turgor. Patients with DKA will commonly demonstrate deep breathing or Kussmaul respirations, a fruity odor to their breath, and abdominal tenderness. Patients with HHS may present with profound neurologic changes including focal deficits,

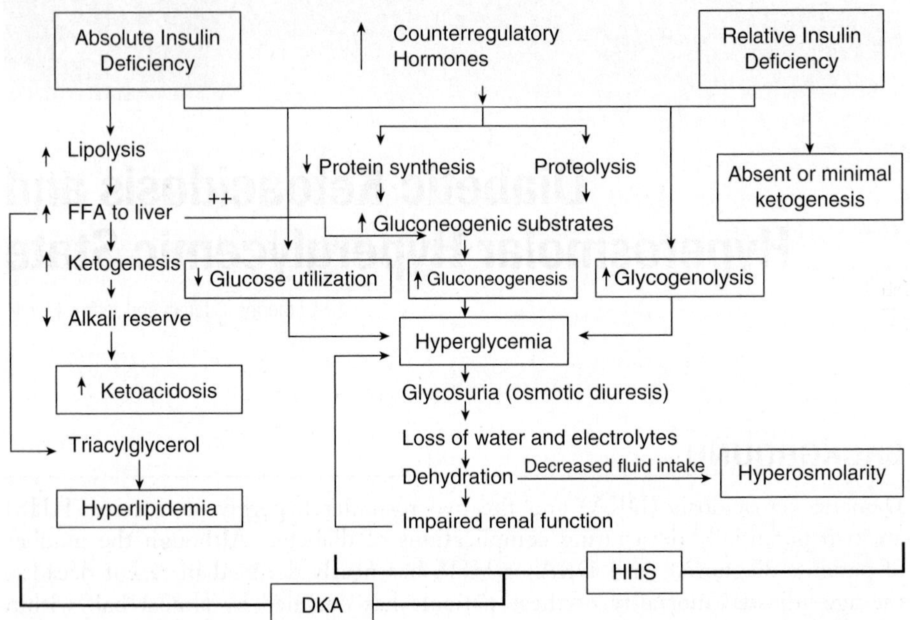

FIGURE 42.1 Pathogenesis of DKA and HHS. Copyright © 2006 American Diabetes Association From Diabetes Care Vol 29, Issue 12, 2006. Information updated from Kitabchi AE, Umpierrez GE, Miles JM, et al. Hyperglycemic crises in adult patients with diabetes. *Diabetes Care.* 2009;32:1335. From American Diabetes Association. FFA, free fatty acids.

seizures, or coma. The most common insult precipitating both conditions is infection. Other triggers include insufficient insulin, drugs, and other severe physiologic stresses such as myocardial ischemia, stroke, and pancreatitis.[3]

DIAGNOSTIC EVALUATION

When DKA or HHS is suspected, the laboratory evaluation should include plasma glucose, basic metabolic panel, serum osmolarity, venous blood gas, serum lactate, and detection of ketones. A complete blood count, urinalysis, blood and urine cultures, chest radiograph, and electrocardiogram may help detect coexisting or triggering illness.

Hyperglycemia is a cardinal feature of both conditions and is typically more profound in patients with HHS (Table 42.1). Patients with DKA may however present with serum glucose <300 mg/dL; therefore, in a patient clinically suspected of having DKA, laboratory evaluation should always include calculation of the anion gap (AG) and serum ketones.[3,4]

Ketones

In the patient with DKA, hepatic fatty acid oxidation produces ketone bodies, specifically acetoacetic acid, beta-hydroxybutyric acid, and acetone. The standard laboratory test used to detect serum ketones uses a nitroprusside reagent. While widely available,

TABLE 42.1 Diagnostic Criteria for DKA and HHS

	DKA			HHS
	Mild (Plasma Glucose >250 mg/dL)	Moderate (Plasma Glucose >250 mg/dL)	Severe (Plasma Glucose >250 mg/dL)	Plasma Glucose >600 mg/dL
Arterial pH	7.25–7.30	7.00 to <7.24	<7.00	>7.30
Serum bicarbonate (mEq/1)	15–18	10 to <15	<10	>18
Urine ketone[a]	Positive	Positive	Positive	Small
Serum ketone[a]	Positive	Positive	Positive	Small
Effective serum osmolality[b]	Variable	Variable	Variable	>320 mOsm/kg
Anion gap[c]	>10	>12	>12	Variable
Mental status	Alert	Alert/drowsy	Stupor/coma	Stupor/coma

[a]Nitroprusside reaction method.
[b]Effective serum osmolality: 2[Measured Na^+ (mEq/L)] + Serum Glucose (mg/dL)/18.
[c]Anion gap: $Na^+ - [(Cl^- + HCO_3^-$ (mEq/L)]. Na^+, sodium; Cl–, chloride; HCO_3–, bicarbonate.
Adapted from Adrogué HJ, Lederer ED, Suki WN, Eknoyan G. Determinants of plasma potassium levels in diabetic ketoacidosis. *Medicine (Baltimore).* 1986;65(3):163.
 Information updated from Kitabchi AE, Umpierrez GE, Miles JM, et al. Hyperglycemic crises in adult patients with diabetes. *Diabetes Care.* 2009;32:1335. From American Diabetes Association.

this test does not detect beta-hydroxybutyric acid and thus may yield a false-negative result. To avoid false-negative results, serum beta-hydroxybutyric acid should be measured directly, when possible.

Anion Gap Metabolic Acidosis

Patients with DKA will have a metabolic acidosis, with an arterial pH, by definition, of <7.3, and an elevated AG.

$$AG = Na^+ - \left(Cl^- + HCO_3^-\right)$$

The AG reflects the difference between measured cations and anions and is elevated in DKA due to the presence of the ketoacids. Normal AG values are 7 to 11, with >12 considered elevated. Patients with hypoalbuminemia will have a factitiously lower AG due to the partial loss of negatively charged albumin particles.[5] The AG should be corrected in patients with hypoalbuminemia using the following calculation:

$$\text{Corrected Anion Gap} = AG + \left[2.5 \times (4 - \text{Albumin})\right]$$

Arterial versus Venous Blood Gas

Recent studies demonstrate that peripheral venous blood gas (VBG) samples can be used to accurately assess the degree of acidosis in patients presenting to the emergency department.[6–8] Compared with an arterial blood gas (ABG), the VBG will be lower by approximately 0.02 to 0.04 pH units. In general, VBGs and ABGs agree, but periodic correlation should be performed if serial VBGs are being used to monitor a patient's acid–base status.

Osmolarity

Unlike patients with DKA, patients with HHS will present with significantly elevated serum osmolarity. Hyperosmolarity is primarily due to the marked free water loss associated with glucose-induced osmotic diuresis. Serum osmolarity is calculated as follows:

$$\text{Serum osmolarity} = \left[2 \times \text{Na}^{+}\ (\text{meq/L})\right] + \left[\text{Glucose}\ (\text{mg/dL})/18\right] + \left[\text{BUN}/2.8\right] + \left[\text{EtOH}/4.6\right]$$

A serum osmolarity >320 can result in mental status changes, including stupor and coma. In patients with HHS presenting with neurologic impairment but normal serum osmolarity, a rigorous search for alternative explanations of their altered mental status is required.[9,10]

Potassium

Despite presenting with elevated serum potassium levels, patients with DKA and HHS will often have a potassium deficit ranging between 3 and 5 mg/kg.[11,12] The potassium deficit is multifactorial and can be attributed to decreased intake and increased urinary and gastrointestinal losses.[12] Elevated serum potassium is mechanistically related to insulin deficiency, hyperglycemia, and acidosis, which decrease its regular cellular uptake.[12] As patients receive treatment for DKA and HHS, potassium uptake resumes and serum levels will rapidly fall, placing patients at risk for cardiac dysrhythmias and respiratory muscle weakness. Potassium levels should be followed closely at every stage of treatment to prevent these treatment complications.[11] Protocols for management of DKA (Table 42.2) include components for potassium replacement and to withhold insulin therapy until serum potassium levels are >3.3 mEq/L.[3]

Sodium

The hyperglycemia present in both DKA and HHS will initially create an osmotic gradient that draws water from the cellular space, effectively lowering the measured serum sodium. This osmotic effect of glucose on serum sodium should be corrected using the following calculation:

$$\text{Corrected Na}^{+} = \text{Measured Na}^{+} + 0.016 \times (\text{Serum Glucose} - 100)$$

The finding of hypernatremia in either DKA or HHS indicates that a significant free water deficit exists.

Phosphate

Serum phosphate may be normal or elevated in patients with DKA or HHS due to extracellular shifts; however, patients are typically phosphate depleted due to urinary loss and decreased intake.[13] As with potassium, insulin therapy will unmask this deficit as it drives phosphate back into the cells. Although phosphate replacement has yet to demonstrate clinical benefit in patients with DKA, patients should be administered

TABLE 42.2 Management Guidelines

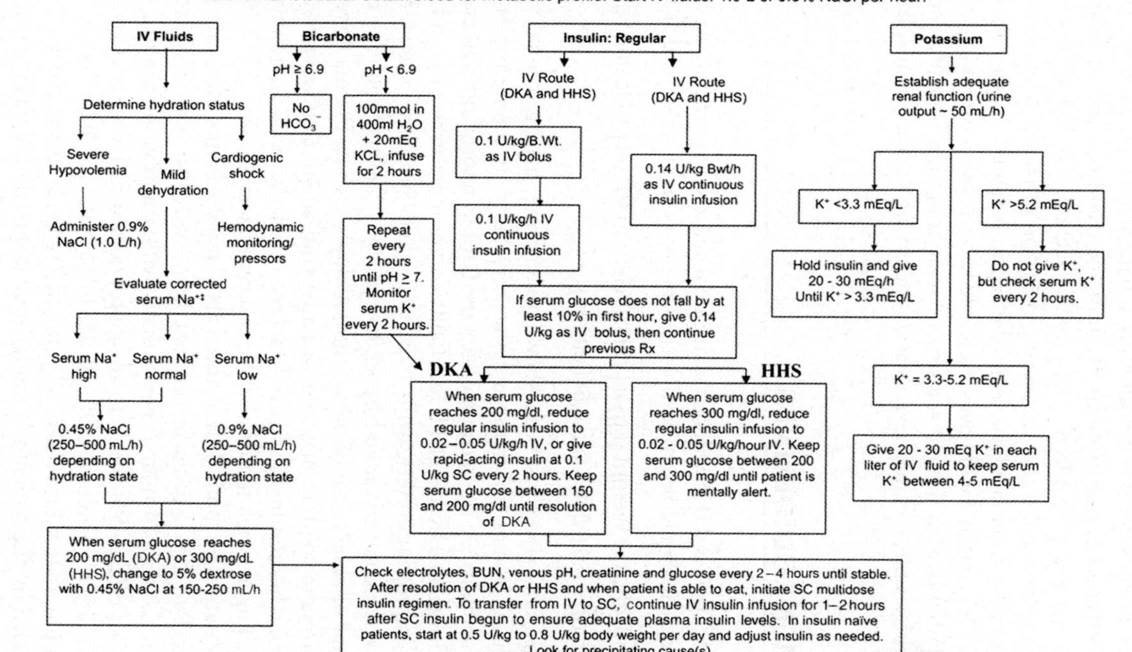

DKA diagnostic criteria: blood glucose 250 mg/dL, arterial pH < 7.3, bicarbonate 15 mEq/L, and moderate ketonuria or ketonemia. HHS diagnostic criteria: serum glucose >600 mg/dL, arterial pH > 7.3, serum bicarbonate > 15 mEq/L, and minimal ketonuria and ketonemia.

[a]15–20 mL/kg/h.

[b]Serum Na should be corrected for hyperglycemia (for each 100 mg/dL glucose > 100 mg/dL, add 1.6 mEq to sodium value for corrected serum value).

Bwt, body weight; IV, intravenous; SC, subcutaneous.

phosphorus when cardiac dysfunction, anemia, or respiratory depression is present, or when phosphate levels are <1 mg/dL.[3,14,15]

DIFFERENTIAL DIAGNOSIS

Other diagnoses to consider when evaluating a patient with an elevated AG acidosis include lactic acidosis, starvation or alcoholic ketoacidosis, uremic acidosis, and toxic ingestion. Patents with DKA may produce lactate, but will have a predominance of ketone bodies and a less significant elevation of lactate when compared to patients with primary lactic acidosis (e.g., the septic patient). Patients with starvation or alcoholic ketoacidosis will have detectable ketones but without hyperglycemia or glycosuria. Patients with uremic acidosis or toxic ingestion may present with an elevated AG acidosis but will not have the accompanying hyperglycemia, ketonemia, or glycosuria.

MANAGEMENT GUIDELINES

Fluid

All patients with DKA or HHS will be volume depleted and require fluid resuscitation. The free water deficit should be replaced within 24 hours and is calculated as follows:

$$\text{Free Water Deficit} = \text{Weight (kg)} \times \left[\left(\text{Serum Na}^+ / 140\right) - 1\right] \times \text{Dosing Factor}$$

$$\text{Dosing Factor} = 0.6\ (\text{Male}) \text{ and } 0.5\ (\text{Female})$$

Fluid resuscitation alone has been shown to improve hyperglycemia, as well as decrease peripheral insulin resistance and the availability of counterregulatory hormones.[16] Isotonic fluids are the recommended medium to restore intravascular volume and tissue perfusion in DKA and HHS.[3] Colloids are more expensive and have not been shown to improve mortality, while hypertonic fluids have been shown to worsen hyperosmolarity, hypernatremia, and hyperchloremia.[17–19] Normal saline is the initial resuscitative fluid of choice; use of other isotonic fluids such as Plasma-Lyte, lactated Ringer's or Hartmann solution may benefit patients in whom aggressive resuscitation with normal saline has resulted in hyperchloremic metabolic acidosis; however, robust evidence compelling a switch to one of these choices is lacking.[20–22]

Fluid resuscitation in both DKA and HHS should begin at a rate of 15 to 20 mL/kg/h or 1 to 1.5 L given in the first hour, with the goal of correcting free water deficits in the first 24 hours.[3] For patients with a normal or elevated corrected sodium >140 mg/dL, 0.45% NaCl is an appropriate initial resuscitative fluid. For patients with a corrected sodium <140 mg/dL, 0.9% NaCl should be used.[3] After the first hour, an appropriate infusion rate of saline will range between 250 and 500 mL/h and will be guided by the patient's hemodynamic status, fluid deficit, urinary output, renal and cardiac function, electrolyte status, and osmolarity correction.[3] When serum glucose levels decrease to 200 mg/dL in DKA and 300 mg/dL in HHS, 5% dextrose should be added to the replacement fluids to avoid hypoglycemia. The insulin infusion should not be stopped until the acidosis is corrected, unless potassium levels drop below 3 mg/dL (Table 42.2).

Insulin

Along with intravenous fluids, insulin is the second essential therapy in DKA and HHS. Regular insulin is typically given as a continuous infusion; a loading dose is not necessary if an initial infusion rate is at least 0.14 units/kg/h.[23] Alternatively, a priming dose of 0.1 units/kg may be given prior to the initiation of an infusion of 0.1 units/kg/h of regular insulin. There is evidence for the administration of subcutaneous rapid-acting insulin analogs in place of intravenous insulin therapy.[24–26] For patients with mild to moderate DKA without severe acidosis, shock, or coma, use of a short-acting insulin such as aspart or lispro given every 1 to 2 hours has been shown to be successful in the treatment of DKA.[24–26] This approach has the advantage of enabling patient management outside of the intensive care unit; however, its use necessitates cautious patient selection, and further research is warranted before it is implemented widely.

A critical aspect in the management of DKA or HHS is the transition from continuous infusion to subcutaneous insulin. In DKA, the hyperglycemia will typically resolve earlier than the metabolic acidosis. Insulin infusion should continue until the resolution of DKA or HHS, with the addition of 5% dextrose to the replacement fluids when the glucose decreases to 200 or 300 mg/dL in DKA and HHS, respectively. According to the American Diabetes Association (ADA), resolution of DKA and HSS is defined when the following goals are achieved[3]:

- HHS: glucose 250 to 300 mg/dL
  - Normal osmolality with normal mental status
- DKA: glucose <200 mg/dL and two of the following:
  - Serum anion gap ≤12 mEq/L
  - Serum bicarbonate ≥15 mEq/L
  - Venous pH >7.30

When these criteria are achieved, the patient should be transitioned to subcutaneous insulin, with overlapping intravenous insulin for 1 to 2 hours. Patients with known diabetes can be given their usual insulin regimen while insulin naïve patients may be started at 0.5 to 0.8 units/kg/d; both regimens must be dosed according to the type of insulin that is used. Types of insulin and their onset, peak effect, duration of action, and dosing time are summarized in Table 42.3.

TABLE 42.3 Types of Insulin

Type of Insulin	Onset	Peak Effect	Duration of Action	Dosing Time
Mealtime Insulin (Short Acting)				
Aspart (Novolog) (rapid acting)	5–15 min	1 h	3–5 h	Within 20 min, before or after a meal
Regular (Humulin R) (short acting)	30 min	2–4 h	5–8 h	30 min before a meal
Basal Insulin (Long Acting)				
Glargine (Lantus)(long acting)	1.5–2 h	No peak	24 h	Usually q 12 or q 24
NPH (Humulin N) (intermediate acting)	1–2 h	4–12 h	12–18 h	Once or Twice daily

Potassium

As noted, patients with DKA or HHS may present as normokalemic or hyperkalemic, despite experiencing overall potassium depletion. The true deficit is unmasked during the treatment of DKA and HHS. Because of this, any patient with an initial serum potassium <3.3 mEq/L should receive potassium replacement prior to the initiation of insulin therapy to avoid triggering cardiac arrhythmias and respiratory muscle weakness.[3,11,12] The ADA recommends maintaining potassium between the range of 4 and 5 mEq/L and replacing potassium for patients with initial level <5 mEq/L.[3]

Bicarbonate

A recent randomized trial failed to show benefit from the administration of bicarbonate to DKA patients with metabolic acidosis and pH levels of 6.9 to 7.14.[27] Similarly, a systematic review examining 44 studies found no evidence of improved glycemic control or clinical improvement with the use of bicarbonate therapy in DKA.[28] Moreover, a retrospective analysis of bicarbonate use for DKA and HHS revealed evidence of harm, including transient paradoxical worsening of ketosis, increased need for potassium supplementation, and, in pediatric patients, increased risk of cerebral edema and prolonged hospitalization.[28] Notably, no prospective randomized trials have studied the use of bicarbonate in DKA patients with pH <6.9. Due to concern about the effects of severe acidosis on vital organ function, the ADA continues to recommend administering 100 mmol of sodium bicarbonate in 400 mL sterile water with 20 mEq KCl at 200 mL/h for 2 hours, or until venous pH is >7.0.[3]

Complications

Common complications in the treatment of DKA and HHS are hypoglycemia and hypokalemia. Patients with these metabolic derangements are best served in the intensive care setting, where clinicians can more easily provide close monitoring of serum electrolytes and glucose. Another common complication is a non-AG hyperchloremic metabolic acidosis, which can follow aggressive resuscitation with normal saline, but is usually self-limited and rarely consequential.[29]

A serious complication of treatment that occurs more frequently in pediatric patients is cerebral edema. Symptoms including headache, lethargy, and depressed mental status present within 12 to 24 hours of treatment and may rapidly progress to include seizures, incontinence, and brain herniation. The mortality associated with cerebral edema is as high as 20% to 40%.[3] The optimal treatment is preventative, with a focus on fluid and sodium replacements in hyperosmolar patients, and the addition of 5% dextrose once glucose levels reach 200 mg/dL (DKA) or 300 mg/dL (HHS).[3] A clinical suspicion for cerebral edema should prompt immediate intensive care unit consultation.

CONCLUSION

All patients with DKA or HHS should be considered for ICU level of care at presentation and aggressively resuscitated. With proper management in the emergency department, patients who approach normalization of AG, have pH > 7.25, and can protect their airway, may be considered for a higher-acuity floor or step-down bed.

Early ICU care should be provided in patients who are severely acidemic or hypokalemic, cannot protect their airway, cannot tolerate fluid resuscitation (e.g., renal or cardiac patients), or have another pathophysiologic process present (e.g., sepsis). In the transfer from the ED to the ICU, important communications include the patients' comorbidities and mental status; their free water deficit and status of fluid resuscitation, insulin requirements and trajectory of AG correction; and electrolyte status and the trajectory of correction.

LITERATURE TABLE

TRIAL	DESIGN	RESULT
Insulin		
Kitabchi et al., *Diabetes Care.* 2008[23]	Prospective randomized study of 37 DKA patients assigned to 1) Insulin 0.07 units/kg load plus 0.07 units/kg/h infusion vs. 2) No load, insulin 0.07 units/kg/h infusion vs. 3) No load, infusion 0.14 units/kg/h	No significant difference in times to resolution of DKA between three groups
Bicarbonate		
Morris et al., *Ann Intern Med.* 1986[26]	Prospective randomized protocol of 21 patients. Various doses of bicarbonate administered based on pH 6.9–7.14 vs. control group who did not receive bicarbonate	No significant difference in rate of change of pH, ketone bodies, bicarbonate, or glucose levels between the two groups
Chua et al., *Ann Intensive Care.* 2011[28]	Systematic review of 44 studies—adults and pediatric patients with DKA, comparing outcomes of patients who received bicarbonate vs. no bicarbonate. No studies involved patients with pH < 6.85	Two RCTs showed transient improvement in acidosis in the first 2 h with bicarbonate treatment, however there was no evidence of improved glycemic control or clinical efficacy. In pediatric patients receiving bicarbonate there was retrospective evidence of increased risk of cerebral edema and prolonged hospitalization, and weak evidence of transient worsening of ketoacidosis and increased need for potassium supplementation

REFERENCES

1. http://www.cdc.gov/diabetes/statistics/dkafirst/fig7.htm (Accessed Feb 20, 2012)
2. Wang J, Williams DE, Narayan KM, et al. Declining death rates from hyperglycemic crisis among adults with diabetes, U.S., 1985–2002. *Diabetes Care.* 2006;29(9):2018.
3. Kitabchi AE, Umpierrez GE, Miles JM, et al. Hyperglycemic crises in adult patients with diabetes. *Diabetes Care.* 2009;32(7):1335.
4. Miles JM, Gerich JE. Glucose and ketone body kinetics in diabetic ketoacidosis. *Clin Endocrinol Metab.* 1983;12:303–319.
5. Feldman M, Soni N, Dickson B. Influence of hypoalbuminemia or hyperalbuminemia on the serum anion gap. *J Lab Clin Med.* 2005;146(6):317.
6. Gokel Y, Paydas S, Koseoglu Z, et al. Comparison of blood gas and acid–base measurements in arterial and venous blood samples in patients with uremic acidosis and diabetic ketoacidosis in the emergency room. *Am J Nephrol.* 2000;20(4):319.
7. Brandenburg MA, Dire DJ. Comparison of arterial and venous blood gas values in the initial emergency department evaluation of patients with diabetic ketoacidosis. *Ann Emerg Med.* 1998;31(4):459.
8. Malatesha G, Singh NK, Bharija A, et al. Comparison of arterial and venous pH, bicarbonate, PCO_2 and PO2 in initial emergency department assessment. *Emerg Med J.* 2007;24(8):569.

9. Umpierrez GE, Kelly JP, Navarrete JE, et al. Hyperglycemic crises in urban blacks. *Arch Intern Med.* 1997;157:669–675.
10. Kitabchi AE, Fisher JN. Insulin therapy of diabetic ketoacidosis: physiologic versus pharmacologic doses of insulin and their routes of administration. In: Brownlee M, ed. *Handbook of Diabetes Mellitus.* New York: Garland ATPM Press; 1981:95–149.
11. Abramson E, Arky R. Diabetic acidosis with initial hypokalemia. Therapeutic implications. *JAMA.* 1966;196(5):401.
12. Adrogué HJ, Lederer ED, Suki WN, et al. Determinants of plasma potassium levels in diabetic ketoacidosis. *Medicine (Baltimore).* 1986;65(3):163.
13. Kebler R, McDonald FD, Cadnapaphornchai P. Dynamic changes in serum phosphorus levels in diabetic ketoacidosis. *Am J Med.* 1985;79(5):571.
14. Fisher JN, Kitabchi AE. A randomized study of phosphate therapy in the treatment of diabetic ketoacidosis. *J Clin Endocrinol Metab.* 1983;57:177–180.
15. Winter RJ, Harris CJ, Phillips LS, et al. Diabetic ketoacidosis: induction of hypocalcemia and hypomagnesemia by phosphate therapy. *Am J Med* 1979;67:897–900.
16. Waldhausl W, Klenberger G, Korn A, et al. Effects of rehydration on endocrine derangements and blood glucose concentration. *Diabetes.* 1979;28:577–584.
17. Martin HE, Smith K, Wilson MI. The fluid and electrolyte therapy of severe diabetic acidosis and ketosis; a study of twenty-nine episodes (twenty-six patients). *Am J Med.* 1958;24:376–389.
18. Perel P, Roberts I. Colloids versus crystalloids for fluid resuscitation in critically ill patients. *Cochrane Database Syst Rev.* 2007;17:CD000567.
19. Bauer M, Kortgen A, Hartog C, et al. Isotonic and hypertonic crystalloid solutions in the critically ill. *Best Pract Res Clin Anaesthesiol.* 2009;23:173–181.
20. Chua HR, Balasubramanian V, Stachowski E, et al. Plasma-lyte 148 vs 0.9% saline for fluid resuscitation in diabetic ketoacidosis. *J Crit Care.* 2012;27:138–145.
21. Van Zyl DG, Rheeder P, Delport E. Fluid management in diabetic-acidosis-Ringer's lactate versus normal saline: a randomized controlled trial. *Q J Med.* 2012;105:337–343.
22. Dhatariya K. Editorial. Diabetic Ketoacidosis. *Brit Med J.* 2007;334:1284–1285.
23. Kitabchi AE, Matteri R, Murphy MB, et al. Is a priming dose of insulin necessary in a low-dose insulin protocol for the treatment of diabetic ketoacidosis? *Diabetes Care.* 2008;31(11):2081–2085.
24. Umpierrez GE, Latif K, Stoever J, et al. Efficacy of subcutaneous insulin lispro versus continuous intravenous regular insulin for the treatment of diabetic ketoacidosis. *Am J Med.* 2004;117:291–296.
25. Umpierrez GE, Latif KA, Cuervo R, et al. Treatment of diabetic ketoacidosis with subcutaneous aspart. *Diabetes Care.* 2004;27:1873–1878.
26. Ersoz HO, Ukinc K, Kose M, et al. Subcutaneous lispro and intravenous regular insulin treatments are equally effective and safe for the treatment of mild and moderate diabetic ketoacidosis in adult patients. *Int J Clin Pract.* 2006;60:429–433.
27. Morris LR, Murphy MB, Kitabchi AE. Bicarbonate therapy in severe diabetic ketoacidosis. *Ann Intern Med.* 1986;105(6):836.
28. Chua HR, Schneider A, Bellomo R. Bicarbonate in diabetic ketoacidosis—a systematic review. *Ann Intensive Care.* 2011;1:23.
29. Adrogue HJ, Wilson H, Boyd AE III, et al. Plasma acid–base patterns in diabetic ketoacidosis. *N Engl J Med.* 1982;307:1603–1610.

43

Adrenal Insufficiency

Thomas B. Perera

BACKGROUND

The adrenal glands are two small, irregularly shaped bodies located superior to each renal pole. Each gland contains two distinct structures, the outer adrenal medulla and the inner adrenal cortex. The adrenal cortex can be divided into three zones: the zona glomerulosa, which produces the mineralocorticoid aldosterone, and the zona fasciculata and zona reticularis, which produce the glucocorticoid cortisol as well as androgens. The outer medulla is responsible for catecholamine production, including epinephrine and norepinephrine.

Cortisol has multiple effects, including increasing blood glucose and gluconeogenesis, suppressing the immune system, decreasing bone formation, and aiding in fat, protein, and carbohydrate metabolism. Aldosterone works on the kidneys to promote reabsorption of sodium and of water and secretion of potassium. Adrenal insufficiency is defined as a condition in which the adrenal glands fail to produce an adequate amount of steroid hormones to meet the needs of the body. Adrenal insufficiency can be a devastating complication of critical illness and, in high-risk patients (e.g., those with hypotension, shock, sepsis), has an incidence of approximately 30% to 40%.[1]

Adrenal gland production of cortisol is regulated through the hypothalamus–pituitary–adrenal gland axis. The hypothalamus responds to external stimuli, including low cortisol levels, by secreting corticotropin-releasing hormone (CRH). This causes the pituitary gland to release corticotropin (adrenocorticotropic hormone [ACTH]), which is the primary regulator of cortisol production and release. Approximately 95% of body cortisol is protein bound; it is the remaining 5% of free cortisol that produces effects in the body. In normal individuals, daily cortisol secretion ranges from 40 to 80 μmol and has a pronounced circadian rhythm. Severe physical or emotional stresses stimulate the secretion of CRH and ACTH, which results in large increases (two- or threefold) in serum cortisol concentrations.

Aldosterone production is mediated by the renin–angiotensin–aldosterone system (RAAS). The RAAS is involved with the regulation of vasoconstriction and extracellular blood volume. Renin is an enzyme secreted by specialized cells that encircle the arterioles at the entrance to the glomeruli of the kidneys. These specialized cells modulate renin production in response to changes in blood flow and blood pressure. Low blood flow to the kidneys from any reason, including low blood pressure, will result in increased renin production and release. Renin promotes conversion of the plasma protein angiotensinogen into angiotensin I, which is subsequently converted into angiotensin II—a potent vasoconstrictor—by the angiotensin-converting enzyme. Angiotensin II acts on receptors in the adrenal glands to stimulate the secretion of aldosterone, which in turn promotes renal resorption of sodium and water.

The adrenal medulla makes up about 10% of the adrenal gland and is an integral part of the sympathetic nervous system. The cells of the medulla, known as chromaffin cells, house chromaffin granules that contain epinephrine, norepinephrine, and dopamine, which are released in response to sympathetic nerve stimulation. In patients with adrenal insufficiency, the adrenal medulla is typically not dysfunctional.

ETIOLOGY

Recognizing adrenal insufficiency is the most challenging aspect of its treatment. The hallmark presentation of this condition is hypotension unresponsive to fluids in a patient with sepsis or another acute stressor; however, its presentation can be much subtler. The provider's goal should be to recognize the disease and start treatment before the patient is in shock; once initiated, treatment is generally straightforward.

In subacute or chronic presentations, the symptoms of adrenal insufficiency may include fatigue, anorexia, nausea, vomiting, muscle aches, weight loss, and a low blood pressure (<110 mm Hg) that may be orthostatic. More than 90% of cases will demonstrate skin hyperpigmentation (due to increased ACTH release) in areas exposed to light, chronic friction, or pressure, as well as the palmar creases.[2]

There are three major types of adrenal insufficiency. Primary adrenal insufficiency is caused by destruction or dysfunction of the adrenal gland itself; this will not manifest until 90% of the gland is destroyed.[3] Because there is direct damage to the gland, glucocorticoid and mineralocorticoid secretion are affected; destruction of the entire gland can affect sympathetic nervous system function as well. In the United States, the most common cause (80%) of primary adrenal insufficiency is autoimmune adrenalitis (Addison disease); half of these cases exist as part of the polyglandular autoimmune syndrome type I or II, which can include diabetes and hypothyroidism in addition to adrenal insufficiency. Worldwide, the most common cause of primary adrenal insufficiency is destruction of the adrenal gland by *Mycobacterium tuberculosis*.

Secondary (and tertiary) adrenal insufficiency results from any process involving the pituitary gland or hypothalamus that interferes with ACTH secretion. Such processes include tumors of the pituitary or hypothalamus, infiltrative processes such as sarcoid or TB, surgery, radiation, trauma, and postpartum pituitary necrosis (Sheehan syndrome). Secondary adrenal insufficiency affects only glucocorticoid production (ACTH only affects cortisol production and release). Mineralocorticoid production and sympathetic function are generally not affected.

By far, the most common etiology of secondary adrenal insufficiency is hypoaldosteronism caused by prolonged glucocorticoid therapy. When exogenous glucocorticoids are administered, the body's production of cortisol can be suppressed, which can lead to decreased adrenal gland responsiveness and atrophy. Inhibition of ACTH secretion depends on the dose, duration, and frequency of glucocorticoid therapy. While there is variation among individual patients, adrenal insufficiency should be considered in symptomatic patients who have received doses of prednisone >7.5 mg per day or

TABLE 43.1 Causes of Adrenal Insufficiency

Primary: Damage to adrenal gland (mineral and glucocorticoid production affected)
- Autoimmune adrenalitis: Isolated or with Polyglandular autoimmune syndrome type I or II
- Infection
  - TB, CMV, Histoplasmosis, Paracoccidioidomycosis, HIV and AIDS, Syphilis
- Adrenal gland destruction
  - Hemorrhage: trauma, coagulants, sepsis, meningococcemia (Waterhouse-Friderichsen)
  - Metastasis: lung breast, colon cancer
  - Bilateral infiltration: lymphoma, sarcoidosis, amyloidosis
- Drug induced
  - Etomidate, ketoconazole, suramin, rifampin, dilantin, barbiturates, Mitotane

Secondary: Interference with ACTH secretion at the pituitary gland (glucocorticoid affected)
- Postpartum pituitary necrosis (Sheehan's syndrome)
- Pituitary tumor, trauma, surgery (Following the cure of Cushing's syndrome)
- Infiltrative diseases- sarcoidosis, TB, eosinophilic granuloma

Tertiary: Interference with corticotropin-releasing hormone (CRH) secretion by the hypothalamus (glucocorticoid affected)
- Glucocorticoid withdrawal after chronic use
- Hypothalamic tumor, trauma, surgery

another steroid equivalent for longer than 3 weeks.[4,5] Inhaled and topical steroids are also demonstrated culprits in adrenal suppression.[6,7] Patients taking medications that inhibit the cytochrome P450 enzyme CYP3A4 (diltiazem, protease inhibitors, azole antifungals, grapefruit juice) will have a prolonged biologic half-life of glucocorticoids and thus an enhanced suppression of adrenal function.[8] The adrenal glands may require 6 to 12 months for full recovery of function following prolonged use of exogenous glucocorticoids.[9] Tertiary adrenal insufficiency results when an insufficient amount of CRH is produced by the hypothalamus (Table 43.1).

SPECIAL CONSIDERATIONS

HIV and AIDS

Adrenal insufficiency has been demonstrated in 5% to 20% of tested patients with HIV.[10] The prevalence increases with the progression of HIV. HIV may result in primary adrenal insufficiency by itself or through associated infection (TB, cytomegalovirus [CMV], Mycobacterium avium-intracellulare (MAI) or malignancy (Kaposi sarcoma, lymphoma). HIV is also associated with secondary adrenal insufficiency through infectious agents that affect the pituitary gland (toxoplasmosis, CMV), drugs that interfere with adrenal function (ketoconazole, megestrol acetate), or drugs that increase degradation of cortisol (rifampin, phenytoin, opiates).[11] Autopsies of patients with AIDS show adrenal injury in over 50% of cases and pituitary involvement injury in 30% of cases.[12]

Etomidate

Etomidate is a first-line anesthetic used in rapid sequence intubation; it is particularly useful in critically ill patients because it is hemodynamically well tolerated. Etomidate, however, decreases available cortisol by inhibiting the 11β-hydroxylase enzyme that converts 11β-deoxycortisol into cortisol in the adrenal gland. Use of continuous etomidate infusion in the critically ill has been associated with an increase in mortality and thus has been curtailed.[13] A single dose of etomidate has been shown to cause laboratory evidence of adrenal suppression for 4 to 24 hours. In one study, 80% of patients showed adrenal suppression when tested at 12 hours after a single dose of etomidate.[14] However, the clinical effects of this effect are still in debate. A multitude of smaller and retrospective studies showed no difference in outcome with etomidate. A large 2012 meta-analysis/systemic review demonstrated that in critically ill patients, the relative risk of death with etomidate use was 1.20 (95% CI 1.04–1.42).[15] Smaller studies have also linked etomidate to a higher risk of pneumonia (56% vs. 26%) in trauma patients.[16] Although evidence is inconclusive, it may be prudent to consider other induction agents if they are available. While some practitioners have opted to give steroids for 24 to 48 hours after an etomidate-assisted intubation in order to compensate for the decreased adrenal function, small studies have failed to demonstrate any changes in patient outcomes with the use of adjunctive steroids.

Sepsis

Infection stimulates an inflammatory, coagulation, and immunologic response that works synergistically to either eliminate or control the infection and to repair associated tissue damage. If left unchecked or unregulated, however, these host defenses may themselves become counterproductive and lead to deterioration in organ function rather than to restoration of homeostasis. It is believed that in some cases of sepsis, it is overaggressive and protracted host defense, rather than the precipitating insult (e.g., pneumonia), that primarily determines outcome.

Infection also stimulates the hypothalamic–pituitary–adrenal axis, causing an increase in glucocorticoid release. Glucocorticoids exert a protective effect by restraining the host defense response at many levels, including suppression of cytokine production. Studies have shown that sepsis nonsurvivors exhibit a persistent and exaggerated increase in circulating inflammatory cytokine concentrations when compared with survivors.[17,18] Research also suggests that cytokines can produce a concentration-dependent resistance to glucocorticoids in target tissues by reducing glucocorticoid receptor binding affinity for cortisol.[19] Finally, inflammatory mediators (including cytokines) are also known to alter the hypothalamic–pituitary–adrenal axis and contribute directly to adrenal insufficiency.

Because of these associations, it was once thought that all patients with severe septic shock should be treated with exogenous steroids. Early treatment and studies used "high-dose" steroids (30 mg/kg methylprednisolone), but showed limited success; subsequent studies of "high-dose" steroids showed at first no improvement, and later, harm.[20,21] The negative effects of glucocorticoid therapy included hyperglycemia, superinfection, muscular weakness, hypernatremia, upper gastrointestinal bleeding, psychosis, and poor wound healing.

More recently, studies have focused on the effect of "low-dose" steroids (e.g., 200 to 300 mg of hydrocortisone or equivalent). Patients considered for exogenous glucocorticoid therapy are those in septic shock who remain unstable after fluid and vasopressor therapy. The endpoints examined were earlier reversal of shock and effect on mortality. A representative study with "low-dose" steroids showed effect on the timing of shock reversal, but no effect at 28-day mortality.[22] A 2002 landmark study separated patients with a normal corticotrophin stimulation (responders) from patients with an abnormally low response (nonresponders). This study showed the 28-day mortality was decreased by corticosteroid therapy in the overall patient population (61% vs. 55%) and in the ACTH nonresponder group of patients (63% vs. 53%), with no increase in adverse events.[23] This study led to the inclusion of steroid therapy in the Surviving Sepsis Campaign in 2004.

An important follow-up trial in 2008 reopened the question of steroids in sepsis.[24] This large study also separated septic shock patients into responders and nonresponders, but found no difference in nonresponders who received glucocorticoids from placebo (39% vs. 36%). Shock reversal did occur more quickly in the treated group (3.3 days vs. 5.8 days); however, no difference in mortality was proven, and the study showed an increase in hyperglycemia, hypernatremia, and superinfections in steroid-treated patients.

Presently, the Surviving Sepsis Campaign 2012 guidelines recommend hydrocortisone at a dose of 200 mg per day for patients who remain hemodynamically unstable after adequate fluid and vasopressor therapy. An ACTH stimulation test is not a prerequisite for initiating steroid therapy (see below).[25]

DIAGNOSTIC EVALUATION

The diagnosis of adrenal insufficiency involves testing cortisol levels. In an unstressed patient, a single morning cortisol level can be sufficient. A level of <3 mcg/dL is diagnostic for adrenal insufficiency, a level of 4 to 10 mcg/dL is suggestive, and a level of >20 mcg/dL excludes the condition. However, as any form of stress increases cortisol levels, this metric is rarely helpful in the emergency or ICU setting. In septic patients, a random level of <10 mcg/dL has been used as an indicator of adrenal insufficiency, while a level of >33 mcg/dL makes the diagnosis unlikely.[26] One study evaluated multiple approaches to diagnosing adrenal insufficiency in critically ill patients with septic shock and concluded that the standard 250 mcg cosyntropin (ACTH) stimulation test—with a result of ≤9 mcg/dL increase from baseline in total cortisol 60 minutes after administration—was the best predictor of decreased adrenal function.[27] A "low-dose" 1 mcg cosyntropin (ACTH) stimulation test has also been in limited use; this more sensitive assay has been shown to be a better predictor of survival, but is not readily available and is not as widely accepted.[28] The American College of Critical Care Medicine currently recommends that adrenal insufficiency in critically ill patients is best identified by an increase in serum cortisol level of <9 mcg/dL after a 250 mg ACTH stimulation test, or a random total cortisol level <10 mcg/dL.[26] It also recommends that these tests be performed only in patients with suspected adrenal insufficiency. This means that not all septic shock patients who are put on steroids require testing.

MANAGEMENT GUIDELINES

In the critical care setting, management of adrenal insufficiency focuses on treating concomitant stresses, resuscitating the patient, and giving glucocorticoids. Hydrocortisone is the glucocorticoid of choice, as it has both glucocorticoid and mineralocorticoid activities; it also adequately treats associated electrolyte disturbances caused by mineralocorticoid deficiency that are seen in primary adrenal insufficiency. Fludrocortisone, a mineralocorticoid, has been studied and is not considered necessary to supplement in the acute setting. Dexamethasone has been suggested for patients who may eventually need an ACTH stimulation test, as it does not interfere with cortisol levels; however, it is not indicated in critically ill patients, especially those with electrolyte disturbances, as it has no mineralocorticoid activity. In all patients receiving hydrocortisone, glucose should be monitored, as hyper- and hypoglycemic episodes are possible. Patients should also be monitored for hypernatremia, and hypertonic saline should generally be avoided.

In patients with acute adrenal crisis, treatment dose hydrocortisone is 50 to 100 mg IV q6h. Alternatively, a dose of hydrocortisone 50 to 100 mg followed by an infusion of 20 mg/hour has been used. Improvement is typically observed within 4 to 6 hours. In the setting of suspected adrenal insufficiency with concomitant septic shock, no standard dosing has been established; a common approach is to give hydrocortisone at a dose of either 200 to 300 mg per day or 50 mg q6h. This is often continued for 5 to 7 days with or without a taper.[25,29] In patients who have a history of adrenal insufficiency who are undergoing an acute stress/procedure, a single dose of 100 mg IV of hydrocortisone has been recommended.

CONCLUSION

Adrenal insufficiency can be a devastating complication of critically illness and is an important entity to consider in the differential diagnosis of patients with persistent hypotension, shock, or sepsis. The use of steroids in sepsis should be strongly considered in patients with vasopressor refractory shock.

LITERATURE TABLE

TRIAL	DESIGN	RESULT
Etomidate		
Chan et al., *Crit Care Med.* 2012[15]	A systematic review of randomized controlled trials and observational studies with meta-analysis assessing the effects of etomidate on adrenal insufficiency (1,303 patients) and mortality (865 patients)	Subjects who received etomidate had an increased risk of adrenal insufficiency (pooled relative risk 1.33; CI 1.22–1.46) and were more likely to die (pooled relative risk 1.20; 95% CI 1.02–1.42)
Asehnoune et al., *Intensive Care Med.* 2012[16]	A sub-study of a randomized, double blind, placebo-controlled trial of hydrocortisone in 149 trauma patients. Patients who received etomidate were compared to controls	Etomidate was associated with hospital-associated pneumonia. 49 (51.6%) of patients with etomidate and 16 (29.6%) patients without etomidate developed with hospital-associated pneumonia by day 28
Sepsis		
The VA Systemic Sepsis Cooperative Study Group. *N Engl J Med.* 1987[20]	RCT of early short-term, high-dose methylprednisolone sodium succinate in 223 patients with septic shock	Mortality not significantly different between the two groups ($p = 0.97$). Resolution of secondary infection within 14 d was significantly lower in the treatment group ($p = 0.03$)
Annane et al., *JAMA.* 2002[23]	RCT comparing hydrocortisone and fludrocortisone or placebo for 7 d in 299 patients separated into two groups by response to a standard 250 mcg ACTH stimulation test	In ACTH stimulation test nonresponders, treated patients had a decrease in mortality 63%–53% ($p = 0.02$) and showed earlier vasopressor withdrawal ($p = 0.001$)

LITERATURE TABLE (*Continued*)		
TRIAL	**DESIGN**	**RESULT**
Sprung et al., *N Engl J Med.* 2008[24] CORTICUS	RCT comparing hydrocortisone or placebo for 5 d and a 6-d taper in 499 patients separated into two groups by response to a standard 250 mcg ACTH stimulation test	No difference in survival or reversal of shock in patients with septic shock, either overall or in nonresponders. Hydrocortisone did hasten reversal of shock in patients in whom shock was reversed
Fludrocortisone		
The COIITSS Study Investigators. *JAMA.* 2010[29]	RCT evaluating tight glycemic control and the addition of fludrocortisone in 509 septic shock patients treated with hydrocortisone	No difference in mortality in patients treated with fludrocortisone ($p = 0.50$)

CI, confidence interval.

REFERENCES

1. Gary P, Zaloga MD, Paul Marik MD. Hypothalamic-Pituitary-adrenal insufficiency. *Crit Care Clin.* 2001;17:25–41.
2. Dunlop D. Eighty-six cases of addison's disease. *Br Med J.* 1963;2(5362):887.
3. Munver R, Volfson IA. Adrenal insufficiency: diagnosis and management. *Curr Urol Rep.* 2006;7:80–85.
4. Bouillon R. Acute adrenal insufficiency. *Endocrinol Metab Clin North Am.* 2006;35:76797.
5. Marik PE. Critical illness-related corticosteroid insufficiency. *Chest.* 2009;135:181–193.
6. Hengge UR, Ruzicka T, Schwartz RA, et al. Adverse effects of topical glucocorticosteroids. *J Am Acad Dermatol.* 2006;54(1):1–15.
7. Zollner EW. Hypothalamic-pituitary-adrenal axis suppression in asthmatic children on inhaled corticosteroids (Part 2). *Pediatr Allergy Immunol.* 2007;18:469.
8. Varis T, Kivisto KT, Backman JT, et al. The cytochrome P450 3A4 inhibitor itraconazole markedly increases the plasma concentrations of dexamethasone and enhances its adrenal-suppressant effect. *Clin Pharmacol Ther.* 2000;68:487–494.
9. Axelrod L. Perioperative management of patients treated with glucocorticoids. *Endocrinol Metab Clin North Am.* 2003;32:367–383.
10. Masharani U, Schambelan M. The endocrine complications of acquired immunodeficiency syndrome. *Adv Intern Med.* 1993;38:323–336.
11. Prasnthai V, Sunthornyothin S, Phowthongkum P, et al. Prevalence of adrenal insufficiency in critically ill patients with AIDS. *J Med Assoc Thai.* 2007;90:1768.
12. Eledrisi MS, Verghese AC. Adrenal Insufficiency in HIV Infection: a review and recommendations. *Am J Med Sci.* 2001;321(2):137–144.
13. Wagner RL, White PF, Kan PB, et al. Inhibition of adrenal steroidogenesis by the anesthetic etomidate. *N Engl J Med.* 1984;310:1415–1421.
14. Vinclair M, Broux C, Faure P, et al. Duration of adrenal inhibition following a single dose of etomidate in critically ill patients. *Intensive Care Med.* 2008;34:714–719.
15. Chan CM, Mitchell AL, Shorr AF. Etomidate is associated with mortality and adrenal insufficiency in sepsis: a meta-analysis*. *Crit Care Med.* 2012;40(11):2945–2953.
16. Asehnoune K, Mahe PJ, Seguin P. Etomidate increases susceptibility to pneumonia in trauma patients. *Intensive Care Med.* 2012;38(10):1673–1678.
17. Hermus ARMM, Sweep CGJ. Cytokines and the hypothalamic-pituitary-adrenal axis. *J Steroid Biochem Mol Biol.* 1990;37:867–871.
18. Damas P, Ledoux D, Nys M, et al. Cytokine serum level during severe sepsis in human IL-6 as a marker of severity. *Ann Surg.* 1992;215:356–362.
19. Kam JC, Szefler SJ, Surs W, et al. Combination IL-2 and IL-4 reduces glucocorticoid receptor-binding affinity and T cell response to glucocorticoids. *J Immunol.* 1993;151:3460–3466.
20. The Veterans Administration Systemic Sepsis Cooperative Study Group. Effect of high-dose glucocorticoid therapy on mortality in patients with clinical signs of systemic sepsis. *N Engl J Med.* 1987;317:659–665.

21. Cronin L, Cook DJ, Carlet J, et al. Corticosteroid treatment for sepsis: a critical appraisal and meta-analysis of the literature. *Crit Care Med.* 1995;24:1430–1439.
22. Cicarelli DD, Viera JE, Martin Besenor FE. Early dexamethasone treatment for septic shock patients: a prospective randomized clinical trial. *Sao Paulo Med J.* 2007;125:237–241.
23. Annane D, Sebille V, Charpentier C, et al. Effect of treatment with low doses of hydrocortisone and fludrocortisone on mortality in patients with septic shock. *JAMA.* 2002;288:862–870.
24. Sprung CL, Annane D, et al. Hydrocortisone therapy for patients with septic shock. *N Engl J Med.* 2008;10;358:111–124.
25. Dellinger P, Levy M, Rhodes A. Surviving sepsis campaign: international guidelines for management of severe sepsis and septic shock: 2012. *Crit Care Med.* 2013;41:580–637.
26. Marik PE, Pastores SM, Annane D, et al. Recommendations for the diagnosis and management of corticosteroid insufficiency in critically ill adult patients: consensus statements from an international task force by the American College of Critical Care Medicine. *Crit Care Med.* 2008;36:1937–1949.
27. Salgado DR, Verdeal JCR, Rocco JR. Adrenal function testing in patients with septic shock. *Crit Care.* 2006;10:R149.
28. Siraux V, De Backer D, Yalavatti G. Relative adrenal insufficiency in patients with septic shock: comparison of low-dose and conventional corticotropin tests. *Crit Care Med.* 2005;33:2479–2486.
29. The COIITSS Study Investigators. Corticosteroid treatment and intensive insulin therapy for septic shock in adults: randomized controlled trial. *JAMA.* 2010;303:341–348.

44

Thyroid Storm and Myxedema Coma

James Lantry III, John E. Arbo, and Geoffrey K. Lighthall

BACKGROUND

Thyrotoxicosis and myxedema coma are life-threatening syndromes representing the extremes of thyroid dysfunction. The rapid deterioration seen in these two conditions can result in significant morbidity and mortality if not promptly recognized.[1] Delays in diagnosis and treatment are attributable in part to the nonspecific symptoms found in each condition.[2] Success in management depends on developing a high level of suspicion for these disease processes, initiating early patient transfer to an intensive care setting, and delivering prompt targeted treatment.[3,4]

THYROTOXICOSIS

Hyperthyroidism refers to any state of elevated production of thyroid hormone; thyrotoxicosis is defined as a pathologic process that results from excess hormone secretion.[3] The overall prevalence of hyperthyroidism in the United States is approximately 1.3%.[2,5,6] Only 0.5% of this population will demonstrate the symptoms of thyrotoxicosis.[5] In the thyrotoxic population, 1% to 2% will progress to a severe, exaggerated, and life-threatening manifestation of thyrotoxicosis called thyrotoxic crisis or thyroid storm.[7,8] The point at which thyrotoxicosis becomes thyroid storm is controversial and somewhat subjective. Efforts to standardize a definition of thyroid storm include a scoring system that evaluates degrees of dysfunction in affected systems (thermoregulatory, cardiac, gastrointestinal, and neurologic).[9] In clinical practice, patients presenting with symptoms of thyrotoxicosis should always be evaluated for impending thyroid storm (Table 44.1).

The most common cause of thyrotoxicosis is Graves disease, a condition in which autoantibodies bind to and stimulate thyroid-stimulating hormone (TSH) receptors on the surface of thyroid follicular cells, leading to unregulated release of the thyroid hormones triiodothyronine (T_3) and thyroxine (T_4).[3] Graves disease occurs most commonly in adults 30 to 40 years of age and is associated with other autoimmune diseases, such as rheumatoid arthritis, as well as with tobacco use, emotional stress, and infection with *Yersinia enterocolitica.*[7] Studies in twins suggest that approximately 80% of susceptibility to Graves disease is driven by genetics.[3] The second most common cause of thyrotoxicosis is excess hormone production by a thyroid nodule, either a solitary toxic adenoma or a toxic multinodular goiter (TMNG). The prevalence of TMNG is higher in women and increases with age.[3]

TABLE 44.1 Diagnostic Criteria for Thyroid Storm

Diagnostic Parameters	Scoring System
Thermoregulatory Dysfunction	
Temperature	
99–99.9	5
100–100.9	10
101–101.9	15
102–102.9	20
103–103.9	25
≥104	30
Central Nervous System effects	
Absent	0
Mild (agitation)	10
Moderate (delirium, psychosis, extreme lethargy)	20
Severe (seizures, coma)	30
Gastrointestinal-hepatic dysfunction	
Absent	0
Moderate (diarrhea, nausea, vomiting, abdominal pain)	10
Severe (unexplained jaundice)	20
Cardiovascular dysfunction	
Tachycardia (beats/min)	
90–109	5
110–119	10
120–129	15
130–139	20
≥140	25
Congestive heart failure	
Absent	0
Mild (pedal edema)	5
Moderate (bibasilar rales)	10
Severe (pulmonary edema)	15
Atrial fibrillation	
Absent	0
Present	10
Precipitating event	
Absent	0
Present	10

Scoring system: A score of 45 or greater is highly suggestive of thyroid storm; a score of 25–44 is suggestive of impending storm, and a score below 25 is unlikely to represent thyroid storm.
Adapted from Burch HB, Wartofsky L. Life-threatening thyrotoxicosis. Thyroid storm. *Endocrinol Metab Clin North Am.* 1993;22(2):263–277.

The prevalence of both Graves disease and TMNG in a population is determined by dietary iodine content.[10] In populations with adequate iodine intake, Graves disease represents nearly 80% of cases of thyrotoxicosis; in populations with inadequate iodine intake, the incidence of TMNG increases and can be responsible for half of all clinical cases.[10,11] Approximately 10% of cases of thyrotoxicosis are linked to thyroid cell inflammation, or thyroiditis, triggers for which include radiation, drug side effects, and autoantibodies as seen with Hashimoto thyroiditis.[1] Subacute thyroiditis, or de Quervain thyroiditis, is a transient hyperthyroid state associated with upper respiratory infections; it presents with neck swelling, malaise, and fatigue. Thyrotoxicosis can be seen in up to 50% of patients with de Quervain thyroiditis, and typically resolves within 8 months of the inciting illness.[10] Postpartum thyroiditis—another cause of transient hyperthyroidism—affects 5% to 10% of women in the first 3 to 6 months after delivery.[12] Finally, thyrotoxicosis can be attributed to exogenous thyroid hormone use in the treatment of hypothyroid disease.[13,14]

Of the numerous causes of thyrotoxicosis, Graves disease is the most common condition associated with thyroid storm.[15] However, thyroid storm can result in any patient from excessive thyroid hormone release of any cause, including excessive iodine exposure from radiocontrast dye or iodine-containing drugs such as amiodarone.[1] The only impetus required to induce thyroid storm from an otherwise stable thyrotoxic state is a stressful event, most commonly from infection or surgery.[10] A recent study of Japanese hospitalized patients estimates the overall incidence of thyroid storm to be 0.2 per 100,000 patients per year; however, the true incidence remains unknown due to significant underdiagnosis.[16]

Physiology and Organ-Specific Effects

Pituitary-derived TSH induces the release of both T_3 and T_4.[2] Both hormones regulate basal metabolism, but T_3 is three to four times more potent than T_4.[3] TSH-induced release accounts for only 20% of circulating T_3; the remainder occurs through peripheral conversion of T_4 to T_3 by the liver and kidney.[5,17] The excess circulating thyroid hormone in a thyrotoxic state can produce a range of detrimental systemic effects, the degree and extent of which determine the presence of thyroid storm (Table 44.1).

Excess thyroid hormone activity produces an adrenergic state characterized by tachycardia, nervousness, and anxiety.[15] This increase in metabolic activity can manifest as heat intolerance, increased perspiration, and lipolysis, eventually leading to as much as a 15% loss of basal body weight.[7]

Cardiovascular manifestations can include tachycardia and other atrial and ventricular arrhythmias, as well as systolic hypertension and widening of pulse pressure.[18] New-onset dilated cardiomyopathy and congestive heart failure have also been reported in previously healthy patients with thyrotoxicosis.[1] These hyperadrenergic effects can lead to increased myocardial oxygen demand and/or coronary artery vasospasm, producing angina and even myocardial infarctions. The thyrotoxic state may also have metabolic consequences, such as acidemia resulting from lipolysis and ketogenesis and tissue acidosis from mismatch between oxygen demand and supply.[1]

Respiratory signs include dyspnea and orthopnea from respiratory muscle weakness, high output cardiac failure, and engorgement of the pulmonary vasculature.[15] A more common finding, however, is tachypnea at rest, which can herald impending respiratory fatigue and collapse.[1,7] Higher respiratory demand may be the result of either adrenergic stimulation or compensation for acidemia.[1]

Gastrointestinal symptoms include hypermotility, which can lead to diarrhea, nausea, and vomiting.[8] Concomitant loss of fluid can exacerbate postural hypotension and vascular collapse and can precipitate a state of shock.[1] Impairment of neurologic regulation of gastric and intestinal activity can lead to gastroparesis and/or pseudo-obstruction.[7]

Hematologic changes include hypercoagulability, leukocytosis, and anemia. Hypercoagulability results from higher concentrations of fibrinogen, factors VIII and IX, plasminogen activator inhibitor 1, and von Willebrand factor.[1] Moderate leukocytosis with a left shift is common, and approximately 22% of patients will suffer from symptomatic anemia.[3] There is also an increase in red blood cell mass secondary to increased erythropoietin levels and an augmentation of platelet plug formation.[19] Thromboembolic complications are responsible for 18% of thyrotoxicosis-related deaths.[18]

Thyrotoxic periodic paralysis (TPP) is an unusual complication of thyrotoxicosis seen in only 0.1% to 0.2% of thyrotoxic patients, with increased incidence in Asians (1.8% to 2.0%) and males (20:1).[1,20] TPP is characterized by transient but recurrent flaccid paralysis of the proximal extremities, decreased deep tendon reflexes, and cardiac conduction abnormalities including atrioventricular blocks and asystole.[20] The specific distribution of muscular findings in TPP contrasts with the generalized myopathy affecting approximately 50% of thyrotoxic patients, where fatigability and global weakness are the main findings.[7] Proximal muscle weakness can also be characteristic of a thyrotoxic state, but to a lesser degree than with TPP.[21]

History and Physical Exam

Thyroid storm occurs most frequently in patients with either undiagnosed or poorly controlled thyrotoxicosis who are exposed to a systemic insult or stress.[14,15] Infection is the most common inciting event; however, case reports have implicated nearly all known forms of physiologic stress.[1] Regardless of the inciting event, untreated thyroid storm is uniformly fatal; even with appropriate treatment, the mortality rate is nearly 50%.[8] The significant morbidity and mortality result from serial decompensation of multiple organ systems.[13]

The four principle findings of thyroid storm are (1) fever out of proportion to infection accompanied by significant diaphoresis, (2) sinus tachycardia or supraventricular arrhythmia (paroxysmal atrial tachycardia or atrial flutter or atrial fibrillation) leading to congestive heart failure, (3) gastrointestinal symptoms (vomiting, diarrhea, or bowel obstruction), and (4) central nervous system symptoms (agitation, restlessness, confusion, delirium or coma).[1,7,22] The diagnosis is made clinically, as laboratory tests and imaging are not specific.

On examination, the thyroid gland will be enlarged and, depending on the etiology of thyrotoxicosis, may contain nodules; additionally, a bruit may be present because of increased thyroid vascularity.[15] The skin will be warm, moist, and velvety, with softening of the hair and nails often leading to nail bed separation (onycholysis) and alopecia.[2,7] Significant hyperpigmentation and raised, asymmetric lesions of the skin may be present.[23] These plaques are often located on the lower extremities and accompanied by significant pretibial myxedema.[7] Hands and feet are frequently swollen and may be accompanied by clubbing.[18] In Graves disease, ophthalmopathy may be observed (lid lag, lid retraction, and proptosis) leading to burning and irritation with blurring of the vision and diplopia.[15] Difficulty with eye closure can lead to corneal ulceration or vision loss unless properly treated.[24] Impairment of mental status, including psychosis and delirium, may also be observed.[11] Patients may appear restless and complain of heat intolerance, palpitations, anxiety, and fatigue and may demonstrate a fine, rapid tremor at rest.[10] Finally, patients may report weight loss despite a significant appetite (Table 44.2).[15]

TABLE 44.2 Clinical Manifestations of Thyrotoxicosis

Organ System	Symptoms	Signs
Neuropsychiatric	Anxiety Fatigue Insomnia Confusion Emotional lability Coma	Hyperreflexia Fine tremor Muscle wasting Weakness Periodic paralysis
Cardiovascular	Palpitations Chest pain	Sinus tachycardia Atrial fibrillation Congestive heart failure Hyperdynamic precordium
Pulmonary	Dyspnea	Rales
Gastrointestinal	Weight loss Dysphagia Hyperphagia Hyperdefecation Diarrhea	Increased bowel sounds
Genitourinary	Decreased libido Oligomenorrhea Amenorrhea	Gynecomastia Spider angiomas
Ophthalmologic	Diplopia Retrobulbar pressure Eye irritation	Exophthalmos Ophthalmoplegia Conjunctival injection
Dermatologic	Hair loss	Palmar erythema Onycholysis Pretibial myxedema Warm, moist, smooth skin
Endocrine	Heat intolerance Neck fullness	Thyroid enlargement

Laboratory Testing and Imaging

Emergency department (ED) laboratory testing for suspected thyrotoxicosis should include a TSH level and a free T_4. TSH levels will often be undetectable (<0.01 microIU/L) due to negative feedback from excess thyroid hormone.[3] The TSH assay is reported in a logarithmic scale, such that a small change in T_4 levels can lead to a larger change in measured TSH; thus, the assay has a high sensitivity to thyroid hormone excess.[25] If thyrotoxicosis is suspected, testing both TSH and free serum T_4 improves diagnostic accuracy by allowing confirmation that the drop in TSH is due to thyroid dysfunction and not due to indirect causes (e.g., glucocorticoid or dopamine use).[3,10] A rise in T_4 is seen in 95% of patients suffering from thyrotoxicosis, with the remaining 5% experiencing an increased free T_3 and normal T_4 levels.[7] This latter pattern can develop in early Graves disease or TMNG; thus, experts recommend checking free T_3 levels to increase sensitivity if thyrotoxicosis figures prominently on the differential diagnosis.[10] The ratio of free T_3 to T_4 helps distinguish increased and decreased thyroid gland metabolism.[18] Patients with Graves disease or TMNG will have an increased ratio of free T_3/T_4 (>20); by contrast, patients with thyroiditis will have a decreased ratio (<20).[15] Testing for total T_3 or T_4 is no longer recommended as liver disease, exogenous hormone use, or pregnancy can cause unreliable protein binding of free thyroid hormones (Fig. 44.1).[7]

Other laboratory abnormalities may include an initial hyperglycemia, mediated by increased glycogenolysis and an increase in insulin clearance; profound hypoglycemia can subsequently result from this depletion of glycogen stores.[1] Hepatic dysfunction can lead to accumulation of lactate dehydrogenase, aspartate aminotransferase, and bilirubin.[7] Acidemia may occur due to lipolysis and dehydration ketosis.[26] Hypercalcemia, the result of hemoconcentration from fluid shifts and an increase in bone resorption, is also common.[15] This increase in osteoblastic bone activity can also lead to elevations in alkaline phosphatase.[15]

Prevention of thyroid storm is dependent on early detection of thyrotoxicosis. While thyroid storm is a clinical diagnosis, thyrotoxicosis is confirmed when laboratory findings corroborate suspicion developed from the history and physical exam.[1] While the trigger of a patient's thyroid storm (e.g., infection) may not be evident initially, clinical stabilization should proceed at the same time as the diagnostic evaluation.[27] Testing for thyroid receptor antibody levels is rarely needed for evaluation of thyrotoxicosis; however, in the pregnant patient, who cannot undergo radionucleotide scanning, the level can help distinguish between Graves disease and gestational thyrotoxicosis.[11,28] Additionally, maternal TSH can cross the placental barrier and have a direct effect on the fetus; it is therefore recommended that TSH levels be drawn between 22 and 26 weeks of gestation in order to determine need for aggressive neonatal monitoring.[3] Finally, 10% of patients with proptosis will be diagnosed with Graves disease by antibody levels alone, as TSH and T_4 may not be abnormal.[15]

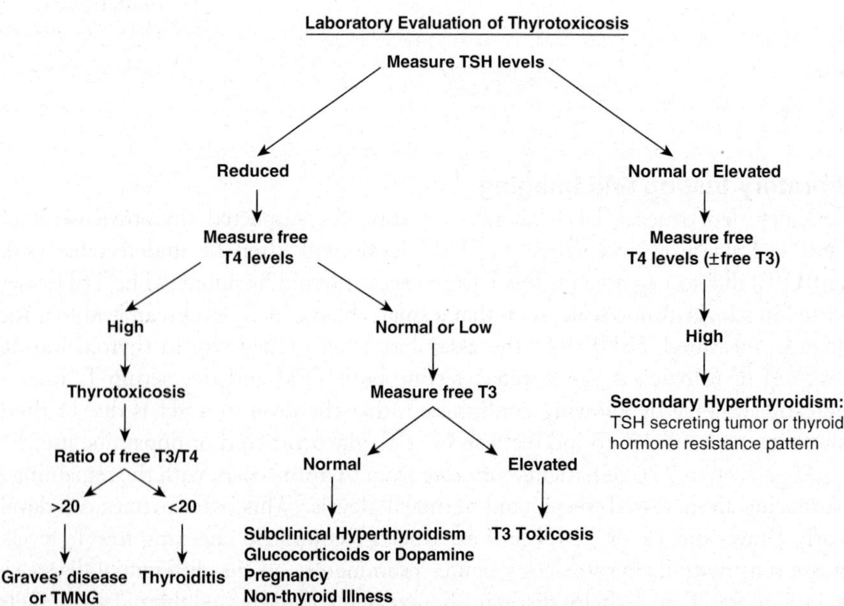

FIGURE 44.1 Laboratory evaluation of thyrotoxicosis. From references Franklyn JA, Boelaert K. Thyrotoxicosis. *Lancet*. 2012;379:1155–1166.; Reid JR, Wheeler SF. Hyperthyroidism: diagnosis and treatment. *Am Fam Physician*. 2005;72(4):623–630.

Radionucleotide testing and ultrasound can help differentiate between thyrotoxicosis caused by hyperthyroidism (i.e., Graves disease or TMNG) and thyrotoxicosis not caused by hyperthyroidism (i.e., thyroiditis or ingestion of exogenous thyroid hormone).[3,15] Radioactive iodine uptake (RAIU) uses either technetium-99m (Tc 99m) or radioiodine[29] to assess the activity of the sodium/iodide symporter on the thyroid gland.[17] Each molecule has advantages in testing: radioiodine is incorporated into hormone production and is thought to be more reflective of true physiology, while Tc 99m requires less acquisition time for similar results—but at the cost of an increased exposure to radiation.[10] Uptake measurements are taken at 4 hours and 24 hours after administration.[29] The pattern of uptake reflects the cause of thyrotoxicosis and helps narrow the differential diagnosis.[3] With ultrasonography, an increase in thyroid total area blood flow (calculated as thyroid artery blood flow/glandular area) of 4% to 8% can differentiate Graves disease from destructive thyroiditis with sensitivity and specificity of 84% and 90%, respectively.[10] This diagnostic approach is operator dependent but is a viable option for patients who cannot tolerate radioactive screening, such as those who are pregnant or breast-feeding.[22]

Differential Diagnosis

Thyroid storm should be suspected in patients with mental status changes, hyperadrenergic state, and any of the systemic manifestations noted above.[8] The differential diagnosis includes generalized infections and sepsis, anxiety, depression, pheochromocytoma, atrial fibrillation/flutter, chronic fatigue syndrome, Plummer-Vinson syndrome, as well as various malignancies.[2,8,11,18] Use of methamphetamine, cocaine, or other nutritional supplements can confuse the clinical picture and should be excluded.[30] In most cases, thyroid testing will help narrow the differential; however, certain medical conditions, such as euthyroid sick syndrome, pregnancy, and hyperemesis gravidarum, will lower TSH levels and affect T_4 assays.[2,7,22] Additionally, the use of glucocorticoids, dopamine, and heparin will lower the TSH level and can confound the diagnosis.[22]

Management Guidelines

Treatment of thyrotoxicosis in the acute care setting focuses on attenuating the hyperadrenergic state, controlling the production and release of thyroid hormone, inhibiting peripheral conversion of T_4 to T_3, and treating the precipitating cause.[12,27] Definitive therapy is achieved with radioactive iodine or surgery (e.g., subtotal thyroidectomy).

Beta-blockers are the primary agents used to attenuate the cardiovascular complications of thyrotoxicosis; propranolol is a first-line agent because of its additional ability to reduce peripheral conversion of T_4 to T_3.[8] The application of adrenergic blockage leads to an improvement in heart rate and cardiac output and a decrease in cardiac oxygen consumption.[27] In patients with preexisting heart failure, because of the concern for abrupt clinical deterioration, continuous cardiac monitoring and, in some cases, a screening echocardiography are required prior to initiation of beta-blocker therapy.[31] When beta-blockers are used in patients with a history of obstructive lung disease, including asthma and COPD, there exists an additional risk of reactive airway disease exacerbation.[15] In these patients, a beta-1–selective agent, such as metoprolol or esmolol, is a reasonable alternative to propranolol. Amiodarone should always be avoided as an antidysrhythmic because of its iodine content.

Thionamides have been successfully used for over 70 years to decrease circulating hormone levels.[15] Propylthiouracil (PTU) and methimazole (MMI) are available in the United States, while Carbimazole (CBZ, metabolized peripherally to MMI) is available in Europe and Asia.[3,7,27] All three agents inhibit the intrathyroid hormone synthesis and have high oral bioavailability, leading to effects within 1 to 2 hours of ingestion.[32] PTU has the added effect of inhibiting peripheral conversion of T_4 to T_3, reducing the concentration of the active hormone.[12] MMI has the advantage of allowing once-daily dosing, which improves compliance, and is 10 to 12 times more potent than PTU, leading to more rapid normalization of thyroid function.[27] All three agents also have an immunomodulatory effect and decrease both natural killer and T-cell substrates and autoantibodies, which may be relevant in patients with Graves disease.[32]

Several randomized trials have examined the efficacy of differing doses of and combinations of these treatments. In one RCT that assessed the treatment efficacy of 10 versus 40 mg of MMI in patients with Graves disease, both groups achieved acceptable levels of euthyroidism within 6 weeks (85% and 92%, respectively), but the higher dose was associated with an increased rate of complications (25% vs. 15.5%).[33] In another RCT of patients with newly diagnosed Graves disease, the clinical efficacy of 15 mg and 30 mg MMI versus 300 mg PTU was assessed over a period of 12 months. For mild or moderate disease (Free T4 (FT_4) < 7 ng/dL), efficacy was the same in all three groups. For severe disease (FT_4 > 7 ng/dL), MMI 30 mg was more efficacious than PTU or lower-dose MMI.[34]

Side effects of PTU and MMI occur in 14% to 52% of patients; they are dose dependent, usually limited to fever, rash, urticaria, and arthralgias, and are typically resolved by switching from one agent to the other.[33,34] One severe side effect, agranulocytosis, affects 0.5% of patients treated with any of the three medications and requires immediate cessation of all thionamides.[27] This complication usually occurs within the first 3 months of treatment, and patients are advised to monitor for oropharyngeal infections commonly associated with this development.[18] Other, less common side effects, including hepatotoxicity and anti-neutrophil cytoplasmic antibody (ANCA)-mediated vasculitis, also require the cessation of thionamides.[32] For these reasons, thionamides are used as primary treatment of thyrotoxicosis only in select populations in whom surgical resection or radiation therapy is undesirable: young patients with mild to moderate illness; patients with only a slight increase in glandular volume; pediatric or adolescent patients; and pregnant or breastfeeding patients.[3] Otherwise, these agents are primarily used as the initial medical therapy for patients awaiting definitive treatment with radioactive iodine or surgical resection.[32] Patients with TMNG benefit greatly from premedication (prior to RAIU or surgery) with thionamides because any delay in treatment leads to high rates of relapse.[32] Caution should be taken with continued use of MMI or PTU in the week prior to radioiodine therapy as either medication can decrease the iodine uptake into the thyroid gland and lead to treatment failure.[35] This decreased in iodine uptake, however, exerts a small protective effect against long-term hypothyroidism by minimizing damage to healthy thyroid tissue.[35]

For those patients unable to tolerate the thionamides, lithium is an alternative agent that blocks thyroid hormone release.[8] Lithium is taken up by the thyroid gland in a manner similar to iodine[32]; however, its effects are transient, and the value of long-term use is undefined.[18]

Other medications are available for short-term symptomatic relief.[7] Glucocorticoids may be used to inhibit the peripheral conversion of T_4 to T_3 and are useful in cases associated with secondary adrenal insufficiency.[32] Graves ophthalmopathy is also improved with long-term (6 to 8 weeks) treatment with glucocorticoids.[3] Cholestyramine is an anion-exchange resin that binds thyroid hormones in the enterohepatic circulation and can increase their fecal excretion.[8] Potassium perchlorate, a competitive inhibitor of iodine transport into the thyroid, is used in patients with iodine-induced thyrotoxicosis.[31] In extreme cases, peritoneal dialysis, plasma exchange, or hemodialysis can be utilized to abruptly lower thyroid hormone concentrations.[18]

Essential supportive care includes antipyretics, cooling, and correction of intravascular fluid deficits.[8] For fever, acetaminophen is the medication of choice, as salicylates decrease thyroid-binding protein and increase free thyroid levels.[7,15] To avoid Wernicke encephalopathy, a condition associated with thyrotoxicosis, thiamine should be given along with a general multivitamin.[26] Treatment of infection, myocardial injury, and other stressors should proceed according to best practices.[27]

Special Populations

The Pregnant Patient

One in 500 pregnancies is complicated by Graves disease, which can lead to significant morbidity including miscarriage, premature labor, low birth weight, and eclampsia.[3,11] Pregnant patients presenting with >5% weight loss, goiter, ophthalmopathy, or onycholysis will require a thorough evaluation for Graves disease.[7,11] Normal hormonal changes in pregnancy can make diagnosis challenging: increased thyroid-binding globulin production will lower free T_4 levels; and human chorionic gonadotropin will lower TSH production in the first trimester. In addition, several classic signs of thyrotoxicosis may be present in normal pregnancy, including a widened pulse pressure and heat intolerance.[3,7,28] Treatment of pregnant patients is difficult, as both PTU and MMI cross the placenta and can cause fetal hypothyroidism and goiter.[27] Of the two, PTU is a better choice; it is more protein bound, slightly reducing its ability enter the fetal circulation[18] and does not carry the same increased risk that MMI does of causing fetal cutis aplasia and gastrointestinal atresia.[31] Treatment aims to use the lowest effective dose of PTU to keep T_4 levels in a high-normal to slightly thyrotoxic range.[27] The level of thyrotoxicosis can wane during pregnancy, and up to 30% of women discontinue use of thionamides in the third trimester.[11] Thyroidectomy is reserved for the second-trimester or for severely decompensated patients, as there is an increased risk of miscarriage.[27] In women with previous thyroid dysfunction, 10% will experience thyrotoxicosis in the postpartum period.[3] Additionally, 80% of women whose pregnancies are complicated by Graves disease will have a relapse in future pregnancies, with 50% developing permanent thyrotoxicosis.[3]

The Elderly

Thyrotoxicosis in the elderly is difficult to diagnose because suggestive symptoms, such as hyperkinesis and ophthalmopathy, are often lacking, and because clinical manifestation is often limited to a single organ system (e.g., heart failure or atrial fibrillation).[7] Up to 70% of elderly patients with thyrotoxicosis demonstrate no clinical signs or symptoms of a goiter and may even have depressive signs, such as apathy and fatigue.[7] This genre of clinical symptoms is termed "apathetic hyperthyroidism" and is often diagnosed after a lengthy workup for cardiotonic-resistant cardiovascular disease.[36]

Amiodarone

Amiodarone, an iodine-containing antiarrhythmic agent, will induce thyrotoxicosis in approximately 6% to 10% of patients.[3] This condition doubles the adverse cardiac effects of the drug and can lead to even worse outcomes in patients with preexisting thyroid disease.[37] Diagnosis is similar to other forms of thyrotoxicosis; however, conditions such as atrial and ventricular arrhythmias, for which the patient would normally take amiodarone, need to be carefully differentiated from thyroid hormone excess.[3] There are two types of amiodarone-related thyroid disease.[38] Type 1 is an iodine-induced thyrotoxicosis that occurs in individuals with preexisting nodules or autoimmune thyroid disease. Type 2 is an amiodarone-induced destruction of the thyroid gland itself.[3,38] Color-flow Doppler will show increased uptake in type 1, which is treated with thionamides and potassium perchlorate.[11,37] Glucocorticoids are the preferred medication for type 2 and often lead to complete resolution.[10] Since the subtype is not always apparent, experts recommend a combination of the three drugs for 6 to 12 months; ongoing consultation by cardiology and endocrinology is recommended because of the long half-life of amiodarone and the complex disease states that it treats.[37]

MYXEDEMA COMA

Hypothyroidism affects approximately 4.6% of the US population and is characterized by a generalized slowing of the body's metabolic processes leading to an overall depression of both physical and mental activity.[39] Myxedema coma is a rare complication of untreated hypothyroidism and describes a state of severely decompensated hypothyroidism in which the body cannot maintain thermal energetic homeostasis.[40] Hypothyroidism is four times more common in women than in men, and 80% of all reported cases of myxedema coma occur in females, a majority over the age of 60.[40] Hallmarks of laboratory diagnosis are severely depressed levels of T_4 and T_3 and an elevation in TSH[41]; however, lab values correlate poorly with the severity of the clinical disease.[42] In the past, their poor predictive value contributed to delays in diagnosis and a mortality rate of 60% to 70%.[41] More recently, advances in physician education have resulted in earlier recognition of this disease and an improved patient mortality rate of 20% to 25%.[31,41] A recent review of risk factors showed higher mortality rates associated with advanced age, hemodynamic instability, severe bradycardia, respiratory failure (requiring intubation), hypothermia, sepsis, depressed Glasgow Coma Scale (GCS), and a higher APACHE II score.[43] This same study also showed that the sequential organ failure assessment (SOFA) score offered the most effective prediction model, with baseline and 3-day SOFA scores of 6 or greater predicting mortality with a sensitivity and specificity of 91.7% and 100%, respectively.

Myxedema coma is most commonly precipitated by a significant systemic stressor in the undiagnosed or poorly managed hypothyroid patient. Infection—notably pneumonia, urinary tract infection, and cellulitis—is the most common trigger.[1] Hypothermia during the winter months is also thought to be responsible for a large number of cases.[44] The seasonal pattern is explained by an age-related loss of temperature regulation coupled with the depressed heat production common to hypothyroidism.[1] Other triggers of myxedema coma include cerebrovascular accidents, congestive heart failure, gastrointestinal bleeds, the use of centrally acting depressants such as sedatives and lithium, or the abrupt discontinuation of thyroid supplements in critically ill patients.[14,26,45] A recent report detailed the development of myxedema crisis following the consumption of raw bok choy, which contains cyanates, nitriles, and oxazolidines that inhibit iodine uptake in the thyroid.[46]

Physiology and Organ-Specific Effects

Thyroid hormones affect the metabolism and development of nearly every cell in the body.[11] In hypothyroidism, there is both an inadequate production of thyroid hormones and decreased peripheral conversion of T_4 to the active hormone T_3.[47] Patients suffering from hypothyroidism rely upon both arms of the autonomic nervous system to maintain circulatory homeostasis and a normal core temperature.[39,48] Any further reduction in intravascular volume (dehydration, blood loss), compromise to ventilation (infection), or insult to the central nervous system (drugs) can overwhelm these mechanisms and lead to myxedema coma.[40]

Clinically, patients will demonstrate global depressed physiologic function manifested as hypothermia, bradycardia, hypertension, respiratory acidosis, and depressed mental status leading to a comatose state.[44] Respiratory failure results from decreased central nervous system sensitivity to hypoxia and hypercarbia, as well as airway problems from macroglossia, respiratory muscle weakness, and nonpitting edema (myxedema) of the nasopharynx.[41] Altered vascular permeability leads to effusions and ascites; renal injury leads to water retention and hyponatremia; and depressed inotropy and chronotropy lead to intractable cardiogenic collapse.[41]

History and Physical Exam

Myxedema coma can be difficult to distinguish from other life-threatening conditions, such as heart failure, hypothermia, or respiratory dysfunction, that present with similar manifestations.[42] Even more difficult is recognizing this disease in an unstable, altered, or septic patient.[41] Providers must maintain a high clinical suspicion, guided by a detailed patient history noting any previous use of thyroid hormones or recent discontinuation of thyroid supplements, to make the diagnosis.[1]

The physical exam should focus on identifying the classic features of hypothyroidism: dry skin, brittle nails, hair loss, delayed tendon reflexes, and goiter.[49] Additionally, mucin deposits can lead to swelling of the hands, ptosis, periorbital edema, macroglossia, laryngeal edema, and other nondependent sites of nonpitting edema.[44,48] In patients with hypothyroidism due to prior treatment for Graves disease, a subtle clue is the presence of Graves orbitopathy, which does not resolve with treatment of the thyrotoxic state and can signal that the patient has previously received thyroid depressant treatments.[41] Providers should also look for signs of prior thyroid surgery, such as a midline incision in the anterior neck or documentation of a previous radioactive iodine ablation.[44]

A comatose state is not required for the diagnosis of myxedema coma, but all patients will demonstrate some degree of central nervous system depression, including diminished cognition, lethargy, and somnolence.[1] This alteration of mental status may be worsened by the presence of concomitant hyponatremia, an electrolyte abnormality common in severe hypothyroidism.[41] The pathogenesis of the depressed neurologic function is thought to be related to a depressed respiratory drive leading to hypercarbia; a decrease in cerebral blood flow; and decreased brain glucose utilization coupled with an overall hypoglycemic state.[48] The depressed cerebral function, hyponatremia, hypoglycemia, hypoxemia, and reduced cerebral blood flow can combine to result in generalized seizures that, without early intervention and treatment, can progress to status epilepticus, further clouding the clinical picture.[41,44]

A decreased physiologic response to hypoxia and hypercarbia results in alveolar hypoventilation in patients with previously healthy lung tissue.[4] Studies have shown that both myxedema coma and brief hypothyroid states produce a depressed hypoxic ventilatory drive that reverses with thyroid hormone replacement; however, the hypercapnic respiratory depression is not affected.[41] Associated hypothermia, obesity hypoventilation syndrome, and macroglossia often contribute to the need for ventilator support.[44] Due to the severity of respiratory failure in myxedema coma—even following the initiation of appropriate treatment with levothyroxine—a 3- to 6-month period of mechanical ventilation may be required.[41]

Effects of a decompensated hypothyroid state on the cardiovascular system include bradycardia, hypertension, and narrowing of the pulse pressure.[41] Common electrocardiogram findings include sinus bradycardia, complete heart blocks, QT prolongation, and nonspecific ST-segment changes.[4] An early echocardiogram is recommended to evaluate for pericardial effusions.[44] Despite an overall reduction in cardiac function, overt heart failure in myxedema coma is uncommon.[41] In extreme cases of decompensated hypothyroidism, dilated cardiomyopathy and associated left ventricular failure may develop.[43] Fortunately, improvement in both cardiac output and ejection fraction is seen with prompt initiation of thyroxine therapy.[48]

Gastrointestinal dysmotility can lead to constipation and, without treatment, can progress to paralytic ileus.[42] The associated abdominal pain, nausea, and anorexia can mimic the appearance of a surgical abdomen.[4] This devastating complication can lead to unnecessary exploratory surgery, worsening physiologic stress and precipitating further decompensation of the myxedema coma state (Table 44.3).[41]

Laboratory Testing and Imaging

ED laboratory testing in patients with suspected decompensated hypothyroidism should include a TSH level and a free T_4. In early hypothyroid disease, when production of T_3 is decreased, the peripheral conversion of T_4 to T_3 increases in an attempt to maintain physiologic levels.[48] T_3 and T_4 are bound in the peripheral circulation by proteins, including the high-affinity thyroxine-binding globulin (TBG) and lower-affinity but more abundant albumin.[2] Only the free hormone is able to bind to receptors and create biologic activity.[39] In a nondiseased state, approximately 0.03% of T_4 and 0.5% of T_3 are unbound.[48] A clinical picture consistent with hypothyroid disease coupled with low T_4 levels (T_3 is rarely measured directly) typically confirms the diagnosis.[26] However, changes either in the quantity or in the affinity of available binding proteins can effect a pseudonormalization of thyroid hormone levels, clouding the diagnosis.[48] Notably, certain infections, such as hepatitis and HIV, or any increase in estrogen (e.g., pregnancy), will result in an increase in TBG and can mimic the diagnostic criteria for hypothyroidism.[2]

Elevated TSH is a very specific marker of a hypothyroid state.[14] However, TSH levels can be poorly sensitive for hypothyroid disease resulting from secondary or tertiary causes, also known as central hypothyroidism.[49] In this state, hypothalamic–pituitary–thyroid (HPT) axis dysfunction leads to a decrease in the production of thyrotropin-releasing hormone and thus in serum TSH.[48] The most common culprit is direct

TABLE 44.3 Clinical Manifestations of Myxedema Coma

Organ System	Symptoms	Signs
Neuropsychiatric	Altered mental status Delayed reflex relaxation Depression and psychosis Myalgias Weakness	Confusion Lethargy and somnolence Coma Weight gain Fatigue Memory impairment
Cardiovascular	Pericardial effusion Cardiogenic shock Congestive heart failure (late)	Hypodynamic precordium Bradycardia Elevated diastolic pressure (early) Hypotension (late)
Pulmonary	Pleural effusion	Hyperventilation Myxedema of larynx
Gastrointestinal	Decreased motility Paralytic ileus Myxedema megacolon (late) Ascites Neurogenic oropharyngeal dysphagia	Abdominal distension Fecal impaction Constipation Anorexia Nausea
Genitourinary	Bladder dystonia and distension Menorrhagia	Anasarca
Ophthalmologic	Ptosis	Diplopia Periorbital edema Graves orbitopathy
Dermatologic	Alopecia Generalized swelling	Dry, cool, doughy skin Macroglossia Brittle nails Coarse, sparse hair Nonpitting edema
Endocrine	Hypothermia	Cold intolerance Thyroid enlargement

damage to the pituitary gland (e.g., pituitary adenoma), although systemic diseases, including sarcoidosis and hemochromatosis may also damage the HPT axis.[48] Central hypothyroidism accounts for approximately 5% of myxedema coma cases and may present with normal or even low levels of TSH.[4] The use of corticosteroids and vasopressors such as dopamine can also result in decreased TSH secretion.[41]

Other laboratory abnormalities commonly seen in hypothyroid disease include a marked reduction in the glomerular filtration rate (GFR), which occurs because of decreased renal plasma flow and increased vascular resistance in both the afferent and efferent arterioles.[41] Reduced GFR results in creatinine elevation and an increased risk of hyponatremia.[42] This is thought to be due to the loss of the aldosterone-like effect that T_3 and T_4 have on the Na–K channels of proximal tubular cells, leading to increase in sodium excretion.[4] Renal dysfunction also results in impaired free water clearance and the development of myxedema.[44] Thyroxine replacement has been shown to successfully reverse changes in renal function.[41]

Decreased lipid clearance may also be present, leading to hypercholesterolemia and hypertriglyceridemia.[48] Normocytic anemia may develop due to decreased oxygen requirements and decreased levels of erythropoietin, while alteration to von Willebrand factor synthesis, caused by low thyroxine levels, can result in coagulopathies, including prolonged bleeding and clotting times, decreased platelet adhesiveness, and prolongation of aPTT.[1,41] Elevations of creatinine phosphokinase, lactate dehydrogenase, and aspartate transaminase may also be seen, as can hypoglycemia due to decreased gluconeogenesis (Fig. 44.2).[40,45,49]

Differential Diagnosis

Myxedema coma has no classic presentation and will often present simply as a patient with depressed mental status and hemodynamic instability.[39] A broad differential is required on initial presentation, as adrenal insufficiency, congestive heart failure, hepatic encephalopathy, hypothermia, and septic shock can present in similar fashion.[4] The neurologic manifestations of myxedema coma can also be caused by a cerebrovascular accident, status epilepticus, or meningitis.[1]

Management Guidelines

Patients with myxedema coma require prompt admission to an intensive care unit (ICU) and aggressive hemodynamic support.[1] Due to the mortality risks associated with delays in treatment, therapy should begin prior to laboratory confirmation.[31] A three-tiered treatment plan is recommended: early initiation of thyroid replacement, correction of organ-specific dysfunction, and management of the inciting event (most commonly infection or hypothermia).[47]

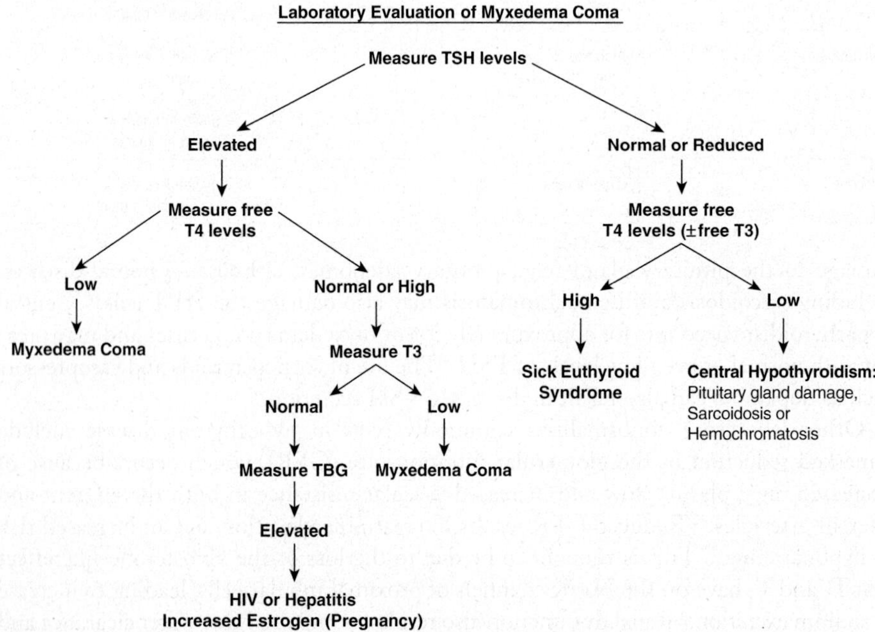

FIGURE 44.2 Laboratory evaluation of myxedema coma. Taken from Sarlis NJ, Gourgiotis L. Thyroid emergencies. *Rev Endocr Metab Disord.* 2003;4:129–136; Bello F, Bakari AG. Hypothyroidism in adults: a review and recent advances in management. *J Diabetes Endocrinol.* 2012;3(5):57–69; Wartofsky L. Myxedema coma. *Endocrinol Metab Clin North Am.* 2006;35:687–698.

Expert consensus is that early thyroid hormone replacement is vital for recovery in uncompensated myxedema coma, but a paucity of clinical trials and a lack of randomized controlled studies have yet to yield censuses on proper timing or dosing.[4,40,41] Timely implementation of therapy should be balanced with close monitoring for the fatal arrhythmias and myocardial ischemia associated with increased oxygen demand from T_3 and T_4 replacement.[1,42] Continuous hemodynamic monitoring is mandatory, as is early cessation of treatment at any signs of instability.[1]

Replacement agents include levothyroxine (LT_4) or liothyronine (LT_3).[4] Parental administration of LT_4 is preferred because unpredictable gastric absorption is common in myxedema coma.[1] Compared to LT_3, LT_4 results in fewer cardiac complications; however, LT_4 requires activation via peripheral 5′-deiodination, a process that can become depressed in severely decompensated patients.[4] Additionally, LT_4 is not well transported across the blood–brain barrier, resulting in slower resolution of neurologic symptoms.[41] Therefore, in the case of a critically ill patient who may have depressed 5′-deiodination, LT_3 is preferred for its immediate bioactivity, faster therapeutic effect, and blood–brain barrier penetration.[1,40,41] Note, however, that LT_3 increases risk of cardiac abnormalities, including ischemia and lethal arrhythmias, which are heightened in the setting of concomitant vasopressor therapy.[42,48]

Some authors have advocated for the use of both agents, combining the quick onset and increased bioavailability of LT_3 with the relative cardiovascular stability associated with LT_4.[1,42] This combination permits lower doses than those would be used in solo therapy, often beginning with intravenous LT_4 and LT_3 and transitioning to oral LT_4 for long-term therapy.[4] Rates of cardiovascular complication are higher with parenteral delivery of either agent, so a prompt transition to oral dosing is advocated once the patient achieves clinical stability.[41]

Controversy over the optimal therapeutic strategy persists, especially regarding dosing.[1] Regardless of therapy used, restoration of hemodynamic stability typically occurs within 24 hours and of thermoregulation within 2 to 3 days.[50] Respiratory dysfunction and kidney injury may take weeks to months to fully resolve.[4] A decline in TSH serves as a marker of clinical recovery and helps to guide further therapy.[41]

Supportive treatment of the patient with myxedema coma can include mechanical ventilation for correction of hypercarbia and support of diaphragmatic weakness; early broad-spectrum antibiotics; aggressive fluid resuscitation; and correction of associated electrolyte disorders (e.g., hyponatremia and hypoglycemia).[48] Care must be taken with treatment of hypothermia, as rapid rewarming can cause peripheral vasodilation and worsening hypotension.[42] Because thyroid hormone therapy results in increased cortisol clearance, all patients treated with LT_3 and LT_4 should be maintained on hydrocortisone until clinically stable.[4] Moreover, the clinical features of myxedema coma and adrenal insufficiency may overlap; if an appropriate response to thyroid hormone therapy is not observed, the provider should assess for, and if present, treat, coexisting adrenal insufficiency.[44,45] Hypotension typically resolves with initiation of thyroid hormone replacement; low-dose vasopressors may be added for additional support.[44]

Special Populations

A rare complication of Hashimoto thyroiditis is Hashimoto encephalopathy.[51] This disease presents as subacute or acute encephalopathy with seizures, stroke-like episodes, myoclonus, and tremor similar to myxedema coma.[52] Lab testing will reveal elevations in thyroid-specific antibodies, elevated cerebrospinal fluid protein without pleocytosis, and an abnormal electroencephalogram.[53] The patient, however, is in a euthyroid state, and steroids are a first-line treatment.[51]

CONCLUSION

Thyroid storm and myxedema coma are disease processes representing the extremes of thyroid dysfunction.[1] Nonspecific presentations and extremely high mortality rates make early recognition essential.[4,7] With early clinical suspicion, prompt laboratory evaluation, and early administration of multifaceted therapies, the morbidity and mortality for both pathologic processes can be lessened substantially.[50] Aggressive hemodynamic and respiratory support in the ED, coupled with referral to an intensive care setting, is imperative to assure successful treatment outcome.[8,47]

LITERATURE TABLE

TRIAL	DESIGN	RESULT
Thyroid Storm		
Hollowell et al., *J Clin Endocrinol Metab.* 2002[6] NHANES III Survey	Survey of 17,353 adult patients representing the geographic and ethnic distribution of the US population	4.6% of population has hypothyroidism (0.3% clinical and 4.3% subclinical). 1.3% of the population has hyperthyroidism (0.5 % clinical and 0.7% subclinical)
Burch et al., *Endocrinol Metab Clin North Am.* 1993[9]	Review of patients with life-threatening thyrotoxicosis	Developed diagnostic scoring system for thyroid storm based on evaluation of fever, presence of precipitating event, and CNS, GI, and cardiac dysfunction. Scores >45 highly suggestive of thyroid storm; 25–44 suggesting of impending storm; and <25 unlikely to represent thyroid storm
Reinwein et al., *J Clin Endocrinol Metab.* 1993[33] European Multicentre Study Group on Antithyroid Drug Treatment	Prospective randomized trial of treatment of 309 patients with Graves disease with 10 mg vs. 40 mg of methimazole (MMI)	Euthyroidism achieved within 6 wk for 85% of patients treated with 10 mg and 92% of patients treated with 40 mg. The higher dose, however, was associated with an increased rate of adverse reactions (25% vs. 15.5%, $p < 0.01$). No changes were noted in the rate of remission
Nakamura et al., *J Clin Endocrinol Metab.* 2007[34]	396 patients with newly diagnosed Graves disease randomized to one of three groups MMI (15 mg and 30 mg) or PTU (300 mg) over 12 mo Study also evaluated the side effect profile of high vs. low-dose MMI and PTU	For mild or moderate disease ($FT_4 < 7$ ng/dL), the efficacy was the same in all three groups ($p < 0.03$). For severe disease ($FT_4 > 7$ ng/dL), MMI 30 mg was more efficacious than PTU or lower-dose MMI ($p < 0.05$) Side effects occurred in 52% of patients treated with 300 mg PTU, 30% of patients treated with 30 mg MMI, and only 14% of patients treated with 15 mg MMI
Walter et al., *BMJ.* 2007[35]	Systematic review and meta-analysis of 14 randomized controlled trials (1306 patients) to determine the effect of adjunctive antithyroid drugs (MMI and PTU) coupled with radioiodine treatment	Adjunctive antithyroid drugs led to increased risk of treatment failure (RR 1.28, $p = 0.006$) but a reduced risk of hypothyroidism (RR 0.68, $p = 0.006$) following radioiodine treatment
Myxedema Coma		
Dutta et al., *Crit Care.* 2008[43]	Observational study of 23 patients to analyze predictors of morbidity and mortality in myxedema coma. Also evaluated efficacy of oral vs. intravenous L-thyroxine	Baseline and day-3 SOFA scores ≥ 6 predicted mortality with a sensitivity of 91.7% and a specificity of 100%. No outcome difference was found between oral and intravenous L-thyroxine

RR, relative risk.

REFERENCES

1. Klubo-Gwiezdzinska J, Wartofsky L. Thyroid emergencies. *Med Clin North Am.* 2012;96:385–403.
2. Pimental L, Hansen KN. Thyroid disease in the emergency department: a clinical and laboratory review. *J Emerg Med.* 2005;28(2):201–209.
3. Franklyn JA, Boelaert K. Thyrotoxicosis. *Lancet.* 2012;379:1155–1166.
4. Wartofsky L. Myxedema coma. *Endocrinol Metab Clin North Am.* 2006;35:687–698.
5. Bahn RS, Burch HB, Cooper DS, et al. Hyperthyroidism and other causes of thyrotoxicosis: management guidelines of the American Thyroid Association and American Association of Clinical Endocrinologists. *Thyroid.* 2011;21(6):593–649.
6. Hollowell JG, Staehling NW, Flanders WD, et al. Serum TSH, T4 and thyroid antibodies in the United States population (1988–1994): National Health and Nutrition Examination Survey (NHANES III). *J Clin Endocrinol Metab.* 2002;87:489–499.
7. McKeown NJ, Tews MC, Gossain VV, et al. Hyperthyroidism. *Emerg Med Clin North Am.* 2005; 23:669–685.
8. Migneco A, Ojetti V, Testa A, et al. Management of thyrotoxic crisis. *Eur Rev Med Pharmacol Sci.* 2005;9:69–74.
9. Burch HB, Wartofsky L. Life-threatening thyrotoxicosis. Thyroid storm. *Endocrinol Metab Clin North Am.* 1993;22(2):263–277.
10. Seigel SC, Hodak SP. Thyrotoxicosis. *Med Clin North Am.* 2012;96:175–201.
11. Cooper DS. Hyperthyroidism. *Lancet.* 2003;362:459–468.
12. Reid JR, Wheeler SF. Hyperthyroidism: diagnosis and treatment. *Am Fam Physician.* 2005;72(4):623–630.
13. Iglesias P, Devora O, Garcia-Arevalo J, et al. Severe hyperthyroidism: etiology, clinical features and treatment outcome. *Clin Endocrinol (Oxf).* 2010;72:551–557.
14. Veloski C, Brennan KJ. Critical care endocrinology. In: Criner GJ, ed. *Critical Care Study Guide.* 2nd ed. New York: Springer; 2010:638–661.
15. Nayak B, Burman K. Thyrotoxicosis and thyroid storm. *Endocrinol Metab Clin North Am.* 2006;35:663–686.
16. Akamizu T, Satoh T, Isozaki O, et al. Diagnostic criteria, clinical features, and incidence of thyroid storm based on nationwide surveys, Japan Thyroid Association, *Thyroid.* 2012;22(7):661.
17. Ross DS. Radioiodine therapy for hyperthyroidism. *N Engl J Med.* 2011;364:542–550.
18. Streetman DD, Khanderia U. Diagnosis and treatment of Graves' disease. *Ann Pharmacother.* 2003;37:1100–1109.
19. Homonick M, Gessl A, Ferlitsch A, et al. Altered platelet plug formation in hyperthyroidism and hypothyroidism. *J Clin Endocrinol Metab.* 2007;92:3006–3012.
20. Pothiwala P, Levine SN. Thyrotoxic periodic paralysis: a review. *J Intensive Care Med.* 2010;25(2):71–77.
21. Lin SH. Thyrotoxic periodic paralysis. *Mayo Clin Proc.* 2005;80(1)99–105.
22. McDermott MT. In the clinic: hyperthyroidism. *Ann Intern Med.* 2012;1:1–16.
23. Dabon-Almirante CL, Surks MI. Clinical and laboratory diagnosis of thyrotoxicosis. *Endocrinol Metab Clin North Am.* 1998;27:25–35.
24. Burch HB, Wartofsky L. Graves' ophthalmopathy: current concepts regarding pathogenesis and management. *Endocr Rev.* 1993;14:747–793.
25. Hadlow NC, Rothacker KM, Wardrop R, et al. The relationship between TSH and free T in a large population is complex and nonlinear and differs by age and sex. *J Clin Endocrinol Metab.* 2013;98(7):2936–2943.
26. Sarlis NJ, Gourgiotis L. Thyroid emergencies. *Rev Endocr Metab Disord.* 2003;4:129–136.
27. Pearce EN, Braverman LE. Hyperthyroidism: advantages and disadvantages of medical therapy. *Surg Clin North Am.* 2004;84:833–847.
28. Varon J, Acosta P. *Handbook of Critical and Intensive Care Medicine.* New York, NY: Springer; 2010.
29. Kusic Z, Becker DV, Saenger EL, et al. Comparison of technetium-99m and iodine 123 imaging of thyroid nodules: correlation with pathologic findings. *J Nucl Med.* 1990;31:393–399.
30. Raptis S, Fekete C, Sarkar S, et al. Cocaine- and amphetamine-regulated transcript co-contained in thyrotropin-releasing hormone (TRH) neurons of the hypothalamic paraventricular nucleus modulates TRH-induced prolactin secretion. *Endocrinology.* 2004;145:1695–1699.
31. Bondugulapati L, Adlan M, Premawardhana L. Review- thyroid emergencies. *Sri Lanka J Crit Care.* 2011;2(1):1–12.
32. Fumarola A, Di Fiore A, Dainelli G, et al. Medical treatment of hyperthyroidism: state of the art. *Exp Clin Endocrinol Diabetes.* 2010;118(10):678–684.
33. Reinwein D, Benker G, Lazarus JH, et al. A prospective randomized trial of antithyroid drug dose in Graves' disease therapy. European Multicenter Study Group on Antithyroid Drug Treatment. *J Clin Endocrinol Metab* 1993;76(6):1516–1521.

34. Nakamura H, Noh JY, Itoh K, et al. Comparison of methimazole and propylthiouracil in patients with hyperthyroidism caused by Graves' disease. *J Clin Endocrinol Metab.* 2007;92(6):2157–2162.
35. Walter MA, Briel M, Christ-Crain M, et al. Effects of antithyroid drugs on radioiodine treatment: systematic review and meta-analysis of randomised controlled trials. *BMJ.* 2007;334(7592):514.
36. Palacious A, Cohen MAA, Cobbs R. Apathetic hyperthyroidism in middle age. *Int J Psychiatry.* 1991;21(4):393–400.
37. Bogazzi F, Bartalena L, Martino E. Approach to the patient with amiodarone-induced thyrotoxicosis. *J Clin Endocrinol Metab.* 2010;95(6):2529–2535.
38. Thomas Z, Bandali F, McCowen K, et al. Drug-induced endocrine disorders in the intensive care unit. *Crit Care Med.* 2010;38(6):S219–S230.
39. Vaidya B, Pearce SH. Management of hypothyroidism in adults. *Br Med J.* 2008;337:284–289.
40. Wall CR. Myxedema coma: diagnosis and treatment. *Am Fam Physician.* 2000;62(11):2485–2490.
41. Kwaku MP, Burman KD. Myxedema coma. *J Intensive Care Med.* 2007;22:224–231.
42. Fliers E, Wiersinga WM. Myxedema coma. *Rev Endocr Metab Disord.* 2003;4:137–141.
43. Dutta P, Bhansali A, Masoodi SR, et al. Predictors of outcome in myxedema coma: a study from a tertiary care center. *Crit Care.* 2008;12:R1.
44. Mathew V, Misgar RA, Ghosh S, et al. Myxedema coma: a new look into an old crisis. *J Thyroid Res.* 2011;2011:493462.
45. Beynon J, Akhtar S, Kearney T. Predictors of outcome in myxoedema coma. *Crit Care.* 2008;12:111.
46. Chu M, Seltzer TF. Myxedema coma induced by ingestion of raw bok choy. *N Engl J Med.* 2010;362(20):1945–1946.
47. Nicoloff JT, LoPresti JS. Myxedema coma. A form of decompensated hypothyroidism. *Endocrinol Metab Clin North Am.* 1993;22:279–290.
48. Bello F, Bakari AG. Hypothyroidism in adults: a review and recent advances in management. *J Diabetes Endocrinol.* 2012;3(5);57–69.
49. Gaitonde DY, Rowley KD, Sweeney LB. Hypothyroidism: an update. *S Afr Fam Pract.* 2012;54(5):384–390.
50. Goldberg PA, Inzucchi SE. Critical issues in endocrinology. *Clini Chest Med.* 2003;24:583–606.
51. Schiess N, Pardo CA. Hashimoto's encephalopathy. *Ann N Y Acad Sci.* 2008;1142:254–265.
52. Mocellin R, Walterfang M, Velakoulis D. Hashimoto's encephalopathy: epidemiology, pathogenesis and management. *CNS Drugs.* 2007;21(10):799–811.
53. Fatourechi V. Hashimoto's encephalopathy: myth or reality? An endocrinologist's perspective. *Best Pract Res Clin Endocrinol Metab.* 2005;19(1):53–66.

SECTION 11
Toxicologic Critical Care

45

Cardiotoxins

Nicholas J. Connors and Silas W. Smith

BACKGROUND

Numerous therapeutic options exist for medical management of dysrhythmia, heart failure, and hypertension. In 2011, more than 42.4 million patients received therapy for hypertension alone, and prescriptions for ACE inhibitors, beta-adrenergic antagonists (BAAs), calcium channel antagonists/"blockers" (CCBs), and angiotensin II inhibitors (alone or in combination) exceeded 509 million.[1] Cardiotoxicity may occur in this setting due to intentional overdose, unintentional therapeutic misadventure, or interaction with other medications.

Cardiotoxicity may also result from noncardiovascular medications with associated sodium or potassium channel antagonism or muscarinic effects; from a variety of systemic pharmaceuticals; and from natural, occupational, or environmental exposures. In the pediatric population, there is risk of unintentional exposure to caregivers' medication or when visiting other households.[2] More than 90,000 incidents involving cardiovascular drugs are reported to poison control centers each year—5.7% and 2.2% of adult and pediatric exposure calls, respectively—accounting for a disproportionate 11% of fatalities.[3] This chapter offers a guide to the diagnostic evaluation and treatment of the cardiotoxins most commonly encountered in the emergency department (ED), namely CCBs, BAAs, cardiac glycosides, and renin–angiotensin system antagonists (RASAs).

HISTORY AND PHYSICAL EXAM

The initial presentation of the cardiotoxic patient may range from asymptomatic to critically ill. Although not always available or reliable, information regarding details of the exposure (agent, intent, dose, formulation, and coingestants), as well as patient-specific factors (age, comorbidities, unique susceptibilities, etc.), should be sought. An appropriate history will consider pertinent cardiovascular symptoms (chest pain, dyspnea, palpitations, etc.) and their onset, as well as any symptoms attributable to other relevant organ systems (central nervous system [CNS], pulmonary, etc.), and more insidious complaints (weakness, nausea, anorexia, fatigue, etc.).

Physical exam should prioritize repeated assessment of vital signs, particularly heart and respiratory rate, blood pressure, and pulse oximetry. The CNS should be assessed for direct or indirect signs of poisoning and/or perfusion abnormalities (agitation, delirium, depression, coma) and seizures (e.g., from bupropion, local anesthetics, methylxanthines, sedative–hypnotic withdrawal, or sympathomimetics). Of note, CCB-poisoned patients may preserve their mental status despite severe hypotension and bradycardia. Rigorous cardiac, pulmonary, vascular, and organ system examinations should evaluate perfusion, failure, and potential reserve. Special attention should be paid to identifying specific patterns of cardiovascular and associated systemic anomalies suggestive of a particular toxidrome, including *cholinergic* (bradycardia with bronchorrhea, bronchospasm, diaphoresis, urination, miosis, lacrimation, emesis), *antimuscarinic* (tachycardia, tachypnea, mydriasis, flushed skin, urinary retention, delirium), and *sympathomimetic* (tachycardia, hypertension, tachypnea, hyperthermia, mydriasis, psychomotor agitation). In addition to a focused physical exam, bedside glucometry (the "sixth vital sign") should be rapidly obtained and addressed. Hyperglycemia may suggest CCB exposure and severity, while hypoglycemia may be seen with BAAs.[4]

DIFFERENTIAL DIAGNOSIS

The number of substances capable of exerting cardiotoxic effects is myriad. Cardiotoxicity is a well-described attribute of abused substances (ethanol, nicotine, etc.), biologicals (aconitine, colchine, ricin, venoms, veratrine, etc.), chemotherapeutics (alkylators, anthracyclines, antimetabolites, monoclonal antibodies, taxanes, vinca alkaloids, etc.), environmental exposures (carbon monoxide, fluorocarbons, particulate air pollution, etc.), metals (arsenic, cadmium, cobalt, lead, etc.), nutritional toxins (thiaminases), and numerous other agents. Toxins that produce acid–base disturbances, autonomic nervous system dysfunction, electrolyte derangement, hematologic dyscrasias, or hypoxia (hypoxemic, histotoxic, or other) may secondarily compromise cardiovascular function. Cardiovascular instability may also accompany toxicologic-associated hyperthermias (anticholinergic crisis, malignant hyperthermia, neuroleptic malignant syndrome, mitochondrial uncoupling, sedative–hypnotic withdrawal, serotonin syndrome, sympathomimetic toxicity, thyroid toxicity, etc.).

Pharmaceuticals that produce hypotension and/or bradycardia include antidysrhythmics, cardiac glycosides (digoxin), BAAs, CCBs, imidazoline derivatives (clonidine, dexmedetomidine, guanfacine, guanabenz, oxymetazoline, and tetrahydrozoline), nitrates, and RASAs. Although uncommon, anticonvulsants (carbamazepine, phenytoin, etc.), barbiturates, and opioids may also cause bradycardia and hypotension. Cardiotoxicity may also arise from medications with sodium channel antagonism (carbamazepine, cocaine, cyclic antidepressants [CAs], local anesthetics, diphenhydramine, lamotrigine, venlafaxine, and others with Vaughan-Williams class IA and IC effects), potassium channel antagonism (antipsychotics, methadone, selective serotonin reuptake inhibitors, etc.), or direct or indirect cholinergic effects.

Sympathomimetics, including adrenergic reuptake inhibitors, amphetamines and their derivatives, cathenones and their analogs, cocaine, phencyclidine (PCP), and piperazines may produce tachycardia and/or hypertension. Methylxanthines (caffeine, theophylline, theobromine), cannabinomimetics, and monoamine oxidase inhibitors may present similarly. Substances with antimuscarinic properties may antagonize vagal effects on cardiac pacemakers, for example, antihistamines, CAs, and scopolamine. Vasodilators such as alpha-blockers, peripherally acting CCBs, and nitrates can result in reflex tachycardia as a compensatory response. Finally, withdrawal from sedative–hypnotics (barbiturates, benzodiazepines, ethanol, gamma hydroxybutyrate [GHB]), opioids, and antihypertensives (clonidine, BAAs, and others) can induce a presentation consistent with sympathomimetic toxicity.

DIAGNOSTIC EVALUATION

An electrocardiogram (ECG) should be rapidly obtained for all cardiotoxic patients. Agents that delay atrial electrical transmission (e.g., quinidine) may produce notched P waves. BAAs, cardiac glycosides, CCBs, cholinergics, and magnesium impair nodal conduction leading to variable blocks. Sodium channel antagonists, such as CAs, and others that compromise myocyte depolarization and disproportionately affect right ventricular depolarization, produce a classic ECG pattern of QRS widening and terminal rightward depolarization of the last 40 milliseconds of the QRS complex, giving rise to an R wave in lead AVR and/or an S wave in leads I and AVL. Hyperkalemia and hypermagnesemia may also cause widening of the QRS complex. Potassium channel antagonism may give rise to an increased QT/QTc interval, yielding a myocardial substrate vulnerable to afterdepolarizations, ventricular tachycardia, and ventricular fibrillation. Although not necessarily indicative of toxicity, digoxin and other cardiac glycosides cause repolarization abnormalities that appear as scooping of the ST segment, or "dig effect." Premature ventricular contractions, representing myocardial irritability, are more ominous and merit consideration for digoxin-specific Fab fragment (DSFab) administration.

Bedside ultrasound is another valuable tool in the hemodynamic status assessment of the cardiotoxic patient.[5] Negative inotrope toxicity may result in global myocardial dysfunction and impaired cardiac output, while a hyperdynamic heart may suggest adrenergic stimulation or represent a reflex to peripherally acting agents. Contemporaneous ultrasound assessment of volume status can also be performed.[6]

Laboratory testing should include serum electrolyte concentrations—particularly sodium, potassium, chloride, and calcium—to help guide repletion or interventions. In acute digoxin ingestions, prior to the availability of DSFab, elevations in serum potassium concentrations (a manifestation of sodium–potassium-ATPase inhibition) between 5 and 5.5 mEq/L were associated with 50% mortality; potassium concentrations above 5.5 mEq/L were associated with 100% mortality.[7] BAA overdose may also elevate serum potassium.[8] Assessment of renal function with urea nitrogen and creatinine may inform anticipated toxicity or duration of effect for renally cleared medications (e.g., atenolol, digoxin). Specific cardiotoxin concentrations are generally unavailable except for digoxin and theophylline, although evaluation of common coingestants (acetaminophen, salicylates, and ethanol) is often warranted.

MANAGEMENT GUIDELINES

Management of cardiotoxic patients requires vigilance on several fronts. Ensuring adequate oxygenation, ventilation, and intravascular volume expansion is essential. Serum glucose levels also require close observation; during periods of stress, myocardial metabolic substrate preference may shift from glucose to fatty acids, which can compromise contractile performance.[9] Toxin-induced hemodynamic instability is not uncommon. Hypertension should be managed with short-acting agents such as nitroglycerine, nitroprusside, or phentolamine. Hypotension should be corrected with titratable, direct-acting inotropic or vasoactive agents, such as norepinephrine, phenylephrine, and epinephrine; these have been proved more effective than indirect agents like dopamine.[10,11]

Decontamination

If not already administered, more definitive antidotal therapy should be considered following hemodynamic stabilization. A risk–benefit assessment should guide the decision to employ adjuncts that alter toxicant pharmacokinetics (e.g., orogastric lavage, activated charcoal, whole-bowel irrigation, urinary alkalinization, extracorporeal removal), particularly in cases of significant gut burden, ongoing absorption, sustained release products, or antimuscarinic or opioid coingestants. For certain potentially severe ingestions, aggressive decontamination with gastric lavage within 1 hour,[12] activated charcoal (1 g/kg),[13] and whole-bowel irrigation (polyethylene glycol electrolyte lavage solution at 1 to 2 L/h until clear rectal effluent)[14] may significantly reduce systemic absorption and alter the disease course.

Adjunct Therapies: Cardiac Pacing, IABP, and ECMO

While atropine and transcutaneous pacing may be employed in the initial management of toxic bradycardias, results are generally unsatisfying due to persistent negative inotropy. As transvenous pacing may actually worsen cardiac glycoside toxicity,[15] this particular condition should be excluded or empirically treated with DSFab prior to any attempts at transvenous pacing. While insufficient data exist regarding the role of intra-aortic balloon pump (IABP) counterpulsation in cardiotoxicity, small series suggest that IABP may be used to support hemodynamics and vital organ perfusion in patients refractory to pharmacologic interventions while toxin metabolism occurs.[16–18] Similarly, case studies have documented successful application of extracorporeal membrane oxygenation (ECMO) cardiopulmonary bypass to treat drug-induced cardiogenic shock and cardiac arrest refractory to traditional interventions.[19]

Specific Antidotes

Relative to the near-inexhaustible list of cardiotoxins, few specific antidotes exist; those that do rarely contain a specific FDA-approved toxicologic indication (e.g., only DSFab of the antidotes below). Given the ethical and practical difficulties in performing randomized or case-controlled trials in overdose victims, high-level evidence is often unavailable. Specific antidotal strategies represent a careful consideration of the medical literature, textbooks, expert opinion, and practice guidelines, although individual and institutional practices vary considerably.

Calcium

Based on anticipated digoxin-induced elevated intracellular Ca^{2+} concentrations and calcium-associated adverse events in digoxin-poisoned canines,[20] calcium should be avoided in hyperkalemia treatment in digoxin toxicity (managed with DSFab). Intravenous calcium is indicated to overcome the direct or indirect antagonism of L-type calcium channels induced by CCB and BAA poisoning. Animal models demonstrate calcium salt benefit in CCB- and BAA-induced deficits in contractility, blood pressure, and cardiac output.[21–23] Human case series and case reports generally support these findings, although conduction deficits and bradycardia may persist, and data for BAA toxicity are less robust.[24,25] Calcium is provided intravenously as 10% calcium gluconate (4.3 mEq elemental calcium per 10 mL), or via a central vein as 10% calcium chloride (13.6 mEq elemental calcium per 10 mL). Both regimens liberate Ca^{2+} rapidly.[26] A reasonable starting dose is 1 g (10 mL) of 10% calcium chloride or 3 g (30 mL) of 10% calcium gluconate, although some practitioners initiate higher doses.[27,28] To sustain therapeutic response, redosing every 20–60 minutes may be required. Ongoing diligent monitoring of calcium, serum phosphate, and hydration status is necessary to mitigate the adverse consequences of hypercalcemia.

Digoxin-Specific Fab Fragments (DSFab)

DSFab is a safe and effective antidote for cardiac glycoside toxicity, and prior to its availability, digoxin toxicity carried a mortality rate exceeding 23% in patients requiring cardiac pacing.[15,29,30] Indications for DSFab therapy include[27]

- Adult ingestions of ≥10 mg of digoxin (4 mg by a child)
- Serum digoxin concentrations ≥15 ng/mL, or concentrations ≥10 ng/mL beyond 6 hours after acute ingestion
- Shock or hemodynamic instability
- Progressive dysrhythmia, bradydysrhythmia refractory to atropine, or evidence of new ventricular ectopy (e.g., PVCs)
- Serum potassium ≥5.0 mEq/L in acute poisoning
- End-organ manifestations (e.g., altered mental status)
- Significant gastrointestinal symptoms or renal impairment in chronic poisoning

DSFab dosing is based either on the digoxin quantity ingested or on postdistributional serum digoxin concentrations:

$$\text{DSFab vials} = (\text{mg ingested} \times 0.8)/(0.5 \text{ mg bound/vial}) \text{ or}$$
$$\text{DSFab vials} = \{[\text{digoxin (ng/mL)}] \times [\text{weight (in kg)}]\}/100$$

The number of vials is rounded up and administered IV over 30 minutes in nonemergent scenarios. Empiric dosing of 10 to 20 vials in acute ingestion, or 3 to 6 vials (1 to 2 vials in children) in chronic ingestion, may be utilized when information is limited or in unstable patients. The rebound in free digoxin concentrations following therapy[31] likely mitigates the exacerbation of heart failure, seen in approximately 3% of patients, due to the sudden lack of inotropic support provided by digoxin.[29] Continued monitoring of electrolytes during DSFab therapy is important, as hypokalemia can develop.

Glucagon

Glucagon binds to G protein receptors, facilitating the production of cyclic adenosine monophosphate (cAMP) and enhancing cardiac inotropy and chronotropy. An increase in cAMP following administration of glucagon occurs independently of beta-adrenergic or calcium channel blockade. In volunteers, glucagon increased heart rate, cardiac index, and mean atrial pressure, but not systemic vascular resistance.[32] Evaluation of glucagon efficacy in BAA or CCB overdose is primarily limited to case series.[33] Dosing strategies typically employ an initial IV bolus of 50 μg/kg (maximum dose, 10 mg), repeatable after 3 to 5 minutes.[28] A continuous infusion of the reversal dose is then provided per hour (e.g., 2 to 5 mg/h to a maximum of 10 mg/h). Nausea and vomiting should be anticipated and mitigated.

High-Dose Insulin Euglycemia (HIE)

Myocardial fuel for oxidative metabolism includes free fatty acids (FFA) at rest, glucose after meals, and lactate and FFA during exercise. During myocardial ischemia, an increase in catecholamine release results in stimulation of adipose release of FFA and decreased excretion of insulin from pancreatic beta cells. Experimental findings correlate elevation of plasma FFA with increased arrhythmias and mortality; insulin and glucose infusion has been found to mitigate this effect by decreasing the uptake of FFA by the myocardium and by enhancing glucose uptake.[34] In dogs poisoned with BAAs or CCBs, HIE outperformed glucagon and epinephrine in mortality benefit and enhanced myocardial contractility.[35,36] Higher insulin dosing (up to 10 units/kg/h) improved mortality and cardiac output in BAA-poisoned pigs compared with placebo or vasopressin plus epinephrine.[37,38] In five patients with refractory, CCB-induced cardiogenic shock, an insulin bolus, followed by infusion at 0.1 to 1.0 units/kg/h, resulted in vasopressor sparing and survival in all.[39] In a prospective observational study of seven patients with severe CCB toxicity given an insulin maintenance infusion of 0.5 to 2.0 units/kg/h, six survived; of these six, those that received an initial insulin bolus also showed improved hemodynamic parameters.[40] A series of patients with cardiogenic shock from BAAs, CAs, and CCBs (alone or in combination) who were treated with HIE (up to 16 units/kg/h) showed survival in 92%, with sufficient hemodynamic improvement to permit vasopressor weaning.[41]

An initial insulin bolus of 0.5 to 1 unit/kg IV with dextrose supplementation as needed is typically followed by an insulin infusion of 1 unit/kg/h; maintenance of euglycemia with a 5% dextrose solution; careful potassium supplementation; and fingerstick glucose measurement every 30 minutes.[40] Titration up to 10 units/kg/h has been described in clinical practice.[42] Insulin's inotropic effect is delayed (approximately 15–45 minutes); therefore, early initiation and concurrent inotrope/vasopressor therapy, with subsequent weaning as tolerated, are recommended. Emergency Department initiation of HIE should be followed by prompt patient transfer to an intensive care setting for rigorous and potentially protracted glucose administration and monitoring.[39]

Intravenous Lipid Emulsion

Intravenous lipid emulsion (ILE) (typically a 20% solution) has emerged as a novel therapy for toxic exposures. ILE's mechanism of action is uncertain, and there are several competing theories to explain its efficacy. These include: creation of an ILE "lipid sink" or "lipid conduit" that isolates xenobiotics (nonnative chemical substances) within the plasma, thereby establishing a gradient that promotes diffusion from target organs and/or enhances elimination or redistribution;[43,44] alteration of myocardial metabolism resulting in increased cardiac FFA metabolism to ATP; or activation of ion channels responsible for cardiac contractility. In vitro models predict ILE efficacy in drugs with more positive partition coefficients (logP) and greater volumes of distribution,[45] although the distribution coefficient (logD, which accounts for ionization, particularly at physiologic pH) is a better descriptor of lipophilicity. Animal studies of ILE demonstrate mortality benefits in rats and dogs exposed to lethal doses of bupivacaine,[43,46] verapamil,[47] and selected other cardiovascular toxins. ILE rescue was first clinically used successfully in a case of seizures and refractory cardiac arrest due to intravenous local anesthetic exposure.[48] Other adult and pediatric case reports suggest benefit in cases of cardiovascular toxicity due to antipsychotics, BAAs, bupropion, CAs, CCBs, cocaine, and local anesthetics.[49–52]

Experts advocate ILE use in bupivacaine toxicity, including in the cases associated with seizures and hemodynamic instability. An ILE bolus of 1.5 mL/kg IV over 1 minute, repeated every 3 to 5 minutes in persistent cardiovascular collapse, is followed by an infusion of 0.25 mL/kg/min (which may be doubled in persistent hypotension) until hemodynamic recovery.[53] This regimen has been generalized for treatment of severe poisoning with other local anesthetics and cardiovascular toxins.

Of note, ILE administration too early after oral poisoning has the potential to facilitate gastrointestinal tract drug absorption or redistribution, exacerbating toxicity and, in theory, compromising the efficacy of lipid-soluble antidotes and concomitant therapies.[54,55] Until further evidence demonstrates ILE superiority, it is used as a last resort when conventional therapies have failed. Potential adverse effects of ILE include hypersensitivity reactions (from egg or soybean allergies), fat embolism and pulmonary toxicity, hyperamylasemia and pancreatitis, acute myocardial infarction, altered coagulation, and laboratory interference with normal serum laboratory testing.

Naloxone

Naloxone has been employed to reverse the effects of clonidine overdose. Naloxone antagonizes the effects of endogenous opioids, particularly in patients with higher baseline concentrations.[56] Although less than half of clonidine-intoxicated patients will respond to naloxone,[57,58] given the potential CNS and hemodynamic benefits, a trial dose may be warranted. High doses may be necessary and should be followed by a continuous infusion.[56] Double-blind controlled studies demonstrate that naloxone pretreatment or coadministration mitigates acute captopril-induced hypotension.[59,60] However, in cases of acute RASA ingestion or in patients with chronic hypertension, naloxone has shown inconsistent efficacy.[61–63]

Sodium Bicarbonate

Sodium bicarbonate exerts two therapeutic effects on the combined sodium channel blockade and QRS widening associated with CAs and other toxins. First, supplemental sodium mitigates channel blockade (as does hypertonic saline). Second, the bicarbonate-induced alkalemia increases the nonionized drug fractions, leading to a decrease in toxin–sodium channel binding.[64] The use of sodium bicarbonate may also mitigate hypoperfusion or seizure-induced acidemia, which can worsen channel blockade. An intravenous bolus of 1 to 2 mEq/kg of 7.5% to 8.4% sodium bicarbonate is followed by an infusion of 132 to 150 mEq in 1 L D5W at a rate of 150 to 200 mL/h, with the goal of narrowing the QRS complex to 100 milliseconds or less and targeting a serum pH 7.45 to 7.55. Rebolusing may be required for recurrent QRS widening. Alkalemia-associated hypokalemia should be anticipated with bicarbonate therapy, and treated appropriately.[65,66]

Experimental Antidotes

Methylene blue, presumably functioning as a nitric oxide scavenger, has anecdotally been employed to reverse refractory vasodilatory shock from BAAs and amlodipine. Dosing has ranged from 1 to 2 mg/kg over 10 to 20 minutes, followed by an infusion of 1 mg/kg/h.[67,68]

CONCLUSION

The treatment of critically ill cardiotoxic patients attempts to identify and reverse the effects of the responsible agent(s), to decontaminate as appropriate, and to provide aggressive supportive care with pharmacologic or adjunctive therapies. Targeted antidotal strategies include calcium, DSFab, glucagon, HIE, ILE, naloxone, or sodium bicarbonate, based on suggestive history or clinical, ECG, or laboratory findings. After initial decontamination and stabilization, patients should be admitted to an intensive care setting for continued monitoring and therapy.

LITERATURE TABLE

TRIAL	DESIGN	RESULT
Calcium		
Ramoska et al., *Ann Emerg Med.* 1993[24]	Case series of 139 CCB overdoses from three regional poison centers	Calcium was administered to 23 patients. 7/11 with sinus node suppression had an increase in heart rate. 16/20 with hypotension had an increase in blood pressure
Howarth et al., *Hum Exp Toxicol.* 1994[25]	Descriptive case study of 15 CCB overdoses	Of the 11 patients who received intravenous calcium, 7 responded with increased heart rate and blood pressure, 3 did not respond, and 1 died
Digoxin-specific Fab fragments		
Antman et al., *Circulation.* 1990[29]	Multicenter open-label study in 150 cardiac glycoside–poisoned patients	80% complete and 10% partial symptom resolution. Of 15 nonresponders, 5 were "moribund" at administration, 4 were inadequately dosed, 5 were absent digoxin toxicity, and 1 was a true nonresponder
Glucagon		
Parmley et al., *N Engl J Med.* 1968[32]	Open-label study of glucagon in 21 volunteers undergoing cardiac catheterization	Increases in heart rate, arterial pressure, and cardiac index were noted after glucagon administration within 1–3 min
Love et al., *Chest.* 1998[33]	Case series of 9 bradycardic patients refractory to atropine	8/9 patients responded to IV glucagon. One who did not was digoxin toxic
High-dose insulin euglycemia		
Kerns et al., *Ann Emerg Med.* 1997[36]	RCT of 27 canines given a propanolol infusion and treated with glucagon, epinephrine, HIE, or saline control	Survival: 6/6 (100%) with HIE, 4/6 with glucagon, 1/6 with epinephrine. HIE increased cardiac contractility
Holger et al., *Clin Toxicol.* 2007[37]	RCT of 10 pigs given IV propranolol and treated with HIE or vasopressin plus epinephrine	Survival: 5/5 (100%) with HIE as high as 10 units/kg/h; 0/5 (0%) with vasopressin and epinephrine past 1.6 h. Cardiac output and heart rate were higher in the HIE group

LITERATURE TABLE *(Continued)*

TRIAL	DESIGN	RESULT
Yuan et al., *Clin Toxicol.* 1999[39]	Case series of 5 patients with refractory cardiogenic shock due to CCB treated with HIE	Patients were treated with insulin 0.1–1 units/kg/h IV. All survived and had evidence of improved hemodynamics while receiving insulin infusions
Holger et al., *Clin Toxicol.* 2011[41]	Observational consecutive case series of 12 patients treated with high-dose insulin protocol for toxin-induced cardiogenic shock (1–10 units/kg/h)	Survival: 11/12 (death in protocol deviation patient with HIE cessation). Hypoglycemia: 6/12. Hypokalemia (<3.0 mEq/L): 8/12
Intravenous lipid emulsion		
Weinberg et al., *Anesthesiology.* 1998[43]	Analysis of 36 rats provided ILE pretreatment and exposure to varying bupivacaine doses or bupivacaine exposure followed by ILE	Bupivacaine LD_{50} increased in proportion to higher concentrations of ILE
French et al., *Clin Toxicol.* 2011[45]	In vitro analysis of xenobiotics possibly affected by ILE	Drugs with a more positive logP (lipophilicity) and higher volume of distribution were more likely to be bound by ILE
Geib et al., *Clin Toxicol.* 2012[50]	Multicenter retrospective chart review of 9 patients treated with ILE-treated drug-induced cardiotoxicity	55% survival in drug-induced cardiovascular collapse, associated with clinically significant adverse effects
Naloxone		
Bamshad et al., *Vet Hum Toxicol.* 1990[57]	Case series of 25 pediatric patients treated for clonidine ingestions	10 were treated with naloxone. 50% improved, and there were no complications with naloxone treatment
Sodium bicarbonate		
Brown et al., *Med J Aust.* 1976[65]	Case series of 11 children with CA exposures	Sodium bicarbonate successfully treated arrhythmias induced by CA exposures
Hoffman et al., *Am J Emerg Med.* 1993[66]	Retrospective study of 91 patients with CA overdose requiring ICU admission treated with sodium bicarbonate	Sodium bicarbonate associated with resolution of hypotension in 20/21 and resolution of QRS prolongation in 39/49 patients. Mental status improved in 40/85 patients

REFERENCES

1. *The Use of Medicines in the United States: Review of 2011.* Parsippany, NJ: IMS Institute for Healthcare Informatics; 2012:1–46.
2. McFee RB, Caraccio TR. "Hang Up Your Pocketbook"—an easy intervention for the granny syndrome: grandparents as a risk factor in unintentional pediatric exposures to pharmaceuticals. *J Am Osteopath Assoc.* 2006;106(7):405–411.
3. Bronstein AC, et al. 2011 Annual Report of the American Association of Poison Control Centers' National Poison Data System (NPDS): 29th Annual Report. *Clin Toxicol (Phila).* 2012;50(10):911–1164.
4. Levine M, et al. Assessment of hyperglycemia after calcium channel blocker overdoses involving diltiazem or verapamil. *Crit Care Med.* 2007;35(9):2071–2075.
5. Dinh VA, et al. Measuring cardiac index with a focused cardiac ultrasound examination in the ED. *Am J Emerg Med.* 2012;30(9):1845–1851.
6. Haydar SA, et al. Effect of bedside ultrasonography on the certainty of physician clinical decision making for septic patients in the emergency department. *Ann Emerg Med.* 2012;60(3):346–358 e4.
7. Bismuth C, et al. Hyperkalemia in acute digitalis poisoning: prognostic significance and therapeutic implications. *Clin Toxicol.* 1973;6(2):153–162.

8. Rosa RM, et al. Adrenergic modulation of extrarenal potassium disposal. *N Engl J Med.* 1980;302(8):431–434.
9. Stanley WC, Recchia FA, Lopaschuk GD. Myocardial substrate metabolism in the normal and failing heart. *Physiol Rev.* 2005;85(3):1093–1129.
10. Knudsen K, Abrahamsson J. Epinephrine and sodium bicarbonate independently and additively increase survival in experimental amitriptyline poisoning. *Crit Care Med.* 1997;25(4):669–674.
11. Teba L, et al. Beneficial effect of norepinephrine in the treatment of circulatory shock caused by tricyclic antidepressant overdose. *Am J Emerg Med.* 1988;6(6):566–568.
12. Vale JA, et al. Position paper: gastric lavage. *J Toxicol Clin Toxicol.* 2004;42(7):933–943.
13. Chyka PA, et al. Position paper: single-dose activated charcoal. *Clin Toxicol (Phila).* 2005;43(2):61–87.
14. Position paper: whole bowel irrigation. *J Toxicol Clin Toxicol.* 2004;42(6):843.
15. Taboulet P, et al. Acute digitalis intoxication—is pacing still appropriate? *J Toxicol Clin Toxicol.* 1993;31(2):261–273.
16. Janion M, et al. Is the intra-aortic balloon pump a method of brain protection during cardiogenic shock after drug intoxication? *J Emerg Med.* 2010;38(2):162–167.
17. Siddaiah L, et al. Intra-aortic balloon pump in toxic myocarditis due to aluminum phosphide poisoning. *J Med Toxicol.* 2009;5(2):80–83.
18. Van Reet B, Dens J. Auto-intoxication with flecainide and quinapril: ECG-changes, symptoms and treatment. *Acta Cardiol.* 2006;61(6):669–672.
19. Johnson NJ, et al. A review of emergency cardiopulmonary bypass for severe poisoning by cardiotoxic drugs. *J Med Toxicol.* 2013;9(1):54–60.
20. Bower JO, Mengle HAK. The additive effect of calcium and digitalis: a warning, with a report of two. *JAMA.* 1936;106(14):1151–1153.
21. Love JN, Hanfling D, Howell JM. Hemodynamic effects of calcium chloride in a canine model of acute propranolol intoxication. *Ann Emerg Med.* 1996;28(1):1–6.
22. Gay R, et al. Treatment of verapamil toxicity in intact dogs. *J Clin Invest.* 1986;77(6):1805–1811.
23. Hariman RJ, et al. Reversal of the cardiovascular effects of verapamil by calcium and sodium: differences between electrophysiologic and hemodynamic responses. *Circulation.* 1979;59(4):797–804.
24. Ramoska EA, et al. A one-year evaluation of calcium channel blocker overdoses: toxicity and treatment. *Ann Emerg Med.* 1993;22(2):196–200.
25. Howarth DM, et al. Calcium channel blocking drug overdose: an Australian series. *Hum Exp Toxicol.* 1994;13(3):161–166.
26. Martin TJ, et al. Ionization and hemodynamic effects of calcium chloride and calcium gluconate in the absence of hepatic function. *Anesthesiology.* 1990;73(1):62–65.
27. Marraffa JM, Cohen V, Howland MA. Antidotes for toxicological emergencies: a practical review. *Am J Health Syst Pharm.* 2012;69(3):199–212.
28. Kerns W II. Management of beta-adrenergic blocker and calcium channel antagonist toxicity. *Emerg Med Clin North Am.* 2007;25(2):309–331; abstract viii.
29. Antman EM, et al. Treatment of 150 cases of life-threatening digitalis intoxication with digoxin-specific Fab antibody fragments. Final report of a multicenter study. *Circulation.* 1990;81(6):1744–1752.
30. Bismuth C, et al. Acute digitoxin intoxication treated by intracardiac pacemaker: experience in sixty-eight patients. *Clin Toxicol.* 1977;10(4):443–456.
31. Ujhelyi MR, Robert S. Pharmacokinetic aspects of digoxin-specific Fab therapy in the management of digitalis toxicity. *Clin Pharmacokinet.* 1995;28(6):483–493.
32. Parmley WW, Glick G, Sonnenblick EH. Cardiovascular effects of glucagon in man. *N Engl J Med.* 1968;279(1):12–17.
33. Love JN, et al. A potential role for glucagon in the treatment of drug-induced symptomatic bradycardia. *Chest.* 1998;114(1):323–326.
34. Oliver EF, Opie LH. Effects of glucose and fatty acids on myocardial ischaemia and arrhythmias. *Lancet.* 1994;343(8890):155–158.
35. Kline JA, et al. Insulin is a superior antidote for cardiovascular toxicity induced by verapamil in the anesthetized canine. *J Pharmacol Exp Ther.* 1993;267(2):744–750.
36. Kerns W, et al. Insulin improves survival in a canine model of acute b-blocker toxicity. *Ann Emerg Med.* 1997;29(6):748–757.
37. Holger JS, et al. Insulin versus vasopressin and epinephrine to treat beta-blocker toxicity. *Clin Toxicol (Phila).* 2007;45(4):396–401.
38. Cole JB, et al. A blinded, randomized, controlled trial of three doses of high-dose insulin in poison-induced cardiogenic shock. *Clin Toxicol (Phila).* 2013;51(4):201–207.

39. Yuan TH, et al. Insulin-glucose as adjunctive therapy for severe calcium channel antagonist poisoning. *J Toxicol Clin Toxicol.* 1999;37(4):463–474.
40. Greene SL, et al. Relative safety of hyperinsulinaemia/euglycaemia therapy in the management of calcium channel blocker overdose: a prospective observational study. *Intensive Care Med.* 2007;33(11):2019–2024.
41. Holger JS, et al. High-dose insulin: a consecutive case series in toxin-induced cardiogenic shock. *Clin Toxicol.* 2011;49(7):653–658.
42. Engebretsen KM, et al. High-dose insulin therapy in beta-blocker and calcium channel-blocker poisoning. *Clin Toxicol (Phila).* 2011;49(4):277–283.
43. Weinberg GL, et al. Pretreatment or resuscitation with a lipid infusion shifts the dose-response to bupivacaine-induced asystole in rats. *Anesthesiology.* 1998;88(4):1071–1075.
44. Shi K, et al. The effect of lipid emulsion on pharmacokinetics and tissue distribution of bupivacaine in rats. *Anesth Analg.* 2013;116(4):804–809.
45. French D, et al. Partition constant and volume of distribution as predictors of clinical efficacy of lipid rescue for toxicological emergencies. *Clin Toxicol (Phila).* 2011;49(9):801–809.
46. Weinberg G, et al. Lipid emulsion infusion rescues dogs from bupivacaine-induced cardiac toxicity. *Reg Anesth Pain Med.* 2003;28(3):198–202.
47. Bania TC, et al. Hemodynamic effects of intravenous fat emulsion in an animal model of severe verapamil toxicity resuscitated with atropine, calcium, and saline. *Acad Emerg Med.* 2007;14(2):105–111.
48. Rosenblatt MA, et al. Successful use of a 20% lipid emulsion to resuscitate a patient after a presumed bupivacaine-related cardiac arrest. *Anesthesiology.* 2006;105(1):217–218.
49. Cave G, Harvey M, Graudins A. Intravenous lipid emulsion as antidote: a summary of published human experience. *Emerg Med Australas.* 2011;23(2):123–141.
50. Geib AJ, Liebelt E, Manini AF. Clinical experience with intravenous lipid emulsion for drug-induced cardiovascular collapse. *J Med Toxicol.* 2012;8(1):10–14.
51. Presley JD, Chyka PA. Intravenous lipid emulsion to reverse acute drug toxicity in pediatric patients. *Ann Pharmacother.* 2013;47(5):735–743.
52. Arora NP, et al. Usefulness of intravenous lipid emulsion for cardiac toxicity from cocaine overdose. *Am J Cardiol.* 2013;111(3):445–447.
53. Neal JM, Mulroy MF, Weinberg GL. American Society of Regional Anesthesia and Pain Medicine checklist for managing local anesthetic systemic toxicity: 2012 version. *Reg Anesth Pain Med.* 2012;37(1):16–18.
54. Perichon D, et al. An assessment of the in vivo effects of intravenous lipid emulsion on blood drug concentration and haemodynamics following oro-gastric amitriptyline overdose. *Clin Toxicol (Phila).* 2013;51(4):208–215.
55. Harvey M, Cave G, Shaw T. Effect of intravenous lipid emulsion and octreotide on enteric thiopentone absorption; a pilot study. *Clin Toxicol (Phila).* 2013;51(2):117–118.
56. Seger DL. Clonidine toxicity revisited. *J Toxicol Clin Toxicol.* 2002;40(2):145–155.
57. Bamshad MJ, Wasserman GS. Pediatric clonidine intoxications. *Vet Hum Toxicol.* 1990;32(3):220–223.
58. Nichols MH, King WD, James LP. Clonidine poisoning in Jefferson County, Alabama. *Ann Emerg Med.* 1997;29(4):511–517.
59. Ajayi AA, et al. Effect of naloxone on the actions of captopril. *Clin Pharmacol Ther.* 1985;38(5):560–565.
60. Millar JA, et al. Attenuation of the antihypertensive effect of captopril by the opioid receptor antagonist naloxone. *Clin Exp Pharmacol Physiol.* 1983;10(3):253–259.
61. Varon J, Duncan SR. Naloxone reversal of hypotension due to captopril overdose. *Ann Emerg Med.* 1991;20(10):1125–1127.
62. Barr CS, Payne R, Newton RW. Profound prolonged hypotension following captopril overdose. *Postgrad Med J.* 1991;67(792):953–954.
63. Bernini GP, et al. Naloxone does not antagonize the antihypertensive effect of chronic captopril therapy in hypertensive patients. *Cardiovasc Drugs Ther.* 1989;3(6):829–833.
64. Sasyniuk BI, Jhamandas V. Mechanism of reversal of toxic effects of amitriptyline on cardiac Purkinje fibers by sodium bicarbonate. *J Pharmacol Exp Ther.* 1984;231(2):387–394.
65. Brown TC. Sodium bicarbonate treatment for tricyclic antidepressant arrhythmias in children. *Med J Aust.* 1976;2(10):380–382.
66. Hoffman JR, et al. Effect of hypertonic sodium bicarbonate in the treatment of moderate-to-severe cyclic antidepressant overdose. *Am J Emerg Med.* 1993;11(4):336–341.
67. Jang DH, Nelson LS, Hoffman RS. Methylene blue in the treatment of refractory shock from an amlodipine overdose. *Ann Emerg Med.* 2011;58(6):565–567.
68. Aggarwal N, et al. Methylene blue reverses recalcitrant shock in beta-blocker and calcium channel blocker overdose. *BMJ Case Rep.* 2013;2013.

46

Pulmonary Toxins

Hong K. Kim and Rama B. Rao

BACKGROUND

The pulmonary system has multiple important physiologic functions. The most essential—oxygenation of hemoglobin—occurs across a layer of endothelial cells in the pulmonary alveoli. Toxins that displace oxygen are termed simple asphyxiants. This group of gases includes hydrocarbons, noble gases, nitrogen, and carbon dioxide. Inhalation of simple asphyxiants reduces the fraction of inspired oxygen (FiO_2) below 21% and lowers the partial pressure of oxygen. These gases leave the pulmonary parenchyma largely intact allowing normal gas exchange to resume once the patient is removed from the toxic environment.

Inhaled toxins that injure or inflame the pulmonary alveoli and result in lung injury are termed pulmonary irritants. These gases disrupt the alveolar epithelial integrity by different mechanisms. Some gases such as chlorine (Cl_2) and ammonia (NH_3) form acids or bases that cause inflammation and disruption of surfactant. Other gases such as ozone (O_3) and oxides of nitrogen (NO_x) produce reactive free radicals or intermediates that result in inflammatory injury, sometimes hours after exposure. These gases are a major contributor to air pollution and high rates of asthma and symptomatic airway disease.

SIMPLE ASPHYXIANTS

Sources of simple asphyxiants include workplace releases of noble gases and agricultural sources such as methane. Iatrogenic asphyxiation may occur in hospitals when nitrous oxide is affixed to a patient's face for prolonged periods, or when a nitrogen line is inadvertently confused for supplemental oxygen. Some simple asphyxiant sources exist in a nongaseous phase (e.g., dry ice [CO_2] in a solid form, or nitrogen [N_2] in liquid form).[1] Asphyxiation from these sources usually occurs in a confined space, requiring phase transition to a gas.[2–4] Occasionally, simple asphyxiants are associated with mass casualties: the large-scale emission of carbon dioxide gas from Lake Nyos, a carbonated volcanic lake in Cameroon, West Africa, asphyxiated more than 1,700 residents and thousands of livestock within a radius of 10 km.[5,6]

Management Guidelines

Because simple asphyxiants reduce the effective fraction of inspired oxygen (FiO_2), the signs and symptoms of toxicity are similar to those of hypoxia; they include altered sensorium, syncope, coma, seizures, and cardiac arrest. Depending on the severity of the global tissue hypoxia, end-organ injury may develop, leading to significant morbidity and mortality. Simple asphyxiants typically do not interfere with ventilation, and with the exception of asphyxia by carbon dioxide, hypercarbia is absent until respiratory depression or arrest occurs. The primary therapeutic intervention in simple asphyxiant toxicity is patient removal from the exposure and restoration of adequate oxygenation and ventilation. In the setting of multiorgan failure from prolonged tissue hypoxia, therapy is limited to supportive care. Given that simple asphyxiants do not cause primary lung injury, recovery is complete provided end-organ damage from tissue hypoxia has not occurred.

PULMONARY IRRITANT GASES

Inhaled pulmonary irritants can destroy the alveolar epithelium, resulting in impaired alveolar gas exchange. The initial disruption of respiratory tract integrity is attributed to one or both of two causes: the acid or base produced when pulmonary irritant gases dissolve in the physiologic alveolar fluid and the generation of free radicals, specifically reactive oxygen species.[7–9] Although the exact mechanism of injury is unknown, the toxic end products of pulmonary irritants are believed to cause direct cellular damage and initiate an inflammatory cascade that can lead to the development of acute respiratory distress syndrome (ARDS). Highly water-soluble toxic gasses such as concentrated ammonia quickly irritate mucous membranes, often prompting rapid retreat from the irritant source. Less water-soluble agents, such as chlorine gas, phosgene, and oxides of nitrogen, do not cause as rapid a reaction and are more likely to result in prolonged exposures.

Two well-known pulmonary irritant gases are chlorine gas [Cl_2] and phosgene [$COCl_2$]. During World War I, both Axis and Allied forces used these agents as chemical weapons; today, they are used in the production of pharmaceuticals, plastics, textiles, and pesticides.[8,10] A majority of exposures to these pulmonary irritants result from mass casualty occupational, industrial, or transportation accidents.[8–14] Domestic exposures—most notably to chlorine gas—do occur occasionally and typically result from unsafe mixing of cleaning agents or from inappropriate use and storage of swimming pool chlorinating solutions (see below).[8,12,15,16]

Chlorine [Cl_2]

While the majority of chlorine gas exposures result from occupational- and industrial-related incidents, nonindustrial exposure can occur when acidic cleaning agents such as hydrochloric acid [HCl] are mixed with sodium hypochlorite [NaOCl], or bleach.[12,15,17,18] Chlorine is a yellowish green gas that has a distinct and readily recognized odor with a density that is twice as heavy as air. It tends to settle near the ground and is dispersed by air movements. The mechanism of injury is the formation of hydrochloric acid, hypochlorous acid, and nascent oxygen [O^-] (oxygen liberated from a chemical reaction) when the chlorine gas dissolves in the alveolar fluid.[8] Complicating this process is nascent oxygen's ability to induce the formation of free radicals, which can cause additional pulmonary injury.

The severity of the toxic effects of chlorine gas inhalation varies from minor respiratory tract irritation to death, depending on ambient concentration of the gas and the duration of exposure.[19] From available data, exposure to 1 to 15 parts per million (ppm) will produce mild to moderate mucous membrane and conjunctival irritation. Inhalation of >30 ppm of chlorine gas results in chest pain, cough, and shortness of breath; chemical pneumonitis and acute pulmonary edema are observed at concentrations between 40 and 60 ppm. Exposure to concentrations above 400 ppm results in death, usually over a period of 30 minutes, while exposure to concentrations >1,000 ppm may be fatal within minutes.[7,8]

The intermediate water solubility of chlorine gas often results in mild or delayed initial symptoms, including conjunctival and nasal irritation, that can contribute to an unintentionally prolonged duration of exposure.[8] A majority of exposures, however, remain brief, with inhalation of low to moderate concentrations resulting in transient symptoms such as cough, shortness of breath, and wheeze.[12,17,19–21] Prolonged exposure can result in severe pulmonary sequelae—often not observed until 4 to 8 hours following inhalation—including pneumonitis, pulmonary edema, and ARDS.[7,9,21]

Chloramines [NH_2Cl, $NHCl_2$, and NCl_3]

Chloramine is produced when chlorine interacts with nitrogen-containing compounds.[22–24] This typically occurs during chlorination of indoor swimming pools where chlorine, in the form of bleach, is used to disinfect both organic (urea and creatinine) and inorganic (ammonia) nitrogen-containing compounds.[23–25] In households, chloramine exposures are reported after two common household cleaning products, bleach and ammonia, are mixed.[23–28] Three different types of chloramines can be generated, depending on the degree of chlorination: monochloramine [NH_2Cl], dichloramine [$NHCl_2$], and trichloramine [NCl_3].[23] The dissolution of chloramine in physiologic fluid (e.g., in the alveoli epithelial layer or mucous membrane) generates hypochlorous acid [HOCl], ammonia, and oxygen radicals—toxic end products that cause irritation of the eyes, respiratory tract, and mucosal membrane. Because chloramines are highly water-soluble, symptom onset is typically immediate, prompting the exposed person to escape to fresh air and minimize prolonged exposure. Significant morbidity, including pneumonitis, has been reported when exposure occurs in a confined space with limited ventilation.[26–28]

Phosgene [$COCl_2$]

Similar to chlorine gas, phosgene has become an important compound in the chemical industry after its debut during World War I. Phosgene is used in the production of organic solvents, dyes, pesticides, and pharmaceuticals.[10,29] The majority of phosgene exposures also occur in the industrial setting.[10,30,31] Phosgene gas may also be emitted by combustion of chlorinated hydrocarbons such as plastic or polyvinyl chloride (e.g., house or vehicle fire).[30]

Contact with phosgene causes tissue injury by two distinct chemical mechanisms: acylation and hydrolysis.[29,32] Acylation (the process of adding an acyl group to a compound) is believed to be the primary mechanism, occurs when phosgene reacts with nucleophilic components of macromolecules (amino, hydroxyl, thiol, and sulfhydryl groups), and produces injury by permanent denaturation of proteins and lipoproteins.[29,32] The second mechanism is the hydrolysis of phosgene in the physiologic fluid of the alveoli, which results in the production of hydrochloric acid [HCl] and carbon dioxide [CO_2] responsible for the initial mucous membrane irritation.[32,33]

The characteristic odor of phosgene gas is described as "fresh hay" (odor threshold 0.4 to 1.5 ppm).[29] This property may contribute to prolonged exposure by inciting deep breathing rather than alarm at the presence of a toxic gas. Moreover, due to phosgene's intermediate water solubility, early symptoms of mucosal irritation are frequently minor, further prolonging exposure and allowing deeper penetration into the lower respiratory tract.[34]

Phosgene toxicity produces three clinical phases: reflex, latent, and delayed pulmonary edema.[35,36] During the initial reflex phase, symptom severity is related to gas concentration.[29,32] Phosgene concentrations of >3 to 5 ppm result in immediate mucous membrane irritation, cough, and chest tightness.[10,29,31,32] Initial exposure stimulates a vagal reflex, which results in decreased vital capacity from rapid shallow breathing, bradycardia, and hypotension.[32,33] In the subsequent latent phase, patients may be asymptomatic for up to 48 hours; in the final, delayed phase, they may develop noncardiogenic pulmonary edema and respiratory distress.[10,29–31,35,37] While the severity of the initial mucosal irritation is dependent on gas concentration, the delayed development of pulmonary edema is correlated with the total dose exposure and reflects a dose–response relationship.[29,32,38,39] Clinically latent pulmonary interstitial inflammation occurs at exposures to 30 to 150 ppm/min, while overt pulmonary edema occurs at exposures to >150 ppm/min. The estimated lethal dose for mortality of 1%, 50%, and 100% is 300 ppm/min, 500 ppm/min, and 1,300 ppm/min, respectively.[32,33]

Management Guidelines

The principle management strategy for pulmonary irritant gas exposure is to remove the patient from the exposure and provide supportive care, including ensuring adequate oxygenation and ventilation. Following removal, patients should be undressed and examined for other potential toxic exposures and traumatic injuries. There is no antidote for pulmonary irritant exposure and no indication for decontamination in setting of acute chlorine, chloramine, and phosgene gas exposure. Decontamination protocols should be considered if dermal or ocular exposure to liquid agents has occurred. Irrigation of the eye and other mucosal surfaces may help reduce irritation, and if respiratory tract irritation is evident, supplemental oxygen and bronchodilators (β-agonists) should be administered.

Several studies have investigated the role of inhaled nebulized sodium bicarbonate in neutralizing the acidic end products of pulmonary irritants and in reducing pulmonary injury.[40–44] In general, chemical neutralization is contraindicated, especially in ingestion of acid or alkali agents, due to its potential to exacerbate the initial caustic injury by producing an exothermic reaction and gas formation. Some practitioners have attempted chemical neutralization of pulmonary irritants, considered safe because the large surface area of the lung and the low concentration of pulmonary irritant end products would allow for the dissipation of the heat and gas produced. To date, however, no convincing evidence exists to support the routine use of inhaled nebulized sodium bicarbonate in pulmonary irritant exposures.[40–44] One case report ($n = 3$) showed immediate relief of symptoms (cough and dyspnea) after 3.75% $NaHCO_3$ nebulized solution was administered following chlorine exposure.[40] However, a small prospective trial ($n = 22$) of 4.2% $NaHCO_3$ nebulized solution for patients with chlorine and chloramine exposures failed to demonstrate any clinical benefit.[42] Chemical neutralization using $NaHCO_3$ has not been studied in gas exposures other than chlorine. Since definitive evidence is lacking, a brief trial of nebulized sodium bicarbonate <4.2% may be attempted in awake patients if tolerated, and continued only if subjective relief occurs, but is unlikely to affect outcome.

The most serious complication of pulmonary irritant exposure is the development of ARDS. In chlorine and phosgene exposure, physical exam findings (rales or crackles) and radiologic signs of pneumonitis or pulmonary edema may not be evident for up to 8 and 48 hours, respectively.[7,9,21,30,31,33,35,45] Although the etiology of ARDS caused by pulmonary irritants is different from the etiology of injury caused by sepsis or trauma, the similarities of the underlying inflammatory response suggest that similar management principles apply. Specifically, targeting tidal volumes of 6 mL/kg and plateau pressure of <30 cm H_2O decreases inflammatory markers and improves survival.[46,47]

In animal model studies, corticosteroids have been shown to improve oxygen delivery and lung compliance and possibly decrease pulmonary injury risk in chlorine gas-induced ARDS and pneumonitis.[48–52] To date, no trials have investigated the role of corticosteroids in countering the inflammatory process during human pulmonary irritant exposure.

Patients exposed to chloramine and chlorine gas who remain asymptomatic after 8 hours of observation may be safely be discharged with adequate follow-up in place. Asymptomatic patients exposed to phosgene should be observed for 24 hours to monitor for delayed onset of pulmonary edema and pneumonitis.

Other Pulmonary Toxins

Although beyond the scope of this chapter, other chemicals, including salicylate, opioids, cocaine, carbon monoxide, and negative inotropic agents (beta-blockers and calcium channel blockers), have also been implicated in pulmonary toxicity/ARDS.[6,53–58] Treatment of lung injury from these agents generally requires supportive care and, in some cases, such as salicylates, treatment to enhance elimination of toxin.

CONCLUSION

Exposure to simple asphyxiants and pulmonary irritants is potentially fatal. Patients exposed to simple asphyxiants who survive to reach medical care generally require only short-term supportive care. Patients surviving pulmonary irritant exposure may present with early and/or late mucosal and respiratory symptoms; for these patients, the specific irritant, duration of exposure, and severity of symptoms will determine the extent of supportive care needed. Although pulmonary toxins are less commonly treated in the ED than many other emergencies, a familiarity with the information presented in this chapter is indispensable for the emergency physician committed to managing the full spectrum of critically ill patients.

LITERATURE TABLE

TRIAL	DESIGN	RESULT
$NaHCO_3$		
Vinsel, *Emerg Med.* 1990[40]	Case report of treatment of acute chlorine gas inhalation with nebulized sodium bicarbonate	Chlorine exposure from swimming pool chlorination system leak. Resolution of symptoms (cough and dyspnea) after treatment with a single nebulized solution of 3.75% $NaHCO_3$ (4 mL)
Douidar, *Pediatr Emerg Care.* 1997[41]	Case report of treatment of acute chlorine gas inhalation with nebulized sodium bicarbonate	Chlorine tablet fume exposure in a 7-year-old girl. Patient received albuterol without symptomatic improvement. Symptoms (hypoxia, coughing, nasal flaring, and subcostal retraction) improved after treatment with a single nebulized solution of 3.75% $NaHCO_3$ (4.25 mL)
Aslan et al., *Inhal Toxicol.* 2006[42]	Double-blind prospective study of $NaHCO_3$ versus control in 44 patients with chlorine gas exposure. All patients also received β-agonist and parenteral steroid as standard therapy	No difference in clinical outcome between $NaHCO_3$ group and control. Force expiratory volume in 1 s (FEV1) was significantly increased in treatment group compared to control ($p < 0.05$)
Bosse, *J Toxicol Clin Toxicol.* 1994[43]	Retrospective review of poison control center (PCC) data in 86 cases of chlorine gas exposure	All patients were recommended to receive treatment with a nebulized solution of 5% $NaHCO_3$ (5 mL) per PCC protocol. Three patients had immediate resolution of symptoms. No pneumonitis and pulmonary edema noted in 17 admitted patients
Corticosteroids		
Wang et al., *Intensive Care Med.* 2002[48]	Animal study. Impact of time to treatment with nebulized budesonide (0.1 mg/kg) following chlorine gas exposure	Significant improvement in lung compliance, pulmonary vascular resistance, and oxygenation when treated with budesonide within 30 min
Wang et al., *Acta Anaesthesiaol Scand.* 2005[49]	Animal study. Efficacy of treatment with IV betamethasone and nebulized budesonide following chlorine gas exposure	Steroid administration improved clinical markers of oxygenation and showed lower histologic injury compared to placebo
Demnati et al., *Toxicol Sci.* 1998[50]	Animal study. Effects of intraperitoneal dexamethasone (300 μg/kg/d × 7 d) on pulmonary function and histologic changes following chlorine gas exposure	Intraperitoneal dexamethasone helped maintain pulmonary function and reduced inflammatory cell count in alveolar fluid 14 d postexposure
Gunnarsson et al., *J Trauma.* 2000[59]	Animal study. Efficacy of treatment with nebulized beclomethasone (20 μg/kg) following chlorine gas exposure	Inhaled beclomethasone immediately after chlorine gas exposure improved lung–thorax compliance and oxygenation
Smith et al., *Mil Med.* 2009[60]	Animal study. Efficacy of treatment with intravenous methylprednisolone (12 mg/kg) and inhaled budesonide (1 mg) following phosgene-induced lung injury in pigs	No change in mortality or incidence of pulmonary edema

REFERENCES

1. Harris PD, Barnes R. The uses of helium and xenon in current clinical practice. *Anaesthesia.* 2008;63(3):284–293.
2. Dunford JV, Lucas J, Vent N, et al. Asphyxiation due to dry ice in a walk-in freezer. *J Emerg Med.* 2009;36(4):353–356.
3. Kim DH, Lee HJ. Evaporated liquid nitrogen-induced asphyxia: a case report. *J Korean Med Sci.* 2008;23(1):163–165.
4. Musshoff F, Hagemeier L, Kirschbaum K, et al. Two cases of suicide by asphyxiation due to helium and argon. *Forensic Sci Int.* 2012;223(1–3):e27–e30.

5. Agency for Toxic Substances and Disease Registry. *Hazardous Substances Emergency Events Surveillance Annual Report*. 2009; http://www.atsdr.cdc.gov/HS/HSEES/annual2009.html. Accessed June 3, 2013.
6. Duberstein JL, Kaufman DM. A clinical study of an epidemic of heroin intoxication and heroin-induced pulmonary edema. *Am J Med.* 1971;51(6):704–714.
7. White CW, Martin JG. Chlorine gas inhalation: human clinical evidence of toxicity and experience in animal models. *Proc Am Thorac Soc.* 2010;7(4):257–263.
8. Winder C. The toxicology of chlorine. *Environ Res.* 2001;85(2):105–114.
9. Van Sickle D, Wenck MA, Belflower A, et al. Acute health effects after exposure to chlorine gas released after a train derailment. *Am J Emerg Med.* 2009;27(1):1–7.
10. Kumar A, Chaudhari S, Kush L, et al. Accidental inhalation injury of phosgene gas leading to acute respiratory distress syndrome. *Indian J Occup Environ Med.* 2012;16(2):88–89.
11. Henneberger PK, Ferris BG Jr, Sheehe PR. Accidental gassing incidents and the pulmonary function of pulp mill workers. *Am Rev Respir Dis.* 1993;148(1):63–67.
12. Cevik Y, Onay M, Akmaz I, et al. Mass casualties from acute inhalation of chlorine gas. *South Med J.* 2009;102(12):1209–1213.
13. Jones RN, Hughes JM, Glindmeyer H, et al. Lung function after acute chlorine exposure. *Am Rev Respir Dis.* 1986;134(6):1190–1195.
14. Wenck MA, Van Sickle D, Drociuk D, et al. Rapid assessment of exposure to chlorine released from a train derailment and resulting health impact. *Public Health Rep.* 2007;122(6):784–792.
15. Deschamps D, Soler P, Rosenberg N, et al. Persistent asthma after inhalation of a mixture of sodium hypochlorite and hydrochloric acid. *Chest.* 1994;105(6):1895–1896.
16. Babu RV, Cardenas V, Sharma G. Acute respiratory distress syndrome from chlorine inhalation during a swimming pool accident: a case report and review of the literature. *J Intensive Care Med.* 2008;23(4):275–280.
17. Gorguner M, Aslan S, Inandi T, et al. Reactive airways dysfunction syndrome in housewives due to a bleach-hydrochloric acid mixture. *Inhal Toxicol.* 2004;16(2):87–91.
18. Mrvos R, Dean BS, Krenzelok EP. Home exposures to chlorine/chloramine gas: review of 216 cases. *South Med J.* 1993;86(6):654–657.
19. Centers for Disease Control and Prevention. Chlorine gas exposure at a metal recycling facility—California, 2010. *MMWR Morb Mortal Wkly Rep.* 2011;60(28):951–954.
20. Agabiti N, Ancona C, Forastiere F, et al. Short term respiratory effects of acute exposure to chlorine due to a swimming pool accident. *Occup Environ Med.* 2001;58(6):399–404.
21. Mohan A, Kumar SN, Rao MH, et al. Acute accidental exposure to chlorine gas: clinical presentation, pulmonary functions and outcomes. *Indian J Chest Dis Allied Sci.* 2010;52(3):149–152.
22. Massin N, Hecht G, Ambroise D, et al. Respiratory symptoms and bronchial responsiveness among cleaning and disinfecting workers in the food industry. *Occup Environ Med.* 2007;64(2):75–81.
23. Levesque B, Duchesne JF, Gingras S, et al. The determinants of prevalence of health complaints among young competitive swimmers. *Int Arch Occup Environ Health.* 2006;80(1):32–39.
24. Kaydos-Daniels SC, Beach MJ, Shwe T, et al. Health effects associated with indoor swimming pools: a suspected toxic chloramine exposure. *Public Health.* 2008;122(2):195–200.
25. Florentin A, Hautemaniere A, Hartemann P. Health effects of disinfection by-products in chlorinated swimming pools. *Int J Hyg Environ Health.* 2011;214(6):461–469.
26. Gapany-Gapanavicius M, Molho M, Tirosh M. Chloramine-induced pneumonitis from mixing household cleaning agents. *BMJ (Clinical research ed.).* 1982;285(6348):1086.
27. Minami M, Katsumata M, Miyake K, et al. Dangerous mixture of household detergents in an old-style toilet: a case report with simulation experiments of the working environment and warning of potential hazard relevant to the general environment. *Hum Exp Toxicol.* 1992;11(1):27–34.
28. Tanen DA, Graeme KA, Raschke R. Severe lung injury after exposure to chloramine gas from household cleaners. *N Engl J Med.* 1999;341(11):848–849.
29. Grainge C, Rice P. Management of phosgene-induced acute lung injury. *Clin Toxicol (Phila).* 2010;48(6):497–508.
30. Gutch M, Jain N, Agrawal A, Consul S. Acute accidental phosgene poisoning. *BMJ Case Rep.* 2012;2012.
31. Lim SC, Yang JY, Jang AS, et al. Acute lung injury after phosgene inhalation. *Korean J Intern Med.* 1996;11(1):87–92.
32. Borak J, Diller WF. Phosgene exposure: mechanisms of injury and treatment strategies. *J Occupgiven Environ Med.* 2001;43(2):110–119.
33. Diller WF. Pathogenesis of phosgene poisoning. *Toxicol Ind Health.* 1985;1(2):7–15.

34. Rodgers GC Jr, Condurache CT. Antidotes and treatments for chemical warfare/terrorism agents: an evidence-based review. *Clin Pharmacol Ther.* 2010;88(3):318–327.
35. Diller WF. Early diagnosis of phosgene overexposure. *Toxicol Ind Health.* 1985;1(2):73–80.
36. Diller WF. Therapeutic strategy in phosgene poisoning. *Toxicol Ind Health.* 1985;1(2):93–99.
37. Diller WF. Late sequelae after phosgene poisoning: a literature review. *Toxicol Ind Health.* 1985;1(2):129–136.
38. Diller WF. Medical phosgene problems and their possible solution. *J Occup Med.* 1978;20(3):189–193.
39. Rinehart WE, Hatch T. Concentration-time product (CT) as an expression of dose in sublethal exposures to phosgene. *Am Ind Hyg Assoc J.* 1964;25:545–553.
40. Vinsel PJ. Treatment of acute chlorine gas inhalation with nebulized sodium bicarbonate. *J Emerg Med.* 1990;8(3):327–329.
41. Douidar SM. Nebulized sodium bicarbonate in acute chlorine inhalation. *Pediatr Emerg Care.* 1997;13(6):406–407.
42. Aslan S, Kandis H, Akgun M, et al. The effect of nebulized NaHCO3 treatment on "RADS" due to chlorine gas inhalation. *Inhal Toxicol.* 2006;18(11):895–900.
43. Bosse GM. Nebulized sodium bicarbonate in the treatment of chlorine gas inhalation. *J Toxicol Clin Toxicol.* 1994;32(3):233–241.
44. Pascuzzi TA, Storrow AB. Mass casualties from acute inhalation of chloramine gas. *Mil Med.* 1998;163(2):102–104.
45. Grainge C, Smith AJ, Jugg BJ, et al. Furosemide in the treatment of phosgene induced acute lung injury. *J R Army Med Corps.* 2010;156(4):245–250.
46. The Acute Respiratory Distress Syndrome Network. Ventilation with lower tidal volumes as compared with traditional tidal volumes for acute lung injury and the acute respiratory distress syndrome. *N Engl J Med.* 2000;342(18):1301–1308.
47. Parsons PE, Eisner MD, Thompson BT, et al. Lower tidal volume ventilation and plasma cytokine markers of inflammation in patients with acute lung injury. *Crit Care Med.* 2005;33(1):1–6; discussion 230–232.
48. Wang J, Zhang L, Walther SM. Inhaled budesonide in experimental chlorine gas lung injury: influence of time interval between injury and treatment. *Intensive Care Med.* 2002;28(3):352–357.
49. Wang J, Winskog C, Edston E, et al. Inhaled and intravenous corticosteroids both attenuate chlorine gas-induced lung injury in pigs. *Acta Anaesthesiol Scand.* 2005;49(2):183–190.
50. Demnati R, Fraser R, Martin JG, et al. Effects of dexamethasone on functional and pathological changes in rat bronchi caused by high acute exposure to chlorine. *Toxicol Sci.* 1998;45(2):242–246.
51. Gunnarsson M, Walther SM, Seidal T, et al. Effects of inhalation of corticosteroids immediately after experimental chlorine gas lung injury. *J Trauma.* 2000;48(1):101–107.
52. Peter JV, John P, Graham PL, et al. Corticosteroids in the prevention and treatment of acute respiratory distress syndrome (ARDS) in adults: meta-analysis. *BMJ.* 2008;336(7651):1006–1009.
53. Ettinger NA, Albin RJ. A review of the respiratory effects of smoking cocaine. *Am J Med.* 1989;87(6):664–668.
54. Fein A, Grossman RF, Jones JG, et al. Carbon monoxide effect on alveolar epithelial permeability. *Chest.* 1980;78(5):726–731.
55. Frand UI, Shim CS, Williams MH Jr. Heroin-induced pulmonary edema. Sequential studies of pulmonary function. *Ann Intern Med.* 1972;77(1):29–35.
56. Heffner J, Starkey T, Anthony P. Salicylate-induced noncardiogenic pulmonary edema. *West J Med.* 1979;130(3):263–266.
57. Heffner JE, Sahn SA. Salicylate-induced pulmonary edema. Clinical features and prognosis. *Ann Intern Med.* 1981;95(4):405–409.
58. Humbert VH Jr, Munn NJ, Hawkins RF. Noncardiogenic pulmonary edema complicating massive diltiazem overdose. *Chest.* 1991;99(1):258–259.
59. Gunnarsson M, Walther SM, Seidal T, et al. Exposure to chlorine gas: effects on pulmonary function and morphology in anaesthetised and mechanically ventilated pigs. *J Appl Toxicol.* 1998;18(4):249–255.
60. Smith A, Brown R, Jugg B, et al. The effect of steroid treatment with inhaled budesonide or intravenous methylprednisolone on phosgene-induced acute lung injury in a porcine model. *Mil Med.* 2009;174(12):1287–1294.

47

Toxicologic Hyperthermic Syndromes

Mai Takematsu and Rama B. Rao

BACKGROUND

Elevations in body temperature may be caused by behavioral factors, exertion, infections, endocrinologic conditions, and environmental exposures; as well as by therapeutic and illicit drugs that disrupt the autonomic nervous system or impair the body's cooling capacity. Core body temperatures in excess of 106°F (41.1°C) precipitate life-threatening hyperthermia—termed heat stroke when the condition is accompanied by altered mental status.

Heat stroke is always a time-sensitive emergency that requires prompt diagnosis and treatment, as its mortality rate is directly related to delays in cooling.[1] Patients subject to such delays are at risk for multisystem organ failure, often heralded by impaired liver synthetic function and disseminated intravascular coagulation (DIC). From 1999 to 2003, a total of 3,442 deaths from heat stroke were reported in the United States; while underlying illnesses contributed to the majority of these deaths, 4.2% were due to toxicologic causes.[2] This chapter reviews some of the common toxicologic hyperthermic syndromes and their management (Table 47.1).

HYPERTHERMIC AGITATED DELIRIUM

Patients with severe hyperthermia may present with agitated delirium—a difficult-to-manage form of heat stroke—that can impair the clinician's ability to obtain vital signs in a timely fashion. When presented with an agitated patient, especially during the summer months, the emergency physician should maintain a high degree of suspicion for a hyperthermic etiology.[3]

History and Physical Exam

Agitated delirium has been used to describe patients with severe agitation who are unresponsive to verbal redirection, are combative, or have altered mental status. Cases are frequently associated with drug use; illicit sympathomimetic agents such as cocaine are common culprits, and patients classically present diaphoretic, tachycardic, hypertensive, and severely agitated (sympathomimetic toxidrome).[4] The use of cocaine or other sympathomimetic agents causes vasoconstriction, which limits effective cooling and simultaneously increases motor tone, generating heat. Data suggest that mortality related to cocaine use increases when ambient temperatures are above 88°F (31.1°C).[5] Centrally

TABLE 47.1 Causes of Toxicologic Hyperthermia

Syndrome	Example	Mechanism
Hyperthermic agitated delirium	Anticholinergic toxicities	Increased tone Impaired sweating
	Sympathomimetic toxicities	Increased tone Impaired vasodilation
Pharmacologic hyperthermic syndromes	Serotonin toxicity NMS MH	Central serotonergic excess Dopaminergic blockade RYR-1 dysfunction
Other causes of drug-induced hyperthermia	Status epilepticus inducing agents, including INH, theophylline, and chloroquine	Increased tone
	Decouplers of oxidative phosphorylation	Conversion of energy to heat

acting anticholinergic agents such as scopolamine can similarly impair cooling and may cause psychomotor agitation. These patients will present with altered mental status, tachycardia, dry skin, pupillary dilation, and urinary retention (anticholinergic toxidrome).[6]

Diagnostic Evaluation

The diagnosis of agitated delirium requires two factors: psychomotor agitation and a reduced ability to focus or shift attention.[4] In addition to toxicologic etiologies, other causes of agitated delirium that should always be considered include infection, postictal states, and endocrinological emergencies. Laboratory assessments should include a basic metabolic panel and urinalysis; blood cultures if etiology of delirium is uncertain; and creatinine kinase to rule out the potential complication of rhabdomyolysis. In addition, liver function tests, a coagulation panel (PT/PTT/INR), and complete blood count should be used to screen for evidence of DIC due to hyperthermic liver injury as well as nonspecific tissue damage, which can lead to consumption of coagulation factors.[7] Arterial/venous blood gas and serum lactate tests should be used to identify acidosis, which commonly accompanies heat stroke. If an intentional self-poisoning is suspected, serum salicylate and acetaminophen concentrations should be obtained.

Management Guidelines

Prompt sedation with benzodiazepines facilitates measurement of body temperature, hemodynamic stabilization, and the rapid cooling that is critical to patient survival. If intravenous access is unavailable, a rapidly sedating benzodiazepine such as midazolam may be administered intramuscularly (10 mg in a 70 kg adult). Lorazepam may also be administered intramuscularly, but its time to peak sedation is typically >15 minutes. In the hyperthermic patient with status epilepticus, however, lorazepam offers equivalent onset for seizure termination with a longer duration of action.

If intravenous access is available, then an adult patient may be administered diazepam in 10 mg aliquots intravenously every 5 minutes until adequate sedation is achieved, which allows for cooling and reduces psychomotor tone. Patients receiving repetitive doses of any intravenous or intramuscular benzodiazepine require close respiratory monitoring. Intramuscular ketamine has been reported for the patient presenting with an agitated delirium, but the data are limited.

Ideally, the hyperthermic patient is cooled using ice water immersion or cold, wet sheets with ice packed across the entire body, with continual fanning. Continuous core temperature monitoring using a rectal probe is preferable. Occasionally, interventions such as intubation and neuromuscular paralysis are required to reduce heat production. Patients can be removed from ice/ice water when the core temperature is 101.3°F (38.5°C) to avoid overshooting normothermia and provoking hypothermia.[8] Cooling is ideally achieved within 15 minutes of presentation to reduce total hyperthermic time.

Invasive cooling methods—including ice water irrigation of the bladder and thoracic and peritoneal cavities—should be avoided, due to their inadequate rate of cooling in patients with hyperthermic emergencies. Similarly, cooling blankets, while low risk, are also inadequate and should also be avoided. Restoration of a patient's intravascular volume may be necessary, with serial evaluations for urine output, assessment of inferior vena cava (IVC) collapse, and lung examinations.[9]

Monitoring

Once cooled, patients should be admitted to an intensive care unit and have serial reassessment of basic laboratory tests. Renal dysfunction and coagulopathy are commonly seen within 24 hours of heat stroke onset and may worsen depending on the duration of hyperthermia; acute renal failure is seen in 30% to 50% of heat stroke patients.[10] Liver function tests may also initially appear normal but worsen as organ dysfunction evolves.

TOXICOLOGIC HYPERTHERMIC SYNDROMES

Serotonin Toxicity

Serotonin toxicity results from excessive stimulation of 5-HT_{1A} and 5-HT_{2A} receptors. It can develop in patients after a large overdose of a single serotonergic agent; in patients taking more than one serotonergic agent; or in individuals who initiate a new serotonergic agent without adequately timed discontinuation of another serotonergic agent[11–15] (Table 47.2).

History and Physical Exam

Serotonin toxicity is often described as a clinical triad of altered mental status, autonomic instability, and muscular hyperactivity.[16] Tremor, shivering, hyperreflexia, and clonus—prominent in the lower extremities and often described as the "dog shakes"—are classic manifestations of this syndrome. Clonus can also be seen in the ocular muscles as a "ping-pong gaze" in which the eyes make horizontal movements. In severe cases, muscle rigidity may lead to hyperthermia, which, when coupled with altered mental status, results in a toxicologic heat stroke.

Life-threatening serotonin toxicity is most often seen in the patient taking a monoamine oxidase inhibitor (MAOI) followed by the ingestion of or iatrogenic administration of a serotonergic drug.[17–19] MAOIs inhibit the presynaptic intracellular breakdown of serotonin, enhancing the amount of serotonin released into the synapse. The subsequent administration of another serotonergic agent can cause excessive receptor stimulation. The onset of life-threatening serotonin syndrome is usually rapid, often within minutes to <2 hours of drug administration.

TABLE 47.2 Substances That Can Contribute to Serotonin Toxicity

Inhibition of serotonin breakdown	MAOI Linezolid Methylene blue
Blockade of serotonin reuptake	SSRI Bupropion Dextromethorphan Cocaine Opioids: fentanyl, meperidine, pentazocine
Serotonin precursors	L-Tryptophan Lysergic acid diethylamide
Serotonin release enhancers	Amphetamine, especially MDMA Buspirone Lithium Mirtazapine

From Vasallo S, Delaney KA. Thermoregulatory principles. In: Nelson LS, Lewin NA, Howland MA, et al., eds. *Goldfrank's Toxicologic Emergencies.* 9th ed. New York: McGraw-Hill Medical Pub.; 2010:228–248.

Diagnostic Evaluation

Serotonin toxicity is a diagnostic challenge; it lacks a specific biomarker, and patients may present within a spectrum of potential signs and symptoms. A milder serotonin toxicity without hyperthermia or autonomic instability may also be difficult to recognize.[16] Such patients can exhibit hyperactivity of the extremities and delirium. Other minor manifestations of serotonin excess—such as diarrhea, hypertension, insomnia, or restlessness—may be present, but mistakenly be attributed to the patient's underlying psychiatric or medical condition.

Unless the patient's presentation follows shortly after an interaction of medications known to precipitate the toxicity, the diagnosis is generally one of exclusion in the differential of hyperthermia. There is no universally accepted diagnostic test; however, the Hunter Serotonin Toxicity Criteria were demonstrated to have a sensitivity and specificity for detecting serotonin toxicity of 84% and 97% respectively. For the screen to be positive, the patient must have taken a serotonergic agent and have any of the five listed symptoms.[20] (Table 47.3). In patients meeting these criteria, the emergency physician should suspect serotonin toxicity and evaluate for complications of hyperthermia, including rhabdomyolysis, renal failure, seizure, DIC, and abnormalities of liver function.[8]

Management Guidelines

When serotonin toxicity presents with severe hyperthermia, cooling should be started as soon as possible, and the offending serotonergic drug should be discontinued.

TABLE 47.3 Hunter Serotonin Syndrome Criteria

Patient must have taken a serotonergic agent and have one of the following:

- Spontaneous clonus
- Inducible clonus and agitation or diaphoresis
- Ocular clonus and agitation or diaphoresis
- Tremor and hyperreflexia
- Increased tone and temperature >38°C and ocular clonus or inducible clonus

Benzodiazepines will relieve most mild to moderate symptoms, including agitation and clonus; in patients with refractory muscle rigidity and hyperthermia, a neuromuscular blockade may be considered for muscle relaxation.[1]

Milder manifestations of serotonin toxicity are generally treated with supportive care and withdrawal or reduction of the responsible serotonergic agent. Evidence supports the use of cyproheptadine—an antihistamine with nonspecific antagonist effects at 5-HT_{1A} and 5-HT_{2A} receptors—for the targeted treatment of the serotonergic excess in patients with mild to moderate symptoms that are insufficiently controlled by sedation. The recommended initial dose is 12 mg followed by 2 mg every 2 hours with a maximum of 32 mg/day until symptoms resolve. A maintenance dose of 8 mg of cyproheptadine every 6 hours can be considered if mild symptoms persist. In case reports, patients responded to 4 mg of cyproheptadine within 2 hours with some requiring one repeat dose.[21,22] There are, however, no definitive data regarding cyproheptadine's utility in severe cases due to the rarity of events and difficulty in randomization.

Neuroleptic Malignant Syndrome

Neuroleptic malignant syndrome (NMS) is a rare but potentially fatal disorder caused by blockade of dopaminergic receptors in the striatum and hypothalamus—such as in patients taking therapeutic antipsychotics—or by withdrawal of therapeutic dopaminergic agents. Reduction of dopamine levels in the hypothalamus changes the core temperature set point, leading to hyperthermia, while blockade of striatal dopamine receptors contributes to muscle rigidity and tremor.[23] Approximately 0.2% to 1.4 % of all patients receiving antipsychotics will develop NMS.[24,25]

History and Physical Exam

Most cases of NMS occur in patients taking therapeutic antipsychotics. The condition is triggered by rapidly escalating dosage, use of high-potency agents such as haloperidol, parenteral administration, and use of depot preparations (intramuscular injections with slow release).[23,24] Atypical antipsychotics may also cause NMS, but less commonly than typical antipsychotics.[26] NMS risk is greatest during the first weeks to months of therapy but can occur anytime during use of neuroleptics. NMS may also be precipitated by cessation of dopamine agonists in patients being treated for Parkinson's, but this is less common.

The four main clinical findings of NMS are: changes in mental status (typically gradual-onset catatonia); increased muscle tone, described as "lead pipe rigidity" and "cogwheeling"; hyperthermia; and autonomic dysfunction presenting as tachycardia with alternating hypotension and hypertension. One study reviewing 340 patients with NMS showed 70.5% of patients developed symptoms in the following order: (1) mental status changes, (2) rigidity, (3) hyperthermia, and (4) autonomic dysfunction. In addition, 83.6% of individual patients demonstrated either altered mental status or rigidity before the onset of hyperthermia or autonomic instability.[24,27,28] NMS is also frequently preceded by the onset of bradykinesis.

Diagnostic Evaluation

In vulnerable patients, NMS can be life threatening; clinicians should maintain a high index of suspicion for hyperthermia when presented with a catatonic, rigid patient, particularly one exposed to elevated ambient temperatures. Like serotonin toxicity, NMS has no diagnostic biomarker. Multiple diagnostic criteria, including the Levenson and Caroff criteria,[27] have been proposed, but none is universally accepted. The most frequently referenced criteria are found in the *Diagnostic and Statistical Manual of Mental Disorders*, 4th ed., which requires the development of severe muscle rigidity and elevated temperature associated with the use of antipsychotic medication, as well as two or more of the following: diaphoresis, elevated blood pressure, tachycardia, incontinence, dysphagia, mutism, tremor, changes in the level of consciousness (ranging from confusion to coma), leukocytosis, and laboratory evidence of muscle injury (elevated creatinine kinase).[29]

Differentiating Serotonin Toxicity from Neuroleptic Malignant Syndrome

Differentiating between NMS and serotonin syndrome can be difficult, since the two syndromes share many clinical features. The following clinical findings can help distinguish them (Table 47.4).

Serotonin toxicity has a rapid onset, within minutes to hours; NMS, by comparison, evolves over days or weeks. Serotonin toxicity carries the additional features of tremors and myoclonus, while NMS is further characterized by bradykinesia, mutism, and gradual-onset catatonia. Finally, in most cases of serotonin syndrome, symptoms resolve within 24 to 72 hours after removal of the offending agent, while in NMS, symptoms may continue for weeks.

Management Guidelines

Patients with NMS who present with life-threatening hyperthermia—that is, heat stroke, or $T > 41.1$°C or 106°F—should be treated aggressively, as outlined in the management section of agitated delirium.[8,30,31] If the syndrome was caused by discontinuation of a dopamine agonist, as with abrupt cessation of Parkinson's medications, the dopaminergic agent should be resumed as soon as possible.

Benzodiazepines are the first-line pharmacologic therapy used to provide sedation and muscle relaxation. Bromocriptine and, rarely, dantrolene may also be used.

TABLE 47.4 Differentiation of Serotonin Toxicity from NMS

	Serotonin Toxicity	NMS
Pathophysiology	Excess stimulation of $5HT_{1A}$ and $5HT_{2A}$ receptors	Dopamine receptor blockade
Time of onset	Minutes to hours	Days to weeks
Resolution of symptoms	24–96 h	Days to weeks
Symptoms	Altered mental status Hyperthermia Autonomic instability Muscle rigidity Tremors ("wet dog shakes"), myoclonus, ocular clonus	Altered mental status Hyperthermia Autonomic instability Muscle rigidity Bradykinesia, mutism, catatonia, severe muscle rigidity ("lead pipe rigidity and cogwheeling")

From Vasallo S, Delaney KA. Thermoregulatory principles. In: Nelson LS, Lewin NA, Howland MA, et al., eds. *Goldfrank's Toxicologic Emergencies*. 9th ed. New York: McGraw-Hill Medical Pub.; 2010:228–248.

Bromocriptine is a central dopamine agonist that can be administered if supportive therapy with benzodiazepines and rapid cooling fail to improve the patient's symptoms. Bromocriptine, however, may lead to a worsening of a patient's underlying psychiatric illness due to dopamine agonism. This effect can be temporized by use of the same benzodiazepines used for muscle relaxation, until the NMS has resolved. Bromocriptine is only available in oral form, and the dose is 2.5 to 10 mg orally three to four times a day. The dosage can be increased with increments of 2.5 mg three times a day every 24 hours until a response is seen or up to a maximum 60 mg per day.[23]

Generally, supportive care, benzodiazepines, and bromocriptine are sufficient to manage muscle rigidity and autonomic dysfunction from NMS; however, patients with severe rigidity unresponsive to benzodiazepines or bromocriptine may require intubation followed by neuromuscular paralysis. Since the clearance of antipsychotics is slow, pharmacological dopaminergic therapies should be continued for at least 10 days after a return to baseline. Premature discontinuation of dopamine agonists may lead to recurrence of NMS. When NMS is related to depot neuroleptics, bromocriptine should be continued for 2 to 3 weeks.[23] Full recovery may take weeks to return to baseline.

Some authors describe the use of dantrolene for treatment of NMS, although data supporting its use are limited, and it is rarely indicated. Dantrolene is more typically used to treat malignant hyperthermia (MH) by inhibiting calcium release from the sarcoplasmic reticulum (see more on "Malignant Hypothermia," below).

Electroconvulsive therapy (ECT) has been suggested as treatment for NMS. ECT is thought to exert its therapeutic effect by enhancing central dopamine activity,[32] and reports have shown that three to four sessions of ECT resolve symptoms of NMS with a mean time from initiation of treatment to resolution of symptoms of 6 days.[33] However, data for ECT are limited, and patients with hyperthermia and organ dysfunction are not candidates for this therapy.

Malignant Hyperthermia

MH is a rare autosomal dominant disorder typically seen in patients who receive inhalational anesthetics or succinylcholine. The incidence of MH in patients exposed to general anesthesia has been reported to be anywhere from 1 in 5,000 to 1 in 62,000.[34,35] In normal muscle, contraction occurs as action potentials open voltage-gated calcium channels, which in turn activate ryanodine receptors (RYR-1) that release calcium for myocyte contraction. The released calcium is recycled by sarcoplasmic Ca^{2+}-ATPase. In MH, this cycling of calcium in the muscle cells becomes disordered.

MH is a form of drug-induced hypermetabolism of skeletal muscle. Patients who are predisposed to MH have mutations of the RYR-1. In susceptible persons, inhalational anesthetic agents and succinylcholine enhance the activity of the defective RYR-1, leading to accelerated release of Ca^{2+} inside the skeletal muscle. Intracellular ATP becomes depleted as the sarcoplasmic Ca^{2+}-ATPase attempts to transport Ca^{2+} back into the sarcoplasmic reticulum of the muscle cells. The result is diffuse, sustained contraction of skeletal muscles, rigidity unresponsive to nondepolarizing neuromuscular blockade, and hyperthermia. This process also leads to anaerobic metabolism with resultant lactic acidosis and an increase in CO_2 production.

History and Physical Exam

Typically, MH symptoms manifest shortly after exposure to an inhalational anesthetic or succinylcholine; however, a delayed onset of up to 7 to 8 hours has been reported.[36] Even among susceptible patients, MH does not always occur with anesthetic drug exposure, so a negative history cannot safely rule out the development of MH with subsequent exposures.[37] The earliest signs of MH are tachycardia, an increase in end-tidal CO_2 concentration, and generalized skeletal muscle rigidity and masseter spasm. Hyperthermia, which is the hallmark of MH, may not be seen until later in the process.

Diagnostic Evaluation

There are no readily available diagnostic tests for MH: diagnosis is suspected when administration of neuromuscular blockers fails to result in paralysis. The gold standard for diagnosing MH is an in vitro contracture test (IVCT). This tests the contracture of muscle fibers in the presence of halothane or caffeine and monitors for abnormal muscle contractility.[35]

The toxicologic differential diagnosis of MH is addressed in Table 47.1. The distinguishing features of MH are exposure to an implicated agent and failure to respond to neuromuscular blockade. Unlike in serotonin syndrome, rigidity in MH is not attended by muscle hyperactivity.

Management Guidelines

When hyperthermia does occur, temperatures will increase by 1°C to 2°C every 5 minutes, and that core temperatures should be continuously monitored.[35] Similar to the treatment of hyperthermic agitated delirium and serotonin toxicity, it is crucial to stop administration of the offending agent. If hyperthermia is present or evolving, cooling should be initiated, as previously outlined.

Dantrolene can be lifesaving and is the definitive therapy for MH. Dantrolene blocks Ca^{2+} release from the skeletal muscle sarcoplasmic reticulum. After the introduction of dantrolene as a therapy, the mortality from MH decreased from 64% to <5%.[38] The starting dose is 2.5 mg/kg IV bolus followed by 2 to 3 mg/kg IV every 15 minutes until resolution of symptoms or to a cumulative dose of 10 mg/kg. To prevent recrudescence, administration of 1 mg/kg IV every 4 to 6 hours for a minimum of 24 to 48 hours is recommended.[35]

Other Drug-Related Hyperthermic Syndromes

Life-threatening hyperthermia may also be triggered when patients generate heat disproportionately to their cooling capacity. Drugs that cause status epilepticus, including isoniazid (INH) theophylline, and chloroquine, can cause excessive heat generation. Termination of convulsions, restoration of adequate ventilation, and rapid cooling are critical interventions. Most toxicologically caused seizures will not respond to traditional anticonvulsant agents such as phenytoin. Benzodiazepines or other sedative hypnotic agents are most efficacious. INH overdose with resultant status epilepticus may require pyridoxine therapy for adequate neurologic inhibition.

Agents that uncouple oxidative phosphorylation, such as salicylates or dinitrophenol (an illegal weight loss agent), may also cause life-threatening hyperthermia. Acidosis evolves as the potential energy unable to be transformed into ATP is dissipated as heat. In each of these cases, the primary intervention is rapid identification of hyperthermia, rapid cooling, and minimization of psychomotor agitation with benzodiazepines, supportive care, and, in extreme cases, intubation with a neuromuscular paralytic agent.

CONCLUSION

Hyperthermic agitated delirium, serotonin syndrome, NMS, and MH share many physical findings. Distinguishing between these syndromes can be difficult and depends on a clear understanding of the patient's pharmacologic history. Essential components of treatment include rapid cooling of life-threatening hyperthermia and supportive care with benzodiazepines. Secondary complications of toxicologic hyperthermic syndromes, which include rhabdomyolysis, acute kidney injury, hyperkalemia, liver injury, and DIC, should be identified and aggressively treated in an intensive care unit.

LITERATURE TABLE

TRIAL	DESIGN	RESULT
Dunkley et al., *QJM.* 2003[20]	Newly created decision rules (Hunter criteria) were applied to prospectively collected dataset and compared with diagnosis by toxicolgist.	Hunter criteria were more sensitive and specific (84% and 97% respectively) than Sternbach criteria (69% and 97%, respectively)
Velamoor et al., *J Nerv Ment Dis.* 1994[28]	Review of 340 case reports to determine the order of symptoms of NMS	70.5% were consistent with sequence of 1) mental status changes, 2) rigidity, 3) hyperthermia, and 4) autonomic dysfunction
Morrison and Serpel, *Eur J Anaesthesiol.* 1998[36]	Reported a case of a 36-y-old man who developed signs of MH as late as 8 h after the initiation of surgery	Emphasizes on the importance of early consideration of diagnosis of MH when increase in end-expiratory CO_2 and tachycardia are observed. Hyperthermia is a late manifestation

REFERENCES

1. Vasallo S, Delaney KA. Thermoregulatory principles. In: Nelson LS, Lewin NA, Howland MA, et al., eds. *Goldfrank's Toxicologic Emergencies.* 9th ed. New York: McGraw-Hill Medical Pub.; 2010:228–248.
2. Anonymous. Heat-related deaths—United States, 1999–2003. *MMWR Morb Mort Wkly.* 2006;55:796–798.
3. Marzuk PM, Tardiff K, Leon AC, et al. Ambient temperature and mortality from unintentional cocaine overdose. *JAMA.* 1998;279:1795–1800.
4. Vilke GM, DeBard ML, Chan TC, et al. Excited elirium Syndrome (ExDS): defining based on a review of the literature. *J Emerg Med.* 2012:897–905.
5. Marzuk PM, Tardiff K, Leon AC, et al. Ambient temperature and mortality from unintentional cocaine overdose. *JAMA.* 1998;279(22):1795–1800.
6. Anonymous. Scopolamine poisoning among heroin users—New York City, Newark, Philadelphia, and Baltimore, 1995 and 1996. *MMWR Morb Mortal Wkly.* 1996;45:457–460.
7. Khatim Y, Mustafa O, Omer M, et al. Blood coagulation and fibrinolysis in heat stroke. *Br J Hematol.* 1985;61:517–523.
8. Proulx CI, Ducharme MB, Kenny GP. Effect of water temperature on cooling efficiency during hyperthermia in humans. *J Appl Physiol.* 2003;94(4):1317–1323.

9. Seraj MA, Channa AB, al Harthi SS, et al. Are heat stroke patients fluid depleted? Importance of monitoring central venous pressure as a simple guideline for fluid therapy. *Resuscitation.* 1991;21:33–39.
10. Yeo TP. Heat stroke: a comprehensive review. *AACN Clin Issues.* 2004;15(2);280–293.
11. Ruiz F. Fluoxetine and the serotonin syndrome. *Ann Emerg Med.* 1994;24(5):983–985.
12. Safferman AZ, Masiar SJ. Central nervous system toxicity after abrupt monoamine oxidase inhibitor switch: a case report. *Ann Pharmacother.* 1992;26(3):337–338.
13. Daniels RJ. Serotonin syndrome due to venlafaxine overdose. *J Accid Emerg Med.* 1998;15(5):333–334.
14. Gill M, LoVecchio F, Selden B. Serotonin syndrome in a child after a single dose of fluvoxamine. *Ann Emerg Med.* 1999;33(4):457–459.
15. Paruchuri P, Godkar D, Anandacoomarswamy D, et al. Rare case of serotonin syndrome with therapeutic doses of paroxetine. *Am J Ther.* 2006;13(6):550–552.
16. Sampson E, Warner JP. Serotonin syndrome: potentially fatal but difficult to recognize. *Br J Gen Pract.* 1999;49(448):867–868.
17. Smilkstein MJ, Smolinske SC, Rumack BH. A case of MAO inhibitor/MDMA interaction: agony after ecstasy. *J Toxicol Clin Toxicol.* 1987;25:1–2.
18. Smith B, Prockop DJ. Central-nervous-system effects of ingestion of l-tryptophan by normal subjects. *N Engl J Med.* 1962;267:1338–1341.
19. Oates JA, Sjoerdsma A. Neurologic effects of tryptophan in patients receiving a monoamine oxidase inhibitor. *Neurology.* 1960;10:1076–1078.
20. Dunkley EJ, Isbister GK, Sibbritt D, et al. The Hunter Serotonin Toxicity Criteria: simple and accurate diagnostic decision rules for serotonin toxicity. *QJM.* 2003;96(9):635–642.
21. Graudins A, Stearman A, Chan B. Treatment of the serotonin syndrome with cyproheptadine. *J Emerg Med.* 1998;16(4):615–619.
22. Lappin RI, Auchincloss EL. Treatment of the serotonin syndrome with cyproheptadine. *N Engl J Med.* 1994;331(15):1021–1022.
23. Bhanushali MJ, Tuite PJ. The evaluation and management of patients with neuroleptic malignant syndrome. *Neurol Clin.* 2004;22(2):389–411.
24. Addonizio G, Susman VL, Roth SD. Neuroleptic malignant syndrome: review and analysis of 115 cases. *Biol Psychiatry.* 1987;22(8):1004–1020.
25. Delay J, Pichot P, Lemperiere T, et al. A non-phenothiazine and non-reserpine major neuroleptic, haloperidol, in the treatment of psychoses. *Ann Med Psychol (Paris).* 1960;118(1):145–152.
26. Kontaxakis VP, Havaki-Kontaxaki BJ, Christodoulou NG, et al. Olanzapine-associated neuroleptic malignant syndrome. *Prog Neuropsychopharmacol Biol Psychiatry.* 2002;26(5):897–902.
27. Caroff SN, Mann SC. Neuroleptic malignant syndrome and malignant hyperthermia. *Med Clin North Am.* 1993;21(4):477–478.
28. Velamoor VR, Norman RM, Caroff SN, et al. Progression of symptoms in neuroleptic malignant syndrome. *J Nerv Ment Dis.* 1994;182(3):168–173.
29. American Psychiatric Association. *Diagnostic and Statistical Manual of Mental Disorders.* 4th ed. Washington, DC; 2000.
30. Armstrong LE, Crago AE, Adams R, et al. Whole-body cooling of hyperthermic runners: comparison of two field therapies. *Am J Emerg Med.* 1996;14(4):355–358.
31. Weiner JS, Khogali M. A physiological body-cooling unit for treatment of heat stroke. *Lancet.* 1980;1(8167):507–509.
32. Hermesh H, Aizenberg D, Weizman A. A successful electroconvulsive treatment of neuroleptic malignant syndrome. *Acta Psychiatr Scand.* 1987;75(3):237–239.
33. Nisijima K, Ishiguro T. Electroconvulsive therapy for the treatment of neuroleptic malignant syndrome with psychotic symptoms: a report of five cases. *J ECT.* 1999;15(2):158–163.
34. Ording H. Incidence of malignant hyperthermia in Denmark. *Anesth Analg.* 1985;64(7):700–704.
35. Rosenberg H, Davis M, James D, et al. Malignant hyperthermia. *Orphanet J Rare Dis.* 2007;2:21.
36. Morrison AG, Serpell MG. Malignant hyperthermia during prolonged surgery for tumour resection. *Eur J Anaesthesiol.* 1998;15(1):114–117.
37. Bendixen D, Skovgaard LT, Ording H, et al. Analysis of anaesthesia in patients suspected to be susceptible to malignant hyperthermia before diagnostic in vitro contracture test. *Acta Anaesthesiol Scand.* 1997;41(4):480–484.
38. Larach MG, Brandom BW, Allen GC, et al. Cardiac arrests and deaths associated with malignant hyperthermia in North America from 1987 to 2006. *Anesthesiology.* 2008;108(4):603–611.

48

Metabolic Inhibitors

Lauren K. Shawn and Lewis S. Nelson

BACKGROUND

The complicated metabolic pathways of the human body present multiple opportunities for poisoning. Toxins can inhibit essential pathways in many ways, such as by blocking enzymes or overwhelming a normal pathway with toxic metabolites. Although there are many known toxins that affect various metabolic pathways, this chapter focuses on those that affect the mitochondria and cause metabolic acidosis, namely, aspirin, cyanide, methanol, and metformin.

ASPIRIN

Aspirin is a common over-the-counter medication used as a cardioprotective agent as well as a pain and fever reducer. Although it is used therapeutically to inhibit platelets and prostaglandins, in overdose, it has neurotoxic effects.

Pathophysiology

Aspirin is a weak acid with a pK_a of 3.5, which means that in a solution with a pH of 3.5, 50% of the aspirin is in an ionized form. When the pH is lower than the pK_a, more of the aspirin is in the nonionized form, which can move more freely through the lipid bilayer of cellular and subcellular membranes. The implication is that at the physiologic pH of tissues and blood, most aspirin is ionized and does not move easily between compartments. However, even at a pH of 7.4, a small amount of aspirin is nonionized (0.004%) and can travel into the brain, and this percentage increases with acidemia.[1] In experimental models, lowering the blood pH produces a shift of salicylate into the tissues, especially the brain[2]; increasing the blood pH with sodium bicarbonate produces a shift in salicylate out of the tissues and into the blood.[2–4] This is a key concept used to manage patients with aspirin toxicity.

In the mitochondria, ionized aspirin binds the hydrogen ions trapped in the intermembrane space and then exits the mitochondria in the nonionized form, preventing the proton motive force from fueling ATP formation (by uncoupling oxidative phosphorylation). Heat, but not energy, is therefore generated, and a low-grade temperature can be seen in patients with significant aspirin toxicity. The brain depends on ATP to pump water out of neurons, and in the absence of ATP, loss of oxidative phosphorylation leads to cerebral edema.

History and Physical Exam

Therapeutic salicylate serum concentrations typically range from 15 to 30 mg/dL. At a serum concentration of approximately 35 mg/dL, aspirin stimulates the brainstem's respiratory center, causing hyperventilation that produces respiratory alkalosis. Some of the earliest signs of aspirin intoxication are tachypnea and hyperpnea; the physical exam of a suspected aspirin toxic patient should include careful attention to the rate and depth of breathing. As a weak acid, aspirin itself causes an anion gap metabolic acidosis at supratherapeutic concentrations. In addition, because of aspirin's ability to impair aerobic metabolism and increase fatty acid metabolism, other organic acids and ketoacids accumulate. The classic blood gas in patients with aspirin toxicity, or salicylism shows a mixed process of respiratory alkalosis with a metabolic acidosis (as opposed to a respiratory compensation for a metabolic acidosis). This acid–base pattern may not be as evident in pediatric exposures, because of their limited ventilatory reserve. Adults who show a "normalization" of their serum pH due to a decreasing respiratory alkalosis are extremely concerning, as this is a sign that respiratory fatigue or lung injury is preventing proper ventilation. Patients with acidemia late in the course of salicylate toxicity are at high risk of permanent neurologic damage and death, as the lowered pH will allow more aspirin to enter the brain.

Tinnitus or the sensation of hearing loss can occur early in toxicity. In the era before immune-modulating drugs, patients with rheumatologic disease were often instructed to titrate their aspirin doses to just below the amount that induced tinnitus.

The most concerning and consequential sign of toxicity is alteration in mental status. This is a sign of cerebral edema and an indication for more aggressive management such as dialysis. Seizures are often a preterminal event. Neuroglycopenia may occur and cause mental status abnormalities even when the serum glucose is within normal limits. The glucose concentration in the cerebral spinal fluid is depleted as salicylate-poisoned neurons utilize more glucose to compensate for the loss of ATP due to uncoupling of oxidative phosphorylation.[5]

The signs and symptoms of chronic salicylism may be more difficult to appreciate, which can delay detection. Furthermore, chronic salicylism is often found in elderly patients, in whom altered mental status, tachypnea, tachycardia, and mild anion gap acidosis may be misinterpreted as resulting from infection, malnourishment, cardiopulmonary disease, or dementia. In one study of 73 consecutive adults hospitalized with salicylate poisoning, 27% were not correctly diagnosed for as long as 72 hours after admission, and the mortality rate associated with this delayed diagnosis was 25%. Many of these patients had neurology consults for altered mental status prior to correct diagnosis.[6]

Aspirin toxicity can increase pulmonary capillary permeability, leading to acute respiratory distress syndrome (ARDS). This pulmonary toxicity can impair ventilation, reducing the respiratory alkalosis and worsening the clinical effects of salicylate toxicity. It can also limit the ability to use sodium bicarbonate infusion as a therapy, since patients with ARDS may not be able to tolerate the fluid load.

Management Guidelines

Initial Resuscitation

Salicylate-poisoned patients can decompensate rapidly if not carefully managed. The hyperpnea, tachypnea, and diaphoresis associated with aspirin toxicity cause a large amount of insensible losses, so fluid status should be monitored and repletion with normal saline should be initiated on arrival. Every patient with suspected salicylate poisoning requires testing of serum salicylate concentration, and repeat levels are needed if the initial concentration is elevated. The frequency of retesting should be based on clinical findings and trends in serum concentration. Additional laboratory testing should include a blood gas (arterial or venous) to monitor pH and pCO_2, serum potassium, serum acetaminophen concentration (in patients with toxicity thought to be due to self-harm), and urine pH every 1 to 2 hours (see Alkalinization below). Given the acid/base physiology of aspirin, a "normal" pH and pCO_2 are not reassuring.

GI Decontamination

Activated charcoal should be administered unless there is a concern for aspiration in a vomiting or altered patient. Whole bowel irrigation should be avoided as it may solubilize an aspirin bezoar and facilitate absorption. If there is concern for a bezoar or the serum salicylate level has plateaued despite alkalinization, multiple doses of activated charcoal may be indicated.

Alkalinization

There is no specific antidote for salicylism, but alkalinization is a mainstay of treatment. Alkalinization of the serum promotes trapping of the ionized salicylate outside the brain. Furthermore, alkaline urine promotes elimination of salicylate; and this effect increases logarithmically as the pH of urine increases from five to eight.[7] There is no specific uptake mechanism in the kidney for salicylate, and passive reabsorption of charged molecules is very limited. Under therapeutic conditions, approximately 10% of salicylates are excreted in the urine as salicylic acid, while the majority of the salicylate is metabolized into a conjugated form in the liver prior to renal elimination. In overdose, the enzymes involved in hepatic metabolism become saturated, and the amount of urinary unconjugated salicylic acid increases. Urine alkalinization does not affect elimination of conjugated salicylate, so serum clearance is less affected. To alkalinize the serum and the urine, sodium bicarbonate is typically dosed as a 1 to 2 mEq/kg bolus, followed by 150 mEq mixed in D5 water at twice maintenance. Titrate with goal of serum pH around 7.5 to 7.55 and urine pH around 8.

Electrolyte Management

Alkalinization will cause potassium to shift intracellularly in order to release hydrogen ions into the serum. The kidneys sense this relative hypokalemia and will begin to reabsorb potassium in exchange for hydrogen ions, preventing proper urine alkalinization despite the sodium bicarbonate infusion. Serum potassium should be repleted to normal levels in order to suppress this physiologic response and maintain urinary alkalinization.

Airway Management

Although many patients with altered mental status are intubated for airway protection, in the case of salicylism, inadequate matching of hyperventilation and subsequent CO_2 retention can be catastrophic because the resulting acidemia will shift more salicylate into the brain.[8] Sedation should be avoided unless the patient is carefully monitored or receiving ventilatory support. In patients receiving mechanical ventilation, every effort should be made to prevent a falling pH and rising PCO_2, which may be done by matching the ventilator settings with the patient's pre-intubation minute ventilation. An experienced operator should perform the intubation, and sodium bicarbonate, 1 to 2 mEq/kg bolus, should be given just prior to intubation to ensure alkalemia during rapid sequence intubation. Patients will require large tidal volumes and a high respiratory rate with the goal of a minute ventilation of 20 to 30 L/min. Despite these steps, patients still may be unable to maintain an appropriate serum pH or may suffer ventilator-associated barotrauma, in which case hemodialysis is indicated.

Hemodialysis

Although some resources and textbooks cite a serum aspirin concentration >100 mg/dL as an absolute indication for dialysis, this does not mean that a patient may not need extracorporeal elimination at lower concentrations. Hemodialysis is indicated when there are signs of end-organ injury or when pulmonary edema and lung injury prevents further use of sodium bicarbonate. This is particularly true in the case of the patient with altered mental status, as serum concentrations may underestimate central nervous system (CNS) concentrations.

CYANIDE

Cyanide is a chemical asphyxiant. It is most commonly encountered clinically in patients who were victims of fires, especially involving the combustion of fabrics and plastics. However, cyanide should be on the differential of a sudden death in an otherwise healthy person because it is such a fast-acting, lethal, and potentially treatable toxin. Cyanide salts such as sodium cyanide and potassium cyanide are used in jewelry making, plastic manufacturing, photography, and other industries. They react with water to form hydrogen cyanide, a gas. Organic compounds containing cyanide also exist. Acetonitrile is methyl cyanide and is commonly found in acrylic nail glue remover and other similar cosmetics. When ingested, it is metabolized by the P450 system to hydrogen cyanide and formaldehyde, causing delayed toxicity.

Iatrogenic cyanide poisoning can occur when nitroprusside is used for the treatment of hypertension. Each nitroprusside molecule contains five cyanide molecules, which may be liberated. After rapid or prolonged infusion, or in malnourished patients, cyanide or its metabolite (thiocyanate) toxicity may occur.

Pathophysiology

Acute cyanide toxicity can occur via inhalational, oral, dermal, and parenteral routes. The dose of cyanide required to produce toxicity is dependent on the form of cyanide and the duration and route of exposure. Hydrogen cyanide gas at concentrations above 270 ppm can be immediately fatal, and ingestion of 200 mg of KCN salt can be fatal within minutes.[9] Cyanide is a very potent toxin and is on a short list of rapidly acting, fatal exposures.

Cyanide is eliminated from the body by multiple pathways. The major route is the enzymatic conversion to thiocyanate by rhodanese (thiosulfate–cyanide sulfurtransferase). This enzyme catalyzes the transfer of a sulfur group from a sulfur donor, such as thiosulfate, to cyanide to form thiocyanate. In acute poisoning, the ability of rhodanese to detoxify cyanide is limited by the endogenous amount of sulfur donor, which is rapidly depleted. Thiocyanate has relatively little inherent toxicity and is eliminated in the urine.

Cyanide inhibits many enzymes, but its most consequential effect is the inhibition of cytochrome oxidase in the mitochondria. Cytochrome oxidase is a key enzyme of the electron transport chain, and oxidative phosphorylation cannot occur without it. Cyanide acts at the cytochrome a3 portion of complex IV of the electron transport chain. As a result, hydrogen ions cannot combine with oxygen to form water, ATP cannot be generated, and oxygen utilization by the tissues is decreased. Cellular asphyxiation occurs despite normal blood oxygen tension, and the excess hydrogen ions cause acidemia. Lactate accumulates because the cessation of the electron transport chain prevents the conversion of nicotinamide adenine dinucleotide (NADH) back into NAD+ and H+, and this favors the conversion of pyruvate to lactate.

History and Physical Exam

Cyanide toxicity can cause rapid and severe neurologic dysfunction and hemodynamic instability. When organic cyanogenic compounds such as acetonitrile are ingested, however, symptoms may be delayed for hours because the parent compound must be metabolized to release cyanide. Cyanide toxicity from a nitroprusside infusion may take hours to days to become clinically apparent.

CNS signs and symptoms of cyanide toxicity are typical of those associated with progressive hypoxia and include headache, anxiety, agitation, confusion, lethargy, seizures, and coma. Centrally mediated tachypnea occurs initially and is followed by bradypnea. Cardiovascular signs can vary early in the clinical course, but bradycardia and hypotension are usually the preterminal findings.

Cyanide victims have classically been described as having cherry red skin coloration, due to increased oxygenation of the venous blood. Cyanide does not typically cause cyanosis despite the similar-sounding names. The word cyanide is derived from the Greek word for blue *kyanos*, due to its liberation from Prussian blue (ferric hexacyanoferrate) upon heating.

Clinicians should have high suspicion for cyanide poisoning in hemodynamically unstable or comatose fire victims, industrial or laboratory workers with sudden collapse, and suicidal patients with rapid collapse and metabolic acidosis following ingestion. Cyanide toxicity should also be considered a potential diagnosis in patients on nitroprusside infusions that develop altered mental status, metabolic acidosis, and abnormal vital signs.

Cyanide and Nitroprusside

Nitroprusside is a nitric oxide–releasing drug and is used as a vasodilator. The standard infusion rate is 3 mcg/kg/min (0.25 mcg/kg/min to 10 mcg/kg/min). The nitroprusside molecule contains five cyanide radicals that are slowly liberated and rapidly metabolized to thiocyanate. In healthy individuals, cyanide detoxification occurs at a rate of about 1 g/kg/min, which corresponds to a sodium nitroprusside infusion rate of 2 g/kg/min.[10] However, critical illness and malnutrition can deplete sulfur stores, so ICU patients are at increased risk for cyanide toxicity. An infusion of nitroprusside at a rate of more than 15 mcg/kg/min administered over a few hours or more than 4 mcg/kg/min for more than 12 hours may overwhelm the capacity of rhodanese for detoxifying cyanide.[11]

Sodium thiosulfate is sometimes coadministered with nitroprusside in order to prevent cyanide toxicity. Dosing of 1 g sodium thiosulfate for every 100 mg of nitroprusside is typically sufficient to prevent cyanide accumulation.[11] However, it is important to note that thiocyanate is renally eliminated and may accumulate in patients with impaired renal function, causing toxicity. The symptoms of thiocyanate toxicity are nonspecific and may include nausea, vomiting, fatigue, dizziness, confusion, delirium, and seizures. Extremely elevated thiocyanate concentrations (>200 g/mL) may produce life-threatening effects, such as hypertension and intracranial pressure elevation. Anion gap metabolic acidosis does not occur with thiocyanate toxicity. Hemodialysis clears thiocyanate from the serum and should be strongly considered in patients with severe clinical manifestations of thiocyanate toxicity.

Laboratory Tests

Laboratory testing for cyanide is not readily available in most clinical settings. In general, the patient's history and physical exam and other ancillary testing will guide management. Expected laboratory findings include an anion gap metabolic acidosis, an elevated lactate concentration, and an elevated venous oxygen saturation.[12] However, none of these findings are specific for cyanide. Other metabolic inhibitors such as carbon monoxide, hydrogen sulfide, and sodium azide, as well as medical conditions such as sepsis, high-output cardiac syndromes, and left-to-right intracardiac shunts, can reduce oxygen extraction. Simultaneous arterial and venous blood gases may show a reduced difference in arterial and venous oxygenation saturation (<10 mm Hg).[13]

A significant association exists between blood cyanide and serum lactate concentrations. In a small group of patients with a strongly suggestive history of cyanide ingestion, a serum lactate concentration above 8 mmol/L was associated with sensitivity of 94%, specificity of 70%, positive predictive value of 64%, and negative predictive value of 98% for a blood cyanide concentration above 1.0 g/mL, which is a toxic concentration.[14] In a case–control study of fire victims, a lactate over 10 mmol/L was a sensitive indicator of cyanide intoxication.[15]

Management Guidelines

Initial Resuscitation

Since cyanide can be so rapidly fatal, there is a limited window to initiate resuscitation. In most cases, empiric administration of antidotes will be required, based on history and clinical appearance. Resuscitation with a focus on airway, breathing, and circulation is the mainstay of treatment, but timely administration of the antidotes is paramount. Patients should be given 100% oxygen. Patients with altered mental status or fire victims with signs of oropharyngeal burns may require intubation in order to protect the airway. Vasopressors may be required to treat persistent hypotension despite adequate intravenous volume resuscitation.

GI Decontamination

Although some in vitro studies suggest that cyanide does not have significant adsorption to activated charcoal, it remains reasonable to administer charcoal to a patient with a protected airway in the setting of potentially toxic ingestion.

Medical Therapy

Either hydroxycobalamin or a cyanide antidote kit should be administered as soon as cyanide poisoning is suspected. Hydroxycobalamin, a vitamin B_{12} precursor, directly binds cyanide (1:1) to form cyanocobalamin (vitamin B_{12}). Hydroxycobalamin has few adverse effects, including a reddish discoloration of the skin, mucous membranes, and urine that can last a few days.[16] Colorimetric laboratory testing can be affected by the red color, and common lab tests, such as serum lactate, may yield inaccurate results. For this reason, blood specimens should be taken for laboratory analysis prior to administering hydroxycobalamin. The package insert lists the lab tests commonly affected and for how long the interference can last. Adult dosing for hydroxycobalamin is 5 g administered as an IV infusion over 15 minutes. Depending on the severity of the poisoning and the clinical response, an additional 5 g may be administered (total dose of 10 g).

The cyanide antidote kit contains three components: amyl nitrite, sodium nitrite, and sodium thiosulfate. Both thiosulfate and nitrite have antidotal efficacy when given alone in animal models of cyanide poisoning, but they have even greater benefit when they are given in combination.[17] Thiosulfate donates the sulfur atoms necessary for rhodanese to convert cyanide to thiocyanate. The nitrites generate methemoglobin, which cyanide binds preferentially over cytochrome a3, leading to improved cytochrome oxidase function. Amyl nitrite is contained within glass pearls that are crushed and intermittently inhaled or introduced into the ventilator. IV sodium nitrite is preferred, and the use of amyl nitrite pearls is reserved for cases in which IV access is delayed or not possible. It is important to note that standard testing for methemoglobin does not detect cyanomethemoglobin. Therefore, it may be difficult to define the optimal methemoglobin concentration to bind cyanide without causing further hypoxia. In addition to excessive methemoglobin formation, other adverse effects of nitrites include hypotension and tachycardia because of its vasodilatory effects. Avoiding rapid infusion, monitoring blood pressure, and adhering to dosing guidelines limit adverse effects.

Sodium thiosulfate is the second component of the cyanide antidote kit, and it works synergistically with both nitrites and hydroxycobalamin in the detoxification of cyanide. Because sodium thiosulfate does not cause methemoglobinemia, it can be used without nitrites in circumstances when the creation of methemoglobinemia would be concerning, such as in patients with high carboxyhemoglobin concentrations. (Adult dosing for sodium thiosulfate: 12.5 g IV over 10 to 30 minutes, adult dosing for amyl nitrite [only if no IV access]: break one ampule in front of mouth and hold for 15 seconds, remove for 15 seconds and repeat as needed until sodium nitrate infusion is begun [if needed]. Adult dosing for sodium nitrite [$NaNO_2$] 3% [30 mg/mL]: 10 mL [300 mg] IV over 2 to 4 minutes.)

METHANOL

Methanol is a common industrial and household product. It can be found in windshield washer fluid, cooking fuel gels for camping and buffet platters (Sterno), gas line antifreeze, photocopier ink, and perfumes. Large outbreaks occur when improper fermentation occurs in illegal ethanol production. Management is often complicated by the inability to obtain serum concentrations in a timely manner.

Pathophysiology

Methanol is rapidly absorbed when ingested. It can also be inhaled and dermally absorbed, but these latter routes are uncommon. Although methanol is not eliminated renally, it can be exhaled—a slow exit route that explains the elimination half-life of almost 30 hours.

Methanol is slowly metabolized to formate through successive oxidation by alcohol dehydrogenase (ADH) and aldehyde dehydrogenase, each of which is coupled to the reduction of NAD+ to NADH and H+.[18] Formate is a mitochondrial toxin that inhibits cytochrome oxidase, interfering with oxidative phosphorylation. The retinal epithelium and optic nerve are especially sensitive to methanol, and affected patients may experience visual impairment ranging from blurry or hazy vision to "snowfield vision" or total blindness.

History and Physical Exam

Toxic alcohols, such as ethylene glycol and methanol, are on the differential diagnosis for anion gap metabolic acidosis. Like ethanol, methanol can cause inebriation, but animal studies suggest that its lower molecular weight makes it less inebriating than other alcohols.[19] Methanol levels of 25 to 50 mg/dL can be toxic, but may not be high enough to cause inebriation, especially in an ethanol-tolerant individual. Lack of inebriation, however, should not be used to rule out toxicity.

The basal ganglia are also uniquely sensitive to formate. Methanol is on a short list of toxins that can cause isolated basal ganglia lesions on CT and MRI.[20] In a comatose patient with an acidemia, isolated basal ganglia infarcts may point to a methanol exposure. In one series, typical radiologic lesions were present in six of nine cases. Other CNS lesions reported include necrosis of the corpus callosum and intracranial hemorrhage.[21]

Laboratory Tests

Local laboratory capabilities greatly affect management of methanol-intoxicated patients. If methanol concentrations can be determined within a clinically reasonable time frame (e.g., within the same day), management and disposition is straightforward. In institutions in which report of serum concentrations takes days to return, physicians often use surrogate tests, which may have significant limitations, to stratify patients.

Methanol and other toxic alcohols are often first considered in the differential of a patient with an unexplained anion gap metabolic acidosis. To help exclude other diagnoses, a serum lactate concentration, serum or urine ketones, salicylate concentration, ethanol concentration, and renal function tests should be assessed. Traditionally, toxic alcohols cause an anion gap acidosis with normal lactate and negative ketones. Once a toxic alcohol is considered on the differential diagnosis, serum concentrations should be sent. Even if the result will not return for days, it can still help guide management.

Often, the diagnostic dilemma in an alcohol user is distinguishing toxic alcohol poisoning from alcoholic ketoacidosis (AKA), since in both cases, an anion gap metabolic acidosis is present. One means of identifying AKA is to note an improvement in the anion gap after administration of intravenous fluids, thiamine, and glucose.

Osmol Gap

Checking an osmol gap historically has been considered an essential part of the evaluation of a potentially toxic alcohol-poisoned patient. However, there are several critical limitations to the test. The osmol gap is defined as the difference between the values for the measured osmolality and the calculated osmolarity. The formula to calculate osmolarity is as follows:

$$\text{Osmolarity} = 2(\text{Na+}) + \text{BUN} / 2.8 + \text{glucose} / 18$$
$$\text{Osmol gap} = \text{measured osmolality} - \text{calculated osmolarity}$$

It is helpful to account for any ethanol in the osmolarity because it may explain the presence of unaccounted osmols:

$$\text{Osmolarity} = 2(\text{Na+}) + \text{BUN} / 2.8 + \text{glucose} / 18 + \text{ethanol} / 4.6$$

In methanol (or any alcohol) poisoning, the toxic molecule has osmotic activity that is measured but not calculated, which creates the osmol gap. The anion gap does not increase until methanol, for example, is metabolized to formate. Although the formate metabolite also has osmotic activity, its activity is accounted for by the sodium ion in the osmolarity calculation because it exists as dissociated sodium formate in solution. As a result, there will be an elevated osmol gap and a normal anion gap initially after the exposure; but as time progresses, the anion gap will increase and the osmol gap will decrease.

A normal osmol gap is approximately -2 ± 6; the range to account for 95% of patient populations is -10 to $+14$.[22] Note that a normal gap measurement can be misleading, since the patient's baseline osmol gap is unknown. For example, a patient with a normal osmol gap of -5, who presents with an osmol gap of 9, has in reality an osmol gap of 14. Since a patient's baseline osmol gap is unknown, it is impossible to know whether the calculated gap during their initial presentation is elevated or not.

Finally, although large osmol gaps may be suggestive of toxic alcohol ingestions, common conditions such as alcoholic ketoacidosis, lactic acidosis, renal failure, and shock are all associated with elevated osmol gaps. ICU patients, regardless of the underlying diagnosis, often have osmol gaps near 20. As a result, a normal osmol gap cannot safely exclude a toxic alcohol exposure, and a mildly elevated one is not specific enough for confirmation. However, a very high osmol gap (>30 mOsm/L) is very suggestive of toxic alcohol poisoning.

Management Guidelines

Medical Therapy

Blocking ADH is the mainstay of treatment in methanol poisoning, since this prevents the production of formate, the toxic metabolite.[18] Blocking ADH can be achieved by the administration of either ethanol or fomepizole. ADH has greater affinity for ethanol than for methanol, and complete blockade occurs with serum ethanol concentrations of approximately 100 mg/dL. Fomepizole is a competitive inhibitor of ADH. Intravenous ethanol is no longer readily available in the United States, but in extreme cases when no other antidote is available and dialysis is delayed, oral ethanol may be used.

Traditionally, intravenous ethanol was the antidote of choice, but its use necessitated an ICU bed, and its administration was complicated by mental status changes, potential loss of airway, and electrolyte changes. The goal of either oral or intravenous administration of ethanol is a serum concentration of 100 mg/dL, which can be inebriating to those without any tolerance to ethanol. Fomepizole is not associated with the mental status or electrolyte changes commonly seen with ethanol administration, and its use may not require an ICU admission.[23] Fomepizole is given as a loading dose of 15 mg/kg, followed by doses of 10 mg/kg every 12 hours for four doses. Importantly, this dosing regimen of fomepizole is based on the pharmacokinetics of ethylene glycol, not methanol. The main limitation of fomepizole is that the half-life of methanol, once ADH is blocked, reaches 50 hours. Methanol is not renally eliminated, but rather is eliminated via exhalation. As a result, a patient may require a week-long course of fomepizole, which can be expensive and require complicated dosing regimens. Fomepizole induces its own metabolism after 48 hours of use by activating the CYP 450 enzyme 2E1. As a result, higher doses (15 mg/kg) may be required when using beyond 48 hours.[24] In this instance, hemodialysis may be a preferred method of treatment.

Hemodialysis

Hemodialysis is indicated in patients with severe acidemia, signs of end-organ injury such as coma or renal failure, and those with methanol concentrations >50 mg/dL. Hemodialysis can clear toxic alcohols and their metabolites and correct any acid–base disturbances. A nephrology consult should be obtained early in the clinical course of any toxic alcohol patient so that that the proper resources can be obtained in a timely manner if needed. In cases of large ingestions resulting in high concentrations of methanol or ethylene glycol, multiple rounds of hemodialysis as well as administration of fomepizole in between sessions may be indicated. Patients should be monitored for recurrent acidosis, abnormal vision changes, and renal failure (in cases of ethylene glycol poisoning) post-dialysis.

Folic Acid

Folate should be administered to any patient with suspected methanol toxicity. Folate is an inexpensive, water-soluble vitamin with minimal associated adverse reactions. Folinic acid (leucovorin) has also been shown to be effective. Animal models show that folic acid and folinic acid enhance formate elimination.[25] Scant human case reports also suggest a benefit. Formate is bound by tetrahydrofolate and then undergoes metabolism by 10-formyltetrahydrofolate dehydrogenase to carbon dioxide and water.

METFORMIN

Metformin is an oral antihyperglycemic agent commonly used to treat diabetes mellitus. Its mechanism of action is inhibition of gluconeogenesis and decreased hepatic glucose production. However, it also enhances peripheral glucose uptake by the GLUT transporters in muscle and adipose cells. Metformin overdose should not cause hypoglycemia unless the patient has increased metabolic demands from being critically ill. The most concerning toxicity involves hyperlactemia and metabolic acidosis, commonly referred to as MALA—metformin-associated lactic acidosis.

It is possible for MALA to develop after a single acute overdose of metformin.[26] More commonly, MALA occurs in patients who are therapeutically on metformin and develop renal impairment. Patients who have unintentional metformin intoxication do poorly compared to those with intentional metformin overdose.[27] This may be due to a delay to diagnosis, inciting medical illness-causing tissue hypoxia or renal failure, or other comorbidities. Patients who are managed on metformin are advised to hold their medication for 72 hours following the administration of iodinated contrast to prevent MALA; however, some authors argue that only diabetics with impaired renal function prior to receiving IV contrast are at risk.[28]

Pathophysiology

Recent animal and in vitro studies show that metformin is a mitochondrial toxin. Metformin decreases lactate uptake and consumption in the hepatocyte. However, metformin also decreases global oxygen consumption and causes mitochondrial dysfunction in nonhepatic tissues as well.[29,30]

The diagnosis of MALA is controversial. The Cochrane Review disputes its existence, but that is likely because any data regarding MALA are derived from case reports and case series rather than randomized controlled trials.[31] Randomized controlled trials of metformin exclude patients with kidney disease and are not assessing for the effects of overdose, so the incidence of MALA in those trials is essentially nonexistent. Based on case reports, case series, and animal models, evidence is overwhelmingly supportive of the existence of MALA, and it should be considered in patients with anion gap metabolic acidosis and elevated lactate concentrations.

History and Physical Exam

MALA can be a fatal, but easily missed, diagnosis. Initial symptoms—which include nausea, lethargy, vomiting, and abdominal pain—can be nonspecific. Careful history should assess for etiology of renal impairment such as dehydration, recent infection, new medication, or a recent IV contrast study. Patients can develop a severe metabolic acidosis and multiorgan dysfunction.

Management Guidelines

Although a sodium bicarbonate infusion may be indicated in patients who have a serum bicarbonate concentration <5 mEq/L, it will likely be insufficient to correct the acid–base abnormalities associated with MALA. Hemodialysis is the mainstay of treatment in those with severe acidemia. Hemodialysis does not effectively remove metformin, but it corrects the acid–base disorder and possibly the renal complications.

CONCLUSION

Mitochondrial toxins can cause severe disruptions in oxidative phosphorylation and ultimately lead to multiorgan failure and death. Initial symptoms are often nonspecific and can be easily overlooked for nontoxicologic etiologies. However, any patient with an anion gap metabolic acidosis, elevated lactate, or suspicious history should be rapidly evaluated for these toxins with judicious use of ancillary testing and antidotes.

LITERATURE TABLE

TRIAL	DESIGN	RESULT
Aspirin		
Hill, *Pediatrics.* 1971[2]	Animal study	Bicarbonate lowered salicylate levels in muscle, brain, and liver. Carbon dioxide had the opposite effect
Rapoport et al., *J Clin Investigations.* 1945[4]	Animal study	Salicylates cause a respiratory alkalosis, sedatives increase toxicity, and bicarbonate infusions increase pH but do not affect pCO_2
Thurston et al., *J Clin Investigation.* 1970[5]	Animal study	Salicylates decrease brain glucose concentration and increase lactate concentration. Administration of glucose improves survival
Stolbach et al., *Acad Emerg med.* 2008[8]	Retrospective chart review of 3,144 patients with salicylate poisoning	Improper mechanical ventilation causes respiratory acidosis, acidemia, and clinical deterioration. All intubated patients had pH <7.4; acidosis correlated with outcome
Cyanide		
Baud et al., *Crit Care Med.* 2002[14]	Retrospective chart review of 11 patients with cyanide poisoning	Serum lactate concentration >8 mmol/L had sensitivity of 94%, specificity of 70%, positive predictive value of 64%, and negative predictive value of 98% for a blood cyanide concentration above 1.0 g/mL
Baud et al., *N Engl J Med.* 1991[15]	Prospective case–control study of serum cyanide levels from 109 patients obtained at the scenes of residential fires prior to medical treatment	Lactate >10 mmol/L sensitive for CN intoxication, lactate elevations correlate with CN more than CO levels
Borron et al., *Ann Emerg Med.* 2007[16]	Prospective, observational case series of 69 patients with cyanide poisoning	67% of confirmed cyanide cases survived after hydroxycobalamin administration; adverse reactions included skin and urine discoloration and hypertension
Methanol		
McMartin et al., *Biochem Med.* 1975[18]	Animal study	Formic acid is responsible for the metabolic acidosis in methanol poisoning. 4-Methylpyrazole can effectively block formate production and prevent acidosis
Hoffman et al., *Clin Tox.* 1993[22]	Prospective, observational study of 321 patients requiring determination of serum ethanol and electrolyte levels	Normal osmol gap is -2 ± 6. Normal osmol gap cannot rule out toxic alcohol ingestion
Brent et al., *N Engl J Med.* 2001[23]	Prospective, observational case series of 11 patients administered fomepizole for treatment of methanol poisoning	Metabolic disturbances resolved in all 11 patients; 9 patients survived. Adverse reactions were minor
McMartin et al., *JPET.* 1977[25]	Animal study	Folate increased formate metabolism to CO_2. Folate deficiency decreased formate metabolism and elimination
Metformin		
Seidowsky et al., *Crit Care Med.* 2009[27]	Retrospective single-center MICU study of 42 patients admitted for metformin-associated lactic acidosis	Intentional metformin overdose had more favorable outcome compared to unintentional intoxication. Multiorgan dysfunction poor prognostic indicator

LITERATURE TABLE *(Continued)*

TRIAL	DESIGN	RESULT
Owen et al., *BioChem J.* 2000[29]	In vitro study	Metformin inhibits gluconeogenesis by inhibiting the respiratory chain
Protti et al., *Crit Care.* 2012[30]	Animal study	Metformin inhibits global oxygen consumption and inhibits complex I of the mitochondria in various tissues including the liver, kidney, and heart
Salpeter et al., *Cochrane database.* 2010[31]	Meta-analysis of 347 prospective trials and observational cohort studies of metformin use in patients with type 2 diabetes	No evidence that metformin causes increased lactic acidosis. Study did not look at patients with impaired renal function or with metformin overdose

REFERENCES

1. Flomenbaum NE. Salicylates. In: Nelson LS, Howland MA, Hoffman RS, et al., eds. *Goldfrank's Toxicologic Emergencies.* 9th ed. New York: McGraw-Hill; 2011.
2. Hill JB. Experimental salicylate poisoning: observations on the effects of altering blood pH on tissue and plasma salicylate concentrations. *Pediatrics.* 1971;47(4):658–665.
3. Hill JB. Salicylate intoxication. *N Engl J Med.* 1973;288(21):1110–1113.
4. Rapoport S, Guest GM. The effect of salicylates on the electrolyte structure of the blood plasma. I. Respiratory alkalosis in monkeys and dogs after sodium and methyl salicylate; the influence of hypnotic drugs and of sodium bicarbonate on salicylate poisoning. *J Clin Invest.* 1945;24(5):759–769.
5. Thurston JH, Pollock PG, Warren SK, et al. Reduced brain glucose with normal plasma glucose in salicylate poisoning. *J Clin Invest.* 1970;49(11):2139–2145.
6. Anderson RJ, Potts DE, Gabow PA, et al. Unrecognized adult salicylate intoxication. *Ann Intern Med.* 1976;85(6):745–748.
7. Kallen RJ, Zaltzman S, Coe FL, et al. Hemodialysis in children: technique, kinetic aspects related to varying body size, and application to salicylate intoxication, acute renal failure and some other disorders. *Medicine.* 1966;45(1):1–50.
8. Stolbach AI, Hoffman RS, Nelson LS. Mechanical ventilation was associated with acidemia in a case series of salicylate-poisoned patients. *Acad Emerg Med.* 2008;15(9):866–869.
9. Kirk MA HC, Isom GE. Cyanide. In: Nelson LS, Howland MA, Hoffman RS, et al., eds. *Goldfrank's Toxicologic Emergencies.* 9th ed. New York: McGraw-Hill; 2011.
10. Schulz V. Clinical pharmacokinetics of nitroprusside, cyanide, thiosulphate and thiocyanate. *Clin Pharmacokinet.* 1984;9:239–251.
11. Rindone JP, Sloane EP. Cyanide toxicity from sodium nitroprusside: risks and management. *Ann Pharmacother.* 1992;26:515–519.
12. Johnson RP, Mellors JW. Arteriolization of venous blood gases: a clue to the diagnosis of cyanide poisoning. *J Emerg Med.* 1988;6(5):401–404.
13. Nelson L. Acute cyanide toxicity: mechanisms and manifestations. *J Emerg Nurs.* 2006;32(4 Suppl):S8–S11.
14. Baud FJ, Borron SW, Megarbane B, et al. Value of lactic acidosis in the assessment of the severity of acute cyanide poisoning. *Crit Care Med.* 2002;30(9):2044–2050.
15. Baud FJ, Barriot P, Toffis V, et al. Elevated blood cyanide concentrations in victims of smoke inhalation. *N Engl J Med.* 1991;325(25):1761–1766.
16. Borron SW, Baud FJ, Barriot P, et al. Prospective study of hydroxocobalamin for acute cyanide poisoning in smoke inhalation. *Ann Emerg Med.* 2007;49(6):794–801, 801 e791–e792.
17. Chen KK, Rose CL. Nitrite and thiosulfate therapy in cyanide poisoning. *J Am Med Assoc.* 1952;149(2):113–119.
18. McMartin KE, Makar AB, Martin G, et al. Methanol poisoning. I. The role of formic acid in the development of metabolic acidosis in the monkey and the reversal by 4-methylpyrazole. *Biochem Med.* 1975;13(4):319–333.
19. Wallgren H. Relative intoxicating effects on rats of ethyl, propyl and butyl alcohols. *Acta pharmacol Toxicol.* 1960;16:217–222.

20. Hantson P, Duprez T, Mahieu P. Neurotoxicity to the basal ganglia shown by magnetic resonance imaging (MRI) following poisoning by methanol and other substances. *J Toxicol Clin Toxicol.* 1997;35(2):151–161.
21. Sefidbakht S, Rasekhi AR, Kamali K, et al. Methanol poisoning: acute MR and CT findings in nine patients. *Neuroradiology.* 2007;49(5):427–435.
22. Hoffman RS, Smilkstein MJ, Howland MA, et al. Osmol gaps revisited: normal values and limitations. *J Toxicol Clin Toxicol.* 1993;31(1):81–93.
23. Brent J, McMartin K, Phillips S, et al. Fomepizole for the treatment of methanol poisoning. *N Engl J Med.* 2001;344(6):424–429.
24. Wiener SW. Toxic alcohols. In: Nelson LS, Lewin N, Howland MA, Hoffman RS, et al., eds. *Goldfrank's Toxicologic Emergencies.* 9th ed. New York: McGraw-Hill; 2011.
25. McMartin KE, Martin-Amat G, Makar AB, et al. Methanol poisoning. V. Role of formate metabolism in the monkey. *J Pharmacol Exp Therap.* 1977;201(3):564–572.
26. Teale KF, Devine A, Stewart H, et al. The management of metformin overdose. *Anaesthesia.* 1998;53(7):698–701.
27. Seidowsky A, Nseir S, Houdret N, et al. Metformin-associated lactic acidosis: a prognostic and therapeutic study. *Crit Care Med.* 2009;37(7):2191–2196.
28. Nawaz S, Cleveland T, Gaines PA, et al. Clinical risk associated with contrast angiography in metformin treated patients: a clinical review. *Clin Radiol.* 1998;53(5):342–344.
29. Owen MR, Doran E, Halestrap AP. Evidence that metformin exerts its anti-diabetic effects through inhibition of complex 1 of the mitochondrial respiratory chain. *Biochem J.* 2000;348(Pt 3):607–614.
30. Protti A, Fortunato F, Monti M, et al. Metformin overdose, but not lactic acidosis per se, inhibits oxygen consumption in pigs. *Crit Care (London, England).* 2012;16(3):R75.
31. Salpeter SR, Greyber E, Pasternak GA, et al. Risk of fatal and nonfatal lactic acidosis with metformin use in type 2 diabetes mellitus. *Cochrane Database Syst Rev (Online).* 2010(4):CD002967.

49

Caustics

Payal Sud and Mark Su

BACKGROUND

In 2010, the American Association of Poison Control Centers documented 201,750 reported exposures to caustic household cleaning substances. Most acid, alkali, and other caustic exposures occur via ingestion: 85% are unintentional, and more than 90% occur in children.[1] Intentional exposures, although less common, are more likely to result in severe damage.[2,3] Immediate risks of caustic exposure include esophageal perforation and death. Delayed risks include stricture formation and esophageal carcinoma.[2,4]

PATHOPHYSIOLOGY

The extent of tissue injury caused by contact with caustics is determined by four factors: the amount of caustic ingested, the specific caustic ingested, the caustic's pH, and its titratable acid/alkaline reserve (TAR).[5,6] Significant damage can be caused by strong acids (pH < 3) and strong bases (pH > 11), as well by certain substances with near-neutral pH, such as phenol, because of high TAR.[6] TAR is defined as the amount of HCl or NaOH needed to titrate a given caustic to a pH of 8, which is close to normal esophageal pH.[5] In evaluating the potential of a substance to cause esophageal injury, TAR may be more accurate than pH; however, TAR values can vary greatly among similar substances and even between solid and liquid forms of the same substance. TAR values may be unavailable to the emergency physician during the initial evaluation of a patient; however, TARs of common household substances are published and can be accessed as needed.[5] While the practical use of TARs in the ED is limited, it is important for the emergency physician to be mindful that a substance can cause significant caustic injury despite having a near-neutral pH.

Alkalis

Strong alkalis (or bases) produce liquefactive tissue necrosis when hydroxide (OH^-) ions penetrate deeply into tissue surfaces. This necrotic tissue is then hydrolyzed by enzymes and forms a soft, purulent fluid mass.[7] Alkalis commonly encountered in the home that can cause significant caustic injury in small amounts include lye-containing liquids typically used in oven cleaners and drain openers (historically composed of potassium hydroxide (KOH), but now more commonly sodium hydroxide (NaOH)). Solid caustics that contain strong alkalis, such as laundry powders and dishwasher detergents, can also cause severe injury in small volumes because of prolonged adherence of the solid to the mucosa.[8] Household strength ammonium hydroxide (NH_4OH, found in multiple household cleaning products) and sodium hypochlorite (NaOCl, found in household bleach) are generally dilute enough not to cause significant esophageal damage except when ingested in large volumes (e.g., in an intentional ingestion).

Liquid detergent capsules, only relatively recently available in North America, deserve special mention for their unique ability to cause serious injury. Introduced in Europe in 2001, these detergent capsules became available in North America in 2011. They contain a concentrated liquid detergent, composed of anionic and ionic detergents, propylene glycol, and ethanol, in a water-soluble polyvinyl alcohol sachet.[9] Although the pH of the detergents is close to physiologic (pH 7 to 9), they have caused severe esophageal, skin, and eye irritation and damage. A recent retrospective review attempted to catalogue the presenting symptoms and outcomes of patients exposed to these capsules.[9] The majority of exposures were unintentional ingestions in children, and vomiting was the most common presenting complaint. Several children presented with severe respiratory distress and central nervous system (CNS) depression, typically shortly after exposure. Consistent follow-up was not possible in a majority of the cases, and thus the long-term effect of these liquid detergent ingestions is unclear; as such, these exposures should be managed cautiously.

Finally, the ingestion of button batteries historically posed a serious threat because of their tendency to leak sodium and potassium hydroxide upon contact with the esophageal mucosa. Newer batteries, although still of clinical concern, are significantly more resistant to leakage.[6]

Acids

Acids dissociate into hydrogen (H^+) ions and cause coagulation necrosis, which results in desiccation of tissues and a firm eschar formation. Eschar formation may, in fact, protect against further injury by limiting deeper penetration of the acid. Common strong household acids include hydrochloric acid (found in toilet bowl cleaners and other cleaning products) and hydrofluoric acid (HF) (present in rust removers and wall and tile cleaners).[1] HF has unique clinical manifestations and management guidelines, which will be discussed at the end of the chapter.

HISTORY AND PHYSICAL EXAM

Alkalis cause liquefactive necrosis, and acids cause coagulation necrosis; however, exposure to both caustics presents similarly. When managing a case of caustic exposure, the EP should obtain a detailed patient history, including intent of ingestion; type, formulation (solid or liquid) and concentration of compound ingested; amount of compound ingested; and time of ingestion. The physical exam should observe for the following:

- Nausea or emesis
- Oropharyngeal edema or burns
- Drooling, hoarseness, or stridor
- Dysphagia or odynophagia
- Epigastric pain or hematemesis

These findings may be indicative of esophageal, gastric, or airway injury.[10] Details of the specific injury patterns associated with each clinical presentation are outlined in the endoscopy and management sections that follow.

DIAGNOSTIC EVALUATION

Laboratory Tests

In addition to the history and physical exam, certain blood tests should be performed. A 2003 study found an arterial pH < 7.22 and a base deficit of 12 to be reliable predictors of severe esophageal injury requiring surgical intervention, such as transhiatal esophagectomy and total gastrectomy.[11] The same study reported a pH < 7.11 and a base deficit of 16.1 to be predictors of death despite intervention, suggesting that severe acidosis correlates well with the degree of tissue necrosis and subsequent lactic acid production.

Imaging

Chest and abdominal x-rays are recommended following any caustic ingestion to exclude obvious esophageal perforation; however, the sensitivity of these tests is limited.[6] Computed tomography (CT) is more sensitive and should be considered in patients with negative x-rays despite a high clinical suspicion for perforation. Contrast esophagography can also be used to detect perforations, which can be visualized on a radiograph as extravasation of the contrast medium. The choice of contrast medium remains controversial; some experts advocate a water-soluble contrast like gastrografin to minimize mediastinal and peritoneal irritation upon extravasation, while others advocate barium, which is less likely to cause aspiration pneumonitis.[6] The appropriate contrast medium should be chosen in conjunction with radiology, toxicology, and gastroenterology consult.

For grading of esophageal injury, recent studies suggest benefits of using CT instead of endoscopy; currently, however, endoscopy remains the current standard.[12,13]

Endoscopy

For the emergency physician, the greatest challenge in treating caustic ingestion is determining which patients require immediate endoscopy. Although it carries a potential risk of further esophageal damage, endoscopic evaluation can differentiate low-grade injuries in patients who may be safely discharged from patients with high-grade injuries requiring more extensive management, including potential surgery or other intervention to reduce the risk of stricture formation.

In the past, endoscopy with rigid endoscopes carried a high risk of perforation. Newer flexible endoscopes have lowered this risk and made endoscopy easier to perform[14]; nevertheless, the indication and timing of the procedure remain controversial. Several studies have evaluated history and physical exam criteria as indicators for emergent endoscopy in patients with caustic ingestions. Their conclusions vary widely. A retrospective review of 378 children found no statistically significant relationship between the presence of symptoms (such as vomiting, excessive drooling, abdominal pain, oropharyngeal burns, dysphagia, nausea and refusal to drink) and the severity of esophageal lesions and thus advocated endoscopy in all ingestions.[15] A second retrospective study of 156 children arrived at similar conclusions, excepting a correlation of vomiting with second- and third-degree esophageal lesions.[16]

Two other studies reported opposite findings in a similar population. In a review of 79 patients younger than 20 years of age, the absence of vomiting, drooling, and stridor was found to have a 100% negative predictive value in identifying esophageal injury, while the presence of two or more of the above three symptoms had a 50% positive predictive value for esophageal injury.[10] Based on these findings, the authors recommended limiting the use of endoscopy to patients with clinical symptoms (vomiting, drooling, stridor) rather than performing endoscopy on all patients. A second prospective study of 85 children likewise reported the absence of symptoms to have a 100% negative predictive value for esophageal injury, and the presence of respiratory symptoms and hematemesis to have a significant positive predictive value for injury.[17] This study also advocated withholding endoscopy in the asymptomatic patient with an unintentional ingestion. These studies did not consider suicidal ingestions, but consensus is that endoscopy is necessary in these cases regardless of symptoms, given the high morbidity associated with intentional ingestions.[1]

Consensus recommendation is that the unintentionally exposed, asymptomatic patient—with no respiratory complaints, drooling, stridor, hoarseness, dysphagia, or vomiting—can be safely discharged after appropriate observation in the ED and a trial of oral intake.[10] Symptomatic patients, whether exposed intentionally or unintentionally, should have formal gastroenterology evaluation for endoscopy. The suicidal patient, regardless of symptoms, deserves consultation for endoscopy.

Timing of Endoscopy

A limited number of studies have considered the time period within which endoscopy should be performed or avoided. Mucosal sloughing typically occurs 4 to 7 days after injury, and collagen deposition does not begin until after 14 days; therefore, the esophagus is considered most vulnerable to endoscopic-induced perforation during the 5- to 15-day period following caustic ingestion.[3,14,18] A 1991 prospective cohort study of 81 patients with caustic ingestions who underwent endoscopy reported that of the 381 total (initial and follow-up) endoscopies performed, no patient experienced perforation in close proximity to endoscopy.[14] Perforation did occur in three patients—on the 9th, 11th, and 15th day following endoscopy, respectively—although these perforations were likely due to the use of rigid endoscopes. The study concluded that endoscopy could safely be performed between 6 and 96 hours following caustic ingestion. Of note, none of the study's patients underwent endoscopy during the 5- to 15-day post-ingestion period due to the assumption of esophageal friability. There are no studies that specifically evaluate endoscopy during the 5- to 15-day interval, and it is recommended to avoid the procedure whenever possible during this time.[3,14,18]

One benefit of early endoscopy is the placement of a nasogastric tube (NGT) (always done under direct visualization), which allows for early enteral nutrition. Early nutrition aids rapid healing of the caustic injury, which in turn reduces hospital length of stay.[19] Enteral nutrition has advantages over parenteral nutrition, including preservation of intestinal mucosa, reduced risk of infection, reduced hepatic and biliary complications, more effective monitoring of electrolytes and nutrients, and more cost-efficient delivery.[19]

Endoscopic Grading System of Esophageal Injuries

Grade I injuries involve superficial tissue damage, such as edema and erythema. These injuries do not progress to stricture formation or carcinoma, and these patients can be discharged safely if able to tolerate a regular diet. No other therapy is required.

Grade IIa injuries involve transmucosal damage with superficial ulceration, sloughing, and mucosal hemorrhage of the esophagus. These patients may be able to tolerate a soft diet, or may need the placement of a NGT for enteral feeding. Grade IIb injuries are similar to IIa injuries, but are circumferential, affecting all sides of the esophagus.

Grade III injuries involve deep ulcerations, tissue necrosis, severe hemorrhage, and perforation. Patients with IIb and III injuries are at a risk of perforation, infection, and stricture formation, and are at a 1,000 times increased risk of developing carcinoma over the following 40-year period.

MANAGEMENT GUIDELINES

Airway Management

Management begins with the airway. Caustics can produce significant airway edema, which can lead to rapid airway compromise. Hoarseness, stridor, and drooling are all signs of upper airway injury and require fiberoptic inspection of the vocal cords by an otolaryngologist in the ED. Although not investigated, the consensus recommendation is to use dexamethasone to treat airway edema at a one-time dose of 10 mg IV.[6] If the edema progresses to airway compromise and respiratory distress, orotracheal intubation must be performed, preferably with a fiberoptic laryngoscope.

Decontamination

Although decontamination is generally contraindicated in caustic ingestions, it is essential in treating caustic exposure to the eye and skin. Dry, powdered caustics should be brushed off the skin before washing, as dissolution of the caustic in water may cause further injury. Ophthalmic exposures should be managed with copious irrigation of the eye using a Morgan lens and normal saline (NS), or lactated Ringer's (LR), until the pH of the eye is close to physiologic pH (7.40). Visual acuity should be assessed after irrigation, and a slit-lamp examination should be performed to look for corneal abrasions and ulcerations. These injuries require ophthalmic antibiotics and timely follow-up with an ophthalmologist.

Activated charcoal, a commonly used gastrointestinal decontaminant, is contraindicated in caustic ingestions. Its use impedes endoscopic visualization of the esophageal mucosa, and it can cause pneumonitis if perforations are present. Ingested caustics should never be neutralized, as this reaction is exothermic and can cause further tissue injury.

Treatment of Esophageal Injury

Surgery

Surgical management is necessary in patients with caustic ingestion who present with perforation, persistent hypotension, and metabolic acidosis.[11,20] Early surgical management (within 24 hours of ingestion) is associated with a lower morbidity and mortality than delayed surgery.[20] Surgery may be also required in grade II and III esophageal injuries.[21]

Steroids

Steroids have been considered for the prevention of caustic ingestion associated esophageal stricture formation, but their use is controversial. A meta-analysis of 361 patients demonstrated a 19% rate of stricture formation in the steroid-treated group and a 41% rate in the untreated group; as a result, the study advocated the use of steroids in high-degree esophageal injuries.[22] They study did not, however, differentiate between grade II and III injuries. Other studies have failed to show a benefit from the use of steroids. A prospective study of 60 children with a range of grade I, II, and III injuries found no statistically significant difference in stricture formation between steroid-treated and untreated groups, even after considering each injury grade separately.[23] A recent review study also reported no difference in stricture formation between steroid-treated and untreated patients.[24] It is important to note that steroid therapy not only lacks proven efficacy but also is potentially harmful, as steroids may suppress immunity in patients with injuries already prone to infection. Current guidelines thus recommend against steroid therapy for prevention of esophageal strictures.[24]

Antibiotics

There are limited data on the use of antibiotics for esophageal injuries. If there is a known source of infection, antibiotics should be administered.[6] Giving antibiotics to patients receiving steroids is reasonable, although in general prophylactic antibiotic therapy is not recommended.

Nasogastric Tube

Placement of a NGT may be necessary to provide enteral nutrition in patients unable to tolerate an oral diet because of esophageal injury. In patients with esophageal injuries, an NGT should be placed only under endoscopic visualization.

Intraluminal Stents

Placement of intraluminal stents, usually made of silicone, may prevent stricture formation and ensure patency of the esophageal lumen.[3,6,25,26] Stents can cause increased trauma at the insertion site and can cause increased gastrointestinal reflux, which may impede healing.[27] Use of stents is decided on a case-by-case basis.

Sucralfate

No significant scientific evidence exists to suggest a benefit of using sucralfate in caustic ingestions.[28]

Proton Pump Inhibitors and H_2 Antagonists

The use of proton pump inhibitors and H_2 antagonists reduces the amount of acid that comes into contact with the esophageal mucosa, aids in healing, and is recommended in all cases.[6]

HYDROFLUORIC ACID

Hydrofluoric acid (HF) is present in multiple products, including oven cleaners, rust removers, aluminum brighteners, heavy-duty cleaners, and laundry detergents. It is also used in plastic dye and electronics manufacturing, as well as in the synthesis of Teflon and Freon.[1,6,29,30] Although technically a weak acid, HF produces a unique systemic toxicity, unrelated to its causticity, which merits special discussion.

Pathophysiology

Aqueous hydrofluoric acid is a weak acid, with a pKa of 3.5.[6] HF toxicity is typically the result of dermal, ocular, or inhalational exposure, although ingestions do also occur. HF penetrates deeply into tissues and dissociates into hydrogen (H^+) and fluoride (F^-) ions. Localized hypocalcemia and hypomagnesemia occur when F^- ions bind to Ca and Mg[6,31–34] and form insoluble salts, such as calcium fluoride (CaF_2), that deposit in the tissues.[31] The pain of HF exposure is due to the corrosive burns of the H^+ ions, as well as the calcium dysregulation, which can result in neuroexcitation and vasospasm with associated pain and ischemia.[6,34]

HF's deep penetration produces systemic toxicity regardless of the route of exposure. In addition to hypocalcemia and hypomagnesemia, hyperkalemia can occur. This is postulated to be due to F^--induced increased intracellular Ca^{2+}, which induces Ca^{2+}-dependent K^+ channels to produce a K^+ efflux.[35] Hypocalcemia, hypomagnesemia, and hyperkalemia can, in turn, cause potentially fatal cardiac dysrhythmias.

History and Physical Exam

Dermal Exposure

Dermal exposure to HF can cause a delayed onset of pain and visible tissue damage. Hyperemia may occur, followed by a white discoloration due to calcium precipitation. Pain may precede tissue changes; therefore, a high level of clinical suspicion is required for the patient who presents with severe hand pain but without obvious skin damage.[6,36–38]

Inhalational Exposure

Inhalational exposure to HF can produce symptoms ranging from mild upper respiratory tract irritation to dyspnea, hypoxemia, and hypocalcemia.[39] A retrospective chart review of 939 patients with inhalational exposure to HF released from a petrochemical plant revealed subjective toxicity including eye and throat irritation, headache, and shortness of breath, as well as objective toxicity, including decreased pulmonary function testing, hypoxemia, and hypocalcemia.[39]

Ingestion

Ingestion of HF results in gastritis and systemic toxicity, including possible cardiac dysrhythmia due to hypocalcemia and hyperkalemia.[40,41] Local tissue damage may result in airway compromise. Intentional ingestion of HF often results in death.[42,43]

Ocular Exposure

HF is highly caustic to the eye; it penetrates deeply and causes corneal stromal edema, conjunctival chemosis, hemorrhage, ischemia, inflammation, and stromal opacification.[44,45] Long-term effects can include corneal revascularization and dry eyes.

Diagnostic Evaluation

Laboratory Tests

Serum calcium, magnesium, and potassium should be monitored. Low serum pH is a sign of worsening systemic toxicity and can be monitored via blood gas analysis.[31] Serum fluoride concentrations are not clinically relevant because of the time it takes to obtain results.[6]

Electrocardiogram

An electrocardiogram should be obtained in all cases of HF exposure to evaluate the effects of hypocalcemia (prolonged QTc) and hyperkalemia (peaked T waves).

Management Guidelines

Decontamination

- *Dermal*: Prompt irrigation with water to limit absorption.
- *Inhalational*: No decontamination possible.
- *Ingestion*: Gastric lavage should be considered, given the high fatality rate with this ingestion.[6] Systemic toxicity from HF is much greater than its caustic potential; thus,

the benefit of removing the gastrointestinal burden of HF outweighs the risk of perforation posed by NGT placement.[46,47] Caution must be exercised to limit exposure of health care personnel to HF, and personal protective equipment should always be worn. Activated charcoal does not bind fluoride ions effectively.[6]

- *Ocular*: Irrigation with NS, LR, or water; prolonged irrigation can be detrimental and should be avoided.[44]

Medical Therapy

- *Dermal*: Topical calcium gel, such as 2.5% calcium gluconate solution (used for IV administration) mixed with a sterile water-soluble lubricant, should be applied over the affected area. Usually, the affected area is the hand, which can then be covered with a glove for 30 minutes to allow absorption of the calcium solution. The calcium from the solution will bind the fluoride ions from the HF, preventing the fluoride ions from depleting the calcium and magnesium stores of the patient.
- *Intradermal*: Injection of dilute calcium gluconate solution into the tissues has been debated, but is no longer recommended as the risk of compartment syndrome, infection, and tissue damage outweighs potential benefit.[6] Intradermal injection of calcium chloride can cause severe tissue necrosis and should always be avoided.
- *Intravenous*: When topical administration fails, 10% intravenous calcium gluconate has been shown to relieve pain and correct hypocalcemia.[36,48,49] There is limited evidence to recommend topical or parenteral magnesium therapy for HF exposures.
- *Intra-arterial*: Intra-arterial infusion of calcium gluconate has been shown to provide rapid analgesia and salvation of tissues.[36,50] The mechanism is thought to be vasodilation, which allows increased delivery of calcium to scavenge the fluoride ions.[36] Adverse effects of this technique include local inflammation, radial artery spasm, and hypomagnesemia.[6,36,50]

All patients with digital exposures require 4 to 6 hours of ED observation to monitor for recurrence of pain and need for repeat calcium administration.[6]

Additional Therapy for Specific Exposures

- *Inhalational*: Treat with nebulized calcium gluconate solution (2.5% to 5%). If laryngeal edema is present, the patient should be intubated with advanced airway techniques, and positive-pressure ventilation should be applied.[6,51,52]
- *Ingestion*: Oral calcium salts have been tested on animals with mixed efficacy; human data are lacking.[53,54]
- *Ocular*: Following copious irrigation, patients should have an ophthalmic examination and ophthalmology consult. The use of 1% calcium gluconate eye drops is controversial because calcium, or magnesium, can cause further ocular irritation.[29,45,51]

Treatment of Severe Toxicity

Cardiac dysrhythmias due to hypocalcemia and hypomagnesemia should be managed with intravenous calcium and magnesium. Hyperkalemia should be aggressively treated using standard therapies. Urinary alkalinization with intravenous sodium bicarbonate can enhance fluoride elimination.[55] Patients who cannot tolerate a large volume load, who are severely ill, or who have renal dysfunction may require hemodialysis for definitive fluoride elimination.[56,57]

CONCLUSION

A majority of lethal caustic exposures are intentional and occur in adults. A majority of accidental caustic exposures occur in children. It is challenging to risk stratify the extent of tissue injury after caustic exposures, and special attention should be directed towards the type of product involved, the intent of exposure, and signs and symptoms such as vomiting, stridor, and drooling. Gastroenterology and surgical consults should be involved early in the care of any significant or symptomatic ingestion. Although decontamination is usually contraindicated in caustic ingestions, it is important in ocular and dermal exposures. Hydrofluoric acid exposures may also require decontamination to prevent systemic toxicity, followed by appropriate calcium therapy.

LITERATURE TABLE

TRIAL	DESIGN	RESULT
Caustics		
Crain et al., *Am J Dis Child.* 1984[10]	Retrospective chart review of 79 patients <20 y old with a history of caustic ingestion	50% of patients with ≥2 signs (vomiting, drooling, stridor) had serious esophageal injury. 0 patients with ≤1 sign had serious esophageal injury. Oropharyngeal burns did not correlate with the degree of esophageal injury
Cheng et al., *Surg Today.* 2003[11]	Retrospective chart review of 129 patients (mean age 42.7) admitted for caustic ingestion	Patients who required surgery had a mean pH of 7.22 ± 0.12, while those that did not require surgery had a mean pH of 7.38 ± 0.06 ($p < 0.001$). Of the patients who underwent surgery, the mean pH of the ones who survived was 7.27 ± 0.09 and that of the ones who died was 7.11 ± 0.11 ($p < 0.001$). Arterial pH < 7.22 indicates severe injury, and emergency surgery must be considered
Zargar et al., *Gastrointest Endosc.* 1991[14]	Prospective observational study of 81 patients with a history of caustic ingestion	Early endoscopy with a flexible endoscopy is safe and does not cause perforations. Endoscopy should be avoided 5–15 d postingestion, as this is the period when the esophagus is the most vulnerable
Lamireau et al., *J Ped Gastroenterol Nutr.* 2001[17]	Prospective cohort study of 85 children admitted for unintentional caustic ingestions	Absence of symptoms has a 100% negative predictive value for esophageal injury in children with unintentional caustic ingestions in developed countries
Peclova and Navratil, *Toxicol Rev.* 2005[24]	Systematic review of 10 studies (2 prospective, 8 retrospective) with a total of 572 patients with 2nd or 3rd degree esophageal burns who either received or did not receive steroid therapy	No difference found in stricture formation between patients who received steroids and those who did not
Hydrofluoric acid		
Hatzifotis et al., *Burns.* 2004[29]	Retrospective chart review of 42 HF burn patients	Mean burn size was 1%; upper limb was most commonly involved, with 64% of cases involving fingers and hand. 17% of patients required surgical debridement; 14% required fingernail removal; no patient died. Hypocalcemia was managed with PO and IV calcium. 5 concise algorithms outlined to manage dermal exposure, inhalational exposure, ingestional exposure, ocular exposure, and systemic toxicity
De Capitani et al., *Sao Paulo Med J.* 2009[36]	Case report of a 41-year-old male with a dermal exposure to 70% HF on his hands	The patient failed topical therapy and required intra-arterial calcium gluconate administration, which resulted in complete recovery from the blanched and edematous finger lesions
Graudins et al., *Ann Emerg Med.* 1997[48]	Case series of a convenience sample of 7 patients with HF burns, in whom topical calcium had failed	IV calcium gluconate with Bier block technique caused complete resolution of pain in 4/7 patients, and the remaining 3/7 patients recovered completely with intra-arterial calcium gluconate. No surgery was required and adverse events were minimal

REFERENCES

1. Bronstein AC, Spyker DA, Cantilena LR, et al. 2010 Annual report of the American Association of Poison Control Centers' National Poison Data System (NPDS): 28th Annual Report. *Clin Tox.* 2011;49:910–941.
2. Gumaste VV, Dave PB. Ingestion of corrosive substances by adults. *Am J Gastroenterol.* 1992;87(1):1–5.
3. Ramasamy K, Gumaste VV. Corrosive Ingestion in Adults. *J Clin Gastroenterol.* 2003;37(2):119–124.
4. Moore WR. Caustic ingestions. Pathophysiology, diagnosis, and treatment. *Clin Pediatr (Phila).* 1986;25(4):192–196.
5. Hoffman RS, Howland MA, Kamerow HN, et al. Comparison of titratable acid/alkaline reserve and pH in potentially caustic household products. *J Toxicol Clin Toxicol.* 1989;27(4–5):241–246.
6. Nelson LS, Lewin NA, Howland MA, et al. *Goldfrank's Toxicologic Emergencies.* 9th ed. New York, NY: McGraw-Hill; 2011.
7. Kumar V, Abbas AK, Fausto N, et al. *Robbins and Cotran Pathological Basis of Disease.* 8th ed. Pennsylvania: Saunders Elseveir; 2010.
8. Kirsh MM, Ritter F. Caustic ingestion and subsequent damage to the oropharyngeal and digestive passages. *Ann Thoracic Surg.* 1976;21:74–82.
9. Williams H, Bateman DN, Thomas SHL, et al. Exposure to liquid detergent capsules: a study undertaken by the UK National Poisons Information Service. *Clin Tox.* 2012;50:776–780.
10. Crain EF, Gershel JC, Mezey AP. Caustic ingestions. Symptoms as predictors of esophageal injury. *Am J Dis Child.* 1984;138(9):863–865.
11. Cheng YJ, Kao EL. Arterial blood gas analysis in acute caustic ingestion injuries. *Surg Today.* 2003;33:483–485.
12. Isbister GK, Page CB. Early endoscopy or CT in caustic injuries: a re-evaluation of clinical practice. *Clin Tox.* 2011;49:641–642.
13. Ryu HH, Jeung KW, Lee BK, et al. Caustic injury: can CT grading system enable prediction of esophageal stricture? *Clin Tox.* 2010;48:137–142.
14. Zargar SA, Kochhar R, Mehta S, et al. The role of fiberoptic endoscopy in the management of corrosive ingestion and modified endoscopic classification of burns. *Gastrointest Endosc.* 1991;37(2):165–169.
15. Gaudreault P, Parent M, McGuigan MA, et al. Predictability of esophageal injury from signs and symptoms: a study of caustic ingestion in 378 children. *Pediatrics.* 1983;71:667–770.
16. Previtera C, Giusti F, Guglielmi M. Predictive value of visible leasions (cheeks, lips, oropharnyx) in suspected caustic ingestion: may endoscopy reasonably be omitted in completely negative pediatric patients? *Pediatr Emerg Care.* 1990;6(3): 176–178.
17. Lamireau T, Rebousissoux L, Denis D, et al. Accidental caustic ingestions in children: is endoscopy always mandatory? *J Pediatr Gastroenterol Nutr.* 2001;33(1):81–4.
18. Cheng HT, Cheng CL, Lin CH, et al. Caustic ingestion in adults: the role of endoscopic classification in predicting outcome. *BMC Gastroenterol.* 2008;8(31).
19. Chibishev A, Simonovska-Veljanovska N, Pereska Z. Artificial nutrition in therapeutic approach of acute caustic poisonings. *Maced J Med Sci.* 2010;3(2).
20. Javed A, Pal S, Krishnan EK, et al. Surgical management and outcomes of severe gastrointestinal injuries due to corrosive ingestion. *World J Gastrointest Surg.* 2012;4(5):121–125.
21. Estrera A, Taylor W, Mills LJ, et al. Corrosive burns of the esophagus and stomach: a recommendation for an aggressive surgical approach. *Ann Thor Surg.* 1986;41:276–283.
22. Howell JM, Dalsey WC, Hartsell FW, et al. Steroids for the treatment of corrosive esophageal injury: a statistical analysis of past studies. *Am J Emerg Med.* 1992;10:421–425.
23. Anderson KD, Rouse TM, Randolph JG. A controlled trial of corticosteroids in children with corrosive injury of the esophagus. *N Engl J Med.* 1990;323(10):637–640.
24. Peclova D and Navratil T. Do corticosteroids prevent oesophageal stricture after corrosive ingestion? *Toxicol Rev.* 2005;24(2):125–129.
25. Berkovits RN, Bose CE, Wijburg FA, et al. Caustic injury of the esophagus. *J Laryngol Otol.* 1996; 110:1041–1045.
26. De Peppo F, Zaccara A, DallOglio L, et al. Stenting for caustic strictures. *J Pediatr Surg.* 1998;22:54–57.
27. Sinar DR, Fletcher JR, Cordova CC, et al. Acute acid-induced esophagitis impairs esophageal persitalsis in baboons. *Gastroenterology.* 1981;80:1286.
28. Reddy AN, Budhraja M. Sucralfate therapy for lye-induced esophagitis. *Am J Gastroenterol.* 1988;83:71–73.
29. Hatzifotis M, Williams A, Muller M, et al. Hydrofluoric acid burns. *Burns.* 2004;30:156–159.
30. Huisman LC, Teijink JAW, Overbosch EH, et al. An atypical chemical burn. *Lancet.* 2001;358:1510.

31. Boink AB, Wemer J, Meulenbelt J, et al. The mechanism of fluoride-induced hypocalcemia. *Hum Exp Toxicol.* 1994;13(3):149–155.
32. Greco RJ, Hartford CE, Haith LR, et al. Hyrdofluoric acid-induced hypocalcemia. *J Trauma* 1988;28:1593–1596.
33. Sanz-Gallen P, Nogue S, Munne P, et al. Hypocalcaemia and hypomagnesaemia due to hydrofluoric acid. *Occup Med.* 2001;51(4):294–295.
34. Thomas D, Jaeger U, Sagoschen I, et al. Intra-arterial calcium gluconate treatment after hydrofluoric acid burn of the hand. *Cardiovasc Intervent Radiol.* 2009;32:155–158.
35. Cummings CC, McIvor ME. Fluoride-induced hyperkalemia: the role of Ca2$^+$-dependent K$^+$ channels. *Am J Emerg Med.* 1988;6(1):1–3.
36. De Capitani EM, Hirano ES, Zuim Ide SC, et al. Fingers burns caused by concentrated hydrofluoric acid, treated with intra-arterial calcium gluconate infusion: case report. *Sao Paolo Med J.* 2009;127(6):379–381.
37. Anderson WJ, Anderson JR. Hydrofluoric acid burns of the hand: mechanism of injury and treatment. *J Hand Surg Am.* 1988;13(1):52–57.
38. Sheridan RL, Ryan CM, Quinby WC Jr, et al. Emergency management of major hydrofluoric acid exposures. *Burns.* 1995;21:62–64.
39. Wing JS, Brender JD, Sanderson LM, et al. Acute health effects in a community after a release of hydrofluoric acid. *Arch Environ Health.* 1991;46(3):155–160.
40. Stremski ES, Grande GA, Ling LJ. Survival following hydrofluoric acid ingestion. *Ann Emerg Med.* 1992;21(11):1396–1399.
41. Yu-Jang S, Li-Hua L, Wai-Mau C, et al. Survival after a massive hydrofluoric acid ingestion with ECG changes. *Am J Emeg Med.* 2001;19(5):458–460.
42. Whiteley P, Aks SE. Case files of the toxicon consortium in Chicago: survival after intentional ingestion of hydrofluoric acid. *J Med Toxicol.* 2010;6:349–354.
43. Kao WF, Dart RC, Kuffner E, et al. Ingestion of low-concentration hydrofluoric acid: an insidious and potentially fatal poisoning. *Ann Emerg Med.* 1999;34(1).
44. McCulley JP, Whiting DW, Petitt MG, et al. Hydrofluoric acid burns of the eye. *J Occup Med.* 1983;25(6):447–450.
45. McCulley JP. Ocular hydrofluoric acid burns: animal model, mechanism of injury and therapy. *Trans Am Ophthalmol Soc.* 1990;88:649–684.
46. Baltazar RF, Mower MM, Reider R, et al. Acute fluoride poisoning leading to fatal hyperkalemia. *Chest.* 1980;78:660–663.
47. Manoguerra AS, Neuman TS. Fatal poisoning from acute hydrofluoric acid ingestion. *Am J Emerg Med.* 1986;4:362–363.
48. Graudins A, Burns MJ, Aaron CK. Regional intravenous infusion of calcium gluconate for hydrofluoric acid burns of the upper extremity. *Ann Emerg Med.* 1997;30(5):604–607.
49. Ryan JM, McCarthy GM, Plunkett PK. Regional intravenous calcium—an effective method of treating hydrofluoric acid burns to limb peripheries. *J Accid Emerg Med.* 1997;14:401–404.
50. Vance MV, Curry SC, Kunkel DB, et al. Digital hydrofluoric acid burns: treatment with intraarterial calcium infusion. *Ann Emerg Med.* 1986;15(8):890–896.
51. Schiettecatte D, Mullie G, Depoorter M. Treatment of hydrofluoric acid burns. *Acta Chir Belg.* 2003;103:375–378.
52. Kono K, Watanabe T, Dote T, et al. Successful treatments of lung injury and skin burn due to hydrofluoric acid exposure. *Int Arch Occup Environ Health.* 2000;73:S93–S97.
53. Heard K, Delgado K. Oral decontamination with calcium or magnesium salts does not improve survival following hydrofluoric acid ingestion. *J Toxicol Clin Toxicol.* 2003;41:789–792.
54. Heard K, Hill RE, Cairns CB, et al. Calcium neutralizes fluoride bioavailability in a lethal model of fluoride poisoning. *J Toxicol Clin Toxicol.* 2001;39(4):349–353.
55. Proudfoot AT, Krenzelok EP, Vale JA. Position paper on urine alkalinization. *J Toxicol Clin Toxicol.* 2004;42:1–26.
56. Berman L, Taves D, Mitra S, et al. Inorganic fluoride poisoning treatment by hemodialysis. *N Engl J Med.* 1973;289:922.
57. Juncos LI, Donadio JV. Renal failure and fluorosis. *JAMA.* 1972;222:783–785.

50

Anticoagulants

Betty C. Chen and Lewis S. Nelson

BACKGROUND

Systemic anticoagulation is widely used to treat patients with or at risk for thromboembolic events. Vitamin K antagonists (VKAs) such as warfarin have been the standard therapy for long-term systemic anticoagulation since the mid-20th century. The discovery of the heparins followed shortly thereafter. Most recently, the development of direct clotting factor antagonists has radically changed the landscape of modern anticoagulation therapy. Although these new anticoagulants boast convenient dosing regimens, their use can result in potentially disastrous bleeding complications. While reversal agents are available for VKAs and certain heparins, no antidotes exist to rapidly reverse anticoagulation with the new direct factor antagonists.

Medical providers and patients must weigh the risks and benefits of systemic anticoagulation. Both spontaneous and traumatic bleeding are the most common and consequential complications of all anticoagulants. Intracranial hemorrhages and bleeding at noncompressible sites, such as the gastrointestinal tract, are examples of life-threatening bleeding events; smaller bleeds are also common and can occur at almost any location.

For the patient who presents with significant blood loss, restoration and maintenance of effective circulating volume is a priority. Although crystalloid infusion and blood transfusion with packed red blood cells (pRBCs) will replace volume, neither reverses medication-induced anticoagulation. Instead, both interventions potentially worsen coagulopathy by producing hypocalcemia from citrate toxicity, dilutional thrombocytopenia, and dilution of existing clotting factors. The use of targeted antidotal therapy depends on the particular anticoagulant involved. Operative or definitive management for the bleeding complications may be necessary in select cases (e.g., drainage of epidural hematomas).

VITAMIN K ANTAGONISTS

Warfarin is the most commonly prescribed oral anticoagulant. It inhibits vitamin K 2,3-epoxide reductase and vitamin K quinone reductase, causing anticoagulation from a depletion of activated factors II, VII, IX, and X.[1,2] In addition to inhibition of these procoagulant clotting factors, VKAs also inhibit anticoagulant factors C and S, which can result in a transient procoagulant state at the initiation of VKA therapy.[2]

History and Physical Exam

Adverse drug events may occur even in VKA-anticoagulated patients who are within therapeutic ranges of anticoagulation. There are many factors that increase the risk for major bleeding in patients treated with the VKAs, including age, comorbid medical problems, labile international normalized ratios (INRs), concomitant ethanol or drug use, and genetic factors.[3,4] Labile INRs are common in patients anticoagulated with the VKAs because of numerous dietary and drug interactions.[2,5]

Bleeding is the most prevalent complication from VKA use, but the emergency physician should also be familiar with a variety of associated nonhemorrhagic complications. Warfarin skin necrosis and purple toe syndrome are uncommon, and providers may misidentify these adverse drug reactions. Warfarin skin necrosis is believed to occur more frequently in patients with deficiencies of protein C, protein S, or antithrombin (AT) III.[6–8] It is thought dermal thrombosis may lead to ischemia, although the mechanism of action is poorly understood.[7,9] Patients typically develop painful and erythematous skin in areas with higher amounts of subcutaneous fat, such as the breasts, abdomen, thighs, and buttocks, within a week of warfarin initiation. These areas progress to necrotic patches that can extend up to 5 cm deep into the tissue.[8,10] In addition, secondary infection is frequently reported as an additional source of morbidity.[11]

Purple toe syndrome is an embolic phenomenon that typically occurs 3 to 8 weeks after initiating treatment with warfarin. It is caused by VKA-induced bleeding into atherosclerotic plaques, with subsequent release of cholesterol emboli.[11]

Diagnostic Evaluation

Prothrombin time (PT) and INR are widely available and inexpensive laboratory tests used to determine warfarin's anticoagulant effect. The PT measures the extrinsic pathway of the coagulation cascade. Because the PT varies due to individual laboratory and reagent variability, the INR is used to standardize results. Each lab calculates an INR based on a PT ratio raised to the lab's unique international sensitivity factor.[12,13] Target INRs typically range between 2 and 3.5, depending on indication for anticoagulation with warfarin.

The PT and INR, however, can be elevated in conditions not specific to warfarin-induced anticoagulation. Hepatic failure, inhibitors to clotting factors, disseminated intravascular coagulation, and a number of other conditions may cause a prolongation of PT and INR. This prolongation does not necessarily reflect anticoagulation.

A mixing study can assist in differentiating between a factor deficiency (such as that created by VKAs) and factor inhibitors (such as heparin). After combining equal volumes of pooled normal plasma and the patient's plasma, failure to correct PT and INR confirms the presence of a clotting factor inhibitor.[14]

Management Guidelines

Reversal of VKA-induced coagulopathy can be achieved by restoration of activated clotting factors II, VII, IX, and X. In patients requiring rapid reversal, such as those with life-threatening bleeding, immediate factor replacement with fresh frozen plasma (FFP) or prothrombin complex concentrates (PCC) rapidly reverses coagulopathy. The American College of Chest Physicians (ACCP) 2012 guideline recommends 4-factor PCC for rapid reversal of VKA-induced coagulopathy in patients with bleeding.[14] The 2012 version recommends PCC over FFP, though there are no large randomized controlled trials that directly compare these reversal strategies. The guideline is based on small, nonblinded, and unevenly matched studies.[15,16] Theoretical advantages for PCC administration include smaller infusion volumes, which decrease time of administration and mitigate risks for volume overload. PCC also obviates the need for cross-matching of blood types, circumvents transfusion reactions, and decreases the risk of viral transmission.[17] However, FFP is more frequently administered to reverse VKA-induced coagulopathy because of lower costs and because 4-factor PCC was unavailable in the United States until its approval in April 2013. Both 3- and 4-factor PCC contain non-activated factors II, VII, IX, and X. However, 3-factor PCC contains reduced amounts of factor VII to decrease thrombogenesis. Some have advocated the use of recombinant activated factor VII (rFVIIa), which is indicated only in patients with hemophilia or inhibitors to factors VIII or IX, for reversal of VKA-induced coagulopathy. However, the latest ACCP guideline explicitly recommends against using rFVIIa for this purpose. The risk of thrombosis following off-label rFVIIa administration may be higher in patients without hemophilia or inhibitors to factor VIII or IX.[18]

Because clotting factors have a definitive half-life, an essential step in reversing VKA-induced coagulopathy is the administration of vitamin K_1 to promote reactivation of inactive vitamin K–dependent clotting factors. Oral administration results in peak plasma concentrations in 3 to 6 hours, whereas intravenous administration results in immediate peak plasma concentrations.[19] Improvement in INR may lag, as clotting factor activation via hepatic gamma–glutamyl carboxylase is the rate-limiting step. In a single study of excessively anticoagulated patients, intravenous administration of vitamin K_1 resulted in return to target INR at 6 hours, while oral administration required 12 hours.[20] Maintaining a normal INR depends on the half-life of vitamin K_1, plasma concentration of vitamin K_1, and the duration of action of the specific VKA. Long-acting VKAs can require repeated doses of vitamin K_1 to prevent excessive anticoagulation.

For adult patients with life-threatening bleeding, 10 mg of vitamin K_1 should be administered intravenously if the benefits of INR normalization outweigh the risks. The rate of infusion should not exceed 1 mg/min, as intravenous administration is associated with anaphylactoid reaction. In nonbleeding patients with an INR >10, small doses of vitamin K_1 (1 to 2.5 mg) should be administered orally. Patients with supratherapeutic INRs <10 can omit their next warfarin dose and recheck their INR if bleeding is not an issue.[14] Subcutaneous administration of vitamin K_1 results in unpredictable absorption kinetics and should be saved for rare occasions when patients are unable to take oral medications.

Patients who develop warfarin skin necrosis should discontinue warfarin therapy, and heparin should be used for systemic anticoagulation. Surgical debridement and amputation of limbs have been reported in severe cases.[11]

HEPARINS

Unfractionated heparin is a mixture of glycosaminoglycans that causes a conformational change in AT, increasing its activity. This inhibits both thrombin and a number of clotting factors, including factors IXa, Xa, XIa, and XIIa.[21] Low molecular weight heparins (LMWHs) are short fragments derived from unfractionated heparin. LMWHs cause distinct conformational changes in AT, which targets inhibition specifically at factor Xa.[22] LMWHs have several potential clinical advantages compared to unfractionated heparin, including longer half-lives and the ability to use fixed-dosing regimens.

Complications of heparin therapy fall into two categories: bleeding complications (expected from any of the anticoagulants) and nonbleeding complications including heparin-induced thrombocytopenia (HIT) and heparin-induced thrombocytopenia and thrombosis syndrome (HIT(T)). It is important to distinguish between postoperative consumptive thrombocytopenia and HIT(T) derived from heparin-induced complications. Postoperative thrombocytopenia usually occurs on postoperative day 1 or 2, followed by an improvement 1 or 2 days later. HIT(T) usually manifests between 5 and 10 days after introduction of heparin. However, an earlier fall in platelet count may occur in patients previously treated with heparin, and this early appearance of thrombocytopenia may confuse providers.[23]

HIT(T) develops as a result of antibodies that recognize a heparin–platelet factor 4 complex. When these antibody–antigen complexes bind to platelets, the consequences are either platelet destruction or platelet activation. HIT occurs when platelets are destroyed without any thrombotic sequelae. HITT occurs when platelets are activated and cause thrombosis. If HIT goes untreated, up to 55% of patients will develop HITT. HIT(T) can also occur with the LMWHs.[23,24]

Diagnostic Evaluation

Activated partial thromboplastin time (aPTT) is the test of choice for monitoring unfractionated heparin's anticoagulant effect. Nomograms can help providers alter heparin dosing based on aPTT results. In patients requiring high-dose heparin, such as those undergoing cardiovascular procedures, activated clotting time can be used instead of aPTT.[25] A subset of patients may manifest heparin resistance, where high doses of heparin cannot achieve aPTTs in the therapeutic range. In these cases, anti-Xa levels may be measured instead of aPTT, which permits lower dosing of heparin while providing similar therapeutic effect and safety profiles.[26]

Patients treated with LMWHs typically do not receive laboratory monitoring.[27] VTE prophylaxis dosing is fixed, while VTE treatment is weight based. Laboratory monitoring with anti-Xa activity measurements should be performed in the case of pregnant patients, obese patients, or those with chronic kidney disease. Therapeutic anti-Xa activity ranges in these populations vary based on indication for anticoagulation.[25]

HIT(T) must be suspected if the platelet count drops below 100×10^9/L or if there is a 40% drop in the platelet count after heparin initiation.[28] Patients who are at highest risk of developing HIT(T) are postoperative patients on either prophylactic or therapeutic heparin. The incidence of HIT(T) in these patients is between 1% and 5%. Cardiac surgery patients also have a higher risk of developing HIT(T) with an incidence between 1 and 3%.[23] In patients with a risk of >1% for developing HIT(T), platelet counts should be monitored every 2 to 3 days starting on day 4 of heparin therapy. If a patient does not develop HIT(T) by day 14 of therapy, then further monitoring is not necessary.[23] HIT antibody assays should be sent to confirm the diagnosis of HIT(T) if the platelet counts drop by the aforementioned amount.

Management Guidelines

For nonsignificant bleeding with an elevated aPTT, cessation of anticoagulation therapy may be sufficient, as unfractionated heparin has a short duration of action between 1 and 2.5 hours, depending on amount administered.[29,30] Significant bleeding, by contrast, may necessitate antidotal therapy. Protamine sulfate binds to heparin and effectively neutralizes its anticoagulant capabilities. One milligram of intravenous protamine neutralizes 100 U of unfractionated heparin, and dosing should reflect the amount of heparin calculated to be present at the time of antidote administration (assume that the half-life of heparin is 60 to 90 minutes).[29] Adverse effects of protamine are numerous. Paradoxical anticoagulation can occur if excessive protamine is administered. Hypotension and bradycardia can occur with correct dosing, but slow infusion helps decrease the risk of these events. Anaphylaxis is also possible, and patients with a history of receiving protamine, fish allergy, or history of vasectomy have a higher risk of developing anaphylaxis to protamine. Because of the risk of anaphylaxis, only patients with life-threatening bleeding should receive protamine.[25]

Protamine is sometimes used to treat patients anticoagulated with LMWHs if they suffer from life-threatening bleeding. There are no proven antidotes for LMWH, but partial reversal may be possible with protamine. One milligram of protamine should be administered per 100 anti–factor Xa units (1 mg enoxaparin is the equivalent to 100 anti–factor Xa units) if LMWH was administered within 8 hours. If bleeding continues, a second dose of protamine at 0.5 mg per 100 anti–factor Xa units can be considered. Smaller doses of protamine should be administered if more than 8 hours has elapsed since LMWH administration.[25]

If HIT(T) is suspected or confirmed in a patient, the most important intervention is cessation of heparin or LMWH therapy. Alternative anticoagulants such as the direct thrombin inhibitors (DTI) argatroban and bivalirudin, or a Xa inhibitor such as danaparoid should be used until a therapeutic INR is achieved with warfarin. Novel oral anticoagulants, such as dabigatran, rivaroxaban, and apixaban, have not been studied for this indication.

DIRECT THROMBIN INHIBITORS

To circumvent the problems associated with the VKAs and the heparins, DTIs have been utilized parenterally, and more recent developments have led to the introduction of oral DTIs. These medications are derived from hirudin, a peptide secreted by the medicinal leech, and they are used to treat acute coronary syndrome and VTE.[31] The most commonly used parenterally administered DTIs are bivalirudin and argatroban. Providers typically use these agents when patients have a contraindication to heparin, such as HIT(T).

Dabigatran, an oral DTI, is currently approved only for VTE and stroke prophylaxis in patients with nonvalvular atrial fibrillation. Initial studies showed favorable results for VTE prophylaxis in patients with nonvalvular atrial fibrillation with lower bleeding and mortality rates.[32] Unfortunately, a higher-than-anticipated bleeding rate associated with dabigatran has been identified in postmarketing analyses and studies.[33,34] A U.S. FDA advisory statement cited dabigatran as the leader in reported adverse drug events in 2012.[35] However, further data in this advisory suggest that risk factors for bleeding include inappropriate renal dosing, age older than 75 years,[33] and use for the wrong indication.[34] In addition, the risk of myocardial infarctions and acute coronary syndrome appeared to be higher in groups treated with dabigatran when compared to patients treated with other anticoagulants.[36]

Diagnostic Evaluation

To estimate the degree of anticoagulation with the DTIs bivalirudin and argatroban, serial aPTT measurements are used most often.[25] Unfortunately, estimates made with aPTT are frequently inaccurate, since the relationship between aPTT and degree of anticoagulation with DTIs is not linear. With dabigatran, the aPTT plateaus when concentrations are over 200 ng/mL, and PT and INR also follow a nonlinear relationship with the serum dabigatran concentration.[37] The use of thrombin time (TT) and ecarin clotting time (ECT), which follow a more linear relationship to DTI concentration, has been proposed as better tests to estimate DTI concentration and anticoagulation.[25,37] With the increased use of DTIs, some laboratories have increased the availability of the TT; ECT still remains largely unavailable for use in real time.

Management Guidelines

The most concerning issue with the DTIs is the absence of a proven reversal agent or strategy. Because the half-lives of the parenteral medications are relatively short, the most critical action is to stop the infusion or administration of the DTI when bleeding is suspected. A single case report describes the use of FFP in a patient who received a 13-fold overdose of argatroban. He was treated with FFP for a prolonged aPTT, which did not normalize. Fortunately, the patient did not suffer any bleeding consequences.[38] Orally administered dabigatran has a half-life of 8 to 12 hours, whereas the parenterally administered DTIs have half-lives of approximately 0.5 to 2 hours.[39] Therefore, bleeding while anticoagulated with dabigatran can be particularly difficult to manage. The manufacturers of dabigatran suggest using supportive care and transfusion of pRBCs and FFP. They also mention that rfVIIa, PCC, and hemodialysis may be considered, although there are no prospective, randomized controlled human studies that show better outcomes with any of these interventions. In a murine study, mice with intracranial bleeds were given increasing doses of 4-factor PCC, which resulted in a dose-dependent response in minimizing hematoma expansion; the mice given PCC at doses of 100 U/kg showed the best response, however, in none of the mice were bleeding times normalized. In the same study, neither rfVIIa nor FFP reduced hematoma expansion.[40] Healthy human volunteers anticoagulated with 2.5 days of dabigatran continued to have abnormal coagulation studies despite treatment with 50 U/kg of 4-factor PCC.[41]

Hemodialysis has been proposed as a possible lifesaving intervention in bleeding patients who are anticoagulated with dabigatran. A single study shows that hemodialysis affords extraction ratios of 62% to 68% at hours 2 and 4 during hemodialysis, respectively, but this study was performed in dialysis-dependent patients who were given a single dose of dabigatran.[42] Unfortunately, further pharmacokinetic characterization published in multiple case reports demonstrates that significant drug rebound, up to 87%, following hemodialysis may limit the effectiveness of hemodialysis. Furthermore, while hemodialysis may decrease serum dabigatran concentrations, it does not necessarily normalize aPTT or TT.[43,44] In addition, providers may be reluctant to place a large-bore hemodialysis catheter in an excessively anticoagulated patient. Despite aggressive intervention in some of these patients, including massive transfusion and hemodialysis, deaths from exsanguination in dabigatran-anticoagulated patients may occur.[43,45]

A monoclonal antibody that neutralizes dabigatran is currently undergoing evaluation for use in patients requiring rapid reversal of anticoagulation.[46,47] Until it or another antidote is approved, providers must make use of imperfectly effective options. From the limited available data, the best choice may be to attempt reversal with PCC in aliquots of 25 U/kg up to a maximum of 100 U/kg. The risk of thrombosis remains and should be weighed against the benefits of treatment in a bleeding patient. 4-factor PCC was utilized in studies that evaluated PCC's ability to reverse dabigatran-induced anticoagulation and is, therefore, preferred over 3-factor PCC if available.[40,41] Hemodialysis may be helpful, particularly in patients with suspected supratherapeutic dabigatran concentrations, assuming that the degree of anticoagulation is directly related to dabigatran concentration. Initiation of hemodialysis should not delay required definitive treatments such as operative intervention to control bleeding.

DIRECT FACTOR Xa INHIBITORS

Rivaroxaban and apixaban are orally active, direct factor Xa inhibitors. They are approved for VTE prophylaxis in patients with atrial fibrillation. Rivaroxaban holds an additional indication for VTE prophylaxis in some postsurgical patients. The factor Xa inhibitors may be safer than the DTIs because they prevent thrombin activation upstream from thrombin itself.[48,49] This indirect inactivation allows downstream administration of clotting factors in bleeding patients. While rivaroxaban is both renally and hepatically eliminated, a large portion of apixaban elimination is fecal.[50,51]

Diagnostic Evaluation

Rivaroxaban inhibits factor Xa activity and prolongs PT and PTT via a dose-dependent relationship.[52–56] The HepTest is a nonapproved assay that measures anti-Xa and anti-IIa activity. It is not widely available, and it has not yet gone through the FDA approval process. Studies show that this assay correlates well with the anticoagulant effect of apixaban.[52,53]

Management Guidelines

Similar to the DTIs, the factor Xa inhibitors have no definitive antidotes. In healthy human volunteers given rivaroxaban for 2.5 days, PT and endogenous thrombin potential, a thrombin generation assay, normalized after 50 U/kg of 4-factor PCC.[41] In a rabbit study, bleeding animals continued to bleed despite treatment with 4-factor PCC and rfVIIa, while a battery of coagulation parameters such as bleeding time, aPTT, anti-Xa activity, and clotting time improved.[57] There are currently no studies that evaluate clinical outcomes associated with antidotal treatment in apixaban-treated patients. Unlike dabigatran, rivaroxaban and apixaban are not amenable to hemodialysis because they are highly protein bound.[58]

Because the anticoagulation effect of these factor Xa inhibitors can last more than 24 hours under certain circumstances, specific interventions to reverse anticoagulation may be necessary if supportive measures with volume resuscitation are not helpful. While PCC may help improve coagulation parameters, there are no randomized controlled outcome studies evaluating this intervention. Under life-threatening circumstances, it is reasonable to administer 4-factor PCC in doses of 25 U/kg to patients anticoagulated with direct factor Xa inhibitors. If necessary, repeated doses up to a total of 100 U/kg may be considered, with the knowledge that an unknown risk of thrombosis is present. If 4-factor PCC is not available, 3-factor PCC may be substituted, but its efficacy is not well studied.

LITERATURE TABLE

TRIAL	DESIGN	RESULT
Direct thrombin inhibitors		
Connolly et al., *N Engl J Med* 2009[32] RE-LY	Prospective RCT of 18,113 patients comparing dabigatran to warfarin in patients with atrial fibrillation	Dabigatran at doses of 110 mg twice daily had similar rates of stroke but lower rates of major bleeding when compared to warfarin cohort. Dabigatran at doses of 150 mg twice daily had lower rates of stroke and similar rates of major hemorrhage when compared to warfarin-treated cohort
Eikelboom et al., *Circulation* 2011[33]	Subgroup analysis of the RE-LY Trial	Dabigatran-anticoagulated patients >75 y of age have a higher risk of extracranial bleeding when compared to warfarin-treated patients
Zhou et al., *Stroke* 2011[40]	Murine study where intracranial hemorrhages were induced in mice treated with dabigatran. Subjects received PCC, FFP, or rFVIIa, and coagulation assays and intracranial hematoma volume were compared	rFVIIa and FFP did not prevent hematoma expansion. PCC prevented hematoma expansion in a dose-dependent fashion. Bleeding time improved in a dose-dependent relationship after PCC administration but did not normalize
Eerenberg et al., *Circulation* 2011[41]	Prospective RCT of 12 healthy patients anticoagulated with dabigatran who received 50 U/kg of PCC	No improvement in coagulation assays after PCC administration
Direct factor Xa inhibitors		
Eerenberg et al., *Circulation* 2011[41]	Prospective RCT of 12 healthy patients anticoagulated with rivaroxaban who received 50 U/kg of PCC	Normalization of PT and endogenous thrombin potential after PCC administration
Patel et al., *N Engl J Med* 2011[48]	Prospective RCT of 14,264 patients comparing rivaroxaban to warfarin in patients with atrial fibrillation	Rivaroxaban had similar rates of stroke, systemic thromboembolism, and major bleeding compared to the warfarin cohort. Intracranial and fatal bleeding was lower in the rivaroxaban group
Granger et al., *N Engl J Med* 2011[49]	Prospective RCT of 18,201 patients comparing apixaban to warfarin in patients with atrial fibrillation	Apixaban had lower rates of stroke and systemic thromboembolism, as well as lower bleeding and mortality rates, when compared to warfarin

REFERENCES

1. Fasco MJ, Hildebrandt EF, Suttie JW. Evidence that warfarin anticoagulant action involves two distinct reductase activities. *J Biol Chem.* 1982;257(19):11210–11212.
2. Ageno W, Gallus AS, Wittkowsky A, et al. Oral Anticoagulant Therapy: Antithrombotic Therapy and Prevention of Thrombosis, 9th ed: American College of Chest Physicians Evidence-Based Clinical Practice Guidelines. *Chest.* 2012;141(2 suppl):e44S–e88S.
3. Pisters R, Lane DA, Nieuwlaat R, et al. A novel user-friendly score (HAS-BLED) to assess 1-year risk of major bleeding in patients with atrial fibrillation: the Euro Heart Survey. *Chest.* 2010;138(5):1093–1100.

4. Lip GY, Frison L, Halperin JL, et al. Comparative validation of a novel risk score for predicting bleeding risk in anticoagulated patients with atrial fibrillation: the HAS-BLED (Hypertension, Abnormal Renal/Liver Function, Stroke, Bleeding History or Predisposition, Labile INR, Elderly, Drugs/Alcohol Concomitantly) score. *J Am Coll Cardiol.* 2011;57(2):173–180.
5. Wells PS, Holbrook AM, Crowther NR, et al. Interactions of warfarin with drugs and food. *Ann Intern Med.* 1994;121(9):676–683.
6. Lacy JP, Goodin RR. Letter: warfarin-induced necrosis of skin. *Ann Intern Med.* 1975;82(3):381–382.
7. Vigano S, Mannucci PM, Solinas S, et al. Decrease in protein C antigen and formation of an abnormal protein soon after starting oral anticoagulant therapy. *Br J Haemat.* 1984;57(2):213–220.
8. Comp PC. Coumarin-induced skin necrosis. Incidence, mechanisms, management and avoidance. *Drug Saf.* 1993;8(2):128–135.
9. McGehee WG, Klotz TA, Epstein DJ, et al. Coumarin necrosis associated with hereditary protein C deficiency. *Ann Intern Med.* 1984;101(1):59–60.
10. Nazarian RM, Van Cott EM, Zembowicz A, et al. Warfarin-induced skin necrosis. *J Am Acad Dermatol.* 2009;61(2):325–332.
11. Peterson CE, Kwaan HC. Current concepts of warfarin therapy. *Arch Intern Med.* 1986;146(3):581–584.
12. Hirsh J. Substandard monitoring of warfarin in North America. Time for change. *Arch Intern Med.* 1992;152(2):257–258.
13. Nichols WL, Bowie EJ. Standardization of the prothrombin time for monitoring orally administered anticoagulant therapy with use of the international normalized ratio system. *Mayo Clinic Proc.* 1993;68(9):897–898.
14. Guyatt GH, Akl EA, Crowther M, et al. Executive Summary: Antithrombotic Therapy and Prevention of Thrombosis, 9th ed: American College of Chest Physicians Evidence-Based Clinical Practice Guidelines. *Chest.* 2012;141(2 suppl):7S–47S.
15. Fredriksson K, Norrving B, Stromblad LG. Emergency reversal of anticoagulation after intracerebral hemorrhage. *Stroke.* 1992;23(7):972–977.
16. Cartmill M, Dolan G, Byrne JL, et al. Prothrombin complex concentrate for oral anticoagulant reversal in neurosurgical emergencies. *Br J Neurosurg.* 2000;14(5):458–461.
17. Ageno W, Garcia D, Aguilar MI, et al. Prevention and treatment of bleeding complications in patients receiving vitamin K antagonists, part 2: Treatment. *Am J Hematol.* 2009;84(9):584–588.
18. O'Connell KA, Wood JJ, Wise RP, et al. Thromboembolic adverse events after use of recombinant human coagulation factor VIIa. *JAMA.* 2006;295(3):293–298.
19. Park BK, Scott AK, Wilson AC, et al. Plasma disposition of vitamin K_1 in relation to anticoagulant poisoning. *Br J Clin Pharmacol.* 1984;18(5):655–662.
20. Lubetsky A, Yonath H, Olchovsky D, et al. Comparison of oral vs intravenous phytonadione (vitamin K_1) in patients with excessive anticoagulation: a prospective randomized controlled study. *Arch Intern Med.* 2003;163(20):2469–2473.
21. Rosenberg RD. Actions and interactions of antithrombin and heparin. *N Engl J Med.* 1975;292(3):146–151.
22. Bounameaux H, Goldhaber SZ. Uses of low-molecular-weight heparin. *Blood Rev.* 1995;9(4):213–219.
23. Linkins L-A, Dans AL, Moores LK, et al. Treatment and prevention of heparin-induced thrombocytopenia: Antithrombotic Therapy and Prevention of Thrombosis, 9th ed: American College of Chest Physicians Evidence-Based Clinical Practice Guidelines. *Chest.* 2012;141(2 suppl):e495S–e530S.
24. Aster RH. Heparin-induced thrombocytopenia and thrombosis. *N Engl J Med.* 1995;332(20):1374–1376.
25. Garcia DA, Baglin TP, Weitz JI, et al. Parenteral Anticoagulants: Antithrombotic Therapy and Prevention of Thrombosis, 9th ed: American College of Chest Physicians Evidence-Based Clinical Practice Guidelines. *Chest.* 2012;141(2 suppl):e24S–e43S.
26. Levine MN, Hirsh J, Gent M, et al. A randomized trial comparing activated thromboplastin time with heparin assay in patients with acute venous thromboembolism requiring large daily doses of heparin. *Arch Intern Med.* 1994;154(1):49–56.
27. Alhenc-Gelas M, Jestin-Le Guernic C, Vitoux JF, et al. Adjusted versus fixed doses of the low-molecular-weight heparin fragmin in the treatment of deep vein thrombosis. Fragmin-Study Group. *Thromb Haemost.* 1994;71(6):698–702.
28. Chong BH, Isaacs A. Heparin-induced thrombocytopenia: what clinicians need to know. *Thromb Haemost.* 2009;101(2):279–283.
29. MacLean JA, Moscicki R, Bloch KJ. Adverse reactions to heparin. *Ann Allergy.* 1990;65(4):254–259.
30. McAvoy TJ. Pharmacokinetic modeling of heparin and its clinical implications. *J Pharmacokinet Biopharm.* 1979;7(4):331–354.

31. Pineo GF, Hull RD. Hirudin and hirudin analogues as new anticoagulant agents. *Curr Opin Hematol.* 1995;2(5):380–385.
32. Connolly SJ, Ezekowitz MD, Yusuf S, et al. Dabigatran versus warfarin in patients with atrial fibrillation. *N Engl J Med.* 2009;361(12):1139–1151.
33. Eikelboom JW, Wallentin L, Connolly SJ, et al. Risk of bleeding with 2 doses of dabigatran compared with warfarin in older and younger patients with atrial fibrillation: an analysis of the randomized evaluation of long-term anticoagulant therapy (RE-LY) trial. *Circulation.* 2011;123(21):2363–2372.
34. Harper P, Young L, Merriman E. Bleeding risk with dabigatran in the frail elderly. *N Engl J Med.* 2012;366(9):864–866.
35. Pradaxa (dabigatran etexilate mesylate): Drug Safety Communication—Safety Review of Post-Market Reports of Serious Bleeding Events. *MedWatch The FDA Safety Information and Adverse Event Reporting Program* 2011; http://www.fda.gov/safety/medwatch/safetyinformation/safetyalertsforhumanmedical-products/ucm282820.htm. Accessed October 12, 2012.
36. Uchino K, Hernandez AV. Dabigatran association with higher risk of acute coronary events: meta-analysis of noninferiority randomized controlled trials. *Arch Intern Med.* 2012;172(5):397–402.
37. van Ryn J, Stangier J, Haertter S, et al. Dabigatran etexilate—a novel, reversible, oral direct thrombin inhibitor: interpretation of coagulation assays and reversal of anticoagulant activity. *Thromb Haemost.* 2010;103(6):1116–1127.
38. Yee AJ, Kuter DJ. Successful recovery after an overdose of argatroban. *Ann Pharmacother.* 2006;40(2):336–339.
39. Stangier J, Rathgen K, Stahle H, et al. The pharmacokinetics, pharmacodynamics and tolerability of dabigatran etexilate, a new oral direct thrombin inhibitor, in healthy male subjects. *Br J Clin Pharmacol.* 2007;64(3):292–303.
40. Zhou W, Schwarting S, Illanes S, et al. Hemostatic therapy in experimental intracerebral hemorrhage associated with the direct thrombin inhibitor dabigatran. *Stroke.* 2011;42(12):3594–3599.
41. Eerenberg ES, Kamphuisen PW, Sijpkens MK, et al. Reversal of rivaroxaban and dabigatran by prothrombin complex concentrate: a randomized, placebo-controlled, crossover study in healthy subjects. *Circulation.* 2011;124(14):1573–1579.
42. Stangier J, Rathgen K, Stahle H, et al. Influence of renal impairment on the pharmacokinetics and pharmacodynamics of oral dabigatran etexilate: an open-label, parallel-group, single-centre study. *Clin Pharmacokinet.* 2010;49(4):259–268.
43. Singh T, Maw TT, Henry BL, et al. Extracorporeal therapy for dabigatran removal in the treatment of acute bleeding: a single center experience. *Clin J Am Soc Nephrol.* 2013;8(9):1533–1539.
44. Chang DN, Dager WE, Chin AI. Removal of dabigatran by hemodialysis. *Am J Kidney Dis.* 2013;61(3):487–489.
45. Chen BC, Viny AD, Garlich FM, et al. Hemorrhagic complications associated with dabigatran use. *Clin Toxicol (Phila).* 2012;50(9):854–857.
46. van Ryn J, Litzenburger T, Waterman A, et al. Dabigatran anticoagulant activity is neutralized by an antibody selective to dabigatran in in vitro and in vivo models. *J Am Coll Cardiol.* 2011;57(14): E1130–E1130.
47. Schiele F, van Ryn J, Canada K, et al. A specific antidote for dabigatran: functional and structural characterization. *Blood.* 2013;121(18):3554–3562.
48. Patel MR, Mahaffey KW, Garg J, et al. Rivaroxaban versus warfarin in nonvalvular atrial fibrillation. *N Engl J Med.* 2011;365(10):883–891.
49. Granger CB, Alexander JH, McMurray JJV, et al. Apixaban versus warfarin in patients with atrial fibrillation. *N Engl J Med.* 2011;365(11):981–992.
50. Raghavan N, Frost CE, Yu Z, et al. Apixaban metabolism and pharmacokinetics after oral administration to humans. *Drug Metab Dispos.* 2009;37(1):74–81.
51. Eriksson BI, Quinla DJ, Weitz JI. Comparative pharmacodynamics and pharmacokinetics of oral direct thrombin and factor Xa inhibitors in development. *Clin Pharmacokinet.* 2009;48(1):1–22.
52. Kubitza D, Becka M, Wensing G, et al. Safety, pharmacodynamics, and pharmacokinetics of BAY 59-7939—an oral, direct Factor Xa inhibitor—after multiple dosing in healthy male subjects. *Eur J Clin Pharmacol.* 2005;61(12):873–880.
53. Kubitza D, Becka M, Voith B, et al. Safety, pharmacodynamics, and pharmacokinetics of single doses of BAY 59-7939, an oral, direct factor Xa inhibitor. *Clin Pharmacol Ther.* 2005;78(4):412–421.
54. He K, Luettgen JM, Zhang D, et al. Preclinical pharmacokinetics and pharmacodynamics of apixaban, a potent and selective factor Xa inhibitor. *Eur J Drug Metab Pharmacoknet.* 2011;36(3):129–139.

55. Mantha S, Cabral K, Ansell J. New avenues for anticoagulation in atrial fibrillation. *Clin Pharmacol Ther.* 2013;93(1):68–77.
56. Wong PC, Crain EJ, Xin B, et al. Apixaban, an oral, direct and highly selective factor Xa inhibitor: in vitro, antithrombotic and antihemostatic studies. *J Thromb Haemost.* 2008;6(5):820–829.
57. Godier A, Miclot A, Le Bonniec B, et al. Evaluation of prothrombin complex concentrate and recombinant activated factor VII to reverse rivaroxaban in a rabbit model. *Anesthesiology.* 2012;116(1):94–102.
58. Weitz JI, Eikelboom JW, Samama MM. New Antithrombotic Drugs: Antithrombotic Therapy and Prevention of Thrombosis, 9th ed: American College of Chest Physicians Evidence-Based Clinical Practice Guidelines. *Chest.* 2012;141(2 suppl):e120S–e151S.

51

Drugs of Abuse

Rana Biary and Jane Marie Prosser

OPIOIDS

Background

Opioids comprise both naturally occurring and synthetic compounds that bind to the μ opioid receptor. μ receptors are located throughout the body, notably in regions of the brain related to analgesia, which include the periaqueductal gray matter, nucleus raphe magnus, and the medial thalamus. They are also found in the respiratory center of the medulla and the gastrointestinal tract.[1] Opioids have been used since ancient times as analgesics, appearing as early as 1500 BC in the *Ebers Papyrus* as a "remedy to prevent excessive crying in children." By the 16th century, there were manuscripts detailing opioid addiction, tolerance, and withdrawal.[2] In 1914, the Harrison Narcotic Act made nonmedical use of opioids illegal in the United States.[1] Heroin is the classic opioid street drug of abuse; however, prescription opioids have become increasingly more common. In New York City, in 2009, prescription opioids surpassed motor vehicle collisions, cocaine, and heroin as the leading cause of accidental death.[3,4]

History and Physical Exam

Opioids can be ingested, injected, insufflated, inhaled, absorbed through the oral and rectal mucosa, or applied topically. The classic clinical presentation—or toxidrome—of an opioid overdose is similar regardless of which opioid is used. It includes miosis, a depressed respiratory rate, and a depressed mental status. Additionally, the patient may have decreased bowel sounds and a mildly decreased blood pressure.[5,6]

Patients with severe overdose may present with hypoxia and crackles on pulmonary exam, consistent with a noncardiogenic pulmonary edema.[5,7] Another, albeit less common presentation, often attributed to rapid bolus injection of fentanyl, is the development of chest wall rigidity.[8,9]

Certain opioids are also known to cause unique complications. The opioid tramadol can cause seizures even in therapeutic doses. Tramadol also causes serotonin syndrome, characterized by hyperthermia, clonus, rigidity, and tremor.[10,11] The synthetic opioids methadone and buprenorphine are known to prolong the QT interval, predisposing patients to torsade de pointes.[12] Intravenous drug users are also at risk for developing complications associated with nonsterile venous puncture, including endocarditis, septic emboli, and epidural abscess.

Differential Diagnosis

Clonidine, an imidazole derivative, is used in the treatment of hypertension, pediatric behavioral disorders, and the treatment of opioid withdrawal. It has some effects on the μ receptor, producing clinical findings resembling opioid overdose, including meiosis and respiratory depression.[1] Clonidine overdoses, by contrast, are usually associated with distinct vital sign abnormalities not common to opiate overdose, including significant bradycardia and hypotension. Benzodiazepines and barbiturates can, like opiates, result in a depressed mental status and respiratory rate.[1] Gamma hydroxybuturate (GHB) may also lead to a depressed respiratory rate and mental status, though its effects are usually transient. The pupils in patients who have overdosed on GHB may also be mitotic and minimally responsive to light.[1] Phencyclidine (PCP), typically described as a stimulant, may in large doses behave as a sedative. Patients will typically have a depressed mental status with mydriasis and rotary nystagmus.

In addition to these drugs, other common etiologies of depressed mental status, including trauma, metabolic disorders (hypoglycemia, hyponatremia), infection, hypoxia, and hypothermia, must always be considered.

Diagnostic Evaluation

Physical exam is the essential tool for the diagnosis of opioid intoxication. As noted, the exam of the patient with opioid intoxication will include pinpoint pupils with a depressed mental status and respiratory rate. Response to naloxone has been suggested to aid in diagnosis but can be associated with complications when used in the undifferentiated patient and is therefore not recommended.

Urine toxicology screens are of limited utility and are therefore not routinely recommended. The urine toxicology screen generally tests for morphine, and because of this, naturally occurring opioids such as heroin and morphine will result in a positive test. Synthetic opioids such as methadone and fentanyl, however, are not metabolized to morphine or its metabolites, and will not result in a positive test. Semisynthetic opioids such as oxycodone and hydrocodone produce variable results. Additionally, a positive result may persist long after acute intoxication. For example, heroin use can result in a positive urine drug screen for up to 4 days post ingestion, giving a potentially misleading explanation for the patient's current symptoms.[13]

Additional testing should include an ECG, liver function tests, and a serum acetaminophen concentration. On the ECG, particular attention should be given to the QTc interval length. Because of the increasing abuse of prescription opioids containing acetaminophen, routine laboratory testing is recommended. In patients who present with crackles, hypoxia, or tachypnea, chest radiography should be performed to look for pulmonary edema.

Management Guidelines

The most common cause of death from opioid overdose is respiratory arrest. The first step in management of a patient with suspected opioid intoxication is to ensure airway management. Administration of naloxone, an opioid antagonist, should be considered in patients with an opioid toxidrome. Studies suggest that naloxone is most likely to be of benefit in those patients whose respiratory rate is <12, or who have significant hypoventilation.[36] To prevent precipitation of withdrawal, a low initial dose of 0.04 to 0.05 mg of naloxone should be administered. The dose can be titrated to an arousable mental status and a respiratory rate of approximately 8 to 10 breaths per minute.[1] Bolus administration can be followed by an infusion, titrated to maintain the same goals. The recommended starting dose for the infusion is two-thirds of the effective bolus dose.[14]

In non–opioid dependent patients, naloxone has few side effects even in high doses.[15] However, injudicious administration in opioid-dependent patients may result in withdrawal including vomiting and diarrhea. This can be harmful in several scenarios. If naloxone is administered to an opioid-dependent patient whose altered mental status is due to a different etiology, vomiting may occur without an increase in mental status, increasing the risk for aspiration. Opiate reversal with naloxone administration in the setting of marked hypoxemia and hypercarbia can also lead to a large catecholamine surge (as an appropriate response to respiratory deficits) and subsequent pulmonary edema. Administration of several breaths via bag valve mask prior to administration will minimize hypoxia and hypercarbia and reduce the likelihood of this response.[16,17]

The duration of action of naloxone is 20 to 90 minutes, shorter than the half-life of most opioids, including heroin.[1] Therefore, patients requiring naloxone should be observed for at least 4 to 6 hours to ensure that they do not develop recurrent respiratory depression. Patients who overdose on long-acting opioids, such as methadone or extended-release oxycodone, will require observation for 24 hours. In patients with a depressed mental status, gastric decontamination with charcoal should be avoided due to the risk of aspiration.

Clinicians must also consider the possibility of unintentional coingestion of adulterants. While classic adulterants included strychnine and quinine, more recently levamisole, caffeine, acetaminophen, phenobarbital, methaqualone, scopolamine, and clenbuterol have also been used.[18]

BENZODIAZEPINES

Background

Benzodiazepines were introduced in the 1960s, as sedatives with a safer side effect profile than that of barbiturates. In Florida, between 2003 and 2009, there was a 233.8% increase in reported deaths caused by alprazolam.[19] A study from the United Kingdom evaluated 1,024 consecutive patients admitted to the hospital, and found that diazepam was the fourth most commonly abused drug overall (third most common among men).[20] Benzodiazepines fall under the category of sedative hypnotics, and act on the $GABA_A$ receptor.[1]

History and Physical Exam

The typical presentation of a benzodiazepine overdose is a depressed mental status with normal vital signs. Patients may also present with slurred speech, gait ataxia, and coma. Respiratory depression is not expected with oral ingestion, unless coingestants such as ethanol or other sedatives have also been consumed.[21] Controversy exists regarding respiratory depression after IV administration, with a few case reports suggesting it may occur.[1]

Another important consideration in cases of intravenous administration of benzodiazepines, particularly in a hospital setting, is the use of diluents. Lorezepam, for example, is typically carried in propylene glycol, which, when administered rapidly, can lead to hypotension. Prolonged exposure to propylene glycol, as occurs with continuous infusions, can lead to an elevated lactate metabolic acidosis.[22]

Differential Diagnosis

The differential diagnosis for benzodiazepines overdose is similar to opioid overdose, and includes any medical condition or toxic ingestion that can result in altered sensorium (e.g., ethanol or opioid ingestion, hypoglycemia, hypoxia, infection).

Diagnostic Evaluation

If the diagnosis is clear on presentation, few tests are likely to add to the clinical picture. As with all overdose patients, acetaminophen and salicylate concentrations and an ECG are useful screening tests to evaluate for potential coingestants.[23] However, if the diagnosis is uncertain, as is often the case, then evaluation of a patient's altered mental status should proceed in the standard fashion, including comprehensive blood testing, head computed tomography, and cerebral spinal fluid (CSF) analysis. As with opioid intoxication, a urine toxicology screen is of limited utility due to false-positive and -negative results.

Management Guidelines

Initial management centers on assessing airway, breathing, and circulation. Intravenous access, cardiac monitoring, and close observation are also indicated. As noted, respiratory depression is not expected with oral benzodiazepine overdose, but sedation and loss of airway protection requiring intubation is possible. Gastric decontamination using charcoal should be avoided due to the risk of aspiration in patients with a depressed mental status.

Flumazenil is a benzodiazepine receptor antagonist and has been used to treat benzodiazepine overdose; however, its use is not routinely recommended due to its risk of precipitating withdrawal, which can be a life-threatening complication.[24] Intubation and mechanical ventilation are generally considered safer than flumazenil in the treatment of benzodiazepine-associated respiratory depression.[25] In circumstances in which the risk of preexisting benzodiazepine dependence is minimal—such as with pediatric patients or patients post procedural sedation—the likelihood of flumazenil precipitating withdrawal will be acceptably low and its use may be reasonable.

Patients with isolated benzodiazepine overdose are expected to have good outcomes, and generally improve with supportive care and close observation. Benzodiazepine withdrawal (covered in the following chapter) can, however, be life threatening.

SYMPATHOMIMETICS

Background

Sympathomimetics are a large category of compounds that cause increased excitatory neurotransmitter release. They include drugs such as amphetamines, phenylethylamines such as MDMA, cocaine, and synthetic cathinone derivatives often referred to as "bath salts." These compounds produce effects specific to each compound; however, common to all is the increased release of epinephrine, norepinephrine, and dopamine, which leads to increased activation of the sympathetic nervous system and euphoria. Certain sympathomimetics, such as the phenylethylamines, also modulate serotonin release.

Patients with sympathomimetic intoxication are at risk for hyperthermia, dysrhythmias, myocardial infarction, strokes, hyponatremia, and death. Stimulants such as ecstasy and bath salts often do not contain the ingredients they are sold as, and may contain different sympathomimetics, caffeine, or even placebo. Furthermore, compounds marketed as "legal highs" may contain illegal substances.[26–29]

History and Physical Exam

Patients with sympathomimetic intoxication present with a variety of issues that occur as a result of increased sympathetic output. The sympathomimetic toxidrome includes mydriasis, hypertension, tachycardia, diaphoresis, hyperthermia, and psychomotor agitation.

The wide range of potential complications associated with sympathomimetic use highlights the importance of a thorough history and physical exam. Signs and symptoms may suggest stroke, seizure (either due to direct sympathomimetic toxicity or from secondary hyponatremia), intracranial hemorrhage, myocardial infarction, and other complications that can accompany increased sympathetic output.

Differential Diagnosis

The differential diagnosis of sympathomimetic toxicity includes any medication capable of causing a sympathomimetic toxidrome including cocaine, PCP/ketamine, amphetamines, and newer synthetic drugs of abuse including bath salts and synthetic cannabis/cannabinoid compounds such as "k2" or "Spice." Patients who are withdrawing from a sedative/hypnotic may also present with altered mental status, diaphoresis, and autonomic instability that can clinically resemble the sympathomimetic toxidrome. As with any suspected overdose that produces a depressed mental status, unless the offending agent is clearly identified, a more comprehensive evaluation is necessary.

Diagnostic Evaluation

Unlike benzodiazepine overdose, patients who present after sympathomimetic intoxication require further diagnostic evaluation, including laboratory evaluation. Laboratory tests should include a basic metabolic panel to evaluate for hyponatremia secondary to drug-induced SIADH and increased free water consumption. Patients may also develop rhabdomyolysis secondary to sympathomimetic ingestion; therefore, a creatinine phosphokinase should be checked, as well as renal function. As in any overdose, acetaminophen and aspirin concentrations should be checked, given the concern for coingestants. As with other ingestions, a urine toxicology screen is of limited utility. Testing should include an ECG to ensure absence of ST-segment changes, as sympathomimetics may be associated with coronary vasospasm. Altered mental status in the setting of sympathomimetic use requires a CT head to rule out stroke, seizure, or intracranial hemorrhage.

Management Guidelines

Prioritization of treatment of sympathomimetic toxicity is guided by patient presentation. In a patient with uncontrolled psychomotor agitation, adequate dosing with benzodiazepines is necessary to ensure that the patient is appropriately sedated and not at risk of harm to self or others. While any benzodiazepine may be used, benzodiazepines with quicker onset, such as midazolam or diazepam, are preferred. Lorazepam, while acceptable, takes approximately 20 minutes to produce peak therapeutic effect.

Hyperthermia is the most common cause of death in patients with sympathomimetic toxicity. High ambient temperatures are known to compound sympathomimetic-induced hyperthermia; in a retrospective review of medical examiner cases from 1990 to 1995, a 33% increase in the mean daily number of cocaine overdose deaths was recorded when ambient temperatures exceeded 31.1°C (2.4 more deaths per day).[30] Initial management should therefore include obtaining a core temperature. If hyperthermia is present, rapid and aggressive treatment is essential. Classically, a "mist and fan" technique has been suggested, although this requires fans of much stronger caliber than are available in most hospitals. For severe hyperthermia, an ice bath is a more efficient intervention. To avoid the risk of overshoot and secondary hypothermia, patients should be removed from the ice bath once core temperatures fall below 38°C.[31]

Because patients with psychomotor agitation and hyperthermia are at risk for muscle breakdown, rhabdomyolysis should be treated empirically with fluid hydration. Urine output should be maintained at a minimum of 1 mL/kg/h.

Patients reporting chest pain should have an ECG performed immediately. Cocaine use can produce coronary vasospasm, as well as increased platelet aggregation and coronary artery atherosclerosis. The management for patients who present with cocaine-induced chest pain parallels the management of ACS with two important exceptions. Cocaine-induced chest pain should be treated with benzodiazepines to decrease the central nervous system release of epinephrine and norepinephrine. Beta-blockers should be avoided, as there is risk not only of worsening the coronary vasospasm but also of further elevating the blood pressure from an unopposed alpha effect.[32] Aspirin should be administered, especially given the increased risk of platelet aggregation that accompanies chronic cocaine use. Nitroglycerin can help with smooth muscle relaxation and may improve coronary vasospasm. In patients with refractory chest pain, phentolamine, an alpha-1 blocker, should be given.[33] Finally, as patients who abuse cocaine and other sympathomimetics are predisposed to coronary artery disease, a cardiac catheterization in patients with ST-segment elevation is indicated.[34]

Seizures may occur in the setting of sympathomimetic overdose because of stimulation of excitatory neurotransmitters; seizures may also occur due to drug-induced hyponatremia.[35] Drugs of abuse, such as MDMA, can lead to hyponatremia through a combination of SIADH and increased free water consumption. Hypertonic saline should be considered in any patient suspected of having ingested MDMA who is actively seizing or who has an altered mental status.

CONCLUSION

Patients with opioid, benzodiazepine, and sympathomimetic overdose commonly present to the ED. Once the emergency physician is familiar with the clinical toxidromes of these overdoses, a focused bedside physical exam will enable formulation of an accurate differential diagnosis and appropriate plan of care.

LITERATURE TABLE		
TRIAL	**DESIGN**	**RESULT**
Opioids		
Duberstein et al., *Am J Med.* 1971[5]	Retrospective study of all heroin overdose cases admitted to two hospitals between July 1, 1968 and November 30, 1970	One hundred and forty-nine patients, all with depressed mental status and depressed respiratory rate. Seventy percent presented with pulmonary edema. Thirteen deaths occurred; all had pulmonary edema
Goldfrank et al., *Ann Emerg Med.* 1986[14]	Two-phase study to determine the pharmacokinetics of naloxone. Developed a continuous dosing nomogram	Continuous infusion of two-thirds of the bolus dose that resulted in reversal should be started for patients requiring continuous infusion
Hoffman et al., *Ann Emerg Med.* 1991[36]	Review of Emergency Medical Service run sheets of 730 patients administered naloxone to determine whether clinical criteria could predict response to naloxone in patients with altered mental status	A respiratory rate <12/min is predictive of a response to naloxone
Benzodiazepines		
Greenblatt et al., *Clin Pharmacol Ther.* 1997[21]	Retrospective review of 773 patients admitted to the Massachusetts General Hospital between 1962 and 1975 with acute overdose on psychotropic drugs	No patient with overdose on oral benzodiazepines alone was observed to have significant toxicity. The frequency and severity of complications (CNS depression, need for assisted ventilation) escalated when benzodiazepines were taken in combination with another medication or drug
Arroliga et al., *Crit Care Med.* 2004[22]	Prospective, observational study of 9 patients receiving high-dose lorazepam infusions (>10 mg/h) to evaluate the relationship between high-dose lorazepam and serum propylene glycol concentrations	Significant laboratory findings consistent with propylene glycol toxicity were present in 6/9 patients at 48 hours as evidenced by an elevated osmolar gap as well as an elevated anion gap. A significant correlation between high-dose lorazepam infusion rate and serum propylene glycol concentration was observed ($r = 0.557$, $p = 0.021$)
Spivey. *Clin Ther.* 1992[24]	Review of 43 patients who developed seizures in proximity to receiving flumazenil	Forty-seven percent of patients had reversal of benzodiazepines suppressing drug-induced seizures. Twelve percent of patients had reversal of benzodiazepines suppressing non–drug-induced seizures. Sixteen percent of patients had reversal of benzodiazepines given for a seizure disorder. Seven percent had reversal of chronic benzodiazepine dependence. Five percent had reversal of benzodiazepines given for conscious sedation. Fourteen percent had no apparent causal relationship
Sympathomimetics		
Baggott et al., *JAMA.* 2000[28]	Ecstasy tablets obtained though an internet site sampled for their contents	One hundred and seven pills were received and assayed, 29% contained identifiable drugs but not MDMA. The most common drug identified was dextromethorphan, although caffeine, ephedrine, and pseudoephedrine were also found. Eight percent of pills had no identifiable drug

(*Continued*)

LITERATURE TABLE (*Continued*)

TRIAL	DESIGN	RESULT
Marzuk et al., *JAMA*. 1998[30]	Retrospective review of 2008 unintentional fatal cocaine overdoses (medical examiner cases, 1990 to 1995)	When ambient temperatures were >31.1°C there was an increase in mean daily number of cocaine overdose deaths of 2.34 (SD 1.68), 33% higher than the mean on days with a maximum temperature of <31.1°C ($p < 0.001$)
Boehrer et al., *Am J Medicine*. 1993[32]	Prospective study of the influence of cocaine on coronary vasoconstriction. Fifteen patients undergoing cardiac catheterization had heart rate, mean arterial pressure, and coronary artery area measured at: (1) baseline, (2) 15 min following administration of intranasal cocaine, and (3) 5 min after saline or labetalol	Intranasal cocaine led to increased myocardial oxygen demand and decreased myocardial oxygen supply through coronary vasoconstriction; labetalol reduced mean arterial pressure ($p = 0.05$), but did not improve coronary vasoconstriction ($p =$ NS)
McCord et al., *Circulation*. 2008[34]	American Heart Association recommendations for management of cocaine-associated chest pain and myocardial infarction based on critical review of the literature form 1960 to 2007	In cocaine-associated chest pain, patients should be treated with aspirin and benzodiazepines; this can be followed by intravenous nitroglycerin or nitroprusside for persistent hypertension (alternative: phentolamine). High-risk patients who present with a ST segment myocardial infarction should undergo catheterization. Beta-blocking agents should be avoided

REFERENCES

1. Lewis S, Nelson NAL, Howland MA, et al. Goldfrank's Toxicologic Emergencies. 9th ed. New York, NY: The McGraw-Hill Companies, Inc.; 2011.
2. Brownstein MJ. A brief history of opiates, opioid peptides, and opioid receptors. *Proc Natl Acad Sci U S A.* 1993;90(12):5391–5393.
3. Tanne JH. Deaths from prescription opioids soar in New York. *BMJ.* 2013;346:f921.
4. Manchikanti L, et al. Opioid epidemic in the United States. *Pain Physician.* 2012;15(3 suppl):ES9–ES38.
5. Duberstein JL, Kaufman DM. A clinical study of an epidemic of heroin intoxication and heroin-induced pulmonary edema. *Am J Med.* 1971;51(6):704–714.
6. Afshari R., Maxwell SR, Bateman DN. Hemodynamic effects of methadone and dihydrocodeine in overdose. *Clin Toxicol (Phila).* 2007;45(7):763–772.
7. Sporer KA, Dorn E. Heroin-related noncardiogenic pulmonary edema: a case series. *Chest.* 2001;120(5):1628–1632.
8. Coruh B, Tonelli MR, Park DR. Fentanyl-induced chest wall rigidity. *Chest.* 2013;143(4):1145–1146.
9. Fahnenstich H, et al. Fentanyl-induced chest wall rigidity and laryngospasm in preterm and term infants. *Crit Care Med.* 2000;28(3):836–839.
10. Abadie D, et al. "Serious" adverse drug reactions with tramadol: a 2010–2011 pharmacovigilance survey in France. *Therapie.* 2013;68(2):77–84.
11. Shadnia S, et al. Recurrent seizures in tramadol intoxication: implications for therapy based on 100 patients. *Basic Clin Pharmacol Toxicol.* 2012;111(2):133–136.
12. Krantz MJ, et al. QTc interval screening in methadone treatment. *Ann Intern Med.* 2009;150(6):387–395.
13. Moeller KE, Lee KC, Kissack JC. Urine drug screening: practical guide for clinicians. *Mayo Clin Proc.* 2008;83(1):66–76.
14. Goldfrank L, et al. A dosing nomogram for continuous infusion intravenous naloxone. *Ann Emerg Med.* 1986;15(5):566–570.

15. Bracken MB, et al. A randomized, controlled trial of methylprednisolone or naloxone in the treatment of acute spinal-cord injury. Results of the Second National Acute Spinal Cord Injury Study. *N Engl J Med.* 1990;322(20):1405–1411.
16. Mills CA, et al. Narcotic reversal in hypercapnic dogs: comparison of naloxone and nalbuphine. *Can J Anaesth.* 1990;37(2):238–244.
17. Mills CA, et al. Cardiovascular effects of fentanyl reversal by naloxone at varying arterial carbon dioxide tensions in dogs. *Anesth Analg.* 1988;67(8):730–736.
18. Hamilton RJ, et al. A descriptive study of an epidemic of poisoning caused by heroin adulterated with scopolamine. *J Toxicol Clin Toxicol.* 2000;38(6):597–608.
19. Centers for Disease, Control and Prevention. Drug overdose deaths—Florida, 2003–2009. *MMWR Morb Mortal Wkly Rep.* 2011;60(26):869–872.
20. Armstrong TM, et al. Comparative drug dose and drug combinations in patients that present to hospital due to self-poisoning. *Basic Clin Pharmacol Toxicol.* 2012;111(5):356–360.
21. Greenblatt DJ, et al. Acute overdosage with benzodiazepine derivatives. *Clin Pharmacol Ther.* 1977;21(4):497–514.
22. Arroliga AC, et al. Relationship of continuous infusion lorazepam to serum propylene glycol concentration in critically ill adults. *Crit Care Med.* 2004;32(8):1709–1714.
23. Lucanie R, Chiang WK, Reilly R. Utility of acetaminophen screening in unsuspected suicidal ingestions. *Vet Hum Toxicol.* 2002;44(3):171–173.
24. Spivey WH. Flumazenil and seizures: analysis of 43 cases. *Clin Ther.* 1992;14(2):292–305.
25. Clemmesen C, Nilsson E. Therapeutic trends in the treatment of barbiturate poisoning. The Scandinavian method. *Clin Pharmacol Ther.* 1961;2:220–229.
26. Ramsey J, et al., Buying "legal" recreational drugs does not mean that you are not breaking the law. *QJM.* 2010;103(10):777–783.
27. Davies S, et al. Purchasing "legal highs" on the Internet—is there consistency in what you get? *QJM.* 2010;103(7):489–493.
28. Baggott M, et al. Chemical analysis of ecstasy pills. *JAMA.* 2000;284(17):2190.
29. Wood DM, et al. Case series of individuals with analytically confirmed acute mephedrone toxicity. *Clin Toxicol (Phila).* 2010;48(9):924–927.
30. Marzuk PM, et al. Ambient temperature and mortality from unintentional cocaine overdose. *JAMA.* 1998;279(22):1795–1800.
31. Costrini A. Emergency treatment of exertional heatstroke and comparison of whole body cooling techniques. *Med Sci Sports Exerc.* 1990;22(1):15–18.
32. Boehrer JD, et al. Influence of labetalol on cocaine-induced coronary vasoconstriction in humans. *Am J Med.* 1993;94(6):608–610.
33. Hollander JE, Carter WA, Hoffman RS. Use of phentolamine for cocaine-induced myocardial ischemia. *N Engl J Med.* 1992;327(5):361.
34. McCord J, et al. Management of cocaine-associated chest pain and myocardial infarction: a scientific statement from the American Heart Association Acute Cardiac Care Committee of the Council on Clinical Cardiology. *Circulation.* 2008;117(14):1897–1907.
35. Ajaelo, I, Koenig K, Snoey E. Severe hyponatremia and inappropriate antidiuretic hormone secretion following ecstasy use. *Acad Emerg Med.* 1998;5(8):839–840.
36. Hoffman JR, et al. The empiric use of naloxone in patients with altered mental status: a reappraisal. *Ann Emerg Med.* 1991;20(3):246–252.

52

Alcohol Withdrawal

Nicole Bouchard

BACKGROUND

Chronic alcoholism and alcohol withdrawal syndrome (AWS) are serious disorders that affect millions of people worldwide. AWS is frequently encountered in hospitalized patients and contributes significantly to patient morbidity and mortality. AWS also imposes a considerable financial burden on hospitals, as these patient visits are often prolonged and not fully reimbursed. In spite of the high volume of medical admissions for moderate to severe AWS, relatively little evidence-based literature addresses its management. This is particularly true in the intensive care unit (ICU), where management varies significantly among institutions.

PATHOPHYSIOLOGY

When the central nervous system is exposed to long-term ethanol use, compensatory changes occur to counter ethanol's depressant effects on the inhibitory centers of the cerebral cortex. The net effect of these compensatory changes is to restore cerebral homeostasis despite the near-constant presence of ethanol. Tolerance to ethanol is an example of such a compensatory changes change. Alcohol potentiates γ-aminobutyric acid ($GABA_A$) signaling by increasing the $GABA_A$ chloride channel opening. With chronic ethanol use, the persistently stimulated inhibitory $GABA_A$ receptors become down-regulated and less sensitive to ethanol.[1–5] Ethanol also inhibits glutamate, the excitatory neurotransmitter that binds to and activates the excitatory *N*-methyl-D-aspartate (NMDA) receptor. In chronic ethanol use, NMDA receptor systems are up-regulated and become more sensitive to glutamate.[6–9] Ethanol use is also associated with increased brain dopamine; this is thought to be a contributing factor to some of its acutely pleasurable effects and addictive qualities.[9–11]

When ethanol exposure is abruptly terminated, there is a loss of homeostasis, and these neurotransmitter systems become imbalanced. This absence of ethanol's depressant effects on the already desensitized, down-regulated GABA system combined with the enhanced NMDA excitatory system and dysregulation of the dopaminergic system is primarily responsible for the development of unopposed CNS excitation and the hyperexcited state associated with AWS.[12–14]

Chronic ethanol use is also thought to desensitize α_2 receptors. The increased dopamine seen with ethanol use is metabolized to norepinephrine (NE) by dopamine-β-hydroxylase, resulting in an increase in available NE. Chronically impaired α_2 receptor activity in the face of increased NE results in adrenergic receptor up-regulation and adrenergic hypersensitivity. These effects may explain the increased sympathetic nervous system activity observed in alcohol withdrawal.[15–17]

HISTORY AND PHYSICAL EXAM

Initial steps in the successful treatment of adult patients at risk of or actively experiencing AWS include early recognition of AWS, appropriate patient disposition, early initiation of symptom-triggered therapy (STT),[18–25] and/or front-loading with benzodiazepines.[26] Early recognition of AWS requires detailed history taking and an awareness of the stages of withdrawal.

Clinical manifestations of alcohol withdrawal occur along a spectrum and often coexist with other pathophysiologic states. Psychological symptoms range from mild anxiety, insomnia, craving, irritability, and labile emotions to significant agitation, trouble thinking clearly, and altered mental status (AMS) or frank delirium. Physical symptoms include headache, diaphoresis, nausea and vomiting, tachycardia, hypertension, tremor, tongue fasciculations, hyperthermia, and seizures.

The typical withdrawal timeline after a patient's last drink is as follows:

- 6 to 12 hours: acute tremulousness ("the shakes"), insomnia, headache
- 12 to 24 hours: visual and/or auditory hallucinations, also known as alcohol hallucinosis
- 6 to 48 hours (or earlier with rapidly declining blood alcohol level [BAL]): seizures ("rum fits") (typically several, usually short and self-terminating)
- 72 to 96 hours: delirium tremens (DT or "DTs") characterized by AMS, delirium, hyperdynamic circulation, hyperventilation, and hyperthermia. DTs may persist for up to 2 weeks (1 week is more common)

Although AWS tends to occur in a temporal progression, there is no fixed sequence. Completion of alcohol withdrawal typically lasts 4 to 7 days; however, significant withdrawal can last up to 2 weeks.[27] Historically, approximately 5% of all patients with AWS will progress to DTs[28]; this number jumps to over 30% for patients who experience withdrawal seizures.[29] In modern times, advances in medical therapy and ICU care have decreased the mortality from AWS with DT from 37% to 5%.[30–33]

DIFFERENTIAL DIAGNOSIS

It is important to consider the complete clinical picture when caring for a patient with AWS. Not only does AWS frequently exist as a result of or in parallel with another pathophysiologic process, but its signs and symptoms can also be masked or complicated by other processes (Table 52.1). Occasionally, symptoms such as isolated tachycardia are wrongly attributed to AWS in the ethanol-dependent patient. Similarly, confounding AWS with other diagnoses (encephalopathy, psychosis, delirium from another cause, CNS injury, infection) can lead to wrong diagnoses, inappropriate sedation, and withheld treatments.[34]

TABLE 52.1 AWS Precipitants and Exacerbating Factors

Category of Precipitant/Complicating Factor	Examples
Comorbid acute medical diagnoses	Trauma, infection, cirrhosis, pancreatitis, gastritis, hepatitis
Comorbid psychiatric diagnoses	Psychosis, suicidality, depression, mania
Other substance addiction or withdrawal	Other benzodiazepines, opioids, cocaine
Iatrogenic causes	Evolution of symptoms while hospitalized, failure of providers to recognize, anticipate, or prevent AWS
Prior AWS episodes	Prior history of significant or undertreated AWS predicts similar or more severe course
Comorbid chronic diagnoses	Medication or treatment nonadherence with coexisting diagnoses, concurrent complicating diagnoses
Comorbid metabolic disarray	Alcohol ketoacidosis, dehydration, electrolyte and vitamin deficiencies

DIAGNOSTIC EVALUATION

A history of physiologic tolerance to ethanol from years of heavy use, coupled with recent cessation or reduction in ethanol intake, places patients at risk for developing AWS, severe AWS, and/or DT. Risk factors for the development of severe AWS and/or DT include duration of ethanol abuse; quantity of ethanol consumed; history of repeated episodes of AWS, DTs, or seizures; withdrawal symptoms with a positive BAL; mild intoxication with BAL >300 to 400 mg/dL; and comorbid infections.[27,35–38] Hypokalemia, thrombocytopenia, and presence of structural brain lesions are additional independent predictors of more severe withdrawal.[36] Certain populations may also be predisposed to severe AWS, and there may be a genetic or racial component (Whites appear more at risk than Blacks for severe AWS).[33,39] When admitted to the hospital, high-risk patients should undergo careful risk assessment, followed by management using an established clinical care pathway. Unrecognized or undertreated withdrawal may progress to more severe withdrawal and exacerbate future episodes of AWS, underscoring the importance of early recognition and treatment.

The most commonly used and highly validated scoring systems for the assessment and STT of AWS are the Clinical Institute Withdrawal Assessment—Alcohol (CIWA-Ar, Ar: Alcohol-revised, and, where available, a new version CIWA-Ad) (Table 52.2).[22,24,26,27,34,40–44] Care must be taken to apply the CIWA score correctly to at-risk patients to avoid erroneous attribution of symptoms to patients not in AWS.[34] Some centers use abridged, institution-specific assessment tools; these may be convenient at a local hospital level but have not been extensively validated.

The strength of the CIWA tools is the ability to detect AWS at an early stage, when treatment will be maximally beneficial. The CIWA-Ar/Ad score becomes more difficult to evaluate in patients with very high scores, DTs, or benzodiazepine-resistant AWS. In these cases, the goal of STT is to maintain light sedation, and an agitation/sedation score such as the Richmond Agitation Sedation Score (RASS) may be a more useful assessment tool (Table 52.3).

TABLE 52.2 Clinical Institute Withdrawal Assessment - Alcohol (CIWA-Ar)

Patient: ____________ **MR #:** ____________ **Date:** (yy/mm/dd) ____/____/____

Time: (24 hr) ________

Pulse or heart rate: ________ **Blood Pressure:** __________ **Temp:** __________

Nausea and Vomiting: Ask *"Do you feel sick to your stomach?" "Have you vomited?"*

Observation:

0 —no nausea and no vomiting
1 —mild nausea with no vomiting
2
3
4 —intermittent nausea with dry heaves
5
6
7 —constant nausea, frequent dry heaves and vomiting

Tremor: Arms extended and fingers spread apart.

Observation:

0 —no tremor
1 —not visible, but can be felt fingertip to fingertip
2
3
4 —moderate, with patient's arms extended
5
6
7 —severe, even with arms not extended

Paroxysmal Sweats:

Observation:

0 —no sweat visible
1 —barely perceptible sweating, palms moist
2
3
4 —beads of sweat obvious on forehead
5
6
7 —drenching sweats

Anxiety: Ask "Do you feel nervous?"

Observation:

0 —no anxiety, at ease
1 —mildly anxious
2
3
4 —moderately anxious, or guarded, so anxiety is inferred
5
6
7 —equivalent to acute panic states as seen in severe delirium or acute schizophrenic reactions

Tactile Disturbances: Ask "Have you any itching, pins and needles sensations, any burning, any numbness, or do you feel bugs crawling on or under your skin?

Observation:

0 —none
1 —very mild itching, pins and needles, burning or numbness
2 —mild itching, pins and needles, burning or numbness
3 —moderate itching, pins and needles, burning or numbness
4 —moderately sever hallucinations
5 —severe hallucinations
6 —extremely severe hallucinations
7 —continuous hallucinations

Auditory Disturbances: Ask "Are you more aware of sounds around you? Are they harsh? Do they frighten you? Are you hearing anything that is disturbing to you? Are you hearing things that you know aren't there?"

Observation:

0 —not present
1 —very mild harshness or ability to frighten
2 —mild harshness or ability to frighten
3 —moderate harshness or ability to frighten
4 —moderately severe hallucinations
5 —severe hallucinations
6 —extremely severe hallucinations
7 —continuous hallucinations

Visual Disturbances: Ask "Does the light appear to be too bright? Is its color different? Does it hurt your eyes? Are you seeing anything that is disturbing you? Are you seeing things that you know aren't there?"

Observation:

0 —not present
1 —very mild sensitivity
2 —mild sensitivity
3 —moderate sensitivity
4 —moderately severe hallucinations
5 —severe hallucinations
6 —extremely sever hallucinations
7 —continuous hallucinations

Headache, Fullness in Head: Ask "Does your head feel different? Does it feel like there is a band around your head?" Do not rate dizziness or lightheadedness. Otherwise, rate severity.

0 —not present
1 —very mild
2 —mild
3 —moderate
4 —moderately severe
5 —severe
6 —very severe
7 —extremely severe

TABLE 52.2 Clinical Institute Withdrawal Assessment–Alcohol (CIWA-Ar) (*Continued*)

Agitation:

Observation:

0 —normal activity
1 —somewhat more than normal activity
2
3
4 —moderately fidgety and restless
5
6
7 —paces back and forth during most of the interview, or constantly thrashes about

Orientation and Clouding of Sensorium: Ask "What day is this? Where are you? Who am I?

0 —oriented and can dp serial additions
1 —cannot do serial additions or is certain about date
2 —disoriented for date by no more than 2 calendar days
3 —disoriented for date by more than 2 calendar days
4 —disoriented for place and/or person

Initial patient classification into mild, moderate, or severe AWD should be based on CIWA-Ar score and clinical picture. At initiation of treatment, CIWA-Ar/Ad/RASS (the latter for ICU patients) should again be assessed. The result of these scores, along with clinical picture, should then guide medication dosing; scoring should be repeated as indicated by the degree of AWS and frequency of medication dosing. No single guideline exists for managing this process; a sample protocol is provided in Figures 52.1–52.3.

MANAGEMENT GUIDELINES

Moderate to severe AWS is most commonly treated with benzodiazepines. Ideal pharmacologic management is tailored to the individual patient and controls hyperadrenergic symptoms, anxiety, agitation, and delirium while minimizing adverse effects. Drug selection and dosing strategy should be informed by the desired pharmacodynamic and pharmacokinetic properties of the drugs, as well as by individual patient characteristics (existing symptoms, underlying illnesses, and/or past episodes of AWS). Ongoing subjective assessments using CIWA-Ar/Ad and RASS scores are essential.

TABLE 52.3 Richmond Agitation Sedation Scale (RASS)

Score	Term	Description
+4	Combative	Overtly combative, violent, immediate danger to staff
+3	Very agitated	Pulls or removes tube(s) or catheter(s); aggressive
+2	Agitated	Frequent nonpurposeful movement, fights ventilator
+1	Restless	Anxious but movements not aggressive vigorous
0	Alert and calm	
−1	Drowsy	Not fully alert, but has sustained awakening (eye-opening/eye contact) to voice (>10 s)
−2	Light sedation	Briefly awakens with eye contact to voice (<10 s)
−3	Moderate sedation	Movement or eye opening to voice (but no eye contact)
−4	Deep sedation	No response to voice, but movement or eye opening to physical stimulation
−5	Unarousable	No response to voice or physical stimulation

When compared to standing doses or continuous infusions of benzodiazepines, well-executed STT with benzodiazepines plus adjunctive agents can decrease total benzodiazepine dose, incidence of intubation and admission to the ICU, and hospital and ICU length of stay (LOS).[18,20–25,42,45–47] In one study, well-executed STT was shown to be comparable to front-loading, an approach in which patients are typically titrated to lid lag, a low CIWA score (<8), or a state of calm.[26] In front-loading, the use of long-acting benzodiazepines with active metabolites can lead to heavier sedation but confers the advantage of autotapering. In the emergency department (ED), front-loading followed by SST is often used in the initial control phase for patients in AWS.[48] Generally speaking, institutional clinical guidelines and individual patient parameters should guide the practitioner's choice of approach.

Benzodiazepines

The five most commonly used benzodiazepines are diazepam, chlordiazepoxide, lorazepam, clonazepam, and oxazepam. There are several important considerations when choosing a pharmacologic agent for a patient in AWD (Table 52.4).

Chlordiazepoxide and diazepam have a longer duration of action due to the presence of active metabolites. This may decrease the rate of breakthrough symptoms and have an autotapering effect.[49,50] Parenteral diazepam has a short onset and is preferred for rapid titration in severe cases; doses of 5 to 20 mg can be given every 5 to 10 minutes. Higher bolus doses can be used if the patient demonstrates tolerance. Oral chlordiazepoxide can be used effectively in moderate withdrawal and can be rapidly titrated at doses of 50 to 100 mg/hour. Patients may also be managed with aggressive oral dosing of chlordiazepoxide. The experience of recent national drug shortages established the efficacy of this approach in patients previously thought to require parenteral medications.[51–53]

Lorazepam, which has a longer time to peak effect (15 to 20 minutes), may lead to iatrogenic oversedation if titrated too rapidly. Lorazepam can be titrated in doses of 1 to 4 mg every 15 to 30 minutes. If higher doses are used, a longer dosing interval is preferred. Due to lorazepam's lack of active metabolites, nondependence on renal or hepatic mechanisms for clearance and predictable $t_{1/2}$, it is preferred over diazepam and chlordiazepoxide for use in patients with COPD, hepatic dysfunction (INR > 1.6), renal dysfunction (Cr_{Cl} < 30 mL/min, S_{Cr} > 2 mg/dL), or age > 65 years.[54] Prolonged lorazepam infusions carry a risk of toxicity from propylene glycol (the diluent in lorazepam infusions) with associated metabolic acidosis and renal failure. Lorazepam is also incompatible with numerous other infusions.

TABLE 52.4 Benzodiazepines for treatment of AWS

Benzodiazepine	PO	IV	Onset	$T_{1/2}$	Comments
Chlordiazepoxide	50 mg	N/A	30–60 min (PO)	5–100 h	Active metabolites
Diazepam	10 mg	5 mg	~5 min (IV)	30–100 h	Active metabolites
Lorazepam	2 mg	1 mg	15–20 min (IV)	10–20 h	No active metabolites
Clonazepam	1 mg	N/A	30–60 min (PO)	20–50 h	No active metabolites
Oxazepam	30 mg	N/A	60 min (PO)	3–25 h	No active metabolites

In general, it is recommended to avoid using different benzodiazepines together (e.g., oral chlordiazepoxide and intravenous benzodiazepines), except during the initial control phase when a patient is progressing from mild to more severe symptoms, or to provide a basis for autotapering (when chlordiazepoxide is added). The deliberate and measured use of different classes of medications based on mechanism of action and synergy can yield good results. Haphazard polypharmacy with benzodiazepines and other sedatives in difficult-to-control patients increases the chances of unexpected synergy and oversedation.

Patients with resistant alcohol withdrawal (defined below) require ICU-level monitoring and a more aggressive pharmacotherapeutic approach. Such patients often require adjunctive therapies like phenobarbital or propofol (see below).

Resistant Alcohol Withdrawal (RAW) is defined as the following:

1. Failure to respond to 200 mg of IV diazepam (or 30 mg lorazepam) in the first 3 hours
2. Failure to respond to 400 mg of IV diazepam (or 60 mg lorazepam) in the first 8 hours
3. Requirement of repeated doses of more than 40 mg of diazepam for control of agitation
4. Persistent CIWA scores of >25 despite aggressive therapy

Barbiturates

Barbiturates are $GABA_A$ agonists and have been employed as monotherapy and, more commonly, as adjuncts in severe DT or RAW.[20,51,52,55–59] The most studied barbiturate in the setting of AWS is phenobarbital, which is typically initiated in a monitored setting when high-dose benzodiazepines have failed to control symptoms. A standard starting dose of phenobarbital of 30 mg can be used, titrated to effect every 30 minutes. As the onset of barbiturates' effect can be delayed, it is prudent to wait approximately 30 minutes before adding an additional agent. The long half-life of barbiturates also confers a beneficial self-tapering effect. One study showed decreased ICU admissions with phenobarbital given as a single dose of 19 mg/kg (vs. placebo) early in the course of treatment.[58] It is unclear, however, whether this outcome demonstrates superiority of loading with a barbiturate, or the benefit of a front-loaded approach in general paired with a less aggressive institutional protocol. In times of nationwide benzodiazepine shortages, the use of barbiturates in the treatment of AWS should be considered a reasonable therapeutic option.[51,52]

Propofol

Propofol is a $GABA_A$ agonist and an NMDA antagonist. It is highly effective at controlling severe AWS symptoms and is generally reserved for cases refractory to high-dose benzodiazepines and barbiturates. Intubation is generally recommended because of propofol's potency and the narrow window between an effective and toxic dose. Propofol's short half-life makes it unsuitable as a primary or exclusive agent. Intubated patients on propofol infusions can be started on a benzodiazepine or chlordiazepoxide via nasogastric tube, in an effort to wean from propofol and establish a base of long-acting benzodiazepines that permit autotapering (see Tapering section).[60,61] Propofol infusions are susceptible to tachyphylaxis and should only be used in a highly monitored setting.[62]

Antipsychotics

In historical studies of AWS, benzodiazepines have been shown far superior to monotherapy with antipsychotics in controlling symptoms and preventing seizures or DT's.[41,63,64] Bolus therapy with the antipsychotic haloperidol, given with clonidine and benzodiazepines, has been described as a successful combination when compared to continuous monotherapy infusions.[24,41,42] It is not clear whether the strength of the treatment reported was the result of attentive STT/bolus therapy, or the combination of the medications used, or both. As a general rule, while there may be a role for antipsychotics in patients in AWS with comorbid psychiatric disorders or pronounced hallucinations, monotherapy with these agents should be avoided.

Anticonvulsants

Some studies have suggested that benzodiazepine use in the treatment of AWS can lead to more craving—of both ethanol and benzodiazepines—and that alternative, non–benzodiazepine-based regimens—such as anticonvulsants—may decrease craving and relapse after detoxification.[65–69] Since these studies considered only short-term outcomes, it is difficult to know whether the effect on craving continues beyond the initial period following detoxification.

The anticonvulsant topiramate is an antiglutaminergic and GABA-enhancing drug, and studies have shown it to attenuate AWS in rodents.[70] Human studies have shown a benefit over placebo for preventing AWS and suggest a possible role for treating ethanol dependence.[9,10,70] Valproic acid,[71–73] gabapentin,[67,74] and carbamazepine[66,71,75] have also been evaluated in the treatment of AWS, primarily in mild to moderate cases in the settings of inpatient and outpatient detoxification units. Studies suggest them to be inadequate as sole agents but potentially more useful in combination therapy.[33,71,76]

A 2010 Cochrane review of anticonvulsants for AWS concluded that there was insufficient evidence in their favor, excepting the use of carbamazepine, which may outperform benzodiazepines in treating some aspects of AWS.[77] Compared to benzodiazepines, carbamazepine appears to have more benefit in symptom control and craving in less medically severe cases and in the outpatient setting, but less benefit in preventing seizures and DTs.[75]

Gamma-hydroxybutyric acid (GHB), also a $GABA_A$ agonist, was found to be comparable, but not superior, to benzodiazepines.[78] GHB has been used more widely in Europe, but concerns for GHB addiction have tempered its use in the United States.[79] Phenytoin has not been shown to be beneficial in seizures related to AWS.[80–82]

Of note, in 2013, an unpublished case series was presented at a national meeting regarding the use of valproic acid or gabapentin with clonidine patches. The investigator described successful detoxification of medically moderate to severe AWS without the use of a benzodiazepine.[53,83] Since the findings remain unpublished, it is difficult to comment on the results, except to say that alternative regimens to benzodiazepines are being explored and discussed.

Clonidine and Dexmedetomidine

Clonidine and dexmedetomidine are centrally acting α_2 agonists. α_2 agonists decrease NE release and reduce symptoms of sympathetic overdrive. These agents have been studied in rodent models for the treatment of AWS[84–87] as well as in a limited number of human trials. The surgical literature has reported the successful use of clonidine with haloperidol and benzodiazepines in the treatment of surgical intensive care unit (SICU) and trauma patients with AWS;[24,41,42,88,89] one randomized controlled trial found transdermal clonidine to be as effective as chlordiazepoxide in the management of mild AWS;[90] and a case series reported using high-dose clonidine patches in combination with valproic acid or gabapentin in the treatment of moderate to severe AWS.[83] Most studies (case reports and uncontrolled case series) of dexmedetomidine in AWS have focused on its use as an adjunctive agent.[91–101] Both clonidine and dexmedetomidine can produce sedation as well as hypotension and bradycardia, and acute withdrawal from dexmedetomodine has been described in patients on prolonged infusions.[102] There is likely a role for clonidine and dexmedetomidine as adjuncts in the treatment of AWS, but more studies are required to fully comment on appropriate case selection, outcomes, and patient safety.[103] At this time, neither agent is recommended for use as monotherapy in AWS.

Baclofen

Baclofen is a stereo-selective agonist of $GABA_B$. It has been shown to be effective in suppressing AWS in rodents[104,105] and, in a small number of human trials, to be comparable, but not superior, to benzodiazepines.[106–108] It is notable that the benzodiazepine doses were low in the human trial comparison groups, suggesting that the study population was experiencing less severe withdrawal. A recent Cochrane review concluded that there were insufficient data to make outcome or safety conclusions regarding baclofen's use for AWS.[109] Baclofen has shown some effect in supporting efforts at alcohol abstinence in alcohol-dependent patients with liver cirrhosis. This application has gained popularity, particularly in Europe, and warrants further study.[106,107,110–113]

Ethanol

Ethanol therapy for AWS (IV or PO) is not recommended due to a high failure rate and potential for complications.[114–117] In both PO and IV forms, alcohol has large free water content, an association with electrolyte and behavioral disturbances, and a tendency to cause hypoglycemia. These factors, as well as difficulties in titration to adequate blood levels, make it an unsuitable choice.[115] In a randomized trial of IV ethanol versus scheduled-dose diazepam in a trauma ICU, IV ethanol was found to be inferior to diazepam and was associated with greater treatment failures.[117] Prophylaxis with ethanol in patients, particularly for elective surgical admissions, is practiced in some centers.[115] A discussion of this is beyond the scope of this chapter, and it remains a controversial practice.

Beta-blockers

Beta-adrenergic agents should not be used to control the hypertension and tachycardia associated with AWS until the underlying cause (i.e., the hyperadrenergic AWS state) is treated. Once fluid status and appropriate sedation are administered, vital sign abnormalities usually normalize. If hypertension coexists, beta-blockers and other antihypertensive agents can be used to control blood pressure. Beta-blockers, by masking abnormal vital signs, can also obscure the diagnosis of delirium tremens.[118]

Tapering

Once initial control of withdrawal symptoms is achieved with benzodiazepines and/or phenobarbital/propofol and a stable clinical trend is established for 24 to 28 hours, a plan for tapering must be implemented. A recommended approach is to taper by approximately 20% per day of total daily benzodiazepine equivalent dose. Taper with chlordiazepoxide when possible (anticipate starting with ≥100 mg chlordiazepoxide PO q2–8h in severe cases). For example, if a patient had a total of 700 mg chlordiazepoxide PO and 8 mg lorazepam IV over 24 hours (equivalent to ~900 mg chlordiazepoxide), then the next day's dose would be 720 mg/day (divided q6–8h). Patients treated with long-acting agents with active metabolites may exhibit varying degrees of an "autotaper" effect while still receiving STT. If during tapering, a patient's CIWA-Ar scores increase to >10, give supplemental medication for breakthrough symptoms and consider a slower taper by increasing the daily dose, that is, tapering by 10% per day. Propofol infusions should be tapered as early as possible (after 2 to 3 days) because of the associated risk of infection and hypertriglyceridemia. Tapering from nonbenzodiazepines is not well described in moderate to severe AWS.

General Supportive Care

The following additional supportive care measures for the patient with AWS should be considered, particularly if the patient is heavily sedated or bedbound.

A. Daily × 7 days: thiamine 100 mg PO/IV, folate 1 mg PO/IV, and MVI PO/IV
B. Careful electrolyte repletion
C. Docusate 100 mg PO/NG/DT/PEG TID and Senna two tablets PO/NG/DT/PEG daily
D. Lacrilube each eye BID or artificial tears two drops each eye QID
E. NPO if compromised mental status, severe agitation, and risk for aspiration
F. Early mobilization from bed whenever possible per ICU/SDU care plan
G. Avoidance of daily interruption of sedation as is routine with other ICU patients
H. Restraints and continuous observation as per hospital policy
I. MICU and psychiatry consult for difficult cases
J. Social Work consult for after care and outpatient detox/rehab follow-up

CONCLUSION

STT with benzodiazepines is currently accepted as best practice in the management of mild to severe AWS. This approach provides the greatest advantage in patients with severe AWS, benzodiazepine-resistant AWS, and DT's, resulting in shorter lengths of stay, decreased complication rates, and lower total medication dose requirements when compared to lower bolus doses or those placed on continuous infusions (especially of benzodiazepines).[35] Propofol and dexmedetomidine are not supported as sole agents or first-line agents, but show promise as rescue medications in benzodiazepine-resistant cases or when intubation is considered imminent. Resource utilization and complications rates remain high for patients with severe AWS, and providers should exercise a low threshold for transfer to the MICU in concerning cases (Figs. 52.2 and 52.3).

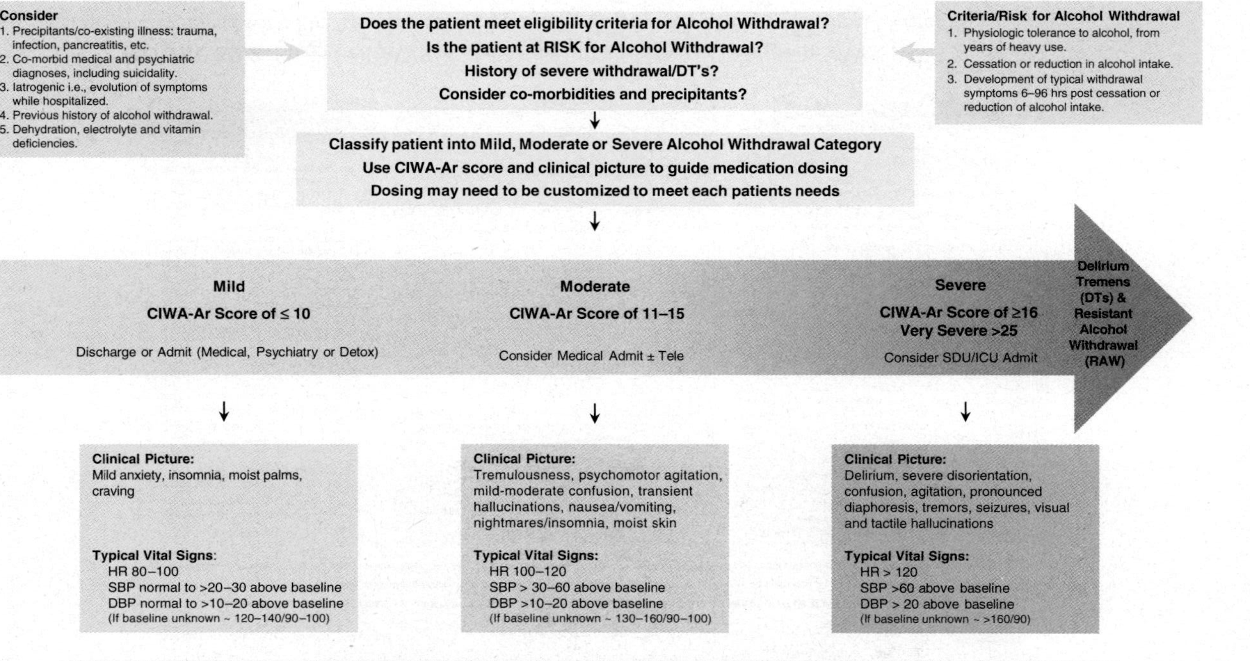

Management of Alcohol Withdrawal: Clinical Guidelines for Medicine and the ED
Always use clinical judgment to customize patient therapy when applying clinical guidelines
Consider
1. Precipitants/co-existing illness: trauma, infection, pancreatitis, etc.
2. Co-morbid medical and psychiatric diagnoses, including suicidality.
3. Iatrogenic i.e., evolution of symptoms while hospitalized.
4. Previous history of alcohol withdrawal.
5. Dehydration, electrolyte and vitamin deficiencies.
Does the patient meet eligibility criteria for Alcohol Withdrawal?
Is the patient at RISK for Alcohol Withdrawal?
History of severe withdrawal/DT's?
Consider co-morbidities and precipitants?
Criteria/Risk for Alcohol Withdrawal
1. Physiologic tolerance to alcohol, from years of heavy use.
2. Cessation or reduction in alcohol intake.
3. Development of typical withdrawal symptoms 6–96 hrs post cessation or reduction of alcohol intake.
Classify patient into Mild, Moderate or Severe Alcohol Withdrawal Category
Use CIWA-Ar score and clinical picture to guide medication dosing
Dosing may need to be customized to meet each patients needs
Mild
CIWA-Ar Score of ≤ 10
Discharge or Admit (Medical, Psychiatry or Detox)
Moderate
CIWA-Ar Score of 11–15
Consider Medical Admit ± Tele
Severe
CIWA-Ar Score of ≥16
Very Severe >25
Consider SDU/ICU Admit
Delirium Tremens (DTs) & Resistant Alcohol Withdrawal (RAW)
Clinical Picture:
Mild anxiety, insomnia, moist palms, craving
Typical Vital Signs:
HR 80–100
SBP normal to >20–30 above baseline
DBP normal to >10–20 above baseline
(If baseline unknown ~ 120–140/90–100)
Clinical Picture:
Tremulousness, psychomotor agitation, mild-moderate confusion, transient hallucinations, nausea/vomiting, nightmares/insomnia, moist skin
Typical Vital Signs:
HR 100–120
SBP > 30–60 above baseline
DBP >10–20 above baseline
(If baseline unknown ~ 130–160/90–100)
Clinical Picture:
Delirium, severe disorientation, confusion, agitation, pronounced diaphoresis, tremors, seizures, visual and tactile hallucinations
Typical Vital Signs:
HR > 120
SBP >60 above baseline
DBP > 20 above baseline
(If baseline unknown ~ >160/90)
The categories are approximations along a continuum/clinical spectrum.
This guideline is intended for use in patients with Alcohol Withdrawal and for patients AT RISK FOR Alcohol Withdrawal.
Consider use of an Alcohol Withdrawal tracking spreadsheet to track CIWA-Ar scores, vital signs and medication requirements over time.

FIGURE 52.1 AWS initial assessment guideline. AWS guidelines codeveloped with Dr. Amy Dzierba, Pharm.D., Columbia University Medical Center.

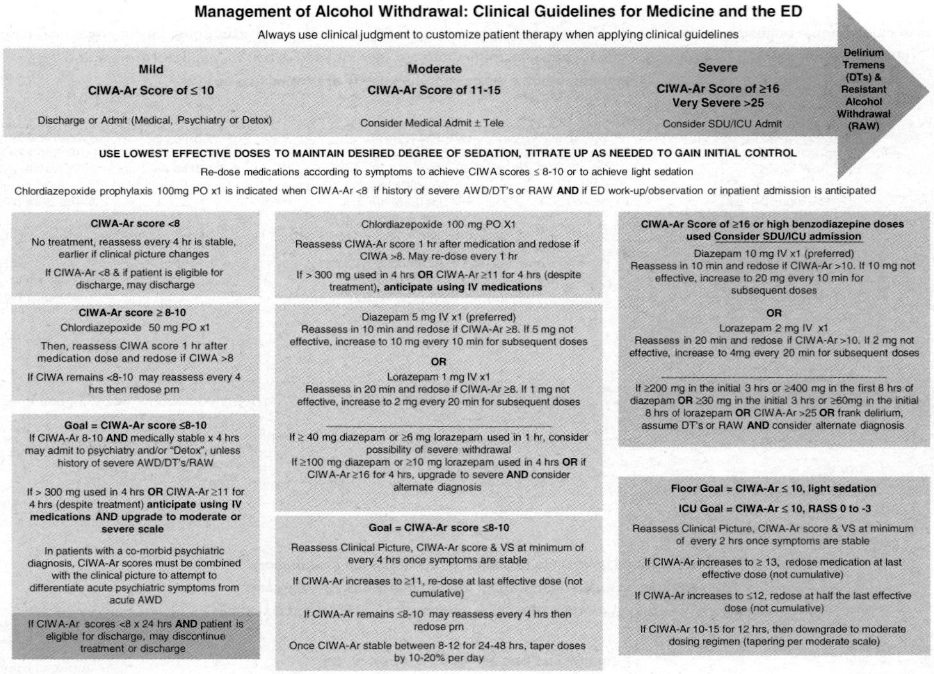

Management of Alcohol Withdrawal: Clinical Guidelines for Medicine and the ED

Always use clinical judgment to customize patient therapy when applying clinical guidelines

Mild
CIWA-Ar Score of ≤ 10
Discharge or Admit (Medical, Psychiatry or Detox)

Moderate
CIWA-Ar Score of 11-15
Consider Medical Admit ± Tele

Severe
CIWA-Ar Score of ≥16
Very Severe >25
Consider SDU/ICU Admit

Delirium Tremens (DTs) & Resistant Alcohol Withdrawal (RAW)

USE LOWEST EFFECTIVE DOSES TO MAINTAIN DESIRED DEGREE OF SEDATION, TITRATE UP AS NEEDED TO GAIN INITIAL CONTROL

Re-dose medications according to symptoms to achieve CIWA scores ≤ 8-10 or to achieve light sedation

Chlordiazepoxide prophylaxis 100mg PO x1 is indicated when CIWA-Ar <8 if history of severe AWD/DT's or RAW **AND** if ED work-up/observation or inpatient admission is anticipated

CIWA-Ar score <8
No treatment, reassess every 4 hr is stable, earlier if clinical picture changes
If CIWA-Ar <8 & if patient is eligible for discharge, may discharge

CIWA-Ar score ≥ 8-10
Chlordiazepoxide 50 mg PO x1
Then, reassess CIWA score 1 hr after medication dose and redose if CIWA >8
If CIWA remains <8-10 may reassess every 4 hrs then redose prn

Goal = CIWA-Ar score ≤8-10
If CIWA-Ar 8-10 **AND** medically stable x 4 hrs may admit to psychiatry and/or "Detox", unless history of severe AWD/DT's/RAW

If > 300 mg used in 4 hrs **OR** CIWA-Ar ≥11 for 4 hrs (despite treatment) **anticipate using IV medications AND upgrade to moderate or severe scale**

In patients with a co-morbid psychiatric diagnosis, CIWA-Ar scores must be combined with the clinical picture to attempt to differentiate acute psychiatric symptoms from acute AWD

If CIWA-Ar scores <8 x 24 hrs **AND** patient is eligible for discharge, may discontinue treatment or discharge

Chlordiazepoxide 100 mg PO X1
Reassess CIWA-Ar score 1 hr after medication and redose if CIWA >8. May re-dose every 1 hr
If > 300 mg used in 4 hrs **OR** CIWA-Ar ≥11 for 4 hrs (despite treatment), **anticipate using IV medications**

Diazepam 5 mg IV x1 (preferred)
Reassess in 10 min and redose if CIWA-Ar ≥8. If 5 mg not effective, increase to 10 mg every 10 min for subsequent doses

OR

Lorazepam 1 mg IV x1
Reassess in 20 min and redose if CIWA-Ar ≥8. If 1 mg not effective, increase to 2 mg every 20 min for subsequent doses

If ≥ 40 mg diazepam or ≥6 mg lorazepam used in 1 hr, consider possibility of severe withdrawal
If ≥100 mg diazepam or ≥10 mg lorazepam used in 4 hrs **OR** if CIWA-Ar ≥16 for 4 hrs, upgrade to severe **AND** consider alternate diagnosis

Goal = CIWA-Ar score ≤8-10
Reassess Clinical Picture, CIWA-Ar score & VS at minimum of every 4 hrs once symptoms are stable
If CIWA-Ar increases to ≥11, re-dose at last effective dose (not cumulative)
If CIWA-Ar remains ≤8-10 may reassess every 4 hrs then redose prn
Once CIWA-Ar stable between 8-12 for 24-48 hrs, taper doses by 10-20% per day

CIWA-Ar Score of ≥16 or high benzodiazepine doses used Consider SDU/ICU admission
Diazepam 10 mg IV x1 (preferred)
Reassess in 10 min and redose if CIWA-Ar >10. If 10 mg not effective, increase to 20 mg every 10 min for subsequent doses

OR

Lorazepam 2 mg IV x1
Reassess in 20 min and redose if CIWA-Ar >10. If 2 mg not effective, increase to 4mg every 20 min for subsequent doses

If ≥200 mg in the initial 3 hrs or ≥400 mg in the first 8 hrs of diazepam **OR** ≥30 mg in the initial 3 hrs or ≥60mg in the initial 8 hrs of lorazepam **OR** CIWA-Ar >25 **OR** frank delirium, assume DT's or RAW **AND** consider alternate diagnosis

Floor Goal = CIWA-Ar ≤ 10, light sedation
ICU Goal = CIWA-Ar ≤ 10, RASS 0 to -3
Reassess Clinical Picture, CIWA-Ar score & VS at minimum of every 2 hrs once symptoms are stable
If CIWA-Ar increases to ≥ 13, redose medication at last effective dose (not cumulative)
If CIWA-Ar increases to ≤12, redose at half the last effective dose (not cumulative)
If CIWA-Ar 10-15 for 12 hrs, then downgrade to moderate dosing regimen (tapering per moderate scale)

FIGURE 52.2 Suggested AWS guideline for mild, moderate, and severe AWS. AWS guidelines codeveloped with Dr. Amy Dzierba, Pharm.D., Columbia University Medical Center.

Management of Alcohol Withdrawal: Clinical Guidelines for Medicine and the ED

Always use clinical judgment to customize patient therapy when applying clinical guidelines

ICU: Delirium Tremens and/or Resistant Alcohol Withdrawal (RAW)

Persistent CIWA-Ar ≥ 25, frank delirium or inability to control symptoms despite medication

AND/OR

≥200 mg in the initial 3 hrs or ≥400 mg of diazepam in the first 8 hrs **OR** ≥30 mg in the initial 3 hrs or ≥60mg of lorazepam in the initial 8 hrs **AND** alternate diagnosis considered **AND ADMIT TO ICU**

USE LOWEST EFFECTIVE DOSES TO MAINTAIN DESIRED DEGREE OF SEDATION, TITRATE UP AS NEEDED TO GAIN CONTROL

Re-dose medications according to symptoms to achieve CIWA scores ≤ 10-15 or to achieve light to moderate sedation (RASS 0 to -3). Score both CIWA and RASS in ICU.

Diazepam is preferred unless: significant COPD, hepatic dysfunction (INR >1.6) and/or renal dysfunction (Cr_{Cl}<30ml.min, S_{Cr} >2mg/dL) and/or age >65.

Increased risk for iatrogenic over-sedation with **lorazepam** secondary to **delayed peak effects** (20-30 mins).

ICU Goal= CIWA-Ar ≤ 10, RASS -1 to -3

Diazepam 20 mg IV x1 (preferred)

Reassess in 10 min and redose at 20 mg if CIWA-Ar ≥13 or RASS ≥1

If ineffective, increase to 40 mg every 10 min for subsequent doses. If CIWA-Ar ≤12 or RASS ≤0 give half the last dose (not cumulative)

OR

Lorazepam 4 mg IV x1

Reassess in 20 min and redose at 4 mg if CIWA-Ar ≥13 or RASS ≥1

If 4 mg not effective, increase to 6 mg every 20 min for subsequent doses. If CIWA-Ar ≤12 or RASS ≤0 give half the last dose (not cumulative)

If ≥200 mg in the initial 3 hrs or ≥400 mg of diazepam in the first 8 hrs **OR** ≥30 mg in the initial 3 hrs or ≥60mg of lorazepam in the initial 8 hrs **AND** alternate diagnosis considered, move to RAW treatment algorithm below.

↓

Continue symptom triggered therapy with high dose diazepam (preferred) or high dose lorazepam (may need to consider lorazepam continuous infusion, this is the least favored option for non-intubated patients and should be reserved for selected patients with above contraindications)

Bolus therapy may reach doses as high as 2000 mg diazepam/day or 200 mg/day or lorazepam

CONSIDER ADDING

1) Phenobarbital (with interspersed benzodiazepines):

Phenobarbital 60 mg IV (bolus) every 30 min – consider halving total daily dose of benzodiazepines if starting phenobarbital and not intubated.

Though the goal of this strategy is to avoid intubation, ***intubation may be required*** due to respiratory depression with concurrent benzodiazepine therapy.

2) Propofol if ≥ 5 doses of phenobarbital over 8 hrs and patient is still having severe symptoms (***intubation usually required***)

Propofol - No Bolus, start drip at 5-10 micrograms/kg/min and titrate to sedation (RASS -3 to -4), maximum dose of 80 micrograms/kg/min.

***3) Lorazepam infusion**- start at 2mg/hr, bolus at 1-2mg every 30 min as necessary and increase drip by 1-2 mg/hr as needed

Reassess Clinical Picture, CIWA-Ar score & VS at minimum of every 1 hr until symptoms are stable. Redose medication at last effective dose if CIWA-Ar ≥13 or RASS ≥1, re-dose at half the last dose for CIWA-Ar ≤12 or RASS ≤0. Hold medication if CIWA-Ar ≤8 or RASS ≤-3 (unless intubated).

ALL patients will require medication TAPERING once stabilized. Begin tapering after 48 hrs or once a stable trends has emerged. Taper by 20% per day.

*If patient requires sedation for co-existing condition, titrate sedation to achieve desired RASS goal and begin tapering when clinically stable (use caution when holding sedation for daily interruption).

FIGURE 52.3 AWS guideline for RAW and DT. AWS guidelines codeveloped with Dr. Amy Dzierba, Pharm.D., Columbia University Medical Center.

LITERATURE TABLE

TRIAL	DESIGN	RESULT
Gold et al., *Crit Care Med.* 2007[20]	Retrospective cohort study of patients treated pre (54 patients) and post (41 patients) the introduction of an AWS guideline for escalating dose therapy in patients admitted to the ICU for the treatment of severe AWS. A previous standard therapy of lower bolus doses and frequent continuous infusions was compared to a strategy of escalating doses of benzodiazepines (primarily diazepam) and adjunctive phenobarbital	Postguideline patients had lower rates of intubation (47% vs. 22%; $p = 0.008$), with trends toward decreased ICU LOS and nosocomial pneumonia
Saitz et al., *JAMA.* 1994[22]	Prospective double-blind RCT of 101 patients with AWS randomized to fixed-dose or symptom triggered-therapy (STT) with chlordiazepoxide	STT therapy, individualized treatment, and decreased both treatment duration ($p < 0.001$) and total dose of medication used ($p < 0.001$)
Spies et al., *Intensive Care Med.* 2003[24]	Prospective double-blind RCT of 44 surgical ICU patients with AWS randomized to either (a) continuous infusion with IV flunitrazepam, clonidine, and haloperidol or (b) the same medications given in a bolus-titrated manner. Severity and duration of AWS was assessed	Bolus-titrated therapy decreased the severity and duration of AWS (median 2 vs. 6 d; $p = \leq 0.01$), total medication requirements, rate of intubation (65% vs. 90%, $p = 0.050$), days of mechanical ventilation (median 6 vs. 12, $p = 0.01$), incidence of pneumonia (43% vs. 26%, $p = \leq 0.01$), and duration ICU length of stay (median 6 vs. 14 d; $p = \leq 0.01$)
Awissi et al., *Intensive Care Med.* 2013[35]	Systematic review of screening tools, prophylaxis, treatment, and outcomes for AWS and DTs in the critically ill	No screening tools have been validated for the ICU. Early and aggressive titration of medication guided by symptoms is the only approach associated with improved outcome. Treatment of AWS is associated with higher ICU complication rates and resource utilization
Sarff and Gold, *Crit Care Med.* 2010[119]	Review article of pathophysiology, diagnosis, and pharmacologic treatment of AWS in critically ill patients	High-dose benzodiazepines, barbiturate, and propofol are supported for the treatment of severe or benzodiazepine-resistant AWS

REFERENCES

1. Cagetti E, Liang J, Spigelman I, et al. Withdrawal from chronic intermittent ethanol treatment changes subunit composition, reduces synaptic function, and decreases behavioral responses to positive allosteric modulators of GABAA receptors. *Mol Pharmacol.* 2003;63:53.
2. Kumar S, Porcu P, Werner DF. The role of GABA receptors in the acute and chronic effects of ethanol: a decade of progress. *Psychopharmacology (Berl).* 2009;205:529.
3. Mihic SJ, Ye Q, Wick MJ, et al. Sites of alcohol and volatile anaesthetic action on GABA(A) and glycine receptors. *Nature.* 1997;389:385.
4. Morrow AL, Suzdak PD, Karanian JW, et al. Chronic ethanol administration alters gamma-aminobutyric acid, pentobarbital and ethanol-mediated $36Cl^-$ uptake in cerebral cortical synaptoneurosomes. *J Pharmacol Exp Ther.* 1988;246:158.
5. Whittemore ER, Yang W, Drewe JA, et al. Pharmacology of the human gamma-aminobutyric acid A receptor alpha 4 subunit expression in *Xenopus laevis* oocytes. *Mol Pharmacol.* 1996;50:1364–1365.
6. Hoffman PL, Grant KA, Snell LD, et al. NMDA receptors: role in ethanol withdrawal seizures. *Ann NY Acad Sci.* 1992;654:52.
7. Tsai G, Gastfriend DR, Coyle JT. The glutamatergic basis of human alcoholism. *Am J Psychiatry.* 1995;152(3):332–340. PMID: 7864257.

8. Tsai G, Coyle JT. The role of glutamatergic neurotransmission in the pathophysiology of alcoholism. *Annu Rev Med.* 1998;49:173–184. PMID: 9509257.
9. Johnson BA, Ait-Daoud N, Bowden CL, et al. Oral topiramate for treatment of alcohol dependence: a randomised controlled trial. *Lancet.* 2003;361(9370):1677–1685. PMID: 12767733.
10. Johnson BA, Swift RM, Ait-Daoud N, et al. Development of novel pharmacotherapies for the treatment of alcohol dependence: focus on antiepileptics. *Alcohol Clin Exp Res.* 2004;28(2):295–301. PMID: 15112937.
11. Swift RM. Topiramate for the treatment of alcohol dependence: initiating abstinence. *Lancet.* 2003;361(9370):1666–1667. PMID: 12767727.
12. Finn DA, Crabbe JC. Exploring alcohol withdrawal syndrome. *Alcohol Health Res World.* 1997;21(2): 149–156. PMID: 15704352.
13. Lingford-Hughes A, Nutt D. Neurobiology of addiction and implications for treatment. *Br J Psychiatry.* 2003;182(2):97–100. PMID: 12562734.
14. Nutt D. Alcohol and the brain: pharmacological insights for psychiatrists. *Br J Psychiatry.* 1999;175(2): 114–119. PMID: 10627792.
15. Borg S, Kvande H, Sedvall G. Central norepinephrine metabolism during alcohol intoxication in addicts and healthy volunteers. *Science.* 1981;213(4512):1135–1137. PMID: 7268421.
16. Linnoila M, Mefford I, Nutt D, et al. NIH conference: alcohol withdrawal and noradrenergic function. *Ann Intern Med.* 1987;107(6):875–889. PMID: 2825572.
17. Sellers EM, Degani NC, Zilm DH, et al. Propranolol-decreased noradrenaline excretion and alcohol withdrawal. *Lancet.* 1976;1(7950):94–95. PMID: 54619.
18. Cassidy EM, O'Sullivan I, Bradshaw P, et al. Symptom-triggered benzodiazepine therapy for alcohol withdrawal syndrome in the emergency department: a comparison with the standard fixed dose benzodiazepine regimen. *Emerg Med J.* 2012;29:802.
19. Daeppen JB, Gache P, Landry U, et al. Symptom-triggered vs fixed-schedule doses of benzodiazepine for alcohol withdrawal: a randomized treatment trial. *Arch Intern Med.* 2002;162:1117. PMID: 12020181.
20. Gold JA, et al. A strategy of escalating doses of benzodiazepines and phenobarbital administration reduces the need for mechanical ventilation in delirium tremens. *Crit Care Med.* 2007;35(3):724–730.
21. Jaeger TM, et al. Symptom-triggered therapy for alcohol withdrawal in medical inpatients. *Mayo Clin Proc.* 2001;76(7):695–701.
22. Saitz R, Mayo-Smith M, Roberts MS, et al. Individualized treatment for ethanol withdrawal. *JAMA.* 1994;272:519–523.
23. See S, Nosal S, Barr WB, et al. Implementation of a symptom triggered benzodiazepine protocol for alcohol withdrawal in family medicine inpatients. *Hosp Pharm.* 2009;44(10):881–887.
24. Spies CD, Otter HE, Hüske B, et al. Alcohol withdrawal severity is decreased by symptom-orientated adjusted bolus therapy in the ICU. *Intensive Care Med.* 2003;29:2230. PMID: 14557857.
25. Stanley KM, Amabile CM, Simpson KN, et al. Impact of an alcohol withdrawal syndrome practice guideline on surgical patient outcomes. *Pharmacotherapy.* 2003;23:843–854. PMID: 12885097.
26. Maldonado JR, Nguyen LH, Schader EM, et al. Benzodiazepine loading versus symptom-triggered treatment of alcohol withdrawal: a prospective, randomized clinical trial. *Gen Hosp Psychiatry.* 2012;34: 611–617. PMID: 22898443.
27. Maldonado JR. An approach to the patient with substance use and abuse. *Med Clin North Am.* 2010;94:1169–1205. PMID: 20951277.
28. Victor M, Adams RD. The effect of alcohol on the central nervous system. In: *Metabolic and Toxic Disease of the Nervous System.* Baltimore, MD: Lippincott Williams & Wilkins. 1953:526–573.
29. Victor M, Brausch C. The role of abstinence in the genesis of alcoholic epilepsy. *Epilepsia.* 1967;8:1–20.
30. Boston LN. Alcohol withdrawal. *Lancet.* 1908;1:18.
31. DeBellis R, Smith BS, Choi S, et al. Management of delirium tremens. *J Intensive Care Med.* 2005;20:164. PMID: 15888905.
32. Pristach CA, Smith CM, Whitney RB. Alcohol withdrawal syndromes—prediction from detailed medical and drinking histories. *Drug Alcohol Depend.* 1983;11:177. PMID: 6861616.
33. Saitz R, O'Malley SS. Pharmacotherapies for alcohol abuse. Withdrawal and treatment. *Med Clin North Am.* 1997;81:881. PMID: 9222259.
34. Hecksel KA, Bostwick JM, Jaeger TM, et al. Inappropriate use of symptom-triggered therapy for alcohol withdrawal in the general hospital. *Mayo Clin Proc.* 2008;83:274–279. PMID: 18315992.
35. Awissi DK, Lebrun G, Coursin DB, et al. Alcohol withdrawal and delirium tremens in the critically ill: a systematic review and commentary. *Intensive Care Med.* 2013;39:16–30. PMID: 23184039.

36. Eyer F, Schuster T, Felgenhauer N, et al. Risk assessment of moderate to severe alcohol withdrawal—predictors for seizures and delirium tremens in the course of withdrawal. *Alcohol Alcohol.* 2011;46:427–433. PMID: 21593124.
37. Monte R, Rabuñal R, Casariego E, et al. Risk factors for delirium tremens in patients with alcohol withdrawal syndrome in a hospital setting. *Eur J Intern Med.* 2009;20(7):690–694. PMID: 19818288.
38. Thiercelin N, Rabiah Lechevallier Z, Rusch E, et al. Risk factors for delirium tremens: a literature review. *Rev Med Interne.* 2012;33:18–22. PMID: 21920639.
39. Chan GM, Hoffman RS, Gold JA, et al. Racial variations in the incidence of severe alcohol withdrawal. *J Med Toxicol.* 2009;5(1):8–14. PMID: 19191209.
40. Nuss MA, Elnicki DM, Dunsworth TS, et al. Utilizing CIWA-Ar to assess use of benzodiazepines in patients vulnerable to alcohol withdrawal syndrome. *W V Med J.* 2004;100:21–25. PMID: 15119493.
41. Spies CD, Dubisz N, Neumann T, et al. Therapy of alcohol withdrawal syndrome in intensive care unit patients following trauma: results of a prospective, randomized trial. *Crit Care Med.* 1996;24:414–422. PMID: 8625628.
42. Spies CD, Rommelspacher H. Alcohol withdrawal in the surgical patient: prevention and treatment. *Anesth Analg.* 1999;88(4):946–954. PMID: 10195555.
43. Sullivan JT, Sykora K, Schneiderman J, et al. Assessment of alcohol withdrawal: the revised clinical institute withdrawal assessment for alcohol scale (CIWA-Ar). *Br J Addict.* 1989;84:1353.
44. Sullivan JT, et al. Benzodiazepine requirements during alcohol withdrawal syndrome: clinical impressions using a standardized withdrawal scale. *J Clin Pharmacol.* 1991;11:291–295.
45. Mayo-Smith MF; for the American Society of Addiction Medicine Working Group on Pharmacological Management of Ethanol Withdrawal. Pharmacological management of ethanol withdrawal: a meta-analysis and evidence based practice guideline. *JAMA.* 1997;278:144–151.
46. Mayo-Smith MF, Beecher LH, Fischer TL, et al. Management of alcohol withdrawal delirium. An evidence-based practice guideline. *Arch Intern Med.* 2004;164:1405.
47. Repper-DeLisi J, Stern TA, Mitchell M, et al. Successful implementation of an alcohol-withdrawal pathway in a general hospital. *Psychosomatics.* 2008;49(4):292–299. PMID: 18621934.
48. Stehman CR, Mycyk MB. A rational approach to treatment of alcohol withdrawal in the ED. *Am J Emerg Med.* 2013;31:734–742. PMID: 23399338.
49. Amato L, Minozzi S, Vecchi S, et al. Benzodiazepines for alcohol withdrawal. *Cochrane Database Syst Rev.* 2010;3:CD005063. doi: 10.1002/14651858.CD005063.pub3.
50. Amato L, Minozzi S, Davoli M. Efficacy and safety of pharmacologic interventions for the treatment of the alcohol withdrawal syndrome. *Cochrane Database Syst Rev.* 2011;CD008537.
51. Hoffman RS. Management of moderate to severe alcohol withdrawal syndromes. UptoDate. http://www.uptodate.com. Accessed September 11, 2013.
52. Miller DG, Weinstein E, Hunter BR. Alcohol, meet benzodiazepine shortage; How to effectively treat alcohol withdrawal during nationwide shortages of benzodiazepines. *Emerg Physic Monthly.* 2012; June.
53. Otto AM. Benzodiazepines discouraged for alcohol withdrawal. *Clinical Psychiatry News.* March 15, 2013. http://www.clinicalpsychiatrynews.com/index.php?id=2407&cHash=071010&tx_ttnews[tt_news]=141547. Accessed April, 2014.
54. Kumar CN, Andrade C, Murthy P. A randomized, double-blind comparison of lorazepam and chlordiazepoxide in patients with uncomplicated alcohol withdrawal. *J Stud Alcohol Drugs.* 2009;70(3):467–474. PMID: 19371497.
55. Hayner CE, Wuestefeld NL, Bolton PJ. Phenobarbital treatment in a patient with resistant alcohol withdrawal syndrome. *Pharmacotherapy.* 2009;29(7):875–878. PMID: 19558262.
56. Hjermø I, Anderson JE, Fink-Jensen A, et al. Phenobarbital vs Diazepam for delirium tremens: a retrospective review. *Dan Med Bull.* 2010;57:A4149.
57. Kramp P, Rafaelsen OJ. Delirium tremends A double blind comparison of diazepam and barbital treatment. *Acta Psychiatr Scand.* 1978;58:174–190.
58. Rosenson J, Clements C, Simon B, et al. Phenobarbital for acute alcohol withdrawal; A prospective randomized double-blind placebo controlled study. *J Emerg Med.* 2013;44:592–598.
59. Young GP, Rores C, Murphy C, et al. Intravenous phenobarbital for alcohol withdrawal and convulsions. *Ann Emerg Med.* 1987;16(8):847–850. PMID: 3619162.
60. Coomes TR, Smith SW. Successful use of propofol in refractory delirium tremens. *Ann Emerg Med.* 1997;30:825. PMID: 9398758.
61. McCowan C, Marik P. Refractory delirium tremens treated with propofol: a case series. *Crit Care Med.* 2000;28:1781. PMID: 10890619.

62. Currier DS, Bevacgua BK. Acute tachyphylaxis to propofol sedation during ethanol withdrawal. *J Clin Anesth.* 1997;9:420–423. PMID: 9257211.
63. Blum K, Eubanks JD, Wallace JE, et al. Enhancement of alcohol withdrawal convulsions in mice by haloperidol. *Clin Toxicol.* 1976;9:427. PMID: 986285.
64. Kaim SC, Klett CJ, Rothfeld B. Treatment of the acute alcohol withdrawal state: a comparison of four drugs. *Am J Psychiatry.* 1969;125(12):1640–1646. PMID: 4890289.
65. Longo LP, Campbell T, Hubatch S. Divalproex sodium (Depakote) for alcohol withdrawal and relapse prevention. *J Addict Dis.* 2002;21(2):55–64. PMID: 11916372.
66. Malcolm R, Myrick H, Roberts J, et al. The effects of carbamazepine and lorazepam on single versus multiple previous alcohol withdrawals in an outpatient randomized trial. *J Gen Intern Med.* 2002;17(5):349–355. PMID: 12047731.
67. Myrick H, Malcolm R, Randall PK, et al. A double-blind trial of gabapentin versus lorazepam in the treatment of alcohol withdrawal. *Alcohol Clin Exp Res.* 2009;33:1582–1588. PMID: 19485969.
68. Zack M, Poulos CX, Woodford TM. Diazepam dose-dependently increases or decreases implicit priming of alcohol associations in problem drinkers. *Alcohol Alcohol.* 2006;41(6):604–610. PMID: 17020910.
69. Poulos CX, Zack M. Low-dose diazepam primes motivation for alcohol and alcohol-related semantic networks in problem drinkers. *Behav Pharmacol.* 2004;15(7):503–512. PMID: 15472572.
70. Cagetti E, Baicy KJ, Olsen RW. Topiramate attenuates withdrawal signs after chronic intermittent ethanol in rats. *Neuroreport.* 2004;15:207–2010. PMID: 15106859.
71. Eyer F, Schreckenberg M, Hecht D, et al. Carbamazepine and valproate as adjuncts in the treatment of alcohol withdrawal syndrome: a retrospective cohort study. *Alcohol Alcohol.* 2011;46:177–184. PMID: 21339186.
72. Lum E, Gorman SK, Slavik RS. Valproic acid management of acute alcohol withdrawal. *Ann Pharmacother.* 2006;40:441–448. PMID: 16507623.
73. Reoux JP, Saxon J, Malte CA. Divalproex sodium in alcohol withdrawal: a randomized double-blind placebo controlled clinical trial. *Alcohol Clin Exp Res.* 2011;25:1324–1329. PMID: 11584152.
74. Bonnet U, Hamzavi-Abedi R, Specka M, et al. An open trial of gabapentin in acute alcohol withdrawal using an oral loading protocol. *Alcohol Alcohol.* 2010;45:143–145. PMID: 20019070.
75. Barrons R, Robertss N. The role of carbamazepine and oxcarbamazepine in alcohol withdrawal syndrome. *J Clin Pharm Ther.* 2010;35:153–167. PMID: 20456734.
76. Hillborn M, Tokola R, Kuusela V, et al. Prevention of alcohol withdrawal seizures in carbamazepine and valproic acid. *Alcohol.* 1989;6:223–226. PMID: 2500138.
77. Minozzi S, Amato L, Vecchi S, et al. Anticonvulsants for alcohol withdrawal. *Cochrane Database Syst Rev.* 2010;CD005064.
78. Addolorato G, Balducci G, Capristo E, et al. Gamma-hydroxybutyric acid (GHB) in the treatment of alcohol withdrawal syndrome: a randomized comparative study versus benzodiazepine. *Alcohol Clin Exp Res.* 1999;23:1596–1604. PMID: 10549990.
79. Addolorato G, Leggio L, Ferrulli A, et al. The therapeutic potential of gamma-hydroxybutyric acid for alcohol dependence: balancing the risks and benefits. A focus on clinical data. *Expert Opin Investig Drugs.* 2009;18:675–686. PMID: 19379123.
80. Alldredge BK, Lowenstein DH, Simon RP. Placebo-controlled trial of intravenous diphenylhydantoin for short-term treatment of alcohol withdrawal seizures. *Am J Med.* 1989;87:645. PMID: 2686433.
81. Chance JF. Emergency department treatment of alcohol withdrawal seizures with phenytoin. *Ann Emerg Med.* 1991;20:520. PMID: 2024792.
82. Rathlev NK, D'Onofrio G, Fish SS, et al. The lack of efficacy of phenytoin in the prevention of recurrent alcohol-related seizures. *Ann Emerg Med.* 1994;23:513. PMID: 8135426.
83. Maldonado JP. *Alcohol Withdrawal Syndrome—Treatment Options Beyond Benzodiazepines.* San Juan, Puerto Rico: ACMT Alcohol Abuse Academy; 2013.
84. Jaatinen P, Riihioja P, Haapalinna A, et al. Prevention of ethanol-induced sympathetic overactivity and degeneration by dexmedetomidine. *Alcohol.* 1995;12(5):439–446. PMID: 8519439.
85. Riihioja P, Jaatinen P, Haapalinna A, et al. Effects of dexmedetomidine on rat locus coeruleus and ethanol withdrawal symptoms during intermittent ethanol exposure. *Alcohol Clin Exp Res.* 1999;23(3):432–438. PMID: 10195815.
86. Riihioja P, Jaatinen P, Oksanen H, et al. Dexmedetomidine alleviates ethanol withdrawal symptoms in the rat. *Alcohol.* 1997;14(6):537–544. PMID: 9401667.
87. Riihioja P, Jaatinen P, Oksanen H, et al. Dexmedetomidine, diazepam, and propranolol in the treatment of ethanol withdrawal symptoms in the rat. *Alcohol Clin Exp Res.* 1997;21(5):804–808. PMID: 9267529.

88. Braz LG, Camacho Navarro LH, Braz JR, et al. Clonidine as adjuvant therapy for alcohol withdrawal syndrome in intensive care unit: case report. *Rev Bras Anestesiol.* 2003;53(6):802–807. PMID: 19471699.
89. Dobrydnjov I, Axelsson K, Berggren L, et al. Intrathecal and oral clonidine as prophylaxis for postoperative alcohol withdrawal syndrome: a randomized double-blinded study. *Anesth Analg.* 2004;98(3):738–744. PMID: 14980929.
90. Baumgartner GR, Rowen RC. Transdermal clonidine vs. chlordiazepoxide in alcohol withdrawal: a randomized controlled clinical trial. *South Med J.* 2001;84(3):312–321. PMID: 2000517.
91. Baddigam K, Russo P, Russo J, et al. Dexmedetomidine in the treatment of withdrawal syndromes in cardiothoracic surgery patients. *J Intensive Care Med.* 2005;20(2):118–123. PMID: 15855224.
92. Cooper L, Castillo D, Martinez-Ruid R, et al. Am Society of Anesthesiology. Adjuvant use of dexmedetomidine may reduce the incidence of endotracheal intubation caused by benzodiazepines in the treatment of delirium tremens [abstract] *Anesthesiology.* 2005;103:A317.
93. Darrouj J, Puri N, Prince E, et al. Dexmedetomidine infusion as adjunctive therapy to benzodiazepines for acute alcohol withdrawal. *Ann Pharmacother.* 2008;42(11):1703–1705. PMID: 18780809.
94. DeMuro JP, Botros DG, Wirkowski E, et al. Use of dexmedetomidine for the treatment of alcohol withdrawal syndrome in critically ill patients: a retrospective case series. *J Anesth.* 2012;26:601–605. PMID: 22584816.
95. Finkel JC, Elrefai A. The use of dexmedetomidine to facilitate opioid and benzodiazepine detoxification in an infant. *Anesth Analg.* 2004;98(6):1658–1659. PMID: 15155322.
96. Kandiah P, Jacob S, Pandya D, et al. Novel use of dexmedetomidine in 7 adults with resistant alcohol withdrawal in the ICU. Poster presented at: The 38th Critical Care Congress of the Society of Critical Care Medicine; January 31–February 4, 2009; Nashville, TN.
97. Maccioli GA. Dexmedetomidine to facilitate drug withdrawal. *Anesthesiology.* 2003;98(2):575–577. PMID: 12552220.
98. Multz AS. Prolonged dexmedetomidine infusion as an adjunct in treating sedation-induced withdrawal. *Anesth Analg.* 2003;96:1054–1055. PMID: 12651659.
99. Prieto MN, Barr J, Tanaka RN, et al.; Am Society of Anesthesiology. Dexmedetomidine: a novel approach to the management of alcohol withdrawal in the ICU. *Anesthesiology.* 2007;107:A1313.
100. Rayner SG, Weinert CR, Peng H, et al. Dexmedetomidine as adjunct treatment for severe alcohol withdrawal in the ICU. *Ann Intensive care.* 2012;23:12. PMID: 22620986.
101. Rovasalo A, Tohmo H, Aantaa R, et al. Dexmedetomidine as an adjuvant in the treatment of alcohol withdrawal delirium: a case report. *Gen Hosp Psychiatry.* 2006;28:362–363. PMID: 16814639.
102. Kukoyi A, Coker S, Lewis L, et al. Two cases of acute dexmedetomidine withdrawal syndrome following prolonged infusion in the intensive care unit: report of cases and review of the literature. *Hum Exp Toxicol.* 2013;32:107–110. PMID: 23111887.
103. Muzyk AJ, Fowler JA, Norwood DK, et al. Role of α2-agonists in the treatment of acute alcohol withdrawal. *Ann Pharmacother.* 2011;45(5):649–657. PMID: 21521867.
104. Colombo G, Serra S, Brunetti G, et al. Suppression by baclofen of alcohol deprivation effect in Sardinian alcohol-preferring (sP) rats. *Drug Alcohol Depend.* 2003;70:105.
105. Humeniuk RE, White JM, Onh J. The effect if GABAB ligands on alcohol withdrawal in mice. *Pharmacol Biochem Behav.* 1994;49:561–566.
106. Addolorato G, Leggio L, Ferrulli A, et al. Effectiveness and safety of baclofen for maintenance of alcohol abstinence in alcohol-dependent patients with liver cirrhosis: randomised, double-blind controlled study. *Lancet.* 2007;370:1915–1922.
107. Addolorato G, Leggio L, Abenavoli L, et al. Baclofen in the treatment of alcohol withdrawal syndrome: a comparative study vs. diazepam. *Am J Med.* 2006;119:276.e13. PMID: 16490478.
108. Lyon JE, Khan RA, Gessert CE, et al. Treating alcohol withdrawal with oral baclofen: a randomized, double-blind, placebo controlled trial. *J Hosp Med.* 2011;6:469–474. PMID: 21990176.
109. Liu J, Wang LN. Baclofen for alcohol withdrawal. *Cochrane Database Syst Rev.* 2013;2:CD008502. PMID: 23450582.
110. Addolorato G, Caputo F, Capristo E, et al. Rapid suppression of alcohol withdrawal syndrome by baclofen. *Am J Med.* 2002;112:226. PMID: 11893350.
111. Addolorato G, Leggio L, Agabio R, et al. Baclofen: a new drug for the treatment of alcohol dependence. *Int J Clin Pract.* 2006;60:1003–1008. PMID: 16893442.
112. Gorsane MA, Kebir O, Hache G, et al. Is baclofen a revolutionary medication in alcohol addiction management? Review and recent updates. *Subst Abuse.* 2012;33:336–349. PMID: 22989277.
113. Leggio L, Garbutt JC, Addolorato G. Effectiveness and safety of baclofen in the treatment of alcohol dependent patients. *CNS Neurol Disord Drug Targets.* 2010;9:33–44. PMID: 20201813.

114. Eggers V, Tio J, Neumann T, et al. Blood alcohol concentration for monitoring ethanol treatment to prevent alcohol withdrawal in the intensive care unit. *Intensive Care Med.* 2002;28:1475–1482. PMID: 12373474.
115. Dissanaike S, Halldorsson A, Frezza EE, et al. An ethanol protocol to prevent alcohol withdrawal syndrome. *J Am Coll Surg.* 2006;203:186–191. PMID: 16864031.
116. Hodges B, Mazur JE. Intravenous ethanol for the treatment of alcohol withdrawal syndrome in critically ill patients. *Pharmacotherapy.* 2004;24:1578. PMID: 15537562.
117. Weinberg JA, Magnotti LJ, Fischer PE, et al. Comparison of intravenous ethanol versus diazepam for alcohol withdrawal prophylaxis in the trauma ICU: results of a randomized trial. *J Trauma.* 2008;64(1):99–104. PMID: 18188105.
118. Zechnich RJ. Beta-blockers can obscure diagnosis of delirium tremens. *Lancet.* 1982;1:1071–1072. PMID: 6122874.
119. Sarff M, Gold JA. Alcohol withdrawal syndromes in the intensive care unit. *Crit Care Med.* 2010; 38(9 Suppl):S494–S501.

SECTION 12

Environmental Critical Care

53

Hypothermia

Morgan Eutermoser and Jay Lemery

BACKGROUND

In 2005, the Centers for Disease Control and Prevention (CDC) Morbidity and Mortality Weekly Report disclosed that 689 deaths per year in the United States were attributable to accidental hypothermia, defined as an involuntary or unintentional drop in core body temperature to <35°C (95°F).[1,2] Heat loss from environmental exposure occurs through four well-known mechanisms: radiation, conduction (which can significantly increase in water and/or wet clothes), convection, and evaporation.[3] Conversely, heat generation occurs through skeletal muscle use as well as through involuntary hypothalamic-mediated shivering.[4] The latter is a neuroendocrine response to mild hypothermia mediated through serotonin, dopamine, norepinephrine, thyroid-stimulating hormone, and thyrotropin-releasing hormone, all of which affect the autonomic nervous system.[3]

Primary hypothermia occurs when an individual's intrinsic compensatory capacity is overwhelmed by cold stress and thus unable to maintain temperature homeostasis. Patients with chronic disease or physiologic vulnerability—such as advanced age, alcohol or drug abuse, and mental impairment—have diminished compensatory capacity and are at greater risk for primary hypothermia.[3,5]

Secondary hypothermia occurs when a person with a systemic illness (e.g., myxedema coma or sepsis) becomes hypothermic due to a pathologic lack of autoregulation. Clinicians should be aware that this may occur even in a warm environment and is a sign of severe physiologic decompensation. This chapter describes the clinically relevant parameters of hypothermia and outlines an appropriate organ system–based approach to diagnosis and management.

DEFINITIONS

Hypothermia is a sign of severe illness and/or significant environmental exposure. Prompt identification is critical for optimal clinical management. Degree of hypothermia is generally stratified to four categories: mild (35°C to 32°C), moderate

(32°C to 28°C), severe (28°C to 20°C), and profound (<20°C).[6] In the absence of an ability to quantify temperature, the Swiss staging system (Table 53.1) may be used to categorize hypothermia severity based on clinical presentation.[7]

PATHOPHYSIOLOGY AND CLINICAL PRESENTATION

Cardiovascular

The initial response to cold stress and mild hypothermia (>33°C) is a norepinephrine (NE)-mediated increase in mean arterial pressure (MAP) and heart rate (HR).[6] These physiologic signs reverse, with a decrease in MAP and HR, when the core temperature falls below 33°C.[6] Sinus bradycardia is an expected finding in hypothermic patients, due to a combination of decreased sympathetic tone and a slowing of spontaneous depolarization of cardiac pacemaker cells.[3] This bradycardia is not vagally mediated, and thus atropine will have limited efficacy in resuscitation. The hypothermic state significantly lowers metabolism, and therefore marked bradycardia is not as detrimental to the body's needs as in a euthermic patient. The hypothermic effect on the myocardium is known to produce an "irritable" state, in which the use of pacing wires and antiarrhythmic drugs during resuscitation has been shown to trigger significant dysrhythmias. These interventions are not supported by available evidence and are not recommended in the current American Heart Association (AHA) guidelines.

The classic ECG finding of hypothermia (<33°C) (Fig. 53.1)—the "J-wave" or "Osborn wave"—is a marked with a dome configuration at the R-ST junction.[8] First characterized in 1953, this EEG morphology was associated by Osborn with the risk of impending ventricular arrhythmias; however, this has since been refuted.[9] J-waves can also be seen in myocardial ischemia, sepsis, and CNS lesions and can be a normal ECG variant in young people.[3] The formation of the J-wave in hypothermia is thought to be due to delayed depolarization or early repolarization of the left ventricular wall.

Atrial fibrillation is quite common at core temperatures below 32°C and will commonly convert spontaneously with rewarming.[3] At 28°C, severe bradycardia (30 to 40 bpm) can be expected.[10] As moderate to severe hypothermia set in, decreased conduction velocity, increased myocardial conduction time, and decreased refractory time can result in the sinus bradycardia degenerating into atrial and ventricular dysrhythmias.[3]

TABLE 53.1 Swiss Staging System

Stage	Clinical Findings	Likely Temperature
I	Alert, shivering	35°C–32°C
II	Drowsy, not shivering	32°C–28°C
III	Unconscious, vital signs present	28°C–24°C
IV	Vital signs absent, appears dead	24°C–13°C
V	Death (irreversible hypothermia)	<13°C

Adapted from Brown Douglas JA, Brugger H, Boyd J, et al. Accidental hypothermia. *N Engl J Med.* 2012;367:1930–1938.

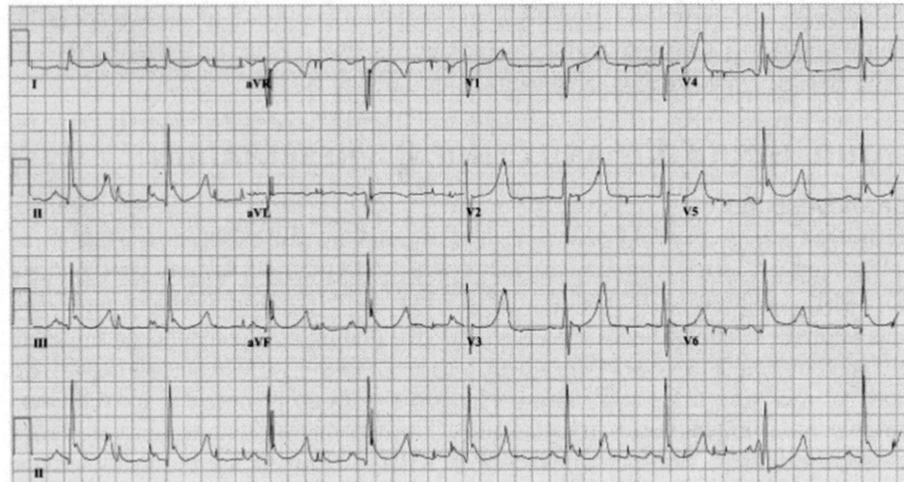

FIGURE 53.1 ECG from a hypothermic patient demonstrating Osborn waves and bradycardia. Reprinted with permission from Dr. Steve Lowenstein, University of Colorado Hospital.

Below 25°C, asystole and ventricular fibrillation occur spontaneously and may be hastened by the jostling of patients by caregivers; therefore, care must be taken when handling these patients.[3]

As previously noted, MAP drops in severe hypothermia, producing an associated significant decrease in global sympathetic tone. Peripheral vasodilation occurs at this time and can result in a warming sensation. When combined with an altered mental status (see neurologic effects below), this warming sensation can lead to "paradoxical undressing," whereby patients may remove clothing in an effort to cool down, compounding environmental hypothermia.[11] During hypothermic resuscitation, IV arterial vasopressor therapies such as vasopressin or phenylephrine may be used to improve peripheral vasomotor tone during rewarming. Careful attention to and correction of any intravascular volume deficit are also important for appropriate resuscitation.

Pulmonary

The initial response to hypothermia is tachypnea driven by the increased metabolic demand from shivering. However, once basal metabolism begins to slow (50% decrease in CO_2 production with an 8°C drop in core temperature), there is a commensurate decrease in minute ventilation. This physiologic change highlights the need to be aware of possible overventilation and subsequent iatrogenic hypocapnia during a hypothermic resuscitation. Direct cold exposure affects pulmonary mechanics through airway congestion, bronchoconstriction, increased secretions, and decreased mucociliary clearance. The primary ventilatory response to cold air is a decrease in baseline ventilation and respiratory chemosensitivity. These responses are thought to provide significant protection against heat loss in animals, although the effect on human physiology is minimal. Cold exposure also elicits an increase in pulmonary vascular resistance. This stimulus is synergistic with hypoxia and may mediate pulmonary hypertension and edema at altitude.[12]

Neurologic

For every 1°C decrease in core body temperature, cerebral metabolism is decreased by 6% to 7%, with EEG silencing typically found at 19°C to 20°C.[3,13] Loss of pupillary light reflex and deep tendon reflexes can be seen in moderate hypothermia.[14] However, in one series of 97 patients with accidental hypothermia, level of consciousness, pupillary reflex, and deep tendon reflexes could not be correlated with temperature even in severe hypothermia.[15] This illustrates an important clinical pearl —patients may appear dead, yet be profoundly hypothermic. Indeed, there have been many case reports of patients who have survived with extremely low core temperatures—as low as 14.2°C in a child and 13.7°C in an adult—thus supporting the maxim patients are not dead until they are warm and dead.[16,17]

Renal

Renal pathology in hypothermia is most commonly due to prerenal failure from cold-induced diuresis and fluid shifts (primary hypothermia) and may be coupled with underlying systemic diseases affecting renal function (secondary).[18] The initial systemic autonomic response to cold stress is that blood flow shifts to the core and away from the periphery.[19] The resulting increased central blood volume and perfusion produce a reduction in CNS release of antidiuretic hormone resulting in renal free water diuresis, a process known as "cold diuresis." This is important to understand during a hypothermic resuscitation, as the patient may have markedly reduced blood volume yet maintain a normal blood pressure due to significant concomitant vasoconstriction. Likewise, when rewarming begins, peripheral vasodilation may lead to core blood redistribution and cardiovascular collapse in the hypothermic dehydrated patient.

Hematologic

Hypothermia causes an increase in blood viscosity, hematocrit, and fibrinogen levels.[13] The normal clotting cascade is also impeded, due to the temperature-mediated inhibition of the catalytic function of multiple clotting cascade components.[20] Severe hypothermia (often with concomitant frostbite) can lead to fulminant disseminated intravascular coagulation from the release of tissue thromboplastin (responsible for catalyzing the conversion of prothrombin to thrombin) from ischemic tissues.[13,21] Cold stress also suppresses bone marrow production, which may lead to thrombocytopenia and cause splenic and hepatic sequestration of platelets.[3] Hypothermia can have significant impact on the care of trauma patients and is considered part of the "lethal triad of trauma" (metabolic acidosis, coagulopathy, and hypothermia).[22]

For every 1°C decline in core temperature, there is a 2% increase in the hematocrit. Anemia in a severely hypothermic patient should therefore raise suspicion and prompt a broader workup.[21] Caution also should be exercised in interpreting prothrombin time and activated partial thromboplastin times. They will not accurately reflect coagulation status because the values are measured at 37°C in the lab rather than the in vivo core body temperature of the patient.

Gastrointestinal

As temperature declines, gut motility begins to slow, often resulting in an ileus at temperatures below 28°C.[13] Decreased hepatic blood flow will cause hepatic impairment, which can result in reduced drug metabolism as well as compromised clearing of lactate.

Pancreatitis is also commonly seen in hypothermia but can be clinically silent, discovered only through elevation of enzymes. Because of this, glucose should be carefully monitored during rewarming.[23]

MANAGEMENT GUIDELINES

Temperature Determination

Optimal clinical management of the hypothermic patient depends on accurate and consistent temperature monitoring. The esophageal probe is the recommended device in a critically hypothermic patient.[24] Temperature determination can be falsely elevated if the patient is intubated or ventilated with heated air, or if the probe is placed too proximally in the esophagus. To avoid this problem, it is recommended to place the probe in the lower third of the esophagus.[25] Rectal temperature measurement is commonly used but has a greater risk of inaccuracy than the esophageal devices. Specifically, rectal temperatures can lag behind true core body temperatures and thus risk accidental overshoot in core temperature during rewarming.[26] Proper placement of the probe is 15 cm into the rectum, avoiding cold feces. Tympanic membrane temperature assessment is cumbersome and not recommended for continuous monitoring, but can effectively and quickly identify core temperature. If used, the ear should be clear of cerumen and shielded from the outside environment.[27] Bladder temperature probes are also not recommended in the severely hypothermic patient and may be confounded if warm saline is instilled into the bladder.

Airway and Breathing

Accurately assessing oxygen saturation in a hypothermic patient can be difficult. The skin surface must be warm and well perfused in order to accurately measure transcutaneous oxygen saturation and is therefore poorly suited to this purpose in the hypothermic patient.[28] Airway management decisions remain the same as in any critically ill patient. Gentle handling of the patient during airway maneuvers is recommended because of a potentially irritable myocardium; however, a multicenter survey that reviewed 117 intubations of hypothermic patients reported no increased complications.[3,29] Endotracheal intubation has an additional benefit of allowing for the inhalation of humidified, heated air. Hypothermic patients are vulnerable to electrolyte imbalances, and succinylcholine should be avoided given its side effect of transient hyperkalemia.[30] In any hypothermic patient with altered mental status, precipitating events, including trauma, infection, and toxic/metabolic disorders, should be carefully assessed.

Medical Therapy

Medications that have temperature-dependent activity may have compromised efficacy in a hypothermic patient. Cold-induced pharmacokinetic changes include increased protein binding and decreased liver metabolism.[31] Advanced Cardiac Life Support (ACLS) drugs given to a hypothermic patient may remain in circulation and subsequently manifest toxic effects during rewarming. Most hypothermic clinical conditions, however, do not require pharmacologic intervention, as rewarming will resolve the majority of cold-induced pathologies (e.g., atrial fibrillation).

High-risk hypothermic patients merit full infectious workups and consideration of broad-spectrum antibiotics. In a retrospective review of 59 patients with accidental hypothermia, 41% also had serious infections with predominance of respiratory and soft tissue infections.[32]

ACLS

ACLS is modified in several protocols. Table 53.2 shows three common transport protocols and recommendations with ACLS modifications. Each patient should be assessed on an individual basis.

Rewarming

Rewarming is divided into three levels: passive external, active external, and active internal/core rewarming.[3] The choice of specific rewarming method(s) should be based on both available resources and specific patient needs.[36] Rescuers should be aware of the phenomenon of afterdrop when extricating a patient from prolonged cold exposure settings (e.g., avalanches). Afterdrop is the decrease in core body temperature during rewarming due to redistribution of peripheral cold blood (also known as core shunting).

TABLE 53.2 ACLS Recommendations in Accidental Hypothermia

State of Alaska Cold Injuries Transport Guidelines[33]	JAMA Guidelines for Cardiopulmonary Resuscitation and Emergency Cardiac Care: Hypothermia[34]	The 2010 American Heart Association Guidelines for Cardiopulmonary Resuscitation and Emergency Cardiovascular Care Science: Cardiac Arrest in Accidental Hypothermia[35]
BLS/ACLS should not be initiated in field if core temperature is <15°C, chest is frozen, victim is underwater for more than an hour, or lethal injury present Signs of life and pulse should be assessed for 45 s before CPR initiated Intubation is safe and needed to give humidified, heated oxygen Maintain the patient in horizontal position Chest compressions should not be performed if there are signs of life Chest compressions should be performed if there are no signs of life. If after 60 min and appropriate CPR and there are still no signs of life, an EMT can discontinue resuscitative efforts Defibrillation and ACLS drugs should only be used if the core temperature is above 86 F One trial of defibrillation can be attempted if temperature is unknown BLS/ACLS procedures should be terminated if there is significant harm/risk to the rescuer or if procedures cause a delay in evacuation IVF should be heated to 42°C–44°C	1. Rescue breaths should be given to the apneic patient 2. Pulse check for 30–45 s prior to initiation of chest compression. Prior recommendations focused on 1- to 2-min check 3. Gentle intubation to avoid ventricular fibrillation 4. Maintain the patient in horizontal position 5. Deliver three shocks for patients in VF; however, if persistent VF, do not shock again until warmed to 30°C 6. Warm oxygen (42°C–46°C) and IVF (43°C) should be started while transporting	1. If no signs of life, begin CPR without delay 2. If VT or VF present, defibrillation should be attempted. No recommendation for ceasing attempts or continued attempts if VT or VF persists 3. Supports advanced airway placement and warmed, humidified oxygen 4. Given animal investigations and vasopressors, reasonable to administer medications according to the standard ACLS algorithm. No formal recommendation to give or withhold ACLS medications 5. Patients should be warm prior to declaration of death

Although some studies[37] show no effect of afterdrop on patients during rewarming, a field study performed in 2010 suggests a significant physiologic effect. In that study, subjects were buried in snow with an esophageal temperature probe in place and wearing an Avalung (a commercially available personal avalanche rescue device to assist in preservation of ventilation). After 60 minutes, subjects were extricated and placed in a warm blanket, subsequently demonstrating a fourfold increase of cooling rate compared to burial cooling rate.[38]

Passive External Rewarming

Passive external rewarming is a noninvasive, spontaneous process that involves removal of wet/cold garments and placement of blankets. Passive rewarming is recommended only for mild hypothermia.

Active External Rewarming

Common methods of active external rewarming include breathing warmed and humidified air, cutaneous warming via localized heating pads, blankets, or commercially available forced-air warmers (e.g., Bair Hugger), and, on occasion, extremity immersion. Heated, humidified air can increase core temperature by 1°C to 2°C/hour.[21] Convection-based forced-air warmers can raise core temperatures 0.9°C/hour. Chemical heat packs or local heating pads can cause thermal injury to skin, especially in an obtunded patient, do not provide core warming, and are not recommended. If available and appropriate for the clinical circumstances, extremity immersion in hyperthermic water has proven utility. In a 1999 study, hypothermic subjects were warmed by either shivering or extremity immersion into 42°C or 45°C water. The subjects in the immersion group achieved a faster rewarming rate.[39]

Active Internal Rewarming

Active internal rewarming techniques have progressed from initial drain placement and warm lavage fluid to cardiopulmonary bypass. A provider's decision to transition from active external to active internal rewarming techniques should be guided by the mental status and hemodynamic stability of the patient, as well as by capacity for close patient monitoring. Rewarming of blood has proven to have superior outcomes than warm lavage of body cavities. There are four techniques to warm blood: cardiopulmonary bypass, arteriovenous rewarming, venovenous rewarming, and hemodialysis. A Swiss review of 32 severely hypothermic young, healthy patients requiring cardiopulmonary bypass yielded 15 long-term survivors with excellent to no cerebral impairment[40] (Table 53.3). Rewarming fluids for all techniques should be calibrated to 40°C to 42°C. Once a patient's core temperature reaches 32°C to 35°C, rewarming should be slowed and stopped completely at 35°C to avoid temperature overshoot.

Termination of Resuscitation

Poor prognostic indicators include serum levels of fibrinogen <50 mg/dL, potassium >10 mEq/L, and ammonia >250 mol/L.[41] One study in 1994 evaluated 22 patients presenting due to hypothermic cardiac arrest. No patient with an arrival potassium level of 9 mEq/L or above survived off of cardiopulmonary bypass.

TABLE 53.3 Active Internal Rewarming Techniques, Advantages, and Rewarming Rates

Technique	Advantages	Rate of Rewarming
Cardiopulmonary bypass	Patients without a perfusing rhythm If cardiac activity lost, flow is preserved. Requires specialized personnel	9.5°C/h
Arteriovenous rewarming	Does not require specialized equipment or personnel Simple Seldinger technique	3°C–4°C/h
Venovenous rewarming	Circuit is not complex, efficient	2°C–3°C/h
Hemodialysis	Portable. Addresses metabolic derangements, renal failure, and dialyzable toxins Catheters are two-way; therefore, only one vessel is needed	2°C–3°C/h

Adapted from Danzl, DF. Hypothermia. *Semin Respir Crit Care Med.* 2002;23:57–68.

These data support the generally accepted recommendation to terminate resuscitation in patients with initial potassium levels of more than 10 mEq/L.[42] The AHA recommends withholding field resuscitation if the body is frozen or the airway is blocked; its 2005 guidelines state, "once the patient is in the hospital, physicians should use their clinical judgment to decide when resuscitative efforts should cease in a victim of hypothermic arrest."[43] However, in the most recent AHA 2010 guidelines, they changed this position to reflect the accepted current view: "Patients should not be considered dead before warming has been provided."[35]

CONCLUSION

Primary hypothermia should be considered in any patient with a history of environmental exposure. Secondary hypothermia should be considered in any chronically ill patient. In primary hypothermia, care will be dictated by the clinical condition of the patient. Understanding the irritability of the myocardium, care should focus on rewarming without invasive procedures or pharmacologic interventions that may do more harm than good.

Clinicians should understand the physiology of core shunting and the potential dangers of afterdrop. Trauma, infection, and toxic/metabolic disarray often exist concomitantly with hypothermia and require comprehensive workup and appropriate supportive care.

Clinicians should be aware of their institution's rewarming capabilities. Passive rewarming is adequate for the vast majority of hypothermic patients. In cases of severe environmental hypothermia, invasive measures involving multiple services (renal, ICU, cardiovascular surgery) may be indicated. In the extreme case of a hypothermic patient without vital signs, clinicians should understand the indications for rewarming and the criteria for cessation of resuscitation.

LITERATURE TABLE

TRIAL	DESIGN	RESULT
Hayward et al., *Resuscitation.* 1984[24]	Controlled observational study that evaluated cardiac, esophageal, rectal, skin, and tympanic temperatures in a patient who was cooled and rewarmed using three different rewarming techniques	During rewarming, divergent temperatures were demonstrated between probe locations. Only esophageal temperature was representative of cardiac temperature
Danzl et al., *Ann Emerg Med.* 1987[29]	Retrospective chart review of 428 cases of hypothermia in 13 emergency departments that assessed outcomes of intubation in 117 patients	Orotracheal intubation performed without complications, including 97 in patients with core temperatures ≤32.2°C
Lewin et al., *Arch Intern Med.* 1981[32]	Retrospective chart review of 59 patients admitted for accidental hypothermia that evaluated infection risk and antibiotic use	Forty-one percent of patients had serious bacterial infections. Infection is frequently masked in hypothermic patients (38% of infections were not diagnosed at time of admission)—study concluded that prompt empiric antibiotic therapy is appropriate
Grissom et al., *Wilderness Environ Med.* 2010[38]	Cohort observational study of six subjects buried in the snow with Avalungs to support breathing to demonstrate the afterdrop phenomenon	Temperature was measured with esophageal probe. The rate of core cooling increased fourfold when subjects were extricated and rewarming was initiated with an insulated wrap compared to burial cooling rate ($p < 0.001$)
Walpoth et al., *N Engl J Med.* 1997[40]	Cohort study of 46 patients with circulatory arrest due to accidental hypothermia	Thirty-two of 46 patients underwent cardiopulmonary bypass with 15 survivors. Follow-up of the 15 survivors showed no hypothermia-related deficits
Mair et al., *Resuscitation.* 1994[42]	Retrospective chart review of 22 patients rewarmed using cardiopulmonary bypass to evaluate poor prognostic indicators	Potassium, pH, and activated clotting time (ACT) values assessed to determine prognostic indicators. Poor prognostic indicators for successful resuscitation: potassium above 9 mmol/L, pH ≤6.50, and ACT above 400s
Schaller et al., *JAMA.* 1990[44]	Retrospective chart review of 24 patients with accidental hypothermia comparing potassium levels and outcomes	No survivors in group with potassium between 6.8 and 24.5 mmol/L compared to complete survival in group with potassium range of 2.7–5.3 mmol/L

REFERENCES

1. Centers for Disease Control and Prevention (CDC). Hypothermia-related deaths—United States, 2003–2004. *MMWR Morb Mortal Wkly Rep.* 2005;54(07):173–175.
2. Brown Douglas JA, Brugger H, Boyd J, et al. Accidental hypothermia. *N Engl J Med.* 2012;367:1930–1938.
3. Danzl DF. Hypothermia. *Semin Respir Crit Care Med.* 2002;23:57–68.
4. Pozos RS, Israel D, McCutcheon R, et al. Human studies concerning thermal-induced shivering, postoperative "shivering," and cold-induced vasodilation. *Ann Emerg Med.* 1987;16:1037–1041.
5. Jurkovich GJ. Environmental cold-induced injury. *Surg Clin North Am.* 2007;87(1):247–267.
6. Chernow B, Lake CR, Zaritsky A, et al. Sympathetic nervous system "switch off" with severe hypothermia. *Crit Care Med.* 1983;11:677–680.
7. Davis PR, Byers M. Accidental hypothermia. *J R Army Med Corps.* 2006;152:223–233.
8. Maruyama M, Kobayashi Y, Kodani E, et al. Osborn waves: history and significance. *Indian Pacing Electrophysiol J.* 2004;4(1):33–39.
9. Osborn JJ. Experimental hypothermia: respiratory and blood pH changes in relation to cardiac function. *Am J Physiol.* 1953;175:389–398.
10. Murphy K, Nowak RM, Tomlanovich MC. Use of bretylium tosylate as prophylaxis and treatment in hypothermic ventricular fibrillation in the canine model. *Ann Emerg Med.* 1986;15(10):1160–1166.

11. Wedin B, Vanggaard L, Hirvonen J. "Paradoxical undressing" in fatal hypothermia. *J Forensic Sci.* 1979;24(3):543–553.
12. Giesbrecht GG. The respiratory system in a cold environment. *Aviat Space Environ Med.* 1995; 66(9):890–902.
13. Mallet ML. Pathophysiology of accidental hypothermia. *QJM.* 2002;95:775–785.
14. Weinberg AD. Hypothermia. *Ann Emerg Med.* 1993;22(2 Pt 2):370–377.
15. Fischbeck KH, Simon RP. Neurologic manifestations of accidental hypothermia. *Ann Neurol.* 1981;10(4):384–387.
16. Dobson JA, Burgess JJ. Resuscitation of severe hypothermia by extracorporeal rewarming in a child. *J Trauma.* 1996;40:483–485.
17. Gilbert M, Busund R, Skagseth A, et al. Resuscitation from accidental hypothermia of 13.7 degrees C with circulatory arrest. *Lancet.* 2000;355(9201):375–376.
18. Kuriyama S, Tomonari H, Numatat M, et al. Clinical characteristics of renal damage in patients with accidental hypothermia. *Nihon Jinzo Gakkai Shi.* 1999;41(5):493–498.
19. Lloyd EL. Accidental hypothermia. *Resuscitation.* 1996;32:111–124.
20. Danzl DF, Pozos RS. Accidental hypothermia. *N Engl J Med.* 1994;331:1756–1760.
21. Cosgriff N, Moore EE, Sauaia A, et al. Predicting life-threatening coagulopathy in the massively transfused trauma patient: hypothermia and acidosis revisited. *J Trauma.* 1997;42:857–861.
22. Moffatt SE. Hypothermia in trauma. *Emerg Med J.* 2013;30(12):989–996.
23. Maclean D, Murison J, Griffiths PD. Acute pancreatitis and diabetic ketoacidosis in accidental hypothermia and hypothermic myxoedema. *Br Med J.* 1973;4(895):757–761.
24. Hayward JS, Eckerson JD, Kemna D. Thermal and cardiovascular changes during three methods of resuscitation from mild hypothermia. *Resuscitation.* 1984;11(1–2):21–33.
25. Danzl DF. Accidental hypothermia. In: Auerbach PS, ed. *Wilderness medicine.* 6th ed. Philadelphia, PA: Mosby; 2012:116–142.
26. Weingart S. Rectal probe temperature lag during rapid saline induction of hypothermia after resuscitation from cardiac arrest. *Resuscitation.* 2009;80:837–838.
27. Walpoth BH, Galdikas J, Leupi F, et al. Assessment of hypothermia with a new "tympanic" thermometer. *J Clin Monit.* 1994;10:91–96.
28. Clayton DG, Webb RK, Ralston AC, et al. A comparison of the performance of 20 pulse oximeters under conditions of poor perfusion [see comments]. *Anaesthesia.* 1991;46:3–10.
29. Danzl DF, Pozos RS, Auerbach PS, et al. Multicenter hypothermia survey. *Ann Emerg Med.* 1987;16(9):1042–1055.
30. Brugger H, et al. Resuscitation of avalanche victims: evidence-based guidelines of the international commission for mountain emergency medicine (ICAR MEDCOM). Intended for physicians and other advanced life support personnel. *Resuscitation.* 2013;84(5):539–546.
31. Wong KC. Physiology and pharmacology of hypothermia. *West J Med.* 1983;138:227–232.
32. Lewin S, Brettman LR, Holzman RS. Infections in hypothermic patients. *Arch Intern Med.* 1981; 141(7):920–925.
33. Transport Guidelines for the Severely Hypothermic. State of Alaska Cold Injuries and Cold Water Near Drowning Guidelines (Rev 01/2005).
34. American Heart Association. Excerpt from Special Situations Section. Guidelines for cardiopulmonary resuscitation and emergency cardiac care. Emergency Cardiac Care Committee and Subcommittees, American Heart Association. Part IV. Special resuscitation situations. *JAMA.* 1992;268(16):2242–2250.
35. Vanden Hoek TL, Morrison LJ, Shuster M, et al. 2010 American Heart Association Guidelines for Cardiopulmonary Resuscitation and Emergency Cardiovascular Care Science. Part 12: Cardiac Arrest in Special Situations. *Circulation.* 2010;122:S829–S861.
36. Rogers I. Which rewarming therapy in hypothermia? A review of the randomized trials. *Emerg Med.* 1997;9:213–220.
37. Kornberger E, Schwarz B, Lindner KH, et al. Forced air surface rewarming in patients with severe accidental hypothermia. *Resuscitation.* 1999;41:105–111.
38. Grissom CK, Harmston CH, McAlpine JC, et al. Spontaneous endogenous core temperature rewarming after cooling due to snow burial. *Wilderness Environ Med.* 2010;21:229–235.
39. Vangaard L, Eyolfson D, Xu X, et al. Arteriovenous anastomoses (AVA) rewarming in 45°C water is effective in moderately hypothermic subjects. *FASEB J.* 1998;12:A90.
40. Walpoth BH, Walpoth-Aslan BN, Mattle HP, et al. Outcome of survivors of accidental deep hypothermia and circulatory arrest treated with extracorporeal blood warming. *N Engl J Med.* 1997; 337(21):1500–1505.

41. Hauty MG, Esrig BC, Hill JG, et al. Prognostic factors in severe accidental hypothermia: experience from the Mt. Hood tragedy. *J Trauma.* 1987;27:1107–1112.
42. Mair P, Korberger E, Furtwaengler W, et al. Prognostic markers in patients with severe accidental hypothermia and cardiocirculatory arrest. *Resuscitation.* 1994;27(1):47–54.
43. 2005 American heart association guidelines for cardiopulmonary resuscitation and emergency cardiovascular care. *Circulation.* 2005;112:IV-136–IV-138.
44. Schaller MD, Fischer AP, Perret CH. Hyperkalemia: a prognostic factor during acute severe hypothermia. *JAMA.* 1990;264(14):1842–1845.

54

Altitude Emergencies

Christopher Davis, Zina Semenovskaya, and Jay Lemery

BACKGROUND

Altitude illness encompasses a spectrum of clinical entities that occur at elevation as a result of hypobaric hypoxia. While a mild case of acute mountain sickness (AMS)—defined as headache with one of the following: nausea, fatigue, dizziness, anorexia, or poor sleep—may be no more than an inconvenience, high-altitude cerebral and pulmonary edema are true emergencies that require critical intervention and stabilization.

Although the concentration of oxygen remains nearly constant at 20.95% up to an elevation of at least 50 km, the partial pressure of oxygen decreases with increasing altitude in logarithmic fashion. With ascent to higher elevations, the lungs experience a decreasing pressure difference between alveolar and pulmonary arterial capillary beds. Without this pressure difference to drive oxygen across the alveolar membrane, tissue oxygen concentrations fall and, with extended time at altitude, result in hypoxia. This decrease begins at 1,500 m above sea level—generally referred to as the physiologic starting point of high altitude. Elevations are further classified as high altitude (1,500 to 3,500 m), very high altitude (3,500 to 5,500 m), and extreme altitude (above 5,500 m)—imprecise categories that loosely correlate to physiologic stress and pathology. While altitude determines the presence and extent of hypobaric hypoxia, increasing latitude, winter season, and the presence of storms driven by lower regional barometric pressure can influence local barometric pressure. These effects may combine to raise the effective altitude by hundreds of meters resulting in significant clinical consequences.

HIGH-ALTITUDE PULMONARY EDEMA

Overview

High-altitude pulmonary edema (HAPE) is a potentially deadly form of noncardiogenic edema driven by hypobaric hypoxia. Ascent to altitude produces an initial hypoxic pulmonary vasoconstrictor response. Although this adaptive response is believed to be useful in mitigating ventilation–perfusion mismatch in disorders such as pneumonia, a global constriction of the pulmonary vascular bed may lead to a pathologic increase in pulmonary artery pressures.[1] While pulmonary artery pressures rise in all individuals with ascent to altitude, HAPE-susceptible individuals manifest an exaggerated response.[2–4]

One theory purports that uneven pulmonary vasoconstriction leads to overperfusion in select areas of the pulmonary vascular bed.[5,6] This unevenly distributed perfusion overloads the pulmonary capillaries, eventually leading to fluid leak and "stress failure" of the alveolar–capillary membrane.[7]

Susceptibility to HAPE is driven by a complex set of factors, including prior history of HAPE, rate of ascent, sleeping altitude, physical exertion, air temperature, concomitant respiratory illness, and individual genetic predisposition or congenital cardiopulmonary abnormalities.[2,8–14] Males were historically considered to be at higher risk for HAPE than females, but this hypothesis may have been influenced by behavioral confounders such as typically faster ascent profiles in males more than innate physiology. One recent study suggests that females may in fact be at higher risk.[15] The incidence of HAPE at moderate elevations of 2,500 m (such as the Rocky Mountains of the American West) is 0.01%. Incidence increases to 2% at 3,600 m and may approach 5% at elevations above 4,300 m.[16] Despite a relatively low incidence, HAPE is believed to be the most common cause of altitude-related death.

Clinical Presentation and Diagnostic Evaluation

The classic victim of HAPE is a young, healthy person who is fit enough to rapidly ascend to high altitude. Symptoms typically develop on the second night of a new and higher sleeping altitude. Development of HAPE after 4 days at a given altitude is rare and should prompt the consideration of alternative diagnoses. Early (and possibly subtle) symptoms include a dry cough and reduced exercise performance. Symptoms may then progress to the more classic findings of dyspnea at rest and cough productive of pink, frothy sputum. The Lake Louise Criteria for the diagnosis of HAPE are based on the patient exhibiting a combination of two cardinal signs along with two symptoms[17] (Table 54.1).

While AMS is present in half of cases, it may notably be absent.[18] Fever is common and does not preclude a diagnosis of HAPE, even in the presence of productive sputum. On chest radiograph, patchy lung infiltrates in the setting of a normal-sized heart confirms the diagnosis. EKG findings suggestive of right heart strain may also be observed. Arterial blood gas analysis reveals respiratory alkalosis with severe hypoxia. Partial pressures of arterial oxygen are typically between 30 and 40 mm Hg.[19] The differential diagnosis for HAPE includes:

TABLE 54.1 Lake Louise Criteria for the Diagnosis of HAPE

Symptoms	Signs
Shortness of breath	Tachycardia
Cough	Tachypnea
Fatigue or weakness	Cyanosis
Decreased exercise performance	Wheezing in at least one lung field
Chest congestions or tightness	Rales in at least one lung field

- Asthma
- Bronchitis
- Heart failure
- Mucus plugging
- Myocardial infarction
- Pneumonia
- Pulmonary embolus

Management Guidelines

As with all altitude illness, the mainstays of treatment are descent and supplemental oxygen. In the field, individuals should descend 500 to 1,000 m or until symptoms resolve.[20] If oxygen is available and symptoms are mild, oxygen may be given to maintain saturations above 90% in lieu of descent.[21] While not systemically studied, simulated descent using a portable hyperbaric chamber can be considered if evacuation and oxygen are unavailable.[22] Clinicians not experienced with these devices should be forewarned that their use may limit ongoing patient contact. More generally, patients should be kept warm and should avoid exertion, as both hypothermia and exercise lead to increased pulmonary artery pressures.[23]

Should weather or logistics preclude the provision of oxygen or descent, pharmacologic pulmonary vasodilators exist that can be used to bridge a patient until evacuation or oxygen is available. These agents are known to reduce pulmonary artery pressures; however, rigorous controlled studies are lacking regarding their efficacy in improving outcome. One study assessed nifedipine in a small cohort and demonstrated a reduction in pulmonary artery pressures and an improvement in arterial oxygenation, albeit with only modest clinical improvement.[24] More recently, phosphodiesterase inhibitors and beta-agonists have shown efficacy in the prevention of HAPE and are commonly used in the field; however, no systematic trials have been performed to demonstrate their use in the acute treatment of HAPE.[25,26] More work is currently needed to determine best pharmacologic practice for the treatment of HAPE; in the interim, it is reasonable to consider use of a pulmonary vasodilator if oxygen and descent are not available.

Once a patient is evacuated to an appropriate medical facility, oxygen should be delivered to maintain saturations above 90%. Positive airway pressure devices may be used to improve oxygenation if available; obtundation due to concomitant high-altitude cerebral edema (HACE) would be a relevant contraindication.[27,28] The need for intubation is rare, but may be necessary for unstable patients with altered mental status or severe hypoxemia not responsive to supplemental oxygen. Patients will typically show clinical improvement within hours after the provision of oxygen. In the acute setting, the addition of a pharmacologic agent to oxygen therapy is reasonable if the patient has stable hemodynamics.

HIGH-ALTITUDE CEREBRAL EDEMA

Overview

HACE is the most critical manifestation of the AMS spectrum. Change in mental status in travelers at high altitude has been observed and documented for over a century,[29] but the first comprehensive review of HACE was not published until 1983.[30] The diagnosis of HACE is most often made clinically and requires mental status changes in individuals exhibiting symptoms of AMS.[31] HACE has been reported to occur in just 1% to 2% of all high-altitude trekkers and in 3.4% of those suffering from AMS.[32,33] Climbers who have developed HAPE have a much higher risk of concomitant HACE while at altitude, with a reported incidence of 13% to 20%; autopsy studies of patients who died of HAPE have shown that up to 50% of those had concurrent HACE.[34]

Although its exact pathophysiology remains unclear, HACE is believed to occur through a cascade of cytotoxic and vasogenic responses resulting in increased cellular permeability, vasoconstriction, and a deleterious rise in intracranial pressure.[35] HACE most commonly occurs at altitudes above 4,700 m; however, it may present at lower altitudes in those already affected by HAPE.[36] It is not known why some individuals are more susceptible than others to developing HACE—rapid ascent, heavy exertion at altitude, and a past history of AMS or HACE remain the most relevant risk factors.[30,31]

Clinical Presentation and Diagnostic Evaluation

Altered mental status and ataxia are pathognomonic for HACE.[30] Typically, individuals report progressively worsening AMS over the preceding 24 to 48 hours. Headache is usually, but not always, present. Early symptoms include drowsiness and subtle psychological and behavioral changes including apathy, social withdrawal, and confusion.[31,37] Ataxia has been reported in approximately 40% to 60%, and papilledema is present in up to 50%.[30] Gastrointestinal symptoms, including anorexia, nausea, and vomiting, may also occur. Visual and auditory hallucinations and seizures are rare. Retinal hemorrhages are associated with HACE but may also be present in climbers unaffected by HACE at higher altitudes. Level of consciousness may progress rapidly to coma, so alertness is a poor prognosticator of disease severity.

In 1991, the International Hypoxia Symposium established a set of guidelines for the clinical diagnosis of HACE. The Lake Louise Criteria for HACE are "the presence of a change in mental status or ataxia in a person with AMS" or "the presence of both a change in mental status and ataxia in a person without AMS."[17] It is critical to maintain a broad differential diagnosis, especially in patients with atypical presentations or those who are not responding to conventional therapy. The differential diagnosis for HACE is broad and includes:

- Hypoglycemia
- Hyponatremia
- Hypothermia
- Central nervous system (CNS) infection
- Seizure
- Migraine
- Psychosis
- CVA
- CNS tumor or hemorrhage
- Carbon monoxide poisoning
- Drugs, alcohol, or toxins

HACE is primarily a clinical diagnosis, with laboratory and imaging studies primarily used to rule out potentially confounding disease processes. Appropriate laboratory studies include an electrolyte panel, complete blood count, glucose, ethanol level, carboxyhemoglobin level, and toxicology screen.[37] Patients with HACE may have a mild leukocytosis, so clinical correlation is necessary to exclude an infectious etiology.[30] A lumbar puncture may be performed if there is sufficient concern for CNS infection or subarachnoid hemorrhage. Typical findings include normal cell counts, but markedly elevated opening pressures as high as 44 to 220 mm H_2O in affected individuals.[38,39] Head computed tomography will show an attenuation of signal in the white matter with compression of sulci and flattening of gyri consistent with cerebral edema. Magnetic resonance imagings (MRIs) will demonstrate increased T2 signaling in the corpus callosum without changes in the gray matter, consistent with the white matter effects of vasogenic edema.[40] Importantly, imaging findings lag behind clinical recovery and can be used to confirm the diagnosis of HACE even after clinical improvement.

Management Guidelines

There is a saying that there are three treatments for HACE: "descent, descent, and descent." All altitude illnesses should be treated primarily by descent to a lower elevation. Current field guidelines recommend descending at least 500 m or to the last known elevation at which the patient was asymptomatic.[41] Delaying descent to wait for aeromedical rescue or to institute pharmacologic treatment can be fatal. If physical descent is impossible due to weather, geography, or severity in a patient's condition, achieving physiologic descent via a portable hyperbaric chamber is also effective.[42] This cylindrical, inflatable pressure bag can simulate descent of over 1,500 m.

Once evacuated to a medical facility, the patient should be placed on high-flow oxygen with a nonrebreather mask. A 10-mg loading dose of dexamethasone may be given intravenously or intramuscularly, depending on available access. Intubation may be required, either for airway control or if there is significant coexisting HAPE. For obtunded patients, a Foley catheter should be placed for bladder decompression. In an effort to reduce intracranial pressure, hyperventilation (following intubation) and hypertonic saline with diuresis have been used for patients with HACE; however, no controlled studies exist to suggest either of these techniques increase survival or improve neurologic outcome. Summary recommendations for treatment of HACE are listed in Table 54.2.

TABLE 54.2 Treatment Strategies for HACE

Treatment	Specifics	Effect
Hyperbaric chamber	1-h segments, 4–6 h total treatment	Physiologic descent, reduces hyperbaric hypoxemia and edema
Oxygen	3 L/min, or to saturation >90%, 4–6 h	Markedly reduces cerebral blood flow and intracranial pressure
Dexamethasone	8–10 mg IM and then 4 mg IM or PO q6h	Improves cognition, possible reduction in edema
Acetazolamide	250–500 mg BID	Increases minute ventilation and oxygenation, decreases CSF volume and ICP

CONCLUSION

HAPE and HACE are medical emergencies that require prompt clinical recognition. Dyspnea at rest is an early sign of HAPE, while ataxia is an important indicator of HACE. Treatment for all altitude emergencies includes descent and oxygen; however, pharmacologic treatment strategies and judicious supportive care may also be necessary.

LITERATURE TABLE

TRIAL	DESIGN	RESULT
Altitude illness		
Sutton et al., *Proceedings from the International Hypoxia Symposium: Hypoxia and Mountain Medicine.* 1991[17]	Consensus guidelines for clinical diagnosis of AMS, HACE, and HAPE	Reference and summary. Subsequent literature uses these criteria for diagnosis of altitude illness
Luks et al., *Wilderness Environ Med.* 2010[41]	Expert panel review of altitude literature graded using the American College of Chest Physicians classification scheme for grading evidence	Evidence-based review of management algorithms for altitude illness including dosing regimens for the treatment and prevention of altitude illnesses
HACE		
Basnyat et al., *Wilderness Environ Med.* 2000[15]	Observational epidemiologic study to determine the incidence of AMS and cerebral edema at 4,300 m	68% of randomly chosen subjects had AMS, and 31% had HACE. Women had a significantly higher rate of HACE (OR 3.15, CI 1.62–6.12)
Hackett et al., *JAMA.* 1998[40]	Case–control study of nine patients with HACE evaluated with MRI showing reversible white matter edema changes	Primary case series supporting an endothelial cytotoxic and vasogenic pathophysiologic basis of HACE. Seven of nine patients showed significant T2 signal in corpus callosum with normal gray matter
HAPE		
Oelz et al., *Lancet.* 1989[24]	Small cohort study of HAPE-susceptible patients taken to altitude to induce HAPE and then given nifedipine	Subjects demonstrated improvements in oxygenation (65 % $\pm$ 11 vs. 73 % $\pm$ 11.4) and decreased pulmonary arterial pressure (133.7 $\pm$ 19.8 vs. 73.7 $\pm$ 13.8 mm Hg) after treatment with nifedipine

CI, confidence interval; OR, odds ratio.

REFERENCES

1. Welling KK, et al. Effect of prolonged alveolar hypoxia on pulmonary arterial pressure and segmental vascular resistance. *J Appl Physiol.* 1993;75:1194–1200.
2. Bartsch P, et al. Prevention of high-altitude pulmonary edema by nifedipine. *N Engl J Med.* 1991;325(18):1284–1289.
3. Hultgren HN, et al. Physiologic studies of pulmonary edema at high altitude. *Circulation.* 1964;29:393–408.
4. Grunig E, et al. Stress Doppler echocardiography for identification of susceptibility to high altitude pulmonary edema + AFs-In Process Citation + AF0. *J Am Coll Cardiol.* 2000;35:980–987.
5. Dawson CA, Linehan JH, Bronowski TA. Pressure and flow in the pulmonary vascular bed. In: Weir KT, Reeves JT, eds. *Pulmonary Vascular Physiology and Pathophysiology.* New York, NY: Marcel Dekker; 1989:51–105.
6. Hultgren HN. High-altitude pulmonary edema: current concepts. *Annu Rev Med.* 1996;47:267–284.

7. West JB, et al. Stress failure in pulmonary capillaries. *J Appl Physiol.* 1991;70:1731–1742.
8. Sophocles AM. High-altitude pulmonary edema in Vail, Colorado, 1975–1982. *West J Med.* 1986;144:569–573.
9. Reeves JT, et al. Seasonal variation in barometric pressure and temperature in Summit County: effect on altitude illness. In: Sutton JR, Houston CS, Coates G, eds. *Hypoxia and Molecular Medicine.* Burlington, VT: Queen City Press; 1993.
10. Nuri M, Khan M, Quraishi M. High altitude pulmonary edema. Response to exercise and cold on systemic and pulmonary vascular beds. *J Pak Med Assoc.* 1988;38:211–217.
11. Yu-Jing S, et al. Endothelial nitric oxide synthase gene polymorphisms associated with susceptibility to high altitude pulmonary edema in Chinese railway construction workers at Qinghai-Tibet over 4 500 meters above sea Level. *Chin Med Sci J.* 2010;25(4):215–222.
12. Hanaoka M, et al. Association of high-altitude pulmonary edema with the major histocompatibility complex. *Circulation.* 1998;97(12):1124–1128.
13. Durmowicz AG, et al. Inflammatory processes may predispose children to high-altitude pulmonary edema. *J Pediatr.* 1997;130(5):838–840.
14. Rios B, Driscoll DJ, McNamara DG. High-altitude pulmonary edema with absent right pulmonary artery. *Pediatrics.* 1985;75:314–317.
15. Basnyat B, et al. Disoriented and ataxic pilgrims: an epidemiological study of acute mountain sickness and high-altitude cerebral edema at a sacred lake at 4300 m in the Nepal Himalayas. *Wilderness Environ Med.* 2000;11(2):89–93.
16. Hall DP, Duncan K, Baillie JK. High altitude pulmonary oedema. *J R Army Med Corps.* 2011;157(1):68–72.
17. Sutton JR, Coates G, Houston CS. Hypoxia and mountain medicine: proceedings of the 7th International Hypoxia Symposium, held at Lake Louise, Canada, February 1991. *Advances in the Biosciences.* 1st ed. Oxford, NY: Pergamon Press; 1992:xi, 330.
18. Viswanathan R, et al. Further studies on pulmonary oedema of high altitude. *Respiration.* 1978;36:216–222.
19. Scherrer U, et al. Inhaled nitric oxide for high-altitude pulmonary edema. *N Engl J Med.* 1996;334:624–629.
20. Marticorena E, Hultgren HN. Evaluation of therapeutic methods in high altitude pulmonary edema. *Am J Cardiol.* 1979;43:307–312.
21. Zafren K, Reeves JT, Schoene R. Treatment of high-altitude pulmonary edema by bed rest and supplemental oxygen. *Wilderness Environ Med.* 1996;7(2):127–132.
22. Freeman K, Shalit M, Stroh G. Use of the Gamow Bag by EMT-basic park rangers for treatment of high-altitude pulmonary edema and high-altitude cerebral edema. *Wilderness Environ Med.* 2004;15(3):198–201.
23. Chauca D, Bligh J. An additive effect of cold exposure and hypoxia on pulmonary artery pressure in sheep. *Res Vet Sci.* 1976;21:123–124.
24. Oelz O, et al. Nifedipine for high altitude pulmonary edema. *Lancet.* 1989;2:1241–1244.
25. Maggiorini M, et al. Both tadalafil and dexamethasone may reduce the incidence of high-altitude pulmonary edema: a randomized trial. *Ann Intern Med.* 2006;145(7):497–506.
26. Swenson ER, Maggiorini M. Salmeterol for the prevention of high-altitude pulmonary edema. *N Engl J Med.* 2002;347(16):1282–1285; author reply 1282–1285.
27. Schoene RB, et al. High altitude pulmonary edema and exercise at 4400 meters on Mt. McKinley: effect of expiratory positive airway pressure. *Chest.* 1985;87:330–333.
28. Koch RO, et al. A successful therapy of high-altitude pulmonary edema with a CPAP helmet on Lenin Peak. *Clin J Sport Med.* 2009;19(1):72–73.
29. Mosso A. *Life of Man in the High Alps.* London, England: T Fisher Unwin; 1898.
30. Dickinson JG. High altitude cerebral edema: cerebral acute mountain sickness. *Semin Respir Med.* 1983;5:151–158.
31. Gallagher SA, Hackett PH. High-altitude illness. *Emerg Med Clin North Am.* 2004;22(2):329–355, viii.
32. Hackett PH, Rennie ID, Levine HD. The incidence, importance, and prophylaxis of acute mountain sickness. *Lancet.* 1976;2:1149–1154.
33. Hochstrasser J, Nanzer A, Oelz O. Das Hoehenoedem in den Schweizer Alpen. *Schweiz Med Wschr.* 1986;116:866–873.
34. Ri-Li G, et al. Obesity: associations with acute mountain sickness. *Ann Intern Med.* 2003;139:253–257.
35. Sutton JR, Lassen N. Pathophysiology of acute mountain sickness and high altitude pulmonary oedema: an hypothesis. *Bull Eur Physiopathol Respir.* 1979;15:1045–1052.
36. Paralikar SJ, Paralikar JH. High-altitude medicine. *Ind J Occup Environ Med.* 2010;14(1):6–12.
37. Hackett PH, Roach RC. High altitude cerebral edema. *High Alt Med Biol.* 2004;5(2):136–146.

38. Milledge JS, West JB, Schoene RB. *High Altitude Medicine and Physiology*. 4th ed. Hodder Arnold, London; 2007.
39. Houston CS, Dickinson JG. Cerebral form of high altitude illness. *Lancet.* 1975;2:758–761.
40. Hackett PH, et al. High-altitude cerebral edema evaluated with magnetic resonance imaging: clinical correlation and pathophysiology. *JAMA.* 1998;280(22):1920–1925.
41. Luks AM, et al. Wilderness Medical Society consensus guidelines for the prevention and treatment of acute altitude illness. *Wilderness Environ Med.* 2010;21(2):146–155.
42. Zafren K. Gamow bag for high-altitude cerebral oedema. *Lancet.* 1998;352(9124):325–326.

55

Drowning

Samuel Gerson and Jose Evangelista III

BACKGROUND

The International Liaison Committee on Resuscitation defines drowning as primary respiratory impairment caused by submersion or immersion in liquid.[1] Updated terminology separates the event into fatal or nonfatal drowning, discouraging the use of ambiguous terms such as near drowning or dry versus wet drowning.[2] Worldwide, drowning accounts for an estimated 388,000 annual deaths, represents 7% of all injury-related fatalities, and is the leading cause of death among young males.[3] In the United States, drowning causes roughly 10 fatalities per day and ranks fifth among leading causes of death from unintentional injury.[4] It is estimated that for every drowning fatality, four nonfatal drowning victims are treated in an emergency department with more than 50% requiring hospital admission; this is compared to a 6% admission rate for all unintentional injuries.[5]

PATHOPHYSIOLOGY

The major pathophysiologic event in drowning is hypoxia secondary to aspiration. Following submersion/immersion, the victim typically passes through the following stages within minutes[6]; breath holding → laryngospasm → aspiration → hypoxia with loss of consciousness and apnea → cardiac arrest. The clinical presentation of drowning results from dysfunction in multiple organ systems including the cardiovascular, pulmonary, and neurologic. As tissue hypoxia and acidemia increase, cardiac rhythm most often progresses from sinus tachycardia, to sinus bradycardia, to pulseless electrical activity (PEA), and eventually to asystole as the terminal event.[7] Regardless of whether salt water or fresh water enters the lung, the resulting injuries are the same: surfactant washout and dysfunction, increased permeability of the alveolar–capillary membrane, decreased lung compliance, and ventilation/perfusion ratio mismatching from areas of unventilated dead space.[8] Depending on the amount of fluid aspirated, pulmonary manifestations range from minor respiratory complaints to fulminant noncardiogenic pulmonary edema consistent with acute respiratory distress syndrome (ARDS).

Neurologic status of the drowning victim depends on the degree and duration of hypoxia prior to successful resuscitation and ranges from awake and alert to comatose in the acute setting.[9] Irreversible brain injury develops within 4 to 10 minutes of tissue hypoxia at normal body temperature, followed by cerebral edema and elevated intracranial pressure (ICP).[10] Hypothermic exposure at the time of drowning may be protective by reducing cerebral oxygen consumption and delaying neuronal death for up to an hour or more.[11] Permanent neurologic sequelae in survivors may vary from minor disorders in memory, movement, and coordination to a more devastating persistent vegetative or comatose state.[9]

PREHOSPITAL AND INITIAL EMERGENCY DEPARTMENT CARE

During the primary response to a drowning incident, respondents should initiate cardiopulmonary resuscitation in a person submerged <60 minutes without clear signs of death.[12] Because respiratory failure is the primary cause of cardiac arrest in drowning, resuscitation begins with rescue breaths or bag–valve–mask (BVM) ventilations in keeping with the traditional protocol of airway, breathing, and circulation (ABC).[13] Providing supplemental oxygen at the highest flow rate available is a critical early action, preferably through a nonrebreather face mask at 15 L/min in the awake, alert patient. If passive measures fail to correct hypoxia, continuous positive airway pressure (CPAP) or bilevel positive airway pressure (BIPAP) may be effective and prevent the need for invasive airway management.[14] However, early intubation and mechanical ventilation with positive end-expiratory pressure (PEEP) is indicated for worsening oxygenation despite noninvasive support or for deterioration of respiratory drive or neurologic status with a goal of maintaining oxygen saturation above 92%.[8] While many drowning accidents involve trauma, cervical spine injuries are rare, and immobilization should only be implemented for cases in which head or neck injury is suspected.[15]

For drowning victims who suffer cardiac arrest, PEA or asystole is managed as per standard advanced cardiovascular life support (ACLS) algorithms. Prompt defibrillation is indicated for rare cases of ventricular fibrillation.[16] As in all hypothermic cases, rewarming the patient to a core temperature above 32°C is essential to optimize resuscitation efforts and prevent dysrhythmias. While there is some debate regarding the duration of resuscitation, most experts agree that efforts should be halted when the patient is rewarmed and is asystolic >20 minutes.[12]

After initial stabilization is achieved and the primary survey completed, further evaluation typically includes chest radiography and arterial blood gas measurements. Lung ultrasound also provides a rapid and effective bedside tool to diagnose, quantify, and monitor pulmonary edema in drowning victims.[17] In patients who remain unresponsive without a clear cause, toxic/metabolic investigation and head/neck imaging are warranted. Use of a validated grading system (See Literature Table for additional details) helps to guide intervention and disposition in the emergency department.[13,18]

- **Grade 1:** No lung findings, normal arterial oxygenation → observation for 6 hours
- **Grade 2:** Scattered pulmonary crackles, stabilized with low flow oxygen → admit for extended observation or discharge if signs of clinical improvement after 6 hours
- **Grades 3 to 6:** Acute pulmonary edema with or without hypotension → ICU admission

MANAGEMENT GUIDELINES

Pulmonary

In drowning victims who require invasive mechanical ventilation, guidelines recommended for ARDS patients (lung-protective ventilation) should be followed:[19]

- Set tidal volumes <6 mL/kg
- Adjust PEEP to optimize alveolar recruitment
- Maintain low plateau pressures
- Minimize suctioning to prevent hypoxia and elevated airway pressures
- Do not attempt to wean prior to 24 hours on mechanical ventilation

Prophylactic antibiotics for pneumonia are advised in cases of exposure to polluted sources; however, they are not routinely indicated for the majority of drowning victims.[20,21] Given the substantially increased risk for translocation of bacteria in the lung in cases of water aspiration (and lung injury), obtaining blood cultures early in the clinical course may be of significant clinical utility. Early respiratory cultures may have diminished utility and are not generally recommended. Glucocorticoids have not been proven to reduce pulmonary injury from drowning, but may be beneficial for bronchospasm poorly controlled by inhaled bronchodilators.[20,22] Exogenous surfactant and inhaled liquid perfluorocarbon use remain controversial, but may be considered in cases that are refractory to standard therapy.[23,24] Finally, extracorporeal membrane oxygenation (ECMO) is indicated with severe ARDS when pulmonary exchange is inadequate to maintain oxygenation.[25,26]

Cardiovascular

In the hypotensive patient, conservative fluid management is recommended to avoid volume overload that could worsen cardiac and pulmonary function.[27] Bedside echocardiography is a useful tool to monitor volume status, identify cardiogenic shock, and guide the use of cardioactive or vasopressor medications.[28] Acute renal failure is uncommon but may result from prerenal (hypovolemia, shock) or renal (anoxic renal tubular injury, rhabdomyolysis) etiologies.[29]

Neurologic

Therapeutic hypothermia in drowning victims is neuroprotective and is supported by extrapolation from randomized clinical trials in cardiac arrest patients,[30,31] and from case reports on drowning.[25,32] While initial resuscitation efforts may require rewarming of a hypothermic patient, core temperature should be maintained at 32°C to 34°C for 24 hours in comatose patients who regain spontaneous circulation. Tight control of blood glucose, arterial oxygenation, and carbon dioxide levels is essential to prevent increases in brain metabolism.[33] Neurologic monitoring techniques—including EEG, MRI, and cerebral biomarkers—provide useful prognostic tools, but have not yet demonstrated an impact on clinical decision-making.[34] Seizures are common after anoxic brain injury and warrant treatment with antiepileptic medications; however, prophylactic anticonvulsants are not currently proven or recommended in drowning victims.[35] Finally, aggressive control of ICP in case reports of pediatric drowning has produced disappointing results and is not considered a management priority.[36]

CONCLUSION

In the United States, drowning ranks fifth among leading causes of death from unintentional injury.[4] Management of the downing victim requires careful evaluation of pulmonary status with use of lung-protective strategies when mechanical ventilation is indicated, conservative fluid management, and consideration of ECMO support in severe cases.

LITERATURE TABLE

TRIAL	DESIGN	RESULT
Szpilman, *Chest.* 1997[18]	Retrospective analysis of 2,304 cases from near-drowning recuperation	1,831 cases included and graded. Gd 1—Normal lung exam = 0% mortality, Gd 2—Scattered rales = 1% mortality, Gd 3—ARDS = 5% mortality, Gd 4—ARDS + low BP = 19% mortality, Gd 5—Respiratory arrest = 44% mortality, and Gd 6—Cardiac arrest = 93% mortality
van Berkel et al., *Intensive Care Med.* 1996[20]	Retrospective analysis of 125 submersion victims	No effect on occurrence of pneumonia with administration of prophylactic antibiotic therapy or prednisolone
Hein et al., *Crit Care.* 2004[32]	Case report of twin toddler drowning victims	Female twin treated with induced hypothermia for 72 h → no neurologic deficits Male twin treated under normothermic conditions → developed apallic syndrome
Guenther et al., *Resuscitation.* 2009[25]	Case report of 2 drowning victims treated with ECMO and prolonged hypothermia	Patients had been submerged >10 min and had severe ARDS and hypotension ECMO/hypothermia maintained for 6 d. Both survived without neurologic deficits

REFERENCES

1. Idris AH, Berg RA, Bierens J, et al. Recommended guidelines for uniform reporting of data from drowning: the "Utstein Style". *Circulation.* 2003;108:2565–2574.
2. Van Beeck EF, Branche CM, Szpilman D, et al. A new definition of drowning: towards documentation and prevention of a global public health problem. *Bull World Health Organ.* 2005;83:801–880.
3. *Media Center: Fact Sheet on Drowning*. Geneva, Switzerland: World Health Organization; 2012 (http://www.who.int/mediacentre/factsheets/fs347/en/index.html).
4. *National Center for Injury Prevention and Control. Web-based Injury Statistics Query and Reporting System (WISQARS).* Atlanta, GA: Centers for Disease Control and Prevention; 2012 http://www.cdc.gov/injury/wisqars).
5. Laosee OC, Gilchrist J, Rudd R. Drowning 2005–2009. *MMWR.* 2012;61(19):344–347.
6. Tipton MJ, Golden FS. A proposed decision-making guide for the search, rescue and resuscitation of submersion (head under) victims based on expert opinion. *Resuscitation.* 2011;82:819–824.
7. Orlowski JP, Abulleil MM, Phillips JM. The hemodynamic and cardiovascular effects of near-drowning in hypotonic, isotonic, or hypertonic solutions. *Ann Emerg Med.* 1989;18:1044–1049.
8. Gregorakos L, Markou N, Psalida V, et al. Near-drowning: clinical course of lung injury in adults. *Lung.* 2009;187:93–97.
9. Conn AW, Montes JE, Barker GA, et al. Cerebral salvage in near drowning following neurological classification by triage. *Can Anaesth Soc J.* 1980;27:201–210.
10. Smith ML, Auer RN, Siesjo BK. The density and distribution of ischemia brain injury in the rat following 2–10 min of forebrain ischemia. *Acta Neuropathol.* 1984;64(4):319–332.
11. Chochinov AH, Baydock BM, Bristow GK, et al. Recovery of a 62-year-old man from prolonged cold water submersion. *Ann Emerg Med.* 1998;31(1):127–131.
12. Vanden Hoek TL, Morrison LJ, Shuster M, et al. Part 12: cardiac arrest in special situations: drowning: 2010 American Heart Association Guidelines for Cardiopulmonary Resuscitation and Emergency Cardiovascular Care. *Circulation.* 2010;122(suppl 3):S847–S848.

13. Spilzman D. Near-drowning and drowning classification: a proposal to stratify mortality based on the analysis of 1831 cases. *Chest.* 1997;122:660–665.
14. Dottorini M, Eslami A, Baglioni S, et al. Nasal-continuous positive airway pressure in the treatment of near-drowning in fresh water. *Chest.* 1996;100(4):1122–1124.
15. Waton RS, Cummings P, Quan L, et al. Cervical spine injuries among submersion victims. *J Trauma.* 2001;51:658–662.
16. Grmec S, Strnad M, Podorsek D. Comparison of the characteristics and outcome among patients suffering out-of-hospital cardiac arrest and drowning victims in cardiac arrest. *Int J Emerg Med.* 2009;2:7–12.
17. Laursen CB, Davidsen JR, Madsen PH. Utility of lung ultrasound in near-drowning victims. *BMJ Case Rep.* 2012;21:2012.
18. Szpilman D, Bierens JJ, Handley AJ, et al. Drowning. *N Engl J Med.* 2012;366(22):2102–2110.
19. Oba Y, Salzman GA. Ventilation with lower tidal volume as compared with traditional tidal volumes for acute lung injury and the acute respiratory distress syndrome. The ACUTE Respiratory Distress Syndrome Network. *N Engl J Med.* 2000;342(18):1301–1308.
20. van Berkel M, Bierens JJ, Lie JJ, et al. Pulmonary oedema, pneumonia and mortality in submersion victims; a retrospective study in 125 patients. *Intensive Care Med.* 1996;22(2):101–107.
21. Wood C. Towards evidence base emergency medicine: best BETs from the Manchester Royal Infirmary: BET 1: prophylactic antibiotics in near-drowning. *Emerg Med J.* 2010;27:393–394.
22. Towards evidence base emergency medicine: best BETs from the Manchester Royal Infirmary: corticosteroids in the management of near-drowning. *Emer Med J.* 2001;18:465–466.
23. Cubattoli L, Franchi F, Coratti G. Surfactant therapy for acute respiratory failure after drowning: two children victims of cardiac arrest. *Resuscitation.* 2009;80:1088–1089.
24. Gauger PG, Pranikoff T, Schreiner RJ, et al. Initial experience with partial liquid ventilation in pediatric patients with acute respiratory distress syndrome. *Crit Care Med.* 1996;24:16–22.
25. Guenther U, Varelmann D, Putensen C, et al. Extended therapeutic hypothermia for several days during extracorporeal membrane oxygenation after drowning and cardiac arrest: two cases of survival with no neurological sequelae. *Resuscitation.* 2009;80:379–381.
26. Thalman M, Trampitsch E, Haberfellner N, et al. Resuscitation in near drowning with extracorporeal membrane oxygenation. *Ann Thorac Surg.* 2001;72:607–608.
27. Wiedemann HP, Wheeler AP, Bernad GR, et al. Comparison of two fluid management strategies in acute lung injury. *N Engl J Med.* 2006;354(24):2564–2575.
28. Perera P, Mailhot T, Riley D, et al. The Rush exam: rapid ultrasound in shock in the evaluation of the critically ill. *Emerg Med Clin North Am.* 2010;28(1):29–56.
29. Spicer ST, Quinn D, Nyi Nyi NN, et al. Acute renal impairment after immersion and near drowning. *J Am Soc Nephrol.* 1999;10:382–386.
30. Hypothermia After Cardiac Arrest Study Group. Mild therapeutic hypothermia to improve the neurological outcome after cardiac arrest. *N Engl J Med.* 2002;346(8):549–556.
31. Bernard SA, Gray TW, Buist MD, et al. Treatment of comatose survivors of out-of- hospital cardiac arrest with induced hypothermia. *M Engl J Med.* 2002;346(8):557–563.
32. Hein OV, Triltsch A, von Buch C. Mild hypothermia after near drowning in twin toddlers. *Crit Care.* 2004;8(5):R353–R357.
33. Warner D, Knape J. Recommendations and consensus brain resuscitation in the drowning victim. In Bierens JJLM, ed. *Handbook on Drowning: Prevention, Rescue, and Treatment.* Berlin: Springer-Verlag; 2006:436–439.
34. Topjian AA, Berg RA, Bierens JJLM, et al. Brain resuscitation in the drowning victim. *Neurocrit Care.* 2012;17:441–467.
35. Abend NS, Topjian A, Ichord R, et al. Electroencephalographic monitoring during hypothermia after pediatric cardiac arrest. *Neurology.* 2009;72(22):1931–1940.
36. Dean JM, McComb JG. Intracranial pressure monitoring in severe pediatric near- drowning. *Neurosurgery.* 1981;9(6):627–630.

SECTION 13
Sedation and Delirium

56

Delirium

Jin H. Han, Eduard E. Vasilevskis, and E. Wesley Ely

BACKGROUND

Delirium is a form of acute brain dysfunction that occurs in 8% to 10% of emergency department (ED) patients.[1,2] By contrast, delirium affects 20% to 70% of intensive care unit (ICU) patients, especially those requiring mechanical ventilation.[3–5] Historically, delirium was considered a normal and transient part of critical illness that posed little consequence to the patient. Evidence collected in the past decade, however, suggests that delirium may affect patient outcomes profoundly. In the critically ill, delirium is an independent risk factor for death, as well as for long-term cognitive impairment, increased ventilator time, prolonged hospitalizations, and increased hospital costs.[6–9]

When present, delirium should be considered a medical emergency, as it can be the sole manifestation of an underlying critical illness. ED management of delirium influences clinical outcomes, and the emergency physician must be adept at detecting delirium, identifying its etiology, and initiating potentially lifesaving therapies. This chapter reviews the definition and risk factors for delirium, validated instruments for its detection, and appropriate diagnostic workup and management in confirmed cases.

DEFINITION

Delirium is an acute reversible disturbance in attention and cognition precipitated by an underlying medical illness not attributable to a preexisting or evolving dementia.[10] Cognitive change in delirium is rapid, occurring over several hours or days and often fluctuating. The core feature of delirium is inattention; other features may include altered consciousness level, disorganized thinking, and sleep–wake cycle disturbances. It is important to note that delirium lies on a continuum of acute brain dysfunction, the most severe form of which is coma (Fig. 56.1).

Delirium is classified into three psychomotor subtypes: hypoactive, hyperactive, and mixed type.[11] Hypoactive or "quiet" delirium is characterized by decreased psychomotor

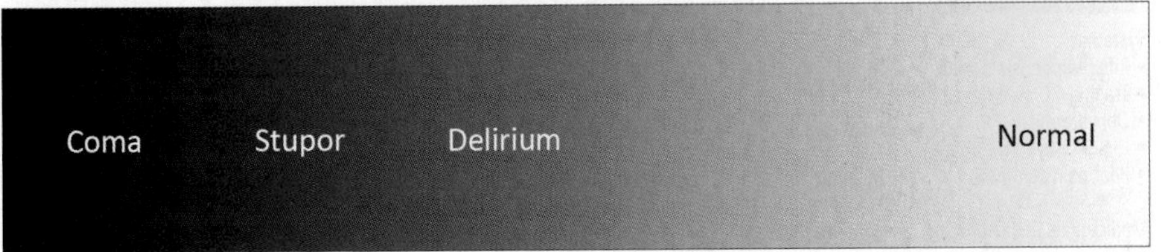

FIGURE 56.1 Spectrum of acute brain dysfunction. Courtesy of Vanderbilt University, Nashville, TN. Copyright © 2012. Used with Permission.

activity and may manifest in a depressed, sedated, somnolent, or lethargic appearance. Its clinical presentation may be subtle, and it is frequently missed or misdiagnosed as depression or fatigue.[12,13] Hyperactive delirium is the most recognizable subtype and is characterized by increased psychomotor activity; patients appear restless, anxious, agitated, and even combative. In mixed-type delirium, patients fluctuate between hypoactive and hyperactive psychomotor activity over a period of minutes to hours. In critically ill patients, hypoactive and mixed type are the commonly observed delirium subtypes; purely hyperactive delirium occurs in <2% of cases.[14,15]

Excited delirium syndrome (ExDS) is an extreme manifestation hyperactive delirium. Patients with ExDS exhibit extreme agitation, aggressiveness, and violent behavior; they also can appear to possess superhuman strength and to be insensitive to pain.[16] Patients with ExDS are an immediate danger to themselves and to the people around them; this unique set of challenges is discussed separately in Chapter 57.

RISK FACTORS FOR DELIRIUM

The onset of delirium involves a complex interaction between patient vulnerability factors and precipitating factors.[17] To establish delirium risk, both sets of factors must be considered. Patients who are vulnerable to developing delirium (e.g., an 89-year-old with severe dementia) require a relatively benign insult (e.g., urinary tract infection without signs of sepsis) to develop delirium. Conversely, patients who are not vulnerable to developing delirium (e.g., a healthy 45-year-old) require higher doses of noxious stimuli (e.g., multifocal pneumonia with septic shock) to develop delirium. Therefore, when a patient with low vulnerability presents to the ED with delirium, the clinician should be vigilant in looking for an underlying life-threatening illness.

Among patient vulnerability factors for delirium, dementia is the most consistent across a variety of clinical settings, including the ED and ICU.[1,18,19] Age, alcohol use, and depression are additional vulnerability factors in the critically ill.[20] Numerous precipitating factors identified in general medical patients are likely equally applicable to the ICU population (Table 56.1). In general, patients with higher illness severity are more likely to develop delirium.[21,22] Drug exposures—notably benzodiazepines, opioids, and medications with anticholinergic properties—may also trigger delirium, as can withdrawal from ethanol and benzodiazepines. Other precipitants, especially in the elderly, include cardiovascular illnesses like congestive heart failure and acute myocardial infarction.[23,24]

TABLE 56.1 Precipitating Factors for Delirium

Systemic • Infection/sepsis • Trauma • Dehydration • Hypo- or hyperthermia • Poor pain control Medications and Drugs • Drug overdoses • Severe ethanol intoxication • Ethanol and benzodiazepine withdrawal • Home medications and medication changes[a] CNS • Meningitis/encephalitis • Cerebrovascular accident • Intracerebral hemorrhage • Subarachnoid hemorrhage • Subdural/epidural hematoma • Nonconvulsive status epilepticus	Metabolic • Thiamine deficiency (Wernicke encephalopathy) • Hypoglycemia/hyperglycemia • Thyroid dysfunction • Hepatic encephalopathy • Renal failure • Hypo- and hypernatremia • Hypo- and hypercalcemia Cardiopulmonary • Hypoxemia • Hypercarbia • Hypertensive encephalopathy • Shock • Acute myocardial infarction[a] • Acute heart failure[a] Iatrogenic • Benzodiazepine • Isolation • Lack of daylight • Physical restraints

[a]More likely to occur in the geriatric patient population, but can occur if the severity of illness is high.

When critically ill patients are boarded for extended periods of time in the ED, emergency physicians become important monitors of potentially preventable iatrogenic risk factors for delirium, specifically the use of deliriogenic medications. Several studies have shown a strong dose–response relationship between benzodiazepine use and the development of delirium in the ICU.[25–27] Opioids may also precipitate delirium, but this relationship is less clear.[5] Since poorly controlled pain can trigger delirium, opioids in some instances may have protective effect; in burn ICU patients, for instance, opioid pain control reduced delirium incidence by 50%.[28,29] Delirium can also be stimulated by negative environmental conditions, such as isolation, lack of daylight, and immobility due to the use of physical restraints.[18]

ASSESSING FOR DELIRIUM

The diagnosis of delirium is commonly missed.[1,12] In the ED, 75% of cases of delirium will go unrecognized; of these, 90% will continue to be overlooked in the inpatient setting.[1] When health care providers fail to identify delirium, it is usually because they are unfamiliar with established diagnostic criteria and rely instead on clinical gestalt and the absence of disorientation, hallucinations, delusions, and agitation—features often absent in patients with delirium.[30]

The American College of Critical Care Medicine, the Society of Critical Care Medicine, and the American Society of Health-System Pharmacists collectively published clinical practice guidelines for pain, agitation, and delirium (2013 PAD Guidelines). The guidelines recommend routine delirium monitoring in critically ill patients, using one of two methods validated in this population: the Confusion Assessment Method for the Intensive Care Unit (CAM-ICU) or the Intensive Care Delirium Screening Checklist (ICDSC).[31]

The CAM-ICU enables assessment of delirium in under a minute—or less if it is performed algorithmically, which allows for early stoppage (Fig. 56.2).[32] The CAM-ICU evaluates four cognitive features: (1) altered mental status or fluctuating course, (2) inattention, (3) altered level of consciousness, and (4) disorganized thinking. Since it does not require the patient to speak, it can be performed in both mechanically ventilated and non–mechanically ventilated patients.[4,33] For a patient to meet criteria for delirium, features 1 and 2, and either feature 3 or feature 4, must be present.

Details on how to perform the CAM-ICU and its training manual are available at www.icudelirium.org. Briefly, feature 1 (altered mental status or fluctuating course) is usually obtained from the family member, friend, or caretaker in the ED. Changes and fluctuations in mental status can also be observed by the health care provider during the ED course. Feature 2 (inattention) uses objective assessments and is comprised of an auditory and visual component. For the auditory component, the patient is given a series

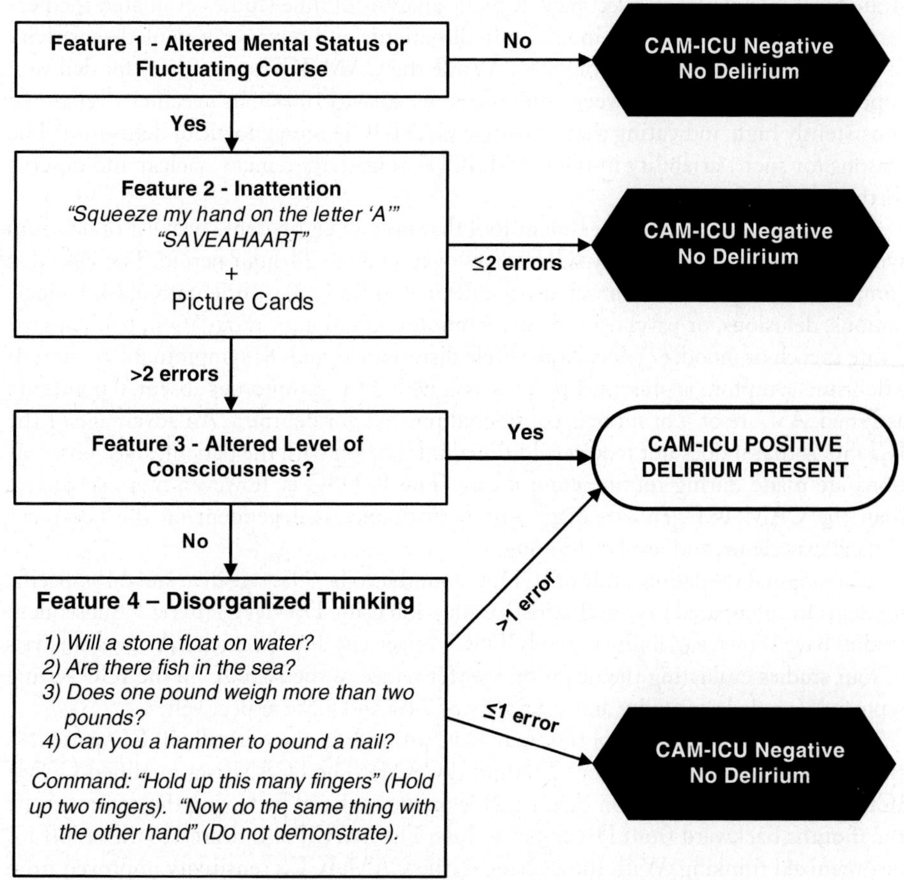

FIGURE 56.2 Confusion Assessment Method for the Intensive Care Unit. Adapted from www.icudelirium.org. Courtesy of Dr. Wes Ely and Vanderbilt University, Nashville, TN. Copyright © 2002. Used with permission.

of 10 letters ("SAVEAHAART") and is asked to squeeze the rater's hand whenever the letter "A" is heard. For the visual component, the patient is asked to remember 5 objects shown on picture cards and then asked to identify the 5 objects from a series of 10 pictures. Patients who are minimally arousable to verbal stimuli and unable to perform the CAM-ICU's inattention tasks are often erroneously classified as "Negative" or "Unable to Assess" for inattention.[34] These patients, however, are actually at the most severe end of the inattention spectrum and should be considered inattentive (feature 2 positive). For feature 3 (altered level of consciousness), a validated arousal scale such as the Richmond Agitation–Sedation Scale is used. For feature 4 (disorganized thinking), the rater asks the patient to answer 4 simple yes/no questions and to perform a simple command.

Initial studies showed the CAM-ICU to have excellent sensitivity (95% to 100%) and specificity (89% to 100%) in detecting delirium in both mechanically ventilated and non–mechanically ventilated patients.[4,33] Because of its ease of use, both nurses and physicians can use it reliably.[4,33] Subsequent validation studies, however, demonstrated variable diagnostic accuracy. A meta-analysis of nine studies evaluated the performance of the CAM-ICU in critically ill patients and reported a pooled sensitivity of 80% and pooled specificity of 96%.[35] While the CAM-ICU's sensitivity for delirium appeared to vary widely between studies (range, 45% to 100%), its specificity remained consistently high, indicating that a positive CAM-ICU is diagnostic of delirium.[35] The reasons for such variability in the CAM-ICU's sensitivity remain unclear and deserve further study.

The ICDSC is another assessment tool that uses an eight-item checklist of delirium symptoms, designed for use by ICU nurses over an 8- to 24-hour period. The checklist comprises (1) altered level consciousness; (2) inattention; (3) disorientation; (4) hallucinations, delusions, or psychosis; (5) psychomotor agitation or retardation; (6) inappropriate speech or mood; (7) sleep/wake cycle disturbance; and (8) symptom fluctuation. If a delirium symptom is present, 1 point is assigned; if the symptom is absent, 0 points are assigned. A score of 4 or more is considered positive for delirium. An advantage of the ICDSC is that it does not require additional interaction with the patient, since observations are made during routine clinical care. The ICDSC is, however, more subjective than the CAM-ICU, and its diagnostic performance is dependent on the observer's clinical experience and level of training.

The original validation study of ICDSC found it to be 99% sensitive and 64% specific for delirium, compared to a psychiatrist's evaluation using DSM-IV criteria.[36] Subsequent studies have shown variability in the ICDSC's sensitivity and specificity. A meta-analysis of four studies evaluating the diagnostic performance of the ICSDC in the ICU setting reported a pooled sensitivity and specificity of 74% and 82%, respectively.[35]

A delirium assessment tool that may have promise in the critically ill ED patient is the Brief Confusion Assessment Method (bCAM). The bCAM is a modified CAM-ICU in which the inattention (feature 2) tasks are replaced by having the patient recite the months backward from December to July. The bCAM also decreases the cutoff for disorganized thinking. With these changes, the CAM-ICU's sensitivity improved from 72% to 84%, without a significant impact on specificity.[37] This study was performed in older ED patients, and its validity in a broader population of critically ill patients may be limited. The bCAM also requires the patient to speak, so this assessment is not useful in mechanically ventilated patients. Future studies are needed to determine the bCAM's diagnostic accuracy in non–mechanically ventilated patients who are critically ill.

TABLE 56.2 Life-Threatening Causes of Delirium
Wernicke disease or ethanol withdrawal
Hypoxia or hypercarbia
Hypoglycemia
Hypertensive encephalopathy
Hyperthermia or hypothermia
Intracerebral hemorrhage
Meningitis/encephalitis
Poisoning (whether exogenous or iatrogenic)
Status epilepticus

Adapted from Caplan GA, et al. Delirium. In: Stern TA, ed. *Massachusetts General Hospital comprehensive Clinical Psychiatry.* 1st ed. Philadelphia, PA: Mosby/Elsevier; 2008.

DIAGNOSTIC EVALUATION

If a patient presents with delirium, or develops delirium during the ED course, aggressive efforts are required to uncover the underlying etiology. Early identification and treatment of delirium reduces hospital costs and improves patient outcomes; each additional day of delirium has been shown to increase risk of 1-year mortality by 10%.[38] Delirium also prolongs the duration of mechanical ventilation and ICU length of stay and accelerates cognitive decline.[7,9]

Life-threatening causes of delirium should be considered first, especially in the otherwise healthy patient (Table 56.2).[39] Many of these processes can be ruled out at the initial assessment, but others, such as meningitis, demand a more extensive evaluation. Once serious causes have been ruled out, precipitating factors listed in Table 56.1 should be considered.

The underlying cause of delirium is best diagnosed via a complete history and physical examination. However, as delirious patients have an acute loss in cognition, obtaining an accurate history can be difficult.[40] It is best to collect collateral patient history from family members or companions as well as an accurate medication history, including any medication or dosing changes (especially in elderly patients). Medication history can be confirmed with the patient's caregiver or pharmacy.[41] If a medication overdose is suspected, every effort should be made to obtain the patient's medication bottles in order to identify the specific medication and amount taken. A careful substance abuse history should also be obtained—preferably from a proxy—as delirium can be precipitated by exposures to, or withdrawal from, benzodiazepines and ethanol.

The physical examination of the delirious patient should be similarly thorough and is summarized in Table 56.3. All patients should be fully exposed to allow for an adequate dermatologic and genitourinary examination looking for signs of infection. Medication patches such as fentanyl and scopolamine should be removed if present.

Routine laboratory testing for patients with delirium includes complete blood count, serum electrolytes, blood urea nitrogen and creatinine, blood glucose, liver function studies, and urinalysis. If the patient is on delirium-inducing medications that are amenable to serum measurement (i.e., anticonvulsants, lithium, theophylline, and digoxin), then these levels should be ordered. Thyroid-stimulating hormone and free T4 levels should be considered to rule out thyroid dysfunction. In patients with respiratory complaints or symptoms, an arterial or venous blood gas should be used to identify hypercarbia. Because sepsis is a major precipitant in delirium, blood and urine and cultures should be considered. A lumbar puncture is not routinely performed, but should be obtained in delirious patients in whom a high clinical suspicion for meningitis or encephalitis exists or if the patient has a fever or

TABLE 56.3 Physical Examination of the Emergency Department Patient with Delirium

Physical Examination	Sign
Head	Soft tissue swelling, ecchymosis, and other signs of trauma looking for traumatic brain injury
Eyes	
Pupil	Mydriasis and miosis may indicate anticholinergic or opioid medication toxicity, respectively
Fundoscopic	Papilledema suggests high intracranial pressure. Retinal subhyaloid hemorrhage suggests subarachnoid hemorrhage
Extraocular muscles	Nystagmus may indicate toxicologic etiology or posterior fossa CNS insult. Ophthalmoplegia may increase the suspicion of Wernicke encephalopathy or increased intracranial pressure
Neck	Meningismus may suggest meningitis or subarachnoid hemorrhage
Respiratory	Look for signs of hypoxemia (cyanosis), respiratory distress, and signs of pneumonia or pulmonary edema
Cardiac	If febrile, new murmurs may indicate endocarditis
Abdomen	Abdominal tenderness may suggest acute surgical emergency such as acute appendicitis, cholecystitis, or diverticulitis
Neurologic	Focal, lateralizing neurologic symptoms may suggest a CNS insult (e.g., cerebrovascular accident, intraparenchymal hemorrhage, or mass effect). If possible, the patient's gait should be assessed; ataxia may indicate Wernicke encephalopathy or medication overdoses
Genitourinary	Look for signs of infection such as perirectal or perianal abscesses or infected decubitus ulcers in paralyzed or bedridden patients
Skin	Look for signs of infection, medication patches (e.g., fentanyl or scopolamine), petechiae, and any sequelae of liver failure

CNS, central nervous system.

leukocytosis without an obvious source.[42,43] Urine drug screens are typically ordered, but a positive result should be interpreted with caution, as it may mislead the clinician and divert attention from an underlying illness. Urine drug screens can produce false-positive and false-negative results and are qualitative and do not provide drug concentrations.[44] In a patient on home opioids or benzodiazepines, it would be difficult to differentiate if positive urine drug screen was the result of an overdose or normal home usage.

If a focal, delirium-inducing process is suspected, imaging is indicated (e.g., chest radiography to evaluate for pneumonia or pulmonary edema in the setting of tachypnea, dyspnea, hypoxemia, or cough). A head CT is not routine, but should be obtained in delirious patients with altered level consciousness, a recent history of a fall or head trauma, or focal neurologic deficits.[45,46] A head CT may also be reasonable if no other etiology for delirium is found. Magnetic resonance imaging of the brain (brain MRI) and electroencephalography are not typically performed in the ED, but may be useful in ruling out cerebrovascular accidents and nonconvulsive status epilepticus, both of which can mimic or precipitate delirium.

PHARMACOLOGIC MANAGEMENT OF DELIRIUM

The pharmacologic management of delirium has three guiding principles: pain control, avoidance of deliriogenic medications, and medical therapy to minimize the time of delirium.

Pain Control

Because inadequate pain control can precipitate delirium, intravenous opioid analgesia may be necessary.[27] Alternative methods for pain control, such as regional or neuraxial (spinal or epidural) anesthesia may also be considered. Importantly, the delirious patient may not be able communicate his or her needs; every effort should be made to identify factors contributing to or aggravating delirium (e.g., urinary retention) while simultaneously treating the patient's discomfort.

Deliriogenic Medications

With the notable exception of patients withdrawing from ethanol (delirium tremens) or benzodiazepines, benzodiazepines should be avoided in the delirious patient because they can increase delirium severity.[47–49] The same holds true for agitated patients, when possible; initial verbal and nonverbal de-escalation techniques should be attempted, including calming the patient environment by dimming or turning off lights, minimizing auditory stimulation from cardiac monitor or intravenous infusion pump alarms, and having family members and familiar objects from home at the patient's bedside. The PAD guidelines also recommend against the use of benzodiazepines to sedate mechanically ventilated patients, endorsing alternative agents less associated with delirium, such as dexmedetomidine or propofol.[31]

Antipsychotics

When nonpharmacologic methods fail, typical (haloperidol) and atypical (olanzapine, ziprasidone, risperidone, quetiapine) antipsychotics may be considered. While some practitioners advocate using antipsychotics for all delirious patients, these medications are typically reserved for delirious patients with agitation or psychotic features (delusions, misperceptions, hallucinations, etc.). Before administering antipsychotic medications, a 12-lead electrocardiogram should be obtained, as these medications can precipitate torsades de pointes in patients with QTc intervals >500 milliseconds.[31] This is especially the case for intravenous haloperidol.[50]

Haloperidol is commonly used in the treatment of delirium and can be given intravenously, intramuscularly, and orally. The 2013 PAD guidelines, however, do not recommend its routine use in the critically ill because of a paucity of supporting data. Only one ICU study—the Modifying the Incidence of Delirium (MIND) Trial—compares haloperidol with placebo for the treatment and prevention of delirium.[51] The trial randomized 103 mechanically ventilated ICU patients to haloperidol (5 mg), ziprasidone (40 mg), or placebo every 6 hours for up to 14 days and demonstrated no differences in days alive without delirium or coma, duration of mechanical ventilation, hospital length of stay, or mortality between the three treatment groups.[51] The trial was, however, intended for use as a pilot study to assess feasibility and was not adequately powered to determine efficacy.

The PAD guidelines support the use of atypical antipsychotics in the treatment of delirium, but this is again based on limited evidence. One small double-blinded randomized control trial compared quetiapine (50 mg q12h, titratable up to 200 mg q12h) with placebo in 36 ICU patients, with both groups receiving additional haloperidol as needed.[52] The quetiapine group had shorter delirium duration and less agitation.[52] A trend toward increased likelihood of hospital discharge to home rather than to rehabilitation was also observed.[52] Atypical antipsychotics are increasingly favored in the treatment of delirium because of a lower association with extrapyramidal side effects.

As new clinical trial data emerge, the PAD recommendations for typical and atypical antipsychotic medications will likely evolve.

Other Agents

Finally, because the pathogenesis of delirium is thought to be due in part to increased anticholinergic central nervous system activity, rivastigmine, a cholinesterase inhibitor, was evaluated for use in elderly patients with delirium. A recent multicenter trial comparing rivastigmine with placebo in critically ill patients was, however, stopped early when the rivastigmine group was noted to have longer duration of delirium and higher mortality.[53]

NONPHARMACOLOGIC MANAGEMENT OF DELIRIUM

Data concerning the nonpharmacologic management of delirium are largely obtained from the geriatric literature, but certain components may be applicable to the critically ill patient. Most of these interventions have multiple components and emphasize (1) encouraging early mobility and avoiding physical restraints; (2) providing a calm and quiet environment, especially at night; (3) reestablishing the sleep–wake cycle reversal commonly observed in delirious patients through environmental modifications (e.g., limit light and noise at night and provide the majority of clinical care during the day) and nonpharmacologic sleep aids (e.g., soothing music, massages, earplugs); (4) reorienting the patient using large clocks or dated whiteboards; (5) performing cognitive stimulating activities such as word games; (6) placing familiar persons or objects near the patient; and (7) reducing sensory deprivation during daytime hours by offering eyeglasses or hearing devices.[54] The efficacy of such bundled protocols in the critically ill, though intuitive, is still not well defined and requires future study. One randomly controlled trial, however, proved the efficacy of the simple and cost-effective earplug in the noisy ED and ICU environment: In 136 critically ill patients, the use of ear plugs at night reduced the onset of delirium by half (hazard ratio 0.47, 95% CI, 0.27 to 0.82).[55]

ABCDE BUNDLE FOR MECHANICALLY VENTILATED PATIENTS

The ABCDE bundle is a recently proposed approach to the management and prevention of delirium in mechanically ventilated patients. The acronym stands for *A*wakening and *B*reathing Coordination, *C*hoice of Medication, *D*elirium monitoring and *E*xercise/*E*arly mobility bundle (ABCDE).[56]

The first two steps of the bundle are the *A*wakening and *B*reathing Coordination, which comprise a daily spontaneous awaking trial (SAT) and spontaneous breath trials (SBT) implemented by bedside nurses and respiratory therapists. Details of these steps are provided in Chapter 58. The key component of the ABC portion of the bundle is the daily interruption of sedation. To pass the SAT, patients must open their eyes to verbal stimuli or tolerate the interruption of sedation for 4 or more hours, without meeting any of the failure criteria. Following a successful SAT, patients proceed to the SBT. Use of this portion of the bundle alone has been shown to decrease both days spent in coma and 1-year mortality.[57]

The third step is *C*hoice of sedation for the mechanically ventilated patient. As previously noted, benzodiazepines should be avoided except in the cases of ethanol or benzodiazepine withdrawal. Preferred alternatives include propofol or dexmedetomidine, both of which have a reduced risk of delirium. Use of dexmedetomidine, when compared to benzodiazepines, is also associated with more ventilator-free days.[58,59]

The fourth step is *D*elirium monitoring. This is particularly important for patients boarded in the ED for prolonged periods. Using validated delirium assessment tools, such as the CAM-ICU or ICDSC in combination with a validated sedation scale (e.g., Richmond Agitation–Sedation Scale), facilitates early delirium recognition and helps tailor sedation management to specific patients' needs. Standardized assessment instruments also provide a structured framework for communication between providers. While the term "altered" may suggest a range of cognitive capacity, "RASS -3 and CAM-ICU positive" provides a clear and succinct description of a patient's mental status.

The fifth step is *E*arly *E*xercise. One randomized controlled trial (RCT) compared mechanically ventilated patients given daily interruptions of sedation with exercise to patients given daily interruption of sedation alone. Patients who received protocolized exercise early in their ICU course experienced an average of two fewer days of delirium, two more ventilator-free days, and a 5-day improvement in time to mobilization out of bed.[60] Patients in the intervention group were also more likely to return to independent functional status at hospital discharge (59% vs. 35%).

A recent study of the ABCDE bundle in 296 mechanically ventilated patients demonstrated more delirium-free and ventilator-free days than historical controls.[61] While these results are encouraging, the study's use of historical controls made it subject to bias from general improvements in care over time; however, obtaining more robust data from randomized controlled trials may not be ethical or feasible.

CONCLUSION

Delirium is a form of acute brain dysfunction that is commonly observed in critically ill patients in the ED. It is associated with accelerated cognitive decline and higher mortality. Delirium follows from a complex interaction between patient vulnerability and precipitating factors and can be diagnosed using a validated assessment such as the CAM-ICU or ICDSC. Once detected, the primary clinical goal is to identify and treat the underlying precipitant. Beyond this, the optimal management of delirium remains unclear. Environmental modifications to calm patients and restore natural sleep cycles may be helpful to all patients. Pharmacologically, benzodiazepines should be avoided whenever possible, including for sedation of mechanically ventilated patients, where alternative sedatives, including propofol or dexmedetomidine, may be used. Atypical antipsychotics, such as quetiapine, may improve outcomes in all critically ill delirious patients, but larger trials are needed to confirm these findings. The ABCDE bundle, which consists of interruption of sedation in mechanically ventilated patients, appropriate choice of medicine, delirium monitoring, and early mobilization, may be a useful model for the treatment and prevention of delirium.

ACKNOWLEDGMENTS

Dr. Han is supported by the National Institutes of Health (K23AG032355). Dr. Vasilevskis is supported by the National Institutes of Health (K23AG040157). Dr. Ely has received grant support and honoraria from Eli Lilly, Hospira, and Pfizer and is supported by the National Institutes of Health (R01 AG035117-02, R01 AG 027472–05). Drs. Ely and Vasilevskis are also supported by the Veterans Affairs Clinical Research Center of Excellence and the Tennessee Valley Geriatric Research, Education and Clinical Center (GRECC).

LITERATURE TABLE		
TRIAL	**DESIGN**	**RESULT**
Delirium and outcomes in critically ill patients		
Ely et al., *JAMA.* 2004[7]	Prospective cohort study that enrolled 275 mechanically ventilated patients. Delirium was ascertained daily using the CAM-ICU. The primary outcome was 6-mo mortality and hospital length of stay. Secondary outcome was duration of mechanical ventilation	Delirium was independently associated with higher 6-mo mortality (hazard ratio 3.2; 95% CI, 1.4–7.7) and longer hospital length of stay (hazard ratio 2.0; 95% CI, 1.4–3.0). Delirium was associated with longer duration of mechanical ventilation (24 d vs. 19 d, *p*-value = 0.03)
Pandharipande et al., *N Engl J Med.* 2013[9]	Prospective cohort study that enrolled 821 medical and surgical ICU patients. Delirium was ascertained daily using the CAM-ICU. The primary outcome was 12-mo global cognition as measured by the RBANS	Of those enrolled, 6% had cognitive impairment at baseline. At 12 months, 34% and 24% had global cognition scores that were similar to patients with moderate traumatic brain injury and mild Alzheimer's disease, respectively. After adjusting for confounders, a longer duration of delirium was independently associated with worse global cognition at 12 months ($p = 0.04$)
CAM-ICU and ICDSC		
Ely et al., *Crit Care Med.* 2001[4]	Prospective observational study that enrolled 38 patients in the ICU, 58% of whom where mechanically ventilated. Two nurses and physician performed the CAM-ICU, and a psychiatrist's DSM-IV assessment was the reference standard for delirium	The CAM-ICU, when performed by nurses, was 95%–100% sensitive and 93% specific. When performed by a physician, the CAM-ICU was 100% sensitive and 89% specific. Interobserver reliability between the nurses and physician was very good
Ely et al., *JAMA.* 2001[33]	Prospective observational study that enrolled 111 mechanically ventilated patients in the ICU. Two nurses performed the CAM-ICU, and a psychiatrist's DSM-IV assessment was the reference standard for delirium	In mechanically ventilated patients, the CAM-ICU was 93%–100% sensitive and 98%–100% specific with excellent interobserver reliability between both nurses. The diagnostic performance was similar in the young and old (≥65 y old), sick and not sick, and in those with and without dementia
Gusmao-Flores et al., *Crit Care.* 2012[35]	Meta-analysis that included 9 studies evaluating the diagnostic performance of the CAM-ICU and 4 studies evaluating the diagnostic performance of the ISCDSC	The CAM-ICU's pooled sensitivity was 80%, and its pooled specificity was 95.9%. The ISCDSC's pooled sensitivity was 74%, and its pooled specificity was 81.9%
Bergeron et al., *Intensive Care Med.* 2001[36]	Prospective observational study that enrolled 93 patients in the medical and surgical ICU	The ICDSC was 99% sensitive and 64% specific
Pharmacologic treatment of delirium		
Girard et al., *Crit Care Med.* 2010[51] The MIND Trial	Blinded RCT that enrolled 103 mechanically ventilated patients. Patients were randomized to receive haloperidol (5 mg), ziprasidone (40 mg), or placebo every 6 h for up to 14 d	There was no difference in the number of days alive without coma or delirium in all three groups. In addition, no differences were observed in ventilator-free days, hospital length of stay, and mortality
Devlin et al., *Crit Care Med.* 2010[52]	Blinded RCT that enrolled 36 ICU patients with delirium. Patients were randomized to receive quetiapine 50 mg q12h (titratable to 200 mg q12h) or placebo. Both groups received adjunctive haloperidol as needed	The quetiapine group had reduced delirium duration (36 vs. 120 h, *p*-value = 0.006), less agitation (*p*-value = 0.02), and a trend toward being more likely to be discharged to home rather than rehabilitation (89% vs. 56%, *p*-value = 0.06). No differences in mortality or ICU LOS were observed

LITERATURE TABLE *(Continued)*

TRIAL	DESIGN	RESULT
ABCDE bundle in mechanically ventilated patients		
Balas et al., *Crit Care Med.* 2014[61]	This was a pre–post study evaluating the effects of implementing the ABCDE bundle that emphasizes interruption of sedation, delirium monitoring, routine delirium screening, and early mobilization. A total of 296 patients were enrolled	The postimplementation group was less likely to experience delirium during their ICU stay (48.7% vs. 62.3%, *p*-value = 0.02) and spent more days breathing without ventilator assistance (median 21 vs. 24 d, *p*-value = 0.04) compared with the preimplementation group. No differences in time to ICU and hospital discharge were observed

95% CI, 95% confidence interval; CAM-ICU, Confusion Assessment Method for the Intensive Care Unit; ICU, intensive care unit; Intensive Care Delirium Screening Checklist, ICDSC; RBANS, Repeatable Battery for the Assessment of Neuropsychological Status; DSM-IV, Diagnostic and Statistical Manual of Mental Disorders, Fourth Edition; LOS, length of stay; RCT, randomized control trial.

REFERENCES

1. Han JH, Zimmerman EE, Cutler N, et al. Delirium in older emergency department patients: recognition, risk factors, and psychomotor subtypes. *Acad Emerg Med.* 2009;16:193–200.
2. Hustey FM, Meldon SW, Smith MD, et al. The effect of mental status screening on the care of elderly emergency department patients. *Ann Emerg Med.* 2003;41:678–684.
3. Dubois MJ, Bergeron N, Dumont M, et al. Delirium in an intensive care unit: a study of risk factors. *Intensive Care Med.* 2001;27:1297–1304.
4. Ely EW, Margolin R, Francis J, et al. Evaluation of delirium in critically ill patients: validation of the Confusion Assessment Method for the Intensive Care Unit (CAM-ICU). *Crit Care Med.* 2001;29:1370–1379.
5. Pandharipande P, Cotton BA, Shintani A, et al. Prevalence and risk factors for development of delirium in surgical and trauma intensive care unit patients. *J Trauma.* 2008;65:34–41.
6. Ely EW, Gautam S, Margolin R, et al. The impact of delirium in the intensive care unit on hospital length of stay. *Intensive Care Med.* 2001;27:1892–1900.
7. Ely EW, Shintani A, Truman B, et al. Delirium as a predictor of mortality in mechanically ventilated patients in the intensive care unit. *JAMA.* 2004;291:1753–1762.
8. Milbrandt EB, Deppen S, Harrison PL, et al. Costs associated with delirium in mechanically ventilated patients. *Crit Care Med.* 2004;32:955–962.
9. Pandharipande PP, Girard TD, Jackson JC, et al. Long-term cognitive impairment after critical illness. *N Engl J Med.* 2013;369:1306–1316.
10. American Psychiatric Association. *American Psychiatric Association. Task Force on DSM-IV. Diagnostic and Statistical Manual of Mental Disorders: DSM-IV*. 4th ed. Washington, DC: American Psychiatric Association; 1994.
11. Meagher DJ, Trzepacz PT. Motoric subtypes of delirium. *Semin Clin Neuropsychiatry.* 2000;5:75–85.
12. Inouye SK, Foreman MD, Mion LC, et al. Nurses' recognition of delirium and its symptoms: comparison of nurse and researcher ratings. *Arch Intern Med.* 2001;161:2467–2473.
13. Nicholas LM, Lindsey BA. Delirium presenting with symptoms of depression. *Psychosomatics.* 1995;36:471–479.
14. Pandharipande P, Cotton BA, Shintani A, et al. Motoric subtypes of delirium in mechanically ventilated surgical and trauma intensive care unit patients. *Intensive Care Med.* 2007;33:1726–1731.
15. Peterson JF, Pun BT, Dittus RS, et al. Delirium and its motoric subtypes: a study of 614 critically ill patients. *J Am Geriatr Soc.* 2006;54:479–484.
16. Vilke GM, Payne-James J, Karch SB. Excited delirium syndrome (ExDS): redefining an old diagnosis. *J Forensic Leg Med.* 2012;19:7–11.
17. Inouye SK, Charpentier PA. Precipitating factors for delirium in hospitalized elderly persons. Predictive model and interrelationship with baseline vulnerability. *JAMA.* 1996;275:852–857.
18. Van Rompaey B, Elseviers MM, Schuurmans MJ, et al. Risk factors for delirium in intensive care patients: a prospective cohort study. *Crit Care.* 2009;13:R77.

19. Pisani MA, Murphy TE, Van Ness PH, et al. Characteristics associated with delirium in older patients in a medical intensive care unit. *Arch Intern Med.* 2007;167:1629–1634.
20. Brummel NE, Girard TD. Preventing delirium in the intensive care unit. *Crit Care Clin.* 2013;29:51–65.
21. Inouye SK, Viscoli CM, Horwitz RI, et al. A predictive model for delirium in hospitalized elderly medical patients based on admission characteristics. *Ann Intern Med.* 1993;119:474–481.
22. Francis J, Martin D, Kapoor WN. A prospective study of delirium in hospitalized elderly. *JAMA.* 1990;263:1097–1101.
23. Kolbeinsson H, Jonsson A. Delirium and dementia in acute medical admissions of elderly patients in Iceland. *Acta Psychiatr Scand.* 1993;87:123–127.
24. Bayer AJ, Chadha JS, Farag RR, et al. Changing presentation of myocardial infarction with increasing old age. *J Am Geriatr Soc.* 1986;34:263–266.
25. Pandharipande P, Shintani A, Peterson J, et al. Lorazepam is an independent risk factor for transitioning to delirium in intensive care unit patients. *Anesthesiology.* 2006;104:21–26.
26. Pisani MA, Murphy TE, Araujo KL, et al. Benzodiazepine and opioid use and the duration of intensive care unit delirium in an older population. *Crit Care Med.* 2009;37:177–183.
27. Agarwal V, O'Neill PJ, Cotton BA, et al. Prevalence and risk factors for development of delirium in burn intensive care unit patients. *J Burn Care Res.* 2010;31:706–715.
28. Vaurio LE, Sands LP, Wang Y, et al. Postoperative delirium: the importance of pain and pain management. *Anesth Analg.* 2006;102:1267–1273.
29. Morrison RS, Magaziner J, Gilbert M, et al. Relationship between pain and opioid analgesics on the development of delirium following hip fracture. *J Gerontol A Biol Sci Med Sci.* 2003;58:M76–M81.
30. Meagher DJ, Moran M, Raju B, et al. Phenomenology of delirium. Assessment of 100 adult cases using standardised measures. *Br J Psychiatry.* 2007;190:135–141.
31. Barr J, Fraser GL, Puntillo K, et al. Clinical practice guidelines for the management of pain, agitation, and delirium in adult patients in the intensive care unit. *Crit Care Med.* 2013;41:278–280.
32. Ely EW, Truman B, Manzi DJ, et al. Consciousness monitoring in ventilated patients: bispectral EEG monitors arousal not delirium. *Intensive Care Med.* 2004;30:1537–1543.
33. Ely EW, Inouye SK, Bernard GR, et al. Delirium in mechanically ventilated patients: validity and reliability of the confusion assessment method for the intensive care unit (CAM-ICU). *JAMA.* 2001;286:2703–2710.
34. Woien H, Balsliemke S, Stubhaug A. The incidence of delirium in Norwegian intensive care units; deep sedation makes assessment difficult. *Acta Anaesthesiol Scand.* 2013;57:294–302.
35. Gusmao-Flores D, Figueira Salluh JI, Chalhub RA, et al. The confusion assessment method for the intensive care unit (CAM-ICU) and intensive care delirium screening checklist (ICDSC) for the diagnosis of delirium: a systematic review and meta-analysis of clinical studies. *Crit Care.* 2012;16:R115.
36. Bergeron N, Dubois MJ, Dumont M, et al. Intensive Care Delirium Screening Checklist: evaluation of a new screening tool. *Intensive Care Med.* 2001;27:859–864.
37. Han JH, Wilson A, Graves AJ, et al. Validation of the Brief Confusion Assessment Method for Older Emergency Department Patients. *Ann Emerg Med.* 2011;60(suppl):S28.
38. Pisani MA, Kong SY, Kasl SV, et al. Days of delirium are associated with 1-year mortality in an older intensive care unit population. *Am J Respir Crit Care Med.* 2009;180:1092–1097.
39. Caplan GA, Cassem NH, Murray GB. Delirium. In: Stern TA, ed. *Massachusetts General Hospital Comprehensive Clinical Psychiatry.* 1st ed. Philadelphia, PA: Mosby/Elsevier; 2008:xvii, 1273.
40. Han JH, Bryce SN, Ely EW, et al. The effect of cognitive impairment on the accuracy of the presenting complaint and discharge instruction comprehension in older emergency department patients. *Ann Emerg Med.* 2011;57:662–671.
41. Mazer M, Deroos F, Hollander JE, et al. Medication history taking in emergency department triage is inaccurate and incomplete. *Acad Emerg Med.* 2011;18:102–104.
42. Warshaw G, Tanzer F. The effectiveness of lumbar puncture in the evaluation of delirium and fever in the hospitalized elderly. *Arch Fam Med.* 1993;2:293–297.
43. Metersky ML, Williams A, Rafanan AL. Retrospective analysis: are fever and altered mental status indications for lumbar puncture in a hospitalized patient who has not undergone neurosurgery? *Clin Infect Dis.* 1997;25:285–288.
44. Moeller KE, Lee KC, Kissack JC. Urine drug screening: practical guide for clinicians. *Mayo Clin Proc.* 2008;83:66–76.
45. Naughton BJ, Moran M, Ghaly Y, et al. Computed tomography scanning and delirium in elder patients. *Acad Emerg Med.* 1997;4:1107–1110.

46. Hardy JE, Brennan N. Computerized tomography of the brain for elderly patients presenting to the emergency department with acute confusion. *Emerg Med Australas.* 2008;20:420–424.
47. Breitbart W, Marotta R, Platt MM, et al. A double-blind trial of haloperidol, chlorpromazine, and lorazepam in the treatment of delirium in hospitalized AIDS patients. *Am J Psychiatry.* 1996;153:231–237.
48. Mayo-Smith MF, Beecher LH, Fischer TL. et al. Management of alcohol withdrawal delirium. An evidence-based practice guideline. *Arch Intern Med.* 2004;164:1405–1412.
49. American Psychiatric Association. Practice guideline for the treatment of patients with delirium. *Am J Psychiatry.* 1999;156:1–20.
50. Hassaballa HA, Balk RA. Torsade de pointes associated with the administration of intravenous haloperidol:a review of the literature and practical guidelines for use. *Expert Opin Drug Saf.* 2003;2:543–547.
51. Girard TD, Pandharipande PP, Carson SS, et al. Feasibility, efficacy, and safety of antipsychotics for intensive care unit delirium: the MIND randomized, placebo-controlled trial. *Crit Care Med.* 2010;38:428–437.
52. Devlin JW, Roberts RJ, Fong JJ, et al. Efficacy and safety of quetiapine in critically ill patients with delirium: a prospective, multicenter, randomized, double-blind, placebo-controlled pilot study. *Crit Care Med.* 2010;38:419–427.
53. van Eijk MMJ, Roes KCB, Honing MLH, et al. Effect of rivastigmine as an adjunct to usual care with haloperidol on duration of delirium and mortality in critically ill patients: a multicentre, double-blind, placebo-controlled randomised trial. *Lancet.* 2010;376:1829–1837.
54. Chong MS, Chan MP, Kang J, et al. A new model of delirium care in the acute geriatric setting: geriatric monitoring unit. *BMC Geriatr.* 2011;11:41.
55. Van Rompaey B, Elseviers MM, Van Drom W, et al. The effect of earplugs during the night on the onset of delirium and sleep perception: a randomized controlled trial in intensive care patients. *Crit Care.* 2012;16:R73.
56. Vasilevskis EE, Pandharipande PP, Girard TD, et al. A screening, prevention, and restoration model for saving the injured brain in intensive care unit survivors. *Crit Care Med.* 2010;38:S683–S691.
57. Girard TD, Kress JP, Fuchs BD, et al. Efficacy and safety of a paired sedation and ventilator weaning protocol for mechanically ventilated patients in intensive care (Awakening and Breathing Controlled trial): a randomised controlled trial. *Lancet.* 2008;371:126–134.
58. Pandharipande PP, Pun BT, Herr DL, et al. Effect of sedation with dexmedetomidine vs lorazepam on acute brain dysfunction in mechanically ventilated patients: the MENDS randomized controlled trial. *JAMA.* 2007;298:2644–2653.
59. Riker RR, Shehabi Y, Bokesch PM, et al. Dexmedetomidine vs midazolam for sedation of critically ill patients: a randomized trial. *JAMA.* 2009;301:489–499.
60. Schweickert WD, Pohlman MC, Pohlman AS, et al. Early physical and occupational therapy in mechanically ventilated, critically ill patients: a randomised controlled trial. *Lancet.* 2009;373:1874–1882.
61. Balas MC, Vasilevskis EE, Olsen KM, et al. Effectiveness and safety of the awakening and breathing coordination, delirium monitoring/management, and early exercise/mobility bundle*. *Crit Care Med.* 2014;42:1024–1036.

57

Sedation of the Agitated Patient

Randall Wood and Jin H. Han

BACKGROUND

Emergency physicians are frequently called upon to provide care to agitated, violent, and combative patients. These patients pose a significant safety threat to themselves and to the providers who care for them; furthermore, their agitation can impede the diagnostic workup and delay potentially lifesaving care. Chemical sedation is often necessary in order to ensure patient and provider safety and to expedite the diagnostic workup.

Acute undifferentiated agitation can be classified broadly into medical, toxicologic, or psychiatric etiologies (Table 57.1). It may present with a wide spectrum of severity; patients may be agitated but cooperative or dangerously combative. Excited delirium syndrome (ExDS), also referred to as agitated delirium, is a recently-recognized syndrome that represents the most severe form of agitation. ExDS can be precipitated by almost any psychiatric or medical condition, drug, toxin, or biochemical or physiologic alteration.[1] Patients with ExDS are typically young males; they present in a hyperadrenergic autonomic state characterized by hyperthermia, tachycardia, insensitivity to pain, and superhuman strength.[1] ExDS is associated with an increase in mortality and represents a true medical emergency that requires immediate attention.

MANAGEMENT GUIDELINES

Although sedation is a critical component of the management of acute agitation in the emergency department (ED), health care professionals should be mindful that these patients are experiencing personal, psychological, and medical crises and that they deserve respect and dignity. Prior to administering sedative agents, de-escalation techniques both verbal and environmental (i.e., turning the lights down, minimizing ambient noise) should be attempted. Such techniques may fail in the severely agitated (or combative) patients, some of whom may require physical restraint prior to chemical sedation. If physical restraint is used, it should be for the shortest time possible; positioning a restrained patient in the prone position should be avoided as this has been associated with increased mortality.[2]

Benzodiazepines and antipsychotic medications are the most commonly-used pharmacologic agents for the sedation of the agitated patient (Table 57.2). Although intravenous (IV) administration of these medications allows for rapid onset, this dosing route may be challenging and unsafe in the combative and uncooperative patient. For this reason, intramuscular (IM) formulations are often used initially until an IV

TABLE 57.1 Differential Diagnosis for Acute Undifferentiated Agitation

- Intoxication (alcohol, stimulant, polysubstance)
- Ethanol or benzodiazepine withdrawal
- Hypoxia
- Electrolyte disturbances
- Hypoglycemia
- CNS infection
- Sepsis
- Thyroid storm
- Head injury or intracranial lesion
- Hypothermia or heat stroke
- Neuroleptic malignant syndrome
- Serotonin syndrome
- Psychosis from psychiatric disease

can be established. Oral administration of benzodiazepines and antipsychotics is rarely given in acutely agitated patients, but can be considered in those who are cooperative.[3]

MEDICATIONS USED FOR SEDATION OF THE SEVERELY AGITATED EMERGENCY DEPARTMENT PATIENT

Benzodiazepines

Benzodiazepines have a long history of use in the treatment of agitation. This drug class binds to the gamma–aminobutyric acid β (GABA-β)-subtype receptor—the primary inhibitory neurotransmitter of the central nervous system—and exerts sedative, hypnotic, anxiolytic, anticonvulsant, amnestic, and muscle relaxant effects.[4] Lorazepam and midazolam are the most commonly used and best studied benzodiazepines for the management of acute agitation because they have predictable onset of action when given in the IM form. Diazepam, chlordiazepoxide, and clonazepam are infrequently used in the acute management of agitation because they have longer half-lives and have

TABLE 57.2 Agents for Acute Undifferentiated Agitation in the Emergency Department

Agent	Formulation	Dose (mg)	Max Daily Dose (mg)
Lorazepam	IV	2	12
	IM	2–4	12
Midazolam	IV	2–5	15
	IM	5	15
Haloperidol	IV	5–10	20–30
	IM	5–10	20–30
Droperidol	IV	2.5–5	15
	IM	2.5–10	15
Olanzapine	IM	5–10	30
	PO	5–10	30

IV, intravenous; IM, intramuscular; PO, oral. Consider using lower doses for elderly patients.
Adapted from Vilke GM, et al. *J Forensic Leg Med.* 2012;19:117–121; and Wilson MP, et al. *West J Emerg Med.* 2012;13:26–34.

inconsistent IM absorption.[5] Midazolam has a faster onset and shorter duration of action than lorazepam, especially when given IM; however, patients receiving midazolam may require more frequent redosing because of its shorter half-life.[6,7]

The dosing of IM and IV midazolam and lorazepam is listed in Table 57.2. Protocols recommend dosing midazolam 2 to 5 mg IV every 5 to 10 minutes.[8,9] Serial dosing, however, must be used cautiously, as it may increase the risk of respiratory depression, which was reported to be as high as 13% with use of this protocol.[9] Fortunately, this serious side effect is usually transient;[5,9,10] it may, however, be more common in patients with ethanol or opiate intoxication and so should be used with caution in this population. Additional side effects of benzodiazepines include ataxia, dizziness, and decreased blood pressure, especially in patients who are hypovolemic.

Benzodiazepines should be reserved for patients whose agitation is severe and who present an immediate threat to themselves or others. They may also be useful in patients who are withdrawing from ethanol or benzodiazepines or those who have taken stimulants such as amphetamines or cocaine.[11] For agitated patients with delirium, the risks and benefits of benzodiazepine use, which can exacerbate delirium, must be carefully weighed.[12]

Typical Antipsychotics

Typical, or first-generation, antipsychotics have a long history of use in the treatment of agitation. Haloperidol and droperidol are high-potency butyrophenone antipsychotics that primarily antagonize the D2 dopamine receptor. Despite their side effects (discussed below), and the availability of newer generation atypical antipsychotics, haloperidol and droperidol are still widely used for the management of agitation. They have relatively little effect on hemodynamics[13] and can be given orally, intramuscularly, and intravenously.

Although haloperidol is more commonly used for agitation, droperidol offers several advantages. Droperidol may have a more rapid onset of action and a shorter half-life when given intramuscularly.[14] In one randomized controlled study comparing droperidol 5 mg IM with haloperidol 5 mg IM, droperidol achieved more rapid control of the patient's agitation without any relative increase in side effects.[15] Compared with IM haloperidol, IM droperidol may also last longer and be less likely to require repeat dosing.[16] The dosages for haloperidol and droperidol are listed in Table 57.2. Serial dosing (i.e., every 5 to 10 minutes) can be required to achieve adequate sedation; total doses exceeding 20 mg are associated with increased side effects and have limited incremental benefit.[6,17,18]

One of the most feared side effects of both droperidol and haloperidol is QT prolongation and torsades de pointes, especially when theses drugs are given intravenously and at higher doses.[19,20] Because of reports of cardiac death secondary to torsades de pointes, the FDA issued a black box warning on droperidol in 2001 that has curtailed its use in the clinical setting. This warning is not without controversy. Many have argued that the adverse events observed with droperidol were at doses much higher than typically used for agitation. Several studies have also shown droperidol to be safe for use at doses typically administered for agitation.[21,22] Regardless, special care should be taken when using either haloperidol or droperidol in patients with a known prolonged QT interval, who take other QT prolonging medications, or have medical conditions that cause QT prolongation. A 12-lead electrocardiogram should be obtained if possible prior to IV administration. If the patient's QTc interval is >500 milliseconds, the IV route should be avoided.

Haloperidol and droperidol can also cause extrapyramidal symptoms (EPS)—including acute dystonic reactions, akathisia, and pseudoparkinsonism—due to their blockade of dopamine receptors in the basal ganglia. Because haloperidol and droperidol have relatively little anticholinergic activity, EPS occurs in up to 20% of patients treated with these medications.[23] Anticholinergic agents such as diphenhydramine (25 to 50 mg), benztropine (1 to 2 mg), and promethazine (25 to 50 mg) are usually effective in treating acute EPS, though severe akathisia may require benzodiazepines.

Droperidol and haloperidol have also been shown to decrease seizure threshold and should be used with caution in patients with a history of seizures. Finally, neuroleptic malignant syndrome (NMS) is a rare but potentially fatal complication of these medications.

Atypical Antipsychotics

Olanzapine, risperidone, aripiprazole, and ziprasidone have been extensively evaluated for the treatment of acute agitation in the psychiatric patients; their role in the ED patient with undifferentiated agitation is less clear. Most atypical antipsychotics have oral and IM formulations, although the IM formulation may be less readily available in the ED.

Compared to typical antipsychotics, second-generation, or atypical, antipsychotics have a favorable side effect profile. Atypical antipsychotics also antagonize the dopamine D2 receptor, but unlike typical psychotics, they also antagonize the serotonin 5-HT2, histamine, alpha, and muscarinic receptors to variable degrees. They are less likely to cause oversedation, EPS, QT prolongation, and vital sign abnormalities. Some concerns, however, have been raised about hypotension and oxygen desaturation caused by parenteral olanzapine used in combination with benzodiazepines, especially in patients intoxicated with ethanol.[25–27] Similar to typical antipsychotics, NMS has also been reported in patients receiving atypical antipsychotics.[28]

CHOICE OF MEDICATION FOR SEDATION OF THE AGITATED PATIENT

The choice of medication for sedating the agitated ED patient can depend on how quickly sedation needs to be achieved and on the desired length of sedation. Several randomized controlled trials of typical antipsychotics have explored how they compare with benzodiazepines as monotherapy for controlling agitation. In one study, 111 ED patients with severe agitation were treated with either midazolam 5 mg IM, lorazepam 2 mg IM, or haloperidol 5 mg IM; midazolam was reported as having the shortest time to adequate sedation and shorter times to awakening compared with haloperidol and lorazepam.[7] A second study compared midazolam 5 gm IV with droperidol 5 mg IV in 153 agitated ED patients and allowed these medications to be redosed every 5 minutes until adequate sedation was achieved.[8] The study observed that more patients in the midazolam group achieved adequate sedation within 5 minutes (45% vs. 17%), suggesting that midazolam may have faster onset of action than droperidol. Both medications had side effects; there was a trend toward increased respiratory depression in the midazolam group (4.1% vs. 0.0%) and dystonic reactions in the droperidol group (0.0% vs. 3.8%). A third study compared droperidol IV (2.5 mg for patients <50 kg, 5.0 mg for patients >50 kg) with lorazepam IV (2.0 mg for patients <50 kg, 4.0 mg for patients >50 kg) in 202 agitated ED patients; repeat dosing was allowed in 30 minutes.[28] Though sedation was similar for both medications at 5 minutes, a larger proportion of the droperidol group achieved adequate sedation at subsequent time intervals. In addition, more patients in the lorazepam arm required redosing compared with the droperidol arm. No major adverse events occurred in either group.

The role of atypical antipsychotics in the management of the acutely agitated ED patient is less well established. To date, most research has been conducted in patients whose agitation has a psychiatric cause; in this population, atypical antipsychotics such as olanzapine, aripiprazole, and risperidone are as effective as haloperidol and show a lower incidence of EPS.[29–31] Only one randomized controlled trial has evaluated the role of atypical antipsychotic medications in the ED patient with undifferentiated agitation. This study randomized 144 agitated ED patients to receive midazolam 5 mg IM, droperidol 5 mg IM, or ziprasidone 20 mg IM.[17] Only 39% of the ziprasidone group achieved adequate sedation within 15 minutes compared to 69% of the midazolam group and 60% of the droperidol group.[17] As result, IM ziprasidone is not recommended for rapid sedation of the agitated patient.

In the agitated patient with a psychiatric etiology, several studies have demonstrated that a butyrophenone in combination with a benzodiazepine results in improved sedation with less EPS than monotherapy.[23,32,33] In ED patients, the role of combination therapy in the patient with undifferentiated agitation remains unclear. One randomized controlled trial compared droperidol 10 mg IM, midazolam 10 mg IM, and the combination of droperidol 5 mg IM + midazolam 5 mg IM in 91 violent and agitated ED patients.[34] The study did not observe any differences in the duration of agitation between the three groups. However, the midazolam group required more redosing to maintain adequate sedation; this group also experienced a nonsignificant tendency to develop oxygen desaturations, especially in patients with ethanol intoxication. A second randomized controlled trial compared midazolam IV alone with midazolam IV used in conjunction with either droperidol 5 mg IV or olanzapine 5 mg IV.[24] The combination of droperidol + midazolam or olanzapine + midazolam was associated with significantly shorter times to adequate sedation compared with midazolam alone. More patients in the midazolam-only group required additional sedation within 60 minutes. There were no differences in adverse events or ED length of stay. Several retrospective studies, however, raise concerns that combining olanzapine with a benzodiazepine may result in lower oxygen saturations when given to patients with ethanol intoxication.[35,36] As a result, additional research is needed to determine the safety and efficacy of combining antipsychotics and benzodiazepine in the treatment of agitation in the ED.

SUMMARY RECOMMENDATIONS

Based on the abovementioned studies, the following general conclusions can be made:

- Droperidol and midazolam appear to achieve fastest onset of sedation; midazolam, however, may require redosing if prolonged sedation is needed.
- Combination therapy with an antipsychotic and a benzodiazepine has been shown to be effective for managing agitation in psychiatric patients, but its effectiveness in the ED patient with undifferentiated agitation is yet to be determined. The use of midazolam in conjunction with droperidol or olanzapine is as effective as monotherapy, but may result in prolonged sedation.

- Midazolam, whether used as monotherapy or in conjunction with an antipsychotic, may cause respiratory compromise in ethanol-intoxicated patients and should be used with caution.
- No droperidol study has reported torsades de pointes, but patients who received droperidol developed longer QTc when compared with midazolam.[8]

Other Agents Used for the Sedation of the Agitated Patient

Ketamine is a dissociative anesthetic that antagonizes the *N*-methyl-*D*-aspartate receptor. It is commonly used in the ED for procedural sedation and induction of intubation and minimally affects respiratory drive. Several case reports have shown that ketamine may be useful in the treatment of severe agitation refractory to antipsychotics or benzodiazepines.[37–39]

Dexmedetomidine is an alpha-2 agonist sedative that produces minimal respiratory depression; an advantage of this agent is that patients remain easily arousable, even while their agitation is adequately controlled. The evidence supporting its use is limited to case reports in patients with delirium tremens.[40] Further research is needed to establish the role and safety of both ketamine and dexmedetomidine in treating agitation in the ED.

CHOICE OF SEDATIVES BASED UPON CAUSE OF AGITATION

Recently, the American Association for Emergency Psychiatry released a consensus statement on the management of agitation in the ED including specific types of agitation that may warrant specific sedatives.[11] In a busy ED, however, it is often challenging to determine the cause of agitation, especially early in a patient's course. With this caveat, for agitation secondary to stimulants, benzodiazepines are considered the first-line agent. Benzodiazepines should also be used for agitation secondary to alcohol and benzodiazepine withdrawal. For alcohol-intoxicated patients, benzodiazepines should be avoided because of increased risk of respiratory depression; haloperidol or a second-generation antipsychotic should be used instead. For agitation secondary to a psychiatric illness, antipsychotics are preferred over benzodiazepines, and atypical antipsychotics are preferred over typical antipsychotics. Benzodiazepines may be used if the initial dose of antipsychotic medications is insufficient to control agitation. For agitation secondary to hyperactive delirium not caused by a stimulant, ethanol withdrawal, or benzodiazepine withdrawal, haloperidol is recommended if immediate pharmacologic control is required. Benzodiazepines can exacerbate the delirium component of hyperactive delirium and should be avoided in those instances.[41]

CONCLUSION

The management of severe acute agitation in the ED is challenging and requires a coordinated effort between emergency physicians, nurses, and staff. When nonpharmacological methods fail to calm the patient, intervention with chemical sedation can to ensure patient and staff safety and facilitate the diagnostic workup. Familiarity with the summary recommendations provided in this chapter can help guide selection of the most appropriate sedative agent.

LITERATURE TABLE

TRIAL	DESIGN	RESULT
Sedation of acute undifferentiated agitation		
Nobay et al., *Acad Emerg Med.* 2004[7]	Blinded RCT comparing midazolam 5 mg IM, lorazepam 2 mg IM, or haloperidol 5 mg IM in 111 violent and severely agitated ED patients	Mean time to adequate sedation was significantly (p-value <0.05) shorter in the midazolam group (18 min) compared with those who received haloperidol (28 min) or lorazepam (32 min). Mean time to awakening was significantly shorter (p-value < 0.05) in the midazolam group (82 min) compared with lorazepam (217 min) and haloperidol (127 min)
Knott et al., *Ann Emerg Med.* 2006[8]	Blinded RCT comparing midazolam 5 mg IV with droperidol 5 mg IV in 153 agitated ED patients; each group could be redosed every 5 min for a total of six doses until adequate sedation was achieved	More patients in the midazolam group achieved adequate sedation within 5 min (45% vs. 17%, p-value < 0.001), but the proportion of patients achieving adequate sedation in 10 min were similar (55% vs. 53%, p-value = 0.91). Three patients in the midazolam group required airway intervention including one intubation
Martel et al., *Acad Emerg Med.* 2005[17]	Blinded RCT comparing droperidol 5 mg IM, ziprasidone 20 mg IM, and midazolam 5 mg IM in 144 ED patients with acute undifferentiated agitation	Fewer patients in the ziprasidone (39%) group were adequately sedated within 15 min compared with the midazolam (69%) and droperidol (60%) groups (p-value = 0.01). However, the midazolam group required more rescue medications (50%) compared with droperidol (10%) or ziprasidone (20%) groups (p-value < 0.05). The proportion of patients with respiratory depression were not significantly different between the three groups
Chan et al., *Ann Emerg Med.* 2013[24]	Multicenter-blinded RCT investigating IV droperidol (5 mg) vs. IV olanzapine (5 mg) vs. IV saline (placebo) in 336 acutely agitated ED patients. These were immediately followed by incremental IV midazolam boluses (2.5–5 mg) titrated until sedation was adequately achieved	Median difference for times to sedation between placebo (midazolam only) and olanzapine + midazolam group was 4 min (95% CI, 1–6 min), and the median difference for times to sedation between placebo and the droperidol + midazolam group was 5 min (95% CI, 1–6 min). More patients in the placebo group required additional sedation in the 60 min. All groups had similar rates of adverse events, and no differences in ED LOS were observed
Richards et al., *J Emerg Med.* 1998[28]	Randomized nonblinded trial comparing droperidol IV (2.5 mg for patients <50 kg, 5.0 mg for patients >50 kg) with lorazepam IV (2.0 mg for patients <50 kg, 4.0 mg for patients >50 kg) in 202 ED agitated patients	Sedation scores were similar at 5 min. The droperidol group, however, had achieved better sedation than lorazepam after 10 min through 60 min. More patients in the lorazepam arm required redosing compared with the droperidol arm
Isbister et al., *Ann Emerg Med.* 2010[34]	Blinded RCT that investigated droperidol 10 mg IM, midazolam 10 mg IM, and the combination of droperidol 5 mg IM + midazolam 5 mg IM in 91 violent and agitated ED patients	No difference in the median duration of agitation between the three treatment arms, but redosing was required more often in patients who received midazolam (62%) compared with droperidol (33%) and combination therapy (41%). Oxygen desaturation was the most common adverse event and occurred with greater frequency in the midazolam group (28%) than with the droperidol group (6%) or the combination group (7%), although this finding did not reach statistical significance. This complication was observed predominantly in patients with ethanol intoxication

RCT, randomized control trials; IV, intravenous; IM, intramuscular; ED, emergency department; 95% CI, 95% confidence intervals; LOS, length of stay.

REFERENCES

1. Vilke GM, DeBard ML, Chan TC, et al. Excited Delirium Syndrome (ExDS): defining based on a review of the literature. *J Emerg Med.* 2012;43:897–905.
2. Chan TC, Vilke GM, Neuman T, et al. Restraint position and positional asphyxia. *Ann Emerg Med.* 1997;30:578–586.

3. Gault TI, Gray SM, Vilke GM, et al. Are oral medications effective in the management of acute agitation? *J Emerg Med.* 2012;43:854–859.
4. Mihic SJ, Harris RA. Chapter 17. Hypnotics and sedatives. In: Goodman LS, Brunton LL, Chabner B, et al., eds. *Goodman and Gilman's the Pharmacological Basis of Therapeutics.* 12th ed. New York: McGraw-Hill; 2011.
5. Battaglia J: Pharmacological management of acute agitation. *Drugs.* 2005;65:1207–1222.
6. Rund DA, Ewing JD, Mitzel K, et al. The use of intramuscular benzodiazepines and antipsychotic agents in the treatment of acute agitation or violence in the emergency department. *J Emerg Med.* 2006;31:317–324.
7. Nobay F, Simon BC, Levitt MA, et al. A prospective, double-blind, randomized trial of midazolam versus haloperidol versus lorazepam in the chemical restraint of violent and severely agitated patients. *Acad Emerg Med.* 2004;11:744–749.
8. Knott JC, Taylor DM, Castle DJ. Randomized clinical trial comparing intravenous midazolam and droperidol for sedation of the acutely agitated patient in the emergency department. *Ann Emerg Med.* 2006;47:61–67.
9. Spain D, Crilly J, Whyte I, et al. Safety and effectiveness of high-dose midazolam for severe behavioural disturbance in an emergency department with suspected psychostimulant-affected patients. *Emerg Med Australas.* 2008;20:112–120.
10. Alexander J, Tharyan P, Adams C, et al. Rapid tranquillisation of violent or agitated patients in a psychiatric emergency setting. Pragmatic randomised trial of intramuscular lorazepam v. haloperidol plus promethazine. *Br J Psychiatry.* 2004;185:63–69.
11. Wilson MP, Pepper D, Currier GW, et al. The psychopharmacology of agitation: consensus statement of the American association for emergency psychiatry project Beta psychopharmacology workgroup. *West J Emerg Med.* 2012;13:26–34.
12. Breitbart W, Marotta R, Platt MM, et al. A double-blind trial of haloperidol, chlorpromazine, and lorazepam in the treatment of delirium in hospitalized AIDS patients. *Am J Psychiatry.* 1996;153:231–237.
13. Foster S, Kessel J, Berman ME, et al. Efficacy of lorazepam and haloperidol for rapid tranquilization in a psychiatric emergency room setting. *Int Clin Psychopharmacol.* 1997;12:175–179.
14. Cressman WA, Plostnieks J, Johnson PC. Absorption, metabolism and excretion of droperidol by human subjects following intramuscular and intravenous administration. *Anesthesiology.* 1973;38:363–369.
15. Thomas H Jr, Schwartz E, Petrilli R. Droperidol versus haloperidol for chemical restraint of agitated and combative patients. *Ann Emerg Med.* 1992;21:407–413.
16. Resnick M, Burton BT. Droperidol vs. haloperidol in the initial management of acutely agitated patients. *J Clin Psychiatry.* 1984;45:298–299.
17. Martel M, Sterzinger A, Miner J, et al. Management of acute undifferentiated agitation in the emergency department: a randomized double-blind trial of droperidol, ziprasidone, and midazolam. *Acad Emerg Med.* 2005;12:1167–1172.
18. Baldessarini RJ, Cohen BM, Teicher MH. Significance of neuroleptic dose and plasma level in the pharmacological treatment of psychoses. *Arch Gen Psychiatry.* 1988;45:79–91.
19. Lawrence KR, Nasraway SA. Conduction disturbances associated with administration of butyrophenone antipsychotics in the critically ill: a review of the literature. *Pharmacotherapy.* 1997;17:531–537.
20. Hassaballa HA, Balk RA. Torsade de pointes associated with the administration of intravenous haloperidol: a review of the literature and practical guidelines for use. *Expert Opin Drug Saf.* 2003;2:543–547.
21. Chase PB, Biros MH. A retrospective review of the use and safety of droperidol in a large, high-risk, inner-city emergency department patient population. *Acad Emerg Med.* 2002;9:1402–1410.
22. Shale JH, Shale CM, Mastin WD. A review of the safety and efficacy of droperidol for the rapid sedation of severely agitated and violent patients. *J Clin Psychiatry.* 2003;64:500–505.
23. Battaglia J, Moss S, Rush J, et al. Haloperidol, lorazepam, or both for psychotic agitation? A multicenter, prospective, double-blind, emergency department study. *Am J Emerg Med.* 1997;15:335–340.
24. Chan EW, Taylor DM, Knott JC, et al. Intravenous droperidol or olanzapine as an adjunct to midazolam for the acutely agitated patient: a multicenter, randomized, double-blind, placebo-controlled clinical trial. *Ann Emerg Med.* 2013;61:72–81.
25. Zacher JL, Roche-Desilets J. Hypotension secondary to the combination of intramuscular olanzapine and intramuscular lorazepam. *J Clin Psychiatry.* 2005;66:1614–1615.
26. Wilson MP, Chen N, Vilke GM, et al. Olanzapine in ED patients: differential effects on oxygenation in patients with alcohol intoxication. *Am J Emerg Med.* 2012;30:1196–1201.
27. Marder SR, Sorsaburu S, Dunayevich E, et al. Case reports of postmarketing adverse event experiences with olanzapine intramuscular treatment in patients with agitation. *J Clin Psychiatry.* 2010;71:433–441.

28. Richards JR, Derlet RW, Duncan DR. Chemical restraint for the agitated patient in the emergency department: lorazepam versus droperidol. *J Emerg Med.* 1998;16:567–573.
29. Breier A, Meehan K, Birkett M, et al. A double-blind, placebo-controlled dose–response comparison of intramuscular olanzapine and haloperidol in the treatment of acute agitation in schizophrenia. *Arch Gen Psychiatry.* 2002;59:441–448.
30. Hsu WY, Huang SS, Lee BS, et al. Comparison of intramuscular olanzapine, orally disintegrating olanzapine tablets, oral risperidone solution, and intramuscular haloperidol in the management of acute agitation in an acute care psychiatric ward in Taiwan. *J Clin Psychopharmacol.* 2010;30:230–234.
31. Tran-Johnson TK, Sack DA, Marcus RN, et al. Efficacy and safety of intramuscular aripiprazole in patients with acute agitation: a randomized, double-blind, placebo-controlled trial. *J Clin Psychiatry.* 2007;68:111–119.
32. Garza-Trevino ES, Hollister LE, Overall JE, et al. Efficacy of combinations of intramuscular antipsychotics and sedative-hypnotics for control of psychotic agitation. *Am J Psychiatry.* 1989;146:1598–1601.
33. Yildiz A, Sachs GS, Turgay A. Pharmacological management of agitation in emergency settings. *Emerg Med J.* 2003;20:339–346.
34. Isbister GK, Calver LA, Page CB, et al. Randomized controlled trial of intramuscular droperidol versus midazolam for violence and acute behavioral disturbance: the DORM study. *Ann Emerg Med.* 2010;56(4):3920491.e1.
35. Wilson MP, MacDonald K, Vilke GM, et al. A comparison of the safety of olanzapine and haloperidol in combination with benzodiazepines in emergency department patients with acute agitation. *J Emerg Med.* 2012;43:790–797.
36. Wilson MP, MacDonald K, Vilke GM, et al. Potential complications of combining intramuscular olanzapine with benzodiazepines in emergency department patients. *J Emerg Med.* 2012;43:889–896.
37. Roberts JR, Geeting GK. Intramuscular ketamine for the rapid tranquilization of the uncontrollable, violent, and dangerous adult patient. *J Trauma.* 2001;51:1008–1010.
38. Hick JL, Ho JD. Ketamine chemical restraint to facilitate rescue of a combative "jumper". *Prehosp Emerg Care.* 2005;9:85–89.
39. Ho JD, Smith SW, Nystrom PC, et al. Successful management of excited delirium syndrome with prehospital ketamine: two case examples. *Prehosp Emerg Care.* 2013;17:274–279.
40. Muzyk AJ, Fowler JA, Norwood DK, et al. Role of alpha2-agonists in the treatment of acute alcohol withdrawal. *Ann Pharmacother.* 2011;45:649–657.
41. Clegg A, Young JB. Which medications to avoid in people at risk of delirium: a systematic review. *Age Ageing.* 2011;40:23–29.

58

Induction of Intubation and Sedation of the Mechanically Ventilated Patient

Jin H. Han and Pratik Pandharipande

BACKGROUND

Sedation is the pharmacologic reduction of agitation and anxiety, and it is an indispensable tool for the clinician treating critically ill emergency department (ED) patients. Sedation is used in the induction of intubation, as well as for maximizing comfort and reducing anxiety in the already intubated patient. Choice of sedative agents in the ED may have ramifications in the intensive care unit (ICU) and hospital course and may affect patient outcomes. This chapter reviews the pharmacologic agents used for the induction for intubation and for the sedation of mechanically ventilated patients.

INDUCTION AGENTS

The ED is frequently tasked with the initial management of a critically ill patient's airway. Induction for endotracheal intubation employs sedatives—called, in this context, induction agents—at doses that typically suppress ventilation. Etomidate, ketamine, barbiturates (methohexital), benzodiazepines (midazolam), and propofol have all been used in this capacity (Table 58.1).

Etomidate

Etomidate is a carboxylated imidazole derivative that is a potent hypnotic and activates the γ-aminobutyric acid type A (GABA) receptors in the brain; it has no analgesic effects.[1] For induction of intubation, the etomidate dose is 0.3 mg/kg given intravenously (IV).[2] Etomidate is an ideal induction agent in the ED because it has rapid and predictable onset of action (5 to 15 seconds), a short duration of action (5 to 14 minutes), negligible effect on spontaneous respiration at lower doses, and no direct effects on cardiac output or vascular resistance.[1,3,4] Etomidate may be particularly useful in patients with suspected traumatic brain injury or intraocular injuries; by reducing cerebral blood flow and oxygen consumption, it can decrease intracranial and intraocular pressure.[3]

It should be noted that etomidate use can lead to adrenal suppression, and as such its safety has come into question. Etomidate inhibits the 11β-hydroxylase enzyme, which is involved in the production of cortisol. A single dose of etomidate can cause adrenal

TABLE 58.1 Induction Agents for Intubation in the Emergency Department

Induction Agent	Dose	May be Beneficial for...	Side Effects	Caution/Contraindications
Etomidate	0.3 mg/kg	Hemodynamically unstable patients	Myoclonus, adrenal suppression	Consider alternative agent in patients with septic shock
Ketamine	1–2 mg/kg	Hemodynamically unstable patients	Increased heart rate and blood pressure	Use with caution in patients who are markedly hypertensive or tachycardic
Methohexital	1–1.5 mg/kg	Head injury patients with increased ICP, actively seizing	Hypotension	Use with caution in patients with hypovolemia. Avoid in hypotensive patients
Midazolam	0.3 to 0.35 mg/kg	Those who are actively seizing	Hypotension rare, but can occur in the setting of hypovolemia	Use with caution in patients with hypovolemia
Propofol	1–2.5 mg/kg		Hypotension	Use with caution in patients with hypovolemia. Avoid in hypotensive patients

ICP, intracranial pressure. Consider using the lowest dose of induction agent possible to minimize precipitating or exacerbating hemodynamic instability.

suppression for up to 72 hours, but whether this has a clinically relevant effect on outcomes has been a source of significant controversy.[5]

A recent meta-analysis that included five studies reported that critically ill patients who were septic and received etomidate were more likely to die (relative risk = 1.20).[6] However, only two of the five studies included in this meta-analysis were primary analyses of randomized controlled trials.[7,8] A recent retrospective cohort study enrolled 2,014 septic patients and reported that one-time etomidate use was not associated with ICU mortality, hospital mortality, vasopressor use, duration of mechanical ventilation, or ICU length of stay (LOS) in the unadjusted and adjusted models.[9] However, the limitations of retrospective studies are well documented, and larger randomized controlled trials comparing etomidate with other induction agents are needed.

Data regarding the safety of etomidate in nonseptic patients are even more uncertain, as there are few rigorously performed randomized controlled trials comparing etomidate to other induction agents. An association between single-dose etomidate and adverse outcomes (mortality, hospital LOS, ventilator days) has been noted in several retrospective cohort studies of critically ill patients.[10,11] One randomized controlled trial enrolled 469 critically patients with and without sepsis and compared etomidate with ketamine.[8] Though the etomidate group was more likely to have adrenal sufficiency, no significant difference in 28-day mortality was observed in the septic and nonseptic groups. There was, however, a trend toward increased vasopressor use in the etomidate group compared with the ketamine group (59% vs. 51%).[8]

Some clinicians have advocated the use of supplemental hydrocortisone and/or fludrocortisone when etomidate is administered for intubation.[12] In a secondary analysis of a major randomized controlled trial comparing the role of corticosteroids in septic shock, it was found that patients who received hydrocortisone and fludrocortisone for 7 days had lower 28-day mortality rates compared with patients who received placebo (55% vs. 76%).[13,14] However, two additional studies compared hydrocortisone with placebo in patients who received etomidate and observed no improvement in mortality in patients with and without septic shock.[15,16]

Based upon these limited data, etomidate should be used judiciously in patients with sepsis; however, given its favorable hemodynamic profile, etomidate is still preferable to propofol or barbiturates in unstable patients. In nonseptic patients, despite the reports of adrenal insufficiency, the effect of etomidate on patient outcomes remains uncertain.

Myoclonus is another, albeit less serious, side effect of etomidate and has been reported to occur in 10% to 80% of patients when a paralytic is not used.[3] For intubations without neuromuscular blockade, premedication with fentanyl or diazepam prior to etomidate administration may help reduce the incidence of myoclonus.[3]

Ketamine

Ketamine is a promising alternative to etomidate since it does not, in most cases, affect blood pressure or cardiac output and can be used safely in patients who are hemodynamically unstable. Ketamine is a dissociative agent that has anesthetic, amnestic, and anxiolytic properties. Unlike most other induction agents, it also provides analgesia. Ketamine noncompetitively inhibits glutamate at the *N*-methyl-d-aspartate receptors and causes dissociation between the thalamoneocortical and limbic regions of the central nervous system (CNS).[2] Ketamine may also have theoretical benefit in patients with asthma exacerbations; it causes an increase in serum catecholamine levels and may cause bronchodilation.[2] Lastly, patients who receive ketamine are typically able to maintain their respiratory effort and have preserved airway reflexes. For intubation, the dose is 1 to 2 mg/kg IV with an onset of action of approximately 30 seconds.[2]

Ketamine stimulates catecholamine release, but it can also cause slight myocardial depression.[17] Typically, the sympathomimetic stimulation overcomes the myocardial depression and causes an increase in heart rate, blood pressure, and cardiac output.[18] Theoretically, patients who have been physiologically stressed for a prolonged period of time may be depleted of endogenous catecholamines, allowing for the myocardial depression to dominate and cause hypotension. Because of this theoretical risk, ketamine should be used cautiously in patients in whom catecholamine depletion is suspected. Because ketamine increases myocardial oxygen demand, it should also be used cautiously in patients with coronary artery disease and avoided in patients who have evidence of myocardial ischemia.[18] Ketamine can also cause an increase in heart rate and blood pressure and should be used cautiously in patients who are hypertensive or tachycardic.

Traditionally, ketamine has also been used with caution in patients with traumatic brain injury because early small observational trials observed an increase in intracranial pressure (ICP).[19] More recent studies have failed to record a statistically significant increase in ICP, but these studies were similarly limited by their small sample sizes.[19] Until more definitive evidence is available, caution should be exercised with ketamine in this population.

Barbiturates

Barbiturates, such as methohexital, are CNS depressants that exert effects on the GABA receptors and have anxiolytic and sedative properties. Because barbiturates decreases cerebral blood flow and the brains' metabolic demands, they may have a protective effect in head injury patients. Barbiturates also have anticonvulsant properties and may be advantageous to patients who are actively seizing or who have a history of seizure disorder. However, since barbiturates can cause myocardial depression and peripheral vasodilatation, they are seldom used for intubation in the ED, where patients needing intubation are frequently hemodynamically unstable.[2] Barbiturates can also induce aminolevulinic acid synthetase and can precipitate acute porphyric crisis and should be avoided in patients with a history of porphyric disorders.[20] Standard induction dose for methohexital is 1 to 1.5mg/kg/IV.[2]

Benzodiazepines

Benzodiazepines also act on the GABA receptor and have sedative, hypnotic, amnestic, anxiolytic, and anticonvulsant properties, but provide no analgesia.[2] Midazolam (0.3 to 0.35 mg/kg) is the most commonly used benzodiazepine for intubation because it has a rapid onset and short duration of action. Although benzodiazepines have minimal cardiovascular effects, they can cause hypotension in patients who are hypovolemic.[2] Benzodiazepines have anticonvulsant activities and may be useful in patients who are actively seizing.

Propofol

Propofol binds to multiple receptors in the CNS including GABA, glycine, nicotinic, and muscarinic receptors. Propofol has sedative, hypnotic, anxiolytic, amnestic, and anticonvulsant properties, but provides no analgesia.[21] The dose for induction is 1 to 2.5 mg/kg IV. Propofol has several appealing characteristics for an induction agent. First, it is highly lipophilic and easily crosses the blood–brain barrier, resulting in rapid onset of sedation (1 to 2 minutes). Second, it is rapidly redistributed into the peripheral tissues, resulting in a short duration of action (2 to 8 minutes) even in the setting of renal or hepatic dysfunction. The primary disadvantage of propofol is its negative inotropic effect, which can lead to decreased systemic vascular resistance and cause pronounced hemodynamic depression.[22] For this reason, propofol should be used with caution in patients who are volume depleted and should be avoided in patients who are hypotensive.[2] Because propofol is dissolved in a 10% lipid emulsion containing egg, soybean oil, and egg lecithin, allergic reactions can be seen in patients with soybean and egg allergies.[21]

CHOICE OF INDUCTION AGENT

The choice of induction should be guided by the patient's underlying illness and comorbid conditions. Etomidate and ketamine are ideal for use in the ED because of their favorable hemodynamic profiles. Etomidate should probably be avoided in septic patients, although the medical community has not uniformly embraced this recommendation; additional trials are needed to clarify etomidate's safety. Ketamine may be a safer alternative, including in head injury patients. Propofol, barbiturates, and to a lesser extent, benzodiazepines can cause potentially fatal decreases in blood pressure, especially in patients who are volume depleted.

Surprisingly little data exist regarding the effect of induction agent on ease of intubation. One trial randomized 469 septic and nonseptic patients to receive either etomidate or ketamine for the induction of intubation and did not observe any difference in intubation conditions (number of attempts, number of operators, number of alternative techniques, glottis visualization, lifting force, use of external laryngeal pressure, and vocal cord position).[8] In a registry study (NEAR II) of 2,380 ED patients who underwent rapid sequence intubation, etomidate, ketamine, and benzodiazepine were associated with a lower likelihood of successful first-attempt intubation compared with barbiturates.[23] The authors concluded that using methohexital and propofol facilitated rapid sequence intubation, but that the benefits of these medications should be weighed against their capacity to produce hemodynamic instability.

ANALGESIA AND SEDATION IN THE MECHANICALLY VENTILATED PATIENT

Once a patient is intubated in the ED, a primary goal is to ensure comfort in as safe a manner possible. Endotracheal intubation (as well as other critical care procedures) can result in significant anxiety and agitation, which can lead a patient to self-remove lifesaving medical devices. Unrelieved pain and anxiety may also have long-term psychological consequences, including posttraumatic stress disorder.[21]

Analgesia and sedation are an integral part to providing comfort to the mechanically ventilated patient (Fig. 58.1). However, special care must be taken to avoid oversedation, which is associated with increased duration of mechanical ventilation, prolonged ICU stays, and delirium.[24] Delirium has gained increased attention in the critical care literature over the past decade; it has been shown to be a predictor of death and leads to increased duration of mechanical ventilation, longer ICU stays, and long-term cognitive impairment.[25,26]

In 2013, the American College of Critical Care Medicine, Society of Critical Care Medicine, and American Society of Health-System Pharmacists released a clinical practice guideline for the management of pain, agitation, and delirium in critically ill patients (PAD guidelines).[21] These guidelines were developed by a 20-person multidisciplinary task force that reviewed the latest critical care literature and provided consensus recommendations for sedation and analgesia. The subsequent paragraphs provide a summary of these guidelines.

Analgesia

Adequate analgesia is essential to minimizing discomfort, agitation, and delirium in the mechanically ventilated patient (Fig. 58.1).[27] Because vital sign abnormalities alone are inaccurate markers for pain, a validated pain assessment should be used for all intubated patients.[21] The Behavioral Pain Scale and Critical-Care Pain Observation Tool are two examples of pain scales validated for this patient population.[28,29] These scales are based upon the health care providers' observations of the patient's facial expression, upper body movements, and compliance with ventilator.

While it is beyond the scope of this chapter to provide a comprehensive review of analgesia for the mechanically ventilated patient, it is important to note that the PAD guidelines recommend IV administration of opioid medications as first-line treatment of pain related to intubation.[21] Longer-acting opioids (such as morphine and hydromorphone) and shorter-acting opioids (such as fentanyl and remifentanil) can be used.[24] Of the opioid medications listed above, fentanyl is the most commonly used because of its rapid onset of action, short duration of action, and minimal histaminic release.[24] Meperidine is generally avoided because it may be deliriogenic and because it is

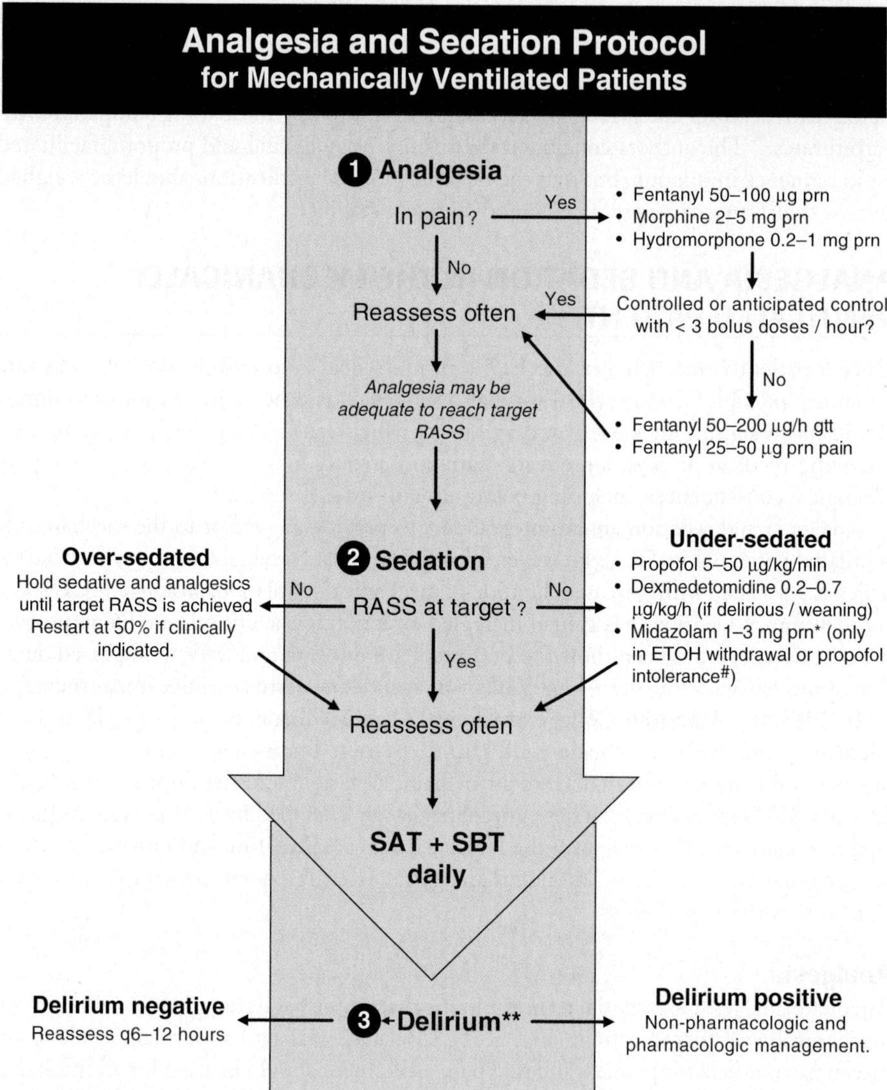

FIGURE 58.1 Empiric Sedation Protocol. *Midazolam 1 to 3 mg/hour gtt may be used if more than three midazolam boluses are given per hour, for propofol intolerance, or if the patient has been on propofol for >96 hours. #Propofol intolerance may be secondary to propofol infusion syndrome. **Delirium monitoring in critically ill patients is reviewed in Chapter 56. RASS, Richmond agitation and sedation scale; gtt, infusion; prn, as needed; ETOH, ethanol; SAT, Spontaneous awakening trial; SBT, Spontaneous breathing trial. Courtesy of icudelirium.org. Used with permission.

metabolized into normeperidine, which is neurotoxic and can cause tremors, myoclonus, and generalized tonic–clonic seizures.[30,31] Morphine has a less clear role in the development of delirium, with studies producing conflicting results. It is possible that opioid medications may be delirium protective when used for pain control, but deliriogenic in higher doses.[32,33] Nonopioid analgesia—such as regional anesthesia, IV acetaminophen, oral, IV or rectal cyclooxygenase inhibitors, or IV ketorolac—can be also used as adjunctive therapy for pain control.[21]

Sedation

After adequate pain control has been achieved, the next step (Fig. 58.1) is to provide sedation, if needed, to further minimize anxiety and agitation. Dosing must be guided by ongoing, accurate assessment of a patient's agitation and depth of sedation. Traditionally, descriptors such as lethargic, drowsy, somnolent, restless, agitated, or combative have been used, but these terms may have different meanings for different health providers; instead, arousal scales with standardized definitions should be utilized. The commonly used Richmond Agitation Sedation Scale (RASS, Table 58.2) ranges from −5 (unresponsive to pain and voice) to +4 (extreme combativeness).[34] Alternatively, the Riker Sedation–Agitation Scale can be used and ranges from 1 (unarousable) to 4 (calm) to 7 (dangerous agitation).[35]

In the time immediately following intubation, it is not uncommon for an ED patient to be overly sedated and minimally responsive to painful stimuli. Prolonged and deep sedation (RASS −3 to −5) within the first 48 hours of mechanical ventilation can lead to delayed extubation times and increased in-hospital and 6-month mortality.[36] Ideally, a lighter degree of sedation (RASS −1 or −2) should be targeted, using the least amount of sedation necessary to control agitation and anxiety while maintaining patient comfort.[21] Traditionally, benzodiazepines have been the sedative of choice for mechanically ventilated patients.[21] Recent evidence, however, suggests that alternative sedative agents such propofol and dexmedetomidine, when available, may improve patient outcomes.

TABLE 58.2 Richmond Agitation Sedation Scale

Score	Term	Description
+4	Combative	Overtly combative, violent, immediate danger to staff
+3	Very agitated	Pulls or removes tube(s) or catheter(s); aggressive
+2	Agitated	Frequent nonpurposeful movement
+1	Restless	Anxious but movements not aggressive vigorous
0	Alert and clam	
−1	Drowsy	Not fully alert, but has sustained awakening (eye opening/eye contact) to voice (>10 s)
−2	Light sedation	Briefly awakens with eye contact to voice (<10 s)
−3	Moderate sedation	Movement or eye opening to voice (but no eye contact)
−4	Deep sedation	No response to voice, but movement or eye opening to physical stimulation
−5	Unarousable	No response to voice or physical stimulation

Monitoring for delirium—which affects up to 80% of mechanically ventilated patients and is associated with adverse outcomes—is an essential component of the pain analgesia and sedation protocol (Fig. 58.1).[37] Delirium can be the initial manifestation of oversedation or of a change in patient status, such as pain, hypoxemia, hypoglycemia, hypotension, or ethanol withdrawal. If a patient is found to be delirious, every effort should be made to uncover the underlying precipitant. Delirium can be monitored using validated assessments such as the Confusion Assessment Method for the Intensive Care Unit or the Intensive Care Delirium Screening Checklist.[37,38] Details of the diagnosis and management of critically ill patients with delirium are described in Chapter 56.

SEDATION AGENTS

Benzodiazepines

Benzodiazepines have been used for sedation for many years in EDs and ICUs. Most benzodiazepines are metabolized by the liver, and their effects can be prolonged in patient with hepatic dysfunction. With the exception of lorazepam, the metabolism of benzodiazepines also produces active metabolites that are renally eliminated. This can result in prolonged sedation in patients with renal dysfunction.[24] For all benzodiazepines, elimination is impaired with increased patient age.

Benzodiazepines can also produce respiratory depression and exacerbate hemodynamic instability, especially in patients with preexisting respiratory or cardiac disease.[21] Although they are in continued widespread use in the ICU setting, benzodiazepines are known to impair quality of sleep, which can increase the risk for delirium and lead to extended mechanical ventilation time and ICU LOS.[24] While there has been a recent push to curtail ICU reliance on benzodiazepines, practice patterns have yet to comply.[24,39]

Propofol

For sedation of the mechanically ventilated patient, propofol is initially given as a bolus injection of 5 μg/kg IV over 5 minutes followed by an infusion of 5 to 50 μg/kg/min.[23] Propofol crosses the blood–brain barrier with ease, and it is rapidly redistributed into the peripheral tissues, causing it to have a rapid onset and short duration of action. For these reasons, propofol is widely used in the ICU setting, especially for patients that require frequent awakenings for neurologic examinations. In addition, it is useful for performing spontaneous awakening and breathing trials. Note that emergence can be delayed with prolonged propofol infusions once the peripheral tissues have been saturated.

Propofol is a sympatholytic and can lead to hypotension and respiratory depression. Its hemodynamic effects are more pronounced in patients with baseline respiratory insufficiency, cardiovascular instability, or significant hypovolemia. Propofol infusion syndrome (PRIS), although less likely to occur early in a patient's ED or ICU course, is a potentially fatal complication of propofol sedation. The clinical features of PRIS are variable, but can include hypotension and bradycardia, metabolic acidosis, and hypertriglyceridemia.[21] Acute kidney injury, hyperkalemia, rhabdomyolysis, and enlarged or fatty liver are also observed.[40] PRIS occurs more frequently in patients receiving prolonged (>48 hours) propofol infusions at higher doses >75 μg/kg/min and in patients with acute neurologic or inflammatory illnesses.[24,41] When large doses of propofol are used in critically ill patients, it is recommended that serum pH, lactate, creatinine kinase, triglyceride levels, and electrocardiograms (Brugada-type changes) be routinely monitored.[24] If PRIS is suspected, treatment consists of discontinuation of the propofol infusion and provision of supportive care.

Dexmedetomidine

Whereas benzodiazepine and propofol are GABA receptor agonists, dexmedetomidine is an alpha-2 receptor agonist. It exerts its effects primarily on the presynaptic neurons within the locus ceruleus and spinal cord. Patients sedated with dexmedetomidine are easily arousable to the point of being interactive, and there is minimal associated respiratory depression.[21] Unlike propofol and benzodiazepines, dexmedetomidine does not have anticonvulsant properties, but does provide analgesia by an unknown mechanism. The loading dose is 1 μg/kg IV over 10 minutes, and maintenance dose is 0.2 to 0.7 μg/kg/h.[21] Studies have shown safety up to 2 g/kg/h but at the expense of increased risk of bradycardia.[42] Because dexmedetomidine is metabolized in the liver, lower doses may be required in patients with hepatic dysfunction. There is no need for dose adjustment for patients with renal dysfunction.[24]

Bradycardia and hypotension are the most common side effects of dexmedetomidine.[42] However, the bradycardia observed with dexmedetomidine typically does not require intervention.[24] Hypertension may also occur, usually during bolus dosing, via stimulation of the postjunctional alpha-2 receptors located on arterial and venous smooth muscle.[24]

CHOICE OF SEDATION AGENT

The PAD guidelines currently recommend nonbenzodiazepines (propofol and dexmedetomidine) for sedation of mechanically ventilated patients.[21] Based on a recent meta-analysis,[43] propofol appears to decrease ICU LOS and slightly decrease the time spent on the ventilator compared with benzodiazepines, but it does not affect mortality. When compared to midazolam, a shorter-acting benzodiazepine, propofol's benefit in reducing ICU LOS disappears.[43] It is unclear whether propofol decreases the risk of delirium when compared with benzodiazepines.

Several recent studies have compared dexmedetomidine with a variety of other sedative agents in mechanically ventilated patients.[21] The MENDS and SEDCOM studies compared dexmedetomidine with lorazepam and midazolam, respectively, and both studies observed that the dexmedetomidine group was less likely to develop delirium.[44,45] Patients receiving dexmedetomidine were also more likely to be close to target sedation compared with patients receiving lorazepam, but no differences were observed when dexmedetomidine was compared with midazolam in this regard. More importantly, the use of dexmedetomidine may facilitate liberation from the ventilator; in the SEDCOM study, patients receiving dexmedetomidine spent a median of two fewer days on the ventilator compared with the midazolam group.[45] Dexmedetomidine may also have some mortality benefit in septic patients. In a secondary analysis of the MENDS trial, dexmedetomidine was observed to reduce the risk of mortality by 70% in septic patients compared with patients who received lorazepam.[46]

More recently, two multicentered randomized controlled trials compared dexmedetomidine with propofol (PRODEX trial) and midazolam (MIDEX trial).[47]

Time at target arousal was similar between the dexmedetomidine and control (midazolam and propofol) groups.[47] Duration of mechanical ventilation was reduced with dexmedetomidine compared with midazolam; no difference was observed with propofol.[47] In both trials, patients on dexmedetomidine were better able to communicate pain than those sedated with midazolam or propofol.[47]

Additional studies are needed to determine if dexmedetomidine should be routinely used for sedation in mechanically ventilated patients and to determine its performance compared with propofol. While there is a push to decrease use of benzodiazepines as the sedation agent of choice, benzodiazepines will continue to play an important role in patients with status epilepticus, or in patients who are withdrawing from ethanol or benzodiazepines.[21]

INTERRUPTION OF SEDATION

Recently, there has been a paradigm shift in sedation protocols for mechanically ventilated patients, with the goal of reducing duration of mechanical ventilation and patient morbidity. The Awakening and Breathing Controlled (ABC) trial evaluated the efficacy and safety of a "Wake Up and Breathe" protocol that paired management of sedation with ventilation management (Fig. 58.2). This protocol combined spontaneous breathing trials (SBTs), which are standard of care in most intensive care units, with spontaneous awakening trials (SATs), which involve routine interruption of the patient's sedation.

The "Wake Up and Breathe" protocol (SAT + SBT) was compared to the standard of care (SBT alone) in a multicenter randomized control trial that enrolled 336 mechanically ventilated patients.[48] Patients who were randomized to the "Wake Up and Breathe" intervention arm spent more days breathing without assistance and had shorter ICU and hospital LOSs. At 1-year follow-up, patients in the intervention arm were less likely to die (44% vs. 58%); for every seven patients treated with the intervention, one life was saved. More patients in the intervention group self-extubated (10% vs. 4%), but there was no difference in patients requiring reintubation. There is natural concern that the SAT may cause undue psychological stress in the patient. However, studies have demonstrated that routine interruption of sedation not only did not result in adverse psychological outcomes but also produced a reduction in symptoms of posttraumatic stress disorder in this population.[49]

The decision of when to begin SAT and SBT is based on the provider's clinical judgment and the patient's severity of illness. A patient mechanically ventilated because of a drug overdose, for example, will likely begin an SAT + SBT trial earlier than a patient intubated because of a massive traumatic brain injury. As a general rule, ventilator weaning should be initiated within 12 to 24 hours—and in certain circumstances may be initiated in the ED.

CONCLUSION

Sedation is an integral part of ED care of the critically ill patient. For induction of intubation, etomidate has been the medication of choice, but its use is controversial, as a one-time dose causes adrenal suppression and may lead to higher mortality, especially in septic patients. Ketamine is a viable alternative induction agent notable for its minimal impact on a hemodynamic status. Propofol, methohexital, and to a lesser extent midazolam are more likely to cause hypotension, especially in patients who are hypovolemic.

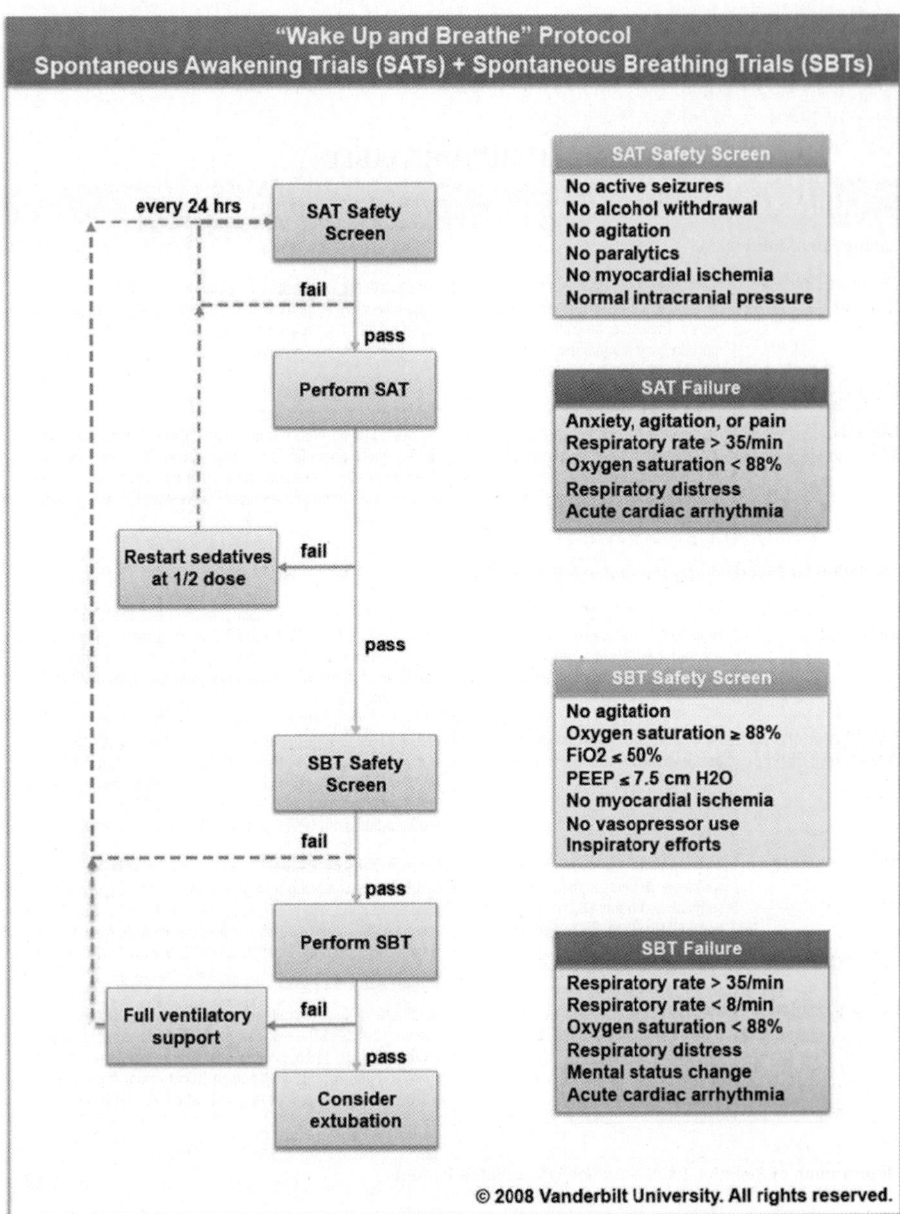

FIGURE 58.2 "Wake Up and Breathe Protocol." SAT, Spontaneous awakening trial; SBT, Spontaneous breathing trial. Courtesy of icudelirium.org. Used with permission.

Once a patient is intubated and on mechanical ventilation, achieving adequate analgesia and sedation is critical to optimizing outcome. For sedation of most patients, propofol and dexmedetomidine should—when available—be used in place of benzodiazepines. If a patient is anticipated to be the ED for more than 12 hours, SAT and SBT trials should be considered, as these can facilitate early extubation and improve mortality.

ACKNOWLEDGMENT

Dr. Han is supported by the National Institutes of Health (K23AG032355).

LITERATURE TABLE

TRIAL	DESIGN	RESULT
Induction of Intubation		
Chan et al., *Crit Care Med.* 2012[8]	Meta-analysis of 5 studies that enrolled 896 critically patients with sepsis. They compared all-cause mortality and adrenal insufficiency in patients who received etomidate with other induction agents	Septic patients who received etomidate for induction of intubation were more likely to die (pooled relative risk 1.20, 95% CI: 1.02–1.42) and were more likely to develop adrenal insufficiency (pooled relative risk 1.33, 95% CI: 1.22–1.46)
Jabre et al., *Lancet.* 2009[10]	Multicenter RCT of 469 septic and nonseptic patients who were randomized to receive either etomidate or ketamine for the induction of intubation	There was no difference in Sequential Organ Failure Assessment scores, which quantifies organ dysfunction. There was also no difference in 28-d mortality, duration of mechanical ventilation, and ICU LOS. Intubating conditions were not different between the two groups
Sedation for Mechanically Ventilated Patients		
SEDCOM Study Group, *JAMA.* 2009[47]	Multicenter RCT of 366 mechanically ventilated patients in medical and surgical ICUs comparing dexmedetomidine and midazolam	Patients receiving dexmedetomidine were less likely to be delirious (54% vs. 77%, $p < 0.001$) and had shorter times to extubation (median 3.7 vs. 5.6 d, $p = 0.01$). No statistically significant differences in time spent at target sedation, ICU LOS, or mortality
Pandharipande et al., *Crit Care Med.* 2010[48]	Multicenter RCT of 103 mechanically ventilated patients in medical and surgical ICUs comparing dexmedetomidine and lorazepam	Patients receiving dexmedetomidine spent less time delirious or comatose than those receiving lorazepam (median 7 d vs. 3 d, $p = 0.01$). Patients on dexmedetomidine spent more time at target sedation. Dexmedetomidine improved 28-d mortality in septic patients only (HR 0.3, 95%CI: 0.1–0.9)
Jakob et al., *JAMA.* 2012[49] MIDEX	Multicenter RCT of 300 mechanically ventilated patients in medical, surgical, and trauma ICUs comparing dexmedetomidine and midazolam	Duration of mechanical ventilation was shorter in the dexmedetomidine group compared with the midazolam group (median 123 h vs. 164 h, $p = 0.03$). Dexmedetomidine also improved the patient's ability to communicate pain. No difference in time spent at target sedation, ICU LOS, hospital LOS, or mortality were observed
Jakob et al., *JAMA.* 2012[49] PRODEX	Multicenter RCT of 298 mechanically ventilated patients in medical, surgical, and trauma ICUs comparing dexmedetomidine and propofol	No difference in time spent on mechanical ventilation was observed between the dexmedetomidine and propofol groups (median 97 h vs. 118 h, p-value = 0.24). The dexmedetomidine group had improved ability to communicate pain. There was no difference in time spent at target sedation, ICU LOS, hospital LOS, and mortality
Interruption of Sedation for Mechanically Ventilated Patients		
Girard et al., *Lancet.* 2008[50] ABC	Multicenter RCT that enrolled 336 patients and compared SAT (daily interruption of sedation) + SBT with SBT alone	The SAT + SBT group had more ventilator-free days (mean difference 3.1 d, p-value = 0.02), shorter ICU LOS (9.1 d vs. 12.9 d, $p = 0.03$), and hospital LOS (14.9 d vs. 19.2 d, $p = 0.04$). Patients in the SAT + SBT group also had lower 1-y mortality rates (44% vs. 58%, $p = 0.01$). There was no difference in reintubation rates

RCT, randomized control trial; CI, confidence interval; HR, hazard ratio; LOS, length of stay.

REFERENCES

1. Forman SA. Clinical and molecular pharmacology of etomidate. *Anesthesiology.* 2011;114:695–707.
2. Mace SE. Challenges and advances in intubation: rapid sequence intubation. *Emerg Med Clin North Am.* 2008;26:1043–1068, x.
3. Bergen JM, Smith DC. A review of etomidate for rapid sequence intubation in the emergency department. *J Emerg Med.* 1997;15:221–230.
4. Zed PJ, Abu-Laban RB, Harrison DW. Intubating conditions and hemodynamic effects of etomidate for rapid sequence intubation in the emergency department: an observational cohort study. *Acad Emerg Med.* 2006;13:378–383.
5. Vinclair M, Broux C, Faure P, et al. Duration of adrenal inhibition following a single dose of etomidate in critically ill patients. *Intensive Care Med.* 2008;34:714–719.
6. Chan CM, Mitchell AL, Shorr AF. Etomidate is associated with mortality and adrenal insufficiency in sepsis: a meta-analysis*. *Crit Care Med.* 2012;40:2945–2953.
7. Tekwani KL, Watts HF, Sweis RT, et al. A comparison of the effects of etomidate and midazolam on hospital length of stay in patients with suspected sepsis: a prospective, randomized study. *Ann Emerg Med.* 2010;56:481–489.
8. Jabre P, Combes X, Lapostolle F, et al. Etomidate versus ketamine for rapid sequence intubation in acutely ill patients: a multicentre randomised controlled trial. *Lancet.* 2009;374:293–300.
9. McPhee LC, Badawi O, Fraser GL, et al. Single-dose etomidate is not associated with increased mortality in ICU patients with sepsis: analysis of a large electronic ICU database. *Crit Care Med.* 2013;41(3):774–783.
10. Warner KJ, Cuschieri J, Jurkovich GJ, et al. Single-dose etomidate for rapid sequence intubation may impact outcome after severe injury. *J Trauma.* 2009;67:45–50.
11. Hildreth AN, Mejia VA, Maxwell RA, et al. Adrenal suppression following a single dose of etomidate for rapid sequence induction: a prospective randomized study. *J Trauma.* 2008;65:573–579.
12. Bloomfield R, Noble D. Etomidate and intensive care physicians. *Intensive Care Med.* 2005;31:1453; author reply 1454.
13. Annane D, Sebille V, Charpentier C, et al. Effect of treatment with low doses of hydrocortisone and fludrocortisone on mortality in patients with septic shock. *JAMA.* 2002;288:862–871.
14. Annane D. Etomidate and intensive care physicians. *Intensive Care Med.* 2005;31:1454.
15. Payen JF, Dupuis C, Trouve-Buisson T, et al. Corticosteroid after etomidate in critically ill patients: a randomized controlled trial. *Crit Care Med.* 2012;40:29–35.
16. Cuthbertson BH, Sprung CL, Annane D, et al. The effects of etomidate on adrenal responsiveness and mortality in patients with septic shock. *Intensive Care Med.* 2009;35:1868–1876.
17. Gelissen HP, Epema AH, Henning RH, et al. Inotropic effects of propofol, thiopental, midazolam, etomidate, and ketamine on isolated human atrial muscle. *Anesthesiology.* 1996;84:397–403.
18. Tweed WA, Minuck M, Mymin D. Circulatory responses to ketamine anesthesia. *Anesthesiology.* 1972;37:613–619.
19. Filanovsky Y, Miller P, Kao J. Myth: ketamine should not be used as an induction agent for intubation in patients with head injury. *CJEM.* 2010;12:154–157.
20. James MF, Hift RJ. Porphyrias. *Br J Anaesth.* 2000;85:143–153.
21. Barr J, Fraser GL, Puntillo K, et al. Clinical practice guidelines for the management of pain, agitation, and delirium in adult patients in the intensive care unit. *Crit Care Med.* 2013;41:278–280.
22. Gauss A, Heinrich H, Wilder-Smith OH. Echocardiographic assessment of the haemodynamic effects of propofol: a comparison with etomidate and thiopentone. *Anaesthesia.* 1991;46:99–105.
23. Sivilotti ML, Filbin MR, Murray HE, et al. Does the sedative agent facilitate emergency rapid sequence intubation? *Acad Emerg Med.* 2003;10:612–620.
24. Hughes CG, McGrane S, Pandharipande PP. Sedation in the intensive care setting. *Clin Pharmacol.* 2012;4:53–63.
25. Girard TD, Jackson JC, Pandharipande PP, et al. Delirium as a predictor of long-term cognitive impairment in survivors of critical illness. *Crit Care Med.* 2010;38:1513–1520.
26. Ely EW, Shintani A, Truman B, et al. Delirium as a predictor of mortality in mechanically ventilated patients in the intensive care unit. *JAMA.* 2004;291:1753–1762.
27. Agarwal V, O'Neill PJ, Cotton BA, et al. Prevalence and risk factors for development of delirium in burn intensive care unit patients. *J Burn Care Res.* 2010;31:706–715.
28. Payen JF, Bru O, Bosson JL, et al. Assessing pain in critically ill sedated patients by using a behavioral pain scale. *Crit Care Med.* 2001;29:2258–2263.
29. Gelinas C, Fillion L, Puntillo KA, et al. Validation of the critical-care pain observation tool in adult patients. *Am J Crit Care.* 2006;15:420–427.

30. Marcantonio ER, Juarez G, Goldman L, et al. The relationship of postoperative delirium with psychoactive medications. *JAMA.* 1994;272:1518–1522.
31. Armstrong PJ, Bersten A. Normeperidine toxicity. *Anesth Analg.* 1986;65:536–538.
32. Dubois MJ, Bergeron N, Dumont M, et al. Delirium in an intensive care unit: a study of risk factors. *Intensive Care Med.* 2001;27:1297–1304.
33. Morrison RS, Magaziner J, Gilbert M, et al. Relationship between pain and opioid analgesics on the development of delirium following hip fracture. *J Gerontol A Biol Sci Med Sci.* 2003;58:M76–M81.
34. Sessler CN, Gosnell MS, Grap MJ, et al. The richmond agitation-sedation scale: validity and reliability in adult intensive care unit patients. *Am J Respir Crit Care Med.* 2002;166:1338–1344.
35. Riker RR, Picard JT, Fraser GL. Prospective evaluation of the Sedation-Agitation Scale for adult critically ill patients. *Crit Care Med.* 1999;27:1325–1329.
36. Shehabi Y, Bellomo R, Reade MC, et al. Early intensive care sedation predicts long-term mortality in ventilated critically ill patients. *Am J Respir Crit Care Med.* 2012;186:724–731.
37. Ely EW, Inouye SK, Bernard GR, et al. Delirium in mechanically ventilated patients: validity and reliability of the confusion assessment method for the intensive care unit (CAM-ICU). *JAMA.* 2001;286:2703–2710.
38. Bergeron N, Dubois MJ, Dumont M, et al. Intensive care delirium screening checklist: evaluation of a new screening tool. *Intensive Care Med.* 2001;27:859–864.
39. Skrobik Y. Counterpoint: should benzodiazepines be avoided in mechanically ventilated patients? No. *Chest.* 2012;142:284–287; discussion 287–289.
40. Kam PC, Cardone D. Propofol infusion syndrome. *Anaesthesia.* 2007;62:690–701.
41. Vasile B, Rasulo F, Candiani A, et al. The pathophysiology of propofol infusion syndrome: a simple name for a complex syndrome. *Intensive Care Med.* 2003;29:1417–1425.
42. Tan JA, Ho KM. Use of dexmedetomidine as a sedative and analgesic agent in critically ill adult patients: a meta-analysis. *Intensive Care Med.* 2010;36:926–939.
43. Ho KM, Ng JY. The use of propofol for medium and long-term sedation in critically ill adult patients: a meta-analysis. *Intensive Care Med.* 2008;34:1969–1979.
44. Pandharipande PP, Pun BT, Herr DL, et al. Effect of sedation with dexmedetomidine vs lorazepam on acute brain dysfunction in mechanically ventilated patients: the MENDS randomized controlled trial. *JAMA.* 2007;298:2644–2653.
45. Riker RR, Shehabi Y, Bokesch PM, et al. Dexmedetomidine vs midazolam for sedation of critically ill patients: a randomized trial. *JAMA.* 2009;301:489–499.
46. Pandharipande PP, Sanders RD, Girard TD, et al. Effect of dexmedetomidine versus lorazepam on outcome in patients with sepsis: an a priori-designed analysis of the MENDS randomized controlled trial. *Crit Care.* 2010;14:R38.
47. Jakob SM, Ruokonen E, Grounds RM, et al. Dexmedetomidine vs midazolam or propofol for sedation during prolonged mechanical ventilation: two randomized controlled trials. *JAMA.* 2012;307:1151–1160.
48. Girard TD, Kress JP, Fuchs BD, et al. Efficacy and safety of a paired sedation and ventilator weaning protocol for mechanically ventilated patients in intensive care (Awakening and Breathing Controlled trial): a randomised controlled trial. *Lancet.* 2008;371:126–134.
49. Kress JP, Gehlbach B, Lacy M, et al. The long-term psychological effects of daily sedative interruption on critically ill patients. *Am J Respir Crit Care Med.* 2003;168:1457–1461.

SECTION 14
Geriatrics and Palliative Care

59

The Geriatric Patient

Mary R. Mulcare, Alexis Halpern, and Michael E. Stern

BACKGROUND

Geriatric patients, or "older adults," are defined chronologically as 65 years and older. They represent a growing percentage not only of our adult patient population but also of those requiring critical care–level interventions within the emergency department (ED). Between 2000 and 2010, the population 65 years and older increased at a faster rate (15.1% over a 10-year period) than the U.S. population as a whole (9.7% over a 10-year period) and currently represents over 13% of the total U.S. population. There was a concomitant increase in persons 85 years and older by a remarkable 29.6% over the same time frame. The older adult population is expected to double to more than 70 million by 2030.[1] A recent retrospective cohort study in the United States showed that older adult patients represent 45.7% of the total intensive care unit (ICU) population (with 10.35% of all patients being over 85 years old).[2] An analysis of over 120,000 ICU patients in Australia and New Zealand demonstrated that 13% of ICU admissions were for patients over 80 years old, with an annual increase in ICU admission in this population of 5.6% per year.[3]

The baseline health and functioning of older adults is improving, as advances in education have yielded changes in lifestyle with respect to diet, exercise, and preventative care. In addition, improvements in pharmacotherapy and health-related technology are enabling this population to live longer and better. With better resources and more effective goal-directed therapy, our ability to resuscitate and care for very sick older adults has also greatly improved, as have clinical outcomes in this population.[4] Age alone, therefore, should no longer be the deciding factor when formulating plans of care for critically ill geriatric patients. Rather, it should be a combination of the severity of the acute medical issue, the biologic and physiologic state of the patient, and the patient's wishes.

GENERAL APPROACH TO THE OLDER ADULTS

The reality of aging is that all persons experience approximately a 1% per year decline in physiologic functioning after age 30.[5,6] However, everyone starts at a different baseline. There are two ways to quantify age: biologic age (physiologic age), often associated with frailty, poor biologic reserve, or impairment of several biologic systems,[4] and chronologic age.[7] The literature differs over whether advanced age should be considered an independent risk factor for mortality,[2,3,8] but several authors have emphasized that advanced age alone does not preclude a successful ICU outcome.[9–12] Aspects of particular importance in surviving critical illness that may be independent of chronologic age include overall physiologic reserve, organ structure and function (e.g., cardiac or renal), pulmonary compliance and vital capacity, and changes in volume of distribution that occur with changes in body composition. Each of these is discussed further in the sections below.

The emergency physician should be cognizant of the following common themes in the management of older adults.

1. *Polypharmacy* is widely prevalent and represents a serious hazard to this population. The decreased functional reserve of major organ systems increases the risk of decompensation in response to certain medications, particularly those affecting the cardiovascular and renal system. Drugs with hepatic clearance, such as diazepam, can also cause significant harm. When considering medical therapy, the mantra "start low and go slow" is well advised in the geriatric population.[13]
2. *Atypical presentations* are the rule, not the exception, in medical, surgical, and trauma patients. While this text does not focus on trauma, clinicians should maintain a high index of suspicion for severe traumatic injuries with even the most minor of mechanisms, such as a fall from standing height. Geriatric patients are more susceptible to intracranial hemorrhage, fractures, and their associated complications, with increased risk for bleeding diatheses given the prevalence of anticoagulant and antiplatelet use. Among patients older than 85 years, trauma is the second most common cause for ICU admission following cardiovascular diagnoses.[2]

With these caveats in mind, the following sections review acute presentations in older adults that require special consideration.

SEPSIS

Severe sepsis continues to carry a high mortality rate despite advances in early detection and goal-directed therapy.[14] Older adults have decreased physiologic reserve, undergo immune system senescence, and are more likely to have multiple comorbidities. It follows that the incidence of sepsis is higher in older adults and that age is an independent predictor of mortality. Older adults have a relative risk of sepsis of 13.1 compared with younger patients.[15] The mortality rate for patients >65 years is 27.7% and close to 40% for those over 85 years.[15] Pneumonia is the most common culprit for infection, followed by urinary tract infections and then bacteremia.[15] Thus, the workup for these patients should always include a chest radiograph, urinalysis, urine culture, and blood cultures; this is true even if a fever is not documented, since a blunted or absent fever response is common in older patients.

As with all patients, early antibiotic coverage is essential, with mortality increasing each hour treatment is delayed.[16] This population is also more susceptible to drug-resistant organisms, as their tendency toward infection leads to frequent antibiotic use, both as outpatients and as inpatients.[17] The following are important considerations when choosing an appropriate antibiotic regimen:

1. Is the patient coming from a nursing home or rehabilitation center?
2. What infections has the patient previously had, and what were the sensitivities on prior cultures?
3. Based on the presentation and exam, what is the most likely source of the infection? (Remember: these patients present atypically)
4. What are the local/regional resistance patterns, including those at the local nursing homes and neighboring communities?

In the absence of specific microbial data indicating a history of resistant organisms, the initial antibiotic regimen should be broad spectrum and then narrowed once further clinical data and culture sensitivities are obtained.

Early goal-directed therapy (EGDT) and aggressive fluid resuscitation have become a mainstay of sepsis therapy.[18] The mean age of the 263 patients included in the EGDT study was 65.7 years (SD 17.2); however, there was no subgroup analysis performed on those patients 65 years and older. To our knowledge, there have been no further studies that specifically explore the use of EGDT in this population. Thus, older adults should receive aggressive fluid resuscitation (a minimum of 30 mL/kg)[19] when indicated based on sepsis markers. As this population has a higher rate of heart failure and, therefore, has difficulty managing fluid balance, the clinician should perform frequent patient reassessments during fluid infusion, paying particular attention to respiratory status.

The use of vasopressors in the older adult population has not been extensively studied. Important factors to consider when deciding to initiate vasopressor support include this group's increased incidence of heart failure and potential need for inotropic support. Confounding this picture is that one-third of heart failure in older patients is primarily diastolic, resulting from impaired ventricular relaxation. These patients are particularly dependent on late diastolic filling in order to maintain adequate preload. As this late-phase filling is provided by atrial contraction, adequate rate control is essential in order to avoid pulmonary congestion. Rate control in a tachycardic patient, however, should not be initiated until initial, yet judicious fluid resuscitation has occurred, as an elevated heart rate is often a necessary compensatory mechanism. When choosing a rate-controlling agent, it is important to remember that as one ages, cardiac output declines and the heart increasingly relies on endogenous catecholamines for inotropic support. Because of this, beta-blocker agents can place older adult patients at greater risk of acute pulmonary edema, and many emergency physicians are therefore more comfortable using calcium channel blockers as the initial rate-controlling agent.

The use of corticosteroids has also not been specifically studied in the older adult population. Studies supporting the use of steroids, including the CORTICUS trial,[20] had a mean patient age of 60.8 years, with 79% of the patients younger than 75, making it difficult to generalize findings to the older adult population.[14]

Abdominal pain is a common presenting complaint in the older adult population. As with other illness, significant abdominal pathology in older adults frequently presents atypically, often without localizing signs on exam and therefore requires comprehensive evaluation with advanced imaging. Of older adults presenting with abdominal pain to the ED, approximately 60% will be admitted, and close to 20% will require invasive procedures or surgery. Approximately 14% of patients with abdominal pain discharged home from the ED, as well as 9% of those discharged from inpatient admissions for abdominal pain, will return to the ED within 2 weeks of the index visit, with a nearly 5% mortality rate if admitted or readmitted to the hospital.[21] Moreover, patients aged 75 years and older are less likely to have an ED diagnosis that is concordant with the final diagnosis than patients who are younger (76% vs. 87%).[21] It is important to remember that diseases such as appendicitis and cholecystitis have a bimodal distribution, with a significant percentage occurring in older adults (14% and 12% to 41%, respectively).[22–24]

CARDIAC DYSFUNCTION

With advanced age, the heart undergoes structural changes—including left ventricular (LV) wall thickening, left atrial and LV cavity dilation, and coronary artery wall thickening—that together result in decreased LV relaxation and diminished functional cardiac reserve. As a result of these changes, the older adult patient typically will have a higher resting systolic blood pressure, decreased intrinsic sinus rate, and increased sympathetic activity but with decreased response to beta-adrenergic stimulation. On electrocardiogram, clinicians will most often find nonspecific ST or T wave changes, decreased QRS voltage, increased ectopic beats, lengthening of the intervals, and bundle branch blocks.

With our aging population, patients admitted to the ICU more frequently demonstrate evidence of these changes in cardiac function, including an increased incidence of heart failure, cardiac arrhythmia, and valvular heart disease. The aging population, conversely, confers a reduced prevalence of diabetic complications, alcohol abuse, chronic obstructive pulmonary disease (COPD), and liver failure.[2] A retrospective cohort study of 1,409 patients confirmed that cardiac patients are the most common ICU admission group in patients >65 years (67.7%), with acute coronary syndrome (ACS) being the most frequent diagnosis (76.7%).[4] A separate study showed that having a cardiac diagnosis on admission correlates significantly with an increased mortality risk.[8]

HEART FAILURE

Congestive heart failure (CHF) is the most common principal diagnosis among all hospital admissions in older adults. In 2009, CHF accounted for 149 hospital stays per 10,000 population among all adults aged 65 to 84 years and for 433 stays per 10,000 population among all adults aged 85 years and older.[25] As an individual ages, the decreased elasticity of the great vessels leads to increased afterload, causing LV hypertrophy, increased coronary artery oxygen consumption, and possible ischemia. Increased afterload is compounded by chronically impaired renal flow, which leads to afferent vasoconstriction and increased fluid retention, exacerbating already compromised cardiac function.[26]

Of note, a CHF patient's ejection fraction, a value often ascertained in the ED through chart review or bedside echocardiography, is frequently normal or even increased. It has been shown that as many as 30% to 50% of heart failure patients have circulatory congestion on the basis of diastolic dysfunction, with impaired ventricular relaxation causing higher LV filling pressures and reduced left ventricular end diastolic pressure (LVEDP).[27,28] This diastolic failure often requires a clinical approach that focuses on afterload reduction while remaining cognizant of the risk of overdiuresis, as is discussed below.

Because CHF is primarily a clinical diagnosis, pertinent findings on a physical exam, including lower extremity edema and crackles in the lung bases, are important to identify. Depending on the degree of heart failure, the patient will present with varying levels of dyspnea, fatigue, and/or orthopnea. In the setting of severe hypoxia, an older adult patient may also present with atypical symptoms including somnolence, confusion, and failure to thrive.

The causes of exacerbations of heart failure in older adults are myriad. Medication and dietary nonadherence are most common, followed by arrhythmias, cardiac ischemia, renal failure, pulmonary embolisms, uncontrolled hypertension, adverse effects of medications, and infection.[26] The key to management beyond the initial presentation is identifying the underlying precipitant. B-type natriuretic peptide (BNP) is a common marker for CHF (90% sensitive, 76% specific); however, plasma BNP levels have been shown to increase with age independent of ejection fraction, decreasing specificity.[29] Other important diagnostic laboratory values include hemoglobin (anemia is an independent prognostic factor in elderly), electrolytes (in particular, hypokalemia from diuretic use), and troponin, which, along with an ECG, is needed to exclude ischemia as a precipitating cause. Chest radiograph and echocardiography can help confirm the diagnosis.

All patients presenting in acute pulmonary edema require immediate intervention. Following assessment and stabilization of the ABCs, first-line therapy includes supplemental oxygen and nitrates. However, when initiating medical therapy for CHF in an older adult, the emergency physician must proceed with an appreciation of the cardiovascular changes that can occur with age. For example, extra care must be taken in patients with severe aortic stenosis (AS), as nitrates can cause an acute and severe drop in blood pressure. It is also imperative to ask patients if they recently have taken Viagra or any other phosphodiesterase type-5 inhibitor, as this combination may also result in rapid hypotension. Intravenous ACE inhibitor (enalaprilat) is an alternative option if nitrates are contraindicated but is used more commonly in chronic management.[30] Diuretics are also effective in the setting of frank volume overload; however, care must be taken not to over diurese and potentially compromise perfusion. Fortunately, in most cases of decompensated heart failure, it is the accompanying sympathetic surge—not a sudden volume overload—that is the primary cause of pulmonary decompensation. Equally challenging are patients with diastolic heart failure who are preload dependent and thus require higher filling pressures due to a stiff LV. As such, if not carefully managed, these patients—following aggressive nitrate and diuretic therapy—can decompensate due to a lack of forward flow. Noninvasive positive pressure ventilation (NIPPV) reduces intubation rates in this population and is discussed further in the next section.

ACS complicated by cardiogenic shock occurs in 5% to 7% of all adult patients with an associated mortality rate >50%.[31] The mortality rate is higher for elderly patients with ACS than for younger patients; however, percutaneous coronary intervention (PCI) appears to provide better long-term survival and quality of life (defined by return to good functional status) for older adults receiving the therapy than for those who do not.[32] For geriatric patients presenting in cardiogenic shock, inotropic assistance may be needed. Dobutamine (beta-1 agonist) and milrinone (phosphodiesterase inhibitor) are the drugs of choice. While emergency physicians have been traditionally more comfortable using dobutamine in the ED setting, it carries a greater risk of ventricular ectopy and tachycardia when compared to phosphodiesterase inhibitors.[33]

CARDIAC ARRHYTHMIAS

Admission to hospitals for cardiac arrhythmias increased by 25% in adults aged 85 years old and above between 1997 and 2009.[25] As people age, there is a stretching and fatiguing of the conduction system, which leads to ectopic beats and altered paths of depolarization. These patients present with a range of symptoms and degree of hemodynamic compromise, which dictates how quickly the emergency physician must act and which strategies are most appropriate. Management beyond the initial resuscitation—which focuses on identifying the underlying etiology of the arrhythmia—requires an appreciation of cardiac and vascular changes that occur in the aging population.

Atrial fibrillation (AF) is the most common sustained arrhythmia in older adults, with a prevalence of 5% and an incidence that doubles with each decade of life.[34] AF leads to 20% of all stroke-related deaths.[35] Acute management of AF with rapid ventricular rate is dictated by the patient's hemodynamic state. If the patient is hypotensive or unstable, immediate cardioversion is required and safe in the elderly, with similar success and complication rates to that of the younger population.[36] Cardioversion for those patients with stable, new-onset AF can also be effective (see Chapter 17).

If the patient is symptomatic and normotensive, rate-controlling agents should be utilized along with anticoagulation. Given the prevalence of heart failure as previously discussed, the emergency physician should presume an abnormal EF if no information is known. Emergency physicians will often use diltiazem, which is a good choice in older adults as it can be titrated with small boluses followed by a drip, allowing for close monitoring of potential hemodynamic compromise. Based on experience with this population, consensus recommendation is to start with 10 mg IV diltiazem and titrate, rather than the recommended 0.25 mg/kg. Amiodarone is the preferred drug in known impaired cardiac function as it causes less hypotension[37]; however, it is harder to titrate. Digoxin is another option for rate control, but its onset of action is significantly delayed and thus not ideal for use in the ED setting. In patients with known normal EF, beta-blockers and verapamil may also be considered. However, verapamil can have altered pharmacokinetics in the elderly due to reliance on hepatic metabolism[38] and therefore should be used cautiously.

If a patient with rapid AF is asymptomatic, the emergency physician has time to investigate the etiology, such as noncompliance with home medications or any of the myriad pathologic causes/triggers of AF. Slowing a patient in AF too quickly may be ill advised if the patient's rate is an appropriate response to an underlying condition such as dehydration, fever, or infection. Administration of intravenous fluids, antibiotics, and antipyretics may lower the heart rate while treating the inciting cause.

Given the prevalence of conduction disease in older adults, sick sinus syndrome and complete heart block are more common in this population and should be considered in any patient with cardiac instability. A 12-lead electrocardiogram is essential for any patient with arrhythmia or derangement in vital signs.

OTHER CARDIAC CONSIDERATIONS

Aortic Stenosis

AS affects nearly 10% of patients over 80 years and is the third most common cause of cardiac death.[39] Symptomatic AS, which often presents in the setting of ACS, acute decompensated heart failure, or syncope, requires treatment that provides necessary afterload reduction while maintaining adequate preload. Nitrates and diuretics should be used judiciously. Aortic valvuloplasty or replacement (AVR) is the definitive treatment for severe AS. Recent studies have shown favorable survival in patients >80 years of age (>50% surviving 6 years) after AVR, with concomitant coronary artery bypass grafting not changing the mean survival rates.[39,40]

Acute Coronary Syndrome

ACS is common in this age group, and older adults with an acute myocardial infarction have a higher mortality risk. Atypical presentations of ACS are commonplace in older adults; over 50% of this population's myocardial infarctions will present without chest pain, or "silent."[41] The differences between men and women in presentation and mortality attenuate with increasing age. There are significant data now showing that fibrinolysis, PCI, and CABG should be considered in even the very old.[31,40,42–44]

RESPIRATORY DISTRESS

The management of respiratory failure in older adults is multifaceted and requires consideration of patient acuity, resource utilization, and the degree of invasiveness of potential interventions. The decision to implement mechanical ventilation can be complex, especially in very chronologically old patients.[45] Studies suggest that age is an independent risk factor for mortality in the setting of mechanical ventilation.[46,47] However, evidence regarding the role of pulmonary physiology—independent of age—is more compelling.

Age-related changes in pulmonary physiology result in a decline in overall patient functioning.[48] Decreased lung compliance and stiffening of costovertebral joint articulations and associated muscles, including the diaphragm, lead to increased risk of complications from mechanical ventilation. There is an increased propensity toward distal airway collapse, with a subsequent decrease in lung surface area, gas exchange, and lung capacity. Reduced peripheral carbon dioxide sensitivity decreases the hypoxic drive and ventilatory response, often most pronounced during sleep. Because of these physiologic impairments, older adults are more likely to develop chronic respiratory failure when recovering from an acute pulmonary illness.

An ARDS network subgroup analysis showed that patients older than 70 years who require endotracheal intubation and mechanical ventilation have an equally effective response to low tidal volume ventilation, despite increased mortality.[49] Further data are needed to determine appropriate ventilatory strategies in older adults, given their higher rates of COPD and primary lung conditions.[14]

NIPPV has an important role in treating mild to moderate respiratory distress in older adults.[48,50] In both younger and older patients, NIPPV is associated with overall less discomfort, fewer complications, and better short-term results than endotracheal ventilation for specific disease processes, described below. NIPPV promotes muscle rest and improves gas exchange by increasing alveolar recruitment and lung volume. The ability of the patient to protect his or her airway is always a concern with NIPPV, especially in older adults with comorbid conditions. Dementia alone should not preclude the use of NIPPV; agitated delirium, however, may limit its use.[51]

NIPPV can be helpful in the management of the following illnesses:

- *Acute exacerbation of COPD*: The success rate of NIPPV in the older adult population is similar to that in the general population.[52] A positive response to NIPPV is defined by improved acidosis, a lower respiratory rate, and decreased hypercapnia, all within 1 to 2 hours (with a maximum response period of up to 4 hours) before additional ventilatory support is needed.[51,52]
- *Acute cardiogenic pulmonary edema*: NIPPV (CPAP in particular) has been shown to improve gas exchange, normalize hemodynamics, and decrease rates of intubation.[53] It should be used with caution in patients with active cardiac ischemic or acute myocardial infarction, as it can increase oxygen demand by coronary arteries, worsening ischemia.[48,54]
- *Pneumonia* (leading infectious cause of death in this age group): NIPPV use is controversial. Limited data suggest NIPPV may be helpful in patients with underlying COPD.[48]
- *End-of-life scenarios*: Consider NIPPV, as it can serve as a palliative measure.

Based on findings from the studies above, if no significant improvement is achieved within 2 hours of NIPPV, endotracheal intubation and ventilation should to be considered in older adults, especially if a reversible condition is causing acute respiratory failure.[51]

DELIRIUM AND AGITATION

Delirium, or an acute change in mental status not caused by underlying dementia, is an often underappreciated consequence of both critical illness and the hospital environment.[55] It is an emergency unto itself, with an in-hospital mortality rate mirroring that of sepsis or acute myocardial infarction.[56] The older adult population is especially at risk of delirium and can present with either a hypoactive (i.e., somnolent, lethargic, stuporous, etc.) or hyperactive (i.e., agitated, etc.) state (discussed in detail below).[57]

Identifying delirium is the first challenge for the emergency physician, especially when the patient's degree of underlying cognitive impairment is unknown. The Confusion Assessment Method (CAM)[58] is the most commonly used tool in critical care settings[59] and is the only validated tool for the ED (86% sensitivity, 100% specificity).[60] The CAM evaluates four elements: (1) acute onset and fluctuating course, (2) inattention, (3) disorganized thinking, and (4) altered level of consciousness. A patient must demonstrate elements 1 and 2 as well as either 3 or 4 to be considered "delirious."[58] The CAM-ICU scale has the potential to be even more applicable in the ED, once validated.[57]

Older adults experience physiologic changes that alter both pharmacokinetics and pharmacodynamics, predisposing them to delirium. Changes in drug distribution (pharmacokinetics) occur due to relatively higher fat stores as compared to lean muscle mass. This increases the absorption of lipophilic drugs and imparts a longer half-life (e.g., propofol, diazepam, midazolam). The lower percentage of muscle mass in an older adult's body decreases the absorption of hydrophilic drugs (e.g., digoxin, theophylline), thereby lowering their effective half-life but raising their peak plasma concentrations and therefore toxicity risk.[38] Older adults are also more likely to have decreased gastrointestinal first-pass metabolism, hepatic metabolism and clearance, and renal clearance. Acute renal failure is also more common in the elderly population,[14] and multiple commonly prescribed drugs—including digoxin, enoxaparin, dabigatran, metformin, lithium, and Parkinson medications such as amantadine—may cause toxicity in this clinical setting. Finally, aging also effects neurohormonal receptors, especially adrenergic receptors, which can alter a drug's effects on the body (pharmacodynamics); however, inadequate evidence exists to provide specific recommendations regarding this process.[14] Medication dosing decisions should take into account the pharmacokinetics and pharmacodynamics of each drug as well as the patient's underlying physiologic functioning.

Delirium has three clinical subtypes: hyperactive, hypoactive, or mixed type. Hyperactive (or agitated) delirium can make evaluation of the underlying precipitant challenging for the emergency physician. Once a patient has been identified as delirious, the next step is the evaluation of the delirium precipitant. Certain causes are often overlooked, yet are more readily reversible than the traditionally considered life-threatening causes, such as infection, stroke, MI, hypoglycemia, and underlying cognitive impairment. These less frequently considered causes include inadequate pain control, urinary retention, constipation, dehydration, polypharmacy, and environmental precipitants in the patient's immediate surrounding.[57]

Delirium can be managed with both nonpharmacologic (preferred) and pharmacologic interventions, although the literature reveals no current standard of practice. Nonpharmacologic strategies include decreasing sensory stimulation, keeping family (or familiar faces) at the bedside or utilizing one to one observation, and choosing a calmer and quieter location for the patient, preferentially by a window, to maintain orientation. Pharmacologic interventions should be reserved for emergencies; in other words, when patient or provider safety is of concern, or if the patient's agitation is impeding the necessary medical care. Benzodiazepines should be avoided, especially as monotherapy, as they may worsen delirium (discussed in detail in Chapter 56). If necessary for minimal sedation, lorazepam is preferred over diazepam because of how they are metabolized in the liver. Haloperidol, a typical antipsychotic, has been the traditional drug of choice in the treatment of delirium, with a prolonged QT interval being the only significant contraindication. Currently, however, the atypical antipsychotics, such as olanzapine, quetiapine, and risperidone, are increasingly used in the management of delirium. Each of these antipsychotic options, however, has limitations, and familiarity with their side effect/safety profiles is necessary. Despite several studies involving atypical antipsychotics, there is no clear evidence to date on the efficacy and safety profile of these drugs for use in managing agitated delirium in the elderly.

CONCLUSION

Admissions to the hospital in general, and ICUs in particular, are increasing more rapidly than our resources can sustain. More than any other demographic, the older adult population is contributing to this complex problem.[3] ICU triage is known to be a subjective process, and literature demonstrates age-discriminatory practices, especially when resources are scarce.[61,62] These age-biased practices are supported by studies showing that patients over 80 years of age have lower short-term survival rates, modified by prehospital function, comorbid illness, surgical status, primary diagnosis, and illness severity. Survivors in this age group are more likely to go to rehab or long-term care facilities.[3]

After correcting for disease severity, however, elderly patients have the greatest mortality benefit when receiving ICU-level care. The older adult patients who are deemed "too well" for the ICU and diverted to lower levels of care suffer the greatest loss. Limited physiologic reserve increases their vulnerability to disease processes. Receiving care in a setting that makes early recognition of decompensation possible has a marked effect on their clinical outcomes.[63] Emergency physicians should advocate for older patients to be triaged to the ICU whenever warranted. Until we have a more reliable way to predict prognosis, these patients need to be treated aggressively, unless their wishes are otherwise.

While the ED will continue to send critically ill older adults to the ICU, the emergency physician can also work to help avert many of the conditions that lead to these admissions. Preventable illnesses such as falls and gastrointestinal bleeds are a source of many ICU admissions in the elderly, especially in individuals over 80 years of age and with the advent of novel anticoagulants. Emergency physicians on the front lines of care for these patients can coordinate preventative measures as part of their purview of care. Good discharge planning and medication reconciliation upon discharge is essential and can help minimize return visits and new illnesses by working to ensure a safer home environment and more coordinated primary care.

LITERATURE TABLE

TRIAL	DESIGN	RESULT
Demographics		
Fuchs et al., *Intensive Care Med.* 2012[2]	Retrospective cohort of 7,265 patients >65 y of age admitted to ICUs assessing admission characteristics and mortality rates	Patients >65 y represent 45.7% of total ICU population (10.35% of total >85 y) with a change in prevalence of admission characteristics with age. Age (especially >75 y) is a significant independent risk factor for mortality for ICU patients at 28 d and 1 y
Bagshaw et al., *Crit Care.* 2009[3]	Retrospective analysis of data from Australian and New Zealand Intensive Care Society Adult Patient Database. Data obtained for 120,123 adult ICU admissions across 57 ICUs to evaluate the rate, characteristics, and outcomes of ICU patients >80 y of age	13% of ICU admissions were very elderly (>80 y), showing annual ICU admission increase of 5.6%/year. Patients >80 y had lower short-term survival modified by preceding functional status and frailty, comorbid illness, primary diagnosis, surgical status, and illness severity. Survivors were more likely to go to rehab or long-term care facilities
Roch et al., *Crit Care.* 2011[8]	Retrospective cohort chart review with prospective follow-up to evaluate short- and long-term survival in 299 adults >80 y after medical ICU admission	In hospital mortality of 55% (46% in ICU), 2-y mortality of 53% of survivors (relative to 18% of general population of age). Mortality most influenced by severity of acute illness, preexistence of underlying disease, and a cardiac diagnosis at the time of admission
Sprung et al, *Crit Care Med.* 2012[63]	Eldicus Trial, Part II: prospective, observational cohort studying triage decision making in European ICUs and the benefit of ICU admission for elderly	8,472 triages in 6,796 patients, of which 82% were accepted to an ICU. Refusal rates (11% for ages 18–44 to 36% for ages >84) and mortality (11% to 48% in respective groups) increased with increasing age. There was a greater mortality reduction in older adults admitted to the ICU when corrected for disease severity (age >65 [OR 0.65, 95% CI 0.55–0.78, $p < 0.0001$]; age <65 [OR 0.74, 95% CI 0.57–0.97, $p = 0.01$])

LITERATURE TABLE *(Continued)*

TRIAL	DESIGN	RESULT
Sepsis		
Martin et al., *Crit Care Med.* 2006[15]	Longitudinal observational study using national hospital discharge data. Data included 10,422,301 adult sepsis patients hospitalized over 24 y	Elderly patients accounted for 12% of population but 64.9% of sepsis cases (RR 13.1 [95% CI 12.6–13.6] compared to younger patients); linear increase in case-fatality rate by age
Lewis et al., *J Gerontol A Biol Sci Med.* 2005[21]	Prospective observational study of 360 patients over 60 years old presenting with nontraumatic abdominal pain to the ED, evaluated for clinical course, diagnosis, and mortality	Mean age 73.2 ± 8 y (66% female, 51% white); 58% admitted; 18% surgical intervention or invasive procedure; 7% readmission rates; 5% mortality at 2 wk. Older patients had higher mortality rates (OR 4.4; 95% CI 1.4–14) and lower diagnostic concordance rates (76% vs. 87%, $p = 0.01$)
Cardiac		
Blancas et al., *Eur Geriatr Med.* 2012[4]	Retrospective cohort study of 1,409 patients >65 y of age admitted to an ICU	Confirmed that cardiac patients are the most common admission group in patients >65 (67.7%), with ACS being most frequent diagnosis (76.7%)
Respiratory		
Ely et al., *Ann Intern Med.* 2002[49]	Retrospective chart review of 902 patients in ARDS network	Age ≥70 was a strong predictor of in-hospital death (hazard ratio 2.5 (CI 2.0–3.2), longer duration of mechanical ventilation, and higher rates of reintubation
Balami et al., *Age Ageing.* 2006[52]	Prospective observational study of 36 patients >65 y with acute COPD exacerbations (defined by acidosis, respiratory rate, and hypercapnia)	Of the 36 patients, 2 failed NIPPV due to inability to tolerate mask. 7 patients did not improve at 4 h. All 9 of these patients died (mortality rate 25%). 27 of 34 patients initiated on NIPPV showed significant improvement (79%) and had no complications
Delirum		
Monette et al., *Gen Hosp Psychiatry.* 2001[60]	Prospective, observational study of 110 elderly patients interviewed by a geriatrician in the ED and a trained nonphysician in CAM methodology	Interrater reliability with Kappa coefficient of 0.91, sensitivity of 0.86, and specificity of 1.00, PPV 1.00, NPV 0.97. Concluded that CAM methodology by trained interviewer is able to detect delirium in ED setting

CI, confidence interval; OR, odds ratio; RR, relative risk.

REFERENCES

1. Werner CA. *The Older Population: 2010*, US Census Bureau, 2011. http://www.census.gov/prod/cen2010/briefs/c2010br-09.pdf. Accessed June 14, 2013.
2. Fuchs L Chronaki CE, Park S, et al. ICU admission characteristics and mortality rates among elderly and very elderly patients. *Intensive Care Med.* 2012;38(10):1654–1661.
3. Bagshaw SM, Webb SA, Delaney A, et al. Very old patients admitted to intensive care in Australia and New Zealand: a multi-centre cohort analysis. *Crit Care.* 2009;13(2):R45.
4. Blancas R, Martinez Gonzalez Ó, Vigil D, et al. Influence of age and intensity of treatment on intra-ICU mortality of patients older than 65 years admitted to the intensive care unit. *Eur Geriatr Med.* 2012;3(5):290–294.
5. Hamel MB, Davis RB, Teno JM, et al. Older age, aggressiveness of care, and survival for seriously ill, hospitalized adults. *Ann Intern Med.* 1999;131:721–728.
6. Schwab CW, Kauder DR. Trauma in the Geriatric Patient. *Arch Surg.* 1992;127(6):701–706.
7. McDermid RC, Bagshaw SM. ICU and critical care outreach for the elderly. *Best Pract Res Clin Anaesthesiol.* 2011;25(3):439–449.

8. Roch A, Wiramus S, Pauly V, et al. Long-term outcome in medical patients aged 80 or over following admission to an intensive care unit. *Crit Care.* 2011;15(1):R36.
9. De Rooij SE, Govers A, Korevaar JC, et al. Short-term and long-term mortality in very elderly patients admitted to an intensive care unit. *Intensive Care Med.* 2006;32(7):1039–1044.
10. Kaarlola A, Tallgren M, Pettila V. Long-term survival, quality of life, and quality-adjusted life-years among critically ill elderly patients, *Crit Care Med.* 2006;34:2120–2126.
11. Nathanson BH, Higgins TL, Brennan MJ, et al. Do elderly patents fare well in the ICU? *Chest.* 2011;139:825–831.
12. Sacanella E, Pérez-Castejón JM, Nicolás JM, et al. Functional status and quality of life 12 months after discharge from a medical ICU in healthy elderly patients: a prospective observational study. *Crit Care.* 2011;15(2):R105.
13. Geriatric Emergency Medicine Task Force. S. o. A. E. M., *Emergency Care of the Elder Person.* Wilton, CT: Beverly Cracom Publications; 1996.
14. Rajapakse S, Rajapakse A. Age bias in clinical trials in sepsis: how relevant are guidelines to older people? *J Crit Care.* 2009;24(4):609–613.
15. Martin GS, Mannino DM, Moss M. The effect of age on the development and outcome of adult sepsis. *Crit Care Med.* 2006;34(1):15–21.
16. Kumar A, Roberts D, Wood KE, et al. Duration of hypotension before initiation of effective antimicrobial therapy is the critical determinant of survival in human septic shock. *Crit Care Med.* 2006;34:1589–1596.
17. Yoshikawa TT. Antimicrobial resistance and aging: beginning of the end of the antibiotic era? *J Am Geriatr Soc.* 2002;50(Suppl 7):S226–S229.
18. Rivers E, Nguyen B, Havstad S, et al.; Early Goal-Directed Therapy Collaborative Group. Early goal-directed therapy in the treatment of severe sepsis and septic shock. *N Engl J Med.* 2001;345:2247–2256.
19. Dellinger RP, Levy MM, Rhodes A, et al., Surviving sepsis campaign: international guidelines for management of severe sepsis and septic shock: 2012. *Crit Care Med.* 2013;41(2):580–637.
20. Sprung CL, Annane D, Keh D, et al.; CORTICUS Study Group. Hydrocortisone therapy for patients with septic shock. *N Engl J Med.* 2008;358:111–124.
21. Lewis LM, Banet GA, Blanda M, et al. Etiology and clinical course of abdominal pain in senior patients: a prospective, multicenter study. *J Gerontol A Biol Sci Med Sci.* 2005;60A(8):1071–1076.
22. Reiss R, Deutsch AA. Emergency abdominal procedures in patients above 70. *J Gerontol.* 1985;40:154.
23. Fenyo G. Acute abdominal disease in the elderly. *Am J Surg.* 1982;143:751.
24. Bugliosi TF, Meloy TD, Vukov LF. Acute abdominal pain in the elderly. *Ann Emerg Med.* 1990;19:1383.
25. AHRQ, C. f. D., Organization, and Markets, Healthcare Cost and Utilization Project, Nationwide Inpatient Sample 1997 and 2009, Most frequent principal diagnoses by age.
26. Gupta R, Kaufman S. Cardiovascular emergencies in the elderly. *Emerg Med Clin North Am.* 2006;24(2):339–370.
27. Ghali JK, Kadakia S, Cooper RS, et al. Bedside diagnosis of preserved versus impaired left ventricular systolic function in heart failure. *Am J Cardiol.* 1991;67:1002.
28. *Merck Manual of Geriatrics.* Whitehouse, NJ: Merck & Co; 2010–2011.
29. Maisel AS, Clopton P, Krishnaswamy P, et al. Impact of age, race and sex on the ability of B-type natriuretic peptide to aid in the emergency diagnosis of heart failure: results from the Breathing Not Properly (BNP) multinational study. *Am Heart J.* 2004;147(6):1078–1084.
30. Sacchetti A, Ramoska E, Moakes ME, et al. Effect of ED management on ICU use in acute pulmonary edema. *Am J Emerg Med.* 1999;17:571–574.
31. Jeger RV, Urban P, Harkness SM, et al. Early revascularization is beneficial across all ages and a wide spectrum of cardiogenic shock severity: a pooled analysis of trials. *Acute Card Care.* 2011;13(1):14–20.
32. Tomassini F, Gagnor A, Migliardi A, et al. Cardiogenic shock complicating acute myocardial infarction in the elderly: predictors of long-term survival. *Catheter Cardiovasc Interv.* 2011;78(4):505–511.
33. Caldicott LD, Hewley K, Heppell R, et al. Intravenous enoximone or dobutamine for severe heart failure after acute myocardial infarction: a randomized double-blinded trial. *Eur Heart J.* 1993;14(5):696–700.
34. Feinberg WM, Blackshear JL, Laupacis A, et al. Prevalence, age distribution, and gender of patients with atrial fibrillation. Analysis and implications. *Arch Intern Med.* 1995;155(5):469–473.
35. American Heart Association. *2005 Heart and Stroke Statistical Update*, Dallas, TX: American Heart Association; 2004.
36. Fumagalli S, Boncinelli L, Bondi E, et al. Does advanced age affect the immediate and longterm results of direct-current external cardioversion of atrial fibrillation. *J Am Geriatr Soc.* 2002;50(7):1192–1197.
37. Kilborn MJ, Rathore SS, Gersh BJ, et al. Amiodarone and mortality among elderly patients with acute myocardial infarction with atrial fibrillation. *Am Heart J.* 2002;144(6):1095–1101.

38. Midlov P, Eriksson T, Kragh A. *Drug-related Problems in the Elderly*. New York: Springer Publishing; 2009.
39. Likosky DS, Sorensen MJ, et al. Long-term survival of the very elderly undergoing aortic valve replacement. *Circulation.* 2009;120:S127–S133.
40. Likosky DS, Dacey LJ, et al. Long-term survival of the very elderly undergoing coronary artery bypass grafting. *Ann Thorac Surg.* 2008;85(4):1233–1237.
41. Canto JG, Rogers WJ, Goldberg RJ, et al. Association of age and sex with myocardial infarction symptom presentation and in-hospital mortality. *JAMA.* 2012;307:813–822.
42. Appleby CE, Ivanov J, MacKie K, et al. In-hospital outcomes of very elderly patients (85 years and older) undergoing percutaneous coronary intervention. *Catheter Cardiovasc Interv.* 2011;77(5):634–641.
43. Bueno H, Betriu A, et al. Primary angioplasty vs. fibrinolysis in very old patients with acute myocardial infarction: TRIANA randomized trial and pooled analysis with previous studies. *Eur Heart J.* 2011;32(1):51–60.
44. Hsieh TH, Wang JD, Tsai LM. Improving in-hospital mortality in elderly patients after acute coronary syndrome-a nationwide analysis of 97,220 patients in Taiwan during 2004–2008. *Int J Cardiol.* 2012;155(1):149–154.
45. Carson S. The epidemiology of critical illness in the elderly. *Crit Care Clin.* 2003;19:605–617.
46. Ely EW, Evans GW, Haponik EF. Mechanical ventilation in a cohort of elderly patients admitted to an intensive care unit. *Ann Intern Med.* 1999;131:96–104.
47. Esteban A, Anzueto A, Frutos F, et al. Characteristics and outcomes in adult patients receiving mechanical ventilation: a 28-day international study. *JAMA.* 2002;287:345–355.
48. Muir J-F, Lamia B, Molano C, et al. Respiratory failure in the elderly patient. *Semin Respir Crit Care Med.* 2010;31(5):634–646.
49. Ely EW, Wheeler AP, Thompson BT, et al. Recovery rate and prognosis in older persons who develop acute lung injury and the acute respiratory distress syndrome. *Ann Intern Med.* 2002;136:25–36.
50. Lightowler JV, Wedzicha JA, Elliott MW, et al. Non-invasive positive pressure ventilation to treat respiratory failure resulting from exacerbations of chronic obstructive pulmonary disease: Cochrane systemic review and meta-analysis. *BMJ.* 2003:326(7382);185.
51. Rozzini R, Sabatini T, Trabucchi M. Non-invasive ventilation for respiratory failure in elderly patients. *Age Ageing.* 2006;35(5):546–547.
52. Balami JS, Packham SM, Gosney MA. Non-invasive ventilation for respiratory failure due to acute exacerbations of chronic obstructive pulmonary disease in older patients, *Age Ageing.* 2006;35(1):75–79.
53. Yan AT, Bradley TD, Liu PP. The role of contiguous positive airway pressure in the treatment of congestive heart failure. *Chest.* 2001;120:1675–1685.
54. Mehta S, Hill NS. Noninvasive ventilation. *Am J Respir Crit Care Med.* 2001;163(2):540–577.
55. Han JH, Wilson A, Ely EW. Delirium in the older emergency department patient: a quiet epidemic. *Emerg Med Clin North Am.* 2010;28:611–631.
56. Inouye SK. Delirium in older persons. *N Engl J Med.* 2006;354:1157–1165.
57. Rosen A, Connors S, Clark S, et al. Agitated delirium in older adults in the emergency department: clinical review and new, evidence-based protocol. [under review], 2013.
58. Inouye SK, van Dyck CH, Alessi CA, et al. Clarifying confusion: the confusion assessment method. A new method for detection of delirium. *Ann Intern Med.* 1990;113:941–948.
59. Wei LA, Fearing MA, Sternberg EJ, et al. The confusion assessment method: a systematic review of current usage. *J Am Geriatr Soc.* 2008;56:823–830.
60. Monette J, Galbaud du Fort G, Fung SH, et al. Evaluation of the Confusion Assessment Method (CAM) as a screening tool for delirium in the emergency room. *Gen Hosp Psychiatry.* 2001;23:20–25.
61. Garrouste-Orgeas M, Montuclard L, Timsit JF, et al. Triaging patients to the ICU: a pilot study of factors influencing admission decisions and patient outcomes. *Intensive Care Med.* 2003;29:774–781.
62. Nuckton TJ, List ND. Age as a factor in critical care unit admissions. *Arch Intern Med.* 1995;155:11087–11092.
63. Sprung CL, Artigas A, Kesecioglu J, et al. The eldicus prospective, observational study of triage decision making in european intensive care units. Part II: Intensive care benefit for the elderly. *Crit Care Med.* 2012;40(1):132–138.

60

Palliative Care in the Emergency Department

Lawrence A. Ho and J. Randall Curtis

BACKGROUND

Emergency medicine is typically characterized as a fast-paced, procedure-based specialty that focuses on the evaluation and stabilization of acutely ill patients. Training of emergency medicine physicians, therefore, is centered on interventions aimed at preserving life and achieving clinical stability. At times, however, when these interventions fail, the core tenets of emergency medicine can appear to be at odds with those of palliative care, which balances quality of life with the burdens of invasive treatment. In the intensive care unit (ICU) setting, successful integration of palliative care has been shown to be associated with a number of key outcomes. These outcomes include improved quality of death and dying, shorter ICU length of stay for patients who die in the ICU, increased family satisfaction, and reductions in family members' psychological symptoms after a patient's death.[1–5]

These benefits have also been recognized in the emergency department (ED), evidenced by positive physicians' attitudes and a growing body of literature regarding palliative care in the ED.[6–11] Hospice and palliative medicine are now also official subspecialties of the American College of Emergency Physicians. Despite these advances, significant challenges remain in the successful integration of palliative care in the ED. These include medicolegal issues (which may lead the emergency physician to favor aggressive over palliative treatment to avoid litigation), a narrow view of the role of the emergency physician (perpetuating the perception that end-of-life issues should be addressed by inpatient teams), and lack of awareness among ED staff about ED palliative care resources.[8,12]

The importance of palliative care and end-of-life decision making in the ED is increasingly evident. The majority of seriously ill patients begin their hospital course in the ED, and decisions made in the ED frequently dictate subsequent medical decisions and therapeutic direction.[13–15] Because patients who die in the ED are often elderly, ED-based end-of-life discussions and decisions are likely to become increasingly important as our population ages.[6] A comprehensive discussion of palliative care in emergency medicine is beyond the scope of this book; therefore, this chapter focuses on the pillar of successful palliative care, namely, communication. In the growing literature on the role of palliative care in the ED, there is little specific guidance for ED-based discussions on end-of-life care. This review, and the recommendations made, is therefore largely extrapolated from the critical care literature.

COMMUNICATION

Deaths in the hospital setting often involve withholding or withdrawing life-supporting treatments. In the ICU, the percentage of such deaths is as high as 90%.[16] Limited data suggest that this proportion is considerably lower in the ED, but decisions to limit life-sustaining treatment in this setting are nevertheless common.

The decision to withhold or withdraw life-sustaining therapies should always involve effective communication, including sharing information about illness and prognosis, offering support, and engaging patients and families in the treatment decision process.[17] Families rate successful communication as one of the most important skills of a quality health care provider, and effective communication has been shown to improve patient and family outcomes.[18–21] Significant barriers to successful communication do exist, however; and when asked, few families consider patient–clinician communication to have been adequate.[22]

General End-of-Life Communication Considerations

End-of-life care in the intensive care or acute care setting typically involves multiple health care professionals from different disciplines. This is true even in the ED, where time from presentation to disposition is typically measured in hours, rather than days. It is important that all team members who communicate directly with patients and families be involved in the end-of-life decision-making process.[23] Clear communication—and, ideally, agreement—within the health care team about appropriate patient care helps prevent conflicting messages to the patient or family, facilitates cooperation among clinicians, and minimizes provider internal conflict and "burnout."[24–28]

Although consensus among providers is very important, the fundamental goal of any end-of-life discussion is to align clinicians', patients', and/or families' views of what is happening to the patient. The most challenging conversations occur when the clinicians' and patients' and/or families' goals of care differ. Although aligning separate viewpoints can be time consuming, these efforts, if successful, greatly facilitate future decisions about end-of-life care.[23] A useful mnemonic that can enhance clinician–family communication is VALUE.[17,29,30]

VALUE: 5-Step Approach to Improving Communication in ICU with Families

- *V*—*Value* family statements
- *A*—*Acknowledge* family emotions
- *L*—*Listen* to the family
- *U*—*Understand* the patient as a person
- *E*—*Elicit* family questions

Reproduced from Curtis et al. Practice guidance for evidenced-based ICU family conferences. *Chest.* 2008;134(4):835–843.

When this mnemonic was used as part of an intervention to improve clinician–family communication in the ICU, it was shown to significantly reduce family symptoms of depression, anxiety, and posttraumatic stress disorder 90 days after the patient's death.[3]

The appropriate time to initiate of end-of-life care conversation can be difficult to gauge. It is generally a good idea to discuss end-of-life issues as soon as possible for the seriously ill patient, although circumstances may dictate different timing.[23] Conversations held early in the ED course often focus on prognosis and treatment options, rather than on withdrawal/withholding of life support and end-of-life care; even so, they can set the stage for subsequent end-of-life care conversations once the patient is admitted to the hospital. For patients with a very poor prognosis or with severe underlying terminal or life-limiting illnesses, discussion of withdrawal/withholding of life support and end-of-life is appropriate in the ED.

A recent qualitative analysis of communication between patients and providers identified six essential themes.[31] These include (1) talking with patients in an honest and straightforward way, (2) being willing to talk about dying, (3) giving bad news in a sensitive way, (4) encouraging questions from patients, (5) being sensitive to when patients are ready to talk about death, and (6) listening to patients. Of these, listening to patients and families is of the greatest importance. Clinicians tend to dominate communication with patients and families; an observational study evaluating audiotapes of family conferences in the ICU found that clinicians spent 70% of time talking and only 30% of the time listening.[30] This study also found that the higher the proportion of time a family spent speaking, the more satisfied the family was with the conference.

Cross-Cultural Communication and Spirituality

Cultural or language barriers may limit successful communication. Family allies, such as religious or community leaders as well as professional interpreters, can be useful in easing these barriers.[32] Unfortunately, even with professional interpreters, communication errors are common and can affect patient and family understanding, emotional support, and decision making.[33,34] To mitigate these errors, clinicians can take several simple steps: include interpreters in a heath care team meeting prior to the family conference; speak slowly to allow time for interpretation and use pictures or drawings when possible; and try to limit simultaneous conversations.[35]

Spiritual care is very important to many patients and their families, but it is an area of palliative care that many clinicians identify as needing improvement.[36] Family satisfaction with care is increased if spiritual care needs are assessed and a spiritual care provider is made available.[37,38] Provision of spiritual care in the ED can be challenging due to time constraints; however, many hospitals have spiritual care providers available on call.

Family Conferences

As patients are often unable to participate in end-of-life discussions in the setting of an acute or critical illness, family conferences are an essential communication tool. Even with the time constraints in the ED, the family conference can be very useful, albeit in often abbreviated form. Family conferences can also provide an opportunity for palliative care consultants to become involved in patient care. Appropriate preparations, including the use of a "preconference" and following a predetermined, semi-structured conversation format can help ensure an efficient and successful conference. It is, however, also important to be able to adapt this structure to met the needs of individual patients and family members.

Prior to leading a family conference, the clinician should encourage all active members of the team to be involved. Team members should meet in a "preconference" to agree on conference goals and to identify issues or conflicts likely to arise either between team members or with the family during the meeting.[23]

Many family conferences follow a similar structure.[39] This structure typically includes (1) individual introductions and a quick discussion of the goals and agenda, (2) asking the family to describe their understanding of what is happening, (3) an information exchange about the illness and treatments (from clinicians, generally) and about the patient's preferences and values (from the family, generally), (4) a discussion of the prognosis for survival and quality of life, and (5) a discussion of the goals of care and decisions that need to be made.

Several studies have shown that certain conference features result in improved ratings for communication and family experience. These include holding the meeting in a private place, consistent communication among all members, assuring families that patients will be kept comfortable and will not be abandoned no matter what treatment path is followed, and the use of empathic statements by the clinicians.[40–42]

At the conclusion of family conferences, it is important that the clinicians make a recommendation. There is a tendency for some clinicians to merely describe the treatment options, but avoid providing a recommendation.[43] In cases of withholding or withdrawing life support, recommendations are often particularly important. It is not uncommon for family members to resist being put in the position of making the decision to "give up" or "pull the plug."

DECISION MAKING

Often, family members must make critical decisions for their loved ones. In this case, it is important for the clinician to understand and convey the principles of surrogate decision making. The surrogate is asked to consider what the patient would want if he or she could speak for himself or herself—and not to weigh his or her own preference for the patients' care—or what he or she would choose if placed in the patient's situation. This clarification can be especially helpful when the surrogate is faced with continuing or discontinuing life-sustaining therapy.

There is a range of potential roles for physicians in the end-of-life decision-making process. Several critical care societies have issued a joint consensus statement advocating a shared decision-making approach,[44] in which the physician and family share their opinions and jointly reach a decision (Fig. 60.1). Family members and patients may prefer varying degrees of involvement in the decision-making process, so it is important for the physician to take time to determine individual family members' preferred roles.[45] It is also important for the physician to understand that the spectrum of preference ranges from allowing the physician to make the decision, to family members assuming full responsibility for the decision. As the prognosis of a patient worsens, the physician's willingness to take on the burden of a decision should increase.

Resuscitation is a common topic of end-of-life discussions and family conferences. Resuscitation following a cardiac arrest should follow the adult cardiac life support (ACLS) algorithm. While it is possible for a family to consider separate components of the ACLS algorithm (chest compressions, intubation, medications, cardioversion, etc.), these discussions can be unnecessarily complex and can lead to unrealistic expectations

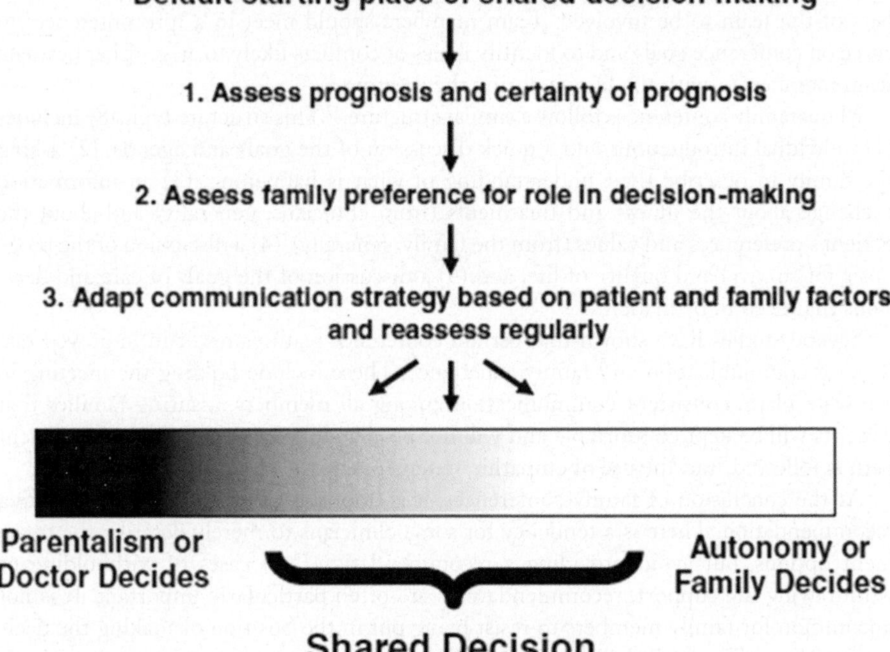

FIGURE 60.1 A schematic for approaching decisions about withholding and withdrawing life support in the ED. Reproduced from Curtis et al. Practice guidance for evidenced-based ICU family conferences. *Chest.* 2008;134(4):835–843.

(e.g., chest compressions and cardioversion, but no intubation). In general, resuscitation should be discussed as a single entity.

FAMILY REACTIONS

The feeling of abandonment, in both patients and families, is common in the end-of-life process. Although patients and families usually do not use the word "abandon," they express this feeling in different ways. Families may either request that everything be done to cure the patient despite overwhelmingly poor chances for survival, or they may express concerns about "letting go" or "giving up."[46] Being aware of these expressions helps the clinician address such concerns. Ensuring that the patient is not suffering and that his or her end-of-life preferences are respected supports nonabandonment. Clinicians should also be mindful of language that may heighten a sense of abandonment. For example, "withdrawal of care" should not be used synonymously with "withdrawal of life support." Following a decision to withdraw or withhold life-sustaining treatments, some patients and families may be worried about transferring to a less intensive care area of the ED; in this case, the clinician should convey that the patient will continue to receive timely and appropriate treatment.

After having an end-of-life conversation with the family, it is imperative to explore the families' reactions and feelings.[39] Several approaches can be used. First, the clinician should summarize what the patient or family has said. This active listening technique verifies to the patient or family that they have been heard; it is especially useful when the clinician and family have differing views. Second—since strong emotions often develop during conversations about prognosis or end-of-life care—the clinician should recognize the family's emotions and explore how and why patients and family members feel the way they do. Exploratory questions, such as "tell me more about that," and reflective statements, such as "it seems to me that you are very upset," can draw out and support family members in the discussion. Finally, once a decision has been made, the clinician can support the family by acknowledging the difficulty of the situation, expressing agreement that the decision is consistent with the patient's values, and voicing appreciation for all family members' comments.

LITERATURE TABLE

TRIAL	DESIGN	RESULT
Decision Making		
Carlet et al., *Intensive Care Med.* 2004[44]	Consensus statement	Advocates shared approach to end-of-life decision making
Communication		
Wenrich et al., *Arch Intern Med.* 2001[31]	20 focus groups consisting of 137 individuals, including patients, family members, and health care professionals analyzing domains of physician skill at end-of-life care	Identified 6 important areas when communicating with dying patients: talking in a straightforward/honest way, willingness to talk about dying, sensitivity in giving bad news, listening, asking questions, and showing sensitivity when patients are ready to talk about dying
Selph et al., *J Gen Intern Med.* 2008[41]	Multicenter prospective study of 51 family conferences that addressed end-of-life decisions	Significant association between empathic statements and family satisfaction with communication ($p = 0.04$)
Family Conferences		
Lautrette et al., *N Engl J Med.* 2007[3]	Multicenter randomized controlled trial surveying families of 126 dying patients in the ICU who received proactive end-of-life conference and brochure vs. customary end-of-life conference	Proactive end-of-life conference using VALUE mnemonic resulted in longer conferences time (30 vs. 20 min, $p < 0.001$) and families having lower symptoms of anxiety, depression, and posttraumatic stress disorder at day 90 ($p \leq 0.02$)
Curtis et al., *Am J Respir Crit Care Med.* 2005[29]	Qualitative study of 51 audiotaped family conferences	29% of family conferences had missed opportunities. Missed opportunities included listening to and responding to the family
McDonagh et al., *Crit Care Med.* 2004[30]	Cross-sectional study reviewing 51 audiotaped conferences in four ICUs	Family members spoke 29% and clinicians spoke 71% of the time. Increased proportion of family speech was significantly associated with increased family satisfaction with physician communication
Stapleton et al., *Crit Care Med.* 2006[42]	Qualitative study of 51 audiotaped family conferences	Increasing frequency of 3 types of clinician statements was associated with increased family satisfaction: assurances that the patient will not be abandoned ($p = 0.015$), assurances that the patient will be comfortable ($p = .029$), and support for family decisions about end-of-life care ($p = 0.005$)
Spiritual Care		
Wall et al., *Crit Care Med.* 2007[37]	Cross-sectional study surveying 356 family members of dying patients about spiritual care	Strong association between satisfaction with spiritual care and satisfaction with total ICU experience ($p < 0.001$)

CONCLUSION

While challenges to successful implementation of palliative care in the ED remain, there is a growing awareness that conducting effective end-of-life discussions is an important component of the ED clinician skill set. Effective communication is a prerequisite to good palliative care, and, although multiple barriers to this goal exist in a busy ED, the evidence-based strategies discussed in this chapter can help clinicians, patients, and their families find common ground.

REFERENCES

1. Campbell ML, Guzman JA. Impact of a proactive approach to improve end-of-life care in a medical ICU. *Chest.* 2003;123:266–271.
2. Curtis JR, Treece PD, Nielsen EL, et al. Integrating palliative and critical care: evaluation of a quality-improvement intervention. *Am J Respir Crit Care Med.* 2008;178:269–275.
3. Lautrette A, Darmon M, Megarbane B, et al. A communication strategy and brochure for relatives of patients dying in the ICU. *N Engl J Med.* 2007;356:469–478.
4. Norton SA, Hogan LA, Holloway RG, et al. Proactive palliative care in the medical intensive care unit: effects on length of stay for selected high-risk patients. *Crit Care Med.* 2007;35:1530–1535.
5. O'Mahony S, McHenry J, Blank AE, et al. Preliminary report of the integration of a palliative care team into an intensive care unit. *Palliat Med.* 2010;24:154–165.
6. Couilliot MF, Leboul D, Douguet F. Palliative care in emergency departments: an impossible challenge? *Eur J Emerg Med.* 2012;19:405–407.
7. Glajchen M, Lawson R, Homel P, et al. A rapid two-stage screening protocol for palliative care in the emergency department: a quality improvement initiative. *J Pain Symptom Manage.* 2011;42:657–662.
8. Grudzen CR, Richardson LD, Hopper SS, et al. Does palliative care have a future in the emergency department? Discussions with attending emergency physicians. *J Pain Symptom Manage.* 2012;43:1–9.
9. Grudzen CR, Stone SC, Morrison RS. The palliative care model for emergency department patients with advanced illness. *J Palliat Med.* 2011;14:945–950.
10. Lamba S, Nagurka R, Walther S, et al. Emergency-department-initiated palliative care consults: a descriptive analysis. *J Palliat Med.* 2012;15:633–636.
11. Rosenberg M, Lamba S, Misra S. Palliative medicine and geriatric emergency care: challenges, opportunities, and basic principles. *Clin Geriatr Med.* 2013;29:1–29.
12. Grudzen CR, Richardson LD, Major-Monfried H, et al. Hospital administrators' views on barriers and opportunities to delivering palliative care in the emergency department. *Ann Emerg Med.* 2013;61:654–660.
13. Meier DE, Beresford L. Fast response is key to partnering with the emergency department. *J Palliat Med.* 2007;10:641–645.
14. Kenen J. Palliative care in the emergency department: new specialty weaving into acute care fabric. *Ann Emerg Med.* 2010;56:A17–A19.
15. Smith AK, Schonberg MA, Fisher J, et al. Emergency department experiences of acutely symptomatic patients with terminal illness and their family caregivers. *J Pain Symptom Manage.* 2010;39:972–981.
16. Prendergast TJ, Luce JM. Increasing incidence of withholding and withdrawal of life support from the critically ill. *Am J Respir Crit Care Med.* 1997;155:15–20.
17. Curtis JR, Patrick DL, Shannon SE, et al. The family conference as a focus to improve communication about end-of-life care in the intensive care unit: opportunities for improvement. *Crit Care Med* 2001;29:N26–N33.
18. Hickey M. What are the needs of families of critically ill patients? A review of the literature since 1976. *Heart Lung.* 1990;19:401–415.
19. Nelson JE. Identifying and overcoming the barriers to high-quality palliative care in the intensive care unit. *Crit Care Med.* 2006;34:S324–S331.
20. Azoulay E, Pochard F, Kentish-Barnes N, et al. Risk of post-traumatic stress symptoms in family members of intensive care unit patients. *Am J Respir Crit Care Med.* 2005;171:987–994.
21. Prendergast TJ, Claessens MT, Luce JM. A national survey of end-of-life care for critically ill patients. *Am J Respir Crit Care Med.* 1998;158:1163–1167.

22. Azoulay E, Chevret S, Leleu G, et al. Half the families of intensive care unit patients experience inadequate communication with physicians. *Crit Care Med.* 2000;28:3044–3049.
23. Curtis JR, Rubenfeld GD. Improving palliative care for patients in the intensive care unit. *J Palliat Med.* 2005;8:840–854.
24. Abbott KH, Sago JG, Breen CM, et al. Families looking back: one year after discussion of withdrawal or withholding of life-sustaining support. *Crit Care Med.* 2001;29:197–201.
25. Tilden VP, Tolle SW, Garland MJ, et al. Decisions about life-sustaining treatment. Impact of physicians' behaviors on the family. *Arch Intern Med.* 1995;155:633–638.
26. Poncet MC, Toullic P, Papazian L, et al. Burnout syndrome in critical care nursing staff. *Am J Respir Crit Care Med.* 2007;175:698–704.
27. Curtis JR, Puntillo K. Is there an epidemic of burnout and post-traumatic stress in critical care clinicians? *Am J Respir Crit Care Med.* 2007;175:634–636.
28. Embriaco N, Azoulay E, Barrau K, et al. High level of burnout in intensivists: prevalence and associated factors. *Am J Respir Crit Care Med.* 2007;175:686–692.
29. Curtis JR, Engelberg RA, Wenrich MD, et al. Missed opportunities during family conferences about end-of-life care in the intensive care unit. *Am J Respir Crit Care Med.* 2005;171:844–849.
30. McDonagh JR, Elliott TB, Engelberg RA, et al. Family satisfaction with family conferences about end-of-life care in the intensive care unit: increased proportion of family speech is associated with increased satisfaction. *Crit Care Med.* 2004;32:1484–1488.
31. Wenrich MD, Curtis JR, Shannon SE, et al. Communicating with dying patients within the spectrum of medical care from terminal diagnosis to death. *Arch Intern Med.* 2001;161:868–874.
32. Kagawa-Singer M, Blackhall LJ. Negotiating cross-cultural issues at the end of life: "You got to go where he lives". *JAMA.* 2001;286:2993–3001.
33. Pham K, Thornton JD, Engelberg RA, et al. Alterations during medical interpretation of ICU family conferences that interfere with or enhance communication. *Chest.* 2008;134:109–116.
34. Thornton JD, Pham K, Engelberg RA, et al. Families with limited English proficiency receive less information and support in interpreted intensive care unit family conferences. *Crit Care Med.* 2009;37:89–95.
35. Norris WM, Wenrich MD, Nielsen EL, et al. Communication about end-of-life care between language-discordant patients and clinicians: insights from medical interpreters. *J Palliat Med.* 2005;8:1016–1024.
36. Ho LA, Engelberg RA, Curtis JR, et al. Comparing clinician ratings of the quality of palliative care in the intensive care unit. *Crit Care Med.* 2011;39:975–983.
37. Wall RJ, Engelberg RA, Gries CJ, et al. Spiritual care of families in the intensive care unit. *Crit Care Med.* 2007;35:1084–1090.
38. Gries CJ, Curtis JR, Wall RJ, et al. Family member satisfaction with end-of-life decision making in the ICU. *Chest.* 2008;133:704–712.
39. Curtis JR, Engelberg RA, Wenrich MD, et al. Studying communication about end-of-life care during the ICU family conference: development of a framework. *J Crit Care.* 2002;17:147–160.
40. Pochard F, Azoulay E, Chevret S, et al. Symptoms of anxiety and depression in family members of intensive care unit patients: ethical hypothesis regarding decision-making capacity. *Crit Care Med.* 2001;29:1893–1897.
41. Selph RB, Shiang J, Engelberg R, et al. Empathy and life support decisions in intensive care units. *J Gen Intern Med.* 2008;23:1311–1317.
42. Stapleton RD, Engelberg RA, Wenrich MD, et al. Clinician statements and family satisfaction with family conferences in the intensive care unit. *Crit Care Med.* 2006;34:1679–1685.
43. Quill TE, Brody H. Physician recommendations and patient autonomy: finding a balance between physician power and patient choice. *Ann Intern Med.* 1996;125:763–769.
44. Carlet J, Thijs LG, Antonelli M, et al. Challenges in end-of-life care in the ICU. Statement of the 5th International Consensus Conference in Critical Care: Brussels, Belgium, April 2003. *Intensive Care Med.* 2004;30:770–784.
45. Heyland DK, Tranmer J, O'Callaghan CJ, et al. The seriously ill hospitalized patient: preferred role in end-of-life decision making? *J Crit Care.* 2003;18:3–10.
46. West HF, Engelberg RA, Wenrich MD, et al. Expressions of nonabandonment during the intensive care unit family conference. *J Palliat Med.* 2005;8:797–807.

SECTION 15

The ED-ICU Transfer of Care

61

ED Evaluation of the Critically Ill Patient

Geoffrey K. Lighthall and John E. Arbo

BACKGROUND

Risk assessment and disposition of the critically ill patient is guided by impression of clinical trajectory as well as presumed diagnosis. While diagnosis is often based on historical information and on physician experience and intuition, the clinical trajectory is dictated by the state of tissue perfusion and the patient's ability to compensate for physiologic perturbations. For example, a patient with a positive troponin, ST changes, and a mean pressure of 65 mm Hg may be having a simple myocardial infarction, while another patient with similar findings may be in cardiogenic shock. Similarly, low blood pressure (BP) in one patient may result from therapeutic lowering of vascular tone (e.g., heart failure), while the same BP in a different individual may signify distributive shock. Differentiating these possibilities enables appropriate disposition and treatment and is essential to the practice of acute care medicine. This chapter focuses on the pathophysiologic roots of organ dysfunction, and demonstrates how an understanding of these principles permits efficient identification of likely diagnoses, institution of timely therapy, and safe patient disposition. Fluency with these principles also enhances communication with other health care providers.

PATHOPHYSIOLOGY OF SHOCK AND ORGAN DYSFUNCTION

Organ dysfunction arising from critical illness can be traced to abnormalities in either one or both of the following physiologic relationships:

1. The autoregulatory curve describing the relationship between organ blood flow and mean arterial pressure (MAP)[1]
2. The relationship between the supply of oxygen to tissues (oxygen delivery or DO_2) and consumption (demand or VO_2)[2–4]

Evaluating these two key homeostatic relationships—MAP/blood flow and oxygen supply/demand (VO_2/DO_2)—is essential in any patient exhibiting distress, organ dysfunction, or hemodynamic instability. Failure to do so commonly results in misdiagnosis and delayed recognition of clinical deterioration.[5–7]

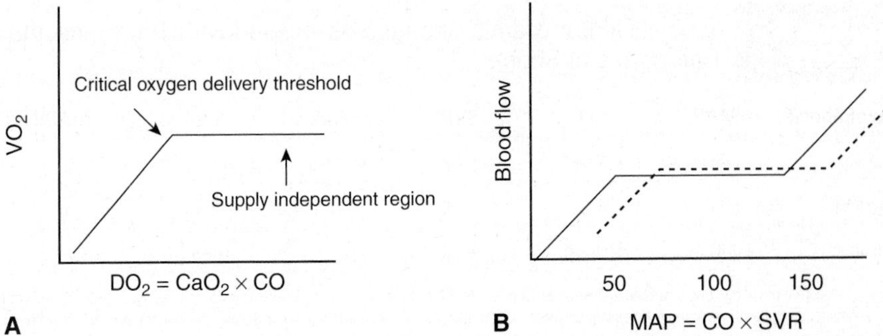

FIGURE 61.1 The key determinants of organ perfusion are depicted. **A:** The relationship between oxygen consumption (VO_2) and delivery (DO_2) is indicated. Patients usually function on the rightward side of the curve where an excess of oxygen is supplied relative to demand. As delivery decreases relative to consumption, the patient moves in a leftward direction on the curve. A decrease in central venous oxygen saturation ($ScvO_2$) accompanies leftward movement on the curve. In severe cases where delivery is unable to meet metabolic demands, the patient slips beneath the critical DO_2 threshold, where VO_2 is limited by delivery. Organ dysfunction and lactic acidosis are regarded as evidence of pathologic oxygen supply. **B:** The autoregulatory curve describing constancy of organ blood flow over a broad range or pressures is shown. Some patients with chronic hypertension have curves shifted to the right relative to the normotensive curve as shown with the dashed line. For both relationships shown, the flat horizontal portions indicate safe ranges, indicative of adequate organ blood flow and intact homeostatic mechanisms. Movement to the down-sloping portions on the left side of the curves indicates decompensation, placing the patient at risk for organ failure. VO_2, oxygen uptake/per minute; CaO_2, oxygen content of arterial blood (mainly hemoglobin); CO, cardiac output; MAP, mean arterial pressure; SVR, systemic vascular resistance; DO_2, oxygen delivery.

Oxygen consumption or demand (VO_2) is determined by physical activity, temperature, and body mass, while oxygen delivery (DO_2) is the product of cardiac output (CO) and the content of arterial oxygen (CaO_2). CO is in turn the product of stroke volume (SV) and heart rate (HR), while arterial oxygen content is primarily determined by hemoglobin concentration and saturation. The graphic representation of these relationships is presented in Figure 61.1. For both curves, the down-sloping limb on the left indicates a region where the patient is at risk for organ failure. Specifically, in curve A, DO_2 below the critical threshold signifies a loss of physiologic reserve and a transition to anaerobic metabolism; in curve B, a MAP below the autoregulatory threshold signifies the inability to maintain a constant blood flow to metabolically active regions with an organ. Appreciating the implication of these curves is essential to understanding the impact of different categories of shock.

For example, the low MAP typically seen in distributive shock becomes life threatening when vascular resistance is unable to maintain MAP above the autoregulatory threshold. Cardiogenic shock may have borderline or low MAP but is differentiated from a simple myocardial infarction by a loss in CO to levels insufficient to meet tissue oxygen demand. Hemorrhagic shock involves both a loss in hemoglobin content and a related loss in ventricular volume—and hence a loss in CO. In severe hemorrhage,

TABLE 61.1 Typical Hemodynamic Changes Associated with Three Accepted Categories of Shock

Type of Shock	MAP	CO	SVR	Preload	DO_2/VO_2	MAP/OBF
Cardiogenic	nl-⇓	⇓⇓⇓*	⇑⇑⇑	nl-⇑⇑	⇓⇓⇓	nl-⇓
Hypovolemic	nl-⇓	⇓	⇑⇑⇑	⇓⇓⇓*	⇓⇓⇓	nl, ⇓
Distributive	⇓⇓	nl, ⇑⇑	⇓⇓⇓*	⇓	nl-⇓	⇓⇓⇓

Arrows show degree of change from baseline in mean arterial pressure (MAP), cardiac output (CO), systemic vascular resistance (SVR), and cardiac preload. Additionally, alterations in the relationship between oxygen delivery and demand (DO_2/VO_2) and mean arterial pressure and organ blood flow (MAP/OBF) are indicated. The asterisk indicates the primary abnormality associated with each shock state.

nl, normal range, arrows showing increases or decreases.

these "two hits" on DO_2 can result in huge derangements in oxidative metabolism. The hemodynamic indices associated with the prototypic shock states are displayed in Table 61.1. As will be shown throughout the chapter, detection of abnormalities in either maintenance of MAP or DO_2 is followed by further differentiation of these parameters as described in Figure 61.2.

EVALUATION OF THE ADEQUACY OF BLOOD PRESSURE

From classic studies, we know that the normotensive brain autoregulates at MAPs between 50 and 150 mm Hg. This corresponds to the flat portion of the curve in Figure 61.1B. A baseline hypertensive patient would operate on a right-shifted antiregulatory curve and may not have normal organ perfusion at mean pressures <65 to 70 mm Hg. Retrospective analyses of trauma registries support the existence of age-related relative hypotension[8] and have demonstrated poorer outcomes in these individuals at MAP values previously considered normal.[9] Based on an aggregate data on patients with septic shock, studies propose that previously normotensive patients should be considered hypotensive if, after receiving 30 mL/kg crystalloid infusion, they still exhibit a decreased systolic pressure (a drop >40 mm Hg) or a decrease in MAP >30 mm Hg.[10] Determination of adequacy of MAP, therefore, often depends upon understanding a patient's usual BP range and the magnitude of acute change. Review of vital signs obtained in the outpatient setting or preoperative visit are helpful in this regard. Patients without clinic notes and charts may be more difficult to evaluate, but the patient history, as well as the presence of renal disease or left ventricular hypertrophy, can provide clues. Pressures noted on admission or obtained in the emergency department are not likely to reflect a patient's true baseline.

EVALUATION OF THE ADEQUACY OF OXYGEN DELIVERY RELATIVE TO DEMAND (VO_2/DO_2)

In many cases, a critically ill patient may arrive at the ED with a BP close to his or her baseline value. It is important to remember that for these patients, evaluation of DO_2/VO_2 is still required. The key question surrounding the status of this relationship is whether the patient's oxygen extraction is abnormally high (a falling DO_2 for a given

Clinical change or suspicion of clinical deterioration

- Change in end organ function
- Significant change in vital signs
- Significant lab abnormality (e.g., lactate, troponin)

Warrants immediate investigation of:

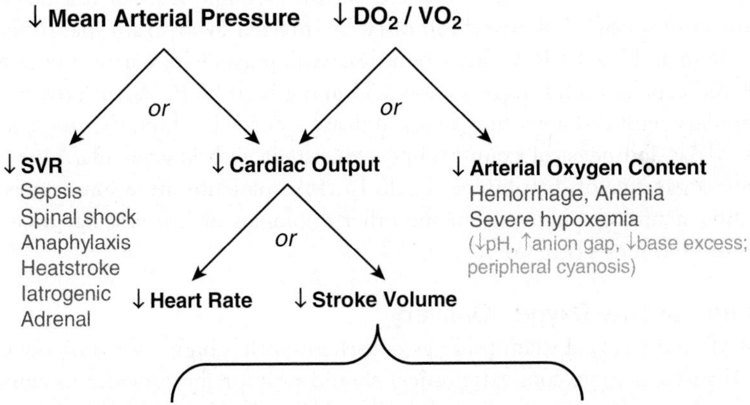

Decreased effective stroke volume—classes of abnormalities

1. Loss of effective circulating volume:
Hypovolemia, hemorrhage (Low JVP, ↓CVP, ↓PaOP, ↑SVR)

2. Adequate circulating volume but inadequate ventricular filling:
PTX, tamponade (↑CVP, var PaOP, ↑SVR)
AV valve stenosis with loss of atrial contraction or filling time

3. Contractility: MI, CHF, Cardio shock (↑CVP, ↑PaOP, ↑SVR)

4. Obstructive: Pulm Embolus (↑CVP, ↑SVR)
High PVR with RV failure (↑CVP, ↑PAP, ↑SVR)
High SVR, or AS with LV failure (↑CVP, ↑PaOP, ↑SVR)

5. Backflow: Mitral regurgitation (↑CVP, ↑PAP, ↑SVR)

FIGURE 61.2 A useful scheme organizing the constituents of MAP and DO_2 in the context of suspected decompensation. For each key abnormality, physiologic variables are indicated in black, along with the main corresponding medical diagnoses indicated in dark gray. For each, key differentiating findings of laboratory or physiologic monitor data are presented in light gray. (VO_2, oxygen uptake; DO_2, oxygen delivery; CO, cardiac output; JVP, jugular venous pressure; MAP, mean arterial pressure; SVR, systemic vascular resistance; CVP, central venous pressure; PAP, pulmonary artery pressure; PaOP, pulmonary artery occlusion (wedge) pressure).

VO_2—moving right to left on that flat portion of the cure in Fig. 61.1A) or whether anaerobic metabolism is already present (an inadequate DO_2 for a given VO_2—the left side downward slope in Fig. 61.1A). Metabolic acidosis, an elevated anion gap, and elevated lactate levels are associated with an oxygen debt and subsequent anaerobic metabolism and can be rapidly identified with point-of-care blood gas analysis. A fall in DO_2 and subsequent abnormal increase in oxygen extraction may be identified by a central venous oxyhemoglobin saturation of <70%. Typically, perturbations in the economy of oxygen extraction result from impaired delivery.

MAKING THE DIAGNOSIS

Evaluation of Low Blood Pressure

A low MAP results from either a low CO or low systemic vascular resistance (SVR). Thus, the etiology of a low MAP can often be inferred by an exam that differentiates between high and low SVR. Cold extremities, weak pulses with narrow pulse pressures, and delayed capillary refill suggest a low CO and a high SVR. Warm extremities with brisk capillary refill and bounding pulses indicate a normal or high CO and a low SVR.

Low MAP and physical exam findings consistent with low vascular tone (i.e., low SVR) are suggestive of distributive shock. In these patients, attention centers on differentiating neurologic injury from the other etiologies of low vascular tone, such as anaphylaxis and sepsis (Fig. 61.2).

Evaluation of Low Oxygen Delivery

Low MAP and physical exam findings consistent with a high SVR and low CO (i.e., increased vascular tone, cool extremities) should prompt the provider to consider the determinants of CO—specifically either a low HR or diminished SV. A key point differentiating causes of low SV is the overall volume status of the patient. Low SV can result from frank hypovolemia as in hemorrhage and severe dehydration, or can exist in the setting of euvolemia or hypervolemia where the low SV results from precardiac obstruction of ventricular filling, poor pump function, postcardiac obstruction, or valvular regurgitation. With hypovolemia, central veins will be collapsed, and peripheral veins may be difficult to locate; findings of hypovolemia should prompt a search for sources of volume loss, particularly bleeding. Low SV from all other causes will be accompanied by normal to large central veins; enlarged central veins should prompt a thorough examination of the chest and echocardiographic examination of the heart. The use of transthoracic echocardiography is increasingly common in ICUs and EDs for focused assessment of these conditions.[11,12] Figure 61.2 provides a systematic approach to the evaluation of the patient with evidence of clinical deterioration or the onset of organ dysfunction. The physiologic parameters incorporated into Figure 61.2 allow consideration of all possibilities for a given category of abnormality, which offers advantages in evaluation of the unstable patient.

Evaluation of Hemorrhage

In a patient in whom blood loss has occurred more than 30 minutes prior to laboratory analysis, interstitial-to-vascular fluid shifts will result in hemodilution and produce an accompanying drop in hematocrit. In this setting, the presence of an elevated lactate or evidence of an imbalance in DO_2/VO_2 would clearly be due to hemorrhage. In hemorrhage, physical exam findings include a weak pulse, narrow pulse pressure, delayed capillary refill, and cold extremities, which suggest that MAP is being maintained by abnormally high vascular resistance. With more rapid or immediate hemorrhage, isovolemic blood loss prior to fluid shifts will fail to reveal a depressed hematocrit, while still yielding findings of increased vascular tone and inadequate DO_2. In the case of low CO suspected to be due to occult hemorrhage (e.g., a retroperitoneal bleed, contained aneurysm rupture, etc.), clinical assessment could still uncover the presence of hemorrhage through exam findings suggestive of a low SV (e.g., flat neck veins).

PROVIDING EMPIRIC THERAPY

Therapy for any shock state involves both targeted interventions as well as empiric resuscitation. The utility of a physiologic evaluation as presented here is its ability to direct therapy appropriate to the class of abnormality while more definitive diagnostic data are being obtained—thereby avoiding undesirable delays in patient care. A hypotensive patient with findings consistent with distributive shock will always require vasopressors and fluids. This intervention can safely take place while the possibilities of allergy and sepsis are investigated and, if present, treated. In a patient with evidence of low CO and compensatory vasoconstriction, the physiologic analysis might encourage use of inotropes and avoidance of additional vasopressors while possibilities of heart failure or outflow tract obstruction are investigated.

END POINTS OF RESUSCITATION

Much controversy exists regarding the desirable end points for resuscitation from shock.[13–17] Rather than target specific numeric indices of DO_2 and CO, a "bare minimum" goal should be to ensure that an adequate MAP has been restored and that DO_2 is not limiting consumption. The concepts presented in this chapter provide a balanced and physiologic approach to achieving these resuscitative goals. From the determinants of MAP, one can see that a MAP that is disproportionately supported by a high vascular resistance will do so at the expense of CO, which can have disastrous consequences DO_2. Similarly, optimization of SV and DO_2 does not guarantee a MAP sufficient to maintain renal and other solid organ function; vasopressors to ensure an adequate SVR may be necessary and may help avoid fluid overload.[18] To achieve these minimum goals, the Society of Critical Care Medicine[19,20] recommends a target MAP of >65 mm Hg and the normalization of central venous oxygen saturation or lactate. Some individualization of the MAP goal may be indicated in patients with known hypertension.

As resuscitation proceeds, it is important to continually reexamine VO_2/DO_2 and adequacy of MAP. If these two physiologic relationships are revisited frequently, missed diagnoses (bleeding, myocardial infarction) and therapeutic mistakes (vasoconstrictors used instead of fluid) can be identified early. For example, in the case of a hypotensive patient given a vasopressor to elevate his or her MAP and subsequently noted to have a rising lactate and falling in pH, evidence would suggest that the initial perception of inadequate vascular tone was incorrect and that correction of MAP would be better served by augmenting CO rather than SVR.

CONCLUSION

The development of shock and organ dysfunction is not a certainty for most medical conditions. Patients progressing to shock are differentiated by the development of abnormalities in at least one of the following two physiologic relationships: (1) the relationship between oxygen supply and demand (DO_2/VO_2) and (2) the relationship between organ blood flow and MAP. Understanding the derivation of these relationships and their significance to overall organ function enables the provider to effectively implement the diagnostic and therapeutic approach outlined in this chapter. Adherence to this approach also ensures the provision of timely and appropriate care; it is comprehensive, efficient, allows prioritization of diagnostic studies, does not delay treatment, helps define end points of resuscitation, and provides a common physiology-based language for enhanced communication with other health care providers.

REFERENCES

1. Granger HJ, Guyton AC. Autoregulation of the total systemic circulation following destruction of the central nervous system in the dog. *Circ Res.* 1969;25(4):379–388.
2. Schumacker PT, Cain SM. The concept of a critical oxygen delivery. *Intensive Care Med.* 1987;13(4):223–229.
3. Shibutani K, Komatsu T, Kubal K, et al. Critical level of oxygen delivery in anesthetized man. *Crit Care Med.* 1983;11(8):640–643.
4. Bredle DL, Samsel RW, Schumacker PT, et al. Critical O2 delivery to skeletal muscle at high and low PO2 in endotoxemic dogs. *J Appl Physiol.* 1989;66(6):2553–2558.
5. Bristow PJ, Hillman KM, Chey T, et al. Rates of in-hospital arrests, deaths and intensive care admissions: the effect of a medical emergency team. *Med J Aust.* 2000;173(5):236–240.
6. Buist MD, Jarmolowski E, Burton PR, et al. Recognising clinical instability in hospital patients before cardiac arrest or unplanned admission to intensive care. A pilot study in a tertiary-care hospital. *Med J Aust.* 1999;171(1):22–25.
7. Schein RM, Hazday N, Pena M, et al. Clinical antecedents to in-hospital cardiopulmonary arrest. *Chest.* 1990;98(6):1388–1392.
8. Edwards M, Ley E, Mirocha J, et al. Defining hypotension in moderate to severely injured trauma patients: raising the bar for the elderly. *Am Surg.* 2010;76(10):1035–1038.
9. Eastridge BJ, Salinas J, McManus JG, et al. Hypotension begins at 110 mm Hg: redefining "hypotension" with data. *J Trauma.* 2007;63(2):291–297; discussion 297–9.
10. Marik PE, Lipman J. The definition of septic shock: implications for treatment. *Crit Care Resusc.* 2007;9(1):101–103.
11. Axler O. Evaluation and management of shock. *Semin Respir Crit Care Med.* 2006;27(3):230–240.
12. Vieillard-Baron A, Charron C, Chergui K, et al. Bedside echocardiographic evaluation of hemodynamics in sepsis: is a qualitative evaluation sufficient? *Intensive Care Med.* 2006;32(10):1547–1552.
13. Elliott DC. An evaluation of the end points of resuscitation. *J Am Coll Surg.* 1998;187(5):536–547.
14. Ivatury RR, Simon RJ, Islam S, et al. A prospective randomized study of end points of resuscitation after major trauma: global oxygen transport indices versus organ-specific gastric mucosal pH. *J Am Coll Surg.* 1996;183(2):145–154.
15. Gattinoni L, Brazzi L, Pelosi P, et al. A trial of goal-oriented hemodynamic therapy in critically ill patients. SvO2 Collaborative Group. *N Engl J Med.* 1995;333(16):1025–1032.
16. Shoemaker WC, Appel PL, Kram HB, et al. Prospective trial of supranormal values of survivors as therapeutic goals in high-risk surgical patients. *Chest.* 1988;94(6):1176–1186.
17. Hayes MA, Timmins AC, Yau EH, et al. Elevation of systemic oxygen delivery in the treatment of critically ill patients. *N Engl J Med.* 1994;330(24):1717–1722.

18. Liu YL, Prowle J, Licari E, et al. Changes in blood pressure before the development of nosocomial acute kidney injury. *Nephrol Dial Transplant.* 2009;24(2):504–511.
19. Rivers E, Nguyen B, Havstad S, et al. Early goal-directed therapy in the treatment of severe sepsis and septic shock. *N Engl J Med.* 2001;345(19):1368–1377.
20. Dellinger RP, Levy MM, Carlet JM, et al. Surviving sepsis campaign: international guidelines for management of severe sepsis and septic shock. 2008. *Crit Care Med.* 2008;36(1):296–327.

62

Severity of Illness Scores and Prognostication

David M. Maslove

The ability to quickly and accurately assess a patient's clinical status is essential to effective triage. This is especially true for patients with critical illness or injury. Severity of illness (SOI) scores help estimate the likelihood of impending clinical deterioration, identify appropriate services for consultation and admission, and enable practitioners to determine which patients will require frequent reassessment; this, in turn, helps guide time management and resource allocation.

In addition to their role in clinical assessment, disease-specific diagnostic and treatment algorithms frequently make use of SOI scores. Likewise, research trials in critical care almost always involve SOI scoring, as a means of both stratifying patients and comparing the results of one trial to another. Finally, some semblance of prognosis, even when imprecise and tentative, can be helpful in addressing the anxiety experienced by patients and families facing the uncertainty of critical illness.

To be useful in a busy emergency department (ED), an SOI score must be easy to use and its parameters should be reliable, objective, unambiguous, limited in number, and available at the time of initial assessment. This poses a challenge; easily obtained clinical parameters like vital signs are prone to disagreement between observers especially in dynamic situations when these signs fluctuate, while more objective laboratory values require additional time and resources to collect and analyze.

The simplest scoring systems use binary variables that are designated a specific cutoff value and then marked as either "present" or "absent." Points assigned to each variable are tallied into an overall integer score that corresponds to a risk category. Traditionally, the most useful SOIs employed a small number of easily remembered parameters, allowing for rapid calculation at the point of care. Increasing adoption of smart phones and other mobile devices in the hospital setting has lessened the importance of simplicity in the scoring system, and SOIs are evolving in response to this technology.

The clinical variables included in SOI scores are determined in numerous ways, ranging from expert opinion to logistic regression. Ideally, scoring systems are derived from data describing one cohort of patients and then validated in a second, independent cohort. Additional studies are often carried out to assess a score's validity under a range of circumstances, such as geographic location or model of health care delivery. In order to maintain score performance, updates are required as practice patterns and case mix evolve.[1]

A score's discrimination refers to its utility in distinguishing patients who experience the outcome of interest, from those who do not. Discrimination is often expressed in terms of sensitivity and specificity, or by a receiver operator characteristics (ROC) curve that relates these terms over a range of cutoff values. Scores are said to be well calibrated if they perform equally well across a range of conditions, including low- and high-risk disease, different diagnoses, and different geographical regions.[2]

Some SOI scores are intended for use with specific clinical presentations and diagnoses, while others are more general. In all cases, prognostic indices and SOI scores must be interpreted with caution; such tools are derived based on population averages and therefore provide only a probabilistic estimate for any given patient. For the most part, SOI scores are meant to help inform clinical decision making, which typically involves many more demographic, physiologic, and psychosocial parameters than can be distilled to a single number.

SYSTEM-SPECIFIC SOI SCORES

Pulmonary

The pneumonia severity index (PSI) for community-acquired pneumonia (CAP) is one of the most familiar disease-specific SOI scores. Also known as the PORT score, (for Pneumonia Patient Outcomes Research Team, the cohort in which it was validated), this SOI was published in 1997 and subsequently validated in several independent studies.[3] Created to standardize admission practices and to identify low-risk patients suitable for home treatment, the PSI generates a score using age and 19 clinical variables recorded as either "present" or "absent." The score, in turn, corresponds to one of five categories predicting risk of death at 30 days (Table 62.1).

Age and comorbidities weigh heavily in the PSI, predisposing the score to overestimate severity in elderly patients with chronic illness and to underestimate severity in young and otherwise healthy patients.[4] In one validation study, only 20% of patients in the highest-risk class (V) were admitted to the ICU, proving that PSI is less useful in prognosticating for ICU admission than for hospital admission.[5] Patients with HIV were excluded from the initial PSI study, and the index was shown to markedly underestimate disease severity in patients with pandemic influenza A(H1N1) during the 2009 outbreak.[6] In a meta-analysis involving 16,519 patients, the PSI was found to be sensitive (pooled sensitivity 90%), but lacked specificity (pooled specificity 53%).[7]

TABLE 62.1 Risk Categories in the Pneumonia Severity Index

Points	Category	30-Day Mortality	Treatment Location
NA[a]	I	0.1%	Outpatient
≤70	II	0.6%	Outpatient
71–90	III	0.9%	Outpatient (consider inpatient)
91–130	IV	9.3%	Inpatient
>130	V	27.0%	Inpatient (consider ICU)

[a]Category I is assigned to patients <50 years of age, with none of the specified coexisting conditions or physical exam findings.
Fine MJ, Auble TE, Yealy DM, et al. A prediction rule to identify low-risk patients with community-acquired pneumonia. *N Engl J Med.* 1997;336:243–250.

With 20 variables to account for, the PSI can be cumbersome to use. A simpler score developed by the British Thoracic Society known as CURB-65 uses only five clinical parameters: confusion, blood urea nitrogen (BUN) level, respiratory rate (RR), blood pressure, and age.[8] One point is assigned for each variable, depending on whether it is present or absent according to a specified cutoff value (Table 62.2). As in the PSI, the total score is then used to assign a risk category that predicts mortality at 30 days. The CURB-65 score is less sensitive than is the PSI (pooled sensitivity 62%), but is more specific (pooled specificity 79%).[7] Other versions of the CURB-65 score include CURB, in which age is omitted, and CRB-65, which does not require the laboratory value of BUN. The exclusion of BUN leads to a decrement in sensitivity (pooled sensitivity 33%), but improves specificity (pooled specificity 92%).[7] Importantly, the original CURB cohorts excluded nursing home residents as well as immunocompromised patients including those with malignancy, HIV, and tuberculosis.

Like the PSI, the CURB-65 score performs poorly in predicting the need for ICU admission. Because delayed ICU admission increases mortality risk in patients with severe CAP, the SMART-COP score was designed to address this issue specifically. This score combines eight clinical characteristics to estimate the risk of requiring intensive respiratory support (either invasive or noninvasive mechanical ventilation) or infusions of vasopressors and can therefore be useful in assigning patients to the appropriate level of care (Table 62.3).[9] A SMART-COP score of ≥3 was found to be more sensitive for the need for ICU-level support than was PSI class IV, PSI class V, or CURB-65 risk category 3 (92.3% vs. 73.6% vs. 38.5%, respectively). ATS/IDSA guidelines on CAP management also offer ICU admission criteria, including the need for invasive mechanical ventilation, septic shock with the need for vasopressors, or any three of a set of minor criteria similar to those used in the aforementioned CAP scores.[10]

Neurologic

In critical neurologic conditions such as subarachnoid hemorrhage (SAH), ischemic stroke, and traumatic brain injury, SOI scores—based on both clinical and imaging characteristics—can be used to estimate prognosis and, in some cases, inform treatment decisions.

TABLE 62.2 CURB-65 Score

Parameters (One Point for Each That Is Present)	Total Score	Risk Category	30-Day Mortality	Treatment Location
• Confusion[a]	0	1	1.5%	Outpatient
• BUN > 7 mmol/L	1			Outpatient
• RR ≥ 30	2	2	9.2%	Consider inpatient
• SBP < 90 mm Hg *or* diastolic blood pressure ≤ 60 mm Hg	3	3	22%	Inpatient
	4			Assess for admission to ICU
• Age ≥ 65	5			

[a]Mental Test Score of 8 or less or new disorientation in person, place, or time.
Lim WS, Van der Eerden MM, Laing R, et al. Defining community acquired pneumonia severity on presentation to hospital: an international derivation and validation study. *Thorax.* 2003;58:377–382.

TABLE 62.3 SMART-COP Score

Parameter	Points
SBP < 90 mm Hg	2
Multilobar involvement on CXR	1
Albumin < 3.5 g/dL	1
Respiratory rate: • ≥25 per minute (for age ≤ 50 y) • ≥30 per minute (for age > 50 y)	1
Tachycardia (HR ≥ 125 bpm)	1
Confusion (new onset)	1
Oxygen low: • For age ≤ 50 years: PaO_2 < 70 mm Hg or O_2 saturation ≤ 93% *or* PaO_2:FiO_2 < 333 • For age > 50 y: PaO_2 < 60 mm Hg or O_2 saturation ≤ 90% *or* PaO_2:FiO_2 < 250	2
Arterial **p**H < 7.35	2

Total score used to predict risk of needing intensive respiratory or vasopressor support.
0–2 points = Low risk.
3–4 points = Moderate risk (1 in 8).
5–6 points = High risk (1 in 3).
≥7 points = Very high risk (2 in 3).
Charles PGP, Wolfe R, Whitby M, et al. SMART-COP: a tool for predicting the need for intensive respiratory or vasopressor support in community-acquired pneumonia. *Clin Infect Dis.* 2008;47:375–384.

Coma

First published in the mid-1970s, the Glasgow Coma Scale (GCS) was initially developed to standardize descriptions of coma. Later, it was modified specifically to evaluate level of consciousness following traumatic brain injury.[11] To calculate the score, points are added for the patient's eye, verbal, and motor responses. Scores range from 3 to 15, with lower scores indicating greater severity of injury (Table 62.4).

Although GCS can be reported as a single sum, this may be less informative than an explicit breakdown of the constituent parts.[11] Common confounders include sedation, analgesia, neuromuscular blockade, delirium, orbital trauma, and intubation, each of which can make it impossible to calculate one or more of the subscores.[12] In intubated patients, for example, the verbal score is often represented by the letter "T," which provides information, but precludes calculation of a total score.[13] Alternative scoring systems, such as the Full Outline of UnResponsiveness (FOUR) score, may be more appropriate in critically ill intubated patients.[14]

In the prehospital setting, GCS is predictive of both death and hospitalization. A GCS of ≤13 in the field is an indication for immediate transport to a specialized trauma center.[15] GCS calculated at ED admission is an independent predictor of mortality[16] as well as of functional status at 6 months.[17] In some studies of the GCS the motor component alone has been shown to correlate with mortality.[16]

In the GCS system, traumatic brain injury is classified as mild (GCS 13 to 15), moderate (GCS 9 to 12), or severe (GCS < 9).[12] A GCS score of 8 or less is often cited as an indication for intubation. Current guidelines from the Eastern Association for the

TABLE 62.4 Glasgow Coma Scale

	Points
Eye Opening	
• Spontaneous	4
• To voice	3
• To pain	2
• None	1
Best Verbal Response	
• Oriented	5
• Confused conversation	4
• Inappropriate words	3
• Incomprehensible sounds	2
• None	1
Best Motor Response	
• Obeys commands	6
• Localizes pain	5
• Withdraws from pain	4
• Abnormal flexion (decorticate)	3
• Extension (decerebrate)	2
• None	1

Sternbach GL. The Glasgow coma scale. *J Emerg Med.* 2000;19:67–71.

Surgery of Trauma recommend endotracheal intubation for patients with GCS ≤ 8, but note that patients with altered mental status and a GCS > 8 often require intubation as well.[18] Airway obstruction, persistent hypoxemia, and hypoventilation should trigger prompt intubation regardless of mental status.

The GCS is likely the most widely used mental status score in the ICU.[11,19] It is easily calculated at the bedside and can be repeatedly measured as a means of tracking the progression of injury and recovery. Interrater agreement depends on provider type and level of experience and is highest when scores are high.[11] The GCS has become integral to other more recently developed SOI scoring systems, including the Acute Physiology and Chronic Health Evaluation (APACHE) and Simplified Acute Physiology Score (SAPS) systems discussed below.

Subarachnoid Hemorrhage

Numerous SOI scores exist for SAH, although most are derived from expert opinion and have only been validated in small cohorts.[20] The most frequently used are the Hunt and Hess scale and the World Federation of Neurological Surgeons (WFNS) scale, which are based on clinical parameters, as well as the Fisher scale, based on computerized tomography (CT) imaging (Table 62.5).

The Hunt and Hess grading system can be difficult to apply consistently; some of its terms are ambiguous, and clinical findings have the potential to span multiple categories. Interrater agreement in applying the score is moderate ($\kappa = 0.48$).[21] The score defines five classes, with a sixth (Hunt and Hess 0) sometimes included for patients with unruptured aneurysms. The Hunt and Hess scale is poorly powered to predict distinct outcomes for each individual class, and as such, classes are sometimes aggregated: Patients are often grouped into low scores (classes 0 to III) versus high scores (classes IV and V) or to "alert" (classes I and II), "drowsy" (classes III and IV), and "comatose" (class V).[20,22] The WFNS comprises a condensed version of the GCS and an additional binary measure for the presence or absence of a focal motor deficit. Its prognostic value is unclear; some studies suggest it correlates with outcome, while others do not.[20,22] The Fisher

TABLE 62.5 Common Scales Used in SAH[25]

	Hunt and Hess	Fisher
Grade I	Asymptomatic or minimal headache and slight nuchal rigidity	No blood visualized
Grade II	Moderate to severe headache, nuchal rigidity, no neurologic deficit other than cranial nerve palsy	Diffuse blood that does not appear dense enough to represent a large, thick homogenous clot
Grade III	Drowsiness, confusion, or mild focal deficit	Dense collection of blood that appears to represent a clot >1 mm thick in the vertical plane or >5 × 3 mm in longitudinal and transverse dimensions in the horizontal plane; severe spasm predicted
Grade IV	Stupor, moderate to severe hemiparesis, possible early decerebrate rigidity, and vegetative disturbances	Intracerebral or intraventricular clots, but with only diffuse blood or no blood in basal cisterns
Grade V	Deep coma, decerebrate rigidity, moribund appearance	

Ferro JM, Canhão P, Peralta R. Update on subarachnoid haemorrhage. *J Neurol.* 2008;255:465–479.

grading system uses CT findings and was initially established to predict the risk of vasospasm; it also has been shown to correlate with outcomes at 1 year and beyond. Patients in Fisher class 3 and 4 have an increased risk of poor outcome or death (relative risk 3.2 to 14.8).[23] Fisher class does not, however, accurately predict long term health-related quality of life.[24] The GCS has also been shown to correlate with outcomes in SAH.[20]

Ischemic Stroke

The National Institutes of Health Stroke Scale (NIHSS) is an 11-part evaluation of neurologic signs and is used for triage and prognostication of ischemic stroke. It incorporates measures of level of consciousness, gaze, visual fields, motor function, ataxia, sensation, speech, language, and neglect. The NIHSS has been shown to correlate with survival, length of stay, discharge destination, and functional status at 1 year.[26] It has been used to identify patients who are appropriate candidates for thrombolytic therapy, with both very high-scoring and very low-scoring patients deemed not suitable for treatment. Patients with profound deficits isolated to a single component of the scale, such as severe aphasia, may score low but should be considered for thrombolysis nonetheless.[27]

Gastrointestinal

Devised in the 1970s to predict complications of acute pancreatitis, the Ranson score is an early example of a disease-specific SOI score.[32] Its use has largely been supplanted by more generalized scoring systems such as APACHE and Sequential Organ Failure Score (SOFA), reflecting the propensity of severe pancreatitis to result in multiple organ dysfunction.[33]

Establishing risk in acute gastrointestinal bleeding can be useful in determining which patients require hospital admission and urgent endoscopy. The Rockall score incorporates age, comorbidities, and the presence of shock to stratify patients according to risk of rebleeding and death.[34] The Glasgow-Blatchford score (GBS) incorporates features of the presentation (melena, syncope), along with heart rate, blood pressure, hemoglobin, BUN, and the presence of cardiac or hepatic disease to derive an integer score.[35] The GBS is predictive of a composite endpoint that includes death; rebleeding; and the need for blood transfusion, endoscopy, or surgery. It has been shown to outperform the Rockall score in a number of prospective evaluations, with an area under the (ROC) of approximately 0.9.[35–37]

TABLE 62.6 King's College Criteria for Liver Transplantation in Acute Liver Failure

Acetaminophen-Induced	Other Causes
• Arterial pH < 7.3	• PTT > 100 s (INR > 6.5)
OR	OR ANY three of the following:
• Grade III or IV encephalopathy AND	• Age < 10 or > 40 y
• PTT > 100 s (INR > 6.5) AND	• Non-A, non-B hepatitis, halothane hepatitis, idiosyncratic drug reactions
• Serum creatinine > 3.4 mg/dL (301 µmol/L)	• Duration of jaundice before onset of encephalopathy >7 days
	• PTT > 50 s (INR > 3.5)
	• Serum bilirubin > 18 mg/dL (308 µmol/L)

Gotthardt D, Riediger C, Weiss KH, et al. Fulminant hepatic failure: etiology and indications for liver transplantation. *Nephrol Dial Transplant.* 2007;22:viii5–viii8.

In patients with acute liver failure (ALF), SOI scoring has been used to estimate the risk of death, so that referral for transplant can be initiated if indicated. The King's College criteria (Table 62.6), developed in the United Kingdom, distinguish between ALF resulting from acetaminophen toxicity and ALF resulting from other causes, many of which portend a worse prognosis.[38] In general, the King's College criteria predict mortality with specificity of approximately 90%, but sensitivity of only approximately 60%.[39,40] This limits the utility of the score somewhat, as many patients who do not meet criteria should still be considered for transplant.[41] The Model for End-Stage Liver Disease (MELD) score is a mathematical combination of the serum bilirubin, creatinine, and INR and is used to evaluate 3-month mortality risk in chronic liver disease. MELD has also been applied to patients with AFL, with a recent prospective analysis showing it to be a better predictor of death than the King's College criteria.[42] In particular, the MELD score improved upon the poor negative predictive value of the King's College criteria, as 20 of the 22 patients who survived without transplantation had a MELD score ≤ 30.

TRAUMA SOI SCORES

Trauma severity scores were initially established for field triage.[28] They have since become important in research, quality of care improvement, and health care administration. Stratifying trauma patients according to severity of injury allows not only the comparison of large and diverse patient groups but also the analysis of trauma outcomes in different settings. Some SOIs are based on anatomical regions of injury or systemic signs of organ dysfunction, while others are designed for specific types of injury.

Anatomical reporting systems allocate points for injuries sustained in distinct body regions. The injury severity score (ISS), one of the first such scores, assigns points based on the Abbreviated Injury Scale (AIS) to each of the six distinct body regions. The ISS is then calculated by adding the squares of the highest AIS values in each of the three most severely injured body regions (Table 62.7). Scores range from 1 to 75, with an AIS of 6 in any single region resulting in an automatic maximal score.

TABLE 62.7 Injury Severity Scale

Abbreviated Injury Scale	ISS Body Regions
1. Minor	1. Head and neck
2. Moderate	2. Face
3. Serious	3. Chest
4. Severe	4. Abdomen
5. Critical	5. Extremity
6. Unsurvivable	6. External

$ISS = A^2 + B^2 + C^2$ where A, B, and C are the highest AIS scores in each of the three most severely injured body regions.

Kim Y-J. Injury severity scoring systems: a review of application to practice. *Nurs Crit Care.* 2012;17:138–150.

The full extent of injury in any given body region is often not known until diagnostic imaging or surgery is performed. The ISS is therefore less useful as a field triage tool than as a means for comparing trauma outcomes in retrospective analyses of clinical and administrative data. An ISS $\geq$ 16 has been correlated with a mortality risk of 10% and is used as a cutoff above which patients should be treated at a specialized trauma center.[28] The ISS may underestimate severity in cases of multiple injuries to the same body region or when significant injuries are sustained in more than three regions.[29] A modification of the ISS, the New Injury Severity Score (NISS) attempts to address this shortcoming by adding the squares of the 3 highest AIS scores, regardless of the body regions in which they occur.[30]

While the ISS and NISS represent injury in purely anatomical terms, other scores incorporate physiologic variables that measure the systemic sequelae of trauma. The Revised Trauma Score (RTS) is one of the most commonly used physiologic scores and is derived from the GCS, systolic blood pressure (SBP), and RR (Table 62.8).[29] The raw score, which is the sum of the coded values of the three variables, can be easily calculated in the field and used for prehospital triage. Values range from 0 to 12, with scores <11 predicting a mortality rate of 12% or greater, suggesting the need for immediate transfer to a trauma center.[28] A weighted version of the RTS can also be calculated, which increases

TABLE 62.8 Revised Trauma Score

GCS	SBP (mm Hg)	RR (per Minute)	Coded Values
13–15	>89	10–29	4
9–12	76–89	>29	3
6–8	50–75	6–9	2
4–5	1–49	1–5	1
3	0	0	0

RTSc = 0.7326 SBP + 0.2908 RR + 0.9368 GCS.

Kim Y-J. Injury severity scoring systems: a review of application to practice. *Nurs Crit Care.* 2012;17:138–150.

the importance of the GCS to reflect the morbidity of isolated severe head injury.[29] The RTS may be difficult to use in patients with unstable or fluctuating vital signs and may underestimate injury severity in patients who have been adequately resuscitated.

Trauma scores that combine anatomical and physiologic components may overcome the limitations of either approach used in isolation. The Trauma and Injury Severity Score (TRISS) is a statistical method of combining the ISS and the RTS to predict mortality risk in either blunt or penetrating trauma.[28] Newer scores, such as the mechanism, GCS, age, and arterial pressure (MGAP) score, incorporate additional clinical and mechanistic features in order to predict mortality.[31]

GENERAL SOI SCORES

Since the early 1980s, a number of multiparameter SOI scoring systems have been designed to estimate mortality in unselected populations of critically ill patients. General SOI scores have been used to enroll patients into clinical trials, to measure disease progression over the course of an ICU stay, and to generate standardized mortality ratios and other measures used in comparing outcomes between ICUs, hospitals, and geographic locales.[43] They are intended to describe groups of patients, with scores predicting average outcomes for the cohort to which they are applied. In the case of a single patient, only a probabilistic estimate of survival can be inferred.[1] Clinicians must therefore exercise caution in applying these scores to individual patients, considering that clinical decisions are informed by significantly more information than is used in SOI scoring, including psychosocial factors and patient preferences.

General SOI scoring systems include the APACHE, the SAPS, and the Mortality Probability Model (MPM), all of which have undergone numerous revisions and reinventions over the last few decades. Clinical variables initially were selected based on expert opinion, but more recently have been determined by logistic regression, applied in some cases to data sets of over 100,000 patients.[44]

The APACHE system is the most popular, with APACHE IV being the most widely used score in the United States and APACHE II the most commonly used worldwide.[43,44] APACHE II incorporates age, operative status (emergency vs. elective), and the presence of severe chronic organ dysfunction or immune suppression, along with 12 physiologic variables. It produces an estimate of mortality based on a mathematical combination of weighted variables.[45] APACHE III is broken down into 3 constituent subscores (age, acute physiology, and chronic health evaluation) and is designed to predict mortality for each of 78 distinct diagnostic categories as well as risk-adjusted ICU length of stay.[2,43] The latest iteration, APACHE IV, uses 142 clinical variables, 115 of which are admission diagnoses, and is used in approximately 7% of the entire United States ICU population.[2,44] Both APACHE III and APACHE IV rely on proprietary algorithms to generate a final score and are made available as commercial services. All APACHE scores are based on the most abnormal values collected during the first 24 hours of the ICU stay.

Some of the newer general SOI scores, such as SAPS 3 and MPM II, are based on values collected at the time of ICU admission, rather than during the first 24 hours. As such, they may be more applicable to the period of ED management prior to transfer to the ICU. SAPS 3 requires input for 20 parameters, including age, comorbidities, pre-ICU clinical status, reasons for ICU admission, and physiologic measures.[46] It has been shown in one large study to overestimate mortality risk as compared to its predecessor, SAPS II.[47] The MPM_0 III (the subscript "0" refers to the time relative to ICU admission that the score is calculated) includes 3 physiologic parameters, along with 13 other features related to chronic conditions, acute conditions, and other demographic and clinical features. It is an update of the MPM_0 II, based on a new retrospective analysis of 124,855 patients in 135 ICUs.[48] The APACHE, SAPS, and MPM models all exhibit good discrimination for predicting mortality, with areas under the ROC curve of between 0.8 and 0.9.[2,44] Calibration for severity levels tends to be worse at the extremes. Calibration for different diagnoses is better for scores such as APACHE IV that incorporate diagnosis explicitly,[49] while calibration for geographic region can be improved by local customization.[43]

In addition to general SOI scores such as those described above, there are a number of scores designed to measure degrees of organ dysfunction in critical illness. These scores, which include the Logistic Organ Dysfunction Score (LODS), the Multiple Organ Dysfunction Score (MODS), and the SOFA, are intended to be more descriptive than predictive. Each uses a similar panel of clinical variables to categorize degrees of perturbation in the neurologic, cardiovascular, respiratory, renal, hematologic, and hepatic organ systems. Scores can be used to convey the extent of organ dysfunction and to track progression of illness. For example, an increasing SOFA score over the first 48 hours of ICU admission has been shown to portend a twofold increase in mortality risk, as compared to a decreasing score (50% vs. 27%).[43]

FUTURE DIRECTIONS

The modern complement of SOI scores includes those used for specific disease conditions, those designed to predict functional status and mortality, and those intended to provide standardized descriptors of disease severity and organ dysfunction. While some scores (APACHE, SAPS, MPM) are of limited use in individualized treatment decisions, they can help provide a framework in which to compare populations of critically ill patients. Importantly, all SOI scores provide a common language, so that clinicians can quickly and efficiently convey disease severity to consultants and colleagues, even across different facilities.

Newer SOI scores will focus on predicting key outcomes not only for the patient but also for the health care system in which they are treated. The PREEDICCT project proposes to develop decision support tools for triage in pandemic and mass casualty situations or in other situations in which resources are constrained.[50] These new scores will reflect the importance of resource allocation in decision making and the need to establish standardized practices that can apply equally in all settings.

Increasingly SOI scores are based on modern statistical techniques and rely less on expert opinion. As electronic medical record coverage expands, new opportunities will emerge to apply real-time data mining algorithms to the derivation and application of SOI scoring. This transformation has immense potential to improve both the precision and calibration of scores, which could in theory be customized even at the level of the individual hospital. Larger data sets could enable outcome prediction for rare conditions that might not otherwise have been captured by existing scoring systems.[51] Better prognostication stands to benefit not only a wider range of patients but also the health systems that care for them.

LITERATURE TABLE

TRIAL	DESIGN	RESULT
Loke et al., *Thorax.* 2010[7]	Meta-analysis of 23 prospective studies (22,753 patients) evaluating the performance of CAP severity scores	PSI was found to be more sensitive but less specific than CURB-65 for prediction of death (pooled sensitivity 90% vs. 62%, pooled specificity 53% vs. 79%)
Husson et al., *J Rehab Med.* 2010[17]	Meta-analysis of 28 prospective studies of early determinants of functional outcome after traumatic brain injury	GCS at the time of ED admission was a strong predictor of poor outcome at 6 mo (assessed mostly by GOS)
Kwakkel et al., *J Neurol Sci.* 2010[26]	Prospective study of the predictive value of the NIHSS in 188 patients with ischemic stroke	The NIHSS score at days 2, 5, and 9 post-stroke were highly predictive of neurologic outcome at 6 mo (as measured by Barthel Index)
Craig et al. *Aliment Pharmacol Ther.* 2010[40]	Systematic review of 14 studies (1,960 patients) evaluating prognostic criteria in acute liver failure due to acetaminophen toxicity	Pooled analysis showed King's College Criteria to have high specificity (94.6%) but poor sensitivity (58.2%)

REFERENCES

1. Keegan MT, Gajic O, Afessa B. Severity of illness scoring systems in the intensive care unit. *Crit Care Med.* 2011;39:163–169.
2. Strand K, Flaatten H. Severity scoring in the ICU: a review. *Acta Anaesthesiol Scand.* 2008;52:467–478.
3. Fine MJ, Auble TE, Yealy DM, et al. A prediction rule to identify low-risk patients with community-acquired pneumonia. *N Engl J Med.* 1997;336:243–250.
4. Pereira J, Paiva J, Rello J. Assessing severity of patients with community-acquired pneumonia. *Semin Respir Crit Care Med.* 2012;33:272–283.
5. Valencia M, Badia JR, Cavalcanti M, et al. Pneumonia severity index class V patients with community-acquired pneumonia: characteristics, outcomes, and value of severity scores. *Chest.* 2007;132:515–522.
6. Brandão-Neto RA, Goulart AC, Santana ANC, et al. The role of pneumonia scores in the emergency room in patients infected by 2009 H1N1 infection. *Eur J Emerg Med.* 2012;19:200–202.
7. Loke YK, Kwok CS, Niruban A, et al. Value of severity scales in predicting mortality from community-acquired pneumonia: systematic review and meta-analysis. *Thorax.* 2010;65:884–890.
8. Lim WS, Van der Eerden MM, Laing R, et al. Defining community acquired pneumonia severity on presentation to hospital: an international derivation and validation study. *Thorax.* 2003;58:377–382.
9. Charles PGP, Wolfe R, Whitby M, et al. SMART-COP: a tool for predicting the need for intensive respiratory or vasopressor support in community-acquired pneumonia. *Clin Infect Dis.* 2008;47:375–384.
10. Mandell LA, Wunderink RG, Anzueto A, et al. Infectious Diseases Society of America/American Thoracic Society consensus guidelines on the management of community-acquired pneumonia in adults. *Clin Infect Dis.* 2007;44(suppl 2):S27–S72.
11. Zuercher M, Ummenhofer W, Baltussen A, et al. The use of Glasgow Coma Scale in injury assessment: a critical review. *Brain Inj.* 2009;23:371–384.
12. Teasdale GM, Murray L. Revisiting the Glasgow Coma Scale and Coma Score. *Intensive Care Med.* 2000;26:153–154.
13. Sternbach GL. The Glasgow coma scale. *J Emerg Med.* 2000;19:67–71.
14. Sadaka F, Patel D, Lakshmanan R. The FOUR score predicts outcome in patients after traumatic brain injury. *Neurocrit Care.* 2012;16:95–101.
15. Sasser SM, Hunt RC, Faul M, et al. Guidelines for field triage of injured patients: recommendations of the National Expert Panel on Field Triage, 2011. *MMWR Recomm Rep.* 2012;61:1–20.
16. Gabbe BJ. The status of the Glasgow Coma Scale. *Emerg Med.* 2003;15:353–360.
17. Husson EC, Ribbers GM, Willemse-van Son AHP, et al. Prognosis of six-month functioning after moderate to severe traumatic brain injury: a systematic review of prospective cohort studies. *J Rehabil Med.* 2010;42:425–436.

18. Mayglothling J, Duane TM, Gibbs M, et al. Emergency tracheal intubation immediately following traumatic injury: an Eastern Association for the Surgery of Trauma practice management guideline. *J Trauma Acute Care Surg.* 2012;73:S333–S340.
19. Fischer M, Rüegg S, Czaplinski A, et al. Inter-rater reliability of the Full Outline of UnResponsiveness score and the Glasgow Coma Scale in critically ill patients: a prospective observational study. *Crit Care.* 2010;14:R64.
20. Rosen DS, Macdonald RL. Subarachnoid hemorrhage grading scales: a systematic review. *Neurocrit Care.* 2005;2:110–118.
21. Degen LAR, Dorhout Mees SM, Algra A, et al. Interobserver variability of grading scales for aneurysmal subarachnoid hemorrhage. *Stroke.* 2011;42:1546–1549.
22. Cavanagh SJ, Gordon VL. Grading scales used in the management of aneurysmal subarachnoid hemorrhage: a critical review. *J Neurosci Nurs.* 2002;34:288–295.
23. Ogilvy CS, Carter BS. A proposed comprehensive grading system to predict outcome for surgical management of intracranial aneurysms. *Neurosurgery.* 1998;42:959–968; discussion 968–970.
24. Kapapa T, Tjahjadi M, König R, et al. Which clinical variable influences health-related quality of life the most after spontaneous subarachnoid hemorrhage? Hunt and Hess Scale, Fisher Score, World Federation of Neurosurgeons Score, Brussels Coma Score, and Glasgow Coma Score Compared. *World Neurosurg.* 2013;80:853–858.
25. Ferro JM, Canhão P, Peralta R. Update on subarachnoid haemorrhage. *J Neurol.* 2008;255:465–479.
26. Kwakkel G, Veerbeek JM, Van Wegen EEH, et al. Predictive value of the NIHSS for ADL outcome after ischemic hemispheric stroke: does timing of early assessment matter? *J Neurol Sci.* 2010;294:57–61.
27. Wechsler LR. Intravenous thrombolytic therapy for acute ischemic stroke. *N Engl J Med.* 2011;364:2138–2146.
28. Senkowski CK, McKenney MG. Trauma scoring systems: a review. *J Am Coll Surg.* 1999;189:491–503.
29. Chawda MN, Hildebrand F, Pape HC, et al. Predicting outcome after multiple trauma: which scoring system? *Injury.* 2004;35:347–358.
30. Kim Y-J. Injury severity scoring systems: a review of application to practice. *Nurs Crit Care.* 2012;17:138–150.
31. Sartorius D, Le Manach Y, David J-S, et al. Mechanism, Glasgow coma scale, age, and arterial pressure (MGAP): a new simple prehospital triage score to predict mortality in trauma patients. *Crit Care Med.* 2010;38:831–837.
32. Imrie CW. Prognostic indicators in acute pancreatitis. *Can J Gastroenterol.* 2003;17:325–328.
33. Rau BM. Predicting severity of acute pancreatitis. *Curr Gastroenterol Rep.* 2007;9:107–115.
34. Rockall TA, Logan RF, Devlin HB, et al. Risk assessment after acute upper gastrointestinal haemorrhage. *Gut.* 1996;38:316–321.
35. Blatchford O, Murray WR, Blatchford M. A risk score to predict need for treatment for upper-gastrointestinal haemorrhage. *Lancet.* 2000;356:1318–1321.
36. Laursen SB, Hansen JM, Schaffalitzky de Muckadell OB. The Glasgow Blatchford score is the most accurate assessment of patients with upper gastrointestinal hemorrhage. *Clin Gastroenterol Hepatol.* 2012;10:1130–1135.e1.
37. Schiefer M, Aquarius M, Leffers P, et al. Predictive validity of the Glasgow Blatchford Bleeding Score in an unselected emergency department population in continental Europe. *Eur J Gastroenterol Hepatol.* 2012;24:382–387.
38. Gotthardt D, Riediger C, Weiss KH, et al. Fulminant hepatic failure: etiology and indications for liver transplantation. *Nephrol Dial Transplant.* 2007;22:viii5–viii8.
39. Blei AT. Selection for acute liver failure: have we got it right? *Liver Transpl.* 2005:S30–34.
40. Craig DGN, Ford AC, Hayes PC, et al. Systematic review: prognostic tests of paracetamol-induced acute liver failure. *Aliment Pharmacol Ther.* 2010;31:1064–1076.
41. Yu AS, Ahmed A, Keeffe EB. Liver transplantation: evolving patient selection criteria. *Can J Gastroenterol.* 2001;15:729–738.
42. Yantorno SE, Kremers WK, Ruf AE, et al. MELD is superior to King's college and Clichy's criteria to assess prognosis in fulminant hepatic failure. *Liver Transpl.* 2007;13:822–828.
43. Vincent J-L, Moreno R. Clinical review: scoring systems in the critically ill. *Crit Care.* 2010;14:207.
44. Breslow MJ. Severity scoring in the critically ill: part 1—interpretation and accuracy of outcome prediction scoring systems. *Chest.* 2012;141:245.
45. Knaus WA, Draper EA, Wagner DP, et al. APACHE II: a severity of disease classification system. *Crit Care Med.* 1985;13:818–829.

46. Moreno RP, Metnitz PGH, Almeida E, et al. SAPS 3—from evaluation of the patient to evaluation of the intensive care unit. Part 2: development of a prognostic model for hospital mortality at ICU admission. *Intensive Care Med.* 2005;31:1345–1355.
47. Poole D, Rossi C, Latronico N, et al. Comparison between SAPS II and SAPS 3 in predicting hospital mortality in a cohort of 103 Italian ICUs. Is new always better? *Intensive Care Med.* 2012;38:1280–1288.
48. Higgins TL, Teres D, Copes WS, et al. Assessing contemporary intensive care unit outcome: an updated Mortality Probability Admission Model (MPM0-III). *Crit Care Med.* 2007;35:827–835.
49. Breslow MJ, Badawi O. Severity scoring in the critically ill: part 2: maximizing value from outcome prediction scoring systems. *Chest.* 2012;141:518–527.
50. Christian MD, Fowler R, Muller MP, et al.; PREEDICCT Study Group. Critical care resource allocation: trying to PREEDICCT outcomes without a crystal ball. *Crit Care.* 2013;17:107.
51. Frankovich J, Longhurst CA, Sutherland SM. Evidence-based medicine in the EMR era. *N Engl J Med.* 2011;365:1758–1759.

63

Indications for Contact and Respiratory Isolation

Chanu Rhee and Michael Klompas

BACKGROUND

Emergency and intensive care department health care providers often encounter patients with suspected or confirmed infections due to transmissible organisms. Isolation of patients who are infected or colonized with selected high-risk organisms is a cost-effective means of reducing rates of nosocomial infection and is a core component of infection control programs.[1,2] Isolation and precaution guidelines were first issued in 1970 by the Centers for Disease Control and were last updated in 2007.[3] A basic understanding of infection control terminology and practice is an essential skill for the emergency physician caring for critically ill patients.

In addition to standard precautions, which are recommended in the care of all hospitalized patients, there are three isolation categories—contact, droplet, and airborne spread—that reflect the major modes of transmission of microorganisms in health care settings. This chapter summarizes the key components and indications for each type of isolation precaution. We also include an overview of empiric isolation precautions for common clinical syndromes for use when the pathogen is unknown.

STANDARD PRECAUTIONS

Standard precautions are recommended in the care of all hospitalized patients, in order to reduce the risk of transmission of infectious agents between patients and health care workers. Standard precautions include the following:

- Practice hand hygiene before and after every patient contact.
- Use gloves, gowns, and eye protection when exposure to body secretions or blood is likely.
- Safely dispose of sharp instruments and needles in puncture-resistant containers.
- Carefully handle soiled patient care materials and linens so as to avoid skin and mucous membrane exposures. Store soiled linens in impervious bags.
- Use safe injection practices.
- Practice respiratory hygiene and cough etiquette, which involves covering the nose and mouth when coughing, prompt disposal of tissues, and hand hygiene after contact with respiratory secretions. This also applies to all patients and accompanying family/friends with signs of respiratory illness (cough, congestion, rhinorrhea).

Hand hygiene is the single most important measure for reducing transmission of microorganisms.[4] Hand cleansing with alcohol-containing disinfectants is more efficient than hand washing with soap and water. Note, however, that alcohol-based disinfectants are not effective against *Clostridium difficile* spores.[5,6]

CONTACT PRECAUTIONS

Contact precautions prevent transmission of infectious agents, which may colonize patients' skin, wounds, and mucous membranes, as well as the inanimate environment. Contact precautions are applied to patients with multidrug-resistant bacteria (such as methicillin-resistant *Staphylococcus aureus* [MRSA], vancomycin-resistant *Enterococcus* [VRE], and some Gram negatives), diarrheal illnesses, draining wounds or abscesses, selected respiratory pathogens, and vesicular rashes (Table 63.1). Contact precautions are necessary every time a provider enters a patient room, regardless of whether or not

TABLE 63.1 Indications for Contact Precautions

Condition/Pathogen	Duration of Precautions and Comments
Multidrug-resistant organisms (infection or colonization): methicillin-resistant *S. aureus*, vancomycin-intermediate and vancomycin-resistant *S. aureus*, vancomycin-resistant *Enterococcus*, multidrug-resistant Gram negatives (e.g., extended-spectrum beta-lactamase–producing and carbapenemase-producing organisms)	Specific types of organisms that warrant precautions and criteria for discontinuing precautions may vary between different geographic areas and institutions
Clostridium difficile	Optimal duration of isolation not well defined, but at the minimum until diarrhea has completely resolved. Hand washing with soap and water is preferred over alcohol (which lacks sporicidal activity)
Respiratory and enteric viral infections: adenovirus, enterovirus, coxsackie virus, rotavirus, human metapneumovirus, parainfluenza, poliomyelitis, respiratory syncytial virus, SARS, MERS-CoV	Generally until resolution of symptoms, but prolonged shedding of viruses tends to occur in immunocompromised patients. Adenovirus also requires droplet precautions
Enteric infections in incontinent or diapered patients: toxin-producing *Escherichia coli* strains (0157:H7), noroviruses, *Giardia lamblia, Salmonella, Shigella, Vibrio parahaemolyticus, Yersinia enterocolitica*, and hepatitis A	Until resolution of symptoms. Can also place in contact isolation for nonincontinent or nondiapered patients for control of institutional outbreaks
Cutaneous viral infections: *varicella–zoster*, severe mucocutaneous disseminated *herpes simplex*	Until lesions are completely crusted over and no new lesions. Susceptible health care workers should not enter the room if immune caregivers are available. Place on airborne precautions as well if patient has disseminated zoster or is immununocompromised (due to high risk of dissemination)
Major draining abscess or infected pressure ulcer (if unable to adequately dress or contain drainage)	Until drainage stops or can be contained by dressing
Burkholderia cepacia infection or colonization in patients with cystic fibrosis	Optimal duration unknown. Avoid exposure to other patients with cystic fibrosis
Staphylococcal scalded skin syndrome or major Staphylococcal or group A streptococcal wound	For staphylococcal scalded skin syndrome, contact precautions should continue for the duration of illness. For staph/strep wound infections, duration is until 24 h of appropriate antibiotic therapy
Extrapulmonary tuberculosis with a draining lesion	Until patient is improving clinically and drainage stops or three consecutive negative cultures from drainage
Cutaneous diphtheria	Until two cultures taken 24 h apart are negative. Pharyngeal diphtheria requires droplet precautions
Head lice	Until after 24 h of appropriate therapy

he or she plans to touch the patient, since inanimate objects in the patient's environment are as likely to harbor pathogens as the patient himself.

Contact precautions include the following steps:

- Use gloves and gowns for all contact with patients and their environment. Remove both gloves and gowns prior to leaving the patient's room.
- Wash hands before entering and after leaving patient rooms. Hands must still be washed before and after donning or removing gloves.
- Place patients in a private room whenever possible. If this is not possible, cohort infected patients with other patients on contact precautions for the same organism.
- Dedicate inexpensive items, such as stethoscopes, to a single patient.

There is some controversy regarding the use of contact precautions for drug-resistant pathogens like MRSA and VRE. Health care workers spend less time in the rooms of patients on contact precautions, compared to those on standard precautions, and this may impair the quality of care.[7] In addition, a recent cluster-randomized trial involving multiple ICUs compared an intervention of enhanced surveillance for MRSA and VRE (through serial nasal and stool/perianal cultures) to standard care.[8] Despite increased use of contact precautions in the intervention group (due to more patients being identified as being colonized with MRSA or VRE), there was no significant change in incidence rates of ICU infection or colonization with those pathogens. The study, however, was confounded by long turnaround times for screening results and suboptimal compliance with hand hygiene and contact precautions. On the other hand, implementation of a multifaceted MRSA "prevention bundle" that included contact precautions as well as universal surveillance, culture change, and emphasis on hand hygiene was associated with a significant decline in healthcare-associated MRSA infections at Veterans Affairs hospitals across the country.[9]

Emerging data suggest that an alternate strategy involving universal decolonization of all critically ill patients with nasal mupirocin and chlorhexidine baths is superior to screening and isolation or targeted decolonization (i.e., screening, isolation, and decolonization of MRSA carriers) in reducing the presence of MRSA and rates of all bloodstream infections.[10] For now, however, practitioners are advised to refer to their local institution's policies.

DROPLET PRECAUTIONS

Droplet precautions prevent transmission of pathogens spread through respiratory secretions. These pathogens are predominantly viral, but include notable bacterial pathogens such as *Neisseria meningitidis*, *Haemophilus influenzae* type B, invasive group A streptococcal infections, and diphtheria (Table 63.2). Droplets are particles of respiratory secretions with mean diameter of larger than 5 μm. They remain suspended in the air only for limited periods and so are generally infectious over short distances (typically less than 3 feet). Unlike airborne pathogens, droplets do not require special air handling and ventilation to prevent transmission. Note that some organisms, such as respiratory viruses, can be transmitted by both droplets and direct patient contact; these require both droplet and contact precautions. Droplet precautions entail the following:

- Wear a mask for close contact with patients (within 3 feet). A respirator (such as an N95 mask) is not necessary.

TABLE 63.2 Indications for Droplet Precautions

Condition/Pathogen	Duration of Precautions and Comments
Influenza	5 d from onset of symptoms, except in immunocompromised patients in whom duration cannot be defined (due to prolonged viral shedding). Health care workers should wear a face mask when entering the room and N95 respirators when performing aerosol-generating procedures (e.g., intubation, bronchoscopy, sputum induction, suctioning of airways, chest compressions)
Neisseria meningitidis: meningitis, pneumonia, or bacteremia	24 h after initiation of appropriate antibiotic therapy
Haemophilus influenzae type B: epiglottitis or meningitis	24 h after initiation of appropriate antibiotic therapy
Mycoplasma pneumoniae: pneumonia	Until illness has resolved
Bordetella pertussis (whooping cough)	5 d after initiation of appropriate antibiotic therapy
Diphtheria (pharyngeal)	Until two cultures 24 h apart are negative
Pneumonic plague (*Yersinia pestis*)	48 h after initiation of appropriate antibiotic therapy
Mumps (infectious parotitis)	9 d after onset of swelling (5 d may be appropriate in community settings)
Rubella	7 d after onset of rash. Susceptible health care workers should not enter the room if immune caregivers are present
Adenovirus pneumonia	Until illness resolved, except in immunocompromised patients in whom duration cannot be defined. Adenovirus also requires contact precautions
Parvovirus B19 (erythema infectiosum)	For the entire hospitalization in immunocompromised patients with chronic disease and 7 d in patients with transient aplastic or red cell crisis
Group A streptococcal disease: serious invasive disease, pneumonia, or major wounds	24 h after initiation of appropriate antibiotic therapy. Contact precautions should also be used if skin lesions are present
Rhinovirus	Until illness resolved
Viral hemorrhagic fevers (Lassa, Ebola, Marburg, Crimean-Congo fever viruses)	Until illness resolved. Patients also require contact precautions

- Place the patient in a private room if possible. If cohorting of patients possessing the same pathogens is necessary, place patient beds at least 3 feet apart and draw the curtains between beds.
- Place a mask on the patient during transport.

For influenza, studies have specifically compared the use of N95 respirators to standard masks and have found no difference in rates of transmission.[11,12]

AIRBORNE PRECAUTIONS

Airborne precautions prevent transmission of pathogen-laden droplets that can remain suspended in the air for prolonged periods. Airborne droplet nuclei are particles of respiratory secretions with mean diameter of 1 to 5 μm. In contrast to contact and droplet precautions, the list of pathogens that require airborne precautions is short: suspected or confirmed tuberculosis, measles, *varicella–zoster*, smallpox, and severe acute respiratory syndrome (SARS). In addition, a novel coronavirus (now designated as the Middle East respiratory syndrome coronavirus, or MERS-CoV) has recently emerged that, similar to SARS, can cause severe lower respiratory tract infection. While the exact nature of exposure causing infection in the MERS-CoV is not known at this time, human-to-human transmission has been observed, including health care–associated clusters of infection. Clinicians should suspect MERS-CoV in patients (or their close contacts) who developed fever and an acute lower respiratory illness within 14 days after traveling from countries in areas involved in the outbreak (which currently includes countries in the Arabian Peninsula). Currently, the recommended infection control policy is the same as that for SARS and includes both airborne and standard precautions.[13] Airborne precautions entail the following:

- Place the patient into an airborne infection isolation room. This means a single-patient, negative pressure room with at least 6 to 12 air exchanges per hour. The air should be exhausted directly to the outside or recirculated through HEPA filters before return.
- Wear a certified respirator (e.g., N95 mask or powered air-purifying respirator) when entering the room. Health care providers need to be fit tested for N95 masks annually. Providers unable to establish an adequate fit with an N95 mask must wear a powered air-purifying respiratory mask instead.
- When possible, assign immune health care workers to care for patients with vaccine-preventable airborne diseases: measles, varicella, and smallpox.
- Minimize patient transport; if this is unavoidable, place a mask on the patient (a regular surgical mask is adequate).

Tuberculosis is the most important pathogen requiring airborne precautions, and it should be suspected in any patient with fever, cough, and upper lobe infiltrate. The threshold for airborne isolation should be very low in patients with HIV/AIDS presenting with fever and a pulmonary infiltrate, especially as they are much more likely to have an atypical appearance on chest radiography. Note that although guidelines recommend discontinuation of airborne precautions once patients are smear negative on three consecutive samples, transmission can still occur in these situations (although at a much lower rate) (Tables 63.3 and 63.4).[14]

TABLE 63.3 Indications for Airborne Precautions

Condition/Pathogen	Duration of Precautions and Comments
Tuberculosis: pulmonary or extrapulmonary with draining lesions	Until patient is improving on effective therapy and has 3 sputum smears negative for acid–fast bacilli (acquired on different days). Contact precautions also required for extrapulmonary TB with draining lesions (see Table 63.1)
Varicella zoster: disseminated or cutaneous in an immunocompromised host	Until lesions are completely crusted over and no new lesions are appearing
Measles (rubeola)	Until 4 d after onset of rash or until illness resolves completely in immunocompromised patients. Susceptible health care workers should not enter the room if immune caregivers are present
Smallpox	Until all scabs have crusted and separated (usually 3–4 wk). Also requires contact precautions. Smallpox has been eradicated, but threat of bioterrorism still exists
SARS (severe acute respiratory syndrome) and MERS-CoV (Middle East respiratory syndrome coronavirus)	Until illness resolved, plus 10 d after resolution of fever. Patients also require contact precautions. There have been no cases of SARS reported since 2004. Current recommendations regarding MERS-CoV are based on scant clinical data, and the period of quarantine considered safe is uncertain

TABLE 63.4 Common Clinical Syndromes That Warrant Empiric Precautions

Clinical Syndrome	Potential Pathogens That Warrant Precautions	Empiric Precautions
Respiratory infections: Fever, cough, upper lobe pulmonary infiltrate (or any lung location in an HIV-infected patient)	*M. tuberculosis*, respiratory viruses, group A streptococcus, methicillin-resistant *S. aureus* Also: SARS, MERS-CoV, or avian influenza if recent travel to countries with active outbreaks	Airborne + contact Use eye/face protection if aerosol-generating procedure performed or contact with respiratory secretions anticipated (e.g., intubation)
Diarrhea: Acute diarrhea likely due to infectious agent in an incontinent or diapered patient	Enteric pathogens (e.g., *E. coli* 0157:H7, *Shigella*, hepatitis A, norovirus, rotavirus, *C. difficile*)	Contact
Rash: 1. Petechial or ecchymotic 2. Vesicular 3. Maculopapular with cough, coryza, and fever	1. *Neisseria meningitidis*, viral hemorrhagic fevers if travel to endemic area (Ebola, Lassa, Marburg viruses) 2. *Varicella zoster, herpes simplex* 3. *Rubeola* (measles)	1. Droplet (for first 24 h of antimicrobial therapy), if viral hemorrhagic fever possible, use droplet + contact precautions 2. Airborne + contact (contact alone adequate if herpes simplex or localized zoster in immunocompetent host) 3. Airborne
Meningitis in adults	*Neisseria meningitidis, Haemophilus influenzae* type B, *M. tuberculosis*	Droplet (for first 24 h of antimicrobial therapy) Airborne if pulmonary infiltrate
Skin or wound infection: Abscess or draining wound that cannot be covered	*S. aureus* (methicillin-sensitive or resistant), group A streptococcus	Contact. Add droplet for the first 24 h of antimicrobial therapy if invasive group A streptococcal disease is suspected

LITERATURE TABLE

TRIAL	DESIGN	RESULT
Methicillin-resistant *Staphylococcus aureus* and vancomycin-resistant *Enterococcus*		
Huskins et al., *NEJM.* 2011[8]	Cluster randomized trial evaluating the effect of universal surveillance for MRSA and VRE with expanded use of barrier precautions, vs. existing practice	During 6-mo intervention period, no significant difference in rates of colonization or infection with MRSA or VRE, but confounded by long turnaround time for screening results (~5 d) and suboptimal compliance with interventions (~69% for hand hygiene, 77% for gowns, and 82% for gloves)
Jain et al., *NEJM.* 2011[9]	Comparison of rates of health care–associated MRSA infection rates before and after national implementation of a MRSA prevention bundle (universal surveillance with nasal cultures or polymerase chain reaction, contact precautions, hand hygiene, culture change) at acute care VA hospitals	After implementation of the MRSA bundle, rates of health care–associated MRSA infections fell by 62% in ICUs and 45% in non-ICUs ($p < 0.001$ for trend)

LITERATURE TABLE *(Continued)*

TRIAL	DESIGN	RESULT
Huang et al., *NEJM.* 2013[10]	Multicenter cluster randomized trial involving 74,256 ICU patients, evaluating universal decolonization (no screening and decolonization of all patients with nasal mupirocin and chlorhexidine baths) vs. screening and isolation alone, vs. targeted decolonization (screening, isolation, and decolonization of MRSA carriers)	After a 12-month baseline period and 18-month intervention period, universal decolonization of all ICU patients was the most effective strategy, reducing the hazard of MRSA-positive clinical cultures by 37% vs. baseline period, compared to 25% for targeted decolonization, and 8% for screening and isolation ($p = 0.01$ for 3-group comparison). Universal decolonization also reduced the hazard of bloodstream infections from any pathogen by 44%, compared to 22% for targeted decolonization, and 1% for screening and isolation respectively ($p < 0.001$ for 3-group comparison)
Influenza		
Loeb et al., *JAMA.* 2009[11]	Randomized trial during 2008–2009 influenza season of fit-tested N95 respiratory vs. surgical mask in 446 health care workers	Surgical masks were noninferior to N95 in terms of rates of laboratory-confirmed influenza
Tuberculosis		
Tostmann et al., *Clin Infec Dis.* 2008[14]	Retrospective study of patients with culture-confirmed TB in the Netherlands from 1996 to 2004, using molecular linkage studies	Patients with smear-negative, culture-positive TB were responsible for 13% of TB transmissions. The relative transmission rate among those with smear-negative TB (vs. smear-positive TB) was 0.24

REFERENCES

1. Haley RW, Culver DH, White JW, et al. The efficacy of infection surveillance and control programs in preventing nosocomial infections in US hospitals. *Am J Epidemiol.* 1985;121(2):182.
2. Kaye KS, Engemann JJ, Fulmer EM, et al. Favorable impact of an infection control network on nosocomial infection rates in community hospitals. *Infect Control Hosp Epidemiol.* 2006;27(3):228.
3. Siegel JD, Rhinehart E, Jackson M, et al.; Healthcare Infection Control Practices Advisory Committee. 2007. *Guideline for Isolation Precautions: Preventing Transmission of Infectious Agents in Healthcare Settings.* http://www.cdc.gov/ncidod/dhqp/pdf/isolation2007.pdf
4. Pittet D, Allegranzi B, Sax H, et al.; WHO Global Patient Safety Challenge, World Alliance for Patient Safety. Evidence-based model for hand transmission during patient care and the role of improved practices. *Lancet Infect Dis.* 2006;6(10):641.
5. Jabbar U, Leischner J, Kasper D, et al. Effectiveness of alcohol-based hand rubs for removal of *Clostridium difficile* spores from hands. *Infect Control Hosp Epidemiol.* 2010;31(6):565.
6. Oughton MT, Loo VG, Dendukuri N, et al. Hand hygiene with soap and water is superior to alcohol rub and antiseptic wipes for removal of *Clostridium difficile. Infect Control Hosp Epidemiol.* 2009;30(10):939.
7. Morgan DJ, Pineles L, Shardell M, et al. The effect of contact precautions on healthcare worker activity in acute care hospitals. *Infect Control Hosp Epidemiol.* 2013;34(1):69–73.
8. Huskins CW, Huckabee CM, O'Grady NP, et al.; for the STAR*ICU Investigators. Intervention to reduce transmission of resistant bacteria in intensive care. *N Engl J Med.* 2011;364:1407–1418.
9. Jain R, Kralovic SM, Evans ME, et al. Veterans Affairs initiative to prevent methicillin-resistant *Staphylococcus aureus* infections. *N Engl J Med.* 2011;364(15):1419.
10. Huang SS, Septimus E, Kleinman K, et al. Targeted versus universal decolonization to prevent ICU infection. *N Engl J Med.* 2013;368(24):2255–2265.
11. Loeb M, Dafoe N, Mahony J, et al. Surgical mask vs N95 respiratory for preventing influenza among health care workers: a randomized trial. *JAMA.* 2009;302(17):1865.
12. Johnson DF, Druce JD, Birch C, et al. A quantitative assessment of the efficacy of surgical and N95 masks to filter influenza virus in patients with acute influenza infection. *Clin Infect Dis.* 2009;49(2):275.
13. CDC. *Interim Infection Prevention and Control Recommendations for Hospitalized Patients with Middle East Respiratory Syndrome Coronavirus (MERS-CoV).* June 2013. Retrieved from http://www.cdc.gov/coronavirus/mers/interim-recommendations-patients-2013.html
14. Tostmann A, Kik SV, Kalisvaart NA, et al. Tuberculosis transmission by patients with smear-negative pulmonary tuberculosis in a large cohort in the Netherlands. *Clin Infect Dis.* 2008;47(9):1135.

EPILOGUE

Scott Weingart

Emergency medicine in the United States is at a crossroads. The purpose of the emergency physician is being determined as we speak by legislators and hospital administrators. Our role in the hospital is slowly being forced to evolve to that of a provider of primary care, available without appointment, 24 hours a day. This is laudable and a boon for patients; it is, however, very different than the original purpose of our specialty.

Many of the founders of our specialty envisioned emergency physicians as the ideal managers of critically ill patients during their initial resuscitation. In the time between caring for these sick patients, the department could also see patients with non–life-threatening complaints. It was understood that these latter patients could wait for care if a critically ill patient arrived, thereby maximizing treatment to the group whose lives depended on our interventions.

During the past decade, this system has been turned around. Now, in many departments, it is the noncrashing patient who takes priority. The wait time of patients with primary care complaints has become a rubric by which an emergency physician is judged. This year, the postvisit reviews of the patients discharged from the emergency department (ED) will be a pay-for-performance measure; not the reviews of patients we admitted to the hospital and not the reviews of the patients we brought back from near-death and sent to the intensive care unit (ICU) markedly improved due to our resuscitation.[1] This is a clear message from the shapers of health care policy: the ED must prioritize the noncrashing patient over the crashing one.

Despite these pressures, we will still always manage airway, breathing, and circulation for the first 10 to 20 minutes of a patient's ED course, but after that, the feeling in some departments is that these high-risk patients should become someone else's problem. The ICU doctors should take these patients upstairs or come manage them in the ED. Unfortunately, waits of 24 to 48 hours for an ICU bed are not uncommon, and a dire shortage of intensivists makes their caring for critical patients in the ED untenable in most hospitals.

But someone must take care of critically ill patients in the ED. These patients must not be left to languish with anything less than the equivalent care they will receive when their ICU bed becomes available. That someone could be an inpatient intensivist, an ED intensivist, or an emergency physician. All three are capable, but if the emergency physician cedes this role, then our profession has become very different than the specialty I hoped for when I was a medical student choosing my future career.

This handbook offers the knowledge and techniques necessary to care for the critically ill patient in the ED. It will guide you through the initial resuscitation and the continued management of these patients during their first 24 hours of intensive care. A wealth of experience is encompassed in the pages of this monograph. It extends the already strong foundations of resuscitation that are the core of our specialty. Please seize the knowledge contained here and use it.

Use it to take back the role of the emergency physician as the ultimate resuscitationist. Use it to care for patients during their most vulnerable moments. Use it to heal and to relieve suffering when we cannot heal. Just because the intubated patients cannot verbalize their complaints and misery, do not let their needs be drowned out by a patient who needs a medication refill. All patients deserve rapid, optimal care, but the purpose of an emergency physician is to provide maximally aggressive care to patients at their sickest. Everything else fills the time until the next crashing patient arrives.

REFERENCES

1. Patient Satisfaction. From ACEP.org (http://www.acep.org/patientsatisfaction/). Accessed March 1, 2013.

INDEX

Note: Page numbers followed by *f* indicate figures and those followed by *t* indicate tables

F

G

R

S

T

U

V

W